AF726114

Neal Halfon • Christopher B. Forrest
Richard M. Lerner • Elaine M. Faustman
Editors

Handbook of Life Course Health Development

Editors
Neal Halfon
Department of Pediatrics
David Geffen School of Medicine
UCLA, Los Angeles, CA, USA

Department of Health Policy
and Management
Fielding School of Public Health
UCLA, Los Angeles, CA, USA

Department of Public Policy
Luskin School of Public Affairs
UCLA, Los Angeles, CA, USA

Center for Healthier Children
Families, and Communities
UCLA, Los Angeles, CA, USA

Richard M. Lerner
Tufts University
Medford, MA, USA

Christopher B. Forrest
Applied Clinical Research Center
Children's Hospital of Philadelphia
Philadelphia, PA, USA

Elaine M. Faustman
Institute for Risk Analysis and Risk
Communication
Department of Environmental and
Occupational Health Sciences
School of Public Health
University of Washington
Seattle, Washington, USA

DOI 10.1007/978-3-319-47143-3

Preface

Maternal and Child Health, Life Course Health Development, and the Life Course Research Network

Prior to 1900, the health of mothers and children was considered a domestic concern. Childbirth was often supervised by untrained birth attendants such as family members; basic care of sick children was rudimentary and undeveloped, with the unfortunate but all-too-real expectation that some children would not survive into adulthood (Rosenfeld and Min 2009). With the advent of scientific medicine in the nineteenth century, discoveries in bacteriology, and other sanitary reforms, childbirth came under greater medical scrutiny, and pediatric hospitals were established to care for ailing children. A greater focus on maternal nutrition, the spread of scientifically supported birthing practices, and other newly minted public health practices – along with improved social and living conditions – led to dramatic decreases in infant mortality rates and to improved child survival. In 1912, the Children's Bureau was established in the United States as a federal agency with responsibility for assuring the health of mothers and children. In 1935, Title V of the Social Security Act established the Maternal and Child Health Bureau (MCHB), which today administers a broad range of programs to address the health needs of the nation's maternal and child health (MCH) population.

For most of the twentieth century, MCH programs and policies continued to focus on two basic areas: (1) promoting healthy births by preventing maternal and infant mortality and, more recently, (2) preventing premature births and providing medical care for children with long-term medical and developmental disorders. Success was marked by decreasing rates of maternal and infant mortality but was challenged by persistent disparities in outcomes, especially differences in infant mortality between White and African-American children. Similarly, while great strides were made in reducing child deaths due to infectious disease and improving the effectiveness, availability, and quality of medical interventions for a range of childhood conditions from hemophilia to complex congenital heart diseases, the number of children reported as being disabled due to a chronic health problem rose dramatically from 2% in 1960 to over 8% in 2011 (Halfon et al. 2012).

In the late 1980s, a new and rapidly converging set of research findings from the life course health sciences began to recast the importance of early life on lifelong health (Ben-Shlomo and Kuh 2002; Halfon and Hochstein 2002). Research that was particularly relevant to the MCH field revealed how:

- Preconception health and perinatal risk can impact birth outcomes and have a sustained and long-term impact on child and adult health several decades later.
- Susceptibility and sensitivity of the developing brain to adversity, as well as to supportive and caring relationships, can be measured not only in brain morphology but also using functional measures of cognitive and emotional performance, including school readiness, academic performance, and long-term mental health.
- Risky and chaotic family environments, and toxic and unpredictable social environments, are transduced into a child's biology, manifesting as disease and causing changes in immune, inflammatory, and metabolic function that can be linked with childhood health conditions like obesity and ADHD and adult conditions like diabetes, hypertension, and heart disease, to name a few.

These and other research findings also suggested new explanatory mechanisms for seemingly intractable problems such as the persistent racial and ethnic gaps in infant mortality. The dominant biomedical approach to treating infant mortality focused on prenatal care and the prevention of pathological signs and symptoms (e.g., eclampsia), but what the findings from the life course health sciences began to suggest is that women's preconception reproductive capacity – including neuroendocrine response patterns, vascular health, and stress reactivity – could condition their response to pregnancy, the timing of parturition, and the likelihood of prematurity (Lu and Halfon 2003). This work suggested that in addition to improving technical interventions to pathophysiological responses that emerge during pregnancy by providing access to high-quality prenatal care, more attention should be focused on improving (if not optimizing) health during the preconception and interconception periods. This idea led to a set of new initiatives focused on girls' and women's reproductive health trajectories, including public health strategies to improve preconception health and research strategies to better understand how adversity impacts reproductive health across the life course.

For the past two decades, there has been a growing recognition across the MCH community that life course health science is building an important evidence base about the central and vital role of health during the prenatal period and the early years on subsequent lifelong health (Halfon and Hochstein 2002; Galobardes et al. 2004 and 2008; Power and Kuh 2013). Research on the changing epidemiology of childhood chronic illness and the growing number of longitudinal studies documenting the legacy of chronic illness in childhood on patterns of adult health, morbidity, and mortality are also connecting the dots between child health and the potential for healthy aging (Halfon 2012; Wise 2004; Wise 2016). As the United States experiences rapidly rising healthcare costs due to rapidly increasing rates of chronic disease and multi-morbidity, life course health science is shining a light on the early part of the life-span when preventable risks are setting in motion the inflammatory, neuroendocrine, and metabolic processes that predispose an individual to degenerative chronic disorders manifested decades later. The recent IOM report *Shorter Lives, Poorer Health* that explores why the United States is the sickest of rich nations also highlights that the health of children in the United States falls far behind the health of children in other nations and that these life course determinants cannot be ignored (Woolf and Aron 2013).

Perhaps the most salient and obvious reason for MCH to adopt a life course perspective has come from the epidemic of childhood obesity, which has demonstrated how childhood growth can influence rates of the most common and costly adult health conditions, including diabetes and cardiovascular disease (Gillman 2004). It has also shown how a mother's prenatal health, along with her preconception weight, influences pregnancy outcomes, the likelihood that an infant will be obese, and the potential for lifelong obesity and resultant comorbidities (Oken and Gillman 2003; Gillman et al. 2008).

For at least the past two decades, life course health science research has been reframing our approach to many persistent health and health-care issues, from infant mortality to obesity, and from school readiness to lifelong cognitive potential and reserves. This research has influenced thought leaders, researchers, policymakers, and service providers to consider the importance and essential role of MCH as a vehicle for improving health outcomes for mothers and children and, ultimately, for the population as a whole. In 2010, as MCHB celebrated its 75th birthday, Peter Van Dyck, the Associate Administrator of the Health Resources and Services Administration and Director of MCHB, announced that the Bureau intended to launch a national dialogue about the importance of life course health science in reaching MCH goals. He also highlighted how MCH could use this science to help research, programs, policies, and partnerships coalesce around moving life course theory into life course practice. The transformation would be accomplished by an integrative approach to understanding how health and disease develop. However, although this transformation is aimed at creating a rigorous approach to the study of the development of heath across the life-span, there is no doubt that there are still many outstanding questions about the relationship between early experiences and lifelong health and well-being, and about how existing and emerging knowledge can be applied to the development of evidence-based practice and policy.

Unfortunately, the lack of a strong research and data infrastructure, coupled with limits on funding currently available in the United States to support the development of new methodologies and collaborative approaches, has hampered the production of the transformative, transdisciplinary, and translational research that is needed to advance the emerging field we have termed "life course health development" (LCHD). Moreover, the fact that researchers who are interested and engaged in LCHD research continue to work in discipline-specific silos has been a significant impediment to rapid progress. In recognition of and response to these challenges, in 2010, MCHB issued a Request for Proposals to develop a Maternal and Child Health Life Course Research Network (LCRN) that would be charged with providing a virtual platform and undertaking a set of activities that would together serve as a new infrastructure for catalyzing progress and enhancing funding to support basic, theoretical, and applied and translational LCHD research of relevance to MCH practice and policy.

The UCLA Center for Healthier Children, Families, and Communities – with the support and participation of a diverse array of colleagues from around the United States – submitted a successful application to establish an LCRN with the following goals:

1. Engage a diverse, active, and sustainable community of LCHD stakeholders.
2. Increase capacity for, engagement in, and production of LCHD research.
3. Catalyze the translation and application of LCHD research to practice and policy.

To launch the LCRN, the UCLA team initiated a strategic network design process that engaged individuals with substantial expertise in health development, as well as those with deep knowledge of the science of network development and facilitation. This strategic design process included a series of interviews with key informants (see http://www.lcrn.net/tag/expert-interviews), as well as an in-person meeting of the network's 30-member design team that resulted in the approval of the LCRN charter (see http://www.lcrn.net/wp-content/uploads/2012/07/LCRN-charter-2.pdf), the development of a scope of work comprised of specific activities intended to achieve the network's aims, a concept for the network's online presence including a website and social networking platform, and the constitution of an advisory committee that would provide UCLA project staff with guidance for the duration of the project (see http://www.lcrn.net/about).

Following the design meeting, project staff undertook a process to develop a series of background papers that would serve as the basis for the MCH Life Course Research Agenda-Setting Meeting that took place in February of 2013 in order to achieve the following aims:

1. Catalyze a paradigm shift in how researchers, practitioners, and policymakers think about, understand, and promote LCHD.
2. Evaluate, refine, and determine the utility of the seven proposed principles of LCHD.
3. Identify the ways in which the topics discussed at the meeting are converging and/or diverging across disciplines.
4. Identify knowledge that is ready for application in order to assist MCH and other practitioners in taking advantage of what we know now and speeding the progression from research to translation.
5. Provide recommendations that will enable the LCRN to develop an MCH Life Course Research Agenda (LCRA) that includes priorities in the areas of basic research, translational research, and methods and data development.
6. Provide background paper authors with input that will advance their papers toward completion and publication.
7. Identify next steps for both the LCRN and the LCHD field as a whole.

Background paper topics were selected by project staff with the input of the LCRN advisory committee and MCHB staff, and included topics that were selected strategically due to their potential to enhance our understanding of health development and advance the LCHD field, as well as topics that were selected more opportunistically when researchers learned of the project and wanted to ensure that the issues of importance to them had a chance of making it into the preliminary version of the LCRA, version 1.0 (see concluding chapter of this volume).

The 2013 agenda-setting meeting brought together 90+ invited stakeholders including researchers, practitioners, policymakers, funders, and other thought leaders from the United States, Canada, and the United Kingdom. Over the 2-day meeting, participants engaged in a highly facilitated process of reviewing the evidence base and providing the background paper authors with the feedback they would need to complete their research and develop a set of recommended research priorities. A highlight of the meeting was to critically examine the seven proposed principles of LCHD (see Halfon and Forrest in this volume) that were intended to provide a more unified theoretical foundation and a more consistent set of terminology for this emerging field.

Following the agenda-setting meeting and in response to the enormous amount of momentum and enthusiasm generated among the participants, UCLA staff, again with the guidance of the LCRN advisory committee and representatives from MCHB, began to pursue development and publication of a volume that would contain revised versions of the background papers, as well as several chapters to be commissioned based on gaps identified at the agenda-setting meeting, plus a preliminary version of the LCRA. To this end, a four-member LCRN editorial team was constituted and charged with working closely with the background paper authors to ready their drafts – with a particular focus on trying to align the chapters with regard to the terminology and, more importantly, the conceptual frameworks underlying the writings – for inclusion in the Handbook of Life Course Health Development, and develop additional chapters and material as needed.

Concurrent with the preparation of this volume, the LCRN has produced three unique webinar series, organized research nodes focused on particular topic areas, developed strategic partnerships aimed at enabling the translation of LCHD research to practice and policy, and produced several peer-reviewed publications, among other activities. We invite readers to learn more about the LCRN – including how to join – at lcrn.net.

References

Ben-Shlomo, Y., & Kuh, D. (2002). A life course approach to chronic disease epidemiology: conceptual models, empirical challenges and interdisciplinary perspectives. *International journal of epidemiology*, *31*(2), 285293.

Galobardes, B., Lynch, J. W., & Davey Smith, G. (2004). Childhood socioeconomic circumstances and cause-specific mortality in adulthood: systematic review and interpretation. *Epidemiology Reviews*, *26*, 7–21.

Galobardes, B., Lynch, J. W., & Smith, G. D. (2008). Is the association between childhood socioeconomic circumstances and cause-specific mortality established? Update of a systematic review. *Epidemiology and Community Health*, *6*(2), 387–90.

Gillman, M. W. (2004). A life course approach to obesity. A life course approach to chronic disease epidemiology. *1*, 473.

Gillman, M. W., Rifas-Shiman, S. L., Kleinman, K., Oken, E., Rich-Edwards, J. W., & Taveras, E. M. (2008). Developmental origins of childhood overweight: potential public health impact. *Obesity*, *16*(7), 1651–6.

Halfon, N., & Hochstein, M. (2002). Life course health development: an integrated framework for developing health, policy, and research. *Milbank Quarterly, 80*(3), 433–79. iii.

Halfon, N., Houtrow, A., Larson, K., & Newacheck, P. W. (2012). The changing landscape of disability in childhood. *The Future of Children*, *22*(1), 13–42.

Lu, M. C., & Halfon, N. Racial and ethnic disparities in birth outcomes: a life-course perspective. *Maternal and Child Health*, *7*(1), 13–30.

Oken, E., & Gillman, M. W. (2003). "Fetal origins of obesity." *Obesity research, 11.4,* 496–506.

Power, C., Kuh, D., & Morton, S. (2013). From developmental origins of adult disease to life course research on adult disease and aging: insights from birth cohort studies. *Annual Review of Public Health*, *34*, 7–28.

Rosenfeld, A., & Min, C. J. (2009). *A history of international cooperation in maternal and child health. Maternal and child health (pp. 3–17).* US: Springer.

Wise, P. H. (2004). The transformation of child health in the United States. *Health Affairs*, *23*(5), 9–25.

Wise, P. H. (2016). Child poverty and the promise of human capacity: childhood as a foundation for healthy aging. *Academic Pediatrics, 16*(3), S37–45.

Woolf, S. H., & Aron, L, (Eds). (2013) US health in international perspective: Shorter lives, poorer health. National Academies Press.

Acknowledgments

This project is supported by the Health Resources and Services Administration (HRSA) of the US Department of Health and Human Services (HHS) under grant number UA6MC19803. This information or content and conclusions are those of the author(s) and should not be construed as the official position or policy of, nor should any endorsements be inferred by, HRSA, HHS, or the US Government.

Contents

The original version of this book was revised. An erratum to this book can be found at https://doi.org/10.1007/978-3-319-47143-3_27

About the Editors

Neal Halfon, MD, MPH is the Director of the UCLA Center for Healthier Children, Families, and Communities. He is also a Professor of pediatrics in the David Geffen School of Medicine at UCLA, of health policy and management in the UCLA Fielding School of Public Health, and of public policy in the UCLA Luskin School of Public Affairs. Dr. Halfon's research has spanned clinical, health services, epidemiologic, and health policy domains. For more than a decade, he has worked with national, state, and local initiatives aimed at improving early childhood systems. Dr. Halfon has also played a significant role in developing new conceptual frameworks for the study of health and health care, including the Life Course Health Development (LCHD) framework. In 2006, Halfon received the Academic Pediatric Associations Annual Research Award for his lifetime contributions to child health research. He received his MD at the University of California, Davis, and MPH at the University of California, Berkeley. He completed his pediatric residency at the University of California, San Diego, and the University of California, San Francisco. Dr. Halfon was also Robert Wood Johnson Clinical Scholar at the University of California, San Francisco.

Christopher B. Forrest, MD, PhD is Professor of Pediatrics and Health Care Management at the Children's Hospital of Philadelphia (CHOP) and the University of Pennsylvania. He is the Director of the CHOP Center for Applied Clinical Research, which uses life course health development science to advance clinical and health services research in pediatrics. Dr. Forrest serves as the Principal Investigator of the PEDSnet (pedsnet.org), a national consortium of children's hospitals (>5 million children) that conducts patient-centered outcomes research among children and youth. He is the Chair of the Research Committee for PCORnet, the national clinical research network funded by PCORI. He also chairs the Steering Committee for the NIH program called PEPR, which is conducting longitudinal studies on person-reported outcome measures in children with chronic conditions. Dr. Forrest received his BA and MD degrees from Boston University and completed his PhD in Health Policy and Management at Johns Hopkins School of Public Health.

Richard M. Lerner, PhD is the Bergstrom Chair in Applied Developmental Science and the Director of the Institute for Applied Research in Youth Development at Tufts University. He went from kindergarten through PhD within the New York City public schools, completing his doctorate at the City

University of New York in 1971 in developmental psychology. Dr. Lerner has more than 700 scholarly publications, including 80 authored or edited books. He was the Founding Editor of the *Journal of Research on Adolescence* and *Applied Developmental Science*, which he continues to edit. He was a 1980–1981 fellow at the Center for Advanced Study in the Behavioral Sciences and is a fellow of the American Association for the Advancement of Science, the American Psychological Association, and the Association for Psychological Science. Dr. Lerner is known for his theory of relations between life-span human development and social change and for his research about the relations between adolescents and their peers, families, schools, and communities. His work integrates the study of public policies and community-based programs with the promotion of positive youth development and youth contributions to civil society. He is married to Dr. Jacqueline V. Lerner, Professor in the Department of Applied Developmental and Educational Psychology in the Lynch School of Education at Boston College. They live in Wayland, Massachusetts. They have three children: Justin, a Director and Screenwriter living in Los Angeles; Blair, an Advertising Executive at Media Contacts in Boston; and Jarrett, a Novelist and Editor living in Boston.

Elaine M. Faustman, PhD, DABT is Professor in the Department of Environmental and Occupational Health and Director of the Institute for Risk Analysis and Risk Communication at the School of Public Health and Community Medicine at the University of Washington. She directs the NIEHS- and EPA-funded Center for Child Environmental Health Risks Research and led the Pacific Northwest Center for the National Children's Study. She is an elected fellow of both the American Association for the Advancement of Science and the Society for Risk Analysis. Dr. Faustman is an Affiliate Professor in the School of Public Affairs at the University of Washington and has been an Affiliate Professor in the Department of Engineering and Public Policy at Carnegie-Mellon University. She has served on the National Toxicology Program Board of Scientific Counselors, the National Academy of Sciences Committee on Toxicology, the Institute of Medicine Upper Reference Levels Subcommittee of the Food and Nutrition Board, and numerous editorial boards. Dr. Faustman chaired the National Academy of Sciences Committee on Developmental Toxicology. She has or is currently serving on the executive boards of the Society of Toxicology, the Society for Risk Analysis, and NIEHS Council. She is past President of the Teratology Society. Her research interests include understanding mechanisms that put children and the public at risk of environmental agents. Currently she is serving on the Committee on NAS Gulf War and Health, Volume 11: Generational Health Effects of Serving in the Gulf War. In particular, Dr. Faustman is interested in the molecular and cellular mechanisms of developmental and reproductive toxicants, characterizing in vitro techniques for developmental toxicology assessment, and development of biologically based dose-response models for non-cancer risk assessment. Dr. Faustman's research expertise includes development of decision-analytic tools for communicating and translating new scientific findings into risk assessment and risk management decisions.

Contributors

Sarah E. Anderson, PhD The Ohio State University, College of Public Health, Columbus, OH, USA

David Askenazi, MD University of Alabama Children's Hospital, Pediatric Nephrology, Birmingham, AL, USA

Susan P. Bagby, MD Division of Nephrology & Hypertension, Department of Medicine, Moore Institute for Nutrition and Wellness, Oregon Health & Science University, Portland, OR, USA

Tami R. Bartell, BA Stanley Manne Children's Research Institute, Ann & Robert H Lurie Children's Hospital of Chicago, Chicago, IL, USA

Milena Batanova, PhD Institute for Applied Research in Youth Development, Tufts University, Medford, MA, USA

Ashley Bennett, MD Department of Pediatrics, USC, Los Angeles, CA, USA

Robert Wm. Blum, MD, MPH, PhD Johns Hopkins Bloomberg School of Public Health, Baltimore, MD, USA

Ed Bowers Clemson University, Youth Development Leadership, Clemson, SC, USA

Claire D. Brindis, DrPH University of California-San Francisco (UCSF), Philip R. Lee Institute for Health Policy Studies and the Adolescent and Young Adult Health National Resource Center, San Francisco, CA, USA

Patrick D. Brophy, MD, MHCDS University of Iowa Stead Family Children's Hospital, Pediatric Nephrology, Iowa City, IA, USA

J. Bryan Carmody, MD University of Virginia, Department of Pediatrics, Division of Nephrology, Charlottesville, VA, USA

Stephen L. Buka Department of Epidemiology, Brown University, Providence, RI, USA

Claire Cameron University at Buffalo, SUNY, Learning and Instruction, Buffalo, NY, USA

Janet M. Catov Department of Obestetrics and Gynecology, University of Pittsburgh, Pittsburgh, PA, USA

University of Pittsburgh, Department of Epidemiology, Pittsburgh, PA, USA

Magee-Womens Research Institute, Pittsburgh, PA, USA

Jennifer R. Charlton, MD, MSc University of Virginia, Department of Pediatrics, Division of Nephrology, Charlottesville, VA, USA

Edith Chen Department of Psychology and Institute for Policy Research, Northwestern University, Evanston, IL, USA

Tina L. Cheng, MD, MPH Department of Pediatrics, Johns Hopkins University School of Medicine, Baltimore, MD, USA

Elizabeth C. Cooksey Center for Human Resource Research, The Ohio State University, Columbus, OH, USA

James J. Crall Division of Public Health and Community Dentistry, University of California Los Angeles (UCLA) School of Dentistry, Los Angeles, CA, USA

Tara Crapnell, OTD, OTR/L UCLA, Department of Pediatrics, Los Angeles, CA, USA

Adrian Davis University College London, NHS Newborn Hearing Screening Program, London, UK

Amelia Dmowska Section of Developmental and Behavioral Pediatrics, University of Chicago Comer Children's Hospitals, Chicago, IL, USA

Irene E. Drmic Hospital for Sick Children, Toronto, ON, Canada

Angela Duckworth University of Pennsylvania, Department of Psychology, Philadelphia, PA, USA

Gary W. Evans Department of Design and Environmental Analysis, Department of Human Development, Cornell University, Ithaca, NY, USA

Elaine M. Faustman, PhD Institute for Risk Analysis and Risk Communication, Department of Environmental and Occupational Health Sciences, School of Public Health, University of Washington, Seattle, WA, USA

Maria Ferris, MD, PhD, MPH UCLA, Department of Pediatrics, Los Angeles, CA, USA

Glenn Flores, MD, FAAP Medica Research Institute, Division of Health Policy and Management, University of Minnesota School of Public Health, Minneapolis, MN, USA

Paula Fomby Survey Research Center, Institute for Social Research, University of Michigan, Ann Arbor, MI, USA

Christopher B. Forrest, MD, PhD Applied Clinical Research Center, Children's Hospital of Philadelphia, Philadelphia, PA, USA

Abigail Fraser Medical Research Council Integrative Epidemiology Unit at the University of Bristol, University of Bristol, Bristol, UK

John Geldhof Oregon State University, Human Development and Family Sciences, Corvallis, OR, USA

Amanda Geller New York University, New York, NY, USA

Steinunn Gestsdóttir University of Iceland, Department of Psychology, Reykjavik, Iceland

Matthew W. Gillman Harvard Medical School and Harvard Pilgrim Health Care Institute, Boston, MA, USA

Marco DelGiudice Department of Psychology, University of New Mexico, Albuquerque, NM, USA

Elizabeth Goodman, MD Division of General Academic Pediatrics, Mass General Hospital for Children, Department of Pediatrics, Harvard Medical School, Boston, MA, USA

Jennie Grammer University of California, Los Angeles, Graduate School of Education and Information Studies, Los Angeles, CA, USA

Neal Halfon, MD, MPH Department of Pediatrics, David Geffen School of Medicine, UCLA, Los Angeles, CA, USA

Department of Health Policy and Management, Fielding School of Public Health, UCLA, Los Angeles, CA, USA

Department of Public Policy, Luskin School of Public Affairs, UCLA, Los Angeles, CA, USA

Center for Healthier Children, Families, and Communities, UCLA, Los Angeles, CA, USA

Lyndsay Harshman, MD University of Iowa Children's Hospital, Pediatrics, Iowa City, IA, USA

Summer Sherburne Hawkins Boston College, Chestnut Hill, MA, USA

Dena Herman Department of Family and Consumer Sciences, California State University Northridge, Northridge, CA, USA

Clyde Hertzman Human Early Learning Partnership, School of Population and Public Health, University of British Columbia, Vancouver, BC, Canada

Dennis Hogan, PhD Sociology and Demography, Population Research and Training Center, Brown University, Providence, RI, USA

Kate Jaeger Princeton University, Princeton, NJ, USA

Robert S. Kahn, MD, MPH Division of General and Community Pediatrics, Cincinnati Children's Hospital Medical Center, University of Cincinnati College of Medicine, Cincinnati, OH, USA

Manmohan K. Kamboj, MD The Ohio State University, College of Medicine, Endocrinology, Metabolism and Diabetes, Nationwide Children's Hospital, Columbus, OH, USA

Pilyoung Kim Department of Psychology, University of Denver, Denver, CO, USA

Alice Kuo, MD, PhD UCLA, Department of Pediatrics, Los Angeles, CA, USA

Mary E. Lacy Department of Epidemiology, Brown University, Providence, RI, USA

Michelle Lampl, MD, PhD Department of Anthropology, Emory University, Atlanta, GA, USA

Center for the Study of Human Health, Emory University, Atlanta, GA, USA

Kandyce Larson, PhD Department of Research, American Academy of Pediatrics, Elk Grove Village, IL, USA

Lynette Lau, PhD UCLA, Department of Pediatrics, Los Angeles, CA, USA

Deborah A. Lawlor Medical Research Council Integrative Epidemiology Unit at the University of Bristol, University of Bristol, Bristol, UK

Richard M. Lerner, PhD Tufts University, Medford, MA, USA

Todd Little Texas Tech University, Department of Educational Psychology and Leadership, Lubbock, TX, USA

Debra Lotstein, MD, MPH UCLA, Department of Pediatrics, Los Angeles, CA, USA

Megan McClelland Human Development and Family Sciences, 245 Hallie E. Ford Center for Healthy Children and Families, Oregon State University, Corvallis, OR, USA

Katherine McGonagle Survey Research Center, Institute for Social Research, University of Michigan, Ann Arbor, MI, USA

Gregory Miller Department of Psychology and Institute for Policy Research, Northwestern University, Evanston, IL, USA

Fred Morrison University of Michigan, Department of Psychology, Ann Arbor, MI, USA

Michael E. Msall, MD Developmental and Behavioral Pediatrics University of Chicago, Comer and LaRabida Children's Hospitals, Chicago, IL, USA

JP Kennedy Research Center on Intellectual and Developmental Disabilities, University of Chicago Comer Children's Hospital, Section of Developmental and Behavioral Pediatrics, Chicago, IL, USA

Amanda Mummert, PhD Department of Anthropology, Emory University, Atlanta, GA, USA

Center for the Study of Human Health, Emory University, Atlanta, GA, USA

Emily Oken Harvard Medical School and Harvard Pilgrim Health Care Institute, Boston, MA, USA

Garrett Pace Doctoral Student, School of Social Work, Department of Sociology, University of Michigan, Ann Arbor, MI, USA

Kimberly J. Reidy, MD Albert Einstein College of Medicine, Montefiore Medical Center, Pediatric Nephrology, Bronx, NY, USA

Janet W. Rich-Edwards Connors Center for Women's Health and Gender Biology, Brigham and Women's Hospital, Boston, MA, USA

Harvard Medical School, Boston, MA, USA

Harvard School of Public Health, Boston, MA, USA

Samantha R. Rosenthal Department of Epidemiology, Brown University, Providence, RI, USA

Shirley A. Russ, MD, MPH UCLA Center for Healthier Children, Families and Communities, Department of Pediatrics, David Geffen School of Medicine, UCLA, Los Angeles, CA, USA

Pamela Salsberry, PhD, RN, FAAN College of Public Health, Division of Health Behavior, Health Promotion, Institute for Population Health, The Ohio State University, Columbus, OH, USA

Narayan Sastry Survey Research Center, Institute for Social Research, University of Michigan, Ann Arbor, MI, USA

Meriah Schoen Center for the Study of Human Health, Emory University, Atlanta, GA, USA

Department of Nutrition, Georgia State University, Atlanta, GA, USA

Teresa Seeman David Geffen School of Medicine, University of California – Los Angeles, Los Angeles, CA, USA

Jeffrey Segar, MD University of Iowa Children's Hospital, Neonatology, Iowa City, IA, USA

David Shoham, PhD, MSPH Department of Public Health Sciences, Loyola University Chicago, Maywood, IL, USA

Sarah A. Sobotka, MD, MS Section of Developmental and Behavioral Pediatrics, University of Chicago Comer Children's Hospitals, Chicago, IL, USA

John Son, MPH Center for Healthier Children, Families and Communities, UCLA, Los Angeles, CA, USA

Mary Sullivan, PhD, RN University of Rhode Island, College of Nursing, Women and Infants Hospital, Providence, RI, USA

Peter Szatmari Centre for Addiction and Mental Health, Hospital for Sick Children, University of Toronto, Toronto, ON, Canada

Rika Tanda, PhD, RN College of Health Science and Professions, Ohio University, Athens, OH, USA

Marion Taylor-Baer Department of Community Health Sciences, Fielding School of Public Health, University of California Los Angeles, Los Angeles, CA, USA

W. Thomas Boyce Departments of Pediatrics and Psychiatry, University of California San Francisco, San Francisco, CA, USA

Kelly Tremblay Speech & Hearing Sciences College of Arts & Sciences, University of Washington, Seattle, WA, USA

Ericka Tullis, MPP Center for Healthier Children, Families and Communities, UCLA, Los Angeles, CA, USA

Fred Volkmar Child Study Center, Yale University School of Medicine, New Haven, CT, USA

Guoying Wang, MD, PhD Department of Population, Family and Reproductive Health, Center on the Early Life Origins of Disease, Johns Hopkins University Bloomberg School of Public Health, Baltimore, MD, USA

Xiaobin Wang, MD, MPH, ScD Center on the Early Life Origins of Disease, Department of Population, Family and Reproductive Health, Johns Hopkins University Bloomberg School of Public Health, Baltimore, MD, USA

David Wood, MD, MPH Department of Pediatrics, ETSU College of Medicine, Johnson City, TN, USA

Introduction to the Handbook of Life Course Health Development

Neal Halfon, Christopher B. Forrest, Richard M. Lerner, Elaine M. Faustman, Ericka Tullis, and John Son

1 Introduction

Over the past several decades, countless studies have linked early life events and experiences with adult health conditions, delineating the developmental origins of common chronic health conditions and specifying the processes by which both adversity and opportunity are integrated into developing biobehavioral systems (Baltes et al. 2006; Bronfenbrenner 2005; Elder et al. 2015). As a result, there is a greater understanding of how health and disease develop, which is leading to new kinds of individual- and population-level strategies that have the potential to prevent disease and optimize health by minimizing the impact of adversity, increasing protective factors, and targeting health-promoting interventions to coincide with sensitive periods of health development.

Insights and evidence from life course chronic disease epidemiology have converged with research from the fields of developmental biology, neuroscience, and developmental science, with studies of typical and atypical development and with new findings from research examining the developmental origins of chronic disease. This wide-ranging research, all focused on understanding how health and disease develop, has involved researchers from a wide variety of disciplines. Life-span developmental psychologists,

N. Halfon, MD, MPH (✉)
Department of Pediatrics, David Geffen School of Medicine, UCLA, Los Angeles, CA, USA

Department of Health Policy and Management, Fielding School of Public Health, UCLA, Los Angeles, CA, USA

Department of Public Policy, Luskin School of Public Affairs, UCLA, Los Angeles, CA, USA

Center for Healthier Children, Families, and Communities, UCLA, Los Angeles, CA, USA
e-mail: nhalfon@ucla.edu

C.B. Forrest, MD, PhD
Applied Clinical Research Center, Children's Hospital of Philadelphia, Philadelphia, PA, USA

R.M. Lerner, PhD
Tufts University, Medford, MA, USA

E.M. Faustman, PhD
Institute for Risk Analysis and Risk Communication, Department of Environmental and Occupational Health Sciences, School of Public Health, University of Washington, Seattle, WA 98105, USA

E. Tullis, MPP • J. Son, MPH
Center for Healthier Children, Families and Communities, UCLA, Los Angeles, CA, USA

N. Halfon et al. (eds.), *Handbook of Life Course Health Development*,
DOI 10.1007/978-3-319-47143-3_1

life course-focused sociologists, human capital-focused economists, and political scientists studying the structure of social institutions are not only studying the same developmental processes; they are also working alongside epidemiologists, physicians, and basic scientists to better understand how health develops over the life course and how these health development processes promote human flourishing.

In response to this burgeoning knowledge, there is growing momentum among practitioners and policymakers to "connect the dots" between what we know and what we do, that is, between the rapidly expanding evidence base from the emerging field of life course health development (LCHD) and the practices and policies that are implemented within the fields of medicine, public health, nursing, mental health, education, urban planning, community development, social welfare, and others (Halfon et al. 2014; Kuh et al. 2013; Braveman 2014; Gee et al. 2012; Lappé and Landecker 2015). At the same time, there is a strong impetus among researchers to continue to fill the substantial gaps in our knowledge and to ensure that research findings are appropriately synthesized and translated before being applied in clinical, public health, or public policy contexts.

Comprised of 26 chapters that grew out of the 2013 Maternal and Child Health (MCH) Life Course Research Agenda-Setting Meeting that was organized by the MCH Life Course Research Network (LCRN) and funded by Health Resources and Services Administration-Maternal and Child Health Bureau (HRSA-MCHB), this volume represents a groundbreaking effort to explore the history of the LCHD field, to take stock of what we know and do not know about how health and disease develop, to provide practitioners and policymakers with guidance regarding the kinds of interventions and efforts that can be beneficial, and to lay the foundation for a research agenda that identifies high-priority areas for basic, clinical, population, and translational investigations in order to strategically target resources and efforts and advance the life course health sciences.

Each chapter is written by a team of leading experts that often spans several different disciplines and therefore reflects a wide range of perspectives on how innovative research, practice, and policy can begin to address our most pressing health challenges. Similarly, the volume's four editors represent different disciplines and perspectives that were brought to bear on the process of selecting topics and authors and on ensuring that each chapter makes a substantial contribution to the field.

In this introductory chapter, we begin by providing a rationale for the publication of this volume, including an historical overview that traces the emergence of the LCHD field and provides evidence of a significant, but as yet incomplete, transformation in how we think about and promote health. We go on to describe the purpose, structure, and content of the volume and to examine some of the challenges for further field building in this area. Finally, we provide readers with information about each section and chapter in this volume, including the impressive backgrounds of the various experts who contributed substantial amounts of both time and original thinking in their roles as authors.

2 Rationale

2.1 The Emergence of a New Field

The science of health has been guided for well over 150 years by a mechanical model that views the body and its component cells as machines and views disease as a breakdown in organ structure and function. Person-environment relationships as causes of disease are either ignored or relegated to secondary concerns. Even though the oversimplified perspective of the body as a machine has been largely abandoned, reducing physiologic and behavioral phenomena to their smallest observable constituent parts remains a mainstay of the biomedical model that dominates contemporary health sciences. This reductionist approach may tell us how parts of a neuron work, but it does not provide an appropriate model for understanding how the nervous system works, how we think, or what produces consciousness (Capra 1982). Even fields like human genomics are moving away from the simplistic notion of single-gene causation, which has failed to yield substantial insights into disease causation, to research on genetic networks and epigenetics

(Huang 2012; Lappé and Landecker 2015). Complex disorders that manifest as a spectrum of phenotypic variability – including cardiovascular disease, obesity, diabetes, and autism – are increasingly understood as manifestations of relations among networks of genes and complex gene-environment coactions that are mediated by equally complex time signatures and temporal coupling. Moreover, the mechanical model of health cannot account for placebo effects, the mind's effects on the body, or psychosomatic illness. It presupposes a mind-body dualism and reifies the distinction between physical and mental health, a vestige of the Cartesian mind-body split (Overton 2015). A reductionist approach to understanding health is inadequate for addressing how different molecular, physiologic, social, and environmental networks work together to produce dynamic stability and change, which are the cornerstones of health outcome trajectories.

Many fields of science – including physics, biology, and the social sciences (especially developmental science) – have shifted from a Cartesian-Newtonian mechanistic ontology to a more complex system-oriented ontology (Lerner 2012). The mechanistic view divides the world into separate or split categories (e.g., nature versus nurture) and reduces it into discrete elements (genes, behaviors, molecules) that are combined, added, and assembled to form what we perceive as biological phenotypes, patterns of behavior, and personalities. As Overton (2012) and others have described, this revolutionary shift in the epistemological and ontological foundations of science took place during the twentieth century as Newtonian physics gave way to general relativity theory and as contemporary formulations of knowing the world were shown to lack explanatory power and utility (Aldwin 2014). Thus, the need for new models that explain the complex phenomena of human health development became apparent.

The synthesis of human health development as explained by theories associated with relational developmental systems (RDS) metatheory is replacing the now anachronistic mechanical model of health (Lerner and Overton 2008; Lerner 2012; Overton 2012). Overton (2015) explains that compared to earlier formulations of understanding human development, RDS metatheory focuses on process (systematic changes in the developmental system), becoming (moving from potential to actuality; a developmental process as having a past, present, and future; Whitehead 1929/1978), holism (the meanings of entities and events derive from the context in which they are embedded), relational analysis (assessment of the mutually influential relations within the developmental system), and the use of multiple perspectives and explanatory forms. Within RDS metatheory, the organism is seen as inherently active, self-creating (autopoietic), self-organizing, self-regulating (agentic), nonlinear and complex, and adaptive (Overton 2015).

The RDS metatheory emphasizes the study and integration of different levels of organization ranging from biology and physiology to culture and history as a means to understand life-span human development (Lerner 2006; Overton 2015). Accordingly, the conceptual emphasis in RDS theories is placed on mutually influential relations between individuals and contexts, represented as individual ⇔ context relations. In a bidirectional relational system, the embeddedness within history (temporality) is of fundamental significance (Elder et al. 2015). The presence of such temporality in the developmental system means that there always exists some potential for systematic change and, thus, for (relative) plasticity in human development. In short, potential plasticity in individual ⇔ context relations derives from the "arrow of time" (Lerner 1984; Lerner and Callina 2014; Overton 2015) running through the integrated (relational) developmental system. Such plasticity also suggests that there are multiple developmental pathways, across the life-span.

Similar conceptual advances have also been generated by systems biology, which focuses on the complex interactions of biological systems using a holistic framework and integrative relational strategies rather than traditional reductionist approaches (Kitano 2002; Antony et al. 2012; Schadt and Björkegren 2012, Kandel et al. 2014). This transformation has been catalyzed by a greater appreciation of dynamical system theory and, more specifically, complex adaptive system theory and its application to molecular biology (Huang 2012). Moreover, as our understanding of epigenetics and systems biology has matured, new insights into how complex gene regulatory networks produce multilevel and multidirectional relationships between genotype and phenotype have been elucidated (Foster 2011; Huang 2012; Piro and Di Cunto 2012; Schadt and Björkegren 2012; Greenblum et al. 2012; Davila-Velderrain et al. 2015). This new knowledge would not have been acquired using reductionist statistical models that analyze data by reducing them to their smallest components and estimating marginal effects of linear models.

In summary, the study of human development has evolved from a field dominated by split, reductionist (psychogenic or biogenic) approaches to a multidisciplinary field that integrates observations, evidence, and analysis that spans from biological to cultural and historical levels of organization across the life-span (e.g., Elder et al. 2015; Ford and Lerner 1992; Gottlieb 1998; Lerner and Callina 2014). Reductionist accounts have given way to a more integrated framework associated with RDS metatheory (Overton 2015; Lerner 2006). Across the past several decades, several scholars have provided ideas contributing to the evolution of this metatheory (e.g., Baltes et al. 2006; Bronfenbrenner 2005; Elder et al. 2015; Lerner 2006; and, even earlier, see von Bertalanffy 1933).

For instance, in psychology, the transition away from what some have characterized as the radical empiricism and atomism of the early behaviorist to ideas akin to those associated with RDS-based theories has followed a similar ontological path (Lerner 2006; Lerner and Overton 2008; Overton 2010, 2012). As Arnold Sameroff explains, psychologists were attempting to find and define the laws that explain behavior and how the mind functions (Sameroff 2010). As it became clear that any particular individual- or population-level signal explained very little of the observed variance in behaviors, developmental scientists began to create new techniques for analyzing intraindividual patterns of change that focus on individuals' unique person-environmental interactions and that separate the behavioral signal from the noisy complexity of life, especially for long-term predictive purposes (Molenaar and Newell 2010; Sameroff 2010). Rather than reducing cognitive, emotional, or overall mental function to its mechanistic components, this more holistic approach views psychological functioning as the product of a relational nexus that defines an individual in association with multiple contexts that interact dynamically over time.

In the same way that biology and psychology have faced the limits of reductionist mechanical models, medicine and health sciences are also experiencing the constraints of the biomedical approach that focuses more on the components of the organism than on the totality of human health. While the biomedical model has been remarkably successful in defining the components of human anatomy, physiology, biochemistry, and metabolism, and has provided useful frameworks for understanding simple mechanics of more linear disease processes (such as infectious diseases), it is increasingly challenged by the complexity of health development and by complex disease pathways that emerge out of multilevel and multiphasic processes that include genetic, biological, behavioral, and whole-organism processes (Halfon et al. 2014).

Similarly, at the clinical and population health levels, simple mechanistic biomedical models, or even more multifaceted biopsychosocial models of health, have difficulty explaining a wide variety of health phenomena, such as how integration of body systems and subsystems results in emergent properties of health at the level of the individual; how evolution constrains the timing and plasticity of human health development; how epigenetic processes result in multiple intermediary endophenotypes that may progress to pathological phenotypes, hover in subclinical states, or resolve; how the adaptive capacities of individuals and populations interact with rapidly changing physical, natural, chemical, social, and nutritional environments to reprogram developing physiology and other regulatory processes through epigenetic modulations of previously selected biological and behavioral scripts; and how integration occurs between biological, behavioral, and environmental systems, organized and driven by adaptive routines structured around different developmentally entrained time horizons. These conundrums have challenged health researchers to develop new frameworks to explain how each of these complex processes contributes to the development of health over time (i.e., contribute to health development).

2.2 The Maturation of the LCHD Field

A vast amount of empirical literature investigating the developmental, genomic, and epigenetic origins of health and disease – as well as on the epidemiology of chronic disease across the life course – has been generated in the past two decades (Halfon and Hochstein 2002; Kuh and Ben-Shlomo 2004; Gluckman and Hanson 2004; Gluckman et al. 2008; Kuh et al. 2013; Berkman et al. 2014; Halfon et al. 2014; the evolution of life course health science is reviewed in Halfon and Forrest 2017). New academic research journals and international research organizations have been spawned that focus on the developmental origins of health and disease. Established professional organizations now include life course and epigenetic and developmental origins of health and disease (DOHaD) tracts at their research meetings, and many major scientific journals have published special issues packaging articles that focus on biological embedding, epigenetics, or other disease-causing mechanisms that are framed from a life course perspective. The US National Academy of Sciences and National Academy of Medicine have both issued several reports on the health, social, and behavioral determinants of health, health measurement, health disparities, and health-care improvement that have incorporated a life course perspective, and the recent framework for the US Healthy People 2020 goals was upgraded to include life course as an organizing principle of the overall framework (Committee on Future Directions for Behavioral and Social Sciences Research 2001; Committee on Evaluation of Children's Health 2004; Committee on the Recommended Social and Behavioral Domains and Measures for Electronic Health Records 2015).

Perhaps the biggest stimulus for thinking differently about origins and development of chronic disease came from a series of provocative studies that were conducted by David Barker and his team. Beginning in the 1980s, Barker's studies began to describe how the prevalence of heart disease in specific areas of England was related to the distribution of birth weights in those same regions. Barker and others went on to use longitudinal datasets to solidify these observations that birth weight, and the nutritional environment and exposures of the fetus and infant, had a direct influence on the development of heart disease that was often only clinically recognized many decades later (Barker et al. 1989, 1993; Barker 1995). These startling findings challenged conventional models of direct or cumulative risk that posited that heart disease was the result of either contemporaneous or lifelong risks including poor nutrition, lack of exercise, smoking, or other behaviors and suggested that there were important latent effects of early nutrition that were somehow conditioning later pathological response patterns. Barker's studies brought attention to other research with similar findings that were less dramatic but entirely consistent with the latent lifelong effects that the Barker studies were revealing. As a result, developmental time frames started to become an important consideration, and the timing of exposures and the recognition of sensitive periods of development all took on new salience.

As this new perspective on the developmental origins of chronic disease began to unfold, there was also another emerging set of new constructs coming into play in what is now termed the field of population health. Following on in the tradition of the 1974 Lalonde Report (produced under the aegis of Canadian Minister of National Health and Welfare) that challenged the dominance of the biomedical model and proposed that the health field needed to consider biology, environment, lifestyle, and health-care organization, a broad multidisciplinary team of Canadian researchers led by the economist Robert Evans began to ask: *why are some people healthy and others not*? (Hancock 1986; Evans et al. 1994). This question led not only to a consideration of the crucial influence of upstream social and behavioral determinants on individual and population health but also to a concern about how early social environments can mold lifelong health trajectories.

Leading this exploration of the developmental role that upstream social factors on health and development for the Evans-led team was Clyde Hertzman. Hertzman went on to solidify his analysis about the importance of what at the time he termed "biological embedding" through a series of studies, analyses of other studies, and reinterpretations of existing literature through this new life course health development lens. In addition to publishing several important articles of conceptual synthesis, Hertzman and Daniel Keating edited the volume *Developmental Health and the Wealth of Nations* in which they unpacked the impact of social gradients on health development and began to specify how different time-specific and pathway effects were at play early in development (Hertzman 1999; Keating and Hertzman 1999; Hertzman and Boyce 2010). They synthesized a wealth of evidence on how early experience affects a child's brain development, social and emotional functioning, and overall health capacities (Hertzman 1994; Keating and Hertzman 1999). The Evans and Hertzman work in Canada emerged about the same time that the *Independent Inquiry into Inequalities in Health Report* (1998) led by Sir Donald Acheson was released in the UK (Acheson 1998). This review – whose panel of experts included David Barker, Michael Marmot, and Hilary Graham, among others – very clearly identified how many health inequalities have their roots in the conditions and experience of mothers and children, with impacts that feedforward across the life-span.

Diana Kuh and Yoav Ben-Shlomo edited a volume entitled *A Life Course Approach to Chronic Disease Epidemiology*, first published in 1997, which coined the term "life course epidemiology" and presented for the first time a series of articles that integrated the empirical research on several specific types of disease from a life course perspective (Kuh and Ben-Shlomo 1997). This work was followed by a second edition in 2004 that updated each of the chapters on the life course approach to obesity or the life course approach to cardiovascular disease, and that began to provide an overarching framework including chapters on life course pathways to adult health (Kuh and Ben-Shlomo 2004). In that volume, there were chapters on "Life course approaches to differentials in health" (Davey Smith and Lynch 2004), "A life course approach to obesity" (Gillman 2004), "Socioeconomic pathways between childhood and adult health" (Kuh et al. 2004), and "Should we intervene to improve childhood circumstances" (Boyce and Keating 2004). Kuh and Ben-Shlomo have gone on to edit a series of books on life course chronic disease epidemiology that continue to analyze and synthesize the literature on health development from a life course perspective (Lawlor and Mishra 2009; Kuh et al. 2013).

In 2000 (Halfon et al. 2000) and 2002 (Halfon and Hochstein 2002), Halfon and colleagues reviewed and synthesized several different life course-focused research streams and suggested that beyond its increasingly well-documented importance for understanding the mechanisms involved with the origins and development of health and disease, this new life course approach was of profound importance for a consideration of how health care should be organized, financed, and delivered. They also suggested that some general principles were emerging and beginning to outline a new model or framework that they termed *"life course health development."* At the same time, many other scientists provided their own synthesis of this emerging literature and what they considered to be its implications for health, health-care delivery, and health policy (Ben-Shlomo and Kuh 2002; Halfon and Hochstein 2002; Lu and Halfon 2003; Forrest and Riley 2004; Worthman and Kuzara 2005). These various attempts at synthesizing the evidence from this new field constituted a tipping point, and over the next decade, the number of empirical studies accelerated at a much faster pace as the early objections to the "Barker hypothesis" melted away in the wake of many confirmatory studies, and the explanatory power of this new conceptualization began to take hold.

This early LCHD synthesis highlighted the linked importance of biological conditioning; the role of multiple, ecologically nested risk, protective, and promoting factors in influencing health trajectories; the developmental significance of different time frames; and the evolution of different health development pathways in relationship to particular socially, culturally, and biologically specified transitions and turning points in an individual's life (Halfon and Hochstein 2002). Over the intervening decade, research has continued to accelerate, advancing in the use of more sophisticated methodologies; employing new and rapidly advancing epigenetic, genomic, and other techniques from systems biology; and, at the same time, supporting and providing more concrete evidence on behalf of these early summative concepts. These threads of scientific inquiry have coalesced to form a network of research that has produced a much more robust and integrated conceptual framework.

3 The Purpose, Structure, and Content of This Volume

The absence of an integrative conceptual framework through which scientists could organize and extend the manifold insights about the individual and contextual processes involved in the development of health across the life course was a fundamental challenge constraining the acceptance and understanding of a LCHD perspective (Halfon et al. 2014; Hanson and Gluckman 2014). However, as noted above, empirical and conceptual advances over the last 30 years have crystallized in the generation, and growing acceptance, of just such an integrative perspective. As a result, the life course health sciences are rapidly maturing and progressing, and the life course health development framework is coming into clearer focus. Nevertheless, there remain a number of challenges and growing pains that are evident as scientists, clinicians, and public health professionals from different fields attempt to incorporate LCHD notions into already established areas of scholarship, practice, and policy development.

For example, the definitions of terms are not always clear, some terms are being redefined to be integrated into this new approach, and other concepts and constructs are adopted before their meaning and significance are fully vetted and analyzed. Good examples of these challenges include terms like "sensitive and critical periods," "developmental programming," "biological embedding," "trajectories," and "pathways." Terms like "programming" have been criticized as being too deterministic given the implication that a certain experience or set of risk factors can program a disease pathway; such a term eschews the nature of developmental plasticity and the phenotypic range that can emerge as the organism or individual encounters other experiences. Hanson and Gluckman have suggested that a term like priming, induction, or conditioning be used to describe the process by which an exposure or experience induces a phenotypic alteration that prepares the organism for a similar environmental challenge later in the life course (Hanson and Gluckman 2014). Throughout this volume, we have sought and encouraged the authors to avoid terms like programming and biological embedding in favor of conditioning or priming. Similarly, notions of critical periods have been part of embryology for over a century, and many biologists will refer to critical periods in biological development as a specific time that usually starts and ends abruptly and during which a given event or its absence has a specific impact on development. The experiments by Hubel and Wiesel to examine the development of the visual cortex seemed to indicate that there were critical periods for specific complex neurons to develop (Hubel and Wiesel 1977). However, most developmental science suggests that because of the inherent plasticity in human development and in many specific regulatory systems, the term "sensitive period" is less deterministic and therefore much more appropriate.

In addition to the confusion around terminology, Hanson and Gluckman suggest several other reasons for why the related concept of developmental origins of health and disease has faced challenges, including confusion between factors correlated with disease and those involved in causation, the assumption that the only pathway connecting early exposures and later disease was low birth weight, a lack of plausible biological mechanisms, a failure to recognize developmental origins under normal rather than under extreme conditions, and the lack of evidence of its relative importance in relationship to other risk factors (Hanson and Gluckman 2014). Whereas all of these challenges are important and have begun to be addressed, the relative risk issues have been some of the most daunting since these questions require longitudinal data over very long time horizons to tease out.

This volume is designed to address these challenges and bridge the resultant gaps, including the delay in broad acceptance and understanding of how health develops across the life-span (Hanson and Gluckman 2014), as well as in the translation of that perspective to health practice and policy.

Each of the six sections comprising this volume was conceptualized during the process of planning the LCRN's 2013 MCH Life Course Research Agenda-Setting Meeting, with the ultimate goal of informing the development of an MCH Life Course Research Agenda (LCRA) that would provide MCHB, the National Institutes of Health (NIH), and other funding institutions and organizations with guidance regarding priority research questions and topics worthy of investment. With input from the LCRN advisory committee, project staff determined that the LCRA (Sect. 6), which is in many ways the culmination of the LCRN's 6 years of work to date, would have to address theoretical concerns (Sect. I), specific periods of the life course (Sect. II), specific health conditions (Sect. III) – some common and some rare but nevertheless important because of their severity or their representativeness of a set of conditions sharing similar life course origins and/or implications – cross-cutting topics in LCHD (Sect. IV), and methodological issues (Sect. V) to support researchers in carrying out the kinds of studies the research agenda would call for.

Similarly, the majority of the chapter topics contained in this volume were selected early on in the development of the agenda-setting process. However, as noted in the Preface, several chapters were commissioned following the 2013 agenda-setting meeting in response to identified gaps, and others were selected based on author interest in submitting a chapter for inclusion in the agenda-setting process and/or published volume. The editors acknowledge that several important topics have not been included in this edition of the volume. In some cases, this omission was due to the difficulty of identifying a qualified author/author team willing to develop a chapter on a given topic; in other instances, chapters were commissioned but not completed in time for inclusion in this edition. It is the editors' hope that future editions of this volume will address these worthy topics through new chapters on topics ranging from asthma and ADHD to family experiences, mental health conditions, and LCHD measures and biomarkers, among others. For now, however, it is our hope that readers will appreciate the range of topics included in this edition and the potential for these 26 chapters – all of which synthesize existing LCHD research, identify knowledge gaps, and/or recommend priorities related to future research and efforts to ensure the appropriate and timely translation of that research into practice and policy – to have a significant impact on how LCHD stakeholders think about, study, and work to promote health.

Chapters "Middle Childhood: An Evolutionary-Developmental Synthesis" and "Pregnancy Characteristics and Women's Cardiovascular Health" contain modified versions of previously published reviews and analyses of existing research. Given the relatively recent emergence of the field of LCHD and our goal to further coalesce that field through the publication of this volume, we thought it important to include the content in the handbook so that the important research both chapters contain could be situated firmly within the growing body of LCHD research and have a meaningful influence on the content of the LCRA.

3.1 Section I: Emerging Frameworks

This section contains a single chapter by pediatricians and public health experts Neal Halfon, MD, MPH, and Christopher B. Forrest, MD, PhD, entitled *The Emerging Theoretical Framework of*

Life Course Health Development (Halfon and Forrest 2017). The authors – who also served as two of the editors of the volume – propose a set of principles that together form a more unified theoretical framework for the emerging LCHD field. These principles have the potential to guide future theory building, research, and policy pertaining to optimizing health development in the USA and abroad. Each subsequent chapter refers to the principles when appropriate to demonstrate how they can help to explain empirical findings or set the stage for future inquiry.

3.2 Section II: Life Stages

Section II is comprised of six chapters exploring health development from the preconceptional/prenatal period to early adulthood. Each describes the kinds of experiences and exposures that result in more (or less) optimal outcomes during a given developmental period *and* the importance of that period for outcomes over the remainder of the life course. As such, this section of the volume grounds the literature reviewed about each life stage firmly within the LCHD framework.

Preconception and Prenatal Factors and Metabolic Risk – by pediatrician, MCH researcher, and molecular epidemiologist Xiaobin Wang, MD, MPH, ScD, and colleagues Guoying Wang, MD, PhD, and Tami R. Bartell – examines health during the earliest part of the life course, reviewing what is known about the mechanisms underlying both its sensitivity to alterations in the intrauterine environment. The authors explain the importance of this life period for lifelong and transgenerational health, including links to obesity, diabetes, cardiovascular disease, behavioral and psychiatric disorders, and more (Wang et al. 2017).

Early Childhood Health and the Life Course: The State of the Science and Proposed Research Priorities was authored by social epidemiologist and developmental-behavioral pediatrician W. Thomas Boyce, MD, and the late Clyde Hertzman, MD, MSc, who, as noted in this introduction, played a central role in delineating early childhood development as a determinant of lifelong health. The chapter reviews the literature regarding the susceptibility of young children to social environmental conditions, explains how variation among individuals in terms of both their susceptibility and their exposures helps to explain variation in health development outcomes, and examines the process by which early adversity becomes biologically embedded (Boyce and Hertzman 2017).

Marco Del Giudice's chapter on *Middle Childhood: An Evolutionary-Developmental Synthesis* demonstrates the unique significance of middle childhood by examining – from an evolutionary perspective – the cognitive, behavioral, and hormonal processes that characterize this life stage, as well as its function as a switch point in the adaptive development of life history strategies and the implications for life course health development (DelGiudice 2017).

Adolescent Health Development: A Relational Developmental Systems Perspective is the result of collaboration among experts in developmental psychology, human development, public health, and pediatrics. The authors are Richard M. Lerner, PhD; Claire C. Brindis, DrPH; Milena Batanova, PhD; and Robert Wm. Blum, MD, MPH, PhD. This chapter relates the seven proposed principles of LCHD to the Relational Developmental Systems (RDS) metatheoretical perspective, illustrating their interrelationships and differences. The authors discuss the implications of both conceptual frameworks for studying the life course origins and impact of adolescent health and for promoting thriving during adolescence (Lerner et al. 2017).

Early Adulthood as a Critical Stage in the Life Course was produced by a group of authors with expertise in pediatrics, occupational therapy, psychology, and public health. In this chapter, David Wood, MD, MPH; Tara Crapnell, ORD, OTR/L; Lynette Lau, PhD; Ashley Bennett, MD; Debra Lotstein, MD, MPH; Maria Ferris, MD, PhD, MPH; and Alice Kuo, MD, PhD, employ an ecological approach to examine the period of life from 20 to 30 years of age. The authors also discuss the impact of chronic disease and other factors that affect the transition to adulthood in the educational, employment, and social arenas (Wood et al. 2017).

Epidemiologists Abigail Fraser, MPH, PhD, MRC; Janet Catov, PhD; Debbie Lawlor, MRC; and Janet Rich-Edwards', ScD, MPH, chapter on *Pregnancy Characteristics and Women's Cardiovascular Health* is a unique contribution exploring the link between women's reproductive outcomes and their risk for cardiovascular disease. The chapter presents the implications for research and policy including the potential to identify high-risk women earlier in the life course (Fraser et al. 2017).

3.3 Section III: The Life Course Origins and Consequences of Specific Diseases and Health Conditions

Section III of this volume examines the life course origins and consequences of some of the most common diseases and health conditions facing the US population today, as well as some less common but nevertheless important ones. Each of the eight chapters reviews and synthesizes prior basic and intervention research, points out the gaps in our knowledge, and speaks to the importance of additional research and its application to the policy and practice arenas. Together, these chapters demonstrate the value of the LCHD perspective in understanding and improving outcomes across a variety of populations and challenges.

Social epidemiologist Summer Sherburne Hawkins, PhD, MS, collaborated with pediatrician and prenatal nutrition expert Emily Oken, MD, MPH and pediatrician and preventive cardiology expert Matthew W. Gillman, MD, SM, to produce *Early in the Life Course: Time for Obesity Prevention*. This chapter adopts a multilevel approach in identifying the periods and factors that are the greatest contributors to obesity and explores how innovative research methodologies can be used to demonstrate causality (Hawkins et al. 2017).

Pediatric Type 2 Diabetes: Prevention and Treatment Through a Life Course Health Development Framework was written by Pamela Salsberry, PhD, RN, FAAN; Rika Tanda, PhD, RN; Sarah E. Anderson, PhD; and Manmohan K. Kamboj, MD, an author team representing a range of fields and disciplines including nursing, pediatrics, public health, endocrinology, and epidemiology. Their chapter uses an LCHD perspective to promote a better understanding of the development of pediatric T2DM, as well as a more effective approach to prevention and treatment (Salsberry et al. 2017).

Clinical psychologist Irene E. Drmic, PhD, CPsych, collaborated with psychiatric and genetic epidemiologist Peter Szatmari, MD, MSc, and *Journal of Autism and Developmental Disabilities* editor-in-chief Fred Volkmar, MD, MA, to produce *Life Course Health Development in Autism Spectrum Disorders*. This chapter applies the LCHD framework to autism spectrum disorders (ASD) in order to inform future research and ultimately improve health development for individuals with ASD, as well as their families and communities (Drmic et al. 2017).

Self-Regulation was written by a large and diverse group of experts spanning developmental, quantitative, and educational psychology. Together, Megan McClelland, PhD; John Geldof, PhD; Frederick J. Morrison; Steinunn Gestsdóttir, PhD; Claire Cameron, PhD; Ed Bowers, MEd, PhD; Angela Duckworth, PhD; Todd Little, PhD; and Jennie Grammer, PhD, examine the development and importance of self-regulation through an LCHD lens and from the standpoint of the relational developmental systems (RDS) metatheoretical framework (McClelland et al. 2017).

A Life Course Health Development Perspective on Oral Health was written by James J. Crall, DDS, ScD, and Christopher Forrest, MD, PhD. By applying the LCHD framework and their expertise in pediatric oral health and public health, the authors advance a more contemporary conceptualization and definition of oral health as a more integral and integrated component of overall health and well-being (Crall and Forrest 2017).

Life Course Health Development Outcomes After Prematurity: Developing a Community, Clinical, and Translational Research Agenda to Optimize Health, Behavior and Functioning is the result of a collaboration among pediatrician Michael E. Msall, MD, and a group of colleagues representing nursing, pediatrics, sociology, and demography, including Sarah A. Sobotka, MD, MS; Amelia Dmowska; Dennis Hoga, PhD; and Mary Sullivan, PhD, RN. Together the authors examine the underlying causes of observed disparities in LCHD outcomes among children born prematurely, the value of life course-focused population-level interventions for closing the gap, and the need to improve the availability and systematic provision of such services (Msall et al. 2017).

A Life Course Approach to Hearing Health was written by Shirley A. Russ, MB, ChB, MRCP, FRACP, MCH; Kelly Tremblay, PhD, CCC-A; Neal Halfon, MD, MPH; and Adrian Davis, BSC, MSc, PhD, FFPH, FSS, OBE – an author team representing both pediatrics and speech and hearing. The chapter explores the origins of the full spectrum of hearing loss, including genetic, congenital, and environmental causes, and the mechanisms by which they interact and act upon an individual's hearing health development over the life-span (Russ et al. 2017).

Nephrologists Patrick Brophy, MD; Jennifer R. Charlton, MD, MSc; J. Bryan Carmody, MD; Kimberly J. Reidy, MD; David Askenazi, MD; and Susan P. Bagby, MD, teamed up with pediatrician Lindsay Harshman, MD; neonatologist Jeffrey Segar, MD; and public health expert David Shoham, PhD, MSPH, to produce *Chronic Kidney Disease: A Life Course Health Development Perspective*. In this chapter, the authors find that the LCHD framework is of great value in both elucidating the sequelae of CKD risk and identifying the kinds of early life interventions that have the potential to mitigate it (Brophy et al. 2017).

3.4 Section IV: Cross-Cutting Topics in Life Course Health Development

This section of the volume addresses four key issues – growth, nutrition, adversity, and disparities – that are relevant to understanding and addressing a wide range of diseases and health conditions.

Growth and Life Course Health Development was written by a team of authors spanning medicine, public health, and anthropology. In their chapter, Amanda Mummert, MA, Meriah Schoen, and Michelle Lampl, MD, PhD, employ a systems biology approach to examine the pathways affecting growth and explore auxology's role in a variety of health trends (Mummert et al. 2017).

From Epidemiology to Epigenetics: Evidence for the Importance of Nutrition to Optimal Health Development Across the Life Course was written by nutrition experts Marion Taylor-Baer, PhD, MSNS, RD, and Dena Herman, MSNS, MPH, RD. Their chapter uses the LCHD framework to examine the crucial role that nutrition plays in the development of health potential over the life-span, including the role of evolutionarily driven adaptive responses during the prenatal and early childhood periods (Taylor-Baer and Herman 2017).

In *How Socioeconomic Disadvantages Get Under the Skin and into the Brain to Influence Health Development Across the Lifespan*, developmental psychologists Pilyoung Kim, PhD; Gary Evans, PhD; Edith Chen, PhD; and Gregory Miller, PhD, collaborated with epidemiologist Teresa Seeman, PhD, to explain the neurobiological mechanisms and processes by which SES-related adversity, including chronic stress, affect health trajectories from early life to old age (Kim et al. 2017).

Health sciences researcher Kandyce Larson, PhD, together with pediatricians Shirley A. Russ, MD, MPH; Robert S. Kahn, MD, MPH; Glenn Flores, MD, FAAP; Elizabeth Goodman, MD; Tina L. Cheng, MD, MPH; and Neal Halfon, MD, MPH, produced *Health Disparities: A Life Course Health Development Perspective and Future Research Directions*. This chapter explores the factors and processes that contribute to health disparities across lifetimes and generations from the perspective of life course health development in order to illuminate potential practice and policy solutions to this persistent problem (Larson et al. 2017).

3.5 Section V: Methodological Approaches

Section V is comprised of five chapters that will be of practical use to researchers who are engaged or who would like to engage in future research aimed at enhancing our understanding of how health develops over the life course and/or understanding how practice and policy can optimize health development outcomes. The first two chapters in this section review current research methods and study designs that are of particular value for LCHD research. The remaining three chapters describe existing longitudinal datasets that have the potential to be used to answer the kinds of research questions that are described in the Life Course Research Agenda, Version 1.0 (Halfon et al. 2017).

In *Core Principles of Life Course Health Development Methodology and Analytics*, developmental and educational psychologist and statistician-methodologist Todd Little, PhD, acknowledges the inherent complexity of LCHD studies. He suggests that underutilized techniques, such as structural equation modeling, multilevel modeling, and mixture distribution modeling, as well as new and collaborative team-based research practices, have the potential to rapidly advance the field (Little 2017).

In *Epidemiological Study Designs: Traditional and Novel Approaches to Advance Life Course Health Development Research*, epidemiologists Stephen L. Buka, PhD; Samantha R. Rosenthal, PhD; and Mary E. Lacy explore the benefits and limitations of the various approaches that can be used to study the development of health and disease over the life course (Buka et al. 2017).

Using the National Longitudinal Surveys of Youth (NLSY) to Conduct Life Course Analyses by sociologist Elizabeth Cooksey, PhD, demonstrates how this long-running three-cohort longitudinal study – which provides a wealth of data on health, education, employment, household information, family background, marital history, child care, income and assets, attitudes, substance use, and criminal activity – can be used to explore various LCHD-related research questions (Cooksey 2017).

Sociologist and demographer Narayan Sastry, PhD, worked with research scientists Paula Fomby, PhD, and Katherine McGonagle, PhD, to develop the chapter on *Using the Panel Study of Income Dynamics (PSID) to Conduct Life Course Health Development Analysis*. This chapter explains how this nationally representative longitudinal study – which is the longest-running household panel study in the world, covering 47 years of data on a wide range of economic, demographic, social, and health topics – can be used to examine health development over the life course (Sastry et al. 2017).

In *Using the Fragile Families and Child Wellbeing Study (FFCWS) in Life Course Health Development Research*, sociologist Amanda Geller, PhD, collaborates with FFCWS staff members Kate Jaeger and Garrett Pace to describe this nationally representative birth cohort study that contains both biological and social indicators. The authors provide examples of its use for exploring questions about health development in households with unmarried parents (Geller et al. 2017).

3.6 Section VI: Conclusions

Section VI of this volume contains a single chapter entitled *Life Course Research Agenda (LCRA), Version 1.0* in which editors Neal Halfon, MD, MPH; Christopher B. Forrest, MD, PhD; Richard M. Lerner, PhD; and Elaine Faustman, PhD, together with LCRN staff members Ericka Tullis, MPP, and John Son, MPH, synthesize the recommendations for future research contained in many of the previous chapters and propose a set of priority research types, topics, and questions, as well as a set of activities aimed at improving our ability to carry out this critical research and ensure its timely translation to practice and policy. The authors also recommend strategies that can support the ongoing refinement of the LCHD theoretical framework (Halfon et al. 2017). As this volume goes to press, the LCRN is initiating an inclusive process to review and refine this initial version of the LCRA so that it is sure to guide both researchers and potential funders toward the studies that will be of greatest benefit in terms of enhancing our rapidly growing but as yet incomplete understanding of life course health development.

References

Acheson, D. (1998). *Independent inquiry into inequalities in health report*. Stationery Office.

Aldwin, C. M. (2014). Rethinking developmental science. *Research in Human Development, 11*(4), 247–254.

Antony, P. M., Balling, R., & Vlassis, N. (2012). From systems biology to systems biomedicine. *Current Opinion in Biotechnology, 23*(4), 604–608.

Baltes, P. B., Lindenberger, U., & Staudinger, U. M. (2006). Lifespan theory in developmental psychology. In W. Damon & R. M. Lerner (Eds.), *Handbook of child psychology. Vol. 1: Theoretical models of human development* (6th ed., pp. 569–664). New York: Wiley.

Barker, D. J. (1995). Fetal origins of coronary heart disease. *BMJ, 311*(6998), 171.

Barker, D. J., Osmond, C., Winter, P. D., Margetts, B., & Simmonds, S. J. (1989). Weight in infancy and death from ischaemic heart disease. *The Lancet, 334*(8663), 577–580.

Barker, D. J., Godfrey, K. M., Gluckman, P. D., Harding, J. E., Owens, J. A., & Robinson, J. S. (1993). Fetal nutrition and cardiovascular disease in adult life. *The Lancet, 341*(8850), 938–941.

Ben-Shlomo, B., & Kuh, D. (2002). A life course approach to chronic disease epidemiology: Conceptual models, empirical challenges and interdisciplinary perspectives. *International Journal of Epidemiology, 31*(2), 285–293.

Berkman, L. F., Kawachi, I., & Glymour, M. M. (Eds.). (2014). *Social epidemiology*. Oxford: Oxford University Press.

Braveman, P. (2014). What is health equity: And how does a life-course approach take us further toward it? *Maternal and Child Health Journal, 18*(2), 366–372.

Bronfenbrenner, U. (2005). *Making human beings human*. Thousand Oaks: Sage.

Boyce, T., & Hertzman, C. (2017). Early childhood and the life course: The state of the science and proposed research priorities. In N. Halfon, C. B. Forrest, R. M. Lerner, & E. Faustman (Eds.), *Handbook of life course health development*. New York: Springer.

Boyce, T. W., & Keating, D. P. (2004). Should we intervene to improve childhood circumstances? In D. Kuh & Y. Ben-Shlomo (Eds.), *A life course approach to chronic disease epidemiology* (Vol. 2). New York: Oxford University Press.

Brophy, P. D., Charlton, J. R., Carmody, J. B., Reidy, K. J., Harshman, L., Segar, J., Askenazi, D., & Shoham, D. (2017). Chronic kidney disease: A life course health-development perspective. In N. Halfon, C. B. Forrest, R. M. Lerner, & E. Faustman (Eds.), *Handbook of life course health development*. New York: Springer.

Buka, S. L., Rosenthal, S. R., & Lacy, M. E. (2017). Epidemiological study designs: Traditional and novel approaches to advance life course health-development research. In N. Halfon, C. B. Forrest, R. M. Lerner, & E. Faustman (Eds.), *Handbook of life course health development*. New York: Springer.

Capra, F. (1982). *The turning point: Science, society, and the rising culture*. Toronto: Bantam Books.

Committee on Future Directions for Behavioral and Social Sciences Research., Singer B. H., Ryff, C. D (Eds.). (2001). *New horizons in health: An integrative approach*. Washington, DC: National Academies Press.

Committee on Evaluation of Children's Health; Board on Children, Youth and Families; Division of Behavioral and Social Sciences and Education; National Research Council; Institute of Medicine. (2004). *Children's health, the nation's wealth: Assessing and improving child health*. Washington, DC: National Academies Press.

Committee on the Recommended Social and Behavioral Domains and Measures for Electronic Health Records, Board on Population Health and Public Health Practice, Institute of Medicine. (2015). *Capturing social and behavioral domains and measures in electronic health records: Phase 2*. Washington, DC: National Academies Press (US).

Cooksey, E. (2017). Using the National Longitudinal Surveys of Youth (NLSY) to conduct life course analyses. In N. Halfon, C. B. Forrest, R. M. Lerner, & E. Faustman (Eds.), *Handbook of life course health development*. New York: Springer.

Crall, J. J., & Forrest, C. B. (2017). A life course health-development perspective on oral health. In N. Halfon, C. B. Forrest, R. M. Lerner, & E. Faustman (Eds.), *Handbook of life course health development*. New York: Springer.

Davey Smith, G., & Lynch, J. (2004). Life course approaches to socioeconomic differentials in health. In D. Kuh & Y. Ben-Shlomo (Eds.), *A life course approach to chronic disease epidemiology* (Vol. 2). New York: Oxford University Press.

Davila-Velderrain, J., Martinez-Garcia, J. C., & Alvarez-Buylla, E. R. (2015). Modeling the epigenetic attractors landscape: Toward a post-genomic mechanistic understanding of development. *Frontiers in Genetics, 6*, 160.

DelGiudice, M. (2017). Middle childhood: An evolutionary-developmental synthesis. In N. Halfon, C. B. Forrest, R. M. Lerner, & E. Faustman (Eds.), *Handbook of life course health development*. New York: Springer.

Drmic, I. E., Szatmari, P., & Volkmar, F. (2017). Life course health-development in autism spectrum disorders. In N. Halfon, C. B. Forrest, R. M. Lerner, & E. Faustman (Eds.), *Handbook of life course health development*. New York: Springer.

Elder, G. H., Shanahan, M. J., & Jennings, J. A. (2015). Human development in time and place. In M. H. Bornstein& T. Leventhal (Eds.), *Handbook of child psychology and developmental science. Vol. 4: Ecological settings and processes in developmental systems* (7th ed., pp. 6–54). Editor-in-chief: R.M. Lerner. Hoboken: Wiley.

Evans, R. G., Barer, M. L., & Marmor, T. R. (Eds.). (1994). *Why are some people healthy and others not?: The determinants of health of populations*. New York: Aldine de Gruyter, 1994.

Ford, D. L., & Lerner, R. M. (Eds.). (1992). *Developmental systems theory: An integrative approach*. Newbury Park: Sage.

Forrest, C. B., & Riley, A. W. (2004). Childhood origins of adult health: A basis for life-course health policy. *Health Affairs (Millwood), 23*(5), 155–164.

Foster, K. R. (2011). The sociobiology of molecular systems. *Nature Reviews Genetics, 12*, 193–203.

Fraser, A., Catov, J. M., Lawlor, D. A., Rich-Edwards, J. W. (2017). Pregnancy characteristics and women's cardiovascular health. In N. Halfon, C. B. Forrest, R. M. Lerner, E. Faustman (Eds.), *Handbook of life course health development*. New York: Springer.

Gee, G. C., Walsemann, K. M., & Brondolo, E. (2012). A life course perspective on how racism may be related to health inequities. *American Journal of Public Health, 102*(5), 967–974.

Geller, A., Jaeger, K., & Pace, G. (2017). Using the fragile families and child wellbeing study (FFCWS) in life course health-development research. In N. Halfon, C. B. Forrest, R. M. Lerner, & E. Faustman (Eds.), *Handbook of life course health development*. New York: Springer.

Gillman, M. W. (2004). A life course approach to obesity. In D. Kuh & Y. Ben-Shlomo (Eds.), *A life course approach to chronic disease epidemiology* (Vol. 2). Oxford University Press.

Gluckman, P. D., & Hanson, M. A. (2004). Living with the past: Evolution, development, and patterns of disease. *Science, 305*(5691), 1733–1736.

Gluckman, P. D., Hanson, M. A., Cooper, C., & Thornburg, K. L. (2008). Effect of in utero and early-life conditions on adult health and disease. *New England Journal of Medicine, 359*(1), 61–73.

Gottlieb, G. (1998). Normally occurring environmental and behavioral influences on gene activity: From central dogma to probabilistic epigenesist. *Psychological Review, 105*, 792–802.

Greenblum, S., Turnbaugh, P. J., & Borenstein, E. (2012). Metagenomic systems biology of the human gut microbiome reveals topological shifts associated with obesity and inflammatory bowel disease. *Proceedings of the National Academy of Sciences, 109*(2), 594–599.

Halfon, N., & Forrest, C. B. (2017). The emerging theoretical framework of life course health-development. In N. Halfon, C. B. Forrest, R. M. Lerner, & E. Faustman (Eds.), *Handbook of life course health development*. New York: Springer.

Halfon, N., Forrest, C. B., Lerner, R. M., Faustman, E., Tullis, E., & Son, J. (2017). Life course research agenda (LCRA), version 1.0. In N. Halfon, C. B. Forrest, R. M. Lerner, & E. Faustman (Eds.), *Handbook of life course health development*. New York: Springer.

Halfon, N., & Hochstein, M. (2002). Life course health development: An integrated framework for developing health, policy and research. *The Milbank Quarterly, 80*(3), 433–479.

Halfon, N., Inkelas, M., & Hochstein, M. (2000). The health development organization: An organizational approach to achieving child health development. *The Milbank Quarterly, 78*(3), 447–497.

Halfon, N., Larson, K., Lu, M., Tullis, E., & Russ, S. (2014). Lifecourse health development: Past, present and future. *Maternal and Child Health Journal, 18*(2), 344–365.

Hancock, T. (1986). Lalonde and beyond: Looking back at "a new perspective on the health of Canadians". *Health Promotion International, 1*(1), 93–100.

Hanson, M. A., & Gluckman, P. D. (2014). Early developmental conditioning of later health and disease: Physiology or pathophysiology? *Physiological Reviews, 94*(4), 1027–1076.

Hawkins, S. S., Oken, E., Gillman, M. W. (2017). Early in the life course: Time for obesity prevention. In N. Halfon, C. B. Forrest, R. M. Lerner, E. Faustman (Eds.), *Handbook of life course health development*. New York: Springer.

Hertzman, C. (1994). The lifelong impact of childhood experiences: A population health perspective. *Daedalus, 123*(4), 167–180.

Hertzman, C. (1999). The biological embedding of early experience and its effects on health in adulthood. *Annals of the New York Academy of Sciences, 896*(1), 85–95.

Hertzman, C., & Boyce, T. (2010). How experience gets under the skin to create gradients in developmental health. *Annual Review of Public Health, 31*, 329–347.

Huang, S. (2012). The molecular and mathematical basis of Waddington's epigenetic landscape: A framework for post-Darwinian biology? *BioEssays, 34*(2), 149–157.

Hubel, D. H., & Wiesel, T. N. (1977). Ferrier lecture: Functional architecture of macaque monkey visual cortex. *Proceedings of the Royal Society of London B: Biological Sciences, 198*(1130), 1–59.

Kandel, E. R., Dudai, Y., & Mayford, M. R. (2014). The molecular and systems biology of memory. *Cell, 157*(1), 163–186.

Keating, D. P., & Hertzman, C. (Eds.). (1999). *Developmental health and the wealth of nations: Social, biological, and educational dynamics*. New York: Guilford Press.

Kim, P., Evans, G. W., Chen, E., Miller, G., & Seeman, T. (2017). How socioeconomic disadvantages get under the skin and into the brain to influence health-development across the lifespan. In N. Halfon, C. B. Forrest, R. M. Lerner, & E. Faustman (Eds.),

Handbook of life course health development. New York: Springer.
Kitano, H. (2002). Systems biology: A brief overview. *Science, 295*(5560), 1662–1664.
Kuh, D., & Ben-Shlomo, Y. (Eds.). (1997). *A life course approach to chronic disease epidemiology* (Vol. 1). Oxford: Oxford University Press.
Kuh, D., & Ben-Shlomo, Y. (Eds.). (2004). *A life course approach to chronic disease epidemiology* (Vol. 2). New York: Oxford University Press.
Kuh, D., Cooper, R., Hardy, R., Richards, M., & Ben-Shlomo, Y. (Eds.). (2013). *A life course approach to healthy ageing*. Oxford: Oxford University Press.
Kuh, D., Power, C., Blane, D., & Bartley, M. (2004). Socioeconomic pathways between childhood and adult health. In D. Kuh & Y. Ben-Shlomo (Eds.), *A life course approach to chronic disease epidemiology* (Vol. 2). New York: Oxford University Press.
Lappé, M., & Landecker, H. (2015). How the genome got a life span. *New Genetics and Society., 34*(2), 152–176.
Larson, K., Russ, S. A., Kahn, R. S., Flores, G., Goodman, E., Cheng, T. L., & Halfon, N. (2017). Health disparities: A life course health-development perspective and future research directions. In N. Halfon, C. B. Forrest, R. M. Lerner, & E. Faustman (Eds.), *Handbook of life course health development*. New York: Springer.
Lawlor, D. A., & Mishra, G. D. (Eds.). (2009). *Family matters: Designing, analysing and understanding family based studies in life course epidemiology*. Oxford: Oxford University Press.
Lerner, R. M. (1984). *On the nature of human plasticity*. New York: Cambridge University Press.
Lerner, R. M. (2006). Developmental science, developmental systems, and contemporary theories. In R. M. Lerner (Ed.), *Theoretical models of human development. Volume 1 of Handbook of child psychology* (6th ed.). Editors-in-chief: Damon W & Lerner RM. Hoboken: Wiley.
Lerner, R. M. (2012). Developmental science: Past, present and future. *International Journal of Developmental Science., 6*, 29–36.
Lerner, R. M., & Callina, K. S. (2014). The study of character development: Towards tests of a relational developmental systems model. *Human Development, 57*(6), 322–346.
Lerner, R. M., & Overton, W. F. (2008). Exemplifying the integrations of the relational developmental system: Synthesizing theory, research, and application to promote positive development and social justice. *Journal of Adolescent Research, 23*, 245–255.
Lerner, R. M., Brindis, C. C., Batanova, M., & Blum, R. W. (2017). Adolescent health: A relational developmental systems perspective. In N. Halfon, C. B. Forrest, R. M. Lerner, & E. Faustman (Eds.), *Handbook of life course health development*. New York: Springer.
Little, T. D. (2017). Core principles of life course health-development methodology and analytics. In N. Halfon, C. B. Forrest, R. M. Lerner, & E. Faustman (Eds.), *Handbook of life course health development*. New York: Springer.
Lu, M., & Halfon, N. (2003). Racial and ethnic disparities in birth outcomes: A life-course perspective. *Maternal and Child Health Journal, 7*(1), 13–30.
McClelland, M., Morrison, F., Gestsdóttir, S., Cameron, C., Bowers, E., Duckworth, A., Little, T., & Grammer, J. (2017). Self-regulation. In N. Halfon, C. B. Forrest, R. M. Lerner, & E. Faustman (Eds.), *Handbook of life course health development*. New York: Springer.
Molenaar, P. C., & Newell, K. M. (Eds.). (2010). *Individual pathways of change: Statistical models for analyzing learning and development*. Washington, DC: American Psychological Association.
Msall, M. E., Sobotka, S. A., Dmowska, A., Hoga, D., & Sullivan, M. (2017). Life-course health-development outcomes after prematurity: Developing a community, clinical, and translational research agenda to optimize health, behavior and functioning. In N. Halfon, C. B. Forrest, R. M. Lerner, & E. Faustman (Eds.), *Handbook of life course health development*. New York: Springer.
Mummert, A., Schoen, M., & Lampl, M. (2017). Growth and life course health-development. In N. Halfon, C. B. Forrest, R. M. Lerner, & E. Faustman (Eds.), *Handbook of life course health development*. Springer.
Overton, W. F. (2010). Life-span development: Concepts and issues. In W. F. Overton (Ed.)., Lerner RM (Editor-in-Chief) *Handbook of life-span development, Vol. 1: Cognition, biology, and methods across the lifespan* (pp. 1–29). Hoboken: Wiley.
Overton, W. F. (2012). Evolving scientific paradigms: Retrospective and prospective. In L. L'Abate (Ed.), *The role of paradigms in theory construction* (pp. 31–65). New York: Springer.
Overton, W. F. (2015). Process and relational developmental systems. In W. F. Overton, & P. C. Molenaar (Eds.), *Theory and method*. Volume 1 of the *Handbook of child psychology and developmental science* (7th ed., pp. 9–62) Editor-in-chief: R. M. Lerner. Hoboken: Wiley.
Piro, R. M., & Di Cunto, F. (2012). Computational approaches to disease-gene prediction: Rationale, classification and successes. *The FEBS Journal, 279*(5), 678–696.
Russ, S. A., Tremblay, K., Halfon, N., & Davis, A. (2017). A lifecourse approach to hearing health. In N. Halfon, C. B. Forrest, R. M. Lerner, & E. Faustman (Eds.), *Handbook of life course health development*. New York: Springer.
Salsberry, P., Tanda, R., Anderson, S. E., & Kamboj, M. K. (2017). Pediatric type 2 diabetes: Prevention and treatment through a life course health-development framework. In N. Halfon, C. B. Forrest, R. M. Lerner, & E. Faustman (Eds.), *Handbook of life course health development*. New York: Springer.
Sameroff, A. (2010). A unified theory of development: A dialectic integration of nature and nurture. *Child Development, 81*(1), 6–22.

Sastry, N., Fomby, P., & McGonagle, K. (2017). Using the panel study of income dynamics (PSID) to conduct life course health-development analysis. In N. Halfon, C. B. Forrest, R. M. Lerner, & E. Faustman (Eds.), *Handbook of life course health development*. New York: Springer.

Schadt, E. E., & Björkegren, J. L. (2012). NEW: Network-enabled wisdom in biology, medicine, and health care. *Science Translational Medicine, 4*(115), 115rv1.

Taylor-Baer, M., & Herman, D. (2017). From epidemiology to epigenetics: Evidence for the importance of nutrition to optimal health-development across the lifecourse. In N. Halfon, C. B. Forrest, R. M. Lerner, & E. Faustman (Eds.), *Handbook of life course health development*. New York: Springer.

von Bertalanffy, L. (1933). *Modern theories of development: An introduction to theoretical biology*. London: Oxford University Press.

Wang, G., Bartell, T. R., & Wang, X. (2017). Preconception and prenatal factors and metabolic risk. In N. Halfon, C. B. Forrest, R. M. Lerner, & E. Faustman (Eds.), *Handbook of life course health development*. New York: Springer.

Whitehead, A. N. (1929/1978). *Process and reality: An essay in cosmology*. New York: The Free Press.

Wood, D., Crapnell, T., Lau, L., Bennett, A., Lotstein, D., Ferris, M., & Kuo, A. (2017). Emerging adulthood as a critical state in the life course. In N. Halfon, C. B. Forrest, R. M. Lerner, & E. Faustman (Eds.), *Handbook of life course health development*. New York: Springer.

Worthman, C. M., & Kuzara, J. (2005). Life history and the early origins of health differentials. *American Journal of Human Biology, 17*(1), 95–112.

Part I

Emerging Frameworks

The Emerging Theoretical Framework of Life Course Health Development

Neal Halfon and Christopher B. Forrest

1 Part 1: Context and Background

Over the last century, we have witnessed the power of the biomedical paradigm to treat the sick and prevent diseases from occurring. Conventional health science, as an applied field, has tried to make sense of what constitutes health by exploring the causes of *disease* in individual patients (medicine) and populations (public health). This approach has created a perspective of health as absence of disease or its risk factors and has been unsuccessful at explaining what it means to be healthy, how health develops over the lifespan, and the impact of health on the lives of individuals.

N. Halfon, MD, MPH (✉)
Department of Pediatrics, David Geffen School of Medicine, UCLA, Los Angeles, CA, USA

Department of Health Policy and Management, Fielding School of Public Health, UCLA, Los Angeles, CA, USA

Department of Public Policy, Luskin School of Public Affairs, UCLA, Los Angeles, CA, USA

Center for Healthier Children, Families, and Communities, UCLA, Los Angeles, CA, USA
e-mail: nhalfon@ucla.edu

C.B. Forrest, MD, PhD
Applied Clinical Research Center, Children's Hospital of Philadelphia, Philadelphia, PA, USA

Concepts of what constitutes health, and theories about how health is produced and optimized, are constantly evolving in response to myriad social and cultural expectations shaped by our contemporary worldview, scientific advances, improvements in health interventions, and the changing capacity of the health system. Stimulated originally by a series of studies demonstrating how growth during early life is related to chronic health conditions that emerge many decades later, an eruption of new research is identifying developmental processes that shape long-term health trajectories (Ben-Shlomo and Kuh 2002; Kuh and Ben-Shlomo 2004; Hanson and Gluckman 2014). This research is demonstrating how complex developmental processes integrate a range of behavioral, social, and environmental influences that modify gene expression, modulate physiologic and behavioral function, and dynamically shape different pathways of health production (Halfon and Hochstein 2002; Kuh and Ben-Shlomo 2004; Halfon et al. 2014). These empirical findings are highlighting the limitations of the more mechanistic biomedical and biopsychosocial models of health, which fail to offer comprehensive explanations about such phenomena as the developmental origins of health, how stress affects current and future health, and the consequences of dynamic interactions between individuals and their environments over time.

Informed by new theoretical perspectives emerging from such fields of study as developmental

N. Halfon et al. (eds.), *Handbook of Life Course Health Development*,
DOI 10.1007/978-3-319-47143-3_2

psychology (Lerner 2012), systems biology (Kitano 2002; Antony et al. 2012; Schadt and Bjorkegren 2012), epigenetics (Egger et al. 2004), the developmental origins of chronic disease (Gluckman and Hanson 2006a), and evolutionary developmental biology (West-Eberhard 2003), a transdisciplinary framework (Gatzweller and Baumuller 2013) is emerging which we call *Life Course Health Development* (*LCHD*) (Halfon and Hochstein 2002, Halfon et al. 2014). As a framework, LCHD organizes several different theories and conceptual models in order to make sense of the enormously challenging question of how health develops over the lifespan.

The LCHD framework addresses the developmental origins of health, the role that biological and behavioral plasticity play in facilitating different levels of adaptation, and how mismatches between biological propensity and environmental context interact to produce breakdowns in health, known as *disease*. As a framework that organizes numerous theories and concepts related to how health develops, LCHD is bridging what have sometimes been assumed to be polar opposites: nature versus nurture, mind versus body, individual versus population, and short-term versus long-term change. By unifying these dichotomies, LCHD offers a new perspective that will guide future scientific inquiry on health development and facilitate a long overdue and needed synthesis of medicine and public health—a synthesis that links treatment, prevention, and health promotion and catalyzes more integrated and networked strategies for designing, organizing, and implementing multilevel health interventions that transcend individual and population dichotomies. The LCHD framework will be increasingly useful as the human ecological footprint expands and influences the health development of Earth itself, creating new threats to human health via rapid and disruptive changes in physical environments, geographic dispersion of populations, and changes in social development.

This emergence of LCHD is reflective of larger scientific trends that are transforming research in the physical, natural, and social sciences. The comfort and certainty of simple, linear, and deterministic causal pathways are giving way to the uncomfortable uncertainty of nonlinear causal clusters that are networked together into complex, multilevel, interactive, and relational systems. LCHD embraces this complexity as the salient target of inquiry and requires research to be conducted with teams that are multidisciplinary, often large, networked, and highly collaborative. These shifts in scientific approach are helping us understand how our modern interdependent world is organized, how it functions, and how it contributes to the production of human health.

Given the explosion of life course-focused research in many scientific fields—including chronic disease epidemiology, developmental neuroscience, developmental psychology, evolutionary biology, genetics, epigenetics, environmental health sciences, economics, sociology, and many more—there is a growing need to provide a systematic framework for understanding and organizing this emerging knowledge base (i.e., sense making) so that it can be more effectively applied to solving health problems and guiding new and productive streams of exploration and discovery.

Our intent is not to provide a grand theory of Life Course Health Development. Rather, we seek to establish a set of principles that describe the contours of the rapidly emerging health development knowledge base by organizing many theories and conceptual models into a coherent synthesis. We recognize that LCHD is a work in progress. Our aim is to create conceptual coherence by contextualizing the meaning of disparate research findings, identifying gaps and uncertainties—including how concepts are defined, operationalized, and interpreted—and moving inquiry, application, and implementation forward. We hope that the principles of LCHD presented here, coupled with our explanatory narrative, will encourage theory building and testing, inspire innovative transdisciplinary research, and mature the framework into a scientific model with descriptive, explanatory, and predictive utility. Furthermore, we hope that LCHD will shine a light on the conundrum of how little attributable risk is explained in many studies of chronic disease, how early experience conditions future biological response patterns, and how these early experiences play through complex, environmentally influenced, and developmentally plastic health development pathways (Table 1).

In Part 2 of this chapter, we describe the ontological pathways—including theories, empirical findings, and concepts—that led to the LCHD framework, thereby orienting our view of health development from simple, mechanistic, and reductionist models to contemporary models that are holistic, complex, dynamically relational, and adaptive. In Part 3, we summarize the principles of the LCHD framework, grounding them in a set of transdisciplinary theories, models, and perspectives and addressing their implications for future inquiry (Fig. 1).

Beginning with the simple, mechanical, and mostly linear biomedical model, we chart how it was transformed into a more hierarchical, dynamic, and multiply determined biopsychosocial model, as the result of scientific breakthroughs in the understanding of the contribution of behavioral, social factors and their influence on individuals during specific life stages. This biopsychosocial model has now evolved into a more complex, relational, adaptive, dynamic, and developmental model of Life Course Health Development (LCHD) as result of the influence of scientific breakthroughs in epigenetics, neurodevelopment, and life course chronic disease epidemiology.

Table 1 Principles of the Life Course Health Development Framework

Principle	Brief description
1. Health Development	Health development integrates the concepts of health and developmental processes into a unified whole
2. Unfolding	Health development unfolds continuously over the lifespan, from conception to death, and is shaped by prior experiences and environmental interactions
3. Complexity	Health development results from adaptive, multilevel, and reciprocal interactions between individuals and their physical, natural, and social environments
4. Timing	Health development is sensitive to the timing and social structuring of environmental exposures and experiences
5. Plasticity	Health development phenotypes are systematically malleable and enabled and constrained by evolution to enhance adaptability to diverse environments
6. Thriving	Optimal health development promotes survival, enhances well-being, and protects against disease
7. Harmony	Health development results from the balanced interactions of molecular, physiological, behavioral, cultural, and evolutionary processes

2 Part 2: Emergence of the Life Course Health Development Framework

The LCHD framework has emerged from a network of theories, conceptual models, and empirical findings and provides a more comprehensive description of how health develops over the life course than any single component part. In this section, we describe the streams of scientific inquiry, the key theories and models, and the seminal scientific insights that are brought together by the LCHD framework. Figure 1 provides an epistemological schematic, charting the changing paradigms of health and how different streams of research and their findings influenced the flow of conceptual models.

A few decades ago, research linked fetal development with degenerative diseases of old age (Ben-Shlomo and Kuh 2002), stimulating new ways of thinking about the mechanisms underlying what was originally termed "fetal programming" and other environmentally induced modifications in gene expression that presumably take place early in life. These insights pointed out the need to better characterize interactions between genes and the environment, to better understand gene regulation that occurs in response to environmental signal transduction, and to better integrate into explanatory models the importance of the timing and phasing of these developmental processes. The prevailing epidemiological framework, with its simple additive, exposure-response models of risk accumulation

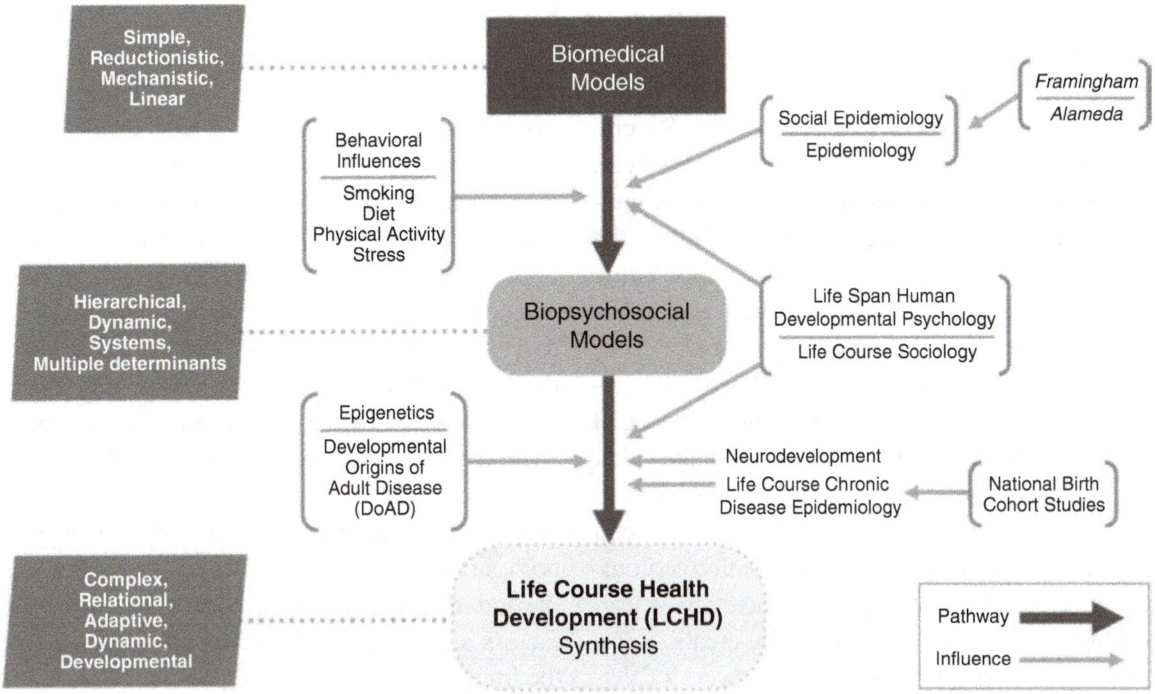

Fig. 1 The evolution of conceptual models of health development

as the etiology for chronic disease in adult life, could not satisfactorily explain these more complex time-dependent phenomena. Instead, a theoretical framework was needed to explain the processes of translating an individual's experiences and exposures into the development of health over the life course.

Two converging streams of biological research and conceptual constructs have contributed to the LCHD framework. The first stream represents the basic biology of human development, informed by the neo-Darwinian synthesis that resulted from the convergence of Darwin's theory of evolution and Mendel's notion of genes as the building blocks of heredity. Although the central dogma of "*genes/DNA → mRNA → proteins*" has served as a foundational construct for modern molecular biology, it led to overly deterministic genotype-to-phenotype models (Huang 2012). Recent advances in panomics (e.g., genomics, epigenomics, proteomics, metabolomics) and systems biology are redefining our understanding of how gene networks are regulated and dynamically interact with each other and the environment, resulting in a new synthesis of biological systems development and functioning (Huang 2012; Forrest 2014; Davila-Velderrain et al. 2015). Breakthroughs in understanding the relationships between evolutionary processes and biological development, and advances in the use of life history theory to explain how mismatches between biological propensities and modern environments influence the onset of disease, have also provided a new way of considering the relationship of an individual's or a population's genetic endowment and the phenotypes that emerge (Del Giudice et al. 2015; Green et al. 2015; Hanson and Gluckman 2014; Lieberman 2014; Gluckman and Hanson 2006a).

The second stream of inquiry, which interacted with genetic concepts and models, represents the evolution of models of disease causation, informed by contributions from basic, clinical, epidemiologic, social, and psychological research disciplines. In the first era of health science, scientific methods applied to medicine resulted in the development of a biomedical framework in which anatomical-pathological disease models, along with other mechanistic constructs, were used to explain why disease develops. One prototypical theoretical construct was germ theory (i.e., germs as the unique causes of infectious diseases) (Stewart 1968). Others included theories of inheritance that were informed by simple and mechanistic notions of genes as the unique causes of inherited disorders and risk status. Several decades of research on the "upstream" social and behavioral determinants of health were stimulated by epidemiologic studies like the Framingham Study and Alameda County Study that highlighted how cardiovascular and other chronic diseases were not caused by bad germs, bad genes, or bad luck, but were related to behaviors like smoking, diet, exercise, and other social factors as well as the metabolic changes that these social and behavioral risk factors induced (Dawber et al. 1974; Haynes 1980; Berkman and Syme 1979). This led to a more dynamic ecological analysis of the multiple risk factors that lead to disease causation, informing the creation of a multi-causal, biopsychosocial framework of disease (Engel 1977). Over the last 20 years, this biopsychosocial model of health has continued to evolve as a result of the integration of concepts from life course research in sociology (Elder 1995; Elder and Shanahan 2007), lifespan developmental research in psychology (Lerner 2012), systems biology (Schadt and Bjorkegren 2012), and longitudinal studies on the origins of chronic disease (Gluckman and Hanson 2004b). The biopsychosocial model undergirds much of the current focus on the social determinants of health and the important role that contextual factors play in shaping health outcomes (McMichael 1999; Krieger 2001).

Midway through the twentieth century, social scientists started examining how the rapidly changing social circumstances of the second industrial revolution were transforming the developmental pathways of different generations. Separate yet related streams of research emerged, converging around notions of the life course, the lifespan, and the human life cycle development. Two lines of investigation in particular have informed recent notions of health development: life course sociology and lifespan human developmental psychology (Diewald and Mayer 2009).

Life course theories emerged in sociology research in the 1960s, championed by Elder, Clausen, and others. These theories distinguished how social institutions and history shape the roles, personal events, transitions, and trajectories of individuals who follow different developmental pathways (Clausen 1986; Elder et al. 2003). Macro-level social processes and social relationships influence interweaving trajectories at different ages, stages, and transitions of development (Elder 1995). Untangling age, period, and cohort effects and understanding the cumulative impact of experience on socially and institutionally constructed life pathways form the basis of life course sociology. For example, the experience of low socioeconomic status, discrimination, and racial segregation may have different effects on health for different cohorts (i.e., groups born at different times), based on prevailing (period effects), compensatory, and mediating factors such as the availability of healthcare or the impact of different social policies (Chen et al. 2010; Masters et al. 2012).

Building on the work of Glen Elder, Duane Alwin (2012) suggested five ways that the term "life course" was used to describe etiologic processes in social and behavioral sciences: (1) lifespan development, humans develop over the life course; (2) agency, individuals construct their lives through choices and actions they take within social structures that provide opportunities and impose constraints; (3) cohort and geographic variation, lives of individuals are embedded and shaped by historical time and place where they live; (4) timing, impact of events, experiences, and transitions are conditional on their timing in a person's life; and, (5) linked lives, people's lives are lived interdependently (e.g., husband and wife, siblings).

Lifespan human developmental psychologists attempt to explain how individual differences emerge at different ages and stages (Lerner 1984; Lerner 2012). These differences are, in part, determined by endogenous characteristics (i.e., each individual's personal adaptability, plasticity, resilience, and reactivity) interacting with exogenous factors (i.e., external physical, social, and psychological environments that promote adaptation). These interactions cause human behavior to continuously change from conception to death (Lerner 1984, 2012). By focusing on the individual's capacity to adapt to events and experiences (Dannefer 1984; Alwin 2012), developmental psychologists have suggested that lifespan human development research concentrates on the plasticity associated with individual development (ontogenesis), whereas life course social sciences researchers emphasize "sociogenesis" or how life pathways are informed and structured by socially constructed developmental scaffolding and constraints. In short, psychologists have tended to focus on how *endogenous or constitutional* ontogenetic processes influence lifelong developmental trajectories, while sociologists have been more concerned with *contextual or exogenous* factors.

Over the past 30 years, there has growing convergence between life course sociology and lifespan human developmental psychology. Research on "linked lives," where the common and differential impact of shared exposures is experienced by individuals whose lives are linked geographically or socially (e.g., spouses, workers in a town, friendship networks) and work on transitions and turning points that are biologically (menarche, menopause) or socially determined (e.g., transitions from preschool to kindergarten, school to work, work to retirement), have each benefited from consideration of endogenous and exogenous factors. As the sociological approaches to life course and psychological approaches to lifespan research converge into a more integrated discipline of developmental science (Cairns et al. 1996; Bornstein and Lamb 2005; Diewald and Mayer 2009), ongoing conceptual and empirical integration is increasingly influenced by the study of nonlinear dynamic systems, including complex adaptive systems theory (Greenberg and Partridge 2010).

Many researchers and thought leaders have contributed to the conceptual evolution and empirical evidence supporting a more integrated developmental systems theory (Sameroff 1975; Bronfenbrenner 1976; Baltes et al. 1980; Lerner 1984; Cicchetti and Cohen 1995; Magnusson 1995; Cairns et al. 1996; Bronfenbrenner and Morris 2006; Sameroff 2010) which built upon earlier behavioral and biological theories (Greenberg and Partridge 2010; Marshall 2014). Overton and Lerner have proposed a theoretical construct that they call "relational developmental systems theory (RDST)" (Lerner 2006; Lerner and Overton 2008). Rejecting what they consider a false dichotomy between individual and context, they suggest that a person's development is embedded in, organized by, and co-regulated by his or her surrounding environments. Developmental regulatory functions are best understood as mutually influential, bidirectional, person-context interactions. RDST sees individuals as active co-developers of their own developmental pathways, adaptively responding to different biological, social, cultural, and physical environmental contexts that they influence and are also influenced by. RDST has been used as a theoretical foundation for research on self-regulation and positive youth development and has added a stronger relational dimension to life course thinking.

Like the converging influences of life course sociology and lifespan human developmental psychology, many fields of the life sciences have also informed this transition toward a life course developmental view of health. Embryologists and teratologists in the first part of the twentieth century understood that environmental insults could disrupt the normal processes of development leading to malformation and other "genetic" abnormalities, and some scientists began to consider how childhood conditions might directly influence adult mortality (Kuh and Davey Smith 2004). But it was not until the 1970s—when Forsdahl suggested a relationship between childhood socioeconomic status and later cardiovascular disease, Barker studied the relationship between birth weight and cardiovascular disease, and Wadsworth observed that other early childhood factors influenced a range of adult health outcomes—that a focus on what is called the developmental origins of adult health and disease (DOHaD) began to emerge (Forsdahl 1977; Arnesen and Forsdahl 1985; Barker et al. 1989a,b; Kuh and Wadsworth 1993).

The receptivity to this new perspective was heightened by a growing number of challenges to the biomedical model of causation. Echoing George Engel and others, social epidemiologists like John Cassel, Leonard Syme, Lisa Berkman, and Michael Marmot and health service researchers like Barbara Starfield began to adopt a more complex, multidimensional "web of causation" construct to explain the origins of disease (Cassel 1964; Starfield 1973; Starfield et al. 1984; Marmot and Syme 1976; Syme and Berkman 1976; Marmot et al. 1978a, b). At the same time, a growing body of new research in psychoneuroimmunology described the "embodiment of disease risk" by demonstrating how different social, cultural, and psychological exposures quite literally "get under the skin" and are encoded or embedded into developing biobehavioral systems (Sapolsky et al. 1985; Maier et al. 1994; Cohen and Herbert 1996; McEwan 1998; Repetti et al. 2002).

Over the past two decades, the Barker hypothesis, as it was commonly referred to, was further elaborated by a series of studies examining the impact of birth weight, fetal growth, placental size, and weight gain in the first year of life on metabolic regulation and cardiovascular disease (Barker et al. 1989a,b, 1993; McMillen and Robinson 2005; Barker et al. 2010). An entire field of life course epidemiology was spawned that has not only confirmed Barker's findings in several other cohorts and settings but vastly expanded the empirical base linking fetal and early childhood growth and nutrition to a growing array of adult health conditions. This work has also gone beyond examining fetal and early childhood origins to explore the developmental origins of health and disease more broadly and has generated various conceptual models to analyze and synthesize results (Schlotz and Phillips 2009; Gluckman et al. 2010; Entringer et al. 2012). A new generation of recent epigenetic studies have begun to provide a stronger biological and theoretical basis for understanding how developmental plasticity is manifested, how gene expression may be modified in response to environmental cues, and how biological and behavioral traits can be perpetuated across multiple generations (Hochberg et al. 2010; Gluckman 2014; Thayer and Kuzawa 2011; Davey Smith 2012; Lillycrop and Burdge 2012; Relton and Davey Smith 2012; Gilbert et al. 2015; Cunliffe 2015).

Complementary studies of the developing brain demonstrated how stress and social adversity influence the biology of human development during sensitive periods (Hertzman 1999; Boyce et al. 2012; Hertzman 2012). Building on earlier studies of experience-dependent and experience-expectant[1] neuronal development, neurodevelopmental research demonstrated how development is guided by the combined and interactive influences of genes and experience (Boyce et al. 2012). Animal models of experience-modified neural development demonstrated how early behavioral experiences of adversity or comfort can lead to different DNA methylation patterns, which are believed to affect gene regulation and result in different functional levels of neurotransmission capacity (Meaney 2001; Szyf et al. 2005; Meaney et al. 2007). Similar methylation alterations have been demonstrated in children who have experienced adversity associated with maternal stress in the early years (Essex et al. 2011). Research on the neurobiology of stress and on the role that cumulative physiologic stress can have on the function of neuroendocrine and neuroimmunologic pathways has provided direct evidence for how exposure to risk and/or highly adverse environments is embedded in lifelong biobehavioral function (Seeman 1997; McEwan 1998; Seeman et al. 2001; Repetti et al. 2011; McEwen 2012). This research on neural development, stress, and biological priming provides an important empirical and conceptual bridge between observed social gradients in health and the experience-dependent conditioning of biobe-

[1]Experience-dependent neuronal development refers to the role that experience plays in fortifying neuronal connections (e.g., a violin player who shows increased synaptic density in the area of the brain corresponding to the motor cortex controlling the fingers, or the hypertrophy of hippocampus in London cab drivers that is associated with improved spatial navigation and spatial memory). Experience-expectant neuronal development refers to brain development that is contingent on experiences that are expected to occur as part of normal development. For example, typical development of the visual cortex occurs in response to visual stimuli that are available in everyday life. If vision is obstructed and the brain does not receive these expected stimuli, the relevant synapses will either not form or will atrophy.

havioral systems that occurs during the process of human development (Hertzman 1999; Keating and Hertzman 1999; Halfon and Hochstein 2002).

In several ways, the converging relationship between life course chronic disease epidemiology, neurodevelopmental, and DOHaD research is analogous to the converging relationship between life course sociology and lifespan human developmental psychology. DOHaD and neurodevelopmental research have focused more on the individual differences in developmental plasticity from early development through old age (ontogenesis), leading to a growing understanding that epigenetic factors influence non-germline heredity. For example, the exposures grandparents experience can influence adaptive responses two generations later. In contrast, life course chronic disease epidemiology has focused more on social class, social gradients, and the social scaffolding of exposures (sociogenesis). New longitudinal cohort studies integrate both perspectives, including not only measures of phenotype but also genetic, epigenetic, and other biobehavioral adaptations (Alfred et al. 2012; Borghol et al. 2012; Elks et al. 2012).

3 Part 3: Principles of the Life Course Health Development Framework

In this section, we present the seven principles of the Life Course Health Development framework that emerged from our analysis of the network of theories, concepts, models, and research findings related to how health develops over the life course.

Each principle is described, connected to relevant theories, models, and perspectives, and discussed in terms of its implications for future research. Together, the principles constitute the LCHD framework, which is proposed as a way of systematically organizing the breadth of theories and conceptual models that help to explain and predict empirical findings on the production of health and disease causation over the life course.

4 Principle 1: Health Development

4.1 What We Mean by "Health Development"

Health development integrates the concepts of health and developmental processes into a unified whole.

We use the term "health development" to signify the framework's central focus, which is the linkage of health and development into a single construct. Health is often understood as a set of instrumental attributes that are employed when individuals pursue goal-directed behavior (Richman 2004; Forrest 2014). These attributes can be thought of as "assets" that are desirable, acquired, optimized, and maintained during the life course, enabling growth of an individual, survival, and adaptation to manifold environments. Examples of health assets that emerge at the level of an individual include motor function (capacity for movement), emotional regulation (capacity to manage emotions during challenges or stressful events), and cognitive function (capacity to perceive, process, and act on information leading to the acquisition of knowledge).

Development, in this context, refers to the processes by which health attributes change (i.e., mature, weather, degrade) during the lifespan. If health is a set of attributes that emerge at the level of the whole individual, development refers to the evolutionarily informed processes by which these attributes enable adaptation to changing social-environmental conditions. Health is the "what" (i.e., what changes) and development is the "how" (i.e., how health attributes change over time) of health development.

As an expression of an organism's livingness and essential adaptive nature, health development is an emergent property of a living system (Forrest 2014). Importantly, because this principle combines both health and development, it blends a temporal dimension into our conceptualization of human health. Health development has time-dependent and transactional connotations and is therefore dynamic.

The health development of an individual at the level of "self" cannot be understood by isolating the biological function (or dysfunction) of an organ system or a particular behavior of an individual—although of course these subsystems have their own unique health development trajectories. The health development of an individual is comprised of an integrated set of capacities that dynamically mature and are involved in managing energy flows; processing and acting on information; recovering from, adapting to, and growing with environmental challenges; learning and forming capabilities; and producing offspring (Forrest 2014). Health development is a life course-informed phenomenon that results from transactions between the organism and its internal (i.e., gene, panomic, organ system, and physiologic networks) and external environments (i.e., family, social, cultural, and physical networks and environments).

4.2 Theories and Frameworks Relevant to Health Development

This principle combines a rich set of theories and conceptual frameworks related to health and development. Conceptualizing health development as an emergent property of an organism differs from earlier linear and reductionistic biomedical models of health and even from multilevel biopsychosocial models. It also sets the stage for considering health development as complex adaptive processes that emerge from living systems interacting with their environments. Its relational ontology implies that other principles contribute to the understanding of this complex emergent process.

The optimization of health development is codependent on several contributing developmental processes and resulting propensities that are highlighted in the other LCHD principles and drawn from relational developmental systems theory (Lerner 2006; Overton 2007), developmental systems theory (Oyama 1985), dynamic systems theory (Spencer et al. 2009), and the unified theory of development (Sameroff 2010).

4.3 Implications of the Health Development Principle

The *health development* principle signals the importance of context and our inability to reduce health to its component parts divorced from the contexts within which they develop. This type of developmental systems thinking requires new typologies to describe health development phenotypes. In effect, a new set of concepts is needed to convey a language of health development as observed and experienced at the level of whole persons in dynamic interaction with their environments. As our understanding of the interrelationships between health development and a range of influential environmental variables matures, health development typologies can become full-fledged ontologies that help explain and predict which relational influences are important and have measurable consequences on health development.

The creation of "whole person" health development metrics that operationalize health development concepts is necessary to capture developmentally influenced continuity, consistency, and variability. To distinguish "health development" from other fields in the developmental sciences, we will need to specify the unique concepts that constitute it and the measures that assess health development's multidimensional functionality (adaptation, energy management, reproduction, information processing, capacity to execute tasks in response, and restoration and their integration) as well as its multilevel (from the molecular to the individual to the environmental) nature. Measures of health development will also need to be informed and reflective of the other LCHD principles outlined below. Such measures will be particularly important in enabling and measuring the contribution of health-producing social systems to the optimization of health development.

5 Principle 2: Unfolding

5.1 What We Mean by "Unfolding"

Health development occurs continuously over the lifespan, from conception to death, and is shaped by prior experiences and environmental interactions.

The *unfolding* principle describes the developmental processes by which expression of a few thousand genes—none of which has a blueprint or roadmap for constituting a viable, living human body—can unfold in an ordered, coherent pattern that has been shaped by the adaptive success of what has worked before. The nonlinear, self-organizing process of development that is made possible by molecule-to-molecule, cell-to-cell, tissue-to-tissue, and human-to-human sensing and communication processes means that health development is neither linear, passive, nor static; rather, it is adaptive, self-organizing, and autocatalytic (Davies 2014).

By "adaptive," we mean those biological, behavioral, and cultural differences that are privileged, prioritized, or selected for because of the advantage they imbue on reproductive fitness and success. Adaptive change occurs at multiple levels, from the biochemical and cellular to behavioral change at the level of individuals to environmental change. For some biological systems, such as neural networks, adaptation occurs quite rapidly, enabling real-time responses to acute environmental challenges and acquisition of novel information. However, some biological and behavioral subsystems change slowly responding to gradual shifts in the intensity and quality of ecological exposures. Thus, the adaptation that characterizes health development transpires over multiple time scales enabling response to both fast- and slow-changing variables. The principles of *complexity* and *timing* will further elaborate on these features of adaptation.

By "self-organizing," we mean the dynamic nonlinear process of self-assembly and self-perpetuation that emerges through multiple relational coactions between the components of a system and its environments. In the case of human health development, it describes how internally determined structures emerge from a genetic code that is regulated by layers of sensing, signaling, and feedback loops that organize the expression of the code based on chemical self-assembly into variable levels and forms of differentiation. Simple differences in external environments (at the cellular, tissue, organ system, organism, or cultural levels) transform the pathways of development from dull uniformity to autocatalytic diversity of forms and function (Davies 2014).

By "autocatalytic," we mean that health development produces the "fuel" that propels it forward (Henrich 2015). Health development dynamically shapes and is shaped by environmental contexts. Today's health development serves as substrate for the emergence of future health development states. The person-environmental transactions that unfold during the life course can influence gene regulation of biobehavioral processes through epigenetic changes. Better characterization of this set of mechanisms is helping to explain how physical and social exposures during childhood affect health and disease during adulthood.

The adaptive, self-organizing, autocatalytic processes of unfolding can help to explain how genes and culture have coevolved. According to Henrich (2015), as humans evolved, cultural information and practices began to accumulate and produce cultural adaptations. These new cultural adaptations feed forward and produce significant selection pressure on genes to improve psychological capacities to further acquire, store, process, and organize an array of fitness-enhancing skills and practices. These new adaptive capacities in turn become increasingly available to others in the same cultural group. So as genetic evolution improves the ability of our brains to learn from others, cultural evolution can generate adaptations (i.e., religions, markets, science) that both enhance function and increase the selective pressure on our brains to effectively navigate these increasingly complex cultural forms.

Life history theory suggests that variation in the process of unfolding result in part from the optimization of fitness that occurs during functionally organized phases of the lifespan. Borrowing from Paul Baltes' lifespan theory (Baltes, Lindenberger, Staudinger 2006), the *unfolding* principle offers a conceptualization of human health development as having four major functional phases:

(1) *Generativity*—the preconception, prenatal, and perinatal periods are dedicated to the formation of the organism.

(2) *Acquisition of capacity*—the early years are dedicated to the acquisition, maturation, and optimization of specific health development capacities.

(3) *Maintenance of capacity*—the middle years are dedicated to maintaining health development capacities in the face of accumulating risks and ongoing weathering.

(4) *Managing decline*—the later years are devoted to managing, adjusting, and adapting to functional decline of various body and regulatory systems, even as other aspects of health development such as stress management and positive psychological functioning may improve with age.

Each of these phases is conceptually distinct but can contain overlapping elements, as is the case when an older individual who is mostly in the process of managing decline can also be acquiring new capacities (e.g., learning to play piano at 70). This becomes an adaptive process of maintaining optimal function in the face of declining capacities.

By reflecting evolutionarily defined developmental processes, levels of plasticity, and variation in expression within and across individuals (and within and across biobehavioral systems in the same individual), these four phases help us to see and understand the patterns and coherence of health development. For example, evolution has ensured that the anatomic and metabolic process of bone development in women produces strong bones that enable additional weight carrying associated with pregnancy, until the age of the fourth and fifth decade when menopause emerges. This is an anticipatory developmental process whereby early anticipatory changes prepare the individual to meet future developmental needs. Optimizing bone metabolism and preventing osteoporosis can take several forms, such as physical activity (particularly on hard surfaces), and include different strategies that can be employed during the phases of acquisition and maintenance of bone metabolism and strength and during the management of decline after menopause.

5.2 Theories and Frameworks Relevant to Unfolding

The concept of health development as a continuously unfolding adaptive and self-organizing process comprised of distinct yet overlapping functional phases provides a framework for considering how evolutionarily defined stages from life history theory (Stearns 1992; Worthman and Kuzara 2005; Del Giudice et al. 2015), psychological constructs from lifespan human development theory (Baltes 1983; Featherman 1983; Lerner et al. 2010), and sociological constructs from life course sociology (Elder 2000; Mayer 2009; Alwin 2012) can be aligned, compared, and potentially integrated. It also provides a better way of articulating and assessing the alignment between biologically, psychologically, socially, and culturally determined transitions and turning points and understanding how they impact health development over the lifespan (Davies 2014; Henrich 2015) (see Principle 4--Timing). For example, the alignment among the biological processes of menarche, the behavioral maturation of reproduction behaviors, and the culturally created process of mating and marriage has dramatically changed as the age of menarche has declined, the age of marriage has increased, and the introduction of sexualized behavioral stimuli has increased through a variety of different media and information platforms.

5.3 Implications of the Unfolding Principle

The adaptive, self-organizing, and autocatalytic way that health development unfolds via complex sensing, communication, and regulatory processes implies that our basic, clinical, and translational research needs to elucidate how these processes influence the adaptive capacity of individuals and populations. A clearer understanding of how similar self-organizing processes unfold from the cellular level to the cultural level could point to new ways of integrating preventive, health promoting and therapeutic interventions designed to optimize health development by embracing a "cells to society" perspective.

We have proposed that there are four major functional phases of LCHD: generativity, acquisition of capacity, maintenance of capacity, and managing decline. Do these four phases provide a logical staging for all aspects of health development? Are there subphases that need to be articulated to help us better understand the dynamics of health development? To address these questions, we need better measurement of the flow of health development, both continuities and discontinuities, and its variation across and within individuals.

Childhood obesity provides a useful example to illustrate the research implications of the *unfolding* principle. To evaluate obesity risk, body mass index (BMI) is assessed at a fixed point in time and contrasted with values obtained with population age-sex-specific norms. Newer statistical methods have been developed that enable analysis of intraindividual trajectories to more accurately characterize the pattern of childhood growth and uncover new associations between the functional form of growth trajectories and future obesity and obesity-related comorbidities (Wen et al. 2012). To apply this sort of methodology to health development more broadly requires precise definitions and frequent assessments of health development measures, as well as an understanding of the expected trajectory of health development for the population. These types of assessments are being made available by electronic health records and other digitized health data collected by healthcare organizations, which are a new and ready data source for health development research.

The interaction between various forms of adversity and health development provides another example. Understanding the effects of social adversity and other environmental exposures on the unfolding of health development entails not only connecting the specific types of adversity to different outcomes but also developing a better understanding of the adaptive and self-organizing neuronal and behavioral processes, pathways, and mechanisms by which these outcomes are affected. These include assessing the relationships between neurodevelopmental correlates of socioeconomic adversity and differential structural and functional changes in different regions of the brain (as measured using functional MRIs) and understanding how these changes feed forward and potentially compound or dissipate over time (Caspi et al. 2003; Evans and Schamberg 2009; Hackman and Farah 2009; Noble et al. 2012; Power et al. 2005a, b; Evans et al. 2012).

The short- and long-term effects of adverse in utero exposures on health development are an area of inquiry that is producing a wealth of information and ripe for expansion (Gluckman et al. 2008). This research includes studies regarding epigenetic programming associated with fetal exposure to chemical compounds, environmental toxicants, and smoking (Skinner et al. 2008; Launay et al. 2009; Perera et al. 2009; Martino and Prescott 2011), as well as studies examining the impact of nutritional stresses on metabolic function and future disease (Li et al. 2010).

Research on the epigenetic effects of adversity on neurodevelopment has exploded in recent years. Beginning with Meaney's pathbreaking work on the impact of maternal behavior on epigenetic mechanisms that influence gene expression and regulation of the endocrine response to stress (including the glucocorticoid receptor and the corticotropin-releasing factor (CRF) systems that regulate the hypothalamic-pituitary-adrenal axis), there have been a large number of studies examining how different experiences, exposures, and influences can lead to epigenetic alterations affecting a wide range of biobehavioral functions (Meaney 2001, 2010; Turecki and Meaney 2016; Lester et al. 2016). One of the most interesting and challenging areas of epigenetic research concerns the trans-generational transmission of exposures and risk through non-germline alterations of genetic information and the persistence of these influences across subsequent generations (Bale 2015).

6 Principle 3: Complexity

6.1 What We Mean by "Complexity"

Health development results from adaptive, multilevel, and reciprocal relations between individuals and their physical, natural, and social environments.

This principle indicates that health development occurs within living systems that are not only adaptive, self-organizing, and autocatalytic but also complex and hierarchically arranged. The topologies of health development phenotypes cannot be fully understood using a traditional biomedical reductionist approach that relies on an analysis and assembly of the parts of subunits. Health development emanates from the hierarchical and relational coactions of the biological and behavioral subsystems and their individual and collective relations with each other and various interconnected external suprasystems (i.e., familial, social, cultural, ecological). Health development phenotypes result from the interplay between the individual and multiple physical, biochemical, psychological, social, and cultural networks that dynamically coact. As in many complex adaptive systems, the directionality of these influences is often context dependent, reciprocal, and influenced by feedback and feedforward influences. On the other hand, small changes in particularly vulnerable parts of a biobehavioral system—or at a specific time-sensitive junction in a cascading process of developmental change—can have profound nonlinear effects on the emergence of a capability or health asset or on the overall robustness or fragility of the health development process.

Transactions between different environments can influence gene expression, and gene expression and resultant phenotype can also influence various environments, which will in turn influence additional gene expression. Processes at the molecular level can dynamically coact with each other, as well as with processes at the social and ecological levels, and everywhere in between. These are not simply hierarchical relationships of dependent parts, but are *holarchical* in the sense that each level is both a part and a whole, nested and hierarchically aligned in the common purpose. In some cases, common purposes are optimizing health development, and in other circumstances, they are aligned to ensure reproductive fitness at the expense of optimal health development (Günther and Folke 1993).

6.2 Theories and Frameworks Relevant to Complexity

The *complexity* principle adds the systems-oriented concepts of complexity, adaptation, emergence, nonlinear change (i.e., small changes can produce large effects and vice versa), and multilevel person-environmental coactions. Key theories, frameworks, and perspectives that support the conceptualization of this principle include general systems theory (von Bertalanffy 1968), chaos theory (Gleick 1987; Lorenz 1993), living systems theory (Miller 1978), human-system framework (Brody 1973; Seeman 1989), and complex adaptive systems theory (Holland 1998). The systems orientation to health development suggests a holistic, integrated view that there is a need to understand the interdependence of the parts that constitute the whole, which is embedded in its natural and social environments.

6.3 Implications of the Complexity Principle

Progress in genomics and network analysis is enabling researchers to interrogate all known gene-disease associations simultaneously and to create a network view of patterns and principles of human disease that would not be apparent by examining genetic associations' one disease at a time (Goh et al. 2007). Extending this approach to health development suggests the need to add environmental exposures, or what has been called the "exposome," to analytic models to engender a better understanding of how networks of genes and networks of environments produce health development phenotypes.

The time-honored scientific approach uses the hypothetico-deductive method that derives its cogency from the certainty of deductive inference and the plausibility of abductive inference. Children exposed to the same interacting family, school, and neighborhood environments experience patterns of risk, protective, and health-promoting influences that emerge out of the complex topography of those person-environmental interactions. By statistically categorizing and analyzing children by their ethnicity, family income, and family structure, the rich interactions of different environmental factors are often lost (Molenaar et al. 2003). Health development is non-ergodic, meaning that each individual's experiences, environmental interactions, and health development phenotypes are unique and that within a population there is marked heterogeneity. Averaging effects across groups tells us something about population effects, but little about individual effects (Molenaar and Campbell 2009). Furthermore, even though individuals may have different life course experiences, they can experience the same health development phenotype, a phenomenon called *equifinality* (Cicchetti and Rogosch 1996).

Systems biology and other systems-oriented sciences offer a set of methods that can address the non-ergodic attribute of health development (Huang 2009). Rather than being hypothesis driven, these methods are systems driven and require a research strategy of interrogating the system at the level of the whole (EA Roberts 2015, 2012). This more complex way of experimenting and generating scientifically valid information bears further discussion and explication. New approaches to study design generation and statistical analysis will be needed to understand how patterns of health development are produced by complex coactions of networks over time. Identifying characteristic health development phenotypes will require nonlinear models that recognize and embrace the complexity of health development. The focus should be on measuring patterns of intraindividual health development, which will require study designs that collect detailed and large volumes of health and environmental information on individuals, forming *big health development data* resources.

Environments coact with individual constitutional factors to produce health development phenotypes within a person. We have only a vague understanding of the specific environmental variables responsible for these interactions. There is an urgent need to create scientifically useful typologies of environmental variables. This will enable research to better understand how health development signals are transduced from the environment to the individual, altering biobehavioral system configuration and function. Better characterization—and, ultimately, standardization—of environmental variables (the exposome) will accelerate research on how an individual's contexts affect the epigenetic topography and organize what complex systems science might refer to as health development attractor[2] states. Standardization of concepts and measures enables synthesis and meta-analyses across studies.

[2]An attractor is the end state of a dynamic system as it moves over time. Once the object or data point goes into the basin of attraction, it does not leave unless a strong force is applied. The set of one or more attractors of a dynamic system can be represented visually or graphically as trajectories in state space, where state space represents the multidimensional, abstract space of all possible system behavior. There are four types of possible attractors: fixed points, limit cycles, toroidal attractors, and chaotic (or strange) attractors. Point attractors are regular, terminating in a single point in state space. Cycle attractors are also regular, sometimes oscillating between two or more fixed points or exhibiting a sinusoidal pattern over time. Toroidal attractors are semi-regular, representing coupled rhythms whose ratio of periodicities terminates in an irrational rather than a rational number and appearing in state space as a donut. Chaotic attractors are fully irregular, represented by an aperiodic trajectory in state space that never repeats or settles to a stable pattern, whose basin of attraction is often fractal in shape; see chaos. Regular point and cycle attractors are characteristics of relatively simple systems. Irregular toroidal and chaotic attractors are more characteristics of complex systems.

We have almost no idea at present how to map or represent multilevel emergence, because the transactional nature of health development is not well specified, measured, analyzed, or interpreted. For example, a child exposed to a stressful stimulus that is repeated in unpredictable and unanticipated ways may experience epigenetic changes in neurotransmitter metabolism that cannot be explained just by measuring the stressful stimulus. The developmental timing of these stressful events, their unpredictable repetition, and the temporal rhythms of restorative processes (e.g., sleep) are also at play, which brings us to the next principle.

7 Principle 4: Timing

7.1 What We Mean by "Timing"

Health development is sensitive to the timing and social structuring of environmental exposures and experiences.

Health development is not a linear process in which exposures to environmental stimuli or internalized experiences have equal effects, regardless of when in the life course they occur. Instead, health development results from nonlinear interactions that are both time-specific and time-dependent. There are sensitive periods of a child's life when the impact of certain exposures can be greater than during other periods (Halfon et al. 2014). Time-specific health development pathways refer to biological conditioning that occurs during these sensitive periods, when developing systems are most adaptable and plastic and exogenous and endogenous influences can result in different adaptive responses. In other words, the same exposures can have very different effects depending on when during the life course they occur. Because childhood is a phase of life when biological and behavioral systems are shaped by environmental exposures and social experiences, the *timing* principle emphasizes the importance of nurturing children when they are most sensitive to these influences (Conti and Heckman 2013). For example, exposure to a rich set of words during the early years of life can greatly improve a child's subsequent language development, with cascading effects on subsequent school performance, health behaviors, and future health status (Hart and Risley 2003).

Time-specific transitions and turning points in health development also result from socially structured pathways that link experiences and exposures in time-influenced ways that create recursive and mutually reinforcing patterns of risk, protection, and promotion. Socially structured pathways have both period-specific and time-dependent (cumulative) characteristics. By arraying risk, protective, and promoting factors into socially constructed and institutionally reinforced pathways that interact with sensitive periods of health development, societies can either support the emergence of positive health development phenotypes or reinforce negative ones. The role, relative dose, duration, and coaction of risk, protective, and promoting factors during formative, maintenance, and declining phases of the life course all influence the slope, shape, and contours of health development trajectories.

Thus, the *timing* principle summarizes a set of models and constructs that elaborate the importance of the time dimension on health development. There are time-specific pathways that refer to sensitive periods when environmental exposures and experiences can influence health development, and there are time-dependent pathways that refer to the accumulation of repeated exposures to the same environmental stimuli that can result in a weathering process that accelerates aging (Geronimus 2013).

7.2 Theories and Frameworks Relevant to Timing

The *unfolding* principle introduced the concept of functional phases or epochs that organize the historical foundations of health development. The *timing* principle adds the concepts of time-dependent and time-sensitive health development pathways that create periods of vulnerability and robustness, as well as social structuring of environmental exposures and experiences. These concepts are drawn from several theories, frameworks, and perspectives including developmental origins of health and disease (Gluckman and Hanson 2006a), life course perspective (Elder 2000; Mayer 2009; Alwin 2012), biological embedding (Hertzman and Boyce 2010), chronobiology (Kreitzman and Foster 2004), developmental time (Kuzawa and Thayer 2011), and adaptive developmental plasticity (Gluckman et al. 2009).

7.3 Implications of the Timing Principle

Scientists have accumulated tantalizing but as yet limited evidence for time-sensitive health development (Hanson and Gluckman 2014; Hertzman 2012; Boyce and Kobor 2015). Progress in this area has been slow in part because of a lack of data systems that integrate large volumes of biological (especially patterns of gene response and epigenetic changes), clinical (such as electronic health records and biosensors), behavioral (self-report questionnaires), and environmental data. Each of these data sources exists in isolation. What is needed is a new field of health development informatics that is devoted to assembling large, integrated, longitudinal data resources and mining them for novel associations between time, environment, and health development outcomes.

Another challenge is the lack of research that establishes the specific time-dependent pathways by which human health development phenotypes are altered or protected by various internal and external factors. A variety of studies suggest that physical and social environments can alter a person's biology via epigenetic pathways that influence regulation of genetic pathways (Hertzman and Boyce 2010). This "embedding" of experience seems to have its largest impact during specific sensitive periods of development. Why the same experience engenders different outcomes among individuals is one of the great mysteries of health development. More work is needed to elucidate these iterative and dynamic pathways that connect environment to gene regulation to physiological states to environmental impact.

8 Principle 5: Plasticity

8.1 What We Mean by "Plasticity"

Health development phenotypes are systematically malleable and are enabled and constrained by evolution to enhance adaptability to diverse environments.

The relative plasticity of these phenotypes is responsive to transactions between evolutionarily selected biological and behavioral conditioning and supportive, challenging, and constraining environments. These phenotypes have evolved to provide adaptive capacity, plasticity (i.e., ability of the organism to systematically alter its phenotype in response to environmental challenges, opportunities, barriers, and constraints), and growth potential, which in aggregate refer to the robustness of an individual's health development. Heredity transmits these evolutionary signals through genetic, epigenetic, behavioral, and cultural dimensions (Jablonka and Lamb 2006), which establish the set of health development phenotypes that, depending on environmental circumstances, may or may not be selected and optimized to produce desirable outcomes. At the microlevel, there are a range of strategies to introduce variable types and levels of plasticity to optimize adaptability from the molecular to the behavioral level. At a macro-level, there are social and cultural strategies that organize the phases and life stages of health development into functionally productive entities.

Because developmental plasticity enables the genome to produce a repertoire of possible phenotypes based on environmental cues, an individual begins their life with the capacity to develop in different ways. Different exposures and experiences select and instruct a developmental pathway to respond based on these evolutionary determined strategies. Underlying many forms of plasticity are epigenetic process and resulting cascades of secondary and tertiary responses. Because plasticity can manifest at different levels, behavioral plasticity may be influenced by neural plasticity, and neural plasticity in turn may be influenced by molecular plasticity influenced by epigenetic mechanisms (Bateson and Gluckman 2011).

8.2 Theories and Frameworks Relevant to Plasticity

Evolution both enables and constrains the portfolio of adaptive plastic responses that an individual may experience in response to environmental interactions. Therefore, plasticity is relative, not absolute. Although Darwin's theory of evolution (Darwin 1859; Huxley 1942) laid the foundation for understanding the principle of *plasticity*, more recent syntheses have expanded our understanding of heredity as including not just genetic change but also epigenetic, behavioral, and cultural phenomena that are transmitted across generations (Waddington 1942; West-Eberhard 2003; Richardson and Boyd 2005; Jablonka and Lamb 2006; Konner 2011; Henrich 2015). These evolutionary forces act at the individual and group level, a perspective known as multilevel selection theory (Okasha 2006).

In some cases, health development outcomes result from the developing individual "predicting" likely future environmental stimuli based on the cues received during sensitive periods of health development. This has been called "predictive adaptive responses" (Gluckman and Hanson 2004). If the developing organism predicts incorrectly—that is, if the environment experienced in the future is not compatible with the cues received during periods of developmental plasticity—health development "mismatches" will occur. This phenomenon can be observed among individuals exposed in utero to maternal malnutrition who later become obese and glucose intolerant, a result of being born into an energy-rich environment (Hales and Barker 1992).

8.3 Implications of the Plasticity Principle

Evolution has acted on body systems in different ways to encode various types and levels of health development plasticity. The formation of some biological subsystems is tightly controlled by time and gene regulation (e.g., cardiovascular), whereas others seem to have a range of phenotypes that can emerge as a result of interactions with the environment (e.g., stress response, executive function). New models are needed to explain the deep archeology of evolution as it relates to the emergence of health development. Fields like comparative biology can test some of these hypotheses by examining the degree to which specific processes and pathways of health development vary or are preserved across species. For example, patterns of sleep have been selected for and preserved across species in ways that affect how sleep is regulated (Tamaki et al. 2016). Moreover, the success of human civilization has removed much of the selection pressure exerted by mortality, so optimization of specific pathways may be more strongly influenced by culture, behavioral, and epigenetic heredity rather than genetic forces (Enriquez and Gullans 2015). This hypothesis should be tested.

The predictive adaptive response hypothesis has accumulated a substantial amount of animal and human evidence for energy regulation (Gluckman and Hanson 2004a,b). This work should be extended to other domains—for example, behavioral health. Just as childhood obesity may result from mismatches between children's energy regulation and exposure to energy-dense environments, it is possible that the proliferation of childhood disorders like attention deficit hyperactivity disorder, anxiety, and learning disabilities may be a consequence of mismatches between predictive adaptive behavioral responses and the demands children face in terms of executive functioning, emotional functioning, and learning in their home, school, and other environments.

9 Principle 6: Thriving

9.1 What We Mean by "Thriving"

Optimal health development promotes survival, enhances well-being, and protects against disease.

Health development bestows upon the individual resources that have instrumental value, enabling an individual to pursue goals and thrive (Seedhouse 2001; Blaxter 2004; Richman 2004; Forrest 2014).

It provides assets that individuals employ to pursue the beings and doings (Sen 1999) that characterize each person's lived experiences. Thus, health development phenotypes are instrumental resources that enable individuals to pursue desired goals and live long, flourishing lives.

Health development phenotypes can be considered optimal according to the degree to which they improve the chances of survival of individuals and groups of individuals, the degree to which they support transmission of heritable information to successor generations, and the degree to which they support physical robustness and psychological flourishing (what we term thriving) across time and within the contexts of its environments.

On the other hand, the pathways by which health development phenotypes are formed can be perturbed to create suboptimal states that are precursors to fully formed disease phenotypes. These so-called endophenotypes represent intermediate, subclinical-phased transitions toward a fully manifest phenotypic expression of a disease or disorder (John and Lewis 1966; Gottesman and Gould 2003). For example, the exposure to unpredictable and uncontrollable stressors during sensitive periods of neural development can influence midbrain development and the functional development of attachment relationships, the prefrontal cortex and the functional development of executive function, and the hypothalamic pituitary axis and the regulation of stress responses (Castellanos and Tannock 2002; Boyce 2016). Endophenotypes characterized by anxious attachment, poor impulse control, and hyperactive stress response can impact health behaviors and mental health and contribute to the development of many different chronic diseases including obesity, diabetes, and cardiovascular disease (Duric et al. 2016).

9.2 Theories and Frameworks Relevant to Thriving

The principle of *health development* articulated the singularity of the concepts of health and development. The principle of *thriving* further clarifies the nature of health development by explicitly characterizing its instrumental nature. That is, health development provides a set of resources that organisms draw on in order to pursue goals, such as surviving, achieving a state of physical robustness and resilience, and psychological flourishing (Seedhouse 2001; Blaxter 2004; Committee on Evaluation of Children's Health 2004; Richman 2004; Forrest 2014). Health development therefore enables the attainment of various beings (states of happiness, life satisfaction, and meaning and purpose) and doings (desired activities that an individual pursues) as individuals pursue their goals over the life course (Sen 1999).

9.3 Implications of the Thriving Principle

LCHD recognizes that phenotype is produced by the continuous coactions of at least five factors: genome, epigenome, environment, developmental time, and life course stage. These coactions do not merely produce single outcomes; instead they produce landscapes of possibilities with peaks and valleys shaped by an individual's life history, evolutionary determined possibilities and constraints, and the five-way interaction. Which "attractor" state (i.e., health development phenotype) an individual settles in is the result of this complex, nonlinear process. We know very little about which attractor states are most likely to produce desirable outcomes (i.e., thriving) for which individuals under which circumstances. As we learn more about the interrelationships among these variables, we will begin to forge an *ontology* that specifies how health development variables interrelate with one another, their subsystems and suprasystem environmental influences, and their consequences. Research is needed that links health development phenotypes, singularly and collectively, that enable individuals with varying personal characteristics and environmental exposures to lead long lives, avoid debilitating disease, and achieve desirable goals and an optimal lived experience.

10 Principle 7: Harmony

10.1 What We Mean by "Harmony"

Health development results from the balanced and coherent relations among molecular, physiological, behavioral, cultural, and evolutionary processes.

Genetic modulations that occur in molecular time frames measured in nanoseconds are linked to biochemical modulation measured in milliseconds, homeostatic mechanisms measured in seconds to days, social norms that evolve or years and decades, cultural processes that change from years to centuries, and ecological processes that until recently took millennia. Harmonious synchronization of these processes produces the rhythms and variability that characterize health development. Loss of coordination of these processes results in less robustness of the human system, with resultant negative consequences. For example, the age of menarche has decreased in response to a variety of environmental changes that have resulted in better health and nutrition. In traditional societies, and until about 100 years ago, menarche coincided with maturation of a repertoire of psychological capabilities. Now, menarche precedes this process of psychological maturation, which has also been altered and extended by other cultural and environmental changes (Gluckman and Hanson 2006b). So the adaptive response of menarche to better nutrition and health has led to a temporal and functional uncoupling of biological and psychological capabilities that had previously been harmonized. This has been associated with a range of maladaptive outcomes (Mendle et al. 2007; Ellis and Essex 2007).

10.2 Theories and Frameworks Relevant to Harmony

The *timing* principle introduced the concepts of time dependence, time sensitivity, and social structuring of exposures. The *harmony* principle extends these concepts by adding the notions of harmonious and balanced relations of the various biological, behavioral, environmental, and cultural systems that an individual is embedded within. Extension of the classic evolutionary modern synthesis—which assumes that phenotypic transitions occur through a series of small steps that result in gradual evolutionary change—has questioned and advanced core assumption about pace of such change. Gradualism has given way in the extended evolutionary synthesis to the notion that evolution can manifest variable rates of change, especially when mutations occur in major regulatory control genes or when developmental process responds to environmental challenges with change in coordinated suites of traits or via nonlinear threshold effects (Laland et al. 2015). Although key theories, frameworks, and models in support of this principle come from chronobiology (Kreitzman and Foster 2004), developmental time (Kuzawa and Thayer 2011), and adaptive developmental plasticity (Gluckman et al. 2009), there is much more theoretical work needed for this principle.

10.3 Implication of the Harmony Principle

According to the principles of *timing* and *plasticity*, we know that there are periods of the life course when environmental influences can have particularly large effects on health development plasticity. The tremendous plasticity of humans contributes to the robustness and the ordinary magic of child health development (Masten 2001). We need better descriptions and conceptualizations of developmental time as it affects all levels and dimensions of health development and how different time frames nest together to produce coherent developmental pathways and robustness and variability in phenotypic expression. This includes a better understanding of how molecular, physiologic, developmental, historical, cultural, and evolutionary time frames independently and in harmony influence phenotypic variation, through genetic, epigenetic, and yet to be determined mechanisms and pathways. Because developmental time is uneven in its potency, intensity of change, and accessibility to environmental influences, there is a great need to better characterize and measure these temporal parameters (Boyce et al. 2012).

11 Summary

Health and development are unified into a single construct (*health development* principle) that adaptively unfolds over the life course (*unfolding* principle) according to the principles of complex adaptive systems (*complexity* principle). Change in health development results from time-specific processes (*timing* principle) that influence biobehavioral systems during sensitive periods when they are most susceptible (*plasticity* principle), and the balanced alignment of molecular, biological, behavioral, cultural, and evolutionary process (*harmony* principle) can result in developmental coherence. Health development provides instrumental assets that enable individuals and populations to pursue desired lived experiences (*thriving* principle).

The Life Course Health Development framework organizes its seven principles into a coherent whole to enable the emergence of a new field of science. The principles should not be viewed as static, independent statements or claims. Instead, they should be considered a set of nodes within a highly interconnected knowledge producing and testing network. We anticipate that these principles will change and evolve as the many fields subsumed by the health development framework themselves mature. Ultimately, we anticipate that the framework will transform into a fully formed theoretical model that enables explanation and prediction of health development phenomena.

References

Alfred, T., Ben-Shlomo, Y., et al. (2012). A multi-cohort study of polymorphisms in the GH/IGF Axis and physical capability: The HALCyon Programme. *PloS One, 7*(1), e29883.

Alwin, D. F. (2012). Integrating varieties of life course concepts. *The Journals of Gerontology. Series B, Psychological Sciences and Social Sciences, 67*(2), 206–220.

Antony, P. M., Balling, R., et al. (2012). From systems biology to systems biomedicine. *Current Opinion in Biotechnology, 23*(4), 604–608.

Arnesen, E., & Forsdahl, A. (1985). The Tromsø heart study: Coronary risk factors and their association with living conditions during childhood. *Journal of Epidemiology and Community Health, 39*(3), 210–214.

Bale, T. L. (2015). Epigenetic and transgenerational reprogramming of brain development. *Nature Reviews Neuroscience, 16*(6), 332–344.

Baltes, P. B. (1983). Life-span developmental psychology: Observations on history and theory revisited. In R. M. Lerner (Ed.), *Developmental Psychology: Historical and philosophical perspectives* (pp. 79–111). Hillsdale: Erlbaum.

Baltes, P. B., Lindenberger, U., & Staudinger, U. M. (2006). *Life span theory in developmental psychology*. New York: John Wiley & Sons, Inc..

Baltes, P. B., Reese, H. W., et al. (1980). Life-span Developmental Psychology. *Annual Review of Psychology, 31*(1), 65–110.

Barker, D. J., Gluckman, P. D., et al. (1993). Fetal nutrition and cardiovascular disease in adult life. *Lancet, 341*(8850), 938–941.

Barker, D. J., Osmond, C., et al. (1989a). Growth in utero, blood pressure in childhood and adult life, and mortality from cardiovascular disease. *BMJ, 298*(6673), 564–567.

Barker, D. J., Osmond, C., et al. (1989b). The intrauterine and early postnatal origins of cardiovascular disease and chronic bronchitis. *Journal of Epidemiology and Community Health, 43*(3), 237–240.

Barker, D. J. P., Thornburg, K. L., et al. (2010). Beyond birthweight: The maternal and placental origins of chronic disease. *Journal of Developmental Origins of Health and Disease, 1*(6), 360–364.

Bateson, P., & Gluckman, P. (2011). *Plasticity, robustness, development and evolution*. Cambridge: Cambridge University Press.

Ben-Shlomo, Y., & Kuh, D. (2002). A life course approach to chronic disease epidemiology: Conceptual models, empirical challenges and interdisciplinary perspectives. *International Journal of Epidemiology, 31*(2), 285–293.

Berkman, L. F., & Syme, S. L. (1979). Social networks, host resistance, and mortality: A nine-year follow-up study of Alameda County residents. *American Journal of Epidemiology, 109*(2), 186–204.

Blaxter, M. (2004). *Health*. Cambridge: Polity Press.

Borghol, N., Suderman, M., et al. (2012). Associations with early-life socio-economic position in adult DNA methylation. *International Journal of Epidemiology, 41*(1), 62–74.

Bornstein, M. H., & Lamb, M. E. (Eds.). (2005). *Developmental science: An advanced textbook* (5th ed.). New York: Psychology Press.

Boyce, W. T., & Kobor, M. S. (2015). Development and the epigenome: the 'synapse'of gene–environment interplay. *Developmental science, 18*(1), 1–23.

Boyce, W. T. (2016). Differential susceptibility of the developing brain to contextual adversity and stress.

Neuropsychopharmacology: Official Publication of the American College of Neuropsychopharmacology, 41(1), 142–162.

Boyce, W. T., Sokolowski, M. B., et al. (2012). Toward a new biology of social adversity. *Proceedings of the National Academy of Sciences of the United States of America, 109*(Suppl 2), 17143–17148.

Brody, H. (1973). The systems view of man: Implications for medicine, science, and ethics. *Perspectives in Biology and Medicine, 17*, 71–92.

Bronfenbrenner, U. (1976). The ecology of human development: History and perspectives [The ecology of human development: History and perspectives]. *Psychologia Wychowawcza 19*(5), 537–549.

Bronfenbrenner, U., & Morris, P. A. (2006). The Bioecological model of human development. In R. M. Lerner & W. Damon (Eds.), *Handbook of child psychology: Theoretical models of human development* (Vol. 1, 6th ed., pp. 793–828). Hoboken: John Wiley & Sons, Inc..

Cairns, R. B., Elder, G. H., et al. (1996). *Developmental science: Cambridge studies in social and emotional development*. New York: Cambridge University Press.

Caspi, A., Sugden, K., et al. (2003). Influence of life stress on depression: Moderation by a polymorphism in the 5-HTT gene. *Science, 301*(5631), 386–389.

Cassel, J. (1964). Social science theory as a source of hypotheses in epidemiological research. *American Journal of Public Health and the Nation's Health, 54*(9), 1482–1488.

Castellanos, F. X., & Tannock, R. (2002). Neuroscience of attention-deficit/hyperactivity disorder: The search for endophenotypes. *Nature Reviews Neuroscience, 3*(8), 617–628.

Chen, F., Yang, Y., et al. (2010). Social change and socioeconomic disparities in health over the life course in China a cohort analysis. *American Sociological Review, 75*(1), 126–150.

Cicchetti, D., & Cohen, D. J. (1995). *Developmental psychopathology: Theory and methods* (Vol. 1). Oxford, UK: John Wiley & Sons.

Cicchetti, D., & Rogosch, F. A. (1996). Equifinality and multifinality in developmental psychopathology. *Development and Psychopathology, 8*(04), 597–600.

Clausen, J. A. (1986). *The life course: A sociological perspective*. Englewood Cliffs: Prentice-Hall.

Cohen, S., & Herbert, T. B. (1996). Health psychology: Psychological factors and physical disease from the perspective of human psychoneuroimmunology. *Annual Review of Psychology, 47*, 113–142.

Committee on Evaluation of Children's Health, N. R. C. (2004). *Children's health, the Nation's wealth: Assessing and improving child health*. Washington, DC: National Academies Press.

Conti, G., & Heckman, J. J. (2013). The developmental approach to child and adult health. *Pediatrics, 131*(Suppl 2), S133–S141.

Cunliffe, V. T. (2015). Experience-sensitive epigenetic mechanisms, developmental plasticity, and the biological embedding of chronic disease risk. *Wiley Interdisciplinary Reviews: Systems Biology and Medicine, 7*(2), 53–71.

Dannefer, D. (1984). The role of the social in life-span developmental psychology, past and future: Rejoinder to Baltes and Nesselroade. *American Sociological Review, 49*(6), 847–850.

Darwin, C. (1859). *On the origin of species by means of natural selection, or the preservation of Favoured races in the struggle for life*. London, UK: John Murray.

Davey Smith, G. (2012). Epigenesis for epidemiologists: Does evo-devo have implications for population health research and practice? *International Journal of Epidemiology, 41*(1), 236–247.

Davies, J. (2014). *Life unfolding: How the human body creates itself*. Oxford, UK: Oxford University Press.

Davila-Velderrain, J., Martinez-Garcia, J. C., & Alvarez-Buylla, E. R. (2015). Modeling the epigenetic attractors landscape: Toward a post-genomic mechanistic understanding of development. *Frontiers in Genetics, 6*, 160.

Dawber, T. R., Kannel, W. B., & Gordon, T. (1974). Coffee and cardiovascular disease: Observations from the Framingham study. *New England Journal of Medicine, 291*(17), 871–874.

Del Giudice, M., Gangestad, S. W., & Kaplan, H. S. (2015). Life history theory and evolutionary psychology. The handbook of evolutionary psychology. John Wiley & Sons, Inc.

Diewald, M., & Mayer, K. U. (2009). The sociology of the life course and life span psychology: Integrated paradigm or complementing pathways? *Advances in Life Course Research, 14*(1), 5–14.

Duric, V., Clayton, S., Leong, M. L., & Yuan, L. L. (2016). Comorbidity factors and brain mechanisms linking chronic stress and systemic illness. *Neural Plasticity, 8*, 2016.

Egger, G., Liang, G., et al. (2004). Epigenetics in human disease and prospects for epigenetic therapy. *Nature, 429*(6990), 457–463.

Elder, G. H., Jr. (1995). The life course paradigm: Social change and individual development. In P. Moen, G. H. Elder Jr., & K. Luscher (Eds.), *Examining lives in context: Perspectives on the ecology of human development* (pp. 101–139). Washington, DC: American Psychological Association.

Elder, G. H., Jr. (2000). The life course. In E. F. Borgatta & R. J. V. Montgomery (Eds.), *Encyclopedia of sociology* (Vol. 3, pp. 1614–1622). New York: Macmillan Reference.

Elder, G. H., & Shanahan, M. J. (2007). The life course and human development. In *Handbook of child psychology*. New York: John Wiley & Sons, Inc.

Elder, G. H., Johnson, M. K., & Crosnoe, R. (2003). The emergence and development of life course theory. *In Handbook of the life course* (pp. 3–19). New York: Springer US.

Elks, C. E., Loos, R. J. F., et al. (2012). Adult obesity susceptibility variants are associated with greater childhood weight gain and a faster tempo of growth: The

1946 British birth cohort study. *American Journal of Clinical Nutrition, 95*(5), 1150–1156.

Ellis, B. J., & Essex, M. J. (2007). Family environments, adrenarche, and sexual maturation: A longitudinal test of a life history model. *Child Development, 78*(6), 1799–1817.

Engel, G. L. (1977). The need for a new medical model: A challenge for biomedicine. *Science, 196*(4286), 129–136.

Enriquez, J., & Gullans, S. (2015). *Evolving ourselves: How unnatural selection and nonrandom mutation are changing life on earth*. New York: Penguin.

Entringer, S., Buss, C., et al. (2012). Fetal programming of body composition, obesity, and metabolic function: The role of intrauterine stress and stress biology. *Journal of Nutrition and Metabolism, 2012*, 632548.

Essex, M. J., Thomas Boyce, W., et al. (2011). Epigenetic vestiges of early developmental adversity: Childhood stress exposure and DNA methylation in adolescence. *Child Development, 84*, 58–75.

Evans, G. W., & Schamberg, M. A. (2009). Childhood poverty, chronic stress, and adult working memory. *Proceedings of the National Academy of Sciences of the United States of America, 106*(16), 6545–6549.

Evans, G. W., Chen, E., et al. (2012). How poverty gets under the skin: A life course perspective. In V. Maholmes & R. B. King (Eds.), *The Oxford handbook of poverty and child development* (pp. 13–100). New York: Oxford University Press.

Featherman, D. L. (1983). Life span perspectives in social science research. In P. B. Baltes & G. Brim (Eds.), *Life-span development and behavior* (Vol. 5, pp. 1–57). New York: Academic Press.

Forrest, C. B. (2014). A living systems perspective on health. *Medical Hypotheses, 82*, 209–214.

Forsdahl, A. (1977). Are poor living conditions in childhood and adolescence an important risk factor for arteriosclerotic heart disease? *British Journal of Preventive & Social Medicine, 31*(2), 91–95.

Gatzweiler, F. W., & Baumüller, H. (2013). Marginality—A framework for analyzing causal complexities of poverty. In J. Braun von & F. W. Gatzweiler (Eds.), *Marginality: Addressing the nexus of poverty, exclusion and ecology* (pp. 27–40). Dordrecht: Springer.

Geronimus, A. T. (2013). Deep integration: Letting the epigenome out of the bottle without losing sight of the structural origins of population health. *American Journal of Public Health, 103*(S1), S56–S63.

Gilbert, S. F., Bosch, T. C., & Ledón-Rettig, C. (2015 Oct 1). Eco-Evo-Devo: Developmental symbiosis and developmental plasticity as evolutionary agents. *Nature Reviews Genetics, 16*(10), 611–622.

Gleick, J. (1987). *Chaos: Making a new science*. New York: Penguin Books.

Gluckman, P. D., & Hanson, M. A. (2004a). Developmental origins of disease paradigm: A mechanistic and evolutionary perspective. *Pediatric Research, 56*(3), 311–317.

Gluckman, P. D., & Hanson, M. A. (2004b). Living with the past: Evolution, development, and patterns of disease. *Science, 305*(5691), 1733–1736.

Gluckman, P. D., & Hanson, M. A. (2004c). The developmental origins of the metabolic syndrome. *Trends in Endocrinology and Metabolism, 15*(4), 183–187.

Gluckman, P. D., & Hanson, M. A. (2006a). *Developmental origins of health and disease*. Cambridge, UK: Cambridge University Press.

Gluckman, P. D., & Hanson, M. A. (2006b). Evolution, development and timing of puberty. *Trends in Endocrinology and Metabolism, 17*(1), 7–12.

Gluckman, P. D., Hanson, M. A., et al. (2008). Effect of in utero and early-life conditions on adult health and disease. *New England Journal of Medicine, 359*(1), 61–73.

Gluckman, P. D., Hanson, M. A., et al. (2009). Towards a new developmental synthesis: Adaptive developmental plasticity and human disease. *The Lancet, 373*(9675), 1654–1657.

Gluckman, P. D., Hanson, M. A., et al. (2010). A conceptual framework for the developmental origins of health and disease. *Journal of Developmental Origins of Health and Disease, 1*(1), 6–18.

Goh, K. I., Cusick, M. E., et al. (2007). The human disease network. *Proceedings of the National Academy of Sciences, 104*(21), 8685–8690.

Gottesman, I. I., & Gould, T. D. (2003). The endophenotype concept in psychiatry: Etymology and strategic intentions. *The American Journal of Psychiatry, 160*(4), 636–645.

Green, S., Fagan, M., & Jaeger, J. (2015). Explanatory integration challenges in evolutionary systems biology. *Biological Theory, 10*(1), 18–35.

Greenberg, G., & Partridge, T. (2010). *Biology, evolution, and psychological development, In The Handbook of life-span development* (pp. 115–148). Hoboken: John Wiley & Sons.

Günther, F., & Folke, C. (1993 Sep). Characteristics of nested living systems. *Journal of Biological Systems, 1*(03), 257–274.

Hackman, D. A., & Farah, M. J. (2009). Socioeconomic status and the developing brain. *Trends in Cognitive Sciences, 13*(2), 65–73.

Hales, C. N., & Barker, D. J. P. (1992). Type 2 (non-insulin dependent) diabetes mellitus: The thrifty phenotype hypothesis. *Diabetologia, 35*, 595–601.

Halfon, N., & Hochstein, M. (2002). Life course health-development: An integrated framework for developing health, policy, and research. *The Milbank Quarterly, 80*(3), 433–479. iii.

Halfon, N., Larson, K., Lu, M., Tullis, E., & Russ, S. (2014). Lifecourse health development: Past, present and future. *Maternal and Child Health Journal, 18*(2), 344–365.

Hanson, M. A., & Gluckman, P. D. (2014). Early developmental conditioning of later health and disease: physiology or pathophysiology? *Physiological Reviews, 94*(4), 1027–1076.

Hart, B., & Risley, T. R. (2003). The early catastrophe: The 30 million word gap by age 3. *American Educator, 27*(1), 4–9.

Haynes, S., Feinleib, M., & Kannel, W. B. (1980). The relationship of psychosocial factors to coronary heart disease in the Framingham Study. III. Eight-year incidence of coronary heart disease. *American Journal of Epidemiology, 111*(1), 37–58.

Henrich, J. (2015). *The secret of our success: how culture is driving human evolution, domesticating our species, and making us smarter*. Princeton: Princeton University Press.

Hertzman, C. (1999). The biological embedding of early experience and its effects on health in adulthood. *Annals of the New York Academy of Sciences, 896*, 85–95.

Hertzman, C. (2012). Putting the concept of biological embedding in historical perspective. *Proceedings of the National Academy of Sciences of the United States of America, 109*(Suppl 2), 17160–17167.

Hertzman, C., & Boyce, T. (2010). How experience gets under the skin to create gradients in developmental health. *Annual Review of Public Health, 31*, 329–347.

Hochberg, Z. E., Feil, R., Constancia, M., Fraga, M., Junien, C., Carel, J. C., Boileau, P., Le Bouc, Y., Deal, C. L., Lillycrop, K., & Scharfmann, R. (2010). Child health, developmental plasticity, and epigenetic programming. *Endocrine Reviews, 32*(2), 159–224.

Holland, J. H. (1998). *Emergence: From chaos to order*. Cambridge, MA: Perseus Books.

Huang, S. (2009). Non-genetic heterogeneity of cells in development: More than just noise. *Development, 136*(23), 3853–3862.

Huang, S. (2012). The molecular and mathematical basis of Waddington's epigenetic landscape: A framework for post-Darwinian biology? *BioEssays: News and Reviews in Molecular, Cellular and Developmental Biology, 34*(2), 149–157.

Huxley, J. (1942). *Evolution: The modern synthesis*. London, UK: Allen & Unwin.

Jablonka, E., & Lamb, K. J. (2006). *Evolution in four dimensions: Genetic, epigenetic, behavioral, and symbolic variation in the history of life*. Cambridge, MA: MIT Press.

John, B., & Lewis, K. R. (1966). Chromosome variability and geographic distribution in insects. *Science, 152*(3723), 711–721.

Keating, D. P., & Hertzman, C. (Eds.). (1999). *Developmental health and the wealth of nations: Social, biological, and educational dynamics*. New York: Guilford Publications.

Kitano, H. (2002). Systems biology: A brief overview. *Science, 295*(5560), 1662–1664.

Konner, M. (2011). *The evolution of childhood: Relationships, emotion, mind*. Cambridge, MA: Belknap Press of Harvard University Press.

Kreitzman, L., & Foster, R. G. (2004). *Rhythms of life: The biological clocks that control the daily lives of every living thing*. New Haven: Yale University Press.

Krieger, N. (2001). Theories for social epidemiology in the 21st century: An ecosocial perspective. *International Journal of Epidemiology, 30*(4), 668–677.

Kuh, D., & Ben-Shlomo, Y. (2004). Introduction. In D. Kuh & Y. Ben-Shlomo (Eds.), *A life course approach to chronic disease epidemiology* (pp. 3–14). New York: Oxford University Press.

Kuh, D., & Davey Smith, G. (2004). The life course and adult chronic disease: An historical perspective with particular reference to coronary heart disease. In *Life course approach to chronic disease epidemiology* (pp. 15–37). Oxford University Press.

Kuh, D. J. L., & Wadsworth, M. E. J. (1993). Physical health status at 36 years in a British national birth cohort. *Social Science & Medicine, 37*(7), 905–916.

Kuzawa, C. W., & Thayer, Z. M. (2011). Timescales of human adaptation: The role of epigenetic processes. *Epigenomics, 3*(2), 221–234.

Laland, K. N., Uller, T., Feldman, M. W., Sterelny, K., Müller, G. B., Moczek, A., Jablonka, E., & Odling-Smee, J. (2015). The extended evolutionary synthesis: Its structure, assumptions and predictions. *Proceedings. Royal Society B, 282*(1813), 20151019.

Launay, J. M., Del Pino, M., et al. (2009). Smoking induces long-lasting effects through a monoamine-oxidase epigenetic regulation. *PloS One, 4*(11), e7959.

Lerner, D. R. M. (1984). *On the nature of human plasticity*. Cambridge: Cambridge University Press.

Lerner, R. M. (2006). Developmental science, developmental systems, and contemporary theories of human development. In W. Damon & R. M. Lerner (Eds.), *Handbook of child psychology, Vol. 1: Theoretical models of human development* (pp. 1–17). Hoboken: Wiley.

Lerner, R. M. (2012). Developmental science: Past, present, and future. *International Journal of Developmental Science, 6*(1), 29–36.

Lerner, R. M., & Overton, W. F. (2008). Exemplifying the integrations of the relational developmental system synthesizing theory, research, and application to promote positive development and social justice. *Journal of Adolescent Research, 23*(3), 245–255.

Lerner, R. M., Overton, W., et al. (2010). Life-span development: Concepts and issues. In *The Handbook of life-span development* (pp. 1–29). Hoboken: Wiley.

Lester, B. M., Conradt, E., & Marsit, C. (2016). Introduction to the special section on epigenetics. *Child Development, 87*(1), 29–37.

Li, C. C., Maloney, C. A., et al. (2010). Epigenetic programming by maternal nutrition: Shaping future generations. *Epigenomics, 2*(4), 539–549.

Lillycrop, K. A., & Burdge, G. C. (2012). Epigenetic mechanisms linking early nutrition to long term health. *Best Practice & Research Clinical Endocrinology & Metabolism, 26*(5), 667–676.

Lieberman, D. (2014). *The story of the human body: evolution, health, and disease*. New York: Vintage Books.

Lorenz, E. (1993). *The essence of chaos*. Seattle: University of Washington Press.

Magnusson, D. (1995). Individual development: A holistic, integrated model. In A. Holistic, P. Moen, G. H. Elder Jr., & K. Luscher (Eds.), *Examining lives in context: Perspectives on the ecology of human development* (pp. 19–60). Washington, DC: American Psychological Association.

Maier, S. F., Watkins, L. R., et al. (1994). Psychoneuroimmunology - the Interface between behavior, brain, and immunity. *American Psychologist, 49*(12), 1004–1017.

Marshall, P. J. (2014). Beyond different levels: embodiment and the developmental system. *Frontiers in Psychology, 5*, 929.

Marmot, M. G., & Syme, S. L. (1976). Acculturation and coronary heart disease in Japanese- Americans. *American Journal of Epidemiology, 104*(3), 225–247.

Marmot, M. G., Adelstein, A. M., et al. (1978a). Changing social-class distribution of heart disease. *British Medical Journal, 2*(6145), 1109–1112.

Marmot, M. G., Rose, G., et al. (1978b). Employment grade and coronary heart disease in British civil servants. *Journal of Epidemiology and Community Health, 32*(4), 244–249.

Martino, D., & Prescott, S. (2011). Epigenetics and prenatal influences on asthma and allergic airways disease. *Chest, 139*(3), 640–647.

Masten, A. S. (2001). Ordinary magic. Resilience processes in development. *The American Psychologist, 56*(3), 227–238.

Masters, R. K., Hummer, R. A., et al. (2012). Educational differences in U.S. adult mortality a cohort perspective. *American Sociological Review, 77*(4), 548–572.

Mayer, K. U. (2009). New Directions in life course research. *Annual Review of Sociology, 35*, 413–433.

McEwan, B. S. (1998). Protective and damaging effects of stress mediators. *New England Journal of Medicine, 338*(3), 171–179.

McEwen, B. S. (2012). Brain on stress: How the social environment gets under the skin. *Proceedings of the National Academy of Sciences of the United States of America, 109*(Suppl 2), 17180–17185.

McMichael, A. J. (1999). Prisoners of the proximate: Loosening the constraints on epidemiology in an age of change. *American Journal of Epidemiology, 149*(10), 887–897.

McMillen, I. C., & Robinson, J. S. (2005). Developmental origins of the metabolic syndrome: Prediction, plasticity, and programming. *Physiological Reviews, 85*(2), 571–633.

Meaney, M. J. (2001). Maternal care, gene expression, and the transmission of individual differences in stress reactivity across generations. *Annual Review of Neuroscience, 24*, 1161–1192.

Meaney, M. J. (2010). Epigenetics and the biological definition of gene x environment interactions. *Child Development, 81*(1), 41–79.

Meaney, M. J., Szyf, M., et al. (2007). Epigenetic mechanisms of perinatal programming of hypothalamic-pituitary-adrenal function and health. *Trends in Molecular Medicine, 13*(7), 269–277.

Mendle, J., Turkheimer, E., & Emery, R. E. (2007). Detrimental psychological outcomes associated with early pubertal timing in adolescent girls. *Developmental Review, 27*(2), 151–171.

Miller, J. G. (1978). *Living systems*. New York: McGraw-Hill.

Molenaar, P. C. M., & Campbell, C. G. (2009). The new person-specific paradigm in psychology. *Current Directions in Psychological Science, 18*(2), 112–117.

Molenaar, P. C. M., Huizenga, H. M., & Nesselroade, J. R. (2003). The relationship between the structure of interindividual and intraindividual variability: A theoretical and empirical vindication of developmental systems theory. In *Understanding Human Development* (pp. 339–360). New York: Springer.

Mortimer, J. T., & Shanahan, M. J. (2007). *Handbook of the life course* New York: Springer Science & Business Media.

Noble, K. G., Houston, S. M., et al. (2012). Neural correlates of socioeconomic status in the developing human brain. *Developmental Science, 15*(4), 516–527.

Okasha, S. (2006). *Evolution and the levels of selection*. New York: NY, Oxford University Press.

Overton, W. F. (2007). A coherent Metatheory for dynamic systems: Relational Organicism- Contextualism. *Human Development, 50*(2–3), 154–159.

Oyama, S. (1985). *The ontogeny of information: Developmental systems and evolution*. Cambridge, UK: Cambridge University Press.

Perera, F., Tang, W. Y., et al. (2009). Relation of DNA methylation of 5′-CpG island of ACSL3 to transplacental exposure to airborne polycyclic aromatic hydrocarbons and childhood asthma. *PloS One, 4*(2), e4488.

Power, C., Graham, H., et al. (2005a). The contribution of childhood and adult socioeconomic position to adult obesity and smoking behaviour: An international comparison. *International Journal of Epidemiology, 34*(2), 335–344.

Power, C., Hypponen, E., et al. (2005b). Socioeconomic position in childhood and early adult life and risk of mortality: A prospective study of the mothers of the 1958 British birth cohort. *American Journal of Public Health, 95*(8), 1396–1402.

Relton, C. L., & Davey Smith, G. (2012). Is epidemiology ready for epigenetics? *International Journal of Epidemiology, 41*(1), 5–9.

Roberts, E. A. (2012). Using metalloproteomics to investigate the cellular physiology of copper in hepatocytes. *Metallomics, 4*(7), 633–640.

Roberts, E. (2015). System-driven research: Legitimate experimental design for biological/biomedical research. Accessed 2017 https://dalspace.library.dal.ca/bitstream/handle/10222/56275/Roberts-Eve-PhD-PHIL-May-2015.pdf?sequence=1&isAllowed=y

Relton, C. L., & Davey Smith, G. (2012). Is epidemiology ready for epigenetics? *International Journal of Epidemiology, 41*(1), 5–9.

Repetti, R. L., Robles, T. F., et al. (2011). Allostatic processes in the family. *Development and Psychopathology, 23*(3), 921–938.

Repetti, R. L., Taylor, S. E., et al. (2002). Risky families: Family social environments and the mental and physical health of offspring. *Psychological Bulletin, 128*(2), 330–366.

Richman, K. A. (2004). *Ethics and the metaphysics of medicine*. Cambridge, MA: The MIT Press.

Richardson, P. J., & Boyd, R. (2005). *Not by genes alone: How culture transformed human evolution*. University of Chicago Press.

Sameroff, A. (1975). Transactional models in early social relations. *Human Development, 18*(1–2), 65–79.

Sameroff, A. (2010). A unified theory of development: A dialectic integration of nature and nurture. *Child Development, 81*(1), 6–22.

Sapolsky, R. M., Krey, L. C., & McEWEN, B. R. U. C. E. S. (1985). Prolonged glucocorticoid exposure reduces hippocampal neuron number: Implications for aging. *The Journal of Neuroscience, 5*(5), 1222–1227.

Schadt, E. E., & Bjorkegren, J. L. (2012). NEW: Network-enabled wisdom in biology, medicine, and health care. *Science Translational Medicine, 4*(115), 115rv111.

Schlotz, W., & Phillips, D. I. (2009). Fetal origins of mental health: Evidence and mechanisms. *Brain, Behavior, and Immunity, 23*(7), 905–916.

Seedhouse, D. D. (2001). *Health: The foundations for achievement*. Hoboken: Wiley.

Seeman, J. (1989). Toward a model of positive health. *The American Psychologist, 44*(8), 1099–1109.

Seeman, T. E. (1997). Price of adaptation--allostatic load and its health consequences. MacArthur studies of successful aging. *Archives of Internal Medicine, 157*(19), 2259–2268.

Seeman, T. E., McEwen, B. S., et al. (2001). Allostatic load as a marker of cumulative biological risk: MacArthur studies of successful aging. *Proceedings of the National Academy of Sciences, 98*(8), 4770–4775.

Sen, A. (1999). *Commodities and capabilities*. Oxford: Oxford University Press.

Skinner, M. K., Anway, M. D., et al. (2008). Transgenerational epigenetic programming of the brain transcriptome and anxiety behavior. *PloS One, 3*(11), e3745.

Spencer, J. P., Thomas, M. S. C., et al. (Eds.). (2009). *Toward a unified theory of development: Connectionism and dynamic systems theory re-considered*. New York: Oxford University Press.

Starfield, B. (1973). Health services research: A working model. *The New England Journal of Medicine, 289*(3), 132–136.

Starfield, B., Katz, H., Gabriel, A., et al. (1984). Morbidity in childhood - a longitudinal view. *The New England Journal of Medicine, 310*(13), 824–829.

Stearns, S. (1992). *The evolution of life histories*. New York: Oxford.

Stewart, G. T. (1968). Limitations of the germ theory. *The Lancet, 291*(7551), 1077–1081.

Syme, S. L., & Berkman, L. F. (1976). Social class, susceptibility and sickness. *American Journal of Epidemiology, 104*(1), 1–8.

Szyf, M., Weaver, I. C. G., et al. (2005). Maternal programming of steroid receptor expression and phenotype through DNA methylation in the rat. *Frontiers in Neuroendocrinology, 26*(3–4), 139–162.

Tamaki, M., Bang, J. W., Watanabe, T., & Sasaki, Y. (2016). Night watch in one brain hemisphere during sleep associated with the first-night effect in humans. *Current Biology, 26*(9), 1190–1194.

Thayer, Z. M., & Kuzawa, C. W. (2011). Biological memories of past environments: Epigenetic pathways to health disparities. *Epigenetics: Official Journal of the DNA Methylation Society, 6*(7), 798–803.

Turecki, G., & Meaney, M. J. (2016). Effects of the social environment and stress on glucocorticoid receptor gene methylation: A systematic review. *Biological Psychiatry, 79*(2), 87–96.

von Bertalanffy, L. (1968). *General system theory: Foundations, development, application*. New York, NY: George Braziller.

Waddington, C. H. (1942). The Epigenotype. *Endeavour, 1*, 18–20.

Wen, X., Kleinman, K., et al. (2012). Childhood body mass index trajectories: Modeling, characterizing, pairwise correlations and socio-demographic predictors of trajectory characteristics. *BMC Medical Research Methodology, 12*, 38.

West-Eberhard, M. J. (2003). *Developmental plasticity and evolution*. New York: Oxford University Press.

Worthman, C. M., & Kuzara, J. (2005). Life history and the early origins of health differentials. *American Journal of Human Biology: The Official Journal of the Human Biology Council, 17*(1), 95–112.

Part II

Life Stages

Preconception and Prenatal Factors and Metabolic Risk

Guoying Wang, Tami R. Bartell, and Xiaobin Wang

1 Introduction

There is growing evidence that early life may have a profound impact on health and disease in later life (Gluckman et al. 2008; Hales et al. 1991). Because this growing evidence about the prenatal and preconception origins of health and disease is vast, this chapter will primarily focused on early life origins of metabolic risk for obesity and type 2 diabetes (T2DM). Obesity and type 2 diabetes affect all age groups including mothers and young children (International Diabetes Federation 2013), especially in poor minority populations (Al-Rubeaan 2015). Increasing evidence points to a profound impact of early life factors (e.g., maternal obesity, diabetes, and unhealthy diet) on offspring metabolic risk (Barbour 2014a), leading to a transgenerational amplification of obesity and diabetes. The period from conception to birth is a time of very rapid growth, cellular differentiation, and functional maturation of organ systems. This early life period is particularly sensitive to alterations of the intrauterine environment including the metabolic milieu. Epigenomic variations (regulation of gene expression) are largely established in utero (Bogdarina et al. 2004) and are particularly sensitive to prenatal environmental factors that may have a lifelong impact on health and disease. Moreover, babies that are large at birth are more likely to be overweight or obese in childhood, with these conditions persisting into adulthood (Knittle et al. 1979; Rolland-Cachera et al. 2006). Recent data suggest that elevated insulin levels may also originate in utero and persist into early childhood (Wang et al. 2014a). Taken together, the prenatal period is a critical developmental stage for obesity and metabolic outcomes (Wang et al. 2014b; Dietz 2004). In light of the global obesity and T2DM epidemic and growing evidence of early life origins of obesity and diabetes, early identification of individuals at high risk and early prevention of obesity and metabolic syndrome are a key to achieve primary prevention and reverse the trends of the obesity and T2DM epidemics.

As illustrated in Fig. 1, human health is interconnected from conception to fetal life to childhood and on into adulthood and influenced by multilevel factors from gene to society. This

G. Wang, MD, PhD
Department of Population, Family and Reproductive Health, Center on the Early Life Origins of Disease, Johns Hopkins University Bloomberg School of Public Health, Baltimore, MD, USA

T.R. Bartell, BA
Stanley Manne Children's Research Institute, Ann & Robert H Lurie Children's Hospital of Chicago, Chicago, IL, USA

X. Wang, MD, MPH, ScD (✉)
Center on the Early Life Origins of Disease, Department of Population, Family and Reproductive Health, Johns Hopkins University Bloomberg School of Public Health, Baltimore, MD, USA
e-mail: xwang82@jhu.edu

N. Halfon et al. (eds.), *Handbook of Life Course Health Development*,
DOI 10.1007/978-3-319-47143-3_3

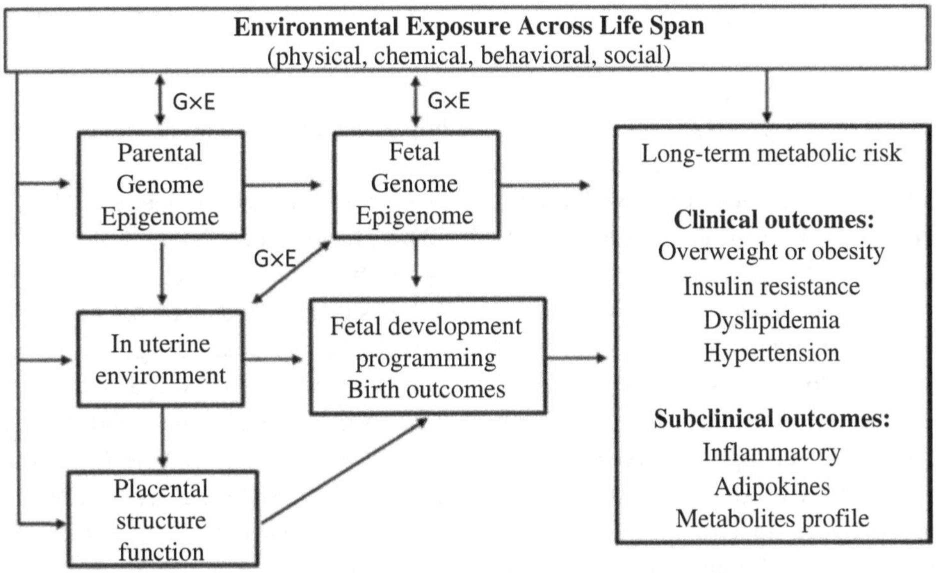

Fig. 1 Conceptual framework for preconceptional and prenatal factors and metabolic risk

chapter will discuss the impact of important preconceptional and prenatal factors, including maternal obesity and/or diabetes, gestational weight gain, and maternal micronutrient status, on in utero and lifelong metabolic outcomes and the possible gene–environment interactions and epigenetic mechanisms underlying early life origins of metabolic risk. Finally, it will provide perspectives on current knowledge gaps and recommendations to advance the field.

2 The Effects of Maternal Preconceptional Obesity and/or Diabetes and Micronutrient Status on Offspring Metabolic Outcomes

Evidence is growing about the associations between early life exposures and later health. Major exposures encompass multilevel and multifactorial influences from the societal level through to individual lifestyle and biological factors. While a discussion of all of the possible risks or protective factors is beyond the scope of this chapter, below we highlight some important preconceptional and prenatal factors, including prepregnancy obesity, excessive weight gain during pregnancy, preexistent or gestational diabetes, and maternal micronutrient status.

2.1 Maternal Prepregnancy Obesity and Gestational Weight Gain

In parallel with the global obesity epidemic, the prevalence of obesity among women of childbearing age has also increased. In 2009–2010, the National Health and Nutrition Examination Survey (NHANES) found that 56% of US women aged 20–39 were overweight or obese (body mass index (BMI) $\geq$ 25 kg/m^2), and in particular, 32% were obese (BMI $\geq$ 30.0 kg/m^2) (Flegal et al. 2012). Thus, more than half of women starting their pregnancy are already overweight or obese, and most of them remain overweight or obese during their entire pregnancy. To further complicate things, women who are overweight or obese going into pregnancy are at an increased risk for developing metabolic disorders, such as gestational diabetes mellitus (GDM) (Torloni et al. 2009), hypertensive disorders of pregnancy (Bautista-Castano et al. 2013), and excessive gestational weight gain (GWG) (Chu et al.

2009). More important, maternal obesity and its relevant metabolic disorders may impact offspring metabolic risk in later life.

Excessive maternal prepregnancy weight and GWG are consistent risk factors for offspring obesity and cardiometabolic risk (Lawlor 2013; Hochner et al. 2012). In the Jerusalem Perinatal Family Follow-Up Study, greater maternal prepregnancy BMI, independent of GWG and confounders, was significantly associated with higher offspring blood pressures, serum insulin and triglyceride concentrations, BMI, waist circumference, and lower high-density lipoprotein cholesterol (Hochner et al. 2012). Of note, the associations between maternal BMI and offspring BP, insulin, and lipids appeared to be largely mediated by offspring concurrent body size (both BMI and waist circumference) (Hochner et al. 2012). This finding emphasizes the impact that maternal adiposity may have through offspring adiposity on various predictors of subclinical and clinical disease, including diabetes mellitus and cardiovascular diseases. A large US cohort study reported that excessive maternal GWG was independently associated with a 46% increased risk of overweight or obesity in offspring at 2–5 years of age (Sridhar et al. 2014). In a retrospective cohort study, excessive maternal GWG had an adverse impact on the risk of childhood overweight and abdominal adiposity (Ensenauer et al. 2013). Kaar et al. further reported that maternal prepregnancy BMI was not only associated with increased general adiposity (BMI) and abdominal adiposity (waist circumference) in offspring but visceral adipose tissue at age 10 years (Kaar et al. 2014). A recent study points to an association between maternal excess weight in pregnancy and offspring BMI increase from adolescence to adulthood (Lawrence et al. 2014). Early pregnancy obesity has also been associated with an increased risk of premature death in adult offspring (Reynolds et al. 2013a). To further the negative impact, maternal prepregnancy BMI was also associated with increased offspring insulin resistance at age 10 years (Kaar et al. 2014) and an increased risk of developing T2DM (Dabelea et al. 2008).

2.2 Preexistent and Gestational Diabetes

In parallel with the obesity epidemic is a diabetes pandemic, which includes an increasing number of women with type 1 diabetes (T1D), T2DM, and GDM (Torloni et al. 2009). A body of studies has established a link between exposure to maternal diabetes in utero and metabolic risk in later life. In a multiethnic population aged 6–13 years, exposure to maternal GDM was associated with higher BMI, waist circumference, and more abdominal fat (Crume et al. 2011). Adjustment for socioeconomic factors, birthweight, gestational age, maternal smoking during pregnancy, diet, and physical activity did not alter the associations; however, adjustment for maternal prepregnancy BMI attenuated all associations (Crume et al. 2011), suggesting that maternal obesity is an important mediator. The studies in Pima Indians of the long-term effects of diabetic pregnancy on offspring revealed that the offspring of women with preexistent diabetes and GDM were more obese and had higher glucose concentrations and more diabetes than the offspring of nondiabetic women or women who developed diabetes after pregnancy (Pettitt et al. 1993). In the Chicago Diabetes in Pregnancy study, offspring of mothers with preexistent diabetes and GDM had significantly higher 2-h blood glucose and insulin levels and rate of impaired glucose tolerance than the control group of nondiabetic mothers (Silverman et al. 1995). In the SEARCH Case–Control Study (Dabelea et al. 2008), maternal diabetes and obesity were associated with 5.7 times and 2.8 times the risk of T2DM in young offspring aged 10–22 years, respectively. Notably, combined prenatal exposure to maternal diabetes and obesity could explain about 47% of the offspring risk of T2DM (Dabelea et al. 2008). Among Pima Indian adults, individuals whose mothers had diabetes during pregnancy had a 40% lower acute insulin response to a 25 g intravenous glucose challenge than those whose mothers developed diabetes at an early age but after the birth of the child (Gautier et al. 2001).

One important mediator is maternal blood glucose level during pregnancy. The Hyperglycemia and Adverse Pregnancy Outcome (HAPO) study demonstrated that maternal glucose levels below those diagnostic of diabetes were positively associated with increased birthweight and cord blood C-peptide levels (Metzger et al. 2008). Poor glycemic control in women with pregestational diabetes increased the risk of congenital malformations and spontaneous abortions (Kendrick 2004; Miller et al. 1981). Although T1D and T2DM have different pathogeneses, the rates of pregnancy loss were similar (Cundy et al. 2007). Another factor related to diabetes is the comorbidities. Diabetic gastropathy, a form of diabetic neuropathy, not only worsens nausea and vomiting but also can cause difficulty with glucose control during pregnancy (Kitzmiller et al. 2008). Reece et al. reviewed the literature and reported that maternal diabetic nephropathy is complicated by hypertension (60%), preeclampsia (41%), premature delivery (22–30%), and fetal growth restriction (16%) (Reece et al. 1998). Taken together, better control of blood glucose levels and diabetic complications may improve prenatal outcomes.

2.3 Maternal Micronutrient Status

Growing evidence suggests that maternal nutrition, through its impact on the fetal intrauterine environment, has a profound and lifelong influence on later health (Barker et al. 1993). Among a number of specific nutrients that have been implicated, folate is particularly important. Folate is an essential vitamin B involved in nucleic acid synthesis, DNA methylation, cellular growth, differentiation, and repair (Crider et al. 2012; Kim 2000). The demand for folate increases during pregnancy due to the need for fetal and placental growth and uterus enlargement (Greenberg et al. 2011). The causal role of folate deficiency in fetal neural tube defects (NTDs) is well established (De Wals et al. 2007). A recent study showed that low maternal folate concentration was associated with higher BMI in offspring at 5–6 years (Krikke et al. 2016). Our study also showed that maternal low folate was not only independently associated with offspring overweight or obesity but also worsened the adverse effects of maternal prepregnancy obesity on offspring metabolic risk (Wang et al. 2016). On the other hand, excess maternal folate status may also link to offspring adverse metabolic outcomes. A study in an Indian population reported a positive association between maternal folate level and offspring homeostatic model assessment-insulin resistance (HOMA-IR) (Krishnaveni et al. 2014). What we gather from the combined results of these studies is that optimizing folate nutrition in women, and especially OWO women, may offer a safe, simple, and effective way to decrease the risk of transgenerational obesity and diabetes.

2.4 Adverse Birth Outcomes

Birthweight reflects cumulative growth in utero. A body of studies has suggested that maternal obesity is associated with a risk for large for gestational age (LGA) or macrosomia in the offspring (Bautista-Castano et al. 2013). In addition, Brumbaugh et al. demonstrated that newborns of obese mothers with GDM showed increased intrahepatic fat at birth (Brumbaugh et al. 2013). Prepregnancy obesity also has been shown to increase the risk of Cesarean section (Martin et al. 2015; Dzakpasu et al. 2014) and preterm birth (Cnattingius et al. 2013). In a case–control study of 914 women with pregestational diabetes and 4000 controls, diabetes was associated with an increased risk of preterm birth (Cnattingius et al. 1994). Maternal diabetes has also been linked to macrosomia and Cesarean section (Barbour 2014b; Koyanagi et al. 2013).

These adverse birth outcomes are also associated with obesity and metabolic syndrome (including hypertension, dyslipidemia, obesity, and insulin resistance/diabetes) in later life. *Hypertension:* Previous studies demonstrated that preterm birth was associated with hypertension in childhood (Sipola-Leppanen et al. 2014) and adulthood (Irving et al. 2000; Johansson et al. 2005). In a prospective study, Irving et al. found that preterm birth was associated with the risk of hypertension and hyperglycemia in adulthood (Irving et al. 2000). A meta-analysis of 27 studies further confirmed that preterm birth was associated with cardiovascular risk factors, such as higher systolic and diastolic blood pressure and low-density lipoprotein cholesterol in adulthood (Parkinson et al. 2013). Even more interesting is that the difference in blood pressure between those born preterm and those born at term may be greater in women than in men (Parkinson et al. 2013). *Dyslipidemia:* A large cohort study reported that boys born early preterm had 6.7% higher total cholesterol, 11.7% higher low-density lipoprotein cholesterol (LDL-C), and 12.3% higher apolipoprotein B concentrations than their term peers (Sipola-Leppanen et al. 2014). *Obesity*: As fat deposition occurs largely during the third trimester of pregnancy, preterm babies are born with low levels of body fat (Rigo et al. 1998; Uthaya et al. 2005). Postnatally, preterm babies are more likely to gain excessive weight, a known risk factor of childhood obesity (Ong et al. 2000), and tend to have a higher proportion of central adiposity (Uthaya et al. 2005). *Insulin resistance/diabetes:* Like children who were born at term and small for gestational age (SGA), children born preterm have lower insulin sensitivity (Wang et al. 2014a; Hofman et al. 2004). Hovi et al. reported that preterm birth itself, independent of birth size, may contribute to insulin resistance, elevated blood glucose, and higher blood pressure (BP) in young adulthood (Hovi et al. 2007). In addition, a Swedish study found that preterm birth was associated with later T2DM: the hazard ratio for T2DM comparing very preterm (≤32 weeks of gestation) with term birth was 1.67 (Kaijser et al. 2009). There is a particular lack of large-scale longitudinal birth cohort studies to examine the effects of preterm birth on metabolic outcomes over critical developmental windows. One prospective birth cohort study found that preterm birth is associated with elevated plasma insulin levels (indirect evidence of insulin resistance) at birth that persist to age 6.5 years (Wang et al. 2014a), suggesting that insulin resistance originates in utero and persists into later life. There is also evidence from a mechanistic study, which revealed that preterm birth increased the risk of T2DM via diminished insulin sensitivity (Pilgaard et al. 2010), and yet another study showed that preterm birth was associated with changes in the cord blood adipokine profile that may contribute to the impairment of glucose metabolism (Bhargava et al. 2004).

3 Mechanisms/Pathways Underlying Early Life Origins of Metabolic Risk

Compelling evidence suggests that prenatal experiences influence metabolic alterations in late life via multiple pathways, including genetic, in utero environment, gene–environment interaction, and epigenetic and shared familial socioeconomic and lifestyle factors (Fig. 1).

3.1 Genetics

Several lines of evidence support that genetics play a key role in the long-term effects of maternal obesity and diabetes on offspring metabolic risk. First, obesity and diabetes tend to aggregate among families. We also know that GDM is associated with a history of T2DM. One study showed that, compared to women with nondiabetic parents, women with any parental history of T2DM experienced a 2.3-fold increased risk of GDM, suggesting that the risk of GDM was positively associated with parental history of T2DM (Williams et al. 2003). Second, the extensive study of genetic variation in obesity and diabetes has led to the identification of numerous candidate genes. Although currently identified genetic markers only explain a small proportion of metabolic risks, twin studies reveal that BMI, body fat, and insulin sensitivity are all highly heritable (Zhang et al. 2009; Ouyang et al. 2010). Finally, some gene variants related to adult diseases have been linked to offspring outcomes. A epidemiological study showed that a genetic risk score (GRS) comprised of SNPs associated with adult obesity-related traits may provide an approach for predicting LGA birth and newborn adiposity beyond established risk factors (Chawla et al. 2014). A genome-wide association study of women of European descent established that common variants near the melanocortin-4 receptor (*MC4R*) influence fat mass, weight and obesity risk and over transmission of the risk allele to obese offspring (Loos et al. 2008). GDM is not only associated with later risk of diabetes in mothers but also with metabolic changes that may lead to the development of diabetes in their offspring (Silverman et al. 1998). Some genes and their interactions in functional networks between the mother and fetus may also play a role in organ development (Charalambous et al. 2007).

Additionally related is the fetal insulin hypothesis proposed by Drs. Hattersley and Tooke, which highlights that fetal genetic factors affect not only insulin-mediated fetal growth by regulating either fetal insulin secretion or insulin sensitivity but also insulin resistance in childhood and adulthood (Hattersley and Tooke 1999). One example is the case in which a mother transmits mutations and pleiotropic effects in the glucokinase gene to her child. The glucokinase gene codes for the glycolytic enzyme glucokinase, which acts as the pancreatic beta-cell glucose sensor (Matschinsky et al. 1993). Such mutations result in mild beta-cell dysfunction with slightly elevated fasting blood glucose concentrations, which is present in early childhood and shows little change with age (Hattersley 1998).

3.2 Intrauterine Environment

Based on observational research, Barker et al. proposed the fetal programming hypothesis, which conceptualized that intrauterine experiences modify fetal systems and influence health in later life (Hales and Barker 1992). Fetal development responds to changes in the in utero environment in response to changing metabolism, hormone production, and tissue sensitivity to hormones (Gluckman et al. 2008). These adaptive changes may influence the relative development of various organs, leading to persistent alterations in physiologic and metabolic homeostasis. *Maternal prepregnancy BMI*: In a large cohort of 4,091 mother–father–offspring trios in Britain, researchers found that the association between parental prepregnancy BMI and offspring adiposity at ages 9–11 years was stronger among mother–offspring pairs than among father–offspring pairs (Lawlor et al. 2008). Given that maternal and paternal prepregnancy BMI are markers of genetic, behavioral, and environmental factors but that only the maternal prepregnancy BMI was reflected in the intrauterine environment, this finding provides some support for the role of the in utero environment in lifelong metabolic risk beyond genetic and shared environmental contributions. *Pregestational and Gestational Diabetes:* A sibling study of Pima Indians showed that the BMI of siblings born after the mother developed T2DM was significantly higher than that of siblings born before their mother developed T2DM (Dabelea et al. 2000). Offspring born to mothers with T2DM or GDM had up to a sixfold higher risk of developing T2DM as young adults compared to offspring born to mothers before they developed T2DM (Dabelea and Crume 2011). Other strong evidence comes from a study in which comparisons were made between sibling groups where one sibling was born before the mother experienced dramatic weight loss after bariatric surgery and the other was born after the surgery (Kral et al. 2006). Siblings born before maternal bariatric surgery were at a much greater risk for obesity than siblings born after the weight loss surgery (Kral et al. 2006). Moreover, infants of mothers who had bariatric surgery before pregnancy were at a reduced risk of being LGA at birth (Johansson et al. 2015) and developing obesity and insulin resistance in childhood and adolescence (Smith et al. 2009). Collectively, these findings support the role of the intrauterine environment in transmitting a risk for obesity beyond that of genetics.

3.3 Gene and Environment Interaction and Epigenetics

Epigenetic mechanisms are critical to normal human development and play an important role in complex human diseases (O'Neill et al. 2014;

Reynolds et al. 2013b; Dolinoy et al. 2007). Both animal models and human studies implicate the intrauterine period as a sensitive time for the establishment of epigenetic variability (Heijmans et al. 2008; Cook et al. 2007; Tang et al. 2012; Radford et al. 2014; Janssen et al. 2013), which in turn influences risk for a range of disorders that develop later in life. In the Boston Birth Cohort, we observed a wide range of interindividual variations in genome-wide methylation at birth (Wang et al. 2012). One possible mechanism by which maternal obesity affects offspring OWO is via alterations in fetal DNA methylation induced by maternal obesity.

Animal studies have shown that certain transient environmental influences in utero can produce persistent changes in epigenetic marks that have lifelong consequences (Sinclair et al. 2007; Anway et al. 2005). In humans, our previous study showed an association between maternal prepregnancy BMI and alterations in fetal DNA methylation (Liu et al. 2014). Other studies also showed the link between maternal obesity and fetal epigenome alterations (Lesseur et al. 2013; Yang et al. 2013). In addition, the use of methyl donor supplementation has been shown to prevent transgenerational obesity (Waterland et al. 2008). A recent study indicated lower DNA methylation plasticity in skeletal muscle among low birthweight vs. normal birthweight men, which potentially contributes to our understanding of the link between low birthweight and an increased risk of T2DM (Jacobsen et al. 2014).

Genes related to metabolic risk are regulated by epigenetic alteration: Evidence suggests that epigenetic mechanisms are involved in the risk of obesity. Current evidence supports the important role of epigenetic regulation in key genes involved in the control of adipogenesis, glucose homeostasis, inflammation, and/or insulin signaling, including *leptin* (Milagro et al. 2009), *peroxisome proliferator-activated receptor gamma* (Noer et al. 2007), *insulin* (Yang et al. 2011), *glucose transporter* (Yokomori et al. 1999), *proliferator-activated receptor-γ* (Fujiki et al. 2009), *lipoprotein lipase* (Noer et al. 2007), and *fatty acid-binding protein 4* (Noer et al. 2007). In addition, greater methylation in the promoter region of the *retinoid X receptor-a* gene was also related to greater adiposity in childhood (Godfrey et al. 2011).

Genes subject to genomic imprinting are predominantly expressed from one of the two parental chromosomes and are often clustered in the genome and epigenetically regulated. The role of imprinted genes in growth control has been apparent since the discovery of imprinting in the early 1980s. A related study found altered methylation at multiple imprint regulatory regions in children born to obese parents compared with children born to nonobese parents (Soubry et al. 2015).

4 Preconception and Prenatal Care

Maternal health is not only important for the mother but also for the fetus and neonate, which makes it critical for women to be and stay healthy during their reproductive years. It is well recognized that optimizing a woman's health and knowledge before planning and conceiving a pregnancy may eliminate or reduce health risks to her and her baby. As emerging clinical and scientific advances come to be realized through a life course health development approach to health optimization, the AAP/ACOG Guidelines for Perinatal Care have shifted from framing preconceptional care as appropriately targeted toward prospective parents who are contemplating pregnancy to an emphasis on the integration of preconception health promotion throughout the lifespan. Taking this approach, all women and men can benefit from preconception health, whether or not they plan to have a baby one day. The implementation of effective interventions that prioritize risk factors and the provision of quality health services during prepregnancy and pregnancy are recommended (Bilano et al. 2014). In a multicenter randomized trial, 1108 overweight (BMI ≥ 25 kg/m^2) women were randomized to a comprehensive dietary and lifestyle intervention. Infants born to women who had received lifestyle advice were significantly less likely to have a birthweight above 4000 g; treatment effect (95%CI):0.82, 0.68–0.99; $P = 0.04$) (Dodd et al. 2014). All women with T2DM should be advised regarding safe, effective contraception and the benefits of optimal glycemic control, folic acid supplementation, and avoidance of potentially harmful medications before attempting pregnancy. Adequate glucose control in a woman with diabetes before conception and throughout pregnancy can decrease maternal morbidity, spontaneous abortion, fetal malformation, fetal macrosomia, intrauterine fetal death, and neonatal morbidity (American College of Obstetricians and Gynecologists 2005).

5 Recommendations for Future Study and Perspectives

5.1 Major Themes and Findings

Growing evidence indicates that preconception and prenatal risk factors may play an important role both in fetal metabolic reprogramming and long-term metabolic disorders in later life. Although the onset of obesity and diabetes may begin later in childhood or adulthood, programming at the earliest ages may contribute a latent susceptibility. In addition to genetic susceptibility, epigenetic alterations may be important molecular mechanisms underlying gene–environment interactions in early life origins of disease. Early identification and intervention may improve long-term health outcomes and help to reverse the obesity and diabetes epidemics during the most sensitive developmental stages, when interventions are likely to be most cost-efficient. Particular attention is required for US urban low-income minority populations that have been disproportionally affected by the obesity and diabetes epidemics, and most likely fall into vicious cycle of transgenerational obesity and diabetes.

5.2 Research Priorities

5.2.1 Epidemiologic research

Despite the notion of early life origins of obesity and T2DM, there is a particular lack of well-powered prospective birth cohort studies to examine to what degree and how early life factors affect pregnancy and infant and child health outcomes across multiple developmental windows in a life course framework, particularly in high-risk US urban low-income minority populations. Findings from this line of research will have important research, clinical, and public health implications.

5.2.2 Mechanism research

In light of growing recognition that epigenetic mechanisms may play an important role in mediating early life origins of diseases and that epigenome is potentially modifiable and reversible, well-designed large-scale prospective birth cohort studies are needed to trace the pathways from early life factors to adverse pregnancy outcomes to postnatal long-term metabolic outcomes and to better understand how epigenome changes from fetal to childhood to adolescence in response to environmental exposures. The role of social and environmental adversity in obesity and diabetes among urban low-income minorities has taken on new urgency given that these populations are disproportionally affected by the obesity and diabetes epidemics. In addition to genetics and epigenetics, the field may also leverage and benefit from the latest advances in other "omics" such as metabolomics and microbiome as well as system sciences and bioinformatics.

5.2.3 Translational research

A particular challenge in preventing childhood obesity is to identify important and modifiable early life risk and protective factors to design safe, effective, and sustainable interventions. Evidence is needed to inform clinical guidelines regarding the optimal age to screen for obesity in children. Conflicting recommendations have been proposed for the starting age: age 6 by the US Preventive Services Task Force (Barton 2010) vs. age 2 by the Expert Committee (Barlow 2007). While low birthweight has been included in current clinical assessment of future metabolic risk, there is a need to consider preterm birth as an important risk factor of future metabolic risk. The American Diabetes Association included histories of SGA and maternal history of diabetes or GDM during the child's gestation as part of their diabetes risk assessment for children

(American Diabetes Association 2014). To date, preterm birth has not been included in the diabetes risk assessment guidelines in children and adults, an area that requires more research given growing evidence linking preterm with subsequent metabolic risk.

5.3 Data and Methods Development Priorities

Advanced analytical methods are needed to comprehensively examine temporal and causal links of multilevel early life factors with metabolic outcomes. Future studies need to fully capture the complex interplay of broad environmental factors, genome, epigenome, metabolome, and microbiome that affect metabolic outcomes across lifespan and generations. While some systems models exist to help characterize particular sub-systems of the complex set of factors that influences children's bodyweight, none have tried to comprehensively represent the relationship between early life factors and the subsequent development of childhood metabolic risk across critical developmental stages.

6 Conclusions

There is growing evidence that preconceptional and prenatal factors play an important role in fetal metabolic programming and metabolic risk in later life. More research is needed to identify important and modifiable early life risk and protective factors and underlying mechanisms, which will pave the road for developing cost-effective early screening, prevention, and treatment strategies to halt and reverse the obesity and T2DM epidemics in the US, in particular among the most vulnerable populations (urban low-income minorities).

7 Source of Funding

Drs. Xiaobin Wang and Guoying Wang are supported in part by the National Institutes of Health (NIH) grant R01HD086013 (PI: X Wang).

References

Al-Rubeaan, K. (2015). National surveillance for type 1, type 2 diabetes and prediabetes among children and adolescents: A population-based study (SAUDI-DM). *Journal of Epidemiology and Community Health*. doi:10.1136/jech-2015-205710.

American College of Obstetricians and Gynecologists. (2005). ACOG Practice Bulletin. Clinical Management Guidelines for Obstetrician-Gynecologists. Number 60, March 2005. Pregestational diabetes mellitus. *Obstetrics and Gynecology, 105*(3), 675–685.

American Diabetes Association. (2014). Diagnosis and classification of diabetes mellitus. *Diabetes Care, 37*(Suppl 1), S81–S90.

Anway, M. D., Cupp, A. S., Uzumcu, M., & Skinner, M. K. (2005). Epigenetic transgenerational actions of endocrine disruptors and male fertility. *Science, 308*(5727), 1466–1469.

Barbour, L. A. (2014a). Changing perspectives in pre-existing diabetes and obesity in pregnancy: Maternal and infant short- and long-term outcomes. *Current Opinion in Endocrinology, Diabetes, and Obesity, 21*(4), 257–263.

Barbour, L. A. (2014b). Changing perspectives in pre-existing diabetes and obesity in pregnancy: Maternal and infant short- and long-term outcomes. *Current Opinion in Endocrinology, Diabetes, and Obesity, 21*(4), 257–263.

Barker, D. J., Gluckman, P. D., Godfrey, K. M., Harding, J. E., Owens, J. A., & Robinson, J. S. (1993). Fetal nutrition and cardiovascular disease in adult life. *Lancet, 341*(8850), 938–941.

Barlow, S. E. (2007). Expert committee recommendations regarding the prevention, assessment, and treatment of child and adolescent overweight and obesity: Summary report. *Pediatrics, 120*(Suppl 4), S164–S192.

Barton, M. (2010). Screening for obesity in children and adolescents: US Preventive Services Task Force recommendation statement. *Pediatrics, 125*(2), 361–367.

Bautista-Castano, I., Henriquez-Sanchez, P., Aleman-Perez, N., et al. (2013). Maternal obesity in early pregnancy and risk of adverse outcomes. *PLoS One, 8*(11), e80410.

Bhargava, S. K., Sachdev, H. S., Fall, C. H., et al. (2004). Relation of serial changes in childhood body-mass index to impaired glucose tolerance in young adulthood. *The New England Journal of Medicine, 350*(9), 865–875.

Bilano, V. L., Ota, E., Ganchimeg, T., Mori, R., & Souza, J. P. (2014). Risk factors of pre-eclampsia/eclampsia and its adverse outcomes in low- and middle-income countries: A WHO secondary analysis. *PLoS One, 9*(3), e91198.

Bogdarina, I., Murphy, H. C., Burns, S. P., & Clark, A. J. (2004). Investigation of the role of epigenetic modification of the rat glucokinase gene in fetal programming. *Life Sciences, 74*(11), 1407–1415.

Brumbaugh, D. E., Tearse, P., Cree-Green, M., et al. (2013). Intrahepatic fat is increased in the neonatal offspring of obese women with gestational diabetes. *The Journal of Pediatrics, 162*(5), 930–936; e931.

Charalambous, M., da Rocha, S. T., & Ferguson-Smith, A. C. (2007). Genomic imprinting, growth control and the allocation of nutritional resources: Consequences for postnatal life. *Current Opinion in Endocrinology, Diabetes, and Obesity, 14*(1), 3–12.

Chawla, R., Badon, S. E., Rangarajan, J., et al. (2014). Genetic risk score for prediction of newborn adiposity and large-for-gestational-age birth. *The Journal of Clinical Endocrinology and Metabolism, 99*(11), E2377–E2386.

Chu, S. Y., Callaghan, W. M., Bish, C. L., D'Angelo, D. (2009). Gestational weight gain by body mass index among US women delivering live births, 2004-2005: Fueling future obesity. *American Journal of Obstetrics and Gynecology,. 200*(3), 271; e271–277.

Cnattingius, S., Berne, C., & Nordstrom, M. L. (1994). Pregnancy outcome and infant mortality in diabetic patients in Sweden. *Diabetic Medicine, 11*(7), 696–700.

Cnattingius, S., Villamor, E., Johansson, S., et al. (2013). Maternal obesity and risk of preterm delivery. *JAMA, 309*(22), 2362–2370.

Cook, J. D., Davis, B. J., Goewey, J. A., Berry, T. D., & Walker, C. L. (2007). Identification of a sensitive period for developmental programming that increases risk for uterine leiomyoma in Eker rats. *Reproductive Sciences, 14*(2), 121–136.

Crider, K. S., Yang, T. P., Berry, R. J., & Bailey, L. B. (2012). Folate and DNA methylation: A review of molecular mechanisms and the evidence for folate's role. *Advances in Nutrition, 3*(1), 21–38.

Crume, T. L., Ogden, L., West, N. A., et al. (2011). Association of exposure to diabetes in utero with adiposity and fat distribution in a multiethnic population of youth: The Exploring Perinatal Outcomes among Children (EPOCH) Study. *Diabetologia, 54*(1), 87–92.

Cundy, T., Gamble, G., Neale, L., et al. (2007). Differing causes of pregnancy loss in type 1 and type 2 diabetes. *Diabetes Care, 30*(10), 2603–2607.

Dabelea, D., & Crume, T. (2011). Maternal environment and the transgenerational cycle of obesity and diabetes. *Diabetes, 60*(7), 1849–1855.

Dabelea, D., Hanson, R. L., Lindsay, R. S., et al. (2000). Intrauterine exposure to diabetes conveys risks for type 2 diabetes and obesity: A study of discordant sibships. *Diabetes, 49*(12), 2208–2211.

Dabelea, D., Mayer-Davis, E. J., Lamichhane, A. P., et al. (2008). Association of intrauterine exposure to maternal diabetes and obesity with type 2 diabetes in youth: The SEARCH Case-Control Study. *Diabetes Care, 31*(7), 1422–1426.

De Wals, P., Tairou, F., Van Allen, M. I., et al. (2007). Reduction in neural-tube defects after folic acid fortification in Canada. *The New England Journal of Medicine, 357*(2), 135–142.

Dietz, W. H. (2004). Overweight in childhood and adolescence. *The New England Journal of Medicine, 350*(9), 855–857.

Dodd, J. M., Turnbull, D., McPhee, A. J., et al. (2014). Antenatal lifestyle advice for women who are overweight or obese: LIMIT randomised trial. *BMJ, 348*, g1285.

Dolinoy, D. C., Weidman, J. R., & Jirtle, R. L. (2007). Epigenetic gene regulation: Linking early developmental environment to adult disease. *Reproductive Toxicology, 23*(3), 297–307.

Dzakpasu, S., Fahey, J., Kirby, R. S., et al. (2014). Contribution of prepregnancy body mass index and gestational weight gain to caesarean birth in Canada. *BMC Pregnancy and Childbirth, 14*, 106.

Ensenauer, R., Chmitorz, A., Riedel, C., et al. (2013). Effects of suboptimal or excessive gestational weight gain on childhood overweight and abdominal adiposity: Results from a retrospective cohort study. *International Journal of Obesity, 37*(4), 505–512.

Flegal, K. M., Carroll, M. D., Kit, B. K., & Ogden, C. L. (2012). Prevalence of obesity and trends in the distribution of body mass index among US adults, 1999-2010. *JAMA, 307*(5), 491–497.

Fujiki, K., Kano, F., Shiota, K., & Murata, M. (2009). Expression of the peroxisome proliferator activated receptor gamma gene is repressed by DNA methylation in visceral adipose tissue of mouse models of diabetes. *BMC Biology, 7*, 38.

Gautier, J. F., Wilson, C., Weyer, C., et al. (2001). Low acute insulin secretory responses in adult offspring of people with early onset type 2 diabetes. *Diabetes, 50*(8), 1828–1833.

Gluckman, P. D., Hanson, M. A., Cooper, C., & Thornburg, K. L. (2008). Effect of in utero and early-life conditions on adult health and disease. *The New England Journal of Medicine, 359*(1), 61–73.

Godfrey, K. M., Sheppard, A., Gluckman, P. D., et al. (2011). Epigenetic gene promoter methylation at birth is associated with child's later adiposity. *Diabetes, 60*(5), 1528–1534.

Greenberg, J. A., Bell, S. J., Guan, Y., & Yu, Y. H. (2011). Folic Acid supplementation and pregnancy: More than just neural tube defect prevention. *Reviews in Obstetrics & Gynecology, 4*(2), 52–59.

Hales, C. N., & Barker, D. J. (1992). Type 2 (non-insulin-dependent) diabetes mellitus: The thrifty phenotype hypothesis. *Diabetologia, 35*(7), 595–601.

Hales, C. N., Barker, D. J., Clark, P. M., et al. (1991). Fetal and infant growth and impaired glucose tolerance at age 64. *BMJ, 303*(6809), 1019–1022.

Hattersley, A. T. (1998). Maturity-onset diabetes of the young: Clinical heterogeneity explained by genetic heterogeneity. *Diabetic Medicine, 15*(1), 15–24.

Hattersley, A. T., & Tooke, J. E. (1999). The fetal insulin hypothesis: An alternative explanation of the association of low birthweight with diabetes and vascular disease. *Lancet, 353*(9166), 1789–1792.

Heijmans, B. T., Tobi, E. W., Stein, A. D., et al. (2008). Persistent epigenetic differences associated with prenatal exposure to famine in humans. *Proceedings of the National Academy of Sciences of the United States of America, 105*(44), 17046–17049.

Hochner, H., Friedlander, Y., Calderon-Margalit, R., et al. (2012). Associations of maternal prepregnancy body mass index and gestational weight gain with adult offspring cardiometabolic risk factors: The Jerusalem Perinatal Family Follow-up Study. *Circulation, 125*(11), 1381–1389.

Hofman, P. L., Regan, F., Jackson, W. E., et al. (2004). Premature birth and later insulin resistance. *The New England Journal of Medicine, 351*(21), 2179–2186.

Hovi, P., Andersson, S., Eriksson, J. G., et al. (2007). Glucose regulation in young adults with very low birth weight. *The New England Journal of Medicine, 356*(20), 2053–2063.

International Diabetes Federation. IDF Diabetes Atlas, 5th ed. 2013.; http://www.idf.org/diabetesatlas. Accessed July 19, 2013.

Irving, R. J., Belton, N. R., Elton, R. A., & Walker, B. R. (2000). Adult cardiovascular risk factors in premature babies. *Lancet, 355*(9221), 2135–2136.

Jacobsen, S. C., Gillberg, L., Bork-Jensen, J., et al. (2014). Young men with low birthweight exhibit decreased plasticity of genome-wide muscle DNA methylation by high-fat overfeeding. *Diabetologia, 57*(6), 1154–1158.

Janssen, B. G., Godderis, L., Pieters, N., et al. (2013). Placental DNA hypomethylation in association with particulate air pollution in early life. *Particle and Fibre Toxicology, 10*, 22.

Johansson, S., Iliadou, A., Bergvall, N., Tuvemo, T., Norman, M., & Cnattingius, S. (2005). Risk of high blood pressure among young men increases with the degree of immaturity at birth. *Circulation, 112*(22), 3430–3436.

Johansson, K., Cnattingius, S., Naslund, I., et al. (2015). Outcomes of pregnancy after bariatric surgery. *The New England Journal of Medicine, 372*(9), 814–824.

Kaar, J. L., Crume, T., Brinton, J. T., Bischoff, K. J., McDuffie, R., & Dabelea, D. (2014). Maternal obesity, gestational weight gain, and offspring adiposity: The exploring perinatal outcomes among children study. *The Journal of Pediatrics, 165*(3), 509–515.

Kaijser, M., Bonamy, A. K., Akre, O., et al. (2009). Perinatal risk factors for diabetes in later life. *Diabetes, 58*(3), 523–526.

Kendrick, J. M. (2004). Preconception care of women with diabetes. *The Journal of Perinatal & Neonatal Nursing, 18*(1):14–25; quiz 26–17.

Kim, Y. I. (2000). Methylenetetrahydrofolate reductase polymorphisms, folate, and cancer risk: A paradigm of gene-nutrient interactions in carcinogenesis. *Nutrition Reviews, 58*(7), 205–209.

Kitzmiller, J. L., Block, J. M., Brown, F. M., et al. (2008). Managing preexisting diabetes for pregnancy: Summary of evidence and consensus recommendations for care. *Diabetes Care, 31*(5), 1060–1079.

Knittle, J. L., Timmers, K., Ginsberg-Fellner, F., Brown, R. E., & Katz, D. P. (1979). The growth of adipose tissue in children and adolescents. Cross-sectional and longitudinal studies of adipose cell number and size. *The Journal of Clinical Investigation, 63*(2), 239–246.

Koyanagi, A., Zhang, J., Dagvadorj, A., et al. (2013). Macrosomia in 23 developing countries: An analysis of a multicountry, facility-based, cross-sectional survey. *Lancet, 381*(9865), 476–483.

Kral, J. G., Biron, S., Simard, S., et al. (2006). Large maternal weight loss from obesity surgery prevents transmission of obesity to children who were followed for 2 to 18 years. *Pediatrics, 118*(6), e1644–e1649.

Krikke, G. G., Grooten, I. J., Vrijkotte, T., van Eijsden, M., Roseboom, T. J., & Painter, R. C. (2016). Vitamin B12 and folate status in early pregnancy and cardiometabolic risk factors in the offspring at age 5-6 years: Findings from the ABCD multi-ethnic birth cohort. *BJOG, 123*(3), 384–392.

Krishnaveni, G. V., Veena, S. R., Karat, S. C., Yajnik, C. S., & Fall, C. H. (2014). Association between maternal folate concentrations during pregnancy and insulin resistance in Indian children. *Diabetologia, 57*(1), 110–121.

Lawlor, D. A. (2013). The Society for Social Medicine John Pemberton Lecture 2011. Developmental overnutrition--an old hypothesis with new importance? *International Journal of Epidemiology, 42*(1), 7–29.

Lawlor, D. A., Timpson, N. J., Harbord, R. M., et al. (2008). Exploring the developmental overnutrition hypothesis using parental-offspring associations and FTO as an instrumental variable. *PLoS Medicine, 5*(3), e33.

Lawrence, G. M., Shulman, S., Friedlander, Y., et al. (2014). Associations of maternal pre-pregnancy and gestational body size with offspring longitudinal change in BMI. *Obesity (Silver Spring), 22*(4), 1165–1171.

Lesseur, C., Armstrong, D. A., Paquette, A. G., Koestler, D. C., Padbury, J. F., & Marsit, C. J. (2013). Tissue-specific Leptin promoter DNA methylation is associated with maternal and infant perinatal factors. *Molecular and Cellular Endocrinology, 381*(1–2), 160–167.

Liu, X., Chen, Q., Tsai, H. J., et al. (2014). Maternal preconception body mass index and offspring cord blood DNA methylation: Exploration of early life origins of disease. *Environmental and Molecular Mutagenesis, 55*(3), 223–230.

Loos, R. J., Lindgren, C. M., Li, S., et al. (2008). Common variants near MC4R are associated with fat mass, weight and risk of obesity. *Nature Genetics, 40*(6), 768–775.

Martin, K. E., Grivell, R. M., Yelland, L. N., & Dodd, J. M. (2015). The influence of maternal BMI and gestational diabetes on pregnancy outcome. *Diabetes Research and Clinical Practice, 108*(3), 508–513.

Matschinsky, F., Liang, Y., Kesavan, P., et al. (1993). Glucokinase as pancreatic beta cell glucose sensor and diabetes gene. *The Journal of Clinical Investigation, 92*(5), 2092–2098.

Metzger, B. E., Lowe, L. P., Dyer, A. R., et al. (2008). Hyperglycemia and adverse pregnancy outcomes. *The New England Journal of Medicine, 358*(19), 1991–2002.

Milagro, F. I., Campion, J., Garcia-Diaz, D. F., Goyenechea, E., Paternain, L., & Martinez, J. A. (2009). High fat diet-induced obesity modifies the methylation pattern of leptin promoter in rats. *Journal of Physiology and Biochemistry, 65*(1), 1–9.

Miller, E., Hare, J. W., Cloherty, J. P., et al. (1981). Elevated maternal hemoglobin A1c in early pregnancy and major congenital anomalies in infants of diabetic mothers. *The New England Journal of Medicine, 304*(22), 1331–1334.

Noer, A., Boquest, A. C., & Collas, P. (2007). Dynamics of adipogenic promoter DNA methylation during clonal culture of human adipose stem cells to senescence. *BMC Cell Biology, 8*, 18.

O'Neill, R. J., Vrana, P. B., & Rosenfeld, C. S. (2014). Maternal methyl supplemented diets and effects on offspring health. *Frontiers in Genetics, 5*, 289.

Ong, K. K. L., Ahmed, M. L., Emmett, P. M., Preece, M. A., Dunger, D. B., & Pregnancy, A. L. S. (2000). Association between postnatal catch-up growth and obesity in childhood: Prospective cohort study. *British Medical Journal, 320*(7240), 967–971.

Ouyang, F., Christoffel, K. K., Brickman, W. J., et al. (2010). Adiposity is inversely related to insulin sensitivity in relatively lean Chinese adolescents: A population-based twin study. *The American Journal of Clinical Nutrition, 91*(3), 662–671.

Parkinson, J. R., Hyde, M. J., Gale, C., Santhakumaran, S., & Modi, N. (2013). Preterm birth and the metabolic syndrome in adult life: A systematic review and meta-analysis. *Pediatrics, 131*(4), e1240–e1263.

Pettitt, D. J., Nelson, R. G., Saad, M. F., Bennett, P. H., & Knowler, W. C. (1993). Diabetes and obesity in the offspring of Pima Indian women with diabetes during pregnancy. *Diabetes Care, 16*(1), 310–314.

Pilgaard, K., Faerch, K., Carstensen, B., et al. (2010). Low birthweight and premature birth are both associated with type 2 diabetes in a random sample of middle-aged Danes. *Diabetologia, 53*(12), 2526–2530.

Radford, E. J., Ito, M., Shi, H., et al. (2014). In utero effects. In utero undernourishment perturbs the adult sperm methylome and intergenerational metabolism. *Science, 345*(6198), 1255903.

Reece, E. A., Leguizamon, G., & Homko, C. (1998). Pregnancy performance and outcomes associated with diabetic nephropathy. *American Journal of Perinatology, 15*(7), 413–421.

Reynolds, R. M., Allan, K. M., Raja, E. A., et al. (2013a). Maternal obesity during pregnancy and premature mortality from cardiovascular event in adult offspring: Follow-up of 1 323 275 person years. *BMJ, 347*, f4539.

Reynolds, R. M., Jacobsen, G. H., & Drake, A. J. (2013b). What is the evidence in humans that DNA methylation changes link events in utero and later life disease? *Clinical Endocrinology, 78*(6), 814–822.

Rigo, J., Nyamugabo, K., Picaud, J. C., Gerard, P., Pieltain, C., & De Curtis, M. (1998). Reference values of body composition obtained by dual energy X-ray absorptiometry in preterm and term neonates. *Journal of Pediatric Gastroenterology and Nutrition, 27*(2), 184–190.

Rolland-Cachera, M. F., Deheeger, M., Maillot, M., & Bellisle, F. (2006). Early adiposity rebound: Causes and consequences for obesity in children and adults. *International Journal of Obesity, 30*(Suppl 4), S11–S17.

Silverman, B. L., Metzger, B. E., Cho, N. H., & Loeb, C. A. (1995). Impaired glucose tolerance in adolescent offspring of diabetic mothers. Relationship to fetal hyperinsulinism. *Diabetes Care, 18*(5), 611–617.

Silverman, B. L., Rizzo, T. A., Cho, N. H., & Metzger, B. E. (1998). Long-term effects of the intrauterine environment. The Northwestern University Diabetes in Pregnancy Center. *Diabetes Care, 21*(Suppl 2), B142–B149.

Sinclair, K. D., Allegrucci, C., Singh, R., et al. (2007). DNA methylation, insulin resistance, and blood pressure in offspring determined by maternal periconceptional B vitamin and methionine status. *Proceedings of the National Academy of Sciences of the United States of America, 104*(49), 19351–19356.

Sipola-Leppanen, M., Vaarasmaki, M., Tikanmaki, M., et al. (2014). Cardiovascular risk factors in adolescents born preterm. *Pediatrics, 134*(4), e1072–e1081.

Smith, J., Cianflone, K., Biron, S., et al. (2009). Effects of maternal surgical weight loss in mothers on intergenerational transmission of obesity. *The Journal of Clinical Endocrinology and Metabolism, 94*(11), 4275–4283.

Soubry, A., Murphy, S. K., Wang, F., et al. (2015). Newborns of obese parents have altered DNA methylation patterns at imprinted genes. *International Journal of Obesity, 39*(4), 650–657.

Sridhar, S. B., Darbinian, J., Ehrlich, S. F., et al. (2014). Maternal gestational weight gain and offspring risk for childhood overweight or obesity. *American Journal of Obstetrics and Gynecology, 211*(3):259; e251–258.

Tang, W. Y., Morey, L. M., Cheung, Y. Y., Birch, L., Prins, G. S., & Ho, S. M. (2012). Neonatal exposure to estradiol/bisphenol A alters promoter methylation and expression of Nsbp1 and Hpcal1 genes and transcriptional programs of Dnmt3a/b and Mbd2/4 in the rat prostate gland throughout life. *Endocrinology, 153*(1), 42–55.

Torloni, M. R., Betran, A. P., Horta, B. L., et al. (2009). Prepregnancy BMI and the risk of gestational diabetes: A systematic review of the literature with meta-analysis. *Obesity Reviews, 10*(2), 194–203.

Uthaya, S., Thomas, E. L., Hamilton, G., Dore, C. J., Bell, J., & Modi, N. (2005). Altered adiposity after extremely preterm birth. *Pediatric Research, 57*(2), 211–215.

Wang, D., Liu, X., Zhou, Y., et al. (2012). Individual variation and longitudinal pattern of genome-wide DNA methylation from birth to the first two years of life. *Epigenetics: Official Journal of the DNA Methylation Society, 7*(6), 594–605.

Wang, G., Divall, S., Radovick, S., et al. (2014a). Preterm birth and random plasma insulin levels at birth and in early childhood. *JAMA, 311*(6), 587–596.

Wang, G., Chen, Z., Bartell, T., & Wang, X. (2014b). Early Life Origins of Metabolic Syndrome: The Role of Environmental Toxicants. *Current Environmental Health Reports*. doi:10.1007/s40572-013-0004-6.

Wang, G., Hu, F., Mistry, K., et al. (2016). Maternal Prepregnancy BMI, Plasma Folate Level and Child Metabolic Risk. *JAMA Pediatrics. 170*(8), e160845.

Waterland, R. A., Travisano, M., Tahiliani, K. G., Rached, M. T., & Mirza, S. (2008). Methyl donor supplementation prevents transgenerational amplification of obesity. *International Journal of Obesity, 32*(9), 1373–1379.

Williams, M. A., Qiu, C., Dempsey, J. C., & Luthy, D. A. (2003). Familial aggregation of type 2 diabetes and chronic hypertension in women with gestational diabetes mellitus. *The Journal of Reproductive Medicine, 48*(12), 955–962.

Yang, B. T., Dayeh, T. A., Kirkpatrick, C. L., et al. (2011). Insulin promoter DNA methylation correlates negatively with insulin gene expression and positively with HbA(1c) levels in human pancreatic islets. *Diabetologia, 54*(2), 360–367.

Yang, Q. Y., Liang, J. F., Rogers, C. J., Zhao, J. X., Zhu, M. J., & Du, M. (2013). Maternal obesity induces epigenetic modifications to facilitate Zfp423 expression and enhance adipogenic differentiation in fetal mice. *Diabetes, 62*(11), 3727–3735.

Yokomori, N., Tawata, M., & Onaya, T. (1999). DNA demethylation during the differentiation of 3T3-L1 cells affects the expression of the mouse GLUT4 gene. *Diabetes, 48*(4), 685–690.

Zhang, S., Liu, X., Brickman, W. J., et al. (2009). Association of plasma leptin concentrations with adiposity measurements in rural Chinese adolescents. *The Journal of Clinical Endocrinology and Metabolism, 94*(9), 3497–3504.

Early Childhood Health and the Life Course: The State of the Science and Proposed Research Priorities

A Background Paper for the MCH Life Course Research Network

W. Thomas Boyce and Clyde Hertzman

But Laura lay awake a little while, listening to Pa's fiddle softly playing and to the lonely sound of the wind in the Big Woods. She looked at Pa sitting on the bench by the hearth, the firelight gleaming on his brown hair and beard and glistening on the honey-brown fiddle. She looked at Ma, gently rocking and knitting.
She thought to herself, 'This is now.'
She was glad that the cozy house, and Pa and Ma and the firelight and the music, were now. They could not be forgotten, she thought, because now is now. It can never be a long time ago.

Little House in the Big Woods
Laura Ingalls Wilder (1932)

1 Introduction: What's So Special About the Early Years?

In these lines from the *Little House* book series recalling her early years in a nineteenth-century pioneer family, Laura Ingalls Wilder evoked what we deem a timeless and evocative, if modestly sentimental, image of childhood: children's dependency upon the reliable and protective presence of parents, children's uniquely vulnerable and consequential sensibilities, their openness to the character and "feel" of the physical and social worlds, and their singular immersion in the present, the moment at hand. The overarching goals of this chapter are to survey extant literature examining evidence for these special susceptibilities of children to social-environmental conditions, to show how variation in life course health development is attributable to interactive differences in constitutional susceptibility and contextual exposure, and to summarize lacunae in our collective vision of how early adversity becomes biologically embedded in the course of individual health development.

Wilder's portrait of early childhood is the same image promulgated in the eighteenth century writings of Jean Jacque Rousseau, who affirmed children's inherent goodness and receptivity to the social world and educational institutions' responsibility never to impede children's natural independence and curiosity (see *Émile, or Treatise*

W. Thomas Boyce (✉)
Departments of Pediatrics and Psychiatry, University of California San Francisco, San Francisco, CA, USA
e-mail: istom.boyce@ucsf.edu

C. Hertzman
Human Early Learning Partnership, School of Population and Public Health, University of British Columbia, Vancouver, BC, Canada

N. Halfon et al. (eds.), *Handbook of Life Course Health Development*,
DOI 10.1007/978-3-319-47143-3_4

on Education). Such an image of childhood is also wholly commensurate with twenty-first century visions of youth as a season of special vulnerability within the human life course health development—a developmental discontinuity from the less susceptible, more defended reaches of adulthood and life in an adult society. Some historians of childhood have claimed that these visions of children's special sentience and fragility are social constructions—products of the temporal and cultural epoch in which we now live. Philippe Ariès in his *Centuries of Childhood* (Ariès 1962) and Edward Shorter in *The Making of the Modern Family* (Shorter 1975) argued, for example, that prior to the seventeenth and eighteenth centuries, fewer distinctions were made between children and their adult counterparts in their needs, capacities, and proclivities. They further held that, as a consequence of the extraordinary rates of infant mortality at the time (25–50%; King 2007), parents were less likely to make strong emotional investments in children. Other scholars have judged such claims hyperbolic, however, discerning evidence for qualitative differentiation between children and adults in ancient Egyptian songs ("Hast thou come to kiss the child?/ I will not let thee kiss him!/ Hast thou come to silence him?/ I will not let thee set silence over him!" (Hrdy 1999)), in the writings of Renaissance Italy and Reformation Germany (King 2007) and in the plays of Shakespeare ("Those that do teach young babes/ Do it with gentle means and easy tasks/ He might ha' chid me so; for, in good faith,/ I am a child to chiding." *Romeo and Juliet*) (Chedgzoy et al. 2007). Cultural historian Peter Stearns (Stearns 2011) thus maintained that a special affection for and attentiveness to children and children's vulnerability are no inventions or fabrications of modernity.

Nonetheless, ethnogeographer Jared Diamond points to the dramatic variation that exists, even in the contemporary world, among parenting practices emanating from this differentiated and particular view of childhood (Diamond 2012). Both Stearns and Diamond cite, for example, the historical and contemporary practice of swaddling infants as an iconic parenting act that is grounded in deep cultural beliefs about the nature of infancy and childhood, about the relationship of children to parents, and about the fundamental nature of the human child. Hrdy shows how extraordinary differences in mothering behavior have occurred, historically and contemporaneously, as a consequence of sociocultural and economic conditions, despite strong, evolutionarily conserved commonalities in innate maternal responses (Hrdy 1999). Further, Barr et al. (1991) demonstrate that developmental and temporal patterns of infant crying are invariant between North American and !Kung San infants, but parental responses to such crying are highly divergent. Though parenting practices come and go and beliefs regarding the consequences of such practices vary by geography and cultural era, most historical and present human societies have attributed to young children a special susceptibility to the character of the social and physical contexts in which they are reared.

There have also been abiding cultural convictions—crossing geography and time—that the special sensibilities of young children, when exposed to psychological and physical adversities, can produce forms of morbidity extending well beyond the exposure itself, into the domain of adult life. We have strongly held beliefs in the continuities—for better and for worse—between childhood and adulthood. John Milton (1608–1674) wrote in *Paradise Regained* that "The childhood shews the man/ As morning shews the day" and William Wordsworth (1770–1850) observed, in *My Heart Leaps Up When I Behold*, that "The Child is father of the Man." Marcel Proust (1871–1922) described, in *Remembrance of Things Past*, the sudden, flooding and vivid awareness of a childhood memory in an ordinary moment of adult life:

> When from a long distant past nothing subsists, after the people are dead, after the things are broken and scattered, taste and smell alone, more fragile but enduring, more unsubstantial, more persistent, more faithful, remain poised a long time, like souls, remembering, waiting, hoping, amid the ruins of all the rest.

In the early and mid-twentieth century, these long held beliefs about childhood's capacity for intrusion into the experiences of adult life began to find their way into the borderlands of emerging science. Freud famously asserted that neurotic behavior and obsessions manifesting in mid-adulthood were often linked, without conscious awareness, to experiences of trauma sustained decades before, in very early life (Freud 1940). Biologist and scholar René Dubos invoked "biological Freudianism" to argue that the adverse exposures of childhood can produce lasting *neurobiological* predispositions that persist even when such exposures are later abated or gone (Dubos et al. 1966). Jerome Kagan (e.g., Brim and Kagan 1980) observed the ways in which human health development is characterized by *both* constancy *and* sometimes remarkable discontinuity across developmental periods. Though the experiences of childhood may not overdetermine or dominate the strengths and liabilities of adult life, our cultural heritage avows not only a child's special receptivity to the provisions and predations of its early world but the lifelong echoes of that receptivity, as well.

2 Susceptibility and Continuity: The Echoes of Childhood

The now thriving science of how early social experience influences lifelong health and development might be legitimately portrayed as building a scientific foundation for these two longstanding tenets of cultural belief. These are the claims (a) that childhood is imbued with a distinctive susceptibility to the character of the social and physical world and (b) that, partially as a consequence of the former, the exposures of early life—those both damaging and sustaining—continue to exert their effects on health and well-being long beyond the childhood years. John Bowlby thus concluded that the infants of all primate species show an evolutionarily conserved predisposition to form powerful emotional attachments to their mothers, striving to stay close to her side at all times and thereby reducing the risks of abandonment or endangerment (Bowlby 1969). Harlow, Suomi, and colleagues, in the nonhuman primate equivalent of Bowlby's work with human children, showed that the drive toward early attachment is so strong that, in the mother's absence, an infant macaque will physically and emotionally bond to an inanimate surrogate but with subsequent behavioral aberrations that extend through the infant's lifetime (Harlow et al. 1971). Over the last two decades, Barker and colleagues produced a large body of findings suggesting that chronic, life-threatening cardiovascular disease in mid- to late life is derived from nutritional deficits and impaired growth occurring in very early, even prenatal life (see, e.g., Barker 1990; Barker and Bagby 2005; Bock and Whelan 1991). Kuh and Ben-Shlomo (2004) outlined a "life course approach" to chronic disease epidemiology, assembling convergent evidence for temporally distant relations between markers of childhood deprivation and compromise and indices of chronic morbidity in adult life. The Human Development Program of the Canadian Institute for Advanced Research (CIFAR) showed how population health and developmental science coincide to reveal powerful societal effects on child development and health and how such effects are transcribed into lifetimes of socially partitioned differences in adult disease (Keating and Hertzman 1999). The American Academy of Pediatrics has recently called public attention to the issue of significant, "toxic" stress and adversity in the lives of young children and asserted that many of the chronic disorders of adult life should now be regarded as "developmental disorders," stemming as they do from adverse childhood experiences and events. Abstracting these and other programs of research, three major reports—in the USA (Shonkoff and Phillips 2000), the UK (Marmot 2010), and Canada (Boivin and Hertzman 2012)—have sought and achieved a multidisciplinary consensus that the experiences of early life, dramatically partitioned by aspects of socioeconomic status (SES) and social position, result in societies with widely divergent developmental and health outcomes. Such societies produce visibly and persistently disadvantaged social groups whose children follow blighted developmental trajectories, acquire chronic disease and disability more frequently and severely, learn and achieve less well, and live substantially shorter, less adaptive lives.

3 Constitution, Context, and the Nonrandom Distribution of Morbidity

Although strong, multinational consensus has been reached on the power and pervasiveness of epidemiologic findings in linking early experience to lifelong disparities in health development and health, urgent and challenging new research questions remain. Among these are the following:

- What is the source of the extensive variability in associations between early adversity and health? Why are some children profoundly affected by early stressors and disadvantage, while others appear to thrive in the face of great risk?
- *How* does it happen? That is, what are mechanisms and mediators by which early exposures become biologically embedded in development, yielding lifelong differences in health? How does adversity "get into the body," altering long-term pathogenic processes that predispose to disease and disorder?
- What role, if any, do constitutional differences in vulnerability—genetic variation, neurobiological response biases, or enduring temperamental attributes—play in the consequences of early life adversity?
- Does the timing, frequency, and persistence of exposure matter? That is, is there unevenness in the effects of adversity by the age of the child or by the intensity and duration of the exposure?
- Are there transgenerational effects of early social adversity? Are the "iniquities of the father visited upon their children, to the second and third generation" (Exodus 34:7)? Are the traumas of a single generation transmitted into the lives of the next?

Such questions are not just scientifically compelling; they do not simply appeal to our twenty-first century zeal to understand nuance, contingency, and mechanism. Conceiving and implementing effective societal interventions to mitigate health disparities will be necessarily conditional upon clear and instructive answers. As an organizational approach to these and other life course health development questions, we propose a useful convergence of *two fundamental principles* emerging from this new science of early childhood experience and development. These are:

Principle 1: Most developmental and health endpoints in human populations are derived from causal interactions between contextual and constitutional factors.

Principle 2: Disordered development and health are nonrandomly distributed by population, space, and time.

Principle 1 affirms a now broadly accepted refutation of earlier claims that maladaptive outcomes are principally genetically or environmentally determined. Incontrovertible evidence now rejects both environmental and genetic determinism and views the genesis of disease as involving a dynamic interplay between environments and genes. Even the simple partitioning of developmental variance into environmental and genetic components falls short of a truly interactive view of the conjoint operation of nurture and nature (Boyce et al. 2012b; Meaney 2010). Importantly, our assertion that causal interactions between contextual and constitutional differences will predominate in the pathogenesis of human morbidities does not entail a claim that no main effects of such differences will be found. Far more research is needed to conclude confidently that gene-environment interplay predominates in the pathogenesis of most human diseases, but such interactive processes appear almost certainly more prevalent and common that was imagined even a decade ago (Dunn et al. 2011; Wright and Christiani 2010). Principle 2 contends, as did Bronfenbrenner's bioecological model (e.g., Bronfenbrenner and Morris 2006), that disorders of health and development are neither evenly nor stochastically distributed within human populations and that such disorders are instead informatively clustered by population (both within and across populations), space (both geography and jurisdiction), and time (both developmental and historical). The maldistribution of disorder within human populations signals important and reliable differences in susceptibility to various forms of morbidity and their causal agents. The aggregation of morbidities by space and time extends beyond conventional understandings of epidemicity to include geographic and mobility effects on morbidity and critical periodicity in developmental processes.

A cross-referencing of these Principles 1 and 2 produces the table below, which divides supportive evidential territory into six domains of research: I. social stratification, poverty, and subordination; II. vulnerability, resilience, and neurobiological susceptibility; III. the topography of vulnerability; IV. marginalization and scapegoating; V. history and affliction; and VI. critical periodicity. These six domains codify the *contextual and constitutional sources of disease maldistribution*, aggregated by population, space, and time. In the sections that follow, we abstract and review each of these arenas of research, which together serve to summarize current and emerging findings on the lifetime effects of early childhood exposures. The crosscutting, confluent cell below the six domains designates a section on interactions between context and constitution, in the form of gene-environment interplay, and their role in the biological embedding of early social adversities and the emergence of what has been called "the social brain." Finally, as indicated in table's bottom cell, we conclude with a specification of missing areas of study, unaddressed questions, and an agenda for future work on the developmental origins of life morbidities (Table 1).

4 Six Domains of Early Developmental Research

4.1 Social Stratification, Poverty, and Subordination

Among the most well-replicated, population-level findings in all of the child health services research is illustrated in Fig. 1. Within childhood populations from a broad diversity of settings, cultures, and societies, a subgroup of 15–20% sustain over half of the populations' morbidities, both biomedical and psychiatric, and are responsible for over half of the health-care utilization (Boyce 1985; Diaz et al. 1986). The public health implications of this finding are self-evident: if we could explain and address the disproportionate morbidity carried by this small subgroup of childhood populations, we might prevent over half of the population's diseases, injuries, and disorders.

The search for an explanation for this highly nonrandom distribution of human morbidity begins and ends with the phenomenon of *social stratification*, that is, the hierarchical social organization that characterizes much of invertebrate to

Table 1 Domains of existing, anticipated, and needed research, organized by Principles 1 and 2

		Principle 1: Developmental and health outcomes stem from interactions between	
		Context	**Constitution**
Principle 2: Disordered outcomes are nonrandomly distributed by	**Population**	I. Social stratification, poverty, and subordination	II. Vulnerability, resilience, and neurobiological susceptibility
	Space	III. The topography of vulnerability	IV. Marginalization and scapegoating
	Time	V. History and affliction	VI. Critical periodicity
		Interactions between context and constitution, gene-environment interplay	
		An Agenda for Future Research	

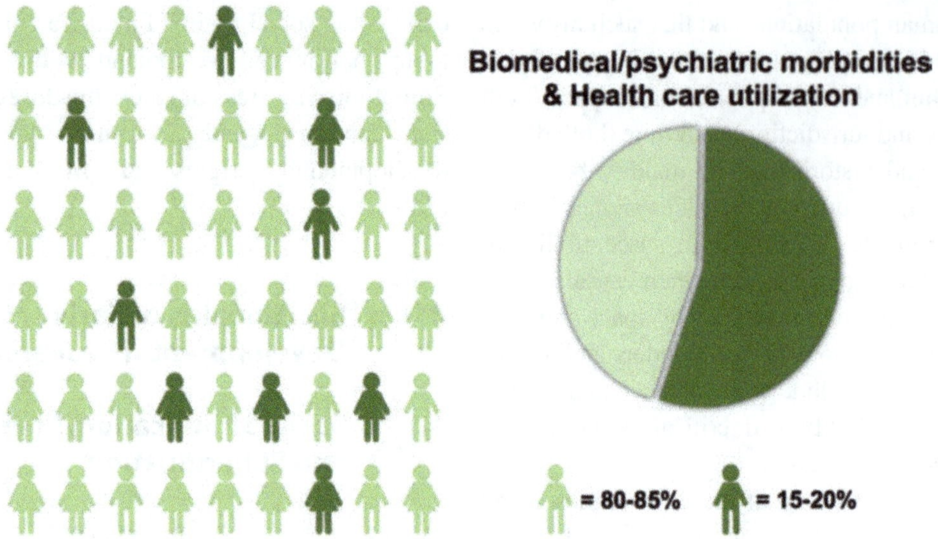

Fig. 1 The nonrandom distribution of biomedical and psychiatric morbidities in child populations

vertebrate phylogeny and manifests as SES within human societies. SES constitutes the single, most powerful epidemiologic determinant of virtually all forms of morbidity, a predictor so potent that we question the authenticity of other associations failing to adjust for SES (Adler et al. 1993, 1994). Beginning early in life, impoverished children and families sustain higher rates of virtually every form of human malady: from low birth weight (Blumenshine et al. 2010) to traumatic injury (Brown 2010), from infectious disease (Dowd et al. 2009) to dental caries (Boyce et al. 2010), and from developmental disability (Msall et al. 1998) to poorer academic achievement (Kawachi et al. 2010). Socioeconomic stratification of developmental psychopathology, moreover, which often emerges in preclinical form in the middle childhood years, exerts lasting influences on academic achievement, employment success, interpersonal relationships, and lifelong well-being (Offord 1995; U.S. Department of Health and Human Services 2011). Figures 2 and 3 show how poor and neglected populations bear disproportionate burdens of disease and disorder throughout the life span (see Marmot 2010)—Fig. 2 showing the graded association between SES and socioemotional adjustment from middle childhood through adolescence and Fig. 3 revealing the same relation with chronic disease at each stage of the life course.

Despite this universality and potency of societal disparities in health, it is only recently that SES has become itself a focus of serious scientific study (Syme 2008). New studies of the SES antecedents of population morbidities have recognized the extended influence of childhood social status on adult disease, even after controlling for SES in adulthood (Cohen et al. 2010; Galobardes et al. 2004; Lawlor et al. 2006). Such evidence for lifelong effects of early disadvantage is rendered still more compelling by research documenting the developmental origins of adult health and disease (Gluckman et al. 2005, 2009) and by epidemiologic work revealing systematic differences in nutrition (Khan and Bhutta 2010), access to medical care (Houweling and Kunst 2010), and physical environmental exposures (Gump et al. 2007) among children of differing social classes.

Although these and other material factors undoubtedly play roles in the origins of health disparities (Hackman et al. 2010), another prominent and increasingly persuasive explanation for such disparities is the SES-stratified differences in early exposures to family adversities and stressors (Brown et al. 2009; Hillis et al. 2004; Wadsworth et al. 2008). Low-SES children live with significantly more family chaos (Evans et al. 2005), sustain more frequent and severe psychological stressors (Evans 2004; Evans and Kim

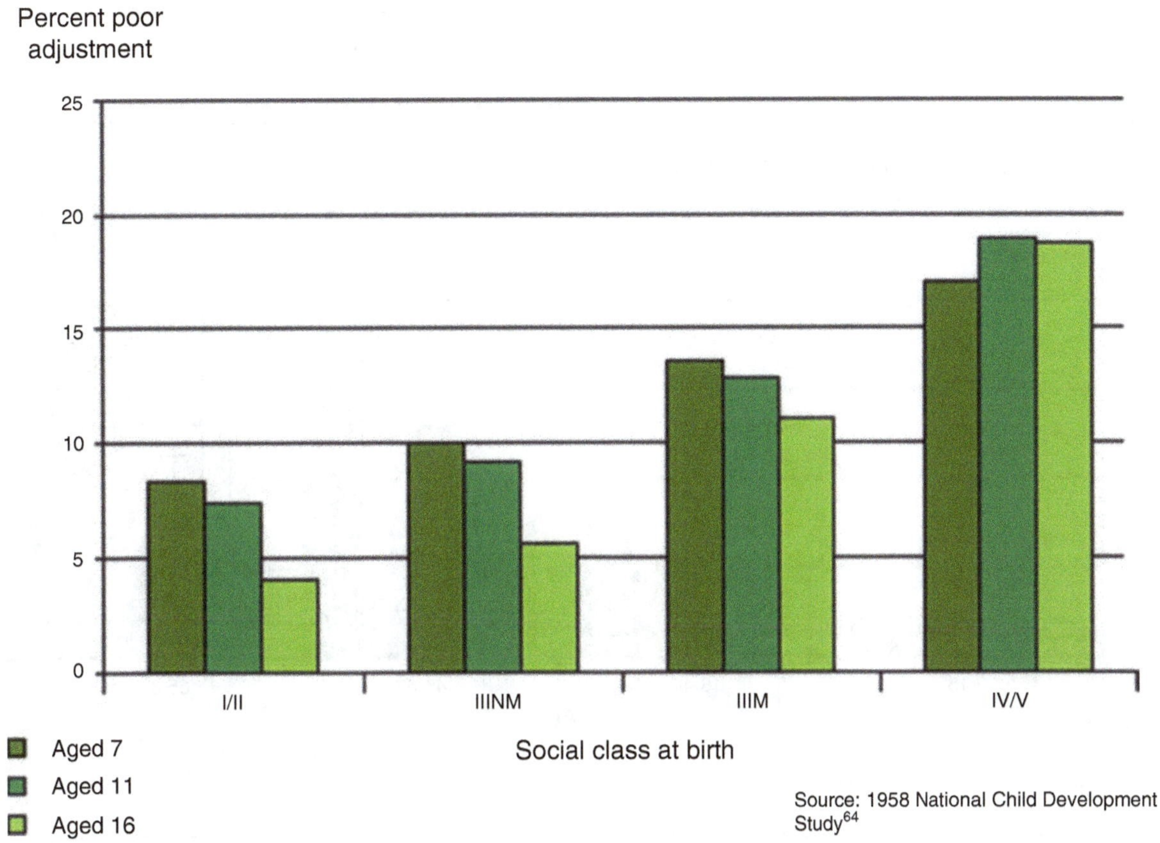

Fig. 2 Rates of poor social/emotional adjustment at ages 7, 11, and 17, by father's social class at birth (Marmot 2010)

2007), and experience fewer supportive parent-child communications (Hart and Risley 1995), relative to their higher SES peers. Low SES children also show greater neurobiological sensitivity to aversive social contexts, in the form of heightened reactivity within the stress-responsive, neuroendocrine pathways, i.e., the hypothalamic-pituitary-adrenocortical (HPA) axis and the autonomic nervous system (ANS) (Boyce et al. 2010; Evans and Kim 2007; Lupien et al. 2001; Steptoe et al. 2002). Further, the exaggerated reactivity of these peripheral stress response systems among disadvantaged youth is subserved by socially partitioned differences in central neural circuits, which also have profound influences on health development, cognitive function, and educational attainment (Curley et al. 2011; Cushing and Kramer 2005; Gianaros and Manuck 2010; Hackman and Farah 2009; MacDonald and Roskams 2009; McEwen and Gianaros 2010).

Influences of childhood SES on health and neurobiological endpoints extend beyond concurrent effects on health and responsivity during childhood to longer-term relations with health status in adult life. Adverse experiences in early childhood, for example, may carry risk effects for coronary artery disease in adult life before the age of 50 years and effects mediated by some form of biological embedding (Kittleson et al. 2006). One important set of candidate mechanisms for such temporally distant effects is the constellation of pro-inflammatory changes that have been shown associated with childhood disadvantage. Programs of work by Miller and Chen (Miller et al. 2009a; Miller et al. 2009b), Cole (Cole 2009; Cole et al. 2007) and others (Danese et al. 2008; McDade 2012), for example, have demonstrated systematic differences in cytokine signaling pathways, transcriptional control, and risk for inflammation- and immune-mediated disease. These studies suggest that changes in immune responsivity and the molecular processes involved in inflammation may be one category of mediating events linking childhood social adversity to adult disease.

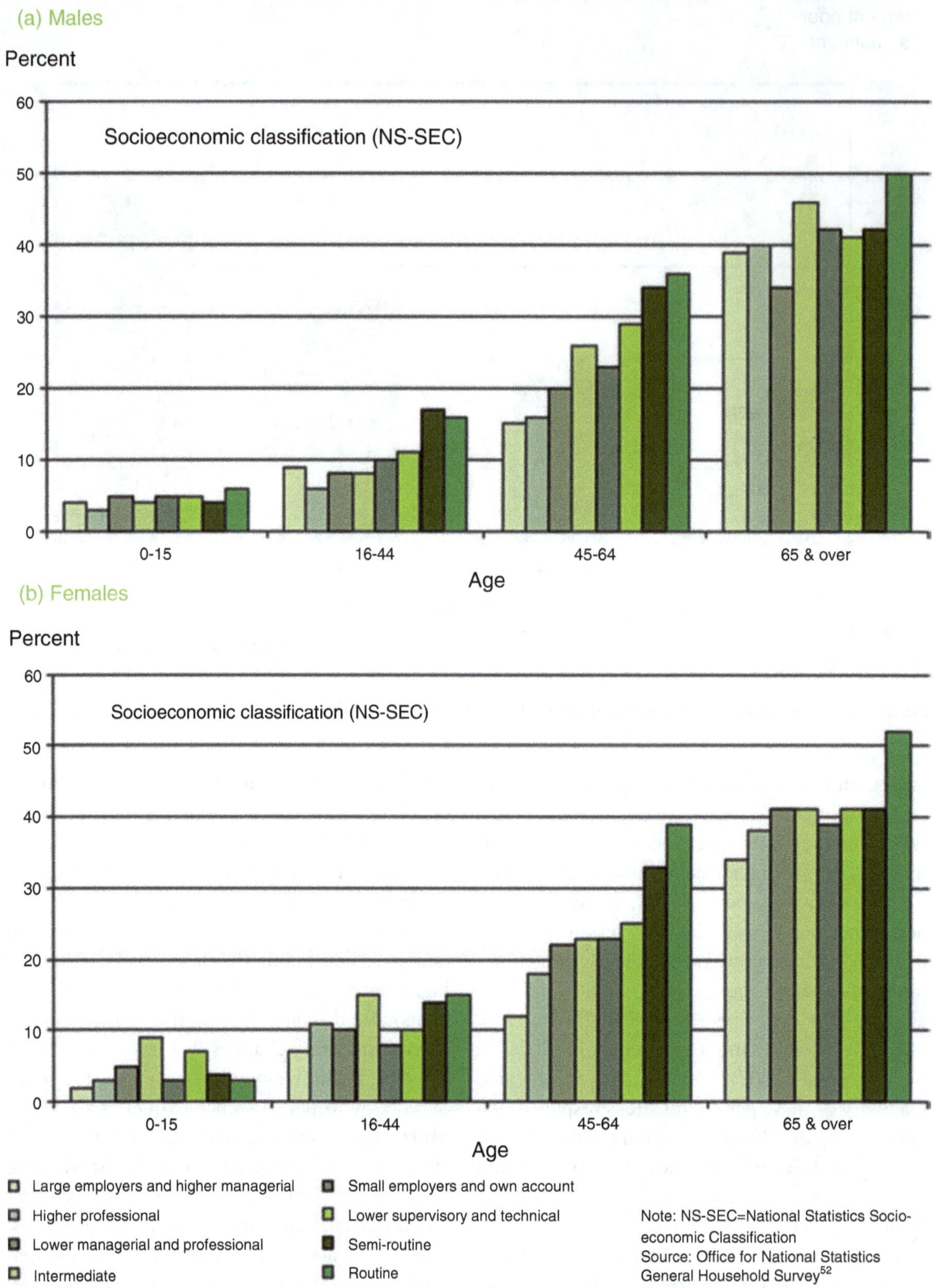

Fig. 3 Percentage of males and females with limiting long-term illness, by age and socioeconomic classification (Marmot 2010)

Finally, there is emerging evidence that experiences of social subordination per se, themselves prevalent sources of human adversity (Keltner et al. 2003), may be related to disorders of mental and physical health, educational failure, and maladaptive behavior, especially in the young. The works of Pellegrini (Pellegrini et al. 2007, 2010), Hawley (Hawley 1999), and Fehr (Fehr et al. 2008) and their colleagues, describing the developmental emergence, behavioral signs, and socioemotional sequelae of childhood dominance and egalitarianism, have offered important "down payments" on such a research agenda. More recently, we have examined linkages between subordination and maladaptive health outcomes in a socioeconomically and ethnically diverse sample of kindergarten children, assessing associations between experiences of dominance-subordination and patterns of maladaptive behavior (Boyce et al. 2012a). As shown in Fig. 4, we found that indicators of mental health in 5-year-old children were stratified within classroom hierarchies in a manner parallel to that seen in larger, adult societies. Children occupying subordinate positions within their classrooms had more depressive symptoms, more frequent episodes of inattention, fewer positive peer relationships, and less evidence of prosocial behavior. Further, we found that the children most likely to show low or diminishing health status were those occupying subordinate social positions who also came from low SES families, and those least likely to show a diminution in health came from classrooms with teachers highly invested in learner-centered pedagogical practices (LCPs). Indeed, as shown in Fig. 4, the link between rank and behavior nearly disappeared in classrooms with strong teacher LCPs, suggesting that classrooms with egalitarian, student-centered "cultures" produced diminished mental health effects of hierarchical social ranks.

Such findings—that social subordination is associated with decrements in mental health, even within hierarchical, early childhood groups—are commensurate, moreover, with prior findings that *subjective* estimates of social class may be a stronger predictor of health outcomes than objective indicators, such as job status, income, or wealth (Adler et al. 2000; Goodman et al. 2003; Ostrove et al. 2000), and that dominance status in *primate* social hierarchies is similarly associated with health, even among captive animals with equal access to food, open environments, and veterinary care (Abbott et al. 2003; Cohen et al. 1997; Kaplan et al. 1982; Sapolsky 2005).

A growing body of research thus demonstrates powerful, graded effects of childhood social stratification and SES on development and health, both in children and their adult counter-

Fig. 4 Depression by social position and learner-centered pedagogical practices (LCPs) at half-SD increments from the mean (−1, −0.5, mean, +0.5, +1 SD) (Boyce et al. 2012a)

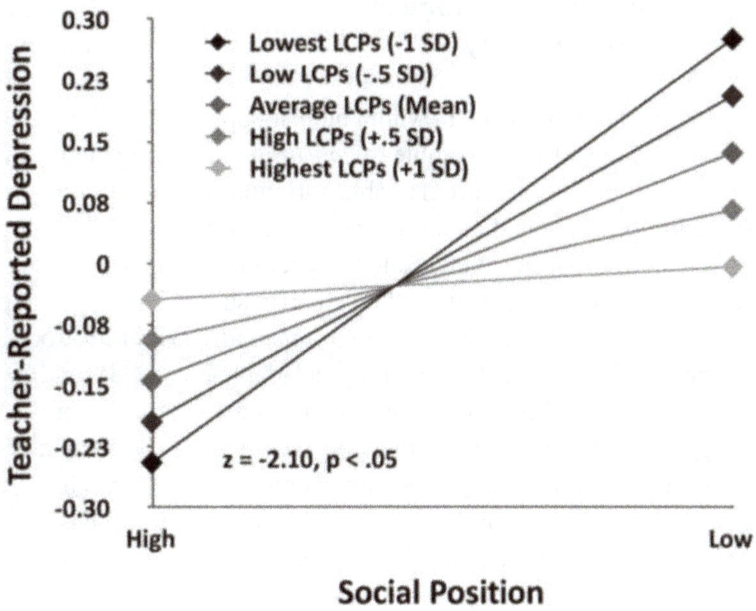

parts. Such effects may account, at least in part, for the strikingly uneven distribution of morbidities within human populations. Nonetheless, as noted by Kessler, Duncan, and colleagues (e.g., Kessler et al. 2014), results of large-scale human experiments challenge assumptions that simply augmenting financial resources or moving children out of high-poverty neighborhoods will have salutary effects on health development. Childhood SES effects are likely mediated by a broad array of factors that include diet, exposures to toxic environmental agents, differences in parenting, and access to health care, but substantial evidence also now implicates differential exposures to stress and adversity as a major mechanism of SES influence. Acquired differences in neurobiological reactivity to stressors and pro-inflammatory shifts in immune signaling pathways may also play an important mediating role in SES-health relations. Lastly, research has also begun to document effects of social subordination per se on childhood health outcomes, independent of family or neighborhood SES. Thus, relations between social position within classroom peer hierarchies and subsequent health outcomes show the same graded associations with morbidity found in studies of nations and large human populations.

4.2 Vulnerability, Resilience, and Neurobiological Susceptibility

The aggregation of ill health within human populations appears also attributable to *constitutional* differences underlying a remarkable variation in susceptibility to social-environmental influence. There is now growing evidence for a generalized sensitivity to social contexts within a human subgroups, i.e., highly sensitive or environmentally "permeable" individuals showing maladaptive outcomes in conditions of adversity but unusually positive outcomes in settings characterized by support, predictability, and protection (see, e.g., Aron et al. 2012; Belsky et al. 2007; Boyce 2016; Boyce and Ellis 2005; Ellis et al. 2011a). Such individuals thus show either the least or most adaptive outcomes within the population, depending upon the character of the proximal social contexts in which they are reared. Studies demonstrating this greater susceptibility of neurobiologically responsive children to both positive and negative aspects of their environments have implicated a wide variety of:

- *Stressors and adversities*, including paternal depression (Cummings et al. 2007), marital conflict (El-Sheikh 2005; El-Sheikh et al. 2007), parental psychopathology (Shannon et al. 2007), and overall family distress (Obradovic et al. 2010)
- *Positive environmental features*, including parental warmth (Ellis et al. 1999), beneficial experiences and exposures (Pluess and Belsky 2013), and supportive interventions (Bakermans-Kranenburg et al. 2008a)
- *Defining biological parameters*, including physiological reactivity (e.g., Alkon et al. 2006; Boyce et al. 1995), differences in brain circuitry (Whittle et al. 2010), and gene polymorphisms (Bakermans-Kranenburg et al. 2008b; Knafo et al. 2011; Manuck et al. 2011)

Most importantly, highly susceptible children (and adults) show bidirectional effects on outcomes in contrasting highly supportive and highly stressful settings—not simply an attenuation of negative effects in low stress circumstances.

Such differences in neurobiological sensitivity—likely based, in part, on genetic and epigenetic variation (Boyce and Kobor 2015)—are figuring prominently in the field's exploration of the biological embedding of early stress. Findings suggesting differential susceptibility have been replicated in many samples of children, a troop of rhesus macaques (Boyce et al. 1998), and in a series of randomized controlled trials of socially supportive interventions (Bakermans-Kranenburg and Van Ijzendoorn 2015; Quas et al. 2004). Neurobiological sensitivity has also been the focus of a ten-paper special section of *Development and Psychopathology*

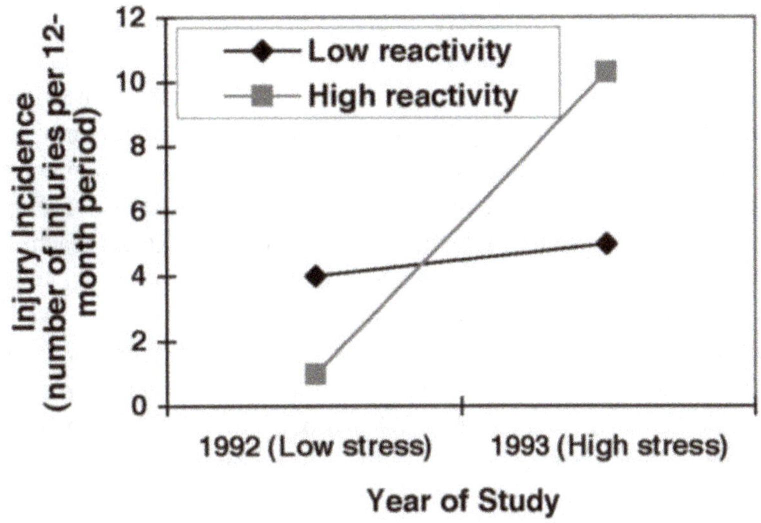

Fig. 5 Incidence of violent injuries in free ranging macaques by confinement stress and reactivity status (Boyce et al. 1998)

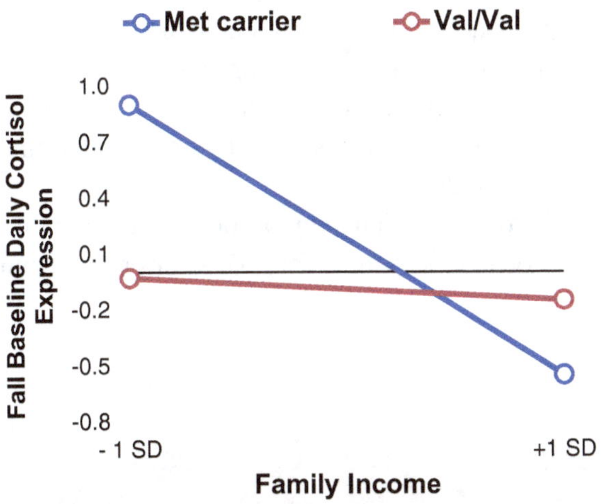

Fig. 6 Daily baseline cortisol expression by family SES and BDNF polymorphism (N. Bush, personal communication, unpublished data, 2017)

(see Ellis et al. 2011a). As shown in the accompanying Figs. 5 and 6, examples have included the differential rates of violent injuries among high and low reactivity rhesus macaques before and during a prolonged period of confinement stress (Fig. 5) and the level of HPA activation among kindergartners by allelic variants in the BDNF gene and family income (Fig. 6). In both cases, the "risky endophenotype" (i.e., high reactivity status or being a Met carrier in the BDNF polymorphism) showed high levels of maladaptive outcomes (injuries or basal cortisol secretion) under stressful conditions but remarkably low levels (lower even than their low-risk counterparts) in positive, low stress settings.

Importantly, strong evolutionary arguments have been made, albeit not without dissension (e.g., Bateson and Gluckman 2011; Overton and Lerner 2014; West-Eberhard 2003) for the conservation of environmental sensitivity within rearing environments of evolutionary adaptedness. Slavich and Cole, for example, have summarized recent evidence on how social-environmental exposures can regulate gene expression, thereby calibrating individual sensitivity to social context (Slavich and Cole 2013). Such sensitivity appears to influence not only the rates and severity of morbidity but also the timing and pace of important developmental transitions, such as puberty (Ellis et al. 2011b). This characteristic, which probably becomes increasingly trait-like over the course of development, appears to emerge as a conditional adaptation, garnering signals from the early social environment about the inherent levels of threat, adversity, support, and nurturance that the growing child is likely to encounter and calibrating stress-responsive biological systems to optimize survival, health, and developmental well-being (Ellis et al. 2006, 2011a; Hane and Fox 2006). Understanding phenotypic variation in environmental susceptibility might logically also play a role in the conceptualization and development of newly individualized approaches to "precision medicine" (Committee on a Framework for Development a New Taxonomy of Disease 2011).

4.3 The Topography of Vulnerability

In addition to their aggregation within *population* subgroups, developmental vulnerability and ill health are also clustered by spatial geography. It is well known, for example, that of the more than 7 million of the world's children less than 5 years of age that die each year, the majority live in the regions of sub-Saharan Africa and South Asia (Liu et al. 2012). Equally familiar is the epidemiologic, small area clustering of neurodevelopmental disorders such as autism spectrum disorder (Mazumdar et al. 2010). Less well known, but equally compelling, are the dramatic differences in developmental vulnerability at primary school entry—differences with major implications for learning and academic success—that are found within major national jurisdictions, such as the Canadian province of British Columbia (see Fig. 7).

Between 2000 and 2011, the provincial BC government, with the assistance and oversight of the Human Early Learning Partnership at UBC Vancouver, completed four population-based assessments of developmental health. Assessments were completed during the kindergarten year, and developmental health was measured using the Early Development Instrument (EDI), a kindergarten teacher-completed checklist for each child based on five scaled measures of development: physical well-being, social competence, emotional maturity, language and cognitive development, and communication and general knowledge (Janus and Offord 2000). The EDI yields, for each child and each scale, a score as "vulnerable" or "not vulnerable." The designation as "vulnerable" is not given directly to the family, however; rather, rates of EDI vulnerability are computed and mapped according to residential neighborhoods where children live. Mapping is done by neighborhoods because local geography defines unique combinations of factors that support or undermine early child development.

Across Canadian neighborhoods, vulnerability rates on one or more of the EDI scales range from

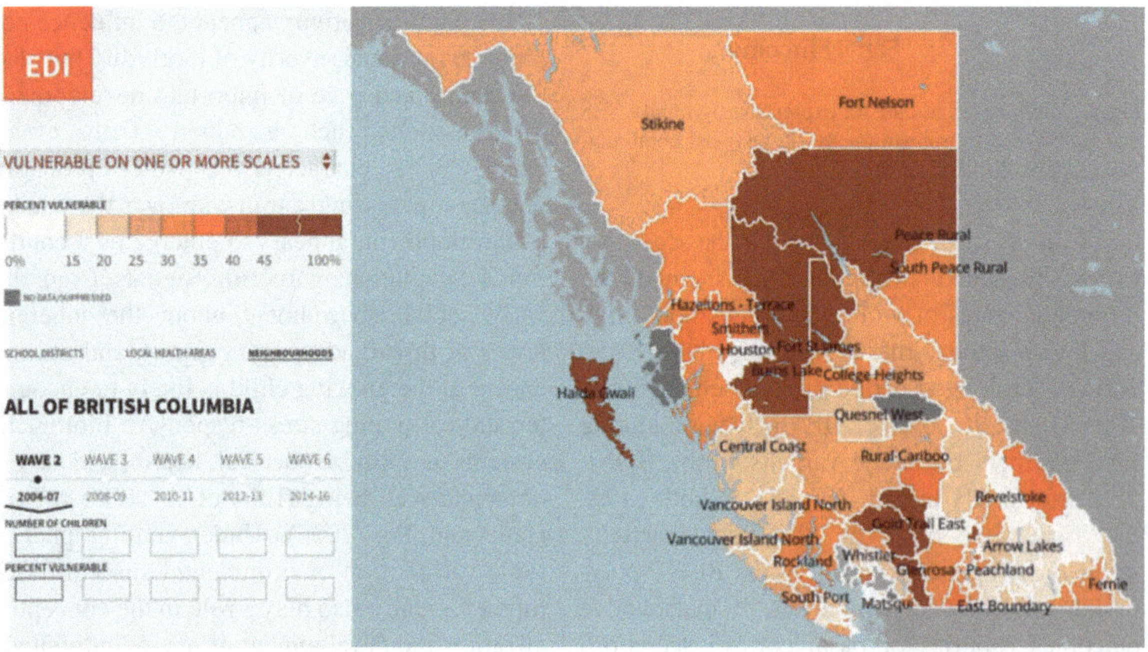

Fig. 7 Neighborhood variation in developmental vulnerability in British Columbia on the early development instrument (http://earlylearning.ubc.ca/interactive-map/)

as low as 4% to as high as 69%, such that there is a more than 17-fold inequality in developmental vulnerability in Canada at the level of the neighborhood. This range is much larger than would be predicted on the basis of random sample surveys of child development, which rarely demonstrate social gradients larger than threefold. Neighborhoods aggregate family environments, reflect broader environments, and have emergent properties, such as safety and social cohesion, that influence developing children. They tend to include families of similar socioeconomic status, unique mixes of relational characteristics (i.e., the factors that shape a family's social identity), and similar levels of access or barriers to programs and services. For analytical purposes, random sample surveys aggregate children from different geographical locales into statistical (rather than real) neighborhoods according to a small number of grouping factors (e.g., median family income or proportion of adults with high school graduation). Such "neighborhood effect" analyses from random sample surveys do not capture the unique circumstances of real neighborhoods. Thus, the 17-fold variation in EDI-estimated developmental health validates this spatial geographic approach to local differences, since only this tactic captures the circumstances of real neighborhoods (Hertzman 2010; Kershaw et al. 2009). Such an approach has been used, for example, to reveal that optimal, area level EDI scores occur within neighborhoods with *mixed*, rather than uniformly affluent, SES representation, i.e., those with relatively equal proportions of affluent and disadvantaged families (Carpiano et al. 2009). Adopted on an even larger scale, such methods are capable of offering social ecological perspectives on the physical, socioeconomic, and social political conditions of children on a global scale (Panter-Brick et al. 2012).

4.4 Marginalization and Scapegoating

Interpersonal marginalization and scapegoating can also contribute to uneven distributions of morbidity and maladaptive development, often based on targeting by individual, constitutional characteristics. Victimization is a well-represented and elemental human behavior, even within groups of very young children. Described by Lord Byron as "the longest pleasure" (*Don Juan*, 13th Canto: "Now hatred is by far the longest pleasure; Men love in haste but they detest at leisure."), hatred and stigmatization have remained, for all of history, a sadly defining feature of human societies. Family systems theory has regarded scapegoating and the designation of an "identified patient" as an effective if personally costly means of securing family solidarity (Vogel and Bell 1961), much as the vilification of Simon in William Golding's *Lord of the Flies* served the cohesion of a marooned band of lost school boys. Behavioral vulnerability stemming from physical weakness, anxiety, poor social skills, or chronic illness has been shown to engender victimization in groups of children (Egan and Perry 1998; Sentenac et al. 2012), and within nonhuman primate troops, the active targeting of highly reactive, more sensitive members has been described during periods of intensive group stress (Boyce et al. 1998). Far from restricted to Western, individualist societies, bullying and victimization are also highly prevalent in more collectivist cultures (Kim et al. 2004). Among human children and youth, such victimization can undermine mental health and lead to poor academic performance (Glew et al. 2005), psychosomatic disorders (Arseneault et al. 2006; Gini and Pozzoli 2009), suicidal ideation behavior (Kim et al. 2009; Turner et al. 2012), and later criminality (Sourander et al. 2007). Among the survivors of population-level genocide, specific genetic variants have been linked to traumatic memory retention and the level of risk for post-traumatic stress disorder (PTSD) (de Quervain et al. 2012). Abusive experiences in children, whether at the hands of family or peers, become itself a social determinant of adult mental and physical health (Greenfield 2010), resulting in the sequestering of morbidities within both perpetrators and their victims.

4.5 History and Affliction

As Kuzawa and Thayer noted (Kuzawa and Thayer 2011), human adaptation to environmental conditions takes place at a variety of timescales, ranging from homeostatic changes that can occur over seconds or minutes to developmental plasticity emerging over months or years to conserved genetic changes that operate on a timescale of millennia. Thus, historical contexts can also concentrate and skew distributions of disease and disorder over epochs of time. For example, prenatal exposures to a natural disaster, such as the 1998 Québec Ice Storm, can contribute to the risk for childhood obesity, even after adjustment for breastfeeding, SES, obstetrical complications, and smoking during pregnancy (Dancause et al. 2012). During historical periods of war, elevated lifetime risks for PTSD are found among children exposed to violent or traumatic events (Javidi and Yadollahie 2012). Researchers have also studied how early life exposures to famine can influence adult health, using historical cohort data from the Finnish crop failure famine of 1866–1868, the Dutch Hunger Winter of 1944–1945, the Siege of Leningrad in 1944, the seasonal famines in the Gambia between 1949 and 1994, and the Chinese Great Leap Forward famine of 1959–1961. Outcomes examined have included adult height and weight, glucose metabolism, blood pressure, lipid profiles, metabolic syndrome, cardiovascular outcomes, self-reported health, mental performance and cognition, mental disorders, and adult mortality (Falconi et al. 2017; Lumey et al. 2011). Exposure episodes related to war, such as the 1944–1945 Dutch Famine of World War II, resulted in elevated odds of developing coronary heart disease in adult life (Painter et al. 2005; Roseboom et al. 2000) and in systematic differences in the epigenetic modification of genes such as insulin-like growth factor (IGF-2) (Heijmans et al. 2008) and aspects of risk that appear capable of crossing into unexposed generations (Painter et al. 2008). Genocide, whether historical in the case of the Holocaust or contemporary, as in the Rwandan atrocities, exerts powerful, lasting damage on children's prospects for health and well-being, both contemporaneous and longitudinal (Hazani and Shasha 2008; Oberg 2008). Each of these examples illustrates how time, in the form of historical period, and context, in the form of broad socioenvironmental perturbations and assaults, converge to influence and bias life course health development.

4.6 Critical Periodicity

Finally, events and exposures within developmental time, rather than historical time, also create constraints and opportunities for healthy development and the avoidance of disorder. The function of neuronal circuits in the brain is guided by experiences in postnatal life that regulate the maturation of inhibitory connections and interneurons (Hensch 2005). Critical periods exist, for example, for the acquisition of language and discrimination of speech sounds in human infants (Weikum et al. 2012), and exposure to music can change auditory preferences in young mice through changes in prelimbic and infralimbic medial prefrontal cortex during an early critical period (Yang et al. 2012). Adult brain plasticity appears to become restricted by structural and functional developmental "brakes," such as perineuronal nets and myelin that inhibit neurite growth and the balance between excitatory and inhibitory circuitries (Bavelier et al. 2010). Genetic, pharmacological, and environmental influences can alter such plasticity, suggesting future opportunities for reopening closed critical periods, such as those for language acquisition or vision, or enhancing recovery from traumatic or cerebrovascular brain injury.

5 Interactions Between Context and Constitution: The Biological Embedding of Early Adversity

These arenas of research, defining the contextual and constitutional origins of disease maldistribution by population, space, and time, converge in a new and growing body of work examining the interplay between genes and environments in determining developmental and health endpoints over the life course. Such research comprises studies of (a) true gene-environment interactions, in which allelic variation moderates primary associations between environmental factors and outcomes, and (b) epigenetic processes, in which exposure-related chemical/structural modifications of chromatin up- or downregulate the transcriptional expression of functionally salient genes. Together, such studies and larger territories of research have begun to advance serious answers, at a variety of analytic levels, to the questions surrounding how socially partitioned early experience "gets under the skin," affecting broad life course trajectories of development and health (Evans et al. 2012; Hertzman and Boyce 2010; Slavich and Cole 2013).

5.1 Chromatin Modification and the Molecular Biology of Epigenesis

As shown in Fig. 8, chromatin is the structural packaging of DNA and its associated proteins into nucleosomes: strands of DNA wrapped around histone protein octamers, like thread around a spool. Nucleosomes in turn form a loosely or tightly wound chromatin "necklace," arrayed like beads on a string. Epigenetics has been defined as a functional modification of DNA that does not involve an alteration of sequence (Meaney 2010). The differentiation of embryonic stem cells into specific tissue lineages, for example, is epigenetically guided by patterns of downregulation and activation of lineage-specific genes (Wu and Sun 2006). Figure 9 shows how DNA methylation changes with development throughout the sequential ontogeny of germ cell development, fertilization, and embryogenesis. The more general processes of gene-environment interplay involve important functional distinctions between gene sequence, epigenetic modifications, and gene expression—variations in each of which may influence individual responses to environmental exposures. Gene sequence variation, for example, has been linked to vulnerability to a variety of maladaptive or disordered health outcomes (Caspi et al. 2002, 2003).

Differences in gene expression have also been associated with disease susceptibility (Liew et al. 2006; Mohr and Liew 2007) and are, in turn, related to a variety of epigenetic, molecular processes, which include DNA methylation, histone modification, production of noncoding microRNAs, presence of various transcription factors, and nucleosome remodeling (Gilbert and Epel 2009). Given the complexities of these chemical mechanisms, however, it is important to understand that (a) DNA methylation is only one form of epigenetic mark, (b) DNA methylation is not the equivalent of gene expression, and (c) it is sometimes unclear whether DNA methylation is a precursor of gene silencing or a marker of such silencing. For purposes of simplicity, the discussion here

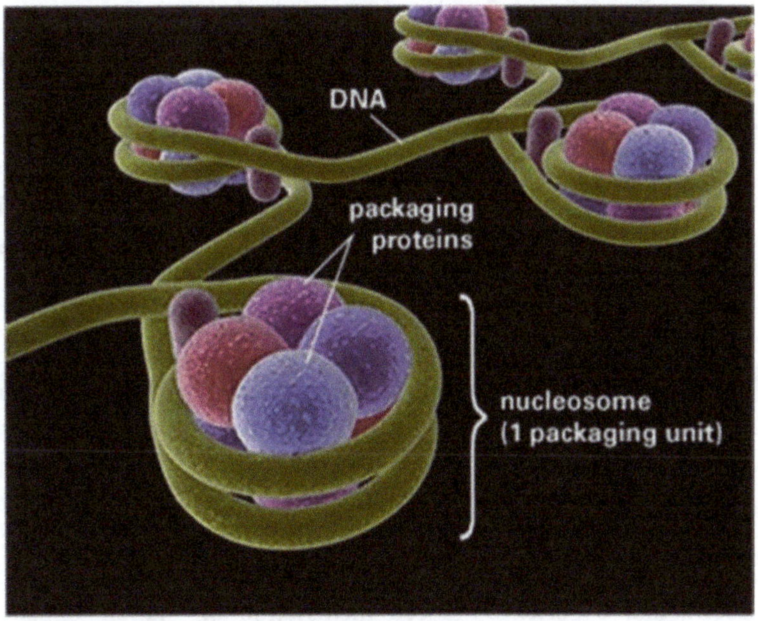

Fig. 8 Chromatin and nucleosome structure (Courtesy of Joseph Roland© 2003 – www.cytographica.com)

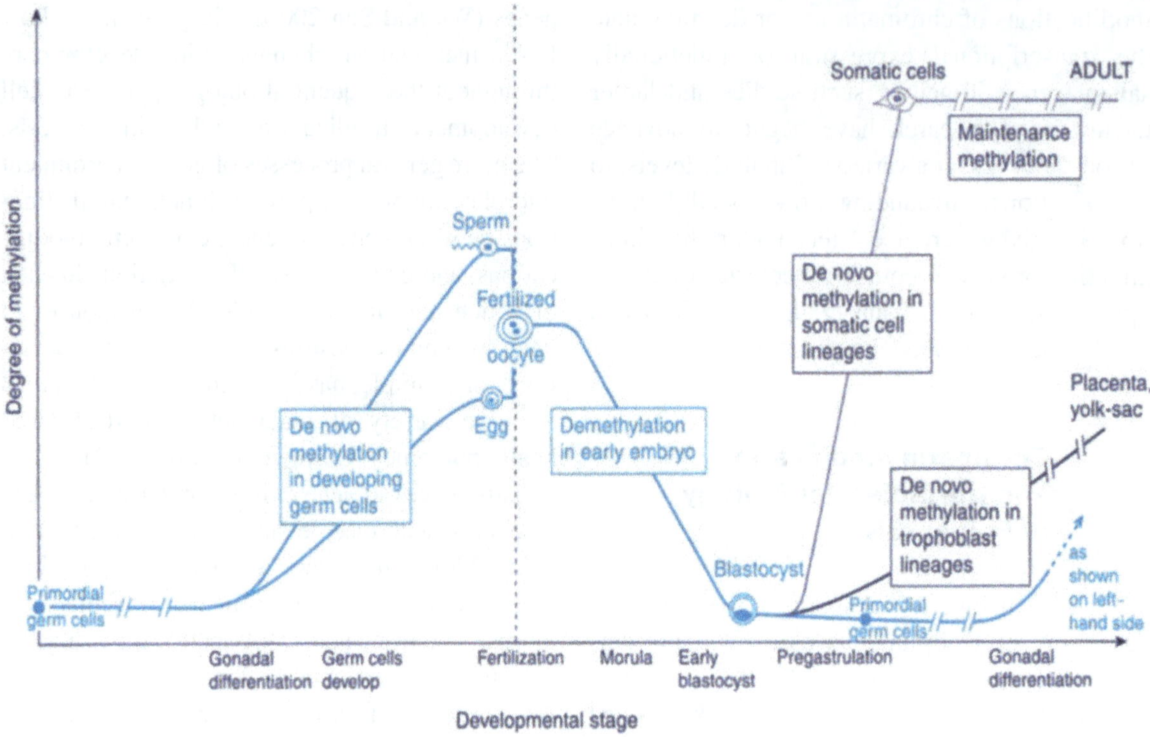

Fig. 9 Epigenetic methylation events in early human gestation (Russo et al. 1999)

focuses primarily upon true gene-environment interactions and a single form of epigenetic modification, the methylation of cytosine-phosphate-guanine (CpG) dinucleotide sites in DNA. The relative stability of DNA methylation suggests that, among epigenetic marks, it may be responsible for longer-term, more developmentally important changes in gene expression.

As shown in Fig. 10, genes have both promoter and coding regions, with the latter demarcated by start and stop sequences recognized by RNA polymerase. RNA polymerase, in association with facilitating transcription factors (i.e., a "transcription complex"), *transcribes* the DNA coding region into messenger RNA, which in turn undergoes ribosomal *translation* into proteins that alter cellular function. Social experiences can result in epigenetic marks, such as CpG methylation, within a gene's promoter region, and the degree of such methylation regulates gene expression, like a dimmer switch regulates light in a room. Transcription start sites and promoters are known to be enriched with CpG sites (areas called "CpG islands") (Turner et al. 2008), and experience-induced methylation of these sites is known to tighten chromatin structure, rendering transcription factor binding sites physically less accessible and interfering with RNA polymerase attachment to the coding start sequence. Thus, the experience-induced methylation of a promoter CpG can effectively silence the gene, altering cellular function and changing physiological processes ranging from neurotransmitter reuptake in neuronal synapses to blood glucose regulation and sympathetic nervous system reactivity.

5.2 The Epigenetics of Social Adversity

Although the study of epigenetics began in the field of cancer biology, research has more recently begun to explore epigenetic processes by which socially stratified exposures to early adversities may condition long-term risks to development and health (Gluckman et al. 2007; Jirtle and Skinner 2007; Tsankova et al. 2007). There is evidence for DNA methylation-associated regulation of adversity-responsive genes in both

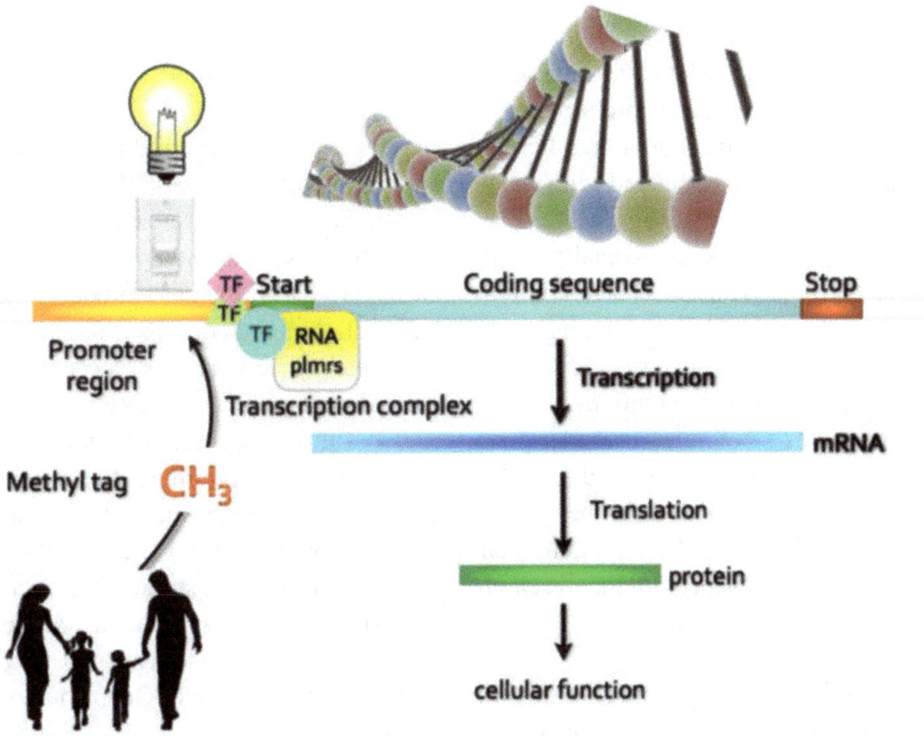

Fig. 10 Simplified representation of epigenetic modification and transcription regulation. *CH_3* methyl group, *Tag* TF transcription factor, *RNA plmrs* RNA polymerase, *mRNA* messenger RNA

laboratory animals (McGowan et al. 2008) and human infants (Oberlander et al. 2008) and for stressor-associated differences in mRNA expression in human subjects (Cole et al. 2007; Morita et al. 2005). Further, the biochemical "markings" of genomic DNA and its associated, nucleosomal histone proteins are the epigenetic mechanisms by which the expression of neuroregulatory genes is controlled (Isles and Wilkinson 2008; Meaney and Ferguson-Smith 2010; Mehler 2008). Epigenetic marks are capable, through this governing of neuroregulatory gene expression, of guiding both neurodevelopment and the function of peripheral and central neural pathways (Liu et al. 2008; MacDonald and Roskams 2009).

The work of Meaney, Szyf, and colleagues (Szyf et al. 2008; Weaver 2009; Weaver et al. 2004; Zhang and Meaney 2010), for example, has demonstrated in the rat pup how maternal licking and grooming in the first several days of life downregulate pups' long-term HPA reactivity through increases in hippocampal glucocorticoid receptor (GR, *NR3C1*) expression and serotonergic tone. Licking and grooming triggers increases in serotonin in the hippocampus, and activation of the 5-HT receptor induces expression of a transcription factor, nerve growth factor-inducible protein-A (NGFI-A). Licking and grooming also facilitates NGFI-A's association with the exon 1_7 GR gene promoter by demethylating a CpG site located in the NGFI-A binding region of this exon. The resulting increased expression of GR results in a downregulation of corticotropin-releasing hormone (CRH) and diminished activation of the HPA axis. Readers are referred to (Hackman et al. 2010) for more detailed description of these molecular events. Other work in rat models of early infant maltreatment has demonstrated enduring methylation of the gene coding for brain-derived neurotrophic factor (BDNF), reduced BDNF expression, and extension of both epigenetic marks and maltreatment of young into a subsequent generation (Roth et al. 2009). Because BDNF is a key mediator of neural plasticity in brain regions such as the prefrontal cortex and hippocampus, such findings might present a legitimate model of the neurocognitive sequelae of transgenerational neglect and abuse of human children. Champagne and colleagues (Champagne et al. 2006) have also shown, in the same model, that the increased estrogen receptor-α (ER-α) expression that occurs in the medial preoptic area of high licking and grooming mothers is associated with cytosine methylation of the ER-α gene promoter.

Nonhuman primate work by Kinnally et al. (Kinnally et al. 2010a, 2010b, 2011) has explored, in infant macaques, interrelations among early stressors (social group vs. nursery rearing and variable foraging vs. control conditions), allelic variation in the *5-HTT* serotonin transporter gene promoter, and both genome-wide and 5-HTT-specific differential methylation in peripheral blood mononuclear cells (PBMCs). Among their findings with direct relevance to the research considered here are the following:

- Higher *5-HTT* CpG methylation, but not sequence variation in the serotonin transporter promoter region, exacerbates the effects of early life stress on behavioral stress reactivity.
- Both greater *5-HTT* and whole-genome methylation level (i.e., 5-methylcytosine content) is associated with enhanced stress reactivity across the subsequent life span.
- When brain tissue is unavailable for methylation analysis, peripheral blood methylation levels may serve as useful surrogates (see also Cupello et al. 2009; Uebelhack et al. 2006).

The Meaney-Szyf research group has also recently advanced evidence, in the postmortem hippocampi of human suicide victims, for hypermethylation of the ribosomal RNA gene and *NR3C1* gene promoters and epigenetic marks suggesting dysregulation in cellular protein synthesis machinery and HPA responsivity (McGowan et al. 2008, 2009). Further, two prospective human studies have now documented differential patterns of DNA methylation conditional upon various aspects of early childhood adversity. First, genome-wide, blood DNA methylation analysis in low- and high-SES subjects from the 1958 British Birth Cohort revealed a cluster of probes obtained from the 500 most variable promoters that was enriched with high-SES individuals, confirming that SES differences contributed to overall epigenetic variation. Methylation levels for 1,252 gene promoters were associated with childhood SES versus 545 promoters for adulthood SES (Borghol et al. 2012). Second, in a subsample of adolescents from the Wisconsin Study of Family and Work birth cohort, Essex et al. (Essex et al. 2013) found differential methylation in 170 CpG sites among participants whose parents reported high levels of stress during their children's early lives. Maternal stressors in infancy and paternal stressors in the preschool years were most strongly predictive of differential methylation, and the patterning of such epigenetic marks varied by children's gender. Both birth cohort studies suggest that epigenetic signatures detectable in adolescence to mid-life are related to early experiences with stressful environments. Other human research has documented:

- Altered DNA methylation of the insulin-like growth factor gene (IGF2) in individuals exposed prenatally to the Dutch Famine of 1944–1945 (Heijmans et al. 2008)
- Increased NR3C1 methylation at an NGFI-A binding site in newborns exposed to mothers' depressed mood in the third trimester of pregnancy (Oberlander et al. 2008)
- Highly variable methylation patterns within the five GR promoters activated in PBMCs, possibly reflecting epigenetic fine-tuning of GR expression by early life experiences (Turner et al. 2008)
- Pro-inflammatory shifts in cytokine expression among young adults with low-SES childhood histories, via transcriptional signaling changes in adrenergic and adrenocortical pathways (Chen et al. 2011; Miller et al. 2009a)
- Both between-tissue and between-individual discordance in epigenetic marks at the insulin-like growth factor, IGF2/H19, locus in multiple tissues at birth, even among monozygotic twins (Ollikainen et al. 2010)
- Differences in risk for psychopathology related to concurrent allelic and epigenetic

variation, such that trauma-related 5-HTT promoter methylation operates as a moderator of the association between the 5-HTT polymorphism and psychological problems (van IJzendoorn et al. 2010)

Taken together, these observations offer evidence for social-environmental regulation of mammalian and human gene expression, at the levels of both whole-genome and candidate gene methylation (Cole 2009). The findings also suggest that divergences in methylation and gene expression begin early in development, even during intrauterine life, and that socially partitioned stress and adversity may be transmuted into mental health risks through molecular modifications of the epigenome. Differential exposures to environmental events may explain, for example, the diverging trajectories of epigenetic profiles found among monozygotic twins over time (Fraga et al. 2005). More broadly, epigenetic remodeling in response to developmentally potent environmental events may serve as a mechanism for neural plasticity and the conditional production of individual differences in attributes and risks for psychopathology (Bagot and Meaney 2010).

5.3 Gene-Environment Interplay in Brain Development

Indeed, there is already emerging evidence that brain processes and neural plasticity may function as key mediators in the linkages between G-E interplay and developmental and health endpoints. Bush et al., for example, have recently shown that the BDNF Val66Met polymorphism confers an increased neuroendocrine sensitivity to socioeconomic context, with Met carriers having the highest and lowest cortisol expression levels, depending on SES (N. Bush, personal communication, unpublished data, 2017). Other findings in the nascent science of "imaging genomics"—a field merging high-throughput genotyping with new brain imaging technologies—are revealing how variations in DNA sequence are associated with structural and functional connectivity in specific brain regions (Thompson et al. 2010). Recent fMRI studies, for example, have demonstrated the heritability of patterns of task-related brain region activation and shown how the COMT val108/158met functional polymorphism is associated with systematic differences in prefrontal cortical physiology and function (Egan et al. 2001). Consistent with the same general hypothesis, Hariri and colleagues (Hariri et al. 2005; Hariri and Weinberger 2003) have found that subjects carrying the less efficient short allele of the 5-HTT gene promoter had an increased amygdalar response to fearful stimuli in comparison with subjects homozygous for the long allele. Even more to the point in regard to the development of brain structures subserving socioemotional development, Alexander et al. (Alexander et al. 2012) recently reported a significant GxE interaction effect on neural response patterns and functional amygdala-hypothalamus connectivity—circuitry that appears closely tied to emotional control and the interpretation of social processes (Blakemore 2010; Norman et al. 2012). Such findings begin to reveal possible neural substrates for previously observed, epidemiological observations linking functional polymorphisms, early stressful events, and vulnerability to psychopathology (Caspi et al. 2003; Moffitt et al. 2005).

Also coming into view through the work of a range of investigators (Adolphs 2009; Blakemore 2010, 2012; Lesch 2007; Norman et al. 2012; Robinson et al. 2005, 2008) is a new corpus of research describing and exploring the *social brain*. Such work has begun to address a neurogenomic basis for complex social cognitions, including the capacities for inferences about others' thoughts and emotions (a cognitive ability referred to in the child development literature as "theory of mind"), recognition of self, processing of facial information, differentiation of social opportunities and challenges, and control of socially evoked emotion. The substrates for these capacities are already known to lie, at the neural circuit level, in functional connectivity between limbic structures, such as the amygdala, hippocampus, and basal ganglia, and prefrontal cortical regions, including the dorsolateral and orbitofrontal cortex, the anterior cingulate and the posterior superior temporal sulcus at the temporoparietal junction. At the molecular level, there is evidence for perturbations in the functionality of such circuits related to allelic and epigenetic variation in genes such as those coding for the serotonin transporter (Lesch 2007), oxytocin (Norman et al. 2012), and endorphins (Keverne et al. 1989). There is to date no single definition of the social brain, but a consensus appears to be forming that a subset of autonomic, neuroendocrine, neural, and genomic processes influence and are influenced by aspects of social cognition and behavior (see Robinson et al. 2005, 2008). Although it will be important to avoid a simplistic attribution of complex cognitive and perceptual events to discrete neural, endocrine, or cellular structures (Norman et al. 2012), there is clearly much to be learned about the nature of sociality, the mechanisms that underpin it, the degree to which these mechanisms are conserved in animal phylogeny, and the implications of perturbations in its development.

In sum, a burgeoning research enterprise is producing evidence, in both animal models and human studies, that many if not most human morbidities have their points of origin in early childhood (Shonkoff and Garner 2012), are the products of gene-environment interplay (Rutter 2006), and influence developing neural circuits that are directly linked to long-term trajectories of health, disease, and life achievement. Although the fields of social epigenetics and developmental neuroscience are yet in their relative infancies, promising advances in both suggest a scientific frontier in which functional interactions among social environments, genetic and epigenetic variation, and the functionality of neural circuits will offer compelling new knowledge of how developmental variation emerges.

6 Summary: What We Know and What We Don't

Deep cultural traditions affirming the special sensibilities of children and the echoing of childhood difficulties and stress into the decades of adult life are becoming now powerfully grounded in a new science describing the biological embedding of early social adversity (Boivin and Hertzman 2012; Boyce et al. 2012a; Hertzman and Boyce 2010). No longer relegated to categories of either unsupported belief or speculative hypothesis, the science of early child development has become a multidisciplinary landscape of novel findings documenting prospective, longitudinal associations, powerful and increasingly causal understandings of mechanism and mediation, and new levels of observation made possible by dramatic technological advances. Among the discrete, foundational discoveries that have become the products of this science are the following:

1. Epidemiologic and population-based studies have soundly documented the propensity for morbidities and difficulties of all kinds—biomedical diseases, psychiatric disorders, injuries, and academic, professional, and personal underachievement—to aggregate by population, space, and time, thereby disproportionately affecting small subgroups of individuals, during constrained periods of historical or developmental time. Thus, especially during periods of strife, war, or economic decline, those people whose health and well-being are most harshly and persistently vulnerable are likely to issue from impoverished, alienated, or otherwise marginalized groups. Misfortune is neither stochastically nor evenly distributed within human populations, and the inequalities that ensue from maldistribution are serious, ethical, and public health challenges to society's commitments to justice and health equity. Our societal aspirations to create a more "empathic civilization" (Rifkin 2009) will demand a more human practice of medicine (Halpern 2001), a broader allegiance to unbiased opportunity (Robert Wood Johnson Foundation Commission to Build a Healthier America 2009), and a deeper commitment to the rich pluripotentiality of young lives (Shonkoff and Phillips 2000).
2. Studies examining the developmental biology of social adversity have positioned this new

science on the cusp of deep mechanistic explanations for the important, earlier insights of Waddington (Waddington 1959, 2012), Gottlieb (Gottlieb 1991), and others (Gilbert 2002; Karmiloff-Smith 2007; Meaney 2010)—insight that organismic development is guided by the *combined, interactive influences of genes and experiences*. We now know that development includes not only gene expression regulation through experiential modification of chromatin structure but also by real GxE interactions and the joint, interactive effects of allelic variation and chromatin modification together (see, e.g., Lam et al. 2012; Pezawas et al. 2005; Rutter 2012). As asserted here and elsewhere, the simple partitioning of developmental variance into genetic and environmentally determined components now falls far short of a truly interactive view of the operation of nature and nurture (Meaney 2010). Coming now steadily into view are the actual molecular mechanisms by which constitution and context conjointly determine differences in health and development, both in childhood and over the lifespan.

3. The origins, dimensions, and consequences of *individual differences in phenotype* are emerging as essential components in a full understanding of the biology of social adversity. Biology is replete with both between- and within-species variation that bears convincing witness to the evolutionary uses of diversity, and elegant ethological and epigenetic work, such as that by Meaney (Meaney 2010), Szyf (McGowan and Szyf 2010), and Suomi (Suomi 2006), reveals the adaptive benefits of phenotypic diversification. There is the nearly tautological reality that the operation of natural selection demands the genetic diversity achieved through spontaneous mutation, but beyond such self-evident principles, there are clear examples of how species diversification enhances survival and fitness. Thus, maternally and epigenetically regulated differentiation of rat pups' adrenocortical responsivity produces a range of low to high reactivity phenotypes, each of which may maximize survival and fitness within particular, early and later life environments (Weaver et al. 2004). Similarly, neither the aggressively uninhibited nor the shy, neophobic phenotypes of young rhesus macaques can be warranted as "normal" or optimal; rather, each has adaptive value within specific social and physical contexts (Cirulli et al. 2009; Stevens et al. 2009). What is salient and important about phenotypic variants is their capacity for enhancing fitness within the diversity of species-typical environments encountered. One illustrative variant are those children and young nonhuman primates that evince an exceptional neurobiological susceptibility to aspects of social settings, a phenotype likely representing a conditional adaptation to early environmental signals (Barr et al. 2004; Belsky 2005; Boyce and Ellis 2005; Ellis et al. 2011a). Such individuals show a heightened risk of morbidity under conditions of stress and adversity but exceptionally good health and positive development in settings characterized by support, nurturance, and stability.
4. Increasingly visible within the emerging literature on the neurobiological consequences of early life adversity is a new collection of studies and papers examining the *social brain* (Adolphs 2009; Blakemore 2010, 2012; Lesch 2007; Norman et al. 2012; Robinson et al. 2005, 2008). The brain has evolved to acquire specific organizational circuits, cortical regions, and subcortical structures dedicated to the detection of survival threats, and social experiences of loneliness, abandonment, or neglect may chronically activate such circuitry, creating long-term perceptual and affective biases and fundamentally altering a child's view of the social world (Eisenberger and Cole 2012). Such circuitry is also represented in the periphery, with both animal (Insel 2010) and human (Norman et al. 2012) studies documenting effects on social affiliative processes mediated in part by hormonal events such as the expression of oxytocin and vasopressin.
5. As also discussed, a remarkable diversity of early, *social environmental dimensions* has been linked to important differences in mental

and physical health, trajectories of development, and individual differences in behavior. Such dimensions include, but are not limited to, acute and chronic stressors, poverty and subjective social marginalization, and the absence of positive contextual factors, such as good parenting or a child-supportive community. Of apparently particular importance to social epidemiologic perspectives on early development are studies describing and documenting the effects of social hierarchies, structural subordination, bullying, discrimination, and victimization. The hierarchical and networked social structures found across phylogeny—literally from fruit flies (fish and primates) to human kindergartners (see Boyce et al. 2012a; Fernald and Maruska 2012; Schneider et al. 2012)—suggest an evolved predisposition with implications for survival, reproduction, and safety. Although such hierarchies may be a heritable legacy from our evolutionary past, promising new work addresses approaches to minimizing the health effects of subordinate social positions at the levels of societies, communities, and schools. Such work also attests to the individual and societal benefits of fostering the development of empathy, altruism, and sociality.

6. The central role of *time*—evolutionary, historical, developmental, neurogenomic, and neurophysiological—in determining phenotypic variation is another recurrent if often implicit theme in emerging developmental science. Much of the biological embedding of current social contexts reflects response predispositions established, selectively and epigenetically, through adaptations to the temporally distant environments of early hominids (Dubos 1965; Nesse and Young 2000). Social disparities in health—products, in part, of the social, economic, and health policies of contemporary societies—wax and wane within historical time according to the era's dominant sociopolitical philosophies (Beckfield and Krieger 2009; Krieger 2001). Further, developmental time is strikingly uneven in its potency, intensity of change, and accessibility to environmental influence. Thus, at quite different levels of temporal resolution, time and timing appear to play crucial, but not yet fully explored, roles in guiding societal, organismic, and neurobiological responses to the conditions of early life.

Taken together, these points of emerging empirical evidence form a constellation of discoveries defining a new and lively research field and the social and developmental biology of early adversity and its influences on life course development and health. Although substantial recent progress has been made within a broad assortment of disciplines, much new research, conceptual integration, and thought remains to be accomplished. The promise of this new field, however, lies in a stunning prospect that understanding the social determinants of morbidities in childhood might unlock new approaches to the prevention and treatment of disorders over the entire life course. A final agenda for future research now outlines a set of proposals for new, promising, and possibly heuristic directions of investigation.

7 An Agenda for Future Research

1. As the fields reporting various forms of interplay between genes and environments exponentially grow, what is now needed are programs of research examining the questions of how and by what mechanisms genes and early social contexts co-determine trajectories of behavioral and biological development. With respect to differences in complex behavior and its disorders, a focus on proximal, neurobiological processes must come strongly to the foreground. Although pursuing the epigenetic pathogenesis of early psychiatric and other disorders is a powerful first step (Docherty and Mill 2008; Robison and Nestler 2011), it must be followed by studies examining the brain structures and neural processes that mediate GxE associations with mental and physical health (Ladd-Acosta et al. 2007; Turecki et al. 2012). As new knowledge of the

interactive genetic and environmental influences on social brain development becomes available, a major challenge will be the integration of mechanistic observations across levels of analysis and scale (Norman et al. 2012).

2. A systematic and useful biology of social adversity will necessarily involve not only a search for the mechanisms (i.e., mediators) underpinning associations among stress, development, and morbidity but also the effects of modifiers (i.e., moderators) that reveal when, at what ages, or in what subgroups such associations hold (Baron and Kenny 1986; Kraemer et al. 2001, 2008). Understanding the mechanistic processes by which an environmental exposure is linked to disordered development can be a powerful aid to elucidating pathogenesis (e.g., the role of high-density lipoprotein transport of cholesterol as a mediator of the association between dietary fat and coronary heart disease (Lloyd et al. 2012)) and imagining novel interventions (e.g., changing mother-infant relationships as a means of altering the association between poverty and child development (Olds et al. 2010)). On the other hand, grasping mediational linkages may be a necessary but insufficient condition for understanding causation, and the parsing of populations into subgroups of varying exposure susceptibility, through the discovery of moderator variables, can also advance comprehension and the tractability of a given association (e.g., changes in the potency of stress-illness associations by differences in individual sensitivity to social contextual effects (Belsky and Pluess 2009; Boyce and Ellis 2005; Ellis et al. 2011a)).
3. As attention to epigenetic development grows, the capacity to place a finer, more exacting point on the specific kinds of environments that interact with particular allelic and epigenetic variants will be important and likely illuminating. Evolutionary perspectives on social adversity will also be essential to understand how difficult "environments of evolutionary adaptedness" shaped human and infra-human biology (e.g., Boyce and Ellis 2005; Sapolsky 2003), how contextual stressors might have generated species diversity (Wolf et al. 2005), and how adversity may have contributed to the emergence of social cooperation (Andras et al. 2007). We need far finer and more precise renditions of the social-environmental dimensions that interact with genes and produce negative and positive outcomes salient to population and public health. An important subtext to such work is the extraordinary value of cross-species, animal-human, comparative studies, which together not only inform the evolutionary biology of social environments and its consequences but also enable experimental studies capable of bolstering the causal inferences disallowed by human research.
4. Successfully pursuing a new developmental science of childhood adversity will surely also involve the perspective of complex adaptive systems. Social causation is nonlinear, rather than Newtonian, in character. Traditional epidemiologic strategies for understanding the health effects of social-environmental factors involve the ascertainment of such factors' "independent" influences on a health endpoint through the use of multiple hierarchical regression models (Diez Roux 2007). Although such an approach allows estimation of the isolated effects of single independent variables, it belies the reality that most human disorders are etiologically complex, with multiple interacting "causes." Even detecting GxE interactions almost certainly underserves the true complexity of pathogenic processes, because allelic variation in a single gene likely interacts with polymorphisms in many other genes, and multiple dimensions of the environment may also interactively influence outcomes. In such circumstances—circumstances that may eventually prove to predominate in disease causation—the use of more sophisticated models and analytic tools may be required to understand the multiply interactive networks of risk factors involved in the ontogeny of disordered development and health (Kauffman 1993; Koopman and Lynch 1999). If so, one such approach with increasingly demonstrable efficacy is the use of complex

systems analysis, involving descriptive inventories of system components, nonlinear mathematical modeling, and the construction of agent-based models of causal networks (Diez Roux 2007; Galea et al. 2010).

5. Finally, as highlighted by Garner, Shonkoff, and others (Garner et al. 2012; Shonkoff 2012), prevention science is powerfully in need of new ideas for and approaches to the design of interventions based on the emerging science of early development. The Nurse-Family Partnership program conceived and elegantly studied by David Olds and colleagues (see http://www.nursefamilypartnership.org), for example, departed dramatically from prior, outmoded early childhood enrichment programs by envisioning the mother-infant dyad as the unit of intervention and by using nurses as home visitors to effectively place the intervention within a medical frame of reference. Nonetheless, even more radical departures are needed from the conventions of traditional early development programs, including careful consideration of how complex dynamic systems thinking might be wed to novel, preventive interventions. Attending closely to discoveries emanating from the disciplines and sciences surveyed here could potentially prompt approaches to targeting and conceiving imaginative interventions with far greater efficacy and whole population effects. However complex and challenging that task might be, all such efforts could be potentially rewarded with a level of health and well-being for our children and grandchildren that is more enduring, robust, and enabling.

The new developmental biology of early life effects on health development over the life course is a now flourishing science, nearing readiness to transform conventional understandings of disease ontogeny, to foster clearer and more vivid perspectives on the temporally distant effects of childhood events, and to broaden and transform approaches to ensuring the health of our children and the developmental sturdiness of their futures. Although much careful and innovative thought will be a prerequisite for such a demanding journey, the road ahead looks promising, indeed.

References

Abbott, D. H., Keverne, E. B., Bercovitch, F. B., Shively, C. A., Mendoza, S. P., Saltzman, W., et al. (2003). Are subordinates always stressed? A comparative analysis of rank differences in cortisol levels among primates. *Hormones and Behavior, 43*(1), 67–82.

Adler, N. E., Boyce, W. T., Chesney, M. A., Folkman, S., & Syme, S. L. (1993). Socioeconomic inequalities in health: No easy solution. *JAMA, 269*(24), 3140–3145.

Adler, N. E., Boyce, W. T., Chesney, M. A., Cohen, S., Folkman, S., Kahn, R. L., & Syme, S. L. (1994). Socioeconomic status and health: The challenge of the gradient. *The American Psychologist, 49*(1), 15–24.

Adler, N. E., Epel, E. S., Castellazzo, G., & Ickovics, J. R. (2000). Relationship of subjective and objective social status with psychological and physiological functioning: Preliminary data in healthy, White women. *Health Psychology, 19*(6), 586–592.

Adolphs, R. (2009). The social brain: Neural basis of social knowledge. *Annual Review of Psychology, 60*, 693–716. doi:10.1146/annurev.psych.60.110707.163514.

Alexander, N., Klucken, T., Koppe, G., Osinsky, R., Walter, B., Vaitl, D., et al. (2012). Interaction of the serotonin transporter-linked polymorphic region and environmental adversity: Increased amygdala-hypothalamus connectivity as a potential mechanism linking neural and endocrine hyperreactivity. *Biological Psychiatry, 72*(1), 49–56. doi:10.1016/j.biopsych.2012.01.030.

Alkon, A., Lippert, S., Vujan, N., Rodriquez, M. E., Boyce, W. T., & Eskenazi, B. (2006). The ontogeny of autonomic measures in 6- and 12-month-old infants. *Developmental Psychobiology, 48*(3), 197–208. doi:10.1002/dev.20129.

Andras, P., Lazarus, J., & Roberts, G. (2007). Environmental adversity and uncertainty favour cooperation. *BMC Evolutionary Biology, 7*, 240. doi:10.1186/1471-2148-7-240.

Ariès, P. (1962). *Centuries of childhood: A social history of family life*. New York: Alfred A. Knopf.

Aron, E. N., Aron, A., & Jagiellowicz, J. (2012). Sensory processing sensitivity: A review in the light of the evolution of biological responsivity. *Personality and Social Psychology Review, 16*(3), 262–282. doi:10.1177/1088868311434213.

Arseneault, L., Walsh, E., Trzesniewski, K., Newcombe, R., Caspi, A., & Moffitt, T. E. (2006). Bullying victimization uniquely contributes to adjustment problems in young children: A nationally representative cohort study. *Pediatrics, 118*(1), 130–138. doi:10.1542/peds.2005-2388.

Bagot, R. C., & Meaney, M. J. (2010). Epigenetics and the biological basis of gene x environment interactions. *Journal of the American Academy of Child and Adolescent Psychiatry, 49*(8), 752–771. doi:10.1016/j.jaac.2010.06.001.

Bakermans-Kranenburg, M. J., & Van Ijzendoorn, M. H. (2015). The hidden efficacy of interventions: Genexenvironment experiments from a differential susceptibility perspective. *Annual*

Review of Psychology, 66, 381–409. doi:10.1146/annurev-psych-010814-015407.

Bakermans-Kranenburg, M. J., Van Ijzendoorn, M. H., Mesman, J., Alink, L. R., & Juffer, F. (2008a). Effects of an attachment-based intervention on daily cortisol moderated by dopamine receptor D4: A randomized control trial on 1- to 3-year-olds screened for externalizing behavior. *Development and Psychopathology, 20*(3), 805–820. doi:10.1017/S0954579408000382.

Bakermans-Kranenburg, M. J., Van Ijzendoorn, M. H., Pijlman, F. T., Mesman, J., & Juffer, F. (2008b). Experimental evidence for differential susceptibility: Dopamine D4 receptor polymorphism (DRD4 VNTR) moderates intervention effects on toddlers' externalizing behavior in a randomized controlled trial. *Developmental Psychology, 44*(1), 293–300. doi:10.1037/0012-1649.44.1.293.

Barker, D. J. (1990). The fetal and infant origins of adult disease. *BMJ, 301*(6761), 1111.

Barker, D. J., & Bagby, S. P. (2005). Developmental antecedents of cardiovascular disease: A historical perspective. *Journal of the American Society of Nephrology, 16*(9), 2537–2544. doi:10.1681/ASN.2005020160.

Baron, R., & Kenny, D. (1986). The moderator-mediator variable distinction in social psychological research: Conceptual, strategic, and statistical considerations. *Journal of Personality and Social Psychology, 51*(6), 1173–1182.

Barr, R. G., Konner, M., Bakeman, R., & Adamson, L. (1991). Crying in !Kung San infants: A test of the cultural specificity hypothesis. *Developmental Medicine and Child Neurology, 33*(7), 601–610.

Barr, C. S., Newman, T. K., Lindell, S., Shannon, C., Champoux, M., Lesch, K. P., et al. (2004). Interaction between serotonin transporter gene variation and rearing condition in alcohol preference and consumption in female primates. *Archives of General Psychiatry, 61*(11), 1146–1152.

Bateson, P., & Gluckman, P. (2011). *Plasticity, robustness, development and evolution*. Cambridge CB2 8RU, UK: Cambridge University Press, The Edinburgh Building.

Bavelier, D., Levi, D. M., Li, R. W., Dan, Y., & Hensch, T. K. (2010). Removing brakes on adult brain plasticity: From molecular to behavioral interventions. *The Journal of Neuroscience, 30*(45), 14964–14971.

Beckfield, J., & Krieger, N. (2009). Epi + demos + cracy: Linking political systems and priorities to the magnitude of health inequities--evidence, gaps, and a research agenda. *Epidemiologic Reviews, 31*, 152–177. doi:10.1093/epirev/mxp002.

Belsky, J. (2005). Differential susceptibility to rearing influence: An evolutionary hypothesis and some evidence. In B. J. Ellis & D. F. Bjorklund (Eds.), *Origins of the social mind: Evolutionary psychology and child development* (pp. 139–163). New York: Guilford.

Belsky, J., & Pluess, M. (2009). Beyond diathesis stress: Differential susceptibility to environmental influences. *Psychological Bulletin, 135*(6), 885–908. doi:10.1037/a0017376.

Belsky, J., Bakermans Kranenburg, M. J., & Van IJzendoorn, M. H. (2007). For better and for worse: Differential susceptibility to environmental influences. *Current Directions in Psychological Science, 16*(6), 300–304.

Blakemore, S. J. (2010). The developing social brain: Implications for education. *Neuron, 65*(6), 744–747. doi:10.1016/j.neuron.2010.03.004.

Blakemore, S. J. (2012). Development of the social brain in adolescence. *Journal of the Royal Society of Medicine, 105*(3), 111–116. doi:10.1258/jrsm.2011.110221.

Blumenshine, P., Egerter, S., Barclay, C. J., Cubbin, C., & Braveman, P. A. (2010). Socioeconomic disparities in adverse birth outcomes: A systematic review. *American Journal of Preventive Medicine, 39*(3), 263–272. doi:10.1016/j.amepre.2010.05.012.

Bock, G. R., & Whelan, J. (Eds.). (1991). *The childhood environment and adult disease*. West Sussez: Ciba Foundation.

Boivin, M., & Hertzman, C. (2012). *Early childhood development: Adverse experiences and developmental health*. Ottawa: Royal Society of Canada.

Borghol, N., Suderman, M., McArdle, W., Racine, A., Hallett, M., Pembrey, M., et al. (2012). Associations with early life socio-economic position in adult DNA methylation. *International Journal of Epidemiology, 41*(1), 62–74.

Bowlby, J. (1969). *Attachment and loss*. London: Hogarth.

Boyce, W. T. (1985). Stress and child health: An overview. *Pediatric Annals, 14*(8), 539–542.

Boyce, W. T. (2016). Differential susceptibility of the developing brain to contextual adversity and stress. *Neuropsychopharmacology Reviews, 41*(1), 142–162.

Boyce, W. T., & Ellis, B. J. (2005). Biological sensitivity to context: I. An evolutionary-developmental theory of the origins and functions of stress reactivity. *Development and Psychopathology, 17*(2), 271–301.

Boyce, W. T., & Kobor, M. S. (2015). Development and the epigenome: The 'synapse' of gene-environment interplay. *Developmental Science, 18*(1), 1–23. doi:10.1111/desc.12282.

Boyce, W. T., Chesney, M., Alkon-Leonard, A., Tschann, J., Adams, S., Chesterman, B., et al. (1995). Psychobiologic reactivity to stress and childhood respiratory illnesses: Results of two prospective studies. *Psychosomatic Medicine, 57*, 411–422.

Boyce, W. T., O'Neill-Wagner, P., Price, C. S., Haines, M., & Suomi, S. J. (1998). Crowding stress and violent injuriesamong behaviorally inhibited rhesus macaques. *Health Psychology, 17*(3), 285–289.

Boyce, W. T., Den Besten, P. K., Stamperdahl, J., Zhan, L., Jiang, Y., Adler, N. E., & Featherstone, J. D. (2010). Social inequalities in childhood dental caries: The convergent roles of stress, bacteria and disadvantage. *Social Science & Medicine, 71*(9), 1644–1652. doi:10.1016/j.socscimed.2010.07.045.

Boyce, W. T., Obradović, J., Bush, N., Stamperdahl, J., Kim, Y. S., & Adler, N. (2012a). Social stratification, classroom 'climate' and the behavioral adaptation of kindergarten children. *Proceedings of the National Academy of Sciences, 109*(Suppl 2), 17168–17173.

Boyce, W. T., Sokolowski, M. B., & Robinson, G. E. (2012b). Toward a new biology of social adversity. *Proceedings of the National Academy of Sciences of the United States of America, 109*(Suppl 2), 17143–17148. doi:10.1073/pnas.1121264109.

Brim, O. G., & Kagan, J. (Eds.). (1980). *Constancy and change in human development*. Cambridge, MA: Harvard University Press.

Bronfenbrenner, U., & Morris, P. A. (2006). The bioecological model of human development. In R. M. Lerner & W. Damon (Eds.), *Handbook of child psychology: Vol. 1. Theoretical models of human development* (6th ed., pp. 793–828). Hoboken: John Wiley & Sons, Inc.

Brown, R. L. (2010). Epidemiology of injury and the impact of health disparities. *Current Opinion in Pediatrics, 22*(3), 321–325. doi:10.1097/MOP.0b013e3283395f13.

Brown, D. W., Anda, R. F., Tiemeier, H., Felitti, V. J., Edwards, V. J., Croft, J. B., & Giles, W. H. (2009). Adverse childhood experiences and the risk of premature mortality. *American Journal of Preventive Medicine, 37*(5), 389–396. doi:10.1016/j.amepre.2009.06.021.

Carpiano, R. M., Lloyd, J. E., & Hertzman, C. (2009). Concentrated affluence, concentrated disadvantage, and children's readiness for school: A population-based, multi-level investigation. *Social Science & Medicine, 69*(3), 420–432. doi:10.1016/j.socscimed.2009.05.028.

Caspi, A., McClay, J., Moffitt, T. E., Mill, J., Martin, J., Craig, I. W., et al. (2002). Role of genotype in the cycle of violence in maltreated children. *Science, 297*(5582), 851–854.

Caspi, A., Sugden, K., Moffitt, T. E., Taylor, A., Craig, I. W., Harrington, H., et al. (2003). Influence of life stress on depression: Moderation by a polymorphism in the 5-HTT gene. *Science, 301*(5631), 386–389.

Champagne, F. A., Weaver, I. C., Diorio, J., Dymov, S., Szyf, M., & Meaney, M. J. (2006). Maternal care associated with methylation of the estrogen receptor-alpha1b promoter and estrogen receptor-alpha expression in the medial preoptic area of female offspring. *Endocrinology, 147*(6), 2909–2915. doi:10.1210/en.2005-1119.

Chedgzoy, K., Greenhalgh, S., & Shaughnessy, R. (2007). *Shakespeare and childhood*. Cambridge, UK: Cambridge University Press.

Chen, E., Miller, G. E., Kobor, M. S., & Cole, S. W. (2011). Maternal warmth buffers the effects of low early-life socioeconomic status on pro-inflammatory signaling in adulthood. *Molecular Psychiatry, 16*(7), 729–737. doi:10.1038/mp.2010.53.

Cirulli, F., Francia, N., Berry, A., Aloe, L., Alleva, E., & Suomi, S. J. (2009). Early life stress as a risk factor for mental health: Role of neurotrophins from rodents to non-human primates. *Neuroscience and Biobehavioral Reviews, 33*(4), 573–585. doi:10.1016/j.neubiorev.2008.09.001.

Cohen, S., Line, S., Manuck, S. B., Rabin, B. S., Heise, E. R., & Kaplan, J. R. (1997). Chronic social stress, social status, and susceptibility to upper respiratory infections in nonhuman primates [see comments]. *Psychosomatic Medicine, 59*(3), 213–221.

Cohen, S., Janicki-Deverts, D., Chen, E., & Matthews, K. A. (2010). Childhood socioeconomic status and adult health. *Annals of the New York Academy of Sciences, 1186*, 37–55. doi:10.1111/j.1749-6632.2009.05334.x.

Cole, S. W. (2009). Social regulation of human gene expression. *Current Directions in Psychological Science, 18*(3), 132–137. doi:10.1111/j.1467-8721.2009.01623.x.

Cole, S. W., Hawkley, L. C., Arevalo, J. M., Sung, C. Y., Rose, R. M., & Cacioppo, J. T. (2007). Social regulation of gene expression in human leukocytes. *Genome Biology, 8*(9), R189. doi:10.1186/gb-2007-8-9-r189.

Committee on a Framework for Development a New Taxonomy of Disease. (2011). *Toward precision medicine: Building a knowledge network for biomedical research and a new taxonomy of disease*. Washington, DC: National Academies Press.

Cummings, E. M., El-Sheikh, M., Kouros, C. D., & Keller, P. S. (2007). Children's skin conductance reactivity as a mechanism of risk in the context of parental depressive symptoms. *Journal of Child Psychology and Psychiatry, 48*(5), 436–445. doi:10.1111/j.1469-7610.2006.01713.x.

Cupello, A., Albano, C., Gatta, E., Scarrone, S., Villa, E., & Zona, G. (2009). Binding of paroxetine to the serotonin transporter in membranes from different cells, subcellular fractions and species. *Neurochemical Research, 34*(2), 255–259. doi:10.1007/s11064-008-9764-z.

Curley, J. P., Jensen, C. L., Mashoodh, R., & Champagne, F. A. (2011). Social influences on neurobiology and behavior: Epigenetic effects during development. *Psychoneuroendocrinology, 36*(3), 352–371. doi:10.1016/j.psyneuen.2010.06.005.

Cushing, B. S., & Kramer, K. M. (2005). Mechanisms underlying epigenetic effects of early social experience: The role of neuropeptides and steroids. *Neuroscience and Biobehavioral Reviews, 29*(7), 1089–1105. doi:10.1016/j.neubiorev.2005.04.001.

Dancause, K. N., Laplante, D. P., Fraser, S., Brunet, A., Ciampi, A., Schmitz, N., & King, S. (2012). Prenatal exposure to a natural disaster increases risk for obesity in 5(1/2)-year-old children. *Pediatric Research, 71*(1), 126–131. doi:10.1038/pr.2011.18.

Danese, A., Moffitt, T. E., Pariante, C. M., Ambler, A., Poulton, R., & Caspi, A. (2008). Elevated inflammation levels in depressed adults with a history of childhood maltreatment. *Archives of General Psychiatry, 65*(4), 409–416.

de Quervain, D. J., Kolassa, I. T., Ackermann, S., Aerni, A., Boesiger, P., Demougin, P., et al. (2012). PKCalpha is genetically linked to memory capacity in healthy subjects and to risk for posttraumatic stress disorder in genocide survivors. *Proceedings of the National Academy of Sciences of the United States of America, 109*(22), 8746–8751. doi:10.1073/pnas.1200857109.

Diamond, J. (2012). *The world until yesterday: What can we learn from traditional societies*. New York: Penguin Group.

Diaz, C., Starfield, B., Holtzman, N., Mellits, E. D., Hankin, J., Smalky, K., & Benson, P. (1986). Ill health and use of medical care: Community-based assessment of morbidity in children. *Medical Care, 24*(9), 848–856.

Diez Roux, A. V. (2007). Integrating social and biologic factors in health research: A systems view. *Annals of Epidemiology, 17*(7), 569–574. doi:10.1016/j.annepidem.2007.03.001.

Docherty, S., & Mill, J. (2008). Epigenetic mechanisms as mediators of environmental risks for psychiatric disorders. *Psychiatry, 7*(12), 500–506.

Dowd, J. B., Zajacova, A., & Aiello, A. (2009). Early origins of health disparities: Burden of infection, health, and socioeconomic status in U.S. children. *Social Science & Medicine, 68*(4), 699–707. doi:10.1016/j.socscimed.2008.12.010.

Dubos, R. J. (1965). *Man adapting*. New Haven: Yale University Press.

Dubos, R., Savage, D., & Schaedler, R. (1966). Biological freudianism. Lasting effects of early environmental influences. *Pediatrics, 38*(5), 789–800.

Dunn, E. C., Uddin, M., Subramanian, S. V., Smoller, J. W., Galea, S., & Koenen, K. C. (2011). Research review: Gene-environment interaction research in youth depression – a systematic review with recommendations for future research. *Journal of Child Psychology and Psychiatry, 52*(12), 1223–1238. doi:10.1111/j.1469-7610.2011.02466.x.

Egan, S. K., & Perry, D. G. (1998). Does low self-regard invite victimization? *Developmental Psychology, 34*(2), 299–309.

Egan, M. F., Goldberg, T. E., Kolachana, B. S., Callicott, J. H., Mazzanti, C. M., Straub, R. E., et al. (2001). Effect of COMT Val108/158 Met genotype on frontal lobe function and risk for schizophrenia. *Proceedings of the National Academy of Sciences of the United States of America, 98*(12), 6917–6922. doi:10.1073/pnas.111134598.

Eisenberger, N. I., & Cole, S. W. (2012). Social neuroscience and health: Neurophysiological mechanisms linking social ties with physical health. *Nature Neuroscience, 15*(5), 669–674. doi:10.1038/nn.3086.

Ellis, B. J., McFadyen-Ketchum, S., Dodge, K. A., Pettit, G. S., & Bates, J. E. (1999). Quality of early family relationships and individual differences in the timing of pubertal maturation in girls: A longitudinal test of an evolutionary model. *Journal of Personality and Social Psychology, 77*(2), 387–401.

Ellis, B. J., Jackson, J. J., & Boyce, W. T. (2006). The stress response systems: Universality and adaptive individual differences. *Developmental Review, 26*(2), 175–212.

Ellis, B. J., Boyce, W. T., Belsky, J., Bakermans-Kranenburg, M. J., & van Ijzendoorn, M. H. (2011a). Differential susceptibility to the environment: An evolutionary--neurodevelopmental theory. *Development and Psychopathology, 23*(1), 7–28. doi:10.1017/S0954579410000611.

Ellis, B. J., Shirtcliff, E. A., Boyce, W. T., Deardorff, J., & Essex, M. J. (2011b). Quality of early family relationships and the timing and tempo of puberty: Effects depend on biological sensitivity to context. *Development and Psychopathology, 23*(1), 85–99. doi:10.1017/S0954579410000660.

El-Sheikh, M. (2005). Stability of respiratory sinus arrhythmia in children and young adolescents: A longitudinal examination. *Developmental Psychobiology, 46*(1), 66–74. doi:10.1002/dev.20036.

El-Sheikh, M., Keller, P. S., & Erath, S. A. (2007). Marital conflict and risk for child maladjustment over time: Skin conductance level reactivity as a vulnerability factor. *Journal of Abnormal Child Psychology, 35*(5), 715–727. doi:10.1007/s10802-007-9127-2.

Essex, M. J., Thomas Boyce, W., Hertzman, C., Lam, L. L., Armstrong, J. M., Neumann, S. M., & Kobor, M. S. (2013). Epigenetic vestiges of early developmental adversity: Childhood stress exposure and DNA methylation in adolescence. *Child Development, 84*(1), 58–75. doi:10.1111/j.1467-8624.2011.01641.x.

Evans, G. W. (2004). The environment of childhood poverty. *The American Psychologist, 59*(2), 77–92.

Evans, G. W., & Kim, P. (2007). Childhood poverty and health: Cumulative risk exposure and stress dysregulation. *Psychological Science, 18*(11), 953–957. doi:10.1111/j.1467-9280.2007.02008.x.

Evans, G. W., Gonnella, C., Marcynyszyn, L. A., Gentile, L., & Salpekar, N. (2005). The role of chaos in poverty and children's socioemotional adjustment. *Psychological Science, 16*(7), 560–565.

Evans, G. W., Chen, E., Miller, G., & Seeman, T. (2012). How poverty gets under the skin: A life-course perspective. In V. Maholmes & R. B. King (Eds.), *The Oxford handbook of poverty and child development* (pp. 13–36). Oxford: Oxford University Press.

Falconi, A. M., Catalano, R., & Boyce, W. T. (2017). Early life predictors of late life health. In W. Satariano & M. Maus (Eds.), *Aging, Place, and Health: A Global Perspective*. Burlington: Jones & Bartlett Learning.

Fehr, E., Bernhard, H., & Rockenbach, B. (2008). Egalitarianism in young children. *Nature, 454*(7208), 1079–1083. doi:10.1038/nature07155.

Fernald, R. D., & Maruska, K. P. (2012). How does social information change the brain? PNAS.

Fraga, M. F., Ballestar, E., Paz, M. F., Ropero, S., Setien, F., Ballestar, M. L., et al. (2005). Epigenetic differences arise during the lifetime of monozygotic twins. *Proceedings of the National Academy of Sciences of the United States of America, 102*(30), 10604–10609.

Freud, S. (1940). An outline of psychoanalysis. In J. Strachey (Ed.), *The standard edition of the complete psychological works of Sigmund Freud* (Vol. 23). London: Hogarth Press.

Galea, S., Riddle, M., & Kaplan, G. A. (2010). Causal thinking and complex system approaches in epidemiology. *International Journal of Epidemiology, 39*(1), 97–106.

Galobardes, B., Lynch, J. W., & Davey Smith, G. (2004). Childhood socioeconomic circumstances and cause-specific mortality in adulthood: Systematic review and interpretation. *Epidemiologic Reviews, 26*, 7–21.

Garner, A. S., Shonkoff, J. P., Siegel, B. S., Dobbins, M. I., Earls, M. F., Garner, A. S., et al. (2012). Early childhood adversity, toxic stress, and the role of the pediatrician: Translating developmental science into lifelong health. *Pediatrics, 129*(1), e224–e231. doi:10.1542/peds.2011-2662.

Gianaros, P. J., & Manuck, S. B. (2010). Neurobiological pathways linking socioeconomic position and health. *Psychosomatic Medicine, 72*(5), 450–461. doi:10.1097/PSY.0b013e3181e1a23c.

Gilbert, S. F. (2002). The genome in its ecological context: Philosophical perspectives on interspecies epigenesis. *Annals of the New York Academy of Sciences, 981*, 202–218.

Gilbert, S. F., & Epel, D. (2009). *Ecological developmental biology: Integrating epigenetics, medicine, and evolution*. Sunderland: Sinauer Associates.

Gini, G., & Pozzoli, T. (2009). Association between bullying and psychosomatic problems: A meta-analysis. *Pediatrics, 123*(3), 1059–1065. doi:10.1542/peds.2008-1215.

Glew, G. M., Fan, M. Y., Katon, W., Rivara, F. P., & Kernic, M. A. (2005). Bullying, psychosocial adjustment, and academic performance in elementary school. *Archives of Pediatrics & Adolescent Medicine, 159*(11), 1026–1031. doi:10.1001/archpedi.159.11.1026.

Gluckman, P. D., Hanson, M. A., & Pinal, C. (2005). The developmental origins of adult disease. *Maternal & Child Nutrition, 1*(3), 130–141.

Gluckman, P. D., Hanson, M. A., & Beedle, A. S. (2007). Non-genomic transgenerational inheritance of disease risk. *BioEssays, 29*(2), 145–154.

Gluckman, P. D., Hanson, M. A., Bateson, P., Beedle, A. S., Law, C. M., Bhutta, Z. A., et al. (2009). Towards a new developmental synthesis: Adaptive developmental plasticity and human disease. *Lancet, 373*(9675), 1654–1657. doi:10.1016/S0140-6736(09)60234-8.

Goodman, E., Adler, N. E., Daniels, S. R., Morrison, J. A., Slap, G. B., & Dolan, L. M. (2003). Impact of objective and subjective social status on obesity in a biracial cohort of adolescents. *Obesity Research, 11*(8), 1018–1026.

Gottlieb, G. (1991). Experiential canalization of behavioral development: Theory. *Developmental Psychology, 27*(1), 4–13.

Greenfield, E. A. (2010). Child abuse as a life-course social determinant of adult health. *Maturitas, 66*(1), 51–55. doi:10.1016/j.maturitas.2010.02.002.

Gump, B. B., Reihman, J., Stewart, P., Lonky, E., Darvill, T., & Matthews, K. A. (2007). Blood lead (Pb) levels: A potential environmental mechanism explaining the relation between socioeconomic status and cardiovascular reactivity in children. *Health Psychology, 26*(3), 296–304. doi:10.1037/0278-6133.26.3.296.

Hackman, D. A., & Farah, M. J. (2009). Socioeconomic status and the developing brain. *Trends in Cognitive Sciences, 13*(2), 65–73. doi:10.1016/j.tics.2008.11.003.

Hackman, D. A., Farah, M. J., & Meaney, M. J. (2010). Socioeconomic status and the brain: Mechanistic insights from human and animal research. *Nature Reviews Neuroscience, 11*(9), 651–659. doi:10.1038/nrn2897.

Halpern, J. (2001). *From detached concern to empathy: Humanizing medical practice*. New York: Oxford University Press.

Hane, A. A., & Fox, N. A. (2006). Ordinary variations in maternal caregiving influence human infants' stress reactivity. *Psychological Science, 17*(6), 550–556. doi:10.1111/j.1467-9280.2006.01742.x.

Hariri, A. R., & Weinberger, D. R. (2003). Imaging genomics. *British Medical Bulletin, 65*, 259–270.

Hariri, A. R., Drabant, E. M., Munoz, K. E., Kolachana, B. S., Mattay, V. S., Egan, M. F., & Weinberger, D. R. (2005). A susceptibility gene for affective disorders and the response of the human amygdala. *Archives of General Psychiatry, 62*(2), 146–152.

Harlow, H. F., Harlow, M. K., & Suomi, S. J. (1971). From thought to therapy: Lessons from a primate laboratory. *American Scientist, 59*(5), 538–549.

Hart, T., & Risley, T. R. (1995). *Meaningful differences in the everyday experience of young American children*. Baltimore, MD: Paul H. Brookes.

Hawley, P. H. (1999). The ontogenesis of social dominance: A strategy-based evolutionary perspective. *Developmental Review, 19*, 97–132.

Hazani, E., & Shasha, S. M. (2008). Effects of the Holocaust on the physical health of the offspring of survivors. *The Israel Medical Association Journal, 10*(4), 251–255.

Heijmans, B. T., Tobi, E. W., Stein, A. D., Putter, H., Blauw, G. J., Susser, E. S., et al. (2008). Persistent epigenetic differences associated with prenatal exposure to famine in humans. *Proceedings of the National Academy of Sciences of the United States of America, 105*(44), 17046–17049. doi:10.1073/pnas.0806560105.

Hensch, T. K. (2005). Critical period plasticity in local cortical circuits. *Nature Reviews. Neuroscience, 6*(11), 877–888. doi:10.1038/nrn1787.

Hertzman, C. (2010). Social geography of developmental health in the early years. *Healthcare Quarterly, 14*(1), 32–40.

Hertzman, C., & Boyce, W. T. (2010). How experience gets under the skin to create gradients in developmental health. *Annual Review of Public Health, 31*, 329–347. 323p following 347. doi:10.1146/annurev.publhealth.012809.103538.

Hillis, S. D., Anda, R. F., Dube, S. R., Felitti, V. J., Marchbanks, P. A., & Marks, J. S. (2004). The association between adverse childhood experiences and adolescent pregnancy, long-term psychosocial consequences, and fetal death. *Pediatrics, 113*(2), 320–327.

Houweling, T. A., & Kunst, A. E. (2010). Socio-economic inequalities in childhood mortality in low- and middle-income countries: A review of the international evidence. *British Medical Bulletin, 93*, 7–26. doi:10.1093/bmb/ldp048.

Hrdy, S. B. (1999). *Mother nature: Maternal instincts and how they shape the human species*. New York: Ballantine Books.

Insel, T. R. (2010). The challenge of translation in social neuroscience: A review of oxytocin, vasopressin, and affiliative behavior. *Neuron, 65*(6), 768–779. doi:10.1016/j.neuron.2010.03.005.

Isles, A. R., & Wilkinson, L. S. (2008). Epigenetics: What is it and why is it important to mental disease? *British Medical Bulletin, 85*, 35–45. doi:10.1093/bmb/ldn004.

Janus, M., & Offord, D. (2000). Reporting on readiness to learn at school in Canada. *Canadian Journal of Policy Research, 1*, 71–75.

Javidi, H., & Yadollahie, M. (2012). Post-traumatic stress disorder. *Journal of Occupational and Environmental Medicine, 3*(1), 2–9.

Jirtle, R. L., & Skinner, M. K. (2007). Environmental epigenomics and disease susceptibility. *Nature Reviews. Genetics, 8*(4), 253–262. doi:10.1038/nrg2045.

Kaplan, J. R., Manuck, S. B., Clarkson, T. B., Lusso, F. M., & Taub, D. M. (1982). Social status, environment, and athersclerosis in cynomolgus monkeys. *Arteriosclerosis, 2*, 359–368.

Karmiloff-Smith, A. (2007). Atypical epigenesis. *Developmental Science, 10*(1), 84–88. doi:10.1111/j.1467-7687.2007.00568.x.

Kauffman, S. A. (1993). *The origins of order: Self-organization and selection in evolution*. New York: Oxford University Press.

Kawachi, I., Adler, N. E., & Dow, W. H. (2010). Money, schooling, and health: Mechanisms and causal evidence. *Annals of the New York Academy of Sciences, 1186*, 56–68. doi:10.1111/j.1749-6632.2009.05340.x.

Keating, D. P., & Hertzman, C. (1999). *Developmental health and the wealth of nations: Social, biological, and educational dynamics*. New York: The Guilford Press.

Keltner, D., Gruenfeld, D., & Anderson, C. (2003). Power, approach, and inhibition. *Psychological Review, 110*(2), 265–284.

Kershaw, P., Forer, B., Lloyd, J. E. V., Hertzman, C., Boyce, W. T., Zumbo, B. D., et al. (2009). The use of population-level data to advance interdisciplinary methodology: A cell-through-society sampling framework for child development research. *International Journal of Social Research Methodology, 12*(5), 387–403.

Kessler, R. C., Duncan, G. J., Gennetian, L. A., Katz, L. F., Kling, J. R., Sampson, N. A., et al. (2014). Associations of housing mobility interventions for children in high-poverty neighborhoods with subsequent mental disorders during adolescence. *JAMA, 311*(9), 937–948. doi:10.1001/jama.2014.607.

Keverne, E. B., Martensz, N. D., & Tuite, B. (1989). Beta-endorphin concentrations in cerebrospinal fluid of monkeys are influenced by grooming relationships. *Psychoneuroendocrinology, 14*(1–2), 155–161.

Khan, Y., & Bhutta, Z. A. (2010). Nutritional deficiencies in the developing world: Current status and opportunities for intervention. *Pediatric Clinics of North America, 57*(6), 1409–1441. doi:10.1016/j.pcl.2010.09.016.

Kim, Y. S., Koh, Y. J., & Leventhal, B. L. (2004). Prevalence of school bullying in Korean middle school students. *Archives of Pediatrics & Adolescent Medicine, 158*(8), 737–741.

Kim, Y. S., Leventhal, B. L., Koh, Y. J., & Boyce, W. T. (2009). Bullying increased suicide risk: Prospective study of Korean adolescents. *Archives of Suicide Research, 13*(1), 15–30. doi:10.1080/13811110802572098.

King, M. L. (2007). Concepts of childhood: What we know and where we might go. *Renaissance Quarterly, 60*(2), 371–407.

Kinnally, E. L., Capitanio, J. P., Leibel, R., Deng, L., LeDuc, C., Haghighi, F., & Mann, J. J. (2010a). Epigenetic regulation of serotonin transporter expression and behavior in infant rhesus macaques. *Genes, Brain, and Behavior, 9*(6), 575–582. doi:10.1111/j.1601-183X.2010.00588.x.

Kinnally, E. L., Karere, G. M., Lyons, L. A., Mendoza, S. P., Mason, W. A., & Capitanio, J. P. (2010b). Serotonin pathway gene-gene and gene-environment interactions influence behavioral stress response in infant rhesus macaques. *Development and Psychopathology, 22*(1), 35–44. doi:10.1017/S0954579409990241.

Kinnally, E. L., Feinberg, C., Kim, D., Ferguson, K., Leibel, R., Coplan, J. D., & John Mann, J. (2011). DNA methylation as a risk factor in the effects of early life stress. *Brain Behavior and Immunity*. doi:10.1016/j.bbi.2011.05.001.

Kittleson, M. M., Meoni, L. A., Wang, N. Y., Chu, A. Y., Ford, D. E., & Klag, M. J. (2006). Association of childhood socioeconomic status with subsequent coronary heart disease in physicians. *Archives of Internal Medicine, 166*(21), 2356–2361.

Knafo, A., Israel, S., & Ebstein, R. P. (2011). Heritability of children's prosocial behavior and differential susceptibility to parenting by variation in the dopamine receptor D4 gene. *Development and Psychopathology, 23*(1), 53–67. doi:10.1017/S0954579410000647.

Koopman, J. S., & Lynch, J. W. (1999). Individual causal models and population system models in epidemiology. *American Journal of Public Health, 89*(8), 1170–1174.

Kraemer, H. C., Stice, E., Kazdin, A., Offord, D., & Kupfer, D. (2001). How do risk factors work together? Mediators, moderators, independent, overlapping and proxy-risk factors. *The American Journal of Psychiatry, 158*, 848–856.

Kraemer, H. C., Kiernan, M., Essex, M., & Kupfer, D. J. (2008). How and why criteria defining moderators and mediators differ between the Baron & Kenny and MacArthur approaches. *Health Psychology, 27*(2 Suppl), S101–S108. doi:10.1037/0278-6133.27.2(Suppl.).S101.

Krieger, N. (2001). Theories for social epidemiology in the 21st century: An ecosocial perspective. *International Journal of Epidemiology, 30*, 668–677.

Kuh, D., & Ben-Shlomo, Y. (2004). *A life course approach to chronic disease epidemiology* (2nd ed.). Oxford: Oxford University Press.

Kuzawa, C. W., & Thayer, Z. M. (2011). Timescales of human adaptation: The role of epigenetic processes. *Epigenomics, 3*(2), 221–234. doi:10.2217/epi.11.11.

Ladd-Acosta, C., Pevsner, J., Sabunciyan, S., Yolken, R. H., Webster, M. J., Dinkins, T., et al. (2007). DNA methylation signatures within the human brain.

American Journal of Human Genetics, 81(6), 1304–1315. doi:10.1086/524110.

Lam, L. L., Emberly, E., Fraser, H. B., Neumann, S. M., Chen, E., Miller, G. E., & Kobor, M. S. (2012). Biological and environmental predictors of variable DNA methylation in a human community cohort. *PNAS*.

Lawlor, D. A., Sterne, J. A., Tynelius, P., Davey Smith, G., & Rasmussen, F. (2006). Association of childhood socioeconomic position with cause-specific mortality in a prospective record linkage study of 1,839,384 individuals. *American Journal of Epidemiology, 164*(9), 907–915. doi:10.1093/aje/kwj319.

Lesch, K. P. (2007). Linking emotion to the social brain. The role of the serotonin transporter in human social behaviour. *EMBO Reports, 8*, S24–S29. doi:10.1038/sj.embor.7401008.

Liew, C. C., Ma, J., Tang, H. C., Zheng, R., & Dempsey, A. A. (2006). The peripheral blood transcriptome dynamically reflects system wide biology: A potential diagnostic tool. *The Journal of Laboratory and Clinical Medicine, 147*(3), 126–132. doi:10.1016/j.lab.2005.10.005.

Liu, L., Li, Y., & Tollefsbol, T. O. (2008). Gene-environment interactions and epigenetic basis of human diseases. *Current Issues in Molecular Biology, 10*(1–2), 25–36.

Liu, L., Johnson, H. L., Cousens, S., Perin, J., Scott, S., Lawn, J. E., et al. (2012). Global, regional, and national causes of child mortality: An updated systematic analysis for 2010 with time trends since 2000. *Lancet, 379*(9832), 2151–2161. doi:10.1016/S0140-6736(12)60560-1.

Lloyd, L. J., Langley-Evans, S. C., & McMullen, S. (2012). Childhood obesity and risk of the adult metabolic syndrome: A systematic review. *International Journal of Obesity, 36*(1), 1–11. doi:10.1038/ijo.2011.186.

Lumey, L. H., Stein, A. D., & Susser, E. (2011). Prenatal famine and adult health. *Annual Review of Public Health, 32*, 237–262. doi:10.1146/annurev-publhealth-031210-101230.

Lupien, S. J., King, S., Meaney, M. J., & McEwen, B. S. (2001). Can poverty get under your skin? Basal cortisol levels and cognitive function in children from low and high socioeconomic status. *Development and Psychopathology, 13*, 653–676.

MacDonald, J. L., & Roskams, A. J. (2009). Epigenetic regulation of nervous system development by DNA methylation and histone deacetylation. *Progress in Neurobiology, 88*(3), 170–183.

Manuck, S. B., Craig, A. E., Flory, J. D., Halder, I., & Ferrell, R. E. (2011). Reported early family environment covaries with menarcheal age as a function of polymorphic variation in estrogen receptor-alpha. *Development and Psychopathology, 23*(1), 69–83. doi:10.1017/S0954579410000659.

Marmot, M. (2010). *Fair society, healthy lives*. Firenze: L.S. Olschki.

Mazumdar, S., King, M., Liu, K. Y., Zerubavel, N., & Bearman, P. (2010). The spatial structure of autism in California, 1993-2001. *Health & Place, 16*(3), 539–546. doi:10.1016/j.healthplace.2009.12.014.

McDade, T. (2012). Early environments and the ecologics of inflammation. *Proceedings of the National Academy of Sciences of the United States of America, 109*(Suppl 2), 17281–17288.

McEwen, B. S., & Gianaros, P. J. (2010). Central role of the brain in stress and adaptation: Links to socioeconomic status, health, and disease. *Annals of the New York Academy of Sciences, 1186*, 190–222. doi:10.1111/j.1749-6632.2009.05331.x.

McGowan, P. O., & Szyf, M. (2010). The epigenetics of social adversity in early life: Implications for mental health outcomes. *Neurobiology of Disease, 39*(1), 66–72. doi:10.1016/j.nbd.2009.12.026.

McGowan, P. O., Sasaki, A., Huang, T. C., Unterberger, A., Suderman, M., Ernst, C., et al. (2008). Promoter-wide hypermethylation of the ribosomal RNA gene promoter in the suicide brain. *PloS One, 3*(5), e2085.

McGowan, P. O., Sasaki, A., D'Alessio, A. C., Dymov, S., Labonte, B., Szyf, M., et al. (2009). Epigenetic regulation of the glucocorticoid receptor in human brain associates with childhood abuse. *Nature Neuroscience, 12*(3), 342–348. doi:10.1038/nn.2270.

Meaney, M. J. (2010). Epigenetics and the biological definition of gene x environment interactions. *Child Development, 81*(1), 41–79. doi:10.1111/j.1467-8624.2009.01381.x.

Meaney, M. J., & Ferguson-Smith, A. C. (2010). Epigenetic regulation of the neural transcriptome: The meaning of the marks. *Nature Neuroscience, 13*(11), 1313–1318. doi:10.1038/nn1110-1313.

Mehler, M. F. (2008). Epigenetic principles and mechanisms underlying nervous system functions in health and disease. *Progress in Neurobiology, 86*(4), 305–341.

Miller, G. E., Chen, E., Fok, A. K., Walker, H., Lim, A., Nicholls, E. F., et al. (2009a). Low early-life social class leaves a biological residue manifested by decreased glucocorticoid and increased proinflammatory signaling. *Proceedings of the National Academy of Sciences of the United States of America, 106*(34), 14716–14721. doi:10.1073/pnas.0902971106.

Miller, A. H., Maletic, V., & Raison, C. L. (2009b). Inflammation and its discontents: The role of cytokines in the pathophysiology of major depression. *Biological Psychiatry, 65*(9), 732–741. doi:10.1016/j.biopsych.2008.11.029.

Moffitt, T. E., Caspi, A., & Rutter, M. (2005). Strategy for investigating interactions between measured genes and measured environments. *Archives of General Psychiatry, 62*(5), 473–481.

Mohr, S., & Liew, C. C. (2007). The peripheral-blood transcriptome: New insights into disease and risk assessment. *Trends in Molecular Medicine, 13*(10), 422–432. doi:10.1016/j.molmed.2007.08.003.

Morita, K., Saito, T., Ohta, M., Ohmori, T., Kawai, K., Teshima-Kondo, S., & Rokutan, K. (2005). Expression analysis of psychological stress-associated genes in peripheral blood leukocytes. *Neuroscience Letters, 381*(1–2), 57–62.

Msall, M. E., Bier, J. A., LaGasse, L., Tremont, M., & Lester, B. (1998). The vulnerable preschool child: The impact of biomedical and social risks on neurodevelopmental function. *Seminars in Pediatric Neurology, 5*(1), 52–61.

Nesse, R. M., & Young, E. A. (2000). Evolutionary origins and functions of the stress response. In G. Fink (Ed.), *Encyclopedia of stress* (Vol. 2, pp. 79–84). San Diego: Academic Press.

Norman, G. J., Hawkley, L. C., Cole, S. W., Berntson, G. G., & Cacioppo, J. T. (2012). Social neuroscience: The social brain, oxytocin, and health. *Social Neuroscience, 7*(1), 18–29. doi:10.1080/17470919.2011.568702.

Oberg, C. (2008). Children of genocide: A legacy of lost dreams. *Pediatrics, 121*(3), 611–615. doi:10.1542/peds.2007-2208.

Oberlander, T. F., Weinberg, J., Papsdorf, M., Grunau, R., Misri, S., & Devlin, A. M. (2008). Prenatal exposure to maternal depression, neonatal methylation of human glucocorticoid receptor gene (NR3C1) and infant cortisol stress response. *Epigenetics, 3*(2), 97–106.

Obradovic, J., Bush, N. R., Stamperdahl, J., Adler, N. E., & Boyce, W. T. (2010). Biological sensitivity to context: The interactive effects of stress reactivity and family adversity on socio-emotional behavior and school readiness. *Child Development, 81*(1), 270–289.

Offord, D. R. (1995). Child psychiatric epidemiology: Current status and future prospects. *Canadian Journal of Psychiatry. Revue Canadienne de Psychiatrie, 40*(6), 284–288.

Olds, D. L., Kitzman, H. J., Cole, R. E., Hanks, C. A., Arcoleo, K. J., Anson, E. A., et al. (2010). Enduring effects of prenatal and infancy home visiting by nurses on maternal life course and government spending: Follow-up of a randomized trial among children at age 12 years. *Archives of Pediatrics and Adolescent Medicine, 164*(5), 419–424. doi:10.1001/archpediatrics.2010.49.

Ollikainen, M., Smith, K. R., Joo, E. J., Ng, H. K., Andronikos, R., Novakovic, B., et al. (2010). DNA methylation analysis of multiple tissues from newborn twins reveals both genetic and intrauterine components to variation in the human neonatal epigenome. *Human Molecular Genetics, 19*(21), 4176–4188. doi:10.1093/hmg/ddq336.

Ostrove, J. M., Adler, N. E., Kuppermann, M., & Washington, A. E. (2000). Objective and subjective assessments of socioeconomic status and their relationship to self-rated health in an ethnically diverse sample of pregnant women. *Health Psychology, 19*(6), 613–618.

Overton, W. F., & Lerner, R. M. (2014). Fundamental concepts and methods in developmental science: A relational perspective. *Research in Human Development, 11*, 63–73.

Painter, R. C., Roseboom, T. J., & Bleker, O. P. (2005). Prenatal exposure to the Dutch famine and disease in later life: An overview. *Reproductive Toxicology, 20*(3), 345–352.

Painter, R., Osmond, C., Gluckman, P., Hanson, M., Phillips, D., & Roseboom, T. (2008). Transgenerational effects of prenatal exposure to the Dutch famine on neonatal adiposity and health in later life. *BJOG: An International Journal of Obstetrics & Gynaecology, 115*(10), 1243–1249.

Panter-Brick, C., Lende, D., & Kohrt, B. (2012). Children in global adversity: Physical health, mental health, behavioral health, and symbolic health. In V. Maholmes & R. B. King (Eds.), *The Oxford handbook of poverty and child development* (pp. 603–621). Oxford: Oxford University Press.

Pellegrini, A. D., Roseth, C. J., Mliner, S., Bohn, C. M., Van Ryzin, M., Vance, N., et al. (2007). Social dominance in preschool classrooms. *Journal of Comparative Psychology, 121*(1), 54–64. doi:10.1037/0735-7036.121.1.54.

Pellegrini, A. D., Van Ryzin, M. J., Roseth, C., Bohn-Gettler, C., Dupuis, D., Hickey, M., & Peshkam, A. (2010). Behavioral and social cognitive processes in preschool children's social dominance. *Aggressive Behavior, 37*(3), 248–257. doi:10.1002/ab.20385.

Pezawas, L., Meyer-Lindenberg, A., Drabant, E. M., Verchinski, B. A., Munoz, K. E., Kolachana, B. S., et al. (2005). 5-HTTLPR polymorphism impacts human cingulate-amygdala interactions: A genetic susceptibility mechanism for depression. *Nature Neuroscience, 8*(6), 828–834.

Pluess, M., & Belsky, J. (2013). Vantage sensitivity: Individual differences in response to positive experiences. *Psychological Bulletin, 139*(4), 901–916. doi:10.1037/a0030196.

Quas, J. A., Bauer, A., & Boyce, W. T. (2004). Physiological reactivity, social support, and memory in early childhood. *Child Development, 75*(3), 797–814.

Rifkin, J. (2009). *The empathic civilization: The race to global consciousness in a world in crisis*. New York: Jeremy P. Tarcher/Penguin.

Robert Wood Johnson Foundation Commission to Build a Healthier America. (2009). Beyond Health Care: New Directions to a Healthier America. Retrieved from Princeton, NJ:

Robinson, G. E., Grozinger, C. M., & Whitfield, C. W. (2005). Sociogenomics: Social life in molecular terms. *Nature Reviews Genetics, 6*, 257–270.

Robinson, G. E., Fernald, R. D., & Clayton, D. F. (2008). Genes and social behavior. *Science, 322*(5903), 896–900. doi:10.1126/science.1159277.

Robison, A. J., & Nestler, E. J. (2011). Transcriptional and epigenetic mechanisms of addiction. *Nature Reviews. Neuroscience, 12*(11), 623–637. doi:10.1038/nrn3111.

Roseboom, T. J., van der Meulen, J. H., Osmond, C., Barker, D. J., Ravelli, A. C., Schroeder-Tanka, J. M., et al. (2000). Coronary heart disease after prenatal exposure to the Dutch famine, 1944-45. *Heart, 84*(6), 595–598.

Roth, T. L., Lubin, F. D., Funk, A. J., & Sweatt, J. D. (2009). Lasting epigenetic influence of early-life adversity on the BDNF gene. *Biological Psychiatry, 65*(9), 760–769. doi:10.1016/j.biopsych.2008.11.028.

Russo, V. E. A., Cove, D. J., Edgar, L. G., Jaenisch, R., & Salamini, F. (Eds.). (1999). *Development: Genetics, epigenetics and environmental regulation*. Berlin: Springer-Verlag.

Rutter, M. (2006). *Genes and behaviour: Nature/nurture interplay explained*. Oxford, UK: Blackwell Publishing.

Rutter, M. (2012). Achievements and challenges in the biology of environmental effects. *PNAS*.

Sapolsky, R. M. (2003). Stress and plasticity in the limbic system. *Neurochemical Research, 28*(11), 1735–1742.

Sapolsky, R. M. (2005). The influence of social hierarchy on primate health. *Science, 308*(5722), 648–652.

Schneider, J., Dickinson, M., & Levine, J. (2012). Social structures depend on innate determinants and chemosensory processing in Drosophila. *PNAS*.

Sentenac, M., Arnaud, C., Gavin, A., Molcho, M., Gabhainn, S. N., & Godeau, E. (2012). Peer victimization among school-aged children with chronic conditions. *Epidemiologic Reviews, 34*(1), 120–128. doi:10.1093/epirev/mxr024.

Shannon, K. E., Beauchaine, T. P., Brenner, S. L., Neuhaus, E., & Gatzke-Kopp, L. (2007). Familial and temperamental predictors of resilience in children at risk for conduct disorder and depression. *Development and Psychopathology, 19*(3), 701–727. doi:10.1017/S0954579407000351.

Shonkoff, J. (2012). Leveraging the biology of adversity and resilience to address the roots of disparities in health and development. *Proceedings of the National Academy of Sciences of the United States of America, 109*(Suppl 2), 17302–17307.

Shonkoff, J. P., & Garner, A. S. (2012). The lifelong effects of early childhood adversity and toxic stress. *Pediatrics, 129*(1), e232–e246. doi:10.1542/peds.2011-2663.

Shonkoff, J. P., & Phillips, D. A. (Eds.). (2000). *From neurons to neighborhoods: The science of early child development*. Washington, DC: National Academy Press.

Shorter, E. (1975). *The making of the modern family*. New York: Basic Books.

Slavich, G. M., & Cole, S. W. (2013). The emerging field of human social genomics. *Clinical Psychological Science: A Journal of the Association for Psychological Science, 1*(3), 331–348.

Sourander, A., Jensen, P., Ronning, J. A., Elonheimo, H., Niemela, S., Helenius, H., et al. (2007). Childhood bullies and victims and their risk of criminality in late adolescence: The Finnish From a Boy to a Man study. *Archives of Pediatrics & Adolescent Medicine, 161*(6), 546–552. doi:10.1001/archpedi.161.6.546.

Stearns, P. N. (2011). *Childhood in world history* (2nd ed.). New York, NY: Routledge.

Steptoe, A., Feldman, P. J., Kunz, S., Owen, N., Willemsen, G., & Marmot, M. (2002). Stress responsivity and socioeconomic status: A mechanism for increased cardiovascular disease risk? *European Heart Journal, 23*, 1757–1763.

Stevens, H. E., Leckman, J. F., Coplan, J. D., & Suomi, S. J. (2009). Risk and resilience: Early manipulation of macaque social experience and persistent behavioral and neurophysiological outcomes. *Journal of the American Academy of Child and Adolescent Psychiatry, 48*(2), 114–127. doi:10.1097/CHI.0b013e318193064c.

Suomi, S. J. (2006). Risk, resilience, and gene x environment interactions in rhesus monkeys. *Annals of the New York Academy of Sciences, 1094*, 52–62. doi:10.1196/annals.1376.006.

Syme, S. L. (2008). Reducing racial and social-class inequalities in health: The need for a new approach. *Health Affairs (Millwood), 27*(2), 456–459. doi:10.1377/hlthaff.27.2.456.

Szyf, M., McGowan, P., & Meaney, M. J. (2008). The social environment and the epigenome. *Environmental and Molecular Mutagenesis, 49*(1), 46–60. doi:10.1002/em.20357.

Thompson, P. M., Martin, N. G., & Wright, M. J. (2010). Imaging genomics. *Current Opinion in Neurology, 23*(4), 368–373. doi:10.1097/WCO.0b013e32833b764c.

Tsankova, N., Renthal, W., Kumar, A., & Nestler, E. J. (2007). Epigenetic regulation in psychiatric disorders. *Nature Reviews. Neuroscience, 8*(5), 355–367. doi:10.1038/nrn2132.

Turecki, G., Ernst, C., Jollant, F., Labonte, B., & Mechawar, N. (2012). The neurodevelopmental origins of suicidal behavior. *Trends in Neurosciences, 35*(1), 14–23. doi:10.1016/j.tins.2011.11.008.

Turner, J. D., Pelascini, L. P., Macedo, J. A., & Muller, C. P. (2008). Highly individual methylation patterns of alternative glucocorticoid receptor promoters suggest individualized epigenetic regulatory mechanisms. *Nucleic Acids Research, 36*(22), 7207–7218. doi:10.1093/nar/gkn897.

Turner, H. A., Finkelhor, D., Shattuck, A., & Hamby, S. (2012). Recent victimization exposure and suicidal ideation in adolescents. *Archives of Pediatrics & Adolescent Medicine*, 1–6. doi:10.1001/archpediatrics.2012.1549.

U.S. Department of Health and Human Services. (2011). *CDC Health Disparities and Inequalities Report—United States, 2011*. Atlanta: U.S. Department of Health and Human Services, Centers for Disease Control and Prevention.

Uebelhack, R., Franke, L., Herold, N., Plotkin, M., Amthauer, H., & Felix, R. (2006). Brain and platelet serotonin transporter in humans-correlation between [123I]-ADAM SPECT and serotonergic measurements in platelets. *Neuroscience Letters, 406*(3), 153–158. doi:10.1016/j.neulet.2006.06.004.

van IJzendoorn, M. H., Caspers, K., Bakermans-Kranenburg, M. J., Beach, S. R., & Philibert, R. (2010). Methylation matters: Interaction between methylation density and serotonin transporter genotype predicts unresolved loss or trauma. *Biological Psychiatry, 68*(5), 405–407. doi:10.1016/j.biopsych.2010.05.008.

Vogel, E. F., & Bell, N. W. (1961). The emotionally disturbed child as the family scapegoat. In N. W. Bell & E. F. Vogel (Eds.), *A Modern introduction to the family*. London: Routledge & Kegan Paul.

Waddington, C. H. (1959). Canalization of development and genetic assimilation of acquired characters. *Nature, 183*(4676), 1654–1655.

Waddington, C. H. (2012). The epigenotype. 1942. *International Journal of Epidemiology, 41*(1), 10–13. doi:10.1093/ije/dyr184.

Wadsworth, M. E., Raviv, T., Reinhard, C., Wolff, B., Santiago, C. D. C., & Einhorn, L. (2008). An indirect effects model of the association between poverty and child functioning: The role of children. *Journal of Loss and Trauma, 30*.

Weaver, I. C. (2009). Epigenetic effects of glucocorticoids. *Seminars in Fetal and Neonatal Medicine, 14*(3), 143–150. doi:10.1016/j.siny.2008.12.002.

Weaver, I. C., Cervoni, N., Champagne, F. A., D'Alessio, A. C., Sharma, S., Seckl, J. R., et al. (2004). Epigenetic programming by maternal behavior. *Nature Neuroscience, 7*(8), 847–854.

Weikum, W. M., Oberlander, T. F., Hensch, T. K., & Werker, J. F. (2012). Prenatal exposure to antidepressants and depressed maternal mood alter trajectory of infant speech perception. *Proceedings of the National Academy of Sciences, 109*(2), 17221–17227. doi:10.1073/pnas.1121263109.

West-Eberhard, M. J. (2003). *Developmental plasticity and evolution*. New York: Oxford University Press.

Whittle, S., Yap, M. B., Sheeber, L., Dudgeon, P., Yucel, M., Pantelis, C., et al. (2010). Hippocampal volume and sensitivity to maternal aggressive behavior: A prospective study of adolescent depressive symptoms. *Development and Psychopathology, 23*(1), 115–129. doi:10.1017/S0954579410000684.

Wolf, D. M., Vazirani, V. V., & Arkin, A. P. (2005). Diversity in times of adversity: Probabilistic strategies in microbial survival games. *Journal of Theoretical Biology, 234*(2), 227–253. doi:10.1016/j.jtbi.2004.11.020.

Wright, R. O., & Christiani, D. (2010). Gene-environment interaction and children's health and development. *Current Opinion in Pediatrics, 22*(2), 197–201. doi:10.1097/MOP.0b013e328336ebf9.

Wu, H., & Sun, Y. E. (2006). Epigenetic regulation of stem cell differentiation. *Pediatric Research, 59*(4 Pt 2), 21R–25R. doi:10.1203/01.pdr.0000203565.76028.2a.

Yang, E.-J., Lin, E. W., & Hensch, T. K. (2012). A critical period for acoustic preference in mice. *Proceedings of the National Academy of Sciences, 109*(Suppl 2), 17213–17220.

Zhang, T. Y., & Meaney, M. J. (2010). Epigenetics and the environmental regulation of the genome and its function. *Annual Review of Psychology, 61*, 439–466, C431–433.. doi:10.1146/annurev.psych.60.110707.163625.

Middle Childhood: An Evolutionary-Developmental Synthesis

Marco DelGiudice

Middle childhood—conventionally going from about 6–11 years of age—is a crucial yet underappreciated phase of human development. On the surface, middle childhood may appear like a slow-motion interlude between the spectacular transformations of infancy and early childhood and those of adolescence. In reality, this life stage is anything but static: the transition from early to middle childhood heralds a global shift in cognition, motivation, and social behavior, with profound and wide-ranging implications for the development of personality, sex differences, and even psychopathology (Table 1).

In the last two decades, converging theories and findings from anthropology, primatology, evolutionary psychology, endocrinology, and behavior genetics have revolutionized our understanding of middle childhood. In this chapter, I show how these diverse contributions can be synthesized into an integrated evolutionary-developmental model of middle childhood. I begin by reviewing the main evolved functions of middle childhood and the cognitive, behavioral, and hormonal processes that characterize this life stage. Then, I introduce the idea that the transition to middle childhood works as a switch point in the development of life history strategies (Del Giudice et al. 2009, 2012; Del Giudice and Belsky 2011) and discuss three insights in the nature of middle childhood that arise from an integrated approach. This chapter was originally published as a short paper in the journal *Child Development Perspectives* (Del Giudice 2014a). It is reprinted here with updated references and a new section on the model's implications for health development in a life course perspective (LCHD).

1 What Is Middle Childhood?

Middle childhood is one of the main stages of human development, marked by the eruption of the first permanent molars around age 6 and the onset of androgen secretion by the adrenal glands at about 6–8 years (Bogin 1997). In middle childhood, body growth slows considerably, usually following a small mid-growth spurt. At the same time, muscularity increases and the body starts accumulating fat (the *adiposity rebound*; Hochberg 2008), while sex differences in body composition become more pronounced (Del Giudice et al. 2009; Wells

This chapter contains a modified version of a previously published review and analysis of existing research, written by Marco Del Giudice, that appeared in *Child Development Perspectives*.
Reprinted with permission from:
Del Giudice, M. (2014), Middle Childhood: An Evolutionary-Developmental Synthesis. Child Dev Perspect, 8: 193–200. doi:10.1111/cdep.12084.

M. DelGiudice (✉)
Department of Psychology, University of New Mexico, Logan Hall, 2001 Redondo Dr. NE, Albuquerque, NM 87131, USA
e-mail: marcodg@unm.edu

N. Halfon et al. (eds.), *Handbook of Life Course Health Development*,
DOI 10.1007/978-3-319-47143-3_5

Table 1 Development in middle childhood

Body growth	Eruption of permanent molars
	Mid-growth spurt, followed by decelerating skeletal growth
	Increased muscle mass
	Increased adiposity and BMI (adiposity rebound)
	Initial development of axillary hair and body odor
	Increased sex differences in adiposity (F > M), bone strength, and muscularity (M > F)
	Emergence of sex differences in vocal characteristics
Brain growth	Approaching peak of overall brain volume
	Peak of gray matter volume
	Continuing increase in white matter volume/integrity
Motor and perceptual skills	Increased gross motor skills (e.g., walking)
	Increased fine motor skills
	Local-global shift in visual processing preferences
Cognitive skills	Increased reasoning and problem-solving skills (e.g., concrete operations)
	Increased self-regulation and executive functions (inhibition, attention, planning, etc.)
	Increased mentalizing skills (multiple perspectives, conflicting goals)
	Increased navigational skills (working memory, ability to understand maps)
Motivation and social behavior	Acquisition of cultural norms (e.g., prosociality)
	Complex moral reasoning (conflicting points of view)
	Increased pragmatic abilities (gossiping, storytelling, verbal competition, etc.)
	Consolidation of status/dominance hierarchies
	Changes in aggression levels (individual trajectories)
	Development of disgust
	Changes in food preferences (e.g., spicy foods)
	Onset of sexual/romantic attraction
	Increased frequency of sexual play
	Increased sense of gender identity
	Peak of sex segregation
	Peak of sex differences in social play (including play fighting vs. play parenting)
	Increased sex differences in physical aggression (M > F)
	Emergence of sex differences in attachment styles
Psychopathology	Early peak of psychopathology onset (externalizing, anxiety, phobias, ADHD)
	Peak onset of fetishistic attractions
	Emergence of sex differences in conduct disorders (M > F)
Social context	Active involvement in caretaking, foraging, domestic tasks, helping
	Expectations of responsible behavior
	Attribution of individuality and personhood ("getting noticed")
Behavior genetics	Increased heritability of general intelligence and language skills
	New genetic influences on general intelligence, language, aggression, and prosociality

See the main text for supporting references
BMI body mass index, *M* male, *F* female, *ADHD* attention deficit hyperactivity disorder

2007). Figure 1 places middle childhood in the broader context of human growth from conception to adolescence.

In biological terms, middle childhood corresponds to human *juvenility*—a stage in which the individual is still sexually immature, but no longer dependent on parents for survival. In social mammals and primates, juvenility is a phase of intense learning—often accomplished through play—in which youngsters practice adult behavioral patterns and acquire essential social and foraging skills. Indeed, the duration of juvenility in

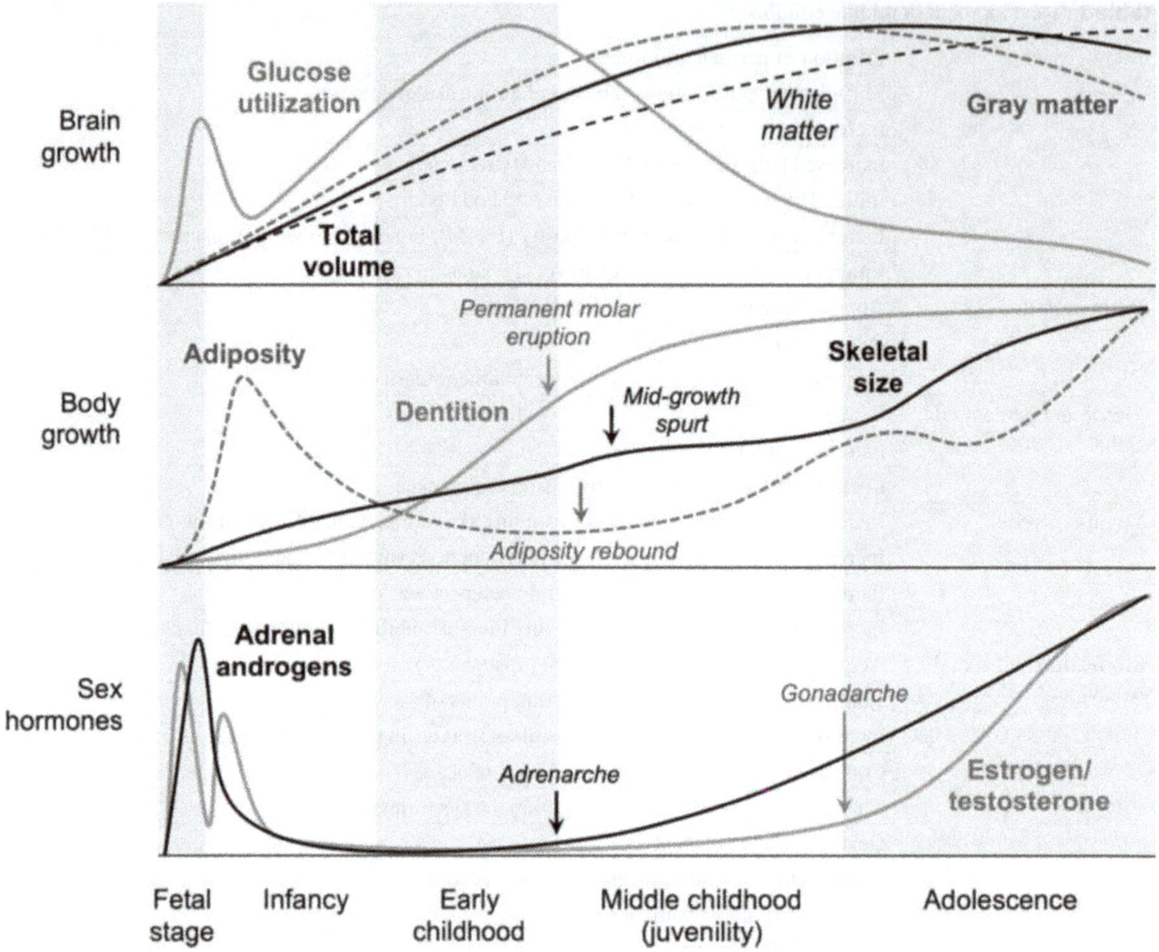

Fig. 1 Developmental trajectories of human growth and sex hormones production, from conception to adolescence. Arrows show the landmark events that characterize middle childhood (Reproduced from Del Giudice 2014a)

primates correlates strongly with the size and complexity of social groups, as well as with cortical brain volume (Joffe 1997). Social learning in juvenility can be understood as investment in *embodied capital*—skills and knowledge that cost time and effort to acquire but increase an individual's performance and reproductive success (Kaplan et al. 2000).

Human children are no exception to this pattern. Social learning is universally recognized as a key evolved function of middle childhood and is enabled by a global reorganization of cognitive functioning known as the *five-to-seven shift* (Weisner 1996). By age 6, the brain has almost reached its maximum size and receives a decreasing share of the body's glucose after the consumption peak of early childhood (Fig. 1; Giedd and Rapoport 2010; Kuzawa et al. 2014). However, brain development proceeds at a sustained pace, with intensive synaptogenesis in cortical areas (gray matter) and rapid maturation of axonal connections (white matter; Lebel et al. 2008). The transition to middle childhood is marked by a simultaneous increase in perceptual abilities (including a transition from local to global visual processing), motor control (including the emergence of adult-like walking), and complex reasoning skills (Bjorklund 2011; Poirel et al. 2011; Weisner 1996). The most dramatic changes probably occur in the domain of self-regulation and executive functions: children become much more capable of inhibiting unwanted behavior, maintaining sustained attention, making and following plans, and so forth (Best et al. 2009; Weisner 1996; see also McClelland et al. 2017). Parallel improvements take place in mentalizing (the ability to understand and represent mental states) and moral reasoning, as children become able to consider multiple perspectives and conflicting goals (Jambon and Smetana 2014; Lagattuta et al. 2009).

In traditional societies, older relatives—especially parents and grandparents—are the main sources of knowledge for juveniles, supplemented by peers and—where available—professional teachers. Storytelling—both fictional and based in real events—is a powerful technology for transmitting knowledge about foraging and social skills, avoidance of dangers, topography, wayfinding, and social roles and norms (Scalise Sugiyama 2011). Storytelling mimics the format of episodic memories, providing the child with a rich source of indirect experience (Scalise Sugiyama 2011). Intriguingly, episodic memory shows dramatic and sustained improvements across middle childhood (Ghetti and Bunge 2012).

However, children at this age are not just learning and playing. Cross-culturally, middle childhood is the time when children are expected to start helping with domestic tasks—such as caring for younger siblings, collecting food and water, tending animals, and helping adults prepare food (Bogin 1997; Lancy and Grove 2011; Scalise Sugiyama 2011; Weisner 1996). In favorable ecologies, juveniles can contribute substantially to family subsistence (Kramer 2011). Thanks to marked increases in spatial cognition—reflected in the emerging ability to understand maps—and navigational skills, children become able to memorize complex routes and find their way without adult supervision (Bjorklund 2011; Piccardi et al. 2014). The important role of juveniles in collecting and preparing food may explain why the emotion of disgust does not fully develop until middle childhood (Rozin 1990a).

The transition to middle childhood is typically associated with a strong separation in gender roles, even in societies where tasks are not rigidly assigned by sex. Spontaneous sex segregation of boys and girls peaks during these years, as does the frequency of sexually differentiated play (Del Giudice et al. 2009). On a broader social level, cross-cultural evidence shows that juveniles start "getting noticed" by adults—that is, they begin to be viewed fully as people with their own individuality, personality, and social responsibility (Lancy and Grove 2011).

In summary, the life stage of juvenility/middle childhood has two major interlocking functions: *social learning* and *social integration* in a system of roles, norms, activities, and shared knowledge. While children are still receiving sustained investment from parents and other relatives—in the form of food, protection, knowledge, and so forth—they also start to actively contribute to their family economy. By providing resources and sharing the burden of child care, juveniles can boost their parents' reproductive potential. The dual nature of juveniles as both *receivers* and *providers* explains many psychological features of middle childhood and has likely played a major role in the evolution of human life history (Kramer 2011).

1.1 Adrenarche

The transition to middle childhood is coordinated by a remarkable endocrinological event: the awakening of the adrenal glands, or *adrenarche* (Auchus and Rainey 2004; Hochberg 2008). Starting at about 6–8 years—with much individual variation and only minor differences between males and females—adrenal glands begin to secrete increasing amounts of androgens (see Fig. 1), mainly dehydroepiandrosterone (DHEA) and its sulfate (DHEAS). Adrenal androgens have only minor effects on physical development, but they have powerful effects on brain functioning. DHEA and DHEAS promote neurogenesis and modulate gamma-aminobutyric acid (GABA) and glutamate receptors; moreover, DHEA can act directly on androgen and estrogen receptors. Even more important, adrenal androgens can be converted to estrogen or testosterone in the brain (Campbell 2006; Del Giudice et al. 2009). As sex hormones, adrenal androgens play a twofold role: They activate sexually differentiated brain pathways that had been previously organized by the hormonal surges of prenatal development and infancy (Fig. 1), and they further organize brain development along sexually differentiated trajectories (Del Giudice et al. 2009).

Adrenal androgens likely provide a major impulse for many of the psychological changes of middle childhood (Campbell 2006, 2011; Del Giudice et al. 2009), including the emergence and intensification of sex differences across domains (see Table 1). Since the age of adrenarche correlates strongly with that of *gonadarche* (the awakening of the testes/ovaries that marks the beginning of puberty; Hochberg 2008), human development shows a peculiar pattern in which sexually differentiated brain pathways are activated several years *before* the development of secondary sexual characteristics. This developmental pattern (shared by chimpanzees and, to a lesser extent, gorillas; Bernstein et al. 2012) results in a temporary decoupling between physical and behavioral development, consistent with the idea of middle childhood as a sexually differentiated phase of social learning and experimentation (Geary 2010). Moreover, adrenal androgens promote extended brain plasticity through synaptogenesis and may play an important role in shifting the allocation of the body's energetic resources away from brain development and toward the accumulation of muscle and fat in preparation for puberty (Campbell 2006, 2011; see also Kuzawa et al. 2014).

2 The Transition to Middle Childhood as a Developmental Switch Point

The evolutionary model of middle childhood sketched in the previous section can be enriched and extended by considering the role of adrenarche as a *developmental switch* (Del Giudice et al. 2009). The concept of a developmental switch was introduced by West-Eberhard (2003); a switch is a regulatory mechanism that activates at a specific point in development, collects input from the external environment or the state of the organism, and shifts the individual along alternative pathways—ultimately resulting in the development of alternative phenotypes (morphological, physiological, or behavioral traits of an organism). For example, a switch may regulate the development of aggressive behavior so that safe conditions entrain the development of low levels of aggression, whereas threatening environments trigger high levels of aggression. Developmental switches enable *adaptive plasticity*—the ability of an organism to adjust its phenotype to match the local environment in a way that promotes biological fitness (West-Eberhard 2003). In other words, plastic organisms track the state of the environment—usually through indirect cues—and use this information to develop alternative phenotypes that tend to promote survival or reproduction under different conditions.

Developmental switches work in a *modular* fashion (see Fig. 2). Activation of a switch leads to the coordinated expression of different genes—both those involved in the regulatory mechanism itself and those involved in the production of the new phenotype. Moreover, alternative phenotypes (A and B in Fig. 2) involve the expression of modular packages of genes specific to each phenotype. Another key aspect of developmental switches is that they integrate variation in the environment with individual differences in the genes that regulate the switch. For example, different individuals may have genetically different thresholds for switching between aggressive and nonaggressive phenotypes. Finally, the embodied effects of past experiences and conditions (e.g., an individual's previous exposure to stress or nutritional conditions early in life) may also modulate how the switch functions, allowing the organism to integrate information over time and across different life stages (Del Giudice 2014b; Ellis 2013). In many instances, the effects of past experience on developmental switches may be mediated by epigenetic mechanisms (see Meaney 2010).

The concept of a developmental switch point resembles that of a *sensitive period*, in that the organism is maximally responsive to some environmental input. The crucial difference is that, because genetic and environmental inputs converge in the regulatory mechanism, a developmental switch amplifies both environmental *and*

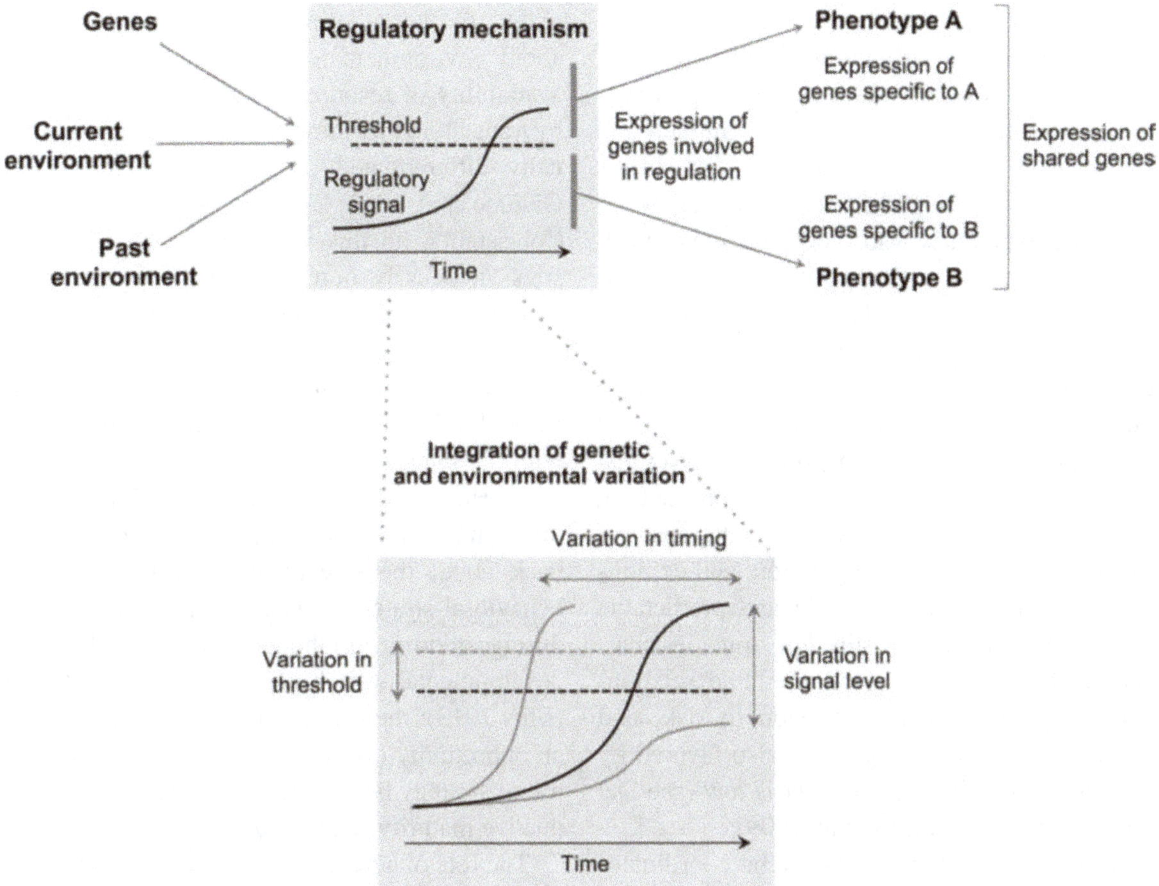

Fig. 2 The concept of a developmental switch. A regulatory mechanism, which may operate through hormonal signals, integrates current and past information from the environment with the individual's genotype. As a result, the individual's developmental trajectory is shifted along alternative pathways—here, A and B—depending on whether a threshold is reached within the mechanism. The location of the threshold, the intensity of the signal, and the timing of the switch point all depend on the joint action of the current state of the environment, the embodied effect of past environmental conditions, and individual variation in the genes involved in the regulatory mechanism. Each alternative pathway involves the modular expression of a set of specific genes, in addition to the shared genes expressed in the new developmental stage. A developmental switch may integrate many sources of input from the environment or produce graded phenotypes rather than discrete alternatives such as A and B

genetic effects on the phenotype (West-Eberhard 2003). Indeed, the activation of a developmental switch exposes many new potential sources of genetic variation, including the genes involved in the regulatory mechanism and in the expression of the new phenotypes (Fig. 2).

2.1 A Switch Point in Life History Development

The role of adrenarche as a developmental switch is not limited to a single trait; in fact, the transition to middle childhood (or *juvenile transition*; Del Giudice et al. 2009) encompasses all the major domains of behavior—from learning and self-regulation to attachment and sexuality (see Table 1). My colleagues and I (Del Giudice and Belsky 2011; Del Giudice et al. 2009, 2012) have argued that the transition to middle childhood is a switch point in the development of *life history strategies*, which are coordinate suites of morphological, physiological, and behavioral traits that determine how organisms allocate their resources to key biological activities such as growth, reproduction, mating, and parenting (for a non-technical overview of life history theory, see Del Giudice et al. 2015). At the level of behavior, individual differences in life history strategy are reflected in patterns of self-regulation, aggression, cooperation and prosociality, attachment, sexuality, and so forth (Del Giudice and Belsky 2011; Del Giudice et al. 2009, 2011; Ellis et al. 2009). Although life history strategies are partly heritable, they also show a degree of plasticity in response to the quality of the environment, including the level of danger and unpredictability –embodied in the experience of early stress—and the availability of adequate nutritional resources. In a nutshell, dangerous and unpredictable environments tend to favor *fast* strategies characterized by early reproduction, sexual promiscuity, unstable relationships, impulsivity, risk taking, aggression, and exploitative tendencies, whereas safe and predictable environments tend to entrain *slow* strategies characterized by late reproduction, stable relationships, high self-control, aversion to risk, and prosociality. Slow strategies are also favored by nutritional scarcity when danger is low (see Del Giudice et al. 2016; Ellis et al. 2009).

Our argument is that adrenarche coordinates the expression of individual differences in life history strategy by integrating individual genetic variation with information about the child's social and physical environment collected throughout infancy and early childhood (Belsky et al. 1991). The stress response system plays a major role in gathering and storing information about environmental safety, predictability, and availability of resources; adrenarche contributes by translating that information into adaptive, sexually differentiated patterns of behavior (Del Giudice et al. 2011; Ellis and Del Giudice 2014). Consistent with this view, both early relational stress and early nutrition have been found to modulate the timing of adrenarche (Ellis and Essex 2007; Hochberg 2008). It is no coincidence that the first sexual and romantic attractions typically develop in middle childhood, in tandem with the intensification of sexual play (Bancroft 2003; Herdt and McClintock 2000). By interacting with peers and adults, juveniles receive feedback about the effectiveness of their nascent behavioral strategies. The information collected during middle childhood feeds into the next developmental switch point, that of gonadarche (Ellis 2013); the transition to adolescence offers an opportunity for youth to adjust or revise their initial strategy before attaining sexual and reproductive maturity (Del Giudice and Belsky 2011).

The role of adrenarche as a switch point in life history development adds another level of complexity to the biological profile of juvenility. Figure 3 outlines an integrated evolutionary-developmental model that brings together the various strands of theory and evidence reviewed in this chapter.

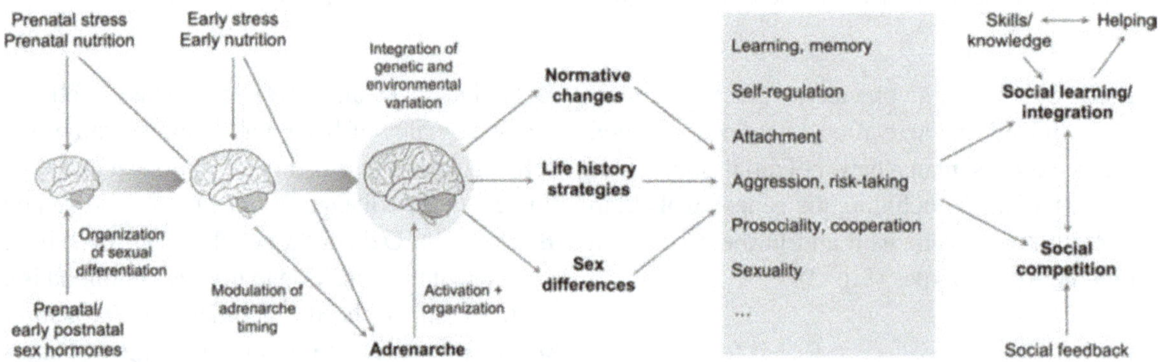

Fig. 3 An integrated evolutionary-developmental model of middle childhood. Adrenarche is shown as a switch in the development of life history strategies, as well as a key mechanism underlying the normative changes of middle childhood and the emergence and intensification of sex differences. At a broader level, development in middle childhood serves two complementary functions, social integration and social competition

3 Three Insights in the Nature of Middle Childhood

3.1 Insight 1: Social Integration and Social Competition Are Complementary Functions of Middle Childhood

Evolutionary accounts of middle childhood typically focus on learning, helping, and other forms of social integration. A life history approach emphasizes the need to consider social competition as a crucial, complementary function of human juvenility. In the peer group, children compete for vital social resources—status, reputation, allies, and friends. While learning and play are relatively risk-free, they are not without consequences. The social position achieved in middle childhood is a springboard for adolescence and adulthood; popularity and centrality within the peer network put a child at a considerable advantage, with potentially long-term effects on mating and reproductive success (Del Giudice et al. 2009).

Physical and relational aggression are obvious tactics for gaining influence, but social competition also occurs through prosocial behaviors such as forming alliances, doing favors, and displaying valuable skills. Indeed, managing the balance between prosocial and coercive tactics is an important part of developing social skills (Hawley 2014). More broadly, competition shapes many aspects of cognitive and behavioral development in middle childhood; for example, increased pragmatic abilities allow children to gossip, joke, tease, and engage in verbal duels—all forms of social competition mediated by language (Locke and Bogin 2006). Intensifying social competition also contributes to explain the early peak of psychopathology onset observed in middle childhood, characterized by increasing rates of externalizing disorders (e.g., conduct disorder), anxiety disorders (including social phobia), and attention deficit hyperactivity disorder (ADHD; Del Giudice et al. 2009).

3.2 Insight 2: Sexual Selection Contributes to the Emergence and Intensification of Sex Differences in Middle Childhood

By determining children's initial place in social networks and hierarchies, competition in middle childhood indirectly affects their ability to attract sexual and romantic partners later. In other words, middle childhood is a likely target for *sexual selection*—that is, natural selection arising from the processes of choosing mates (*mate choice*) and competing for mates (mating *competition*). My colleagues and I (Del Giudice et al. 2009) argued that sexual selection is one reason why sex differences emerge and intensify in middle childhood. In particular, sex differences in physical aggression increase markedly, in tandem with sex differences in muscularity and play fighting. At the same time, attachment styles begin to diverge between males and females, with insecurely attached boys becoming more avoidant and insecure girls becoming more preoccupied/ambivalent (Del Giudice 2009; Del Giudice and Belsky 2010). Different attachment styles are conducive to different social strategies and may be adaptive in regulating children's nascent relationships with peers. There is initial evidence that attachment styles in middle childhood reflect the effects of prenatal sex hormones, which according to our model are activated by adrenal androgens (Del Giudice and Angeleri 2016). Sexual selection also has indirect implications for the development of psychopathology; for example, marked sex differences in the prevalence of conduct disorders become apparent at the beginning of middle childhood, likely reflecting the stronger role of aggression in boys' social competition (see Del Giudice et al. 2009; Martel 2013).

3.3 Insight 3: In Middle Childhood, Heightened Sensitivity to the Environment Goes Hand in Hand with the Expression of New Genetic Factors

When an organism goes through a developmental switch point, inputs from the environment combine with the individual's genotype to determine the resulting phenotype. For example, when adrenal androgens begin to increase during the transition to middle childhood, they activate many hormone-sensitive brain pathways that have been dormant since infancy. In doing so, they release previously hidden genetic variation (Del Giudice et al. 2009). Thus, middle childhood should be characterized by a mixture of heightened sensitivity to the environment—possibly mediated by newly activated epigenetic mechanisms (Meaney 2010) and expression of new genetic factors.

Evidence of increased sensitivity to the environment in middle childhood is not hard to find. Two intriguing and little-known examples concern the development of food preferences and erotic fetishes. In cultures where chili pepper is an essential part of the diet, children tend to dislike spicy food until middle childhood and then increase rapidly their preference for the flavor of chili as a result of social learning (Rozin 1990b). Fetishistic attractions also tend to form in middle childhood, with the onset of pleasurable sensations toward the object of the fetish (e.g., rubber, shoes) that later become fully eroticized (Lawrence 2009). The onset of fetishistic attractions is part of a generalized awakening of sexuality in middle childhood (Table 1) and illustrates the potential for rapid plasticity with long-lasting outcomes. Enhanced sensitivity to the environment extends beyond individual learning to acquiring social norms: for example, cross-cultural differences in prosocial behavior are absent in young children but emerge clearly during middle childhood (House et al. 2013).

On the genetic side of the equation, general intelligence and language skills increase markedly in heritability from early to middle childhood. In both cases, new genetic factors come into play around age 7 (Davis et al. 2009; Hayiou-Thomas et al. 2012). Studies of prosociality and aggression find the same pattern, with new genetic influences on behavior emerging during the transition to middle childhood (Knafo and Plomin 2006; van Beijsterveldt et al. 2003). These genetic findings dovetail with converging evidence that individual changes in levels of aggression are especially frequent during the transition to juvenility (Del Giudice et al. 2009).

4 Implications for Health Development

The main focus of this chapter has been on psychological development, but the implications of the evolutionary-developmental synthesis extend to both mental and physical health. The transition to middle childhood seems to be a switch point for a number of growth and metabolic processes that have long-term impact on health, including the risk for obesity and type 2 diabetes (Hochberg 2008, 2010). These processes become apparent in middle childhood (e.g., anticipated onset of the adiposity rebound, rapid weight gain, onset of insulin resistance), but respond to the accumulated effects of early nutrition and other sources of stress, starting from prenatal life (e.g., intrauterine growth restriction; see Salsberry et al. 2017). From the standpoint of the model presented here, one can predict that metabolic changes in middle childhood will reflect both the "programming" effects of the early environment (Gluckman et al. 2005) and the activation of new genetic factors. Consistent with this view, a recent study has documented significant genetic correlations between puberty timing, insulin levels, type 2 diabetes, and cardiovascular disease (Day et al. 2015). Moreover, some of those factors are likely to be expressed in sexually differentiated ways, and the different patterns of health risk associated with early adrenarche and puberty in boys and girls may be usefully interpreted in light of different constraints on life history trade-offs in the two sexes (see Hochberg 2010). These predictions are consistent with the nonlinear and multilevel nature of developmental processes—one of the guiding principles of LCHD emphasized in this volume.

Another intriguing implication of this perspective is that the juvenile transition may be a promising—and still virtually unexplored—developmental window for intervention. While intervening to change early life conditions may be desirable in view of their long-term effects, this approach is not always possible or realistic. In addition, prenatal factors such as fetal nutrition and gestational stress may be especially difficult to target, as they do not simply mirror the mother's conditions but reflect a complex—and partially conflictual—interplay between fetal and maternal factors (e.g., Del Giudice 2012; Gangestad et al. 2012; Haig 1993). However, the logic of developmental switches (Fig. 2) suggests that the activation of the mechanisms that initiate the switch (e.g., adrenarche) may correspond to a transient phase of instability and openness in the system. If so, it should be possible to exploit that phase to maximize the efficacy of focused interventions—including pharmacological ones. Of course, this would require a better understanding of how different hormonal and neurobiological systems interact during the transition to middle childhood; the existing evidence points to a central role of the hypothalamic-pituitary-adrenal (HPA) axis, the hypothalamic-pituitary-adrenal-thyroid (HPT) axis, and the insulin/insulin-like growth factor 1 (IGF-1) signaling systems as mediators of life history allocations, not just in humans but in other vertebrates as well (see Del Giudice et al. 2015; Ellis and Del Giudice 2014). Those systems might be used as direct targets for intervention, but also as "endophenotypes" or early indicators of the efficacy of interventions. Importantly, neurobiological systems such as the HPA axis regulate both metabolism and behavior—as components of coordinated life history allocations—so that many of the same processes may be relevant to both physical and mental health. The idea that intervening *during* a biological transition may afford more leverage to alter developmental trajectories resonates with two key principles of LCHD, that is, the nonlinearity of developmental processes and their time sensitivity.

Probably the most important take-home point of an evolutionary-developmental approach is that researchers should be more cautious in assuming that undesirable developmental outcomes reflect dysregulation of a biological system (e.g., see Kim et al. 2017) and more open to the possibility that those outcomes may be part of adaptive—or formerly adaptive—strategies for survival and reproduction. As I have argued in detail elsewhere (Del Giudice 2014b, c), a life history framework is especially useful in teasing out the logic of potentially adaptive combinations of traits, highlighting critical factors in the environment, and bridging behavioral development with physical growth trajectories. As an example, consider the association between intrauterine growth restriction and early maturation in children (Hochberg 2008, 2010). This can be interpreted as a manifestation of physiological dysregulation due to prenatal adversity or as an adaptive programming effect on children's metabolic processes and life history trajectories. This alternative interpretation is supported by the association between low birth weight, anticipated puberty, and early childbearing in women (e.g., Nettle et al. 2013). A third possibility is that low birth weight partly reflects reduced energetic and metabolic investment by the mother during pregnancy, which may be adaptive as a component of a fast life history strategy. If so, the association between reduced fetal growth and earlier sexual maturation may not be fully causal, but rather result—at least in part—from shared genetic, or epigenetic, factors that influence life history strategy in both the mother and the offspring. Clearly, the implications for intervention are going to be quite different depending on which of these scenarios apply.

Another recent example is the finding that early adrenarche is associated with reduced white matter volume in the frontal lobe of children (Klauser et al. 2015). Again, the standard interpretation is that early DHEA exposure has a disruptive effect on neurodevelopmental processes; however, it is also possible that different trajectories of brain development—and even associated "symptoms" such as anxiety and aggressive behaviors—may instead reflect alternative strategies on a fast-slow continuum of life history variation. Ellis et al. (2012) present an extended analysis of adolescent risk-taking from this perspective and discuss several implications for the design of interventions. The LCHD principle that evolution both enables and constrains plasticity is especially relevant in this regard; evolutionary scenarios are not just interesting explanatory "stories," but can illuminate limits as well as opportunities for intervention. For example, when considering mother-fetus interactions, the existence of partial conflicts of interest on nutrition, cortisol production, and so on suggests that interventions designed to favor the fetus may sometimes have detrimental side effects for the mother and vice versa (see Del Giudice 2014b; Haig 1993).

In considering potential adaptive explanations for apparently pathological outcomes, it is important to remember that biologically adaptive traits may carry substantial costs. Fitness is ultimately about reproductive success; natural selection does not necessarily promote psychological well-being or physical health and may sacrifice survival in exchange for enhanced reproduction. Moreover, even adaptive developmental processes may result in genuinely maladaptive outcomes for some individuals (Frankenhuis and Del Giudice 2012). It follows that the existence of substantial psychological, social, or health costs does not automatically qualify a trait or behavior as biologically maladaptive (see Del Giudice 2014b; Ellis et al. 2012; Ellis and Del Giudice 2014).

5 Conclusions

We cannot make sense of human development without understanding middle childhood and its many apparent paradoxes. An evolutionary-developmental approach illuminates the complexity of this life stage and shows how different levels of analysis—from genes to society—can be tied together in a coherent synthesis. This emerging view of middle childhood can help developmental scientists appreciate its centrality in the human life history and stimulate ideas for research and intervention. The study of middle childhood may finally be ready to come of age, opening up promising avenues for a better understanding of health development across the life course.

References

Auchus, R. J., & Rainey, W. E. (2004). Adrenarche–physiology, biochemistry and human disease. *Clinical Endocrinology, 60*, 288–296.

Bancroft, J. (Ed.). (2003). *Sexual development in childhood*. Bloomington: Indiana University Press.

Belsky, J., Steinberg, L., & Draper, P. (1991). Childhood experience, interpersonal development, and reproductive strategy: An evolutionary theory of socialization. *Child Development, 62*, 647–670.

Bernstein, R. M., Sterner, K. N., & Wildman, D. E. (2012). Adrenal androgen production in catarrhine primates and the evolution of adrenarche. *American Journal of Physical Anthropology, 147*, 389–400.

Best, J. R., Miller, P. H., & Jones, L. L. (2009). Executive functions after age 5: Changes and correlates. *Developmental Review, 29*, 180–200.

Bjorklund, D. F. (2011). *Children's thinking: Cognitive development and individual differences* (5th ed.). Belmont: Wadsworth.

Bogin, B. (1997). Evolutionary hypotheses for human childhood. *Yearbook of Physical Anthropology, 40*, 63–89.

Campbell, B. C. (2006). Adrenarche and the evolution of human life history. *American Journal of Human Biology, 18*, 569–589.

Campbell, B. C. (2011). Adrenarche and middle childhood. *Human Nature, 22*, 327–349.

Davis, O. S. P., Haworth, C. M. A., & Plomin, R. (2009). Dramatic increase in heritability of cognitive development from early to middle childhood: An 8-year longitudinal study of 8,700 pairs of twins. *Psychological Science, 20*, 1301–1308.

Day, F. R., Bulik-Sullivan, B., Hinds, D. A., Finucane, H. K., Murabito, J. M., Tung, J. Y., et al. (2015). Genetic determinants of puberty timing in men and women: Shared genetic aetiology between sexes and with health-related outcomes. *Nature Communications, 6*, 8842.

Del Giudice, M. (2009). Sex, attachment, and the development of reproductive strategies. *Behavioral and Brain Sciences, 32*, 1–21.

Del Giudice, M. (2012). Fetal programming by maternal stress: Insights from a conflict perspective. *Psychoneuroendocrinology, 37*, 1614–1629.

Del Giudice, M. (2014a). Middle childhood: An evolutionary-developmental synthesis. *Child Development Perspectives, 8*, 193–200.

Del Giudice, M. (2014b). Early stress and human behavioral development: Emerging evolutionary perspectives. *Journal of Developmental Origins of Health and Disease, 5*, 270–280.

Del Giudice, M. (2014c). An evolutionary life history framework for psychopathology. *Psychological Inquiry, 25*, 261–300.

Del Giudice, M., & Angeleri, R. (2016). Digit ratio (2D:4D) and attachment styles in middle childhood: Indirect evidence for an organizational effect of sex hormones. *Adaptive Human Behavior and Physiology, 2*, 1–10.

Del Giudice, M., & Belsky, J. (2010). Sex differences in attachment emerge in middle childhood: An evolutionary hypothesis. *Child Development Perspectives, 4*, 97–105.

Del Giudice, M., & Belsky, J. (2011). The development of life history strategies: Toward a multi-stage theory. In D. M. Buss & P. H. Hawley (Eds.), *The evolution of personality and individual differences*, (pp. 154–176). New York: Oxford University Press.

Del Giudice, M., Angeleri, R., & Manera, V. (2009). The juvenile transition: A developmental switch point in human life history. *Developmental Review, 29*, 1–31.

Del Giudice, M., Ellis, B. J., & Shirtcliff, E. A. (2011). The adaptive calibration model of stress responsivity. *Neuroscience & Biobehavioral Reviews, 35*, 1562–1592.

Del Giudice, M., Angeleri, R., & Manera, V. (2012). Juvenility and the juvenile transition. In R. J. R. Levesque (Ed.), *Encyclopedia of adolescence*, (pp. 1534–1537). New York: Springer.

Del Giudice, M., Gangestad, S. W., & Kaplan, H. S. (2015). Life history theory and evolutionary psychology. In D. M. Buss (Ed.), *The handbook of evolutionary psychology – Vol 1: Foundations* (2nd ed., pp. 88–114). New York: Wiley.

Del Giudice, M., & Angeleri, R. (2016). Digit ratio (2D:4D) and attachment styles in middle childhood: Indirect evidence for an organizational effect of sex hormones. *Adaptive Human Behavior and Physiology, 2*, 1–10.

Ellis, B. J. (2013). The hypothalamic-pituitary-gonadal axis: A switch-controlled, condition-sensitive system in the regulation of life history strategies. *Hormones and Behavior, 64*, 215–225.

Ellis, B. J., & Del Giudice, M. (2014). Beyond allostatic load: Rethinking the role of stress in regulating human development. *Development and Psychopathology, 26*, 1–20.

Ellis, B. J., & Essex, M. J. (2007). Family environments, adrenarche and sexual maturation: A longitudinal test of a life history model. *Child Development, 78*, 1799–1817.

Ellis, B. J., Figueredo, A. J., Brumbach, B. H., & Schlomer, G. L. (2009). The impact of harsh versus unpredictable environments on the evolution and development of life history strategies. *Human Nature, 20*, 204–268.

Ellis, B. J., Del Giudice, M., Dishion, T. J., Figueredo, A. J., Gray, P., Griskevicius, V., et al. (2012). The evolutionary basis of risky adolescent behavior: Implications for science, policy, and practice. *Developmental Psychology, 48*, 598–623.

Frankenhuis, W. E., & Del Giudice, M. (2012). When do adaptive developmental mechanisms yield maladaptive outcomes? *Developmental Psychology, 48*, 628–642.

Gangestad, S. W., Caldwell Hooper, A. E., & Eaton, M. A. (2012). On the function of placental corticotropin-releasing hormone: A role in maternal-fetal conflicts over blood glucose concentrations. *Biological Reviews, 87*, 856–873.

Geary, D. C. (2010). *Male, female: The evolution of human sex differences*. Washington, DC: American Psychological Association.

Ghetti, S., & Bunge, S. A. (2012). Neural changes underlying the development of episodic memory during middle childhood. *Developmental Cognitive Neuroscience, 2*, 381–395.

Giedd, J. N., & Rapoport, J. L. (2010). Structural MRI of pediatric brain development: What have we learned and where are we going? *Neuron, 67*, 728–734.

Gluckman, P. D., Hanson, M. A., & Spencer, H. G. (2005). Predictive adaptive responses and human evolution. *Trends in Ecology & Evolution, 20*, 527–533.

Haig, D. (1993). Genetic conflicts in human pregnancy. *QUARTERLY REVIEW OF BIOLOGY, 68*, 495–532.

Hawley, P. H. (2014). Ontogeny and social dominance: A developmental view of human power patterns. *Evolutionary Psychology, 12*, 318–342.

Hayiou-Thomas, M. E., Dale, P. S., & Plomin, R. (2012). The etiology of variation in language skills changes with development: A longitudinal twin study of language from 2 to 12 years. *Developmental Science, 15*, 233–249.

Herdt, G., & McClintock, M. (2000). The magical age of 10. *Archives of Sexual Behavior, 29*, 587–606.

Hochberg, Z. (2008). Juvenility in the context of life history theory. *Archives of Disease in Childhood, 93*, 534–539.

Hochberg, Z. (2010). Evo-devo of child growth III: Premature juvenility as an evolutionary trade-off. *Hormone Research in Pædiatrics, 73*, 430–437.

House, B. R., Silk, J. B., Henrich, J., Barrett, H. C., Scelza, B. A., Boyette, A. H., et al. (2013). Ontogeny of prosocial behavior across diverse societies. *Proceedings of the National Academy of Sciences USA, 110*, 14586–14591.

Jambon, M., & Smetana, J. G. (2014). Moral complexity in middle childhood: Children's evaluations of necessary harm. *Developmental Psychology, 50*, 22–33.

Joffe, T. H. (1997). Social pressures have selected for an extended juvenile period in primates. *Journal of Human Evolution, 32*, 593–605.

Kaplan, H., Hill, K., Lancaster, J., & Hurtado, A. M. (2000). A theory of human life history evolution: Diet, intelligence, and longevity. *Evolutionary Anthropology, 9*, 156–185.

Kim, P., Evans, G. W., Chen, E., Miller, G., & Seeman, T. (2017). How socioeconomic disadvantages get under the skin and into the brain to influence health development across the lifespan. In N. Halfon, C. B. Forrest, R. M. Lerner, & E. Faustman (Eds.), *Handbook of life course health-development science*. Cham: Springer.

Klauser, P., Whittle, S., Simmons, J. G., Byrne, M. L., Mundy, L. K., Patton, G. C., et al. (2015). Reduced frontal white matter volume in children with early onset of adrenarche. *Psychoneuroendocrinology, 52*, 111–118.

Knafo, A., & Plomin, R. (2006). Prosocial behavior from early to middle childhood: Genetic and environmental influences on stability and change. *Developmental Psychology, 42*, 771–786.

Kramer, K. L. (2011). The evolution of human parental care and recruitment of juvenile help. *Trends in Ecology and Evolution, 26*, 533–540.

Kuzawa, C. W., Chugani, H. T., Grossman, L. I., Lipovich, L., Muzik, O., Hof, P. R., et al. (2014). Metabolic costs and evolutionary implications of human brain development. *Proceedings of the National Academy of Sciences of the United States of America, 111*, 13010–13015.

Lagattuta, K. H., Sayfan, L., & Blattman, A. J. (2009). Forgetting common ground: Six- to seven-year-olds have an overinterpretive theory of mind. *Developmental Psychology, 46*, 1417–1432.

Lancy, D. F., & Grove, M. A. (2011). Getting noticed: Middle childhood in cross-cultural perspective. *Human Nature, 22*, 281–302.

Lawrence, A. A. (2009). Erotic target location errors: An underappreciated paraphilic dimension. *Journal of Sex Research, 46*, 194–215.

Lebel, C., Walker, L., Leemans, A., Phillips, L., & Beaulieu, C. (2008). Microstructural maturation of the human brain from childhood to adulthood. *NeuroImage, 40*, 1044–1055.

Locke, J. L., & Bogin, B. (2006). Language and life history: A new perspective on the development and evolution of human language. *Behavioral and Brain Sciences, 29*, 259–280.

Martel, M. M. (2013). Sexual selection and sex differences in the prevalence of childhood externalizing and adolescent internalizing disorders. *Psychological Bulletin, 139*, 1221–1259.

McClelland, M., Morrison, F., Gestsdóttir, S., Cameron, C., Bowers, E. D., Duckworth, A., Little, T., & Grammer. J. (2017). Self-regulation. In N. Halfon, C. B. Forrest, R. M. Lerner, & E. Faustman (Eds.), *Handbook of life course health-development science*. Cham: Springer.

Meaney, M. J. (2010). Epigenetics and the biological definition of gene x environment interactions. *Child Development, 81*, 41–79.

Nettle, D., Dickins, T. E., Coall, D. A., & de Mornay Davies, P. (2013). Patterns of physical and psychological development in future teenage mothers. *Evolution, Medicine, and Public Health, 2013*, 187–196.

Piccardi, L., Leonzi, M., D'Amico, S., Marano, A., & Guariglia, C. (2014). Development of navigational working memory: Evidence from 6- to 10-year-old children. *British Journal of Developmental Psychology, 32*, 205–217.

Poirel, N., Simon, G., Cassotti, M., Leroux, G., Perchey, G., Lanoë, C., Lubin, A., Turbelin, M. R., Rossi, S., Pineau, A., & Houdé, O. (2011). The shift from local to global visual processing in 6-year-old children is associated with grey matter loss. *PloS One, 6*, e20879.

Rozin, P. (1990a). Development in the food domain. *Developmental Psychology, 26*, 555–562.

Rozin, P. (1990b). Getting to like the burn of chili pepper: Biological, psychological, and cultural perspectives. In B. G. Green, J. R. Mason, & M. R. Kare (Eds.), *Chemical senses – Volume 2: Irritation*. New York: Dekker.

Salsberry, P., Tanda, R., Anderson, S. E., & Kamboj, M. K. (2017). Pediatric type 2 diabetes: Prevention and treatment through a life course health development framework. In N. Halfon, C. B. Forrest, R. M. Lerner, & E. Faustman (Eds.), *Handbook of life course health-development science*. Cham: Springer.

Scalise Sugiyama, M. (2011). The forager oral tradition and the evolution of prolonged juvenility. *Frontiers in Psychology, 2*, 133.

van Beijsterveldt, T. C. E. M., Bartels, M., Hudziak, J. J., & Boomsma, D. I. (2003). Causes of stability of aggression from early childhood to adolescence: A longitudinal genetic analysis in Dutch twins. *Behavior Genetics, 33*, 591–605.

Weisner, T. S. (1996). The 5–7 transition as an ecocultural project. In A. Sameroff & M. Haith (Eds.), *The five to seven year shift: The age of reason and responsibility* (pp. 295–326). Chicago: University of Chicago Press.

Wells, J. C. K. (2007). Sexual dimorphism of body composition. *Best Practice & Research Clinical Endocrinology & Metabolism, 21*, 415–430.

West-Eberhard, M. J. (2003). *Developmental plasticity and evolution*. New York: Oxford University Press.

Adolescent Health Development: A Relational Developmental Systems Perspective

Richard M. Lerner, Claire D. Brindis, Milena Batanova, and Robert Wm. Blum

Consistent with the United Nations Conventions, adolescence encompasses the second decade of life (Lerner and Steinberg 2009). Since the emergence of the study of this portion of the life course (Hall 1904), adolescence has been regarded as a period characterized by purportedly troublesome transformations (e.g., in bodily attributes associated with puberty; Susman and Dorn 2009, 2013) and allegedly problematic transitions (e.g., in regard to socioemotional functions linked to self-definition or identity, Erikson 1959, or to changes in the focus of social relationships, from parents to peers, Freud 1969). When viewed from this "deficit" model, adolescents were seen by both scholars and the general public as both dangerous to themselves and to society (Anthony 1969). They were regarded as "problems to be managed" (Roth and Brooks-Gunn 2003a, b).

Certainly, it may be argued that adolescence is the most profound period of change within the life span. As in infancy and early to middle childhood, the individual's physiological, psychological, behavioral, and social relationship characteristics undergo both quantitative and qualitative changes, that is, transitions and transformations. For instance, changes in the prefrontal cortex, increases in the interconnectivity among brain regions, and increases in dopamine levels provide both vulnerabilities to risk and opportunities for growth in cognitive control (Steinberg 2010). At the same time, most youth in Western societies are experiencing great contextual changes, such as changing schools (e.g., Eccles 2004) and the increased relevance of peer influences on behavior (e.g., Gardner and Steinberg 2005). Moreover, in adolescence, the individual has the cognitive, behavioral, and social relational skills to contribute actively and often effectively to his or her own developmental changes (Lerner 1982; Lerner and Busch-Rossnagel 1981; Lerner and Walls 1999; Ricco and Overton 2011). In contrast to earlier developmental periods, adolescents have a burgeoning capacity

---

The original version of this chapter was revised. An erratum to this chapter can be found at https://doi.org/10.1007/978-3-319-47143-3_27

The writing of this chapter was supported in part by grants from the John Templeton Foundation. We are grateful to Elizabeth Goodman for her comments

R.M. Lerner, PhD (✉)
Tufts University, Medford, MA, USA
e-mail: Richard.lerner@tufts.edu

M. Batanova, PhD
Institute for Applied Research in Youth Development, Tufts University, Medford, MA, USA

C.D. Brindis, DrPH
University of California-San Francisco (UCSF), Philip R. Lee Institute for Health Policy Studies and the Adolescent and Young Adult Health National Resource Center, San Francisco, CA, USA

R.Wm. Blum, MD, MPH, PhD
Johns Hopkins Bloomberg School of Public Health, Baltimore, MD, USA

N. Halfon et al. (eds.), *Handbook of Life Course Health Development*,
DOI 10.1007/978-3-319-47143-3_6

for self-governance, for formulating and taking actions that exert at least some control over their own development. That is, there is uniquely marked development of intentional agency in adolescence. Agency involves self-regulatory skills that include, for instance, the *selection* of goals or the formulation of purposes that are of importance to adolescents' developing senses of self and growing attempts to find a means to "matter" in their world (Eccles 2004; Freund and Baltes 2002; Mascolo and Fischer 2015). There is also growth in the use of executive functioning, strategic thinking, and behavioral skills in recruiting goal-related resources that enable actions *optimizing* the chances of fulfilling their purposes. Furthermore, there is also development of the ability to *compensate* effectively when goals are blocked and/or to select new goals when initial optimization attempts fail and the chances of attaining an initial goal are lost (Gestsdottir and Lerner 2008; McClelland et al. 2015).

In general, scholars who study the adolescent period acknowledge that multiple dimensions of change involving the individual and his or her context characterize this portion of the life span (Lerner et al. 2015; Lerner and Steinberg 2009). However, substantial variation has emerged in scholars' approach to this individual-context relationship. Analogous to interpreting only main effects of statistical analyses framed by the General Linear Model, some scholars have focused on one domain of change (e.g., adolescent identity development) and have not emphasized other levels of organization within the ecology of human development (e.g., see Marcia 1980). Other scholars have taken a reductionist orientation to the phenomena of adolescence and have sought to use biogenic ideas (e.g., genetic or evolutionary biological ideas; see Bjorkland and Ellis, 2005) to interpret all psychological and social relationship phenomena of the period (see Elder 1980, 1998; Elder et al. 2015, for critiques of the main effect or reductionist approaches).

In turn, however, in 2003, Roth and Brooks-Gunn (2003a, b) reviewed the literature on youth development programs aimed at enhancing health and thriving among adolescents. They concluded that adolescents should be regarded not as problems to be managed but, instead, as resources to be developed. Their insight built on at least three sources. First, Larson (2000) provided a compelling vision for research aimed at emphasizing the strengths of adolescence (e.g., involving their burgeoning capacities for intentional self-regulation) and for using these strengths to promote positive youth development (PYD). Instead of health or positive development being conceptualized as the diminution or the absence of disease or of problem behaviors, respectively, the PYD perspective suggested that there were facets of thriving that, when promoted, resulted in healthy and positive development. Second, Eccles and Gootman (2002) edited a field-defining report issued by the National Academy of Sciences about the ways in which community programs for youth development could promote several attributes of psychological and behavioral functioning believed to be indicative of such development. The report included a summary of the attributes of positive development as involving constructs that could be summarized by "Five Cs:" competence, confidence, character, connection, and caring (see too, Lerner et al. 2005). Third, Hamilton (1999) explained that the idea of PYD was being used in the developmental science literature in three ways: (a) as a label for a model of the processes through which health and thriving developed in adolescence, (b) as a philosophy for or an approach to designing community-based programs aimed at promoting thriving, and (c) as instances of such programs.

The emphasis on strengths as compared to deficits and on links between the positive development of youth and their engagement with contextual resources or ecological "developmental assets" (Benson et al. 2006), represented by community-based youth development programs, reflected the spirit of the times (the *zeitgeist*) of developmental science during the latter years of the twentieth century and the first decade of the twenty-first century (Lerner 2012; Lerner et al. 2015). Conceptions of human development, which in earlier periods stressed genetic or maturational determinants of development or approaches to development that reduced human behavior to stimulus-response relations, were being replaced by ideas emphasizing that development involved mutually influential relations among a person's biological and psychological characteristics, social relationships, and influences from families, schools, community institutions, out-of-school-time (OST) programs, and both the designed and natural environment.

Developmental scientists argued that all of these influences, although always present across life, change in their significance across both life and across historical periods (e.g., Bronfenbrenner and Morris 2006; Lerner 2012; Overton 2013, 2015). Indeed, we explain below that, today, these ideas have a new manifestation quite compatible with the PYD perspective: They are found in the seven principles of life course health development (see Halfon and Forrest 2017) that address the conceptualization of the nature and bases of health and positive behavior development across the life span.

Therefore, in the contemporary study of adolescent development, the main effect and reductionist approaches of the past are regarded as anachronistic ideas incapable of producing models that adequately account for the integration of multiple levels of organization within the ecology of human development (Lerner 2015; Lerner and Benson 2013a, b; Lerner et al. 2015). In particular, such traditional approaches overlook the burgeoning information indicating that this integration reflects systemic relations, that is, mutually influential patterns of covariation within and across these levels (e.g., see von Bertalanffy 1933, 1968). At this writing, then, models of adolescent development that are associated with what Overton has explained as a relational developmental systems (RDS) metatheory define the cutting edge of theory-predicated scholarship about adolescent development. This metatheory is derived from a process-relational paradigm (Overton 2015), and the concepts associated with RDS thinking are being used to describe, explain, and optimize the course of development in the second decade of life and, as such, to frame applied research aimed at promoting health and positive development among diverse adolescents (Lerner et al. 2015).

It is not coincidental that concepts associated with the RDS metatheory are entirely consistent with the seven life course health development principles proposed by Halfon and Forrest (2017). This congruence of ideas is based on a few common scholarly roots of these two sets of ideas for understanding human development. For example, the life course conceptions of Elder (1998; Elder et al. 2015), the life span developmental ideas of Baltes (e.g., 1997; Baltes et al. 2006), and the constructs associated with Bronfenbrenner's (1979, 2005; Bronfenbrenner and Morris 2006) bioecological model of human development have shaped both RDS thinking and the life course health development principles. It will be useful, then, to discuss the features of the RDS metatheory and, in this context, point to the compatibility between RDS concepts and the life course health development principles. This discussion will enable us to illustrate how the ideas associated with both approaches to adolescent development can innovatively integrate and extend scholarship about transitions and transformations characterizing the adolescent period. In addition, because of the emphasis in both sets of ideas on the concept of relative *plasticity* in human development—that is, on the potential for systematic changes in the structure and function of health assets across the life course—we will discuss how these two approaches afford optimism that relational changes linked to positive change in the health developmental system can be identified and used to promote thriving in adolescence.

1 Viewing Adolescent Development Through the Lens of the Relational Developmental Systems Metatheory

The study of human development, in general, and adolescent development, more specifically, has evolved from a field dominated by split, reductionist (psychogenic or biogenic) approaches to a multidisciplinary scholarly field (Lerner and Steinberg 2009), one that seeks to integrate variables from biological through cultural and historical levels of organization across the life span into a synthetic, coactional system (e.g., Elder 1998; Ford and Lerner 1992; Gottlieb 1997, 1998; Lerner 2012). Reductionist accounts of development that adhere to a Cartesian dualism pull apart (split) facets of the integrated developmental system (Overton 2015). For instance, reductionist views typically elevate the importance of such split formulations as nature versus nurture, continuity versus discontinuity, stability versus instability, or basic versus applied science (Lerner 2002, 2006).

Split approaches are rejected by proponents of theories derived from an RDS metatheory (e.g., Mistry and Wu 2010; Overton 2013; Overton and Lerner 2014), which in turn are derived from a process-relational paradigm (Overton 2015). Across the past four plus decades, several scholars have provided ideas contributing to the evolution of this paradigm (e.g., Baltes 1997; Baltes, et al., 2006; Brandtstädter 1998; Bronfenbrenner 1979, 2005; Bronfenbrenner and Morris 2006; Elder 1998; Elder et al. 2015; Ford and Lerner 1992; Nesselroade 1988; Overton 1973; Overton and Reese 1981; Riegel 1975, 1976; and, even earlier, see von Bertalanffy 1933).

Overton (e.g., 2013, 2015) has integrated and extended this scholarship. Overton explains that, compared to a Cartesian worldview, the process-relational paradigm focuses on process (systematic changes in the developmental system), becoming (moving from potential to actuality; a developmental process as having a past, present, and future; Whitehead 1929/1978), holism (the meanings of entities and events derive from the context in which they are embedded), relational analysis (assessment of the mutually influential relations within the developmental system), and the use of multiple perspectives and explanatory forms (employment of ideas from multiple theory-based models of change within and of the developmental system) in understanding human development. Within the process-relational paradigm, the organism is seen as inherently active, self-creating (autopoietic), self-organizing, self-regulating (agentic), nonlinear/complex, and adaptive (Overton 2015; see too Sokol et al. 2015). Similarly, these ideas are echoed in the life course health development principles (specifically, Nos. 1 and 3) that health development emerges as a consequence of complex, nonlinear process that results from person⇔environment coactions that are multidimensional, multidirectional, and multilevel.

Accordingly, both within the RDS approach to theory and the life course health development principles, split conceptions are eschewed in favor of a metatheory that emphasizes the study and integration of different levels of organization, ranging from biology/physiology to culture and history, as a means to understand life span human development (Lerner 2006; Overton 2013, 2015), the production of health, and the development of disease. Accordingly, conceptual emphasis is placed on mutually influential relations between individuals and contexts, represented as individual ⇔ context relations.

This representation of the coactions between person and setting within RDS-based models is not meant to convey a person-context interaction—which is typically represented in the developmental literature as person X context. An interaction connotes that the entities involved in the relation are separate and independent (as in a statistical interaction) and that, as such, their association involves a linear combination of discrete and separate variables. Both before and after the interaction, these entities (variables) are independent and unchanged by each other. The bidirectional arrow used in the RDS illustration of person ⇔ context relations is intended to emphasize that the coaction of individual and context involves the entire developmental system. As such, the relations among levels of the autopoietic system, and not independent linear combinatorial attributes, are the focus in such a model. Indeed, the fusion of individual and context within the developmental system means that across ontogeny (across the life span), any portion of the system is inextricably embedded with—or embodied by, in Overton's (2013, 2015) conceptualization—all other portions of the developmental system. Embodiment refers to the way individuals behave, experience, and live in the world by being active agents with particular kinds of bodies; the body is integratively understood as a form (a biological referent), as lived experience (a psychological referent), and as an entity in active engagement with the world (a sociocultural referent) (Overton 2015).

Similarly, within the life course health development perspective, health development is also embodied: It is an emergent property of living systems (Principle 1), and it develops continuously across the life span (Principle 2).

Within the context of such a bidirectional relational system, the embeddedness within history (temporality) is of fundamental significance (Elder 1998; Elder et al. 2015). We may note that the developmental system is embedded in history (temporality). This embeddedness means that change is constant in the developmental system and that, as such, there may be either stochastic or systematic changes in person⇔context relations *across time and place* (Elder 1998; Elder et al. 2015; Misteli 2013). Sensitivity of change to time and place is also a key idea within the life course health development Principle 4, which states that health development is highly sensitive to the timing and social structure of environmental exposures. The presence of such temporality in individual ⇔ context relations within the developmental system means that there always exists some potential for systematic change and, thus, for (relative) plasticity in human development. In short, potential plasticity in individual ⇔ context relations derives from the "arrow of time" (Lerner 1984; Lerner and Benson 2013a, b; Overton 2013) running through the integrated (relational) developmental system.

2 Three Moments of Analysis in an RDS Approach to Adolescent Health Development

To elucidate the role of time and place in contributing to the bidirectional relations of focal concern within RDS metatheory, developmental scientists may focus on either the role of the individual or the context, in particular instantiations of individual⇔context exchanges. This focus may seem contradictory to the fusion among levels of organization emphasized in this approach. However, as we noted earlier, Overton (2015) embeds the RDS metatheory in the process-relational paradigm (see, as well, Sokol et al. 2015). Overton uses this paradigm to explain the possibility of this changing focus in developmental analysis. He notes that the process-relational paradigm involves different moments within a research program.

One moment involves the idea of the identity of opposites, a second moment involves the opposites of identity, and a third (relationally integrative) moment involves the synthesis of wholes. In discussing these three moments of scientific analysis within RDS approaches to developmental science, we point to the predominant trait model of individuality, the Five-Factor Theory (FFT, involving the purported Big Five "personality traits" of conscientiousness, agreeableness, neuroticism, openness to experience, and extraversion; Costa and McCrae 1980, 2006; McCrae et al. 2000). The FFT example is a means to explain these RDS-based moments and to contrast their use with thinking associated with Cartesian, split, reductionist approaches to the study of the individual development.

The first moment recognizes that both individual and context define— and are mutually constituted by—each other in one moment, or point, in a program of developmental inquiry. Overton (2010, p. 14) notes that:

> The principle of the identity of opposites establishes the identity among parts of a whole by casting them not as exclusive contradictions as in the split epistemology, but as differentiated polarities (i.e., coequals) of a unified (i.e., indissociable) inclusive matrix—as a relation. As differentiations, each pole defines and is defined by its opposite.

The identity of opposites, therefore, emphasizes the fused person ⇔ context relationship as the primary unit of analysis for understanding development. As such, in this moment of research, developmental scientists would reject the idea that there are any aspects of human *behavioral* development— for instance, entities such as traits—that "are more or less immune to environmental influences" (McCrae et al. 2000, pp. 175); the idea that such entities are indicators of split notions reflecting "nature over nurture" (McCrae et al. 2000, p. 173) would also be rejected by developmental scientists working within this first moment of analysis.

The second moment that Overton (2010, 2013, 2015; Overton and Müller 2013) discusses is the opposites of identity. This moment allows one, in effect, to hold the other parts of the integrated system in abeyance and focus on one part of the system; however, the ultimate aim is one of reintegrating the part into the whole at a subsequent moment. Overton (2013, pp. 47–48) explains that:

> The limitation of the identity moment of analysis is that, in establishing a flow of categories of one into the other, a stable base for inquiry that was provided by bedrock material atoms of the split metatheory is eliminated...Reestablishing a stable base—not an absolute fixity, nor an absolute relativity, but a relative relativity (Latour 1993)—within relational metatheory requires moving to a second moment of analysis. In this moment of opposition, the law of contradiction is reasserted and categories again exclude each other. As a consequence of this exclusion, parts exhibit unique identities that differentiate each from the other.

Therefore, when functioning within this second moment of analysis, developmental scientists could focus solely on attributes of individuals, for instance, the purported traits of conscientiousness, agreeableness, neuroticism, openness to experience, and extraversion that comprise the Big Five components of the FFT (Costa and McCrae 1980, 2006; McCrae et al. 2000) and, for instance, study the psychometric properties of these constructs to provide "objective," or quantitative, indices of these attributes. Indeed, such psychometric work has often been a part of research programs framed by RDS models (e.g., Damon 2008; Lerner et al. 2015). Thus, working within this second moment of analysis, developmental scientists following an RDS-based model, and social or personality researchers using a Cartesian split model, would be engaging in commensurate work. However, the difference between these two groups of scholars is brought to the fore when the third moment of analysis discussed by Overton (2015) is considered.

The third moment, the synthesis of wholes, occurs when the first two moments are embedded in a multi-perspective process-relational paradigm and are recognized as mutually necessary in a systematic, integrative program of research, wherein one needs both of the first two moments. That is, "A complete relational program requires principles according to which the individual identity of each concept of a formerly dichotomous pair is maintained while simultaneously it is affirmed that each concept constitutes, and is constituted by the other" (Overton and Müller 2013, p. 35).

Accordingly, the developmental scientist working within an RDS model would use an "objective" measure studied within the second moment of analysis within an integrated, relational empirical approach that focused on the individual⇔context relation. Clearly, the trait theorist would not take such a step, given that the work of such scholars is framed by the ideas, noted above, that context is irrelevant to the understanding (i.e., successful prediction) of the life course of the manifestation of traits. Indeed, in their belief "that personality traits are more or less immune to environmental influences" (McCrae et al. 2000, pp. 175), trait theorists maintain that contextual conditions, whether similar or not, are irrelevant to prediction; given the purported biological base of traits, only nature variables have predictive efficacy.

However, there is abundant evidence that purported traits are in fact not "trait-like" at all, that is, these attributes reflect relations between individuals and contexts, as they occur at particular times and places (Ardelt 2000; Block 1995, 2010; Elder 1998; Elder et al. 2015; Roberts et al. 2006). Indeed, methodological work framed by RDS concepts (e.g., Molenaar and Nesselroade 2014, 2015; Nesselroade 1988; Nesselroade and Molenaar 2010) indicates that the purported life span stability of traits, as well as the purported immunity to contextual influences, is empirically counterfactual. Moreover, underscoring the importance of this third moment of analysis discussed by Overton (2015), these methodological innovations demonstrate the ability to index with psychometric precision integrative individual ⇔ context (including individual ⇔ individual) units of analysis (e.g., Molenaar 2014; Molenaar et al. 2014; Molenaar and Nesselroade 2015). This innovation in developmental methodology is important for understanding key features of the individual⇔context relational process propelling developmental change in adolescence.

3 Developmental Regulations, Adaptive Developmental Regulations, and Human Agency in RDS Metatheory

Given the analytic moment of the identity of opposites—that each component of the developmental system constitutes, and is constituted by, the other components of the system—RDS metatheory focuses on the "rules" or processes which govern, or regulate, exchanges between individuals and their contexts. Such processes are the function of the developmental system. An RDS program of research might seek to understand the nature of relations between individuals and their contexts, including the dynamics of those relations across the life course. For instance, RDS-based research might ask how specific features of the individual and specific features of the context coalesce to influence the substantive course of individual⇔individual relations.

Brandtstädter (1998) termed these bidirectional relations "developmental regulations" and noted that, when developmental regulations involve mutually beneficial individual⇔context relations, then these developmental regulations are adaptive. Developmental regulations are the fundamental feature of human life, that is, all human life exists in a context and involves bidirectional exchanges with it (Darwin 1859; Forrest 2014; Tobach and Schneirla 1968). These exchanges involve physiological systems and functions (e.g., respiration, circulation, digestion, reproduction) and behaviors (e.g., social affiliation and cooperation, or aggression and competition, as might be involved in protection, hunting, and scavenging; Johanson and Edey 1981) and involve both organismic self-regulation (e.g., hypothalamic functioning, circadian rhythms) and intentional self-regulation (e.g., goal selection, resource recruitment, and executive functioning; Gestsdóttir and Lerner 2008).

Gestsdóttir et al. (2014) note that self-regulation is a multidimensional construct, involving a range of behaviors, from basic physiological functions to complex intentional cognitive processes (e.g., Bandura 2001; Brandtstädter 1998; McClelland et al. 2015). As such, self-regulation pertains to all aspects of adaption, as people alter their thoughts, attention, emotions, and behaviors to react to contextual events and, as well, to influence selected features of their contexts. Here, culture plays a key moderating role. Trommsdorff (2012) notes that self-regulation "is assumed to develop by organizing inner mental processes and behavior in line with cultural values, social expectations, internalized standards, and one's self-construal" (p. 19).

The developmental course of self-regulation is, in effect, the developmental course of human agency in the context of individual desires, purposes, needs, goals and identity, perceptions of and coactions with other people, the physical ecology, and culture (e.g., Damon 2008; Geldhof et al. 2010; Gestsdóttir and Lerner 2008; Lerner et al. 2001). Agency is a defining feature of the active, self-creating (autopoietic, enactive), and nonlinear adaptive living system (Overton and Lerner 2014; Narvaez 2008; Witherington 2014). Such agency is the individual's contribution to adaptive developmental regulations (Brandtstädter 1998, 1999).

The development of agency begins in early life, primarily with organismic self-regulation processes. However, as we have noted, by the time of adolescence, self-regulation is increasingly intentional and purposeful (Damon 2008) and involves the self-system and the phenomena associated with identity development (Gestsdóttir and Lerner 2008; Lerner et al. 2001). The adolescent instantiation of agency reflects ideas associated with the work of comparative psychologists Tobach and Schneirla (1968), who distinguished between the biosocial functioning of insects (e.g., ants) and the psychosocial functioning of organisms with higher psychological levels, levels that are marked by greater plasticity, rather than stereotypy, in their eventual highest levels of ontogenetic change. Such higher levels provide the physiological base for symbolic functioning.

In turn, reflecting the life course health development principles that evolution enables as well as constrains health development pathways and plasticity (Principle No. 5) and that optimal health development promotes survival, enhances thriving, and protects against disease (Principle No. 6), evolutionary biologists Jablonka and Lamb (2005) note that both psychological processes and cultural processes are integrated with the genetic and epigenetic processes of evolution to make human adaptiveness and contributions qualitatively different than corresponding instances of adaptiveness of social contributions among other organisms. Together, these comparative psychology and evolutionary biology literatures suggest that, among humans, adaptiveness and positive contributions reflect integrated cognitive, emotional, and behavioral processes that involve abstract, symbolic constructs, such as language or moral reasoning, or character virtues (e.g., Lerner and Callina 2014).

4 Implications for Research About Adolescent Health Development

Empirically, indexing such facets of adolescent health development, in general, or the complex dimensions of evolutionary change linked to adolescent health development more specifically (e.g., Gissis and Jablonka 2011; Lerner et al. 2015; Slavich and Cole 2013) may involve both point-in-time (cross-sectional) assessments and historical (longitudinal) assessments (Lerner 2004). Scientists must conduct such assessments within the context of recognizing that contexts are complex (e.g., they exist at multiple levels of organization; Bronfenbrenner 1979). Individuals cannot necessarily act in ways that benefit all levels and all components of the context at all times and places (Elder 1998). Thus, adaption is not treated as a categorical concept (as something that either exists or not) but, instead, as a multivariate concept comprised of ordinal or interval dimensions. Researchers studying adaptation would not ask, then, whether it exists or not; rather, the question would be how beneficial is the developmental regulation (the individual⇔context relation) for specific people or specific social institutions of the context, at specific times and in specific places (e.g., see Bornstein 2006, 2017).

Consistent both with the seventh principle of life course health development, that is, that the cadence of human health development results from the synchronized timing of variables from all levels of the developmental systems—that is, molecular, physiological, behavioral, cultural, and evolutionary processes (e.g., Cole 2014; Meaney 2014; Slavich and Cole 2013)—and with the Bornstein (2017) "specificity principle," we suggest, therefore, that addressing a multipart "what" question is the key to conducting programmatic research about the function, structure, and content of health development in adolescence. In other words, to test RDS-based ideas about the ontogenetically changing structure of adolescent development in general and health development more specifically, researchers need to ascertain answers to the following multipart "what" questions:

1. What specific structure-content relations emerge; at
2. What specific levels of organization within the relational developmental system that are linked to;
3. What specific antecedent and consequent adaptive developmental regulations (to what trajectory of individual⇔context relations); at
4. What specific points in adolescent development; for
5. What specific groups of youth; living in
6. What specific contexts; at
7. What specific points in time (history)?

Such work may have several benefits. Questions about coherence and reliability or consistency of indicators of health development with respect to variation in context may be especially useful for understanding the developmental course of multidimensional, latent variable conceptions of health among diverse adolescents. For instance, are specific indicators of, say, cardiovascular, respiratory, nutritional, or mental health manifested consistently across time and place? To what extent and for whom and under which conditions can biologic propensities to such health developmental challenges be moderated?

Consider nutrition more closely. How do adolescents' diets influence their cardio-metabolic risk as adolescents and adults? Do adolescents maintain a healthy diet across different settings involving peers and family members? Is there age-associated variation in answers to this question, for instance, variation associated with pubertal development or pubertal status/stage (e.g., early, on time, or late)? Do answers to these questions vary in relation to gender? As well, do they vary in relation to normative social transitions (e.g., moving from elementary school to middle school)? How do peer social networks influence these behaviors or family mealtime behaviors? Are answers moderated or changed by the socioeconomic, cultural, religious, or national contexts of youth? In turn, do answers here vary in relation to media exposure about eating and about desirable body types that may be prevalent for youth living in particular settings at particular times in history? Given the synchronization issues raised by the seventh life course health development principle, how are all these answers moderated or changed by what may be nonnormative life or historical events in the lives of adolescents (Baltes et al. 2006)? Examples here may be the death of a parent or deployment in the military (Cozza and Lerner 2013), family disruption due to divorce or separation, or family challenges in the face of environmental tragedies such as weather-related calamities or living in settings beset by violence.

The life course health development principles remind us that health development is highly sensitive to the timing and social structure of environmental events (Principle 4), and these examples of questions reflecting the specificity of health-related individual⇔context relations that may impinge on the thriving of adolescents underscore the subtle and nuanced nature of the developmental system within which adolescent health development is embodied.

The idea of embodiment and of adolescent health development being an emergent property of the living system (Principle 1) underscores that it is insufficient to take a "main effect" approach to the study of even a facet of health development as complex as the effects of nutrition. Scientists and practitioners framing their research and applications, respectively, within RDS-based models and/or life course health development principles must also ask how do answers to all the questions we have posed regarding nutrition covary with comparable questions pertaining to adolescent lifestyle changes (e.g., involving sleep, exercise, or sexual debut), healthy status of bodily systems, and the presence of chronic and acute health challenges, of both more biological (e.g., hormonal changes) and more social origins (e.g., school bullying).

5 Conclusions

The interrelated "what" questions we have presented, illustrated by the example of nutrition's effects on health development, will, then, help developmental and medical science collaborate to understand the assuredly complex questions that need to be addressed in a scholarly agenda that comprehensively describes, explains, and optimizes the course of individual health development across the adolescent period. Developmental scientists know that in some senses each adolescent is like every other adolescent (e.g., there are nomothetic principles that apply to functioning of the physiological and psychological changes prototypic of the period), that each adolescent is like only some other adolescent (e.g., group differential variation exists as, for instance, when both the presence of good health status and healthy disparities vary across gender, race, socioeconomic level, culture, and nation of residence), and that each adolescent is like no other adolescent (e.g., there are idiographic characteristics pertinent to every young person, for instance, resulting from the relations among his/her timing of molecular, physiological, behavioral, cultural, and evolutionary processes brought into high relief by life course health development Principle 7). Therefore, the scholarly agenda brought to the fore by RDS metatheory and by the principles of life course health development will require scholars seeking to understand and to promote adolescent health to accept that their work will be exceedingly more complex than work predicated on main effect or reductionist approaches.

However, the relative plasticity in the development of human health and positive development that is found in studies that have been derived from or associated with RDS-based or life course health development-related scholarship, respectively (e.g., Lerner et al. 2015), is a basis for *optimism* that embracing such complexity is not only the intellectually correct path to take. It is also a feasible approach to adopt. The advances in relational developmental systems-predicated methods that we have discussed (e.g., Molenaar et al. 2014; Molenaar and Nesselroade 2014, 2015; Nesselroade and Molenaar 2010) provide powerful research and data analytic tools enabling such complexity to be integratively assessed.

The adolescent decade is "privileged" because of the generally disease-free status of individuals within it, as compared to subsequent decades of life (e.g., Susman and Dorn 2009; Paus 2009). Nevertheless, application of methods linked to the ideas of RDS metatheory and the principles of life course health development hold the promise of narrowing the disparities that exist across time and place in adolescent health development. In addition, therefore, these conceptions have one other vital asset; their use in research and application will enhance the probability that all youth will transition from adolescence into the adult years in manners that will enable their life course trajectories to more prominently be marked by health and thriving. Such a contribution by these conceptual frameworks will make quite vivid the insight of Lewin (1954) that there is nothing more practical than a good theory.

Acknowledgement Supported (in full or in part) by Grant # U45MC27709 from the Department of Health and Human Services, Health Resources and Services Administration, Maternal and Child Health Bureau (Title V, Social Security Act), Division of Child, Adolescent and Family Health, Adolescent Health Branch.

References

Anthony, E. J. (1969). The reactions of adults to adolescents and their behavior. In G. Caplan & S. Lebovici (Eds.), *Adolescence: Psychosocial perspectives* (p. 77). New York: Basic Books.

Ardelt, M. (2000). Still stable after all these years? Personality stability theory revisited. *Social Psychology Quarterly, 63*(4), 392–405.

Baltes, P. B. (1997). On the incomplete architecture of human ontogeny: Selection, optimization, and compensation as foundations of developmental theory. *American Psychologist, 52*, 366–380.

Baltes, P. B., Lindenberger, U., & Staudinger, U. M. (2006). Lifespan theory in developmental psychology. In W. Damon & R. M. Lerner (Eds.), *Theoretical models of human development. Vol. 1: Handbook of child psychology* (6th ed., pp. 569–664). Hoboken: Wiley.

Bandura, A. (2001). Social cognitive theory: An agentic perspective. *Annual Review of Psychology, 52* 1–26. Palo Alto: Annual Reviews, Inc.

Benson, P. L., Scales, P. C., Hamilton, S. F., & Semsa, A., Jr. (2006). Positive youth development: Theory, research, and applications. In R. M. Lerner (Ed.), *Theoretical models of human development, Volume 1 of handbook of child psychology* (6th ed., pp. 894–941). Editors-in-chief: W. Damon & R. M. Lerner. Hoboken: Wiley.

Bjorklund, D. F., & Ellis, B. J. (2005). Evolutionary psychology and child development: An emerging synthesis. In B. J. Ellis & D. F. Bjorklund (Eds.), *Origins of the social mind: Evolutionary psychology and child development* (pp. 3–18). New York: Guilford.

Block, J. (1995). A contrarian view of the five-factor approach to personality description. *Psychological Bulletin, 117*, 187–215.

Block, J. (2010). The five-factor framing of personality and beyond: Some ruminations. *Psychological Inquiry, 21*(1), 2–25.

Bornstein, M. H. (2006). Parenting science and practice. In K. A. Renninger, & I. E. Sigel (Vol. Eds.), *Handbook of child psychology,* Vol. 4*: Child psychology in practice* (6th ed., pp. 893–949). Editors-in-Chief: W. Damon, & R. M. Lerner. Hoboken: Wiley.

Bornstein, M. H. (2017). The specificity principle in acculturation science. *Perspectives on Psychological Science, 12*(1), 3–45.

Brandtstädter, J. (1998). Action perspectives on human development. In R. M. Lerner (Ed.), *Handbook of child psychology, Vol. 1* (5th ed., pp. 807–866). New York: Wiley.

Brandtstädter, J. (1999). The self in action and development: Cultural, biosocial, and ontogenetic bases of intentional self-development. In J. Brandtstädter & R. M. Lerner (Eds.), *Action and self-development: Theory and research through the life-span* (pp. 37–65). Thousand Oaks: Sage.

Bronfenbrenner, U. (1979). *The ecology of human development*. Cambridge, MA: Harvard University Press.

Bronfenbrenner, U. (2005). *Making human beings human.* Thousand Oaks: Sage Publications.

Bronfenbrenner, U., & Morris, P. A. (2006). The bioecological model of human development. In R. M. Lerner (Ed.), *Theoretical models of human development.* Volume 1 of *Handbook of child psychology* (6th ed., pp. 795–828). Editors-in-chief: W. Damon & R. M. Lerner. Hoboken: Wiley.

Cole, S. W. (2014). Human social genomics. *PLoS Genetics, 10*(8), 1–7.

Costa, P. T., Jr., & McCrae, R. R. (1980). Still stable after all these years: Personality as a key to some issues in adulthood and old age. In P. B. Baltes & O. G. Brim Jr. (Eds.), *Life span development and behavior* (Vol. 3, pp. 65–102). New York: Academic Press.

Costa, P. T., Jr., & McCrae, R. R. (2006). Age changes in personality and their origins: Comment on Roberts,

Walton, and Viechtbauer (2006). *Psychological Bulletin, 132*, 28–30.

Cozza, S. J., & Lerner, R. M. (Eds.). (2013). Military children and families. *The Future of Children, 23*(2), 3–11.

Damon, W. (2008). *The path to purpose: Helping our children find their calling in life*. New York: Simon and Schuster.

Darwin, C. (1859). *The origin of species by means of natural selection or the preservation of favoured races in the struggle for life*. London: J. Murray.

Eccles, J. S. (2004). Schools, academic motivation, and stage-environment fit. In R. M. Lerner & L. Steinberg (Eds.), *Handbook of adolescent psychology* (2nd ed., pp. 125–153). Hoboken: Wiley.

Eccles, J. S., & Gootman, J. A. (Eds.). (2002). *Community programs to promote youth development/committee on community-level programs for youth*. Washington, DC: National Academy Press.

Elder, G. H., Jr. (1980). Adolescence in historical perspective. In J. Adelson (Ed.), *Handbook of adolescent psychology* (pp. 3–46). New York: Wiley.

Elder, G. H., Jr. (1998). The life course and human development. In R. M. Lerner (Ed.), *Handbook of child psychology, Volume 1: Theoretical models of human development* (5th ed., pp. 939–991). Editor-in-chief: W. Damon. New York: Wiley.

Elder, G. H., Jr., Shanahan, M. J., & Jennings, J. A. (2015). Human development in time and place. In M. H. Bornstein and T. Leventhal (Eds.), *Handbook of child psychology and developmental science,* Volume 4: *Ecological settings and processes in developmental systems* (7th ed., pp. 6–54). Editor-in-chief: R. M. Lerner. Hoboken: Wiley.

Ford, D. L., & Lerner, R. M. (1992). *Developmental systems theory: An integrative approach*. Newbury Park: Sage.

Forrest, C. B. (2014). A living systems perspective on health. *Medical Hypotheses, 82*, 209–2143.

Freud, A. (1969). Adolescence as a developmental disturbance. In G. Caplan & S. Lebovici (Eds.), *Adolescence* (pp. 5–10). New York: Basic Books.

Freund, A. M., & Baltes, P. B. (2002). Life-management strategies of selection, optimization and compensation: Measurement by self-report and construct validity. *Journal of Personality and Social Psychology, 82*(4), 642–662.

Gardner, M., & Steinberg, L. (2005). Peer influence on risk taking, risk preference, and risky decision making in adolescence and adulthood: An experimental study. *Developmental Psychology, 41*, 625–635.

Geldhof, G. J., Little, T. D., & Colombo, J. (2010). Self-regulation across the lifespan. In M. E. Lamb & A. M. Freund (Vol. Eds.), *Social and emotional development.* Volume 2 of the *Handbook of lifespan development.* Editor-in-Chief: R. M. Lerner. Hoboken: Wiley.

Gestsdóttir, G., & Lerner, R. M. (2008). Positive development in adolescence: The development and role of intentional self regulation. *Human Development, 51*, 202–224.

Gestsdottir, S., Geldhof, G. J., Paus, T., Freund, A. M., Aðalbjarnardóttir, S., Lerner, J. V., & Lerner, R. M. (2014). Self-regulation among youth in four Western cultures: Is there an adolescence-specific structure of the Selection-Optimization-Compensation (SOC) model? *International Journal of Behavioral Development, 39*(4), 346–358.

Gissis, S. B., & Jablonka, E. (Eds.). (2011). *Transformations of Lamarchism: From subtle fluids to molecular biology*. Cambridge, MA: The MIT Press.

Gottlieb, G. (1997). *Synthesizing nature-nurture: Prenatal roots of instinctive behavior*. Mahwah: Erlbaum.

Gottlieb, G. (1998). Normally occurring environmental and behavioral influences on gene activity: From central dogma to probabilistic epigenesis. *Psychological Review, 105*(4), 792–802.

Halfon, N., & Forrest, C. B. (2017). The emerging theoretical framework of life course health development. In N. Halfon, C. B. Forrest, R. M. Lerner, & E. Faustman (Eds.), *Handbook of life course health-development science*. Cham: Springer.

Hall, G. S. (1904). *Adolescence: Its psychology and its relations to psychology. anthropology, sociology, sex, crime, religion, and education.* New York: Appleton.

Hamilton, S. F. (1999). *A three-part definition of youth development*. Unpublished manuscript. Ithaca: Cornell University College of Human Ecology.

Jablonka, E., & Lamb, M. J. (2005). *Evolution in four dimensions: Genetic, epigenetic, behavioral, and symbolic variation in the history of life*. Cambridge, MA: MIT Press.

Johanson, D. C., & Edey, M. A. (1981). *Lucy: The beginnings of humankind*. New York: Simon & Schuster.

Larson, R. W. (2000). Toward a psychology of positive youth development. *American Psychologist, 55*(1), 170–183.

Latour, B. (1993). *We have never been modern* (trans. Catherine Porter), Cambridge, MA: Harvard University Press.

Lerner, R. M., & Busch-Rossnagel, N. A. (Eds.). (1981). *Individuals as producers of their development: A life-span perspective*. New York: Academic Press.

Lerner, R. M. (1982). Children and adolescents as producers of their own development. *Developmental Review, 2*, 342–370.

Lerner, R. M. (1984). *On the nature of human plasticity*. New York: Cambridge University Press.

Lerner, R. M., & Walls, T. (1999). Revisiting individuals as producers of their development: From dynamic interactionism to developmental systems. In J. Brandtstädter & R. M. Lerner (Eds.), *Action and self-development: Theory and research through the life-span* (pp. 3–36). Thousand Oaks: Sage.

Lerner, R. M. (2002). *Concepts and theories of human development* (3rd ed.). Mahwah: Lawrence Erlbaum Associates.

Lerner, R. M. (2004). *Liberty: Thriving and civic engagement among America's youth.* Thousand Oaks: Sage Publications.

Lerner, R. M., Lerner, J. V., Almerigi, J. B., Theokas, C., Phelps, E., Gestsdottir, S., et al. (2005). Positive Youth Development, Participation in community youth development programs, and community contributions of fifthgrade adolescents: Findings from the first wave of the 4-H study of Positive Youth Development. *Journal of Early Adolescence, 25*(1), 17–71.

Lerner, R. M. (Ed.). (2006). *Theoretical models of human development.* Volume 1 of *Handbook of child psychology* (6th ed.). Editors-in-chief: W. Damon & R. M. Lerner. Hoboken: Wiley.

Lerner, R. M. (2012). Essay review: Developmental science: Past, present, and future. *International Journal of Developmental Science, 6*(1–2), 29–36.

Lerner, R. M., & Callina, K. S. (2014). The study of character development: Towards tests of a relational developmental systems model. *Human Development, 57*(6), 322–346.

Lerner, R. M. (Editor-in-Chief). (2015). *Handbook of child psychology and developmental science* (7th ed.). Hoboken: Wiley.

Lerner, R. M., & Benson, J. B. (Eds.). (2013a). *Embodiment and epigenesis: Theoretical and methodological issues in understanding the role of biology within the relational developmental system. Volume 1: Philosophical, theoretical, and biological dimensions. advances in child development and behavior* (Vol. 44). London: Elsevier.

Lerner, R. M., & Benson, J. B. (Eds.). (2013b). *Embodiment and epigenesis: Theoretical and methodological issues in understanding the role of biology within the relational developmental system. Volume 2: Ontogenetic dimensions. Advances in child development and behavior* (Vol. 45). London: Elsevier.

Lerner, R. M., & Callina, K. S. (2015). The study of character development: Towards tests of a relational developmental systems model. *Human Development, 57*(6), 322–346.

Lerner, R. M., & Steinberg, L. (2009). The scientific study of adolescent development. In R. M. Lerner & L. Steinberg (Eds.), *Handbook of adolescent psychology* (3rd ed., pp. 3–14). Hoboken: Wiley.

Lerner, R. M., Freund, A. M., De Stefanis, I., & Habermas, T. (2001). Understanding developmental regulation in adolescence: The use of the selection, optimization, and compensation model. *Human Development, 44*, 29–50.

Lerner, R. M., Lerner, J. V., Bowers, E., & Geldhof, G. J. (2015). Positive youth development: A relational developmental systems model. In W. F. Overton & P. C. Molenaar (Eds.), *Theory and method.* Volume 1 of the *Handbook of child psychology and developmental science* (7th ed., pp. 607–651). Editor-in-chief: R. M. Lerner. Hoboken: Wiley.

Lewin, K. (1954). Behavior and development as a function of the total situation. In L. Carmichael (Ed.), *Manual of child psychology* (2nd ed.). New York: Wiley.

Marcia, J. E. (1980). Identity in adolescence. In J. Adelson (Ed.), *Handbook of adolescent psychology* (pp. 159–187). New York: Wiley.

Mascalo, M. F., & Fischer, K. W. (2015). The dynamic development of thinking, feeling, and acting: Infancy through adulthood In W. F. Overton & P. C. M. Molenaar (Eds.), *Handbook of child psychology and developmental science* (7th ed.), Volume 1*: Theory and method.* Editor-in-chief: R. M. Lerner. Hoboken: Wiley.

McClelland, M. M., Geldhof, G. J., Cameron, C. E., & Wanless, S. B. (2015). Development and self-regulation. In W. F. Overton & P. C. Molenaar (Eds.), *Theory and method.* Volume 1 of the *Handbook of child psychology and developmental science* (7th ed.). Editor-in-chief: R. M. Lerner. Hoboken: Wiley.

McCrae, R. R., Costa, P. T., Hrebickova, M., Ostendord, F., Angleitner, A., & Avia, M. D. (2000). Nature over nurture: Temperament, personality, and life span development. *Journal of Personality and Social Psychology, 78*(1), 173–186.

Meaney, M. (2014, October 10). *Epigenetics offer hope for disadvantaged children.* [Children and family: Blog]. Retrieved from http://childandfamilyblog.com/epigenetics-offer-hope-disadvantaged-children/

Misteli, T. (2013). The cell biology of genomes: Bringing the double helix to life. *Cell, 152*(6), 1209–1212.

Mistry, J., & Wu, J. (2010). Navigating cultural worlds and negotiating identities: A conceptual model. *Human Development, 53*(1), 5–25.

Molenaar, P. C. (2014). Dynamic models of biological pattern formation have surprising implications for understanding the epigenetics of development. *Research in Human Development, 11*(1), 50–62.

Molenaar, P. C., & Nesselroade, J. R. (2014). New trends in the inductive use of relation developmental systems theory: Ergodicity, nonstationarity, and heterogeneity. In P. C. Molenaar, R. M. Lerner, & K. M. Newell (Eds.), *Handbook of developmental systems and methodology* (pp. 442–462). New York: Guilford Press.

Molenaar, P. C. M., & Nesselroade, J. R. (2015). Systems methods for developmental research. In W. F. Overton & P. C. M. Molenaar (Eds.), *Handbook of child psychology and developmental science* (7th ed.), Volume 1*: Theory and method.* Editor-in-chief: R. M. Lerner. Hoboken: Wiley.

Molenaar, P. C., Lerner, R. M., & Newell, K. M. (2014). Developmental systems theory and methodology: A review of the issues. In P. C. Molenaar, R. M. Lerner, & K. M. Newell (Eds.), *Handbook of developmental systems and methodology* (pp. 3–18). New York: Guilford Press.

Narvaez, D. (2008). Human flourishing and moral development: Cognitive and neurobiological perspectives of virtue development. In L. Nucci & D. Narvaez (Eds.), *Handbook of moral and character education* (pp. 310–327). Oxford: Routledge.

Nesselroade, J. R. (1988). Some implications of the trait-state distinction for the study of development over the life-span: The case of personality. In P. B. Baltes, D. L. Featherman, & R. M. Lerner (Eds.), *Life-span development and behavior* (Vol. 8, pp. 163–189). Hillsdale: Erlbaum.

Nesselroade, J. R., & Molenaar, P. C. M. (2010). Emphasizing intraindividual variability in the study of development over the life span. In W. F. Overton (Ed.), *The handbook of life-span development.* Vol. 1*: Cognition, biology, methods* (pp. 30–54). Editor-in-chief: R. M. Lerner. Hoboken: Wiley.

Overton, W. F. (1973). On the assumptive base of the nature-nurture controversy: Additive versus interactive conceptions. *Human Development, 16*, 74–89.

Overton, W. F. (2010). Life-span development: Concepts and issues. In W. F. Overton (Ed), *Cognition, biology, and methods across the lifespan. Handbook of life-span development*. (Vol. 1, pp. 1–29). Editor-in-chief: R. M. Lerner. Hoboken: Wiley.

Overton, W. F. (2013). Relationism and relational developmental systems; A paradigm for developmental science in the post-Cartesian era. In R. M. Lerner and J. B. Benson (Eds.), *Advances in child development and behavior, volume 44: Embodiment and epigenesis: Theoretical and methodological issues in understanding the role of biology within the relational developmental system, Part A: Philosophical, theoretical, and biological dimensions* (pp. 24–64). London: Elsevier. Development of Character 49.

Overton, W. F. (2015). Process and relational developmental systems. In W. F. Overton & P. C. Molenaar (Eds.), *Theory and method*. Volume 1 of the *Handbook of child psychology and developmental science* (7th ed., pp. 9–62). Editor-in-chief: R. M. Lerner. Hoboken: Wiley.

Overton, W. F., & Lerner, R. M. (2014). Fundamental concepts and methods in developmental science: A relational perspective. *Research in Human Development, 11*(1), 63–73.

Overton, W. F., & Mueller, U. (2013). Meta-theories, theories, and concepts in the study of development. In R. M. Lerner, M A. Easterbrooks, & J. Mistry (Eds.), *Comprehensive handbook of psychology: developmental psychology: Vol. 6*. (pp. 19–58). Editor-in-Chief: Irving B. Weiner. New York: Wiley.

Overton, W. F., & Reese, H. W. (1981). Conceptual prerequisites for an understanding of stability–change and continuity–discontinuity. *International Journal of Behavioral Development, 4*, 99–123.

Paus, T. (2009). Brain development. In R. M. Lerner & L. Steinberg (Eds.), *Handbook of adolescent psychology* (3rd ed., pp. 95–115).

Ricco, R., & Overton, W. F. (2011). Dual systems competence ß-à procedural processing: A relational developmental systems approach to reasoning. *Developmental Review, 31*, 119–150. http://dx.doi.org/10.1016/j.dr.2011.07.005.

Riegel, K. F. (1975). Toward a dialectical theory of human development. *Human Development, 18*, 50–64.

Riegel, K. F. (1976). The dialectics of human development. *American Psychologist, 31*, 689–700.

Roberts, B. W., Walton, K. E., & Viechtbauer, W. (2006). Patterns of mean-level change in personality traits across the life course: A meta-analysis of longitudinal studies. *Psychological Bulletin, 132*(1), 1–25.

Roth, J. L., & Brooks-Gunn, J. (2003a). What is a youth development program? Identification and defining principles. In F. Jacobs, D. Wertlieb, & R. M. Lerner (Eds.), *Enhancing the life chances of youth and families: Public service systems and public policy perspectives: Vol. 2 handbook of applied developmental science: Promoting positive child, adolescent, and family development through research, policies, and programs* (pp. 197–223). Thousand Oaks: Sage.

Roth, J. L., & Brooks-Gunn, J. (2003b). What exactly is a youth development program? Answers from research and practice. *Applied Developmental Science, 7*, 94–111.

Slavich, G. M., & Cole, S. W. (2013). The emerging field of human social genomics. *Clinical Psychological Science, 1*, 331–348.

Sokol, B. W., Hammond, S., Kuebli, J., & Sweetman, L. (2015). The development of agency. In W. F. Overton & P. C. Molenaar (Eds.,) *Theory and method*. Volume 1 of development of the *Handbook of child psychology and developmental science* (7th ed.). Editor-in-chief: R. M. Lerner. Hoboken: Wiley.

Steinberg, L. (2010). A dual systems models of adolescent risk-taking. *Developmental Psychobiology, 52*, 216–224.

Susman, E., & Dorn, L. D. (2009). Puberty: Its role in development. In R. M. Lerner & L. Steinberg (Eds.), *Handbook of adolescent psychology* (3rd ed., pp. 116–151). Hoboken: Wiley.

Susman, E. J., & Dorn, L. D. (2013). Puberty: Its role in development. In R. M. Lerner, M. A., Easterbrooks, & J. Mistry (Eds.), *Handbook of psychology, Volume 6: Developmental psychology* (2nd ed., pp. 289–320). Editor-inchief: I. B. Weiner. Hoboken: Wiley.

Tobach, E., & Schneirla, T. C. (1968). The biopsychology of social behavior of animals. In R. E. Cooke & S. Levin (Eds.), *Biologic basis of pediatric practice* (pp. 68–82). New York: McGraw-Hill.

Trommsdorff, G. (2012). Development of "agentic" regulation in cultural context: The role of self and world views. *Child Development Perspectives, 6*(1), 19–26.

von Bertalanffy, L. (1933). *Modern theories of development*. London: Oxford University Press.

von Bertalanffy, L. (1968). *General systems theory*. New York: Braziller.

Whitehead, A. N. (1929/1978). *Process and reality*. Corrected edn. New York: The Free

Witherington, D. C. (2014). Self-organization and explanatory pluralism: Avoiding the snares of reductionism in developmental science. *Research In Human Development, 11*, 22–36.

Emerging Adulthood as a Critical Stage in the Life Course

David Wood, Tara Crapnell, Lynette Lau, Ashley Bennett, Debra Lotstein, Maria Ferris, and Alice Kuo

1 Introduction to Emerging Adulthood

The path that individuals take from dependency in childhood to independence in adulthood is now a longer and more complicated one than at any other point in history (Arnett 2014). From the mid- to late twentieth century and extending into the twenty-first century, industrial societies have experienced a surge in the concept of individualism and increased salience of self-realization and personal expression (Arnett 1998). Moreover, we have seen a dramatic increase in the number of youth seeking post-high school education, which is required for success as the economy transitions from an industrial to an information-based economy (Rifkin 2011). However, stagnation of wages for low-skilled workers and the lack of work opportunities for youth and young adults, combined with the increased costs of education and independent living, have made the pathway to independence and adulthood prolonged, complex, and varied, creating a new stage in the life course that has been labeled *emerging adulthood* (EA). While not all life course or developmental scientists agree that emerging adulthood constitutes a new developmental stage, there is agreement that social and economic forces have prolonged entry into adulthood and with significant role and developmental challenges beyond the traditional adolescent years (Cote 2014).

At the beginning of this stage, 17–18 years of age, emerging adults are generally dependent, living with their parents or caretakers, beginning to engage in romantic relationships, and attending high school. At the end of this stage, mid- to late 20s, most emerging adults live independently, are in long-term relationships, and have clear career paths ahead of them. How they traverse this life stage is dependent upon the personal, family, and social resources they possess as they enter this stage of life, dynamic and reciprocal interaction between the emerging adult and their environment, and the supports they receive during this stage. The result is that there are many pathways that youth and young adults pursue through this stage to achieve stable adulthood. For example, 40% do not

The original version of this chapter was revised. An erratum to this chapter can be found at https://doi.org/10.1007/978-3-319-47143-3_27

D. Wood, MD, MPH (✉)
Department of Pediatrics, ETSU College of Medicine, PO Box 70578, Johnson City, TN 37614, USA
e-mail: wooddl@etsu.edu

T. Crapnell, OTD, OTR/L • L. Lau, PhD
D. Lotstein, MD, MPH • M. Ferris, MD, PhD, MPH
A. Kuo, MD, PhD
UCLA, Department of Pediatrics, Los Angeles, CA, USA

A. Bennett, MD
Department of Pediatrics, USC, Los Angeles, CA, USA

N. Halfon et al. (eds.), *Handbook of Life Course Health Development*,
DOI 10.1007/978-3-319-47143-3_7

pursue post-high school education. While 60% entered college immediately after graduating high school, many drop out or interrupt their college education with periods of work. Some 33% in this stage remain unmarried; however, 67% of them achieve stable domestic partners. Importantly, only a minority of emerging adults are employed in full-time jobs, limiting the economic opportunities they experience (U.S. Census Bureau. American Community Survey 2006).

Emerging adulthood is considered to be the *volitional years*, as it offers the most opportunity for identity exploration in the areas of love, work, and worldviews (Arnett 2000). During this time, individuals begin to develop the characteristic qualities necessary for becoming self-sufficient, engage in mature, committed relationships, assume more adult roles and responsibilities, and obtain a level of education and training that sets the foundation for work during the adult years. Characterizing emerging adulthood as a stage in the life course has proven to be beneficial to explain the social, cognitive, and psychological development that occurs during this stage. Research demonstrating continued brain development into the late 20s provides further justification for viewing emerging adulthood as a stage in the life course (Spear 2000).

2 Conceptual Framework

The Life Course Health Development (LCHD) model posits that myriad factors (e.g., biological, psychological, cultural) on multiple levels (e.g., micro, meso, macro) interact simultaneously in a transactional fashion to influence an individual's LCHD during each stage to determine a "health developmental" trajectory (see also Halfon and Forrest 2017). The Life Course Health Development (LCHD) model further posits that transitions and pivotal points in an individual's life have the potential to influence and alter an individual's developmental pathways. EA is a life stage characterized by changes in person-context cognitive, emotional, physical, and social domains, and the ultimate pathway achieved by the emerging adults during this stage is determined by the ongoing, dynamic, and reciprocal interactions between the individual and their environment. The degree of agency and role exploration that characterizes EA results in the potential for growth in intellectual and emotional functioning (Arnett 2000). EA represents a broad and diverse but fundamentally important area of consideration by virtue of the multiple avenues through which an individual's developmental trajectories and outcomes may be influenced. Important developmental challenges during EA include the continued formation of identity and values, which occur in the midst of frequent changes in personal relationships, living arrangements, vocational and educational pursuits, and social roles (Shanahan 2000).

No stage in life, other than perhaps infancy, experiences such dynamic and complex changes on the personal, social, emotional, neuroanatomical, and developmental levels. For the 10 years between 18 and 28, the vast majority of emerging adults change living situation, change their primary relationships, complete education or vocational preparation, get married, have children, and transition from adolescent/dependent roles to adult/independent roles. This occurs during often volatile emotional, neurodevelopmental, and social development. Increasing agency occurs at the same time as decreasing institutional and family supports. The theoretical framework developed by Learner and others to create the positive youth development theory nicely explains how the developmental trajectories that emerge during the period of EA are dependent upon multiple influential, bidirectional, person-context coactions. Individuals during emerging adulthood act as co-developers of their own developmental pathways, adaptively responding to different biological, social, cultural, and physical environmental contexts that they influence and are also influenced by (Learner and Overton 2008). Successfully navigating the developmental challenges inherent in EA will likely, in large part, influence the developmental trajectory of adulthood because these challenges ultimately influence the important adult outcomes of independent living, committed intimate relationships, and vocational and educational achievement. Youth and young adults with chronic disease or disabilities face additional challenges (disease management, disease complications, limitations in opportunities, etc.) in the context of these multiple domains of growth and development, which impact their pathway through this stage.

The continued positive trajectory of the emerging adult's mental health, identity formation, education achievement, social relationships, and other developmental areas is somewhat dependent on the degree to which there are matches or mismatches between the individual and his/her resources and the environmental challenges and supports. If the transition, such as school to work, provides a reasonable and developmentally appropriate challenge and the emerging adult successfully navigates that challenge, then the developmental trajectory of the emerging adult will be enhanced. In contrast, if the same transition lacks supports or is an inappropriate match for the emerging adult's abilities (e.g., an inadequate vocational program for an emerging adult with a learning disorder or lack of support for chronic disease management) and the emerging adult experiences failure, then the developmental trajectory may be impaired, resulting in significantly less achievement or developmental progression across the lifespan. A major defining characteristic of the stage of EA is that contexts are changing significantly (family to independence or romantic relationships, school to work or disconnected state, dependent living to independent living arrangements). The changes are so significant that emerging adults need substantial supports to navigate the transition successfully. Emerging adults with disabilities or chronic health conditions require more support to maximize their potential development during EA (Table 1).

Table 1 Principles of the Life Course Health Development framework

Principle	Brief description
1. Health development	Health development integrates the concepts of health and developmental processes into a unified whole
2. Unfolding	Health development unfolds continuously over the lifespan, from conception to death, and is shaped by prior experiences and environmental interactions
3. Complexity	Health development results from adaptive, multilevel, and reciprocal interactions between individuals and their physical, natural, and social environments
4. Timing	Health development is sensitive to the timing and social structuring of environmental exposures and experiences
5. Plasticity	Health development phenotypes are malleable and enabled and constrained by evolution to enhance adaptability to diverse environments
6. Thriving	Optimal health development promotes survival, enhances well-being, and protects against disease
7. Harmony	Health development results from the balanced interactions of molecular, physiological, behavioral, cultural, and evolutionary processes

The above table outlines the seven principles of the Life Course Health Development framework. These principles can be applied to the stage of emerging adulthood in a limited fashion due to the limited research literature focused on this life stage. However, conceptually, using the seven principles to view the stage of emerging adulthood can be instructive and can lead to additional research questions (see end of this article). For example, Principle 5 states that health development expressions are malleable and enable and constrain health development pathways and plasticity. According to Bogin's reserve capacity hypothesis, prolonged childhood into adolescence and perhaps emerging adulthood leads to greater biologic and social resilience in adulthood, which leads to enhanced fertility and greater longevity (Bogin 2013). Principle 4 states that health development is sensitive to life course timing and social structuring of the environment. As we described above, this is particularly true of emerging adulthood, where the interaction between age, personal development, and environment (peers, schools, social institutions, etc.) leads to multiple pathways to identify formation and academic and social achievement during this stage (Benson and Elder 2011; Benson et al. 2012).

Multiple factors can influence the life course during EA, including factors at the macro-level (historical and societal influences), meso-level (parent-child relationship, family environment, and socioeconomic status), and microlevel (individual cognitive, personality, and emotional development). The timing of these exposures during EA, which we consider a critical or sensitive period in the life course development, can significantly impact adult outcomes. For example, an emerging adult that engages in criminal activity and is convicted of a felony will suffer repercussions that will greatly diminish their chances of achieving success in relationships and work. In the sections that follow, we review the macro-, meso-, and microlevel influences occurring during EA for emerging adults generally. Next we explore the additional challenges faced by those with selected chronic health or developmental conditions including mental illness or substance abuse, diabetes, chronic renal failure, and autism, to serve as case studies of the increased complexity faced by emerging adults with chronic disease. Finally, we finish up with a set of questions and issues that are research priorities for developing an LCHD research agenda on the stage of emerging adulthood.

3 Macro-level Influences on the Trajectory of Emerging Adulthood

Emerging adulthood, like many other developmental stages, is a period in the life course that is culturally constructed and not universal (Arnett 1998, 2000). Thus, the very existence and trajectory of EA are dependent on macro-level societal expectations and influences. For many years, it was theorized that an individual transitioned from adolescence (which begins in puberty and ends in the late teens) into young adulthood. Over history and cross-culturally, the length of time during which an individual spends in adolescence has been determined by the age at which the person enters marriage or a committed relationship (Schlegel and Barry III 1991, Gilmore 1990). In fact, human life history posits that the life stage of adolescence came into existence about 75,000 years ago due to changes in human societies and cultures associated with pair bonding and living in large groups (Bogin 2013). So massive culture and reproductive change led to a change in life history with the addition of a new period of development. It is theorized by those promoting emerging adulthood as a new life stage that the same kind of massive cultural and reproductive change is happening once again and new social and cultural demands of adult life necessitate a longer and more complex prologue to adult life.

Although the functional outcome of EA, causing a delayed transition to adulthood, appears relatively novel, this practice of prolonging the transition to adulthood may be dated back to early modern English society from the 1500s to 1700s (Ben-Amos 1994). Similar to what generally occurs during EA today, individuals during that era took part in a "life cycle service" between their late teens and 20s, wherein they would engage in developing important vocational skills (e.g., a trade or craft) and marriage was often postponed until the late 20s for both men and women; adult roles and responsibilities for individuals during that era were provided only gradually, as each individual acquired the desired character qualities deemed appropriate by society (Ben-Amos 1994). It was not until industrialization in America began to emerge in the nineteenth century that the concept of individualism developed and strengthened (Rotundo 1994). The twentieth century marked the first time that an individual could obtain and gain control over the resources that would allow them to choose the timing of major life events and personal expression was valued in society (Modell 1991).

As we move forward into the twenty-first century, individualism in contemporary postindustrial society continues to strengthen, while the age at which individuals marry continues to increase, and individuals increasingly seek to pursue other life course events (Modell 1991; Alwin 1988; Bellah et al. 2007). As a reflection of these trends, recent evidence indicates that contemporary postindustrial society considers marriage status of low importance in the determination of whether or not an individual has reached adulthood; rather, societies in developed countries appear to now consider the acquisition of certain character qualities as the most important indicator of having attained adulthood, the top three character qualities of which include (1) accepting responsibility for oneself, (2) making independent decisions, and (3) assuming financial independence – all of which emphasize an individual's ability to be self-sufficient (Scheer et al. 1996; Greene et al. 1992; Arnett 1997, 1998).

4 Meso-level Influences of Life Trajectories During Emerging Adulthood

Earlier life experiences and family environment can impact one's life trajectory from childhood through EA and into adulthood. Longitudinal studies that span early childhood through EA indicate that there is both continuity and discontinuity of healthy and unhealthy paths and outcomes. (Masten et al. 2006, 2005). In this section, we will be discussing the impact of the parent-child relationship, family environment, and other sociodemographic factors, such as socioeconomic status (SES) and its influence in EA.

4.1 Earlier Parent-Child Relationships

The quality of parent-child relationships during EA is, in large part, a function of the history of early parent-child attachment experiences. Attachment theory suggests that positive bonding with an emotionally available adult during early childhood facilitates the development of the child's capacity to bond with others and respond to stressful events. A history of positive attachment experiences will ultimately provide a foundation for positive interactions with others and foster secure, lasting relationships in EA which subsequently influence the LCHD (Mikulincer M and Shaver PR 2009), whereas insecure attachments can result in mistrust or lack of security and reduced sense of self-efficacy and self-esteem. Simultaneously, social learning theory suggests that styles of family interactions learned in early and middle childhood are carried by emerging adults into adulthood (Whitbeck et al. 1994). Familiar patterns of interaction help individuals deal with new situations and have a significant influence on the emerging adult's capacity to deal with the multiple changes that occur during EA. Alternatively, inadequate parenting, disrupted family bonds, and poverty are environmental risks for childhood-onset conduct, behavioral and emotional problems, and educational underachievement that can persist into adolescence and emerging adulthood (Moffit and Caspi 2001).

Adverse events experienced in childhood such as parental divorce or alcoholism or the experience of abuse are major risk factors for the leading causes of illness and death as well as poor quality of life in adults in the USA. Disruptions in the parent relationship (e.g., divorce) can have strong, negative effects on the parent-child relationship (Aquilino 1994) causing significant emotional impact throughout the life course. Parental divorce may influence the emerging adults' ability to form stable romantic relationships and their decision to marry early or may undermine the emerging adult's financial ability to attend college (Jacquet and Surra 2001, Cherlin et al. 1998).

Importantly, parental acceptance and support for independence have been linked to higher self-esteem, individualism, and feelings of worthiness among emerging adults (Ryan and Lynch 1989). Critical to the emerging adult's achievement of independence are feeling connected, secure, understood, and loved in their families and having the willingness to call on parental resources for help in making choices in educational, relationship, living, and other changes that confront the emerging adult. Persistent connectedness to parents facilitates rather than undermines ongoing identity development in emerging adulthood (Grotevant and Cooper 1986; Ryan and Lynch 1989).

4.2 Childhood Socioeconomic Status

Socioeconomic status (SES), family supports, and the neighborhood environment all can contribute to the positive or negative life trajectory prior to and during EA (Galobardes et al. 2008; Gilman 2012; Gilman and Loucks 2012). Socioeconomic status has been identified as one of the most important health determinants throughout the life course (Miller et al. 2015). Low financial resources and all the other exposures that go along with poverty – poor schools, chaotic families, exposure to violence, and victimization – limit opportunities for growth or acquisition of other resources that enhance quality of life (Wadsworth et al. 2016; Kim et al. 2015).

In addition to being an important predictor of disease-specific morbidity and mortality in adulthood, early childhood poverty has been associated with lower adult educational attainment (Duncan and Brooks-Gunn 2000). Educational achievement has a major influence on the life trajectory, including financial stability and health in EA and onward throughout adulthood. Seventy percent of emerging adults who grow up in poverty delay enrollment in postsecondary education, in comparison to 40% who grow up in household of higher SES. Furthermore, research has indicated that individuals who delay enrollment past the age of 22 are less likely to ever enroll in postsecondary education and less likely to complete a degree (Feliciano and Ashtiani 2012). The result is that only 22% of young adults from low-income families earn college degrees, while 48% of young adults from higher-income families earn at least an associate's degree. Earning a college education results in not only higher lifetime earnings but enhancement of multiple aspects of psychosocial development (Evans and Cassells 2014).

However, while SES has been found to be predictive of educational attainment, the impact of poverty can be mitigated by a number of factors such as individual characteristics of self-efficacy and hope. Students from poor families that have high self-efficacy and a similar concept of hope for educational attainment do equally as well in school as their higher SES peers (Osgood et al. 2005). Recent research by Dweck and colleagues indicates that students' mindsets are critically linked to resilience and achievement and that they can be changed through brief interventions, leading to substantial increases in measures of resilience and achievement (Yeager and Dweck 2012). These studies suggest that in addition to SES, individual characteristics also have a large influence on outcomes of EA and that these characteristics can be influenced through individual interventions. Individual characteristics and development are discussed in the next section.

5 Microlevel Influences on the Trajectories During Emerging Adulthood

As discussed in previous sections, individualism and the qualities of character have become increasingly important in the transition to EA and ultimately reaching full adulthood in postindustrial, developed societies. Studies have shown that the ability to accept responsibility for one's self, make independent decisions, and assume financial independence are the top three most important factors in becoming an adult (Arnett 2014). In order to achieve individualism and obtain these important qualities of character, one needs to reach some degree of cognitive and psychological maturity, as well as possess some level of resilience. These individual factors are discussed in this section.

5.1 Cognitive Development

One of the identified qualities of character that is important in EA and reaching full adulthood is independent decision-making. While the ability to make independent decisions is a reflection of one's psychological and moral identity, it also has to do with cognitive maturity and the ability to weigh a variety of considerations before deciding on a choice. Recent neuroscience research indicates that brain development (particularly in the prefrontal cortex) continues well into the third decade of life, ultimately resulting in the integration and coordination of cognitions, emotion and action, and strategic executive control (Luciana et al. 2005). The continuous unfolding and acquisition of specific neurodevelopmental capacities during adolescences and EA influence the acquisition of goal directedness and future orientation that have been observed behaviorally during EA (Dahl 2004; Nelson et al. 2012; Nurmi 1999; Steinberg et al. 2006). As new capacities emerge, they are available to solve problems, delay gratification, and filter unnecessary input. With maturation of these skills, emerging adults are also more capable of reflecting on the influence of their environment and on their internal state, regulate their emotions, and use problem-solving skills to effectively compromise, which is important for the development of meaningful social interactions and personal relationships as well as in the work environment. These skills also support an emerging adult's capacity for optimally interacting with the health-care system, managing their health-care needs, and making decisions that will influence their long-term health outcomes.

However, the preceding paragraph assumes that the individual has experienced optimal neurodevelopment up to the point that they enter the stage of EA. Studies have demonstrated that exposure to chronic stress during childhood (e.g., poverty) or experiencing adverse childhood events (e.g., child maltreatment, neglect, parental divorce, parental substance abuse) may cause detrimental impact to the developing brain. For example, repeated exposure to stressful events has been associated with structural differences in specific brain regions (i.e., amygdala, hippocampus, and prefrontal cortex), which are in turn associated with functional differences in learning, memory, and aspects of executive functioning. Furthermore, preliminary studies go on to suggest that there may be sensitive periods of brain development with increased susceptibility to the effects of stress and adverse events. These environmentally induced modulations in neurodevelopment can impact an individual's cognitive development and their capacity to develop the necessary skills and relationships that will enable them to thrive.

An emerging adult, who has experienced chronic stress or adverse events earlier in childhood and adolescence and is cognitively immature, is more likely, through adverse interaction with their environment, to suffer secondary effects such as school failure, risky/impulsive behaviors, accidental injury, criminal activity, or substance misuse or overuse. These behaviors may in turn interfere with the ongoing development of an optimal pathway to adulthood. Feelings of isolation and rates of substance abuse in individuals often peak during this period as emerging adults are faced with the stresses of having to navigate societal structures that are not adequately informed or equipped to address the needs of an emerging adult population – all while their brains have yet to reach full maturation (Spear 2000). An impulsive emerging adult fueled by alcohol and despair is at high risk for suicide. It is thus apparent that multiple factors related to an individual's cognitive and emotional development may intersect and interact to multiply the likelihood of adverse or positive health outcomes in EA. It is crucial for service providers to recognize the level of cognitive maturation an emerging adult possesses and tailor their interventions and supports based on this.

5.2 Identity Formation

Identity formation is a major developmental activity during EA. Identity development, occurs in a number of dimensions: (1) psychological dimension, or ego identity via a sense of temporal-spatial continuity and its concomitants; (2) the personal dimension, or a behavioral and character repertoire that differentiates the individuals; and (3) the social dimension, or recognized roles within a community. These components come together during the stage of identity formation (adolescence and EA) and stabilization (EA and young adulthood), and once the identity is considered stable, this is when a relatively firm sense of ego identity is developed, behavior and character become stabilized, and community-sanctioned roles are acquired (2002).

Identity formation during adolescence was thought to be a critical milestone in adolescence; however, it has been recognized that in certain societal contexts, identity formation continues beyond adolescence. In the postindustrial society, with the prolongation of educational and vocational attainment, prolongation of identity exploration in the three main areas of love, work, and worldviews into the 20s has become the norm. Identity formation is critical in EA, as it has direct implications on psychological and moral identity and in achieving the three qualities of character deemed as important in the transition to adulthood.

5.3 Resilience in Emerging Adulthood

Resilience is an individual's capacity to adapt to change in healthy and flexible ways during stressful events (Catalano et al. 2004). Resilience can be measured in various ways, including internal adaption (e.g., well-being, happiness, or self-concept) or external adaption (academic achievement, relationship development) to adverse circumstances, such as how well a person navigates and achieves the developmental tasks presented by the external world (e.g., educational achievement, stable work/career, marriage, etc.). Resiliency in adolescence and young adulthood is higher among youth with higher intellectual resources, optimistic future orientation, the presence of caring relationships with positive adult role models, and opportunities to succeed and serve the community. Emerging adulthood is a particularly important stage in the life course to understand resilience because the important changes in functional capacity, educational achievement, and social roles are large and varied and have a significant influence on life course outcomes.

Key individual characteristics that predict resilience during EA are goal-directed motivation and planfulness about the future. In addition, adult support and mentorship are important factors that help promote resilience (Miller GE 2015; Masten et al. 2005; Arnett 2005). Furstenberg, Brooks-Gunn, and others studied young women who became pregnant during adolescence and found that a small proportion with positive adult relationships had dramatic change in trajectory for the better (Furstenberg 2002). Masten, studying a cohort of low-income youth (beginning at ages 8–12) over a 20-year period, found that a number of factors predict competence in EA including higher intellectual capacity, higher parenting quality, and higher SES (Masten and Coatsworth 1998). When they examined resilience between the 10- and 20-year follow-up, they found that youth doing well in EA was predicted from doing well 10 years earlier. In the context of high adversity, childhood IQ was particularly an important moderator and predictor of resilience. During EA, individuals who were doing well from high-adversity backgrounds had significant personal resources in intelligence and personal competence and a history of receiving high-quality parenting (Masten et al. 2004).

6 Trajectories During Emerging Adulthood for Emerging Adults with Chronic Health Condition

Chronic health conditions can significantly impact the developmental trajectory of emerging adults during this life stage. Many types of chronic conditions, including those that impact physical, intellectual, or emotional functioning, may undermine the assumption of adult roles by the emerging adult, undermine success in school, impair the transition to work, and make living independently more of a challenge. Eighteen percent of youth aged 12–17 in the USA are defined as having a special health-care need, meaning they have a chronic physical, medical, emotional, or developmental condition that requires a more intensive use of health-care and related services. Emerging adults with chronic conditions are at risk for a number of problems during transition to adulthood, including experiencing gaps in needed medical and related services and gaps in health insurance (Lotstein et al. 2008, Reiss et al. 2005). Below we review the impact of several specific chronic conditions on the growth trajectory during emerging adulthood.

6.1 Autism Spectrum Disorders (ASDs)

For youth with autism spectrum disorders (ASDs) and their families, the transition from adolescence to emerging adulthood is a time of uncertainty and loss of entitlement to many services that were available while in the public school system under the Individuals with Disabilities Education Act (IDEA). In comparison to childhood, young adults with autism often experience a dearth of appropriate supports and opportunities. Leaving high school is associated with deterioration in ASD symptom presentation, increase in maladaptive behaviors, and worsening family functioning (Taylor and Seltzer 2010, 2011a, b). Many persons with ASD are able to work successfully within the community (Garcia-Villamisar et al. 2000; Mawhood and Howlin 1999); however, the majority experience difficulty securing meaningful employment (Eaves and Ho 2008; Howlin et al. 2004; Newman et al. 2011). A recent study indicated that only 58% have ever worked for pay. In addition, it was found that only one in five individuals ever lived independently (Roux et al. 2015). Even among those employed, their jobs tended to be low level and low income (Cimera and Cowan 2009; Eaves and Ho 2008; Howlin et al. 2004). Jobs often ended prematurely because of social or behavioral difficulties or other work-related difficulties (Mawhood and Howlin 1999).

Young adults on the autism spectrum are reported to experience difficulties in assuming other important adult roles and responsibilities, including attaining postsecondary education and living independently (Roux et al. 2015). A number of studies (Billstedt et al. 2005; Gillespie-Lynch et al. 2012; Howlin et al. 2004) have found that having an IQ of around 70 seemed to be a critical cutoff point for better outcome (e.g., level of independence). A number of comorbid conditions can complicate the trajectory for youth with intellectual disability through adolescence and EA, such as seizure disorder, which substantially increase in prevalence from childhood through adolescence into adulthood. Adults with ASD and related conditions are more vulnerable to anxiety and depression which can require specific treatments (Skokauskas and Gallagher 2010; White et al. 2009). The majority of young adults with ASD remain dependent on parents for support in living, recreation, and occupational situations. The availability of appropriate resources, services, and supports for the individuals with ASD and their families is key for successful transition into adulthood and better outcomes throughout adult life. The following elements are important for high-quality transition services and associated with improved young adult outcomes: (1) individualized services that reflect the strengths of the individual, (2) positive career development and early work experiences, (3) collaboration and interagency involvement, (4) family supports and expectations, (5) fostering self-determination and independence, (6) social and employment-related skill instruction, and (7) establishment of job-related supports. Therefore, outcomes for emerging adults with ASD could be improved if social and institutional supports available through adolescence continued into adulthood.

6.2 Type 1 Diabetes Mellitus (DM)

The study of emerging adults with type 1 DM has elucidated the potential challenges facing emerging adults with diabetes and other chronic health conditions that have significant self-management burden. Emerging adults with type 1 diabetes face extensive behavioral demands in order to maintain their health, including the necessity for precisely scheduled daily insulin injections, blood glucose monitoring, dietary monitoring, regular physical exercise, and the management of DM-related complications. In early adulthood, frequent changes in roles, living situations, educational routines, jobs, friendships, and romantic relationships are common and can undermine the routines and the resolve needed to maintain metabolic control (Anderson and Wolpert 2004).

The developmental tasks of emerging adulthood may be at odds with maintaining the intensive self-care that is required of those with type 1 diabetes and vice versa. For example, the tasks of establishing autonomy and prevailing egocentrism may be associated with the emerging adult not wanting to follow medical advice or advice of his or her family (Masten et al. 1995). Heightened concern for peer acceptance or the establishment of intimate relationships is characteristic of this period of development. Emerging adults may be reluctant to admit to their significant others that they have type 1 diabetes or any other chronic condition that puts them at risk for being rejected (Madsen et al. 2002). Moreover, the major cognitive developmental milestone during the stage of emerging adulthood is the ability to think abstractly (Erikson 1994). Those who have not yet reached this developmental milestone may struggle with taking responsibility to maintain good disease management and understanding the consequences of poor disease management. Lastly, increased rates of drinking, illicit drug use, or other high-risk behaviors may disrupt the emerging adults' lifestyle and negatively impact self-care management of diabetes, resulting in (Madsen et al. 2002) lack of control of diabetes and the resulting physical and mental consequences of hypo- or hyperglycemia, which undermine emerging adults' abilities to perform in school, maintain relationships, or keep employment.

As has been demonstrated in other chronic childhood conditions, the transition from pediatric- to adult-centered medical care for youth with DM is associated with a decline in DM control (Busse et al. 2007; Oeffinger et al. 2006). Adverse health-related outcomes documented in the young adult population with diabetes include a decline in disease self-care behaviors and an increased risk for diabetes-related complications (Bryden et al. 2001; Fredericks et al. 2010; Yeung et al. 2008). In addition, emerging adults with diabetes are at higher than average risk for psychosocial morbidity including social delays and isolation, impaired social competence, and emotional problems such as depression (Helgeson et al. 2007). As in the case in ASD, additional support for an emerging adult with DM during the transition to adult medical care has been shown to help decrease the adverse outcomes seen with usual practice. For example, DM transition programs that include introductions to new adult care providers or intensive care coordination have been found to be protective (Holmes-Walker et al. 2007).

6.3 Chronic Kidney Disease

Chronic kidney disease (CKD) is a condition characterized by disease progression, significant cardiovascular morbidity, growth failure, neurocognitive impairment, and impaired quality of life changes (Sarnak 2003; Copelovitch et al. 2011; Gerson et al. 2006; McKenna et al. 2006). CKD is divided into five stages based on glomerular filtration rate, with stage 1 being the mildest form and stage 5 the worst form, also called end-stage kidney disease (ESKD), requiring renal replacement therapy (dialysis or transplant) (Hogg et al. 2003). The prevalence of pediatric CKD is unknown as it may be silent in early stages. The prevalence of pediatric ESKD is 15 cases per million population (Saran et al. 2015). African-Americans and Latinos are disproportionately affected by CKD in part due to a higher incidence of glomerular conditions (Ferris et al. 2006). While the 10-year survival for adolescent-onset ESKD is 80–85% (much higher than adult-onset ESKD patients), this still represents a 30-fold increase in mortality compared to the general US adolescent population. Survival is better for younger adolescents, males, Caucasians, Asians, and transplant recipients (2006). However, emerging adults with CKD achieve adult milestones (e.g., employment, marriage) less frequently than their healthy peers (Bartosh et al. 2003).

The burden of care directly correlates with the stage of CKD. Based on the mean number of unique medications, those with CKD stages 1–4 take 6.2 ± 4 of medications, those with peritoneal dialysis (CKD 5) take 8.5 ± 2 medications, those with kidney transplant (CKD 5) take 9.7 ± 4.2 medications, and those on hemodialysis (CKD 5) take 11.3 ± 2.1 (So et al. 2011). The complexity of care also include procedures such as self-catheterization several times per day, fluid and dietary restrictions, blood pressure measurements daily, and injections (erythropoiesis-stimulating agents once to thrice weekly, growth hormone daily, or insulin several times per day). The life course of pediatric-onset CKD-ESKD varies by etiology and age at onset of this condition, but once they reach ESKD, most patients share the same comorbidities (hypertension, anemia, acidosis, metabolic bone disease, and growth delay). Patients with greater level of CKD have a decreased sense of self-worth, perceive a poor future, and feel limited in their physical and psychosocial capacities to have the same potential and opportunity as their healthy peers.

While most children and adolescent patients with ESKD will receive a kidney transplant, they likely will experience dialysis prior to receiving an organ. The most common cause of kidney transplant rejection in adolescents and emerging adults is treatment nonadherence (Andreoni et al. 2013). Adherence among adolescents is compromised by poor understanding and poor consequence recognition leading to an inconsistent commitment to the treatment regimens. Once the kidney transplant is lost, patients return to dialysis and likely will not receive another kidney transplant for many years. As in adult patients, cardiovascular disease (CVD) accounts for a majority of deaths in patients with pediatric-onset CKD, but unlike adults, pediatric-onset CKD patients rarely demonstrate symptomatic atherosclerosis (Shroff et al. 2011). Lastly, survivors of pediatric-onset CKD are at greater risk for malignancies and post-transplant diabetes mellitus (Koukourgianni et al. 2010).

Patients who transfer to adult-focused services without transition preparation and support appear to be at greater risk to lose their kidney transplant (Watson 2000, 2005). The international societies of internal medicine and pediatric nephrology have published position statements and policies to promote health-care transition preparation (Watson 2005; Watson et al. 2011). Strategies to increase patient autonomy, health-care transition, and self-management are needed to achieve successful outcomes at the time of transfer to adult-focused providers.

6.4 Mental Health and Substance Use

Emerging adulthood is a time of increased experimentation with tobacco, drugs, and alcohol (Schulenberg et al. 2004; Schulenberg and Maggs 2002), increasing from rates of 12.2% in adolescence to 40.2% in young adulthood for cigarette smoking, from 10.7% to 41.9% for binge drinking, from 11.2% to 20.3% for illicit drug use, and from 2.6% to 14.9% for heavy alcohol use. While cigarette, alcohol, and drug use are normative during adolescence and emerging adulthood, a number of factors predict excessive use rather than experimentation including genetic (e.g., family history of alcohol abuse), biological (e.g., early puberty timing), family (e.g., low parental monitoring), school (e.g., low grade average, school failure), peer (e.g., peer substance use), and youth personality and psychopathology (e.g., depression) factors (Cicchetti 1999). However, the pattern of use/abuse of these substances is influenced by the experience during the stage of EA. For example, increasing responsibility, work, and marriage all are associated with decreased use of these substances (Masten et al. 1999; Bachman et al. 2014). Again, there is great heterogeneity in the trajectories followed by individuals with regard to substance use during this period, all influenced by the multiplicity of factors listed above.

Among young adults, 13.7% experience serious mental illness such as major depressive disorders, schizophrenia, and bipolar disorder (AmericanPsychiatricAssociation 2013). The neuropsychological pathology that has onset during EA has many of the predisposing factors related to family adversities, such as social disadvantage, divorce, dysfunctional parenting, multiple family changes/moves, and peer group choices. The expanded independence and self-reliance during EA may be difficult to handle for youth with preexisting emotional or social challenges or poor attachment. The decrease in supports from school or family during EA may be even further destabilizing, leading to increased emotional and interpersonal difficulties. Young people with serious mental health conditions have difficulty with impulse control and self-regulation (Walker and Gowen 2011). Their apparent immaturity reflects a delay in social and emotional development and undermines progress toward goals in education, relationships, independence in health, and health-care management.

Three-quarters of lifetime cases of mental, emotional, and behavioral disorders begin by age 24 (Kessler et al. 2005). In emerging adults with social, emotional, and behavioral disorders, much higher risk is associated with onset in early adolescence versus onset in late adolescence (Mofitt and Caspi 2001). Dysfunctional family environments and participation in deviant peer group increase the likelihood of early-onset delinquency followed by a long trajectory of social, emotional, and behavioral problems. Youth with later onset of social, emotional, and behavioral problems are more commonly from relatively healthy family backgrounds and more likely to desist from delinquency by age 23 (Roisman et al. 2004). Similar patterns can be seen for major psychiatric disorders such as depression, with early-onset mood disorders being representative of more severe recurrent forms of mood disorders arising from increased severity and complexity of family and biologic risk factors (Fergusson and Woodward 2002) and later-onset disorders reflecting lower levels of risk factors in childhood.

7 Protective and Risk Factors That Impact Emerging Adulthood

The supports, opportunities, and experiences that occur during the stage of EA greatly influence the ultimate outcome of this stage and the ensuing life trajectory into young adulthood. As discussed in this chapter, critical influences during EA include mentoring relationships, socioeconomic supports, and educational and vocational opportunities. Emerging adulthood typically is accompanied by an increase in agency/independence and decrease in social and institutional support (e.g., schools and family), such that most individuals have more choice in day-to-day activities and life decisions. This increase in choice may result in greater success which will likely contribute to well-being. However, increased freedom can result in poor choices (e.g., drug use, criminal activity) that have a negative impact on the developmental trajectory as well (Schulenberg and Maggs 2002; Schulenberg et al. 2004). For example, many relationships and other aspects of life are so unstable during EA that important and powerful negative experiences can occur such as date rape, school failure, and substance addiction. These experiences can have a lasting, if not lifetime, detrimental impact on the developmental and mental health trajectory of the emerging adult. Similarly, many potential powerful positive influences can occur during this period in life (e.g., marriage, educational achievement, mentoring) that can enhance the developmental and mental health trajectory. Therefore, experiences both distal (early childhood) and proximal (during emerging adulthood) can influence, either positively or negatively, the developmental and mental health trajectory of the emerging adult (Miller et al. 2015).

Practical supports during EA provided by families include financial support for education, transportation, independent living, health insurance, and other necessities. The primary determinant of parental support are the level of parental resources. Emerging adults with wealthier parents and those with fewer siblings receive more financial support for education (Steelman and Powell 1991). Divorced parents provide less financial support than parents with intact marriages (Cooney and Uhlenberg 1992). Support from families by parents and grandparents during EA is also provided in the form of guidance or advice, information, and emotional support. Parents of emerging adults may also help the emerging adult negotiate the health-care system, formulate and carry out educational and vocational goals, and acquire leases for apartments and even provide advice for intimate relationships. In short, continued social and financial connection to parents with adequate emotional and financial resources can be a very significant factor in the positive life trajectory during emerging adulthood (Aquilino 2005). Previous studies have found a high correlation between improved EA outcomes and adolescent hope in the future (Bennett 2014). Hope is a form of personal capital that protects youth from social, emotional, and behavioral disorders and correlates with and predicts the rates of many outcomes, including academic achievement, delay of initiation of early sexual activity, and lower likelihood of violent behavior. Hope requires a sense of self-efficacy and knowledge of alternate outcomes. Hope is reflected in adolescent and young adult goals as they reflect and make ongoing assessments of their current and future selves. Individual goals and aspirations relate to the sense of control an individual feels in relation to a particular domain.

Positive youth development (PYD) programs are approaches that provide supports to adolescents and emerging adults to achieve social, emotional, behavioral, and moral competence, foster self-efficacy, a clear and positive identity, and belief in the future; and reinforce pro-social norms (Catalano et al. 2004). Positive development approaches involve a paradigm shift from targeting the risk factors to enhancing the assets and protective factors. The emphasis on hope, empowerment, and well-being resonates with youth and mental health professionals. The PYD approach outlined above suggests that effective programs to support EA would include an individualized approach supporting young people to identify and move toward personally meaningful goals. This begins with envisioning a positive future identity ("Who do I want to become?"). Pursuing goals promotes a sense of purpose, and making progress toward those goals contributes to building feelings of efficacy, empowerment, and self-determination, enhancing the individual's ability to act as the primary causal agent in pursuing personally meaningful goals (Silbereisen and Lerner 2007).

A PYD perspective further suggests that youth and emerging adults will benefit from learning specific strategies for increasing and maintaining interpersonal support from positive peers, family, providers, and people in the community (Guerra and Bradshaw 2008). Young people can learn specific steps and skills that can help them increase the quality and the extent of their interpersonal networks, as well as the amount of emotional, instrumental, and informational support available to them. Using a PYD perspective suggests that the development of assets is an important recovery-oriented outcome in and of themselves, as well as a mediator of longer-term outcomes related to education, employment, mental health, and general quality of life. Indeed, a review of the available research on community-based programs and interventions for EA reveals a common focus on personal asset building (Lerner 2014). Also consistent with the PYD perspective is that many of the programs and interventions include a focus on changing the meso-environment of youth so that it encourages young people to develop or express strengths and assets.

8 Services and Supports

As we better understand the limits of and issues related to EA, it is imperative that we review and revise policy and current social and medical services and supports so they optimally address the current and future needs of individuals during this life stage. Current medical, mental health, and social service delivery models are geared toward either child or adult populations. In other words, individuals generally seek child-serving services between the ages of 0 and 18, and they are subsequently transferred directly to adult-serving services. However, the various biobehavioral and sociocultural factors discussed above make this direct transition from child to adult-centered care ill-suited for optimally addressing the nuances and challenges that individuals may face during EA. For example, an adult-centered medical doctor may regularly treat patients with fixed habits and lifestyles, who may already suffer from a variety of chronic health conditions. However, many such chronic health conditions in adults represent a culmination of experiences from an individual's earlier years, which may not yet be apparent during EA. It is thus strongly recommended that EA service providers reorient themselves using a prevention-based paradigm and familiarize themselves with the possible antecedents to social, emotional, and medical conditions so that they may make health-care or social service recommendations to minimize risk factors and to maximize strengths and assets to facilitate development along optimal health trajectories. EA presents a unique opportunity for service providers to intervene and influence an individual's LCHD before significant social, emotional, and medical pathology fully develops, utilizing existing knowledge of the skills and capacities associated with EA to inform services and interventions.

In addition to training service providers to reorient their approach to care and become more sensitive to antecedents of chronic health conditions in adulthood, the multifactorial nature of the LCHD model suggests that it would be important for service providers to consider horizontal (i.e., cross sector) and longitudinal (i.e., across the lifespan) service integration. Specifically, the current model posits that myriad factors (e.g., biological, psychological, cultural) on multiple levels (e.g., micro, meso, macro) interact simultaneously in a transactional fashion to influence an individual's LCHD and overall health trajectory. However, most current training models which emphasize specialization in their independent fields and opportunities for cross-disciplinary case conceptualization and collaboration with regard to service delivery – particularly with respect to preventive care, which may be of special importance when considering EA as a sensitive period of development – tend to be rare. Such specialization in service delivery may result in service fragmentation. Additionally, adult service providers generally do not work in tandem with child service providers as individuals transition from one care setting to the next, consequently resulting in potential gaps in service delivery and care, which may be exacerbated as individuals work to rebuild rapport with their new service providers. Moreover, health, mental health, social service, and education professionals rarely collaborate to create comprehensive models across the EA stage. Clearly, the current service delivery infrastructure does not adequately support the needs and challenges unique to emerging adult populations. It is thus important to recognize emerging adults as a unique population requiring additional and specialized skills of service providers and the creation of specific pathways for transition which support continuity of care.

The larger sociopolitical and cultural contexts may also facilitate or create challenges which impact service and intervention efforts directed at emerging adults. The majority of individuals in developed nations transitioning through EA, for instance, may be classified as "digital natives," individuals who have been brought up in environments where exposure to digital technology may be normative and who are therefore familiar with computers and the Internet. As emerging adults increasingly turn to digital and mobile solutions to support and enhance their daily routines, it behooves service providers to creatively explore ways of engaging emerging adult populations using technology. Use of social networks, such as Instagram, Twitter, and Facebook, to advance primary prevention efforts, increase awareness of public health issues, and provide basic health and psychological education affords service providers the opportunity to outreach to unprecedented numbers and populations. Use of text messaging may also be effective as a way of engaging with digital native emerging adult populations and promoting engagement and adherence by emerging adults or to promote youth development programs. Also, as service providers keep pace with technological advancements, they may even begin to explore novel methods of service delivery and intervention using digital or Internet-based platforms, which may increase "buy-in" and potentially preventive service utilization, among digitally native emerging adult populations. For example, service providers might potentially leverage the data that digitally native emerging adults might collect as part of the "quantified self" movement (e.g., pedometer information, weight, blood pressure, etc.) in an effort to inform their ongoing care efforts.

On the other hand, due to clinical billing practices and regulations, as well as patient privacy concerns and regulations (e.g., Health Insurance

Portability and Accountability Act, HIPAA), current service delivery models often tend to operate in a fragmented and siloed fashion, which in turn may limit the ability of service providers to develop a holistic treatment plan to address each individual's needs. Further complicating this fragmentation is the restricted access to health records once an individual turns 18 years of age, when parents who may have been primarily responsible for managing their child's health-care needs no longer are able to access their child's medical records (unless explicit permission is granted by the child, who is now an emerging adult). Depending on each family's cultural context and the relationship between the emerging adult and his or her parents, this transition may be a cause for significant stress and/or strife between family members as they work to renegotiate previously familiar boundaries. Mothers of children with diabetes, for example, have indicated feeling increased stress as their children transitioned from pediatric to adult care, particularly if they perceived that their children were not managing their health-care condition as well as they had been when it was previously under greater parent control (Allen et al. 2011). Such stress might result in familial conflict and dysfunction which could subsequently interfere with the emerging adult's willingness or ability to adequately access services. One potential solution to overcoming the issue of patient privacy may be to implement public health programs and tools to educate and empower individuals with respect to managing and taking an active role in their own care. However, it is important to underscore the need for larger, overall systems to change in order to support service providers in working together with individuals and their families to ensure continuity and comprehensiveness of services and health-related information during the transition.

Finally, the implementation of health-care policies may have important implications for service and intervention delivery with an emerging adult population. With the introduction of the Patient Protection and Affordable Care Act of 2010 (ACA), for example, individuals may now remain on their parents' health insurance plans until they turn 26 years of age. While this theoretically affords emerging adults the opportunity to develop the necessary skills for interacting with the health-care system and managing their own care, research indicates that emerging adults frequently perceived themselves as being at lower risk for health problems and the financial burden of health insurance as lacking in value. Consequently, emerging adults may opt for high-deductible catastrophic insurance which generally costs less compared to other health insurance plans, but translates to fewer opportunities for interaction with the health service sector and fewer opportunities for service providers to intervene early during an individual's LCHD trajectory prior to the onset of chronic adult disease. Importantly, research indicates that despite preventive maintenance health visits being mandatory under the ACA, emerging adults were less likely to request health maintenance visits. Thus, it may be important for public health efforts to determine the underlying factors associated with this diminished utilization of health services by emerging adults and subsequently develop health literacy programs to promote prevention mindedness and service utilization in emerging adults.

9 Recommendations for Research Priorities

The following is a list of issues in life course research that are critical for better understanding the positive supports and challenges that influence the trajectory of development of emerging adults organized along the macro-, meso-, micro-framework.

Macro Issues

- What community supports in emerging adulthood enhance health development into adulthood and improve outcomes for an emerging adult with specific health, mental health, and developmental conditions? Is there an "early intervention model" to optimize outcomes for EA? What model should be used for an

emerging adult with chronic health, mental health, and developmental conditions?
- What are the historical, economic, and cultural influences on the meaning of EA, adaptation, and maladaptation to the stage and expectations for normative transitions? How have these changed over time? How are they different for an emerging adult with social, health, mental health, and developmental problems?
- How have the delays in marriage/relationship commitment impacted adult life trajectories?
- What are the racial and ethnic differences for how these factors interact to support development during EA?
- How has the information economy and the increased demands for education impacted the life course for youth in upper, middle, and lower socioeconomic strata? Are there regional variations in these outcomes and how can they be improved?

Meso Issues

- Earlier childhood development and family environment are predictors of adult outcomes, but it is unclear how optimizing health development can be achieved with supports during EA.
- What is the interaction between health and social system supports, family supports, youth abilities, cognitive and psychological maturity, and EA outcomes for an emerging adult with and without mental or physical disabilities?
- How can the different support systems be integrated to provide seamless services to youth and emerging adults with significant physical, mental health, or intellectual disabilities?
- Using the model below from the work of Masten et al. (2005), how do these different resources, supports, and personal characteristics interact to promote optimal development during EA? (Fig. 1)
- What factors promote resilience for youth during EA who lack family supports?
- What is the role of extended families in support for EA?
- How can studies of conditions and processes that influence development during EA inform educational/vocational/EA support policies?
- How can data be gathered across this stage in the lifespan given that emerging adults leave school and have many changes in living arrangements, education, relationships, and work?

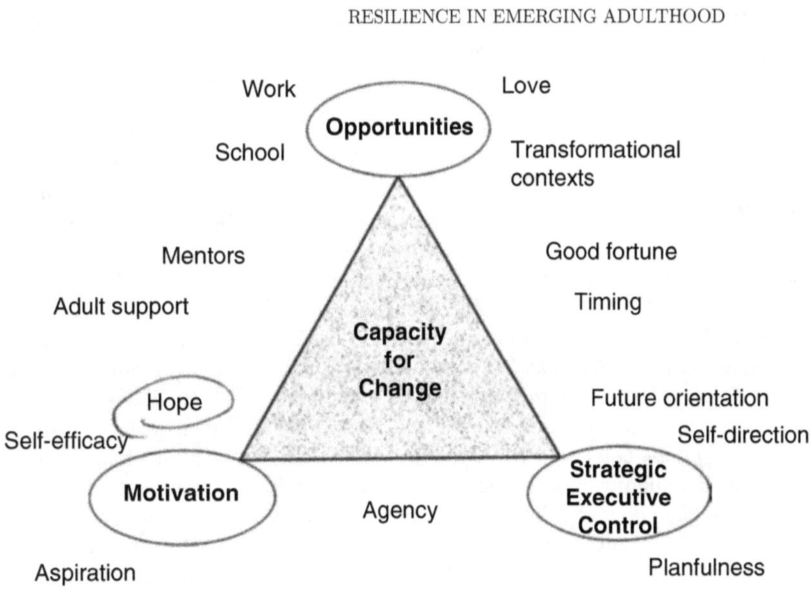

Fig. 1 Moving toward resilience: a model of positive change in emerging adulthood

Micro Issues

- To what degree is cognitive, social, physical, moral, and spiritual development mediated during emerging adulthood? How are these developmental pathways impacted by chronic health, mental health, and developmental conditions?
- How can we optimize the person-context match to promote development during EA with and without chronic health, mental health, and developmental conditions?
- What is the impact of positive turning points in EA compared to early life stages on life trajectories into adulthood?
- During EA, exploration of new experiences is normative. Is more exploration better or worse and for which activities is it better or worse? How is this equation different for an emerging adult with chronic health, mental health, and developmental conditions?
- Do emerging adults with particular health conditions, such as diabetes, spina bifida, solid organ transplant, or cancer survivorship, experience sharply downward trajectories during EA, and what supports are effective to prevent these sharply downward trajectories?
- How does brain development progress during EA? What is the impact of brain development on the factors that influence the developmental trajectory during EA such as executive control (planfulness, future orientation), motivation, self-efficacy, and hope?

References

Allen, D., Channon, S., Lowes, L., Atwell, C., & Lane, C. (2011). Behind the scenes: The changing roles of parents in the transition from child to adult diabetes service. *Diabetic Medicine, 28*(8), 994–1000.

Alwin, D. F. (1988). From obedience to autonomy changes in traits desired in children, 1924–1978. *Public Opinion Quarterly, 52*, 33–52.

American Psychiatric Association. (2013). *Diagnostic and statistical manual of mental disorders*. Arlington: American Psychiatric Publishing.

Anderson, B. J., & Wolpert, H. A. (2004). A developmental perspective on the challenges of diabetes education and care during the young adult period. *Patient Education and Counseling, 53*, 347–352.

Andreoni, K. A., Forbes, R., Andreoni, R. M., Phillips, G., Stewart, H., & Ferris, M. (2013). Age-related kidney transplant outcomes: Health disparities amplified in adolescence. *JAMA Internal Medicine, 173*, 1524–1532.

Aquilino, W. S. (1994). Impact of childhood family disruption on young Adults' relationships with parents. *Journal of Marriage and the Family, 56*, 295–313.

Aquilino, W. S. (2005). Impact of family structure on parental attitudes toward the economic support of adult children over the transition to adulthood. *Journal of Family Issues, 26*, 143–167.

Arnett, J. J. (1997). Young People's conceptions of the transition to adulthood. *Youth & Society, 29*, 3–23.

Arnett, J. J. (1998). Learning to stand alone: The contemporary American transition to adulthood in cultural and historical context. *Human Development, 41*, 295–315.

Arnett, J. J. (2000). Emerging adulthood: A theory of development from the late teens through the twenties. *American Psychologist, 55*, 469.

Arnett, J. J. (2005). The developmental context of substance use in emerging adulthood. *Journal of Drug Issues, 35*, 235–254.

Arnett, J. J. (2014). *Emerging adulthood: The winding road from the late teens through the twenties*. New York: Oxford University Press.

Bachman, J. G., O'malley, P. M., Schulenberg, J. E., Johnston, L. D., Bryant, A. L., & Merline, A. C. (2014). *The decline of substance use in young adulthood: Changes in social activities, roles, and beliefs*. New York: Psychology Press.

Bartosh, S. M., Leverson, G., Robillard, D., & Sollinger, H. W. (2003). Long-term outcomes in pediatric renal transplant recipients who survive into adulthood. *Transplantation, 76*, 1195–1200.

Bellah, E. R. N., Bellah, R. N., Tipton, S. M., Sullivan, W. M., Madsen, R., Swidler, A., Sullivan, W. M., & Tipton, S. M. (2007). *Habits of the heart: Individualism and commitment in American life*. Berkeley: University of California Press.

Ben-Amos, I. K. (1994). *Adolescence and youth in early modern England*. New Haven: Yale University Press.

Bennett, A. (2014). Finding hope in hopeless environments. *International Journal of Child Health And Human Development, 7*, 313.

Benson, J. E., & Elder, G. H. (2011). Young adult identities and their pathways: A developmental and life course model. *Developmental Psychology, 47*, 1646–1657.

Benson, J. E., Johnson, M. K., & Elder, G. H. (2012). The implications of adult identity for educational and work attainment in young adulthood. *Developmental Psychology, 48*(6), 1752.

Billstedt, E., Gillberg, C., & Gillberg, C. (2005). Autism after adolescence: Population-based 13-to 22-year follow-up study of 120 individuals with autism diagnosed in childhood. *Journal of Autism and Developmental Disorders, 35*, 351–360.

Bogin, B. (2013). Chapter 2, Childhood, adolescence and longevity: A chapter on human Evolutionary life history. In B. Hewlett (Ed.), *Adolescent identify: Evolutionary, cultural and developmental perspectives*. New York: Routledge.

Brody, G. H., et al. (2013). Is resilience only skin deep? Rural African Americans' socioeconomic status–related risk and competence in preadolescence and psychological adjustment and Allostatic load at age 19. *Psychological Science*. doi:10.1177/0956797612471954.

Bryden, K. S., Peveler, R. C., Stein, A., Neil, A., Mayou, R. A., & Dunger, D. B. (2001). Clinical and psychological course of diabetes from adolescence to young adulthood a longitudinal cohort study. *Diabetes Care, 24*, 1536–1540.

Busse, F., Hiermann, P., Galler, A., Stumvoll, M., Wiessner, T., Kiess, W., & Kapellen, T. (2007). Evaluation of patients' opinion and metabolic control after transfer of young adults with type 1 diabetes from a pediatric diabetes clinic to adult care. *Hormone Research in Pædiatrics, 67*, 132–138.

Catalano, R. F., Berglund, M. L., Ryan, J. A., Lonczak, H. S., & Hawkins, J. D. (2004). Positive youth development in the United States: Research findings on evaluations of positive youth development programs. *The Annals of the American Academy of Political and Social Science, 591*, 98–124.

Cherlin, A. J., Chase-Lansdale, P. L., & Mcrae, C. (1998). Effects of parental divorce on mental health throughout the life course. *American Sociological Review, 63*(2), 239–249.

Cicchetti, D., et al. (1999). *A developmental psychopathology perspective on drug abuse. Drug abuse: Origins & interventions* (pp. 97–117). Washington, DC: American Psychological Association, xxiii, 492 pp.

Cimera, R. E., & Cowan, R. J. (2009). The costs of services and employment outcomes achieved by adults with autism in the us. *Autism, 13*, 285–302.

Cooney, T. M., & Uhlenberg, P. (1992). Support from parents over the life course: The adult Child's perspective. *Social Forces, 71*, 63–84.

Copelovitch, L., Warady, B. A., & Furth, S. L. (2011). Insights from the chronic kidney disease in children (Ckid) study. *Clinical Journal of the American Society of Nephrology, 6*, 2047–2053.

Cote, J. E. (2014). The dangerous myth of emerging adulthood: An evidence-based critique of a flawed developmental theory. *Applied Developmental Science, 18*(4), 177–188.

Dahl, R. E. (2004). Adolescent brain development: A period of vulnerabilities and opportunities. Keynote address. *Annals of the New York Academy of Sciences, 1021*, 1–22.

Duncan, G. J., & Brooks-Gunn, J. (2000). Family poverty, welfare reform, and child development. *Child Development, 71*, 188–196.

Eaves, L. C., & Ho, H. H. (2008). Young adult outcome of autism Spectrum disorders. *Journal of Autism and Developmental Disorders, 38*, 739–747.

Erikson, E. H. (1994). *Identity: Youth and crisis*. New York: Ww Norton & Company.

Evans, G. W., & Cassells, R. C. (2014). Childhood poverty, cumulative risk exposure, and mental health in emerging adults. *Clinical Psychological Science, 2*(3), 287–296.

Feliciano, C., & Ashtiani, M. (2012). *Postsecondary educational pathways of low-income youth: An analysis of add health data*. Irvine: Uc/Accord.

Fergusson, D. M., & Woodward, L. J. (2002). Mental health, educational, and social role outcomes of adolescents with depression. *Archives of General Psychiatry, 59*, 225–231.

Ferris, M. E., Gipson, D. S., Kimmel, P. L., & Eggers, P. W. (2006). Trends in treatment and outcomes of survival of adolescents initiating end-stage renal disease care in the United States of America. *Pediatric Nephrology, 21*, 1020–1026.

Fredericks, E. M., Dore-Stites, D., Well, A., Magee, J. C., Freed, G. L., Shieck, V., & James Lopez, M. (2010). Assessment of transition readiness skills and adherence in pediatric liver transplant recipients. *Pediatric Transplantation, 14*, 944–953.

Furstenberg, F. F. (2002). How it takes thirty years to do a study. In *Looking at lives: American longitudinal studies of the twentieth century* (pp. 37–57).

Galobardes, B., Lynch, J. W., & Smith, G. D. (2008). Is the Association between childhood socioeconomic circumstances and cause-specific mortality established? Update of a systematic review. *Journal of Epidemiology and Community Health, 62*, 387–390.

Garcia-Villamisar, D., Ross, D., & Wehman, P. (2000). Clinical differential analysis of persons with autism in a work setting: A follow-up study. *Journal Of Vocational Rehabilitation, 14*, 183–185.

Gerson, A. C., Butler, R., Moxey-Mims, M., Wentz, A., Shinnar, S., Lande, M. B., Mendley, S. R., Warady, B. A., Furth, S. L., & Hooper, S. R. (2006). Neurocognitive outcomes in children with chronic kidney disease: Current findings and contemporary endeavors. *Mental Retardation and Developmental Disabilities Research Reviews, 12*(3), 208–215.

Gillespie-Lynch, K., Sepeta, L., Wang, Y., Marshall, S., Gomez, L., Sigman, M., & Hutman, T. (2012). Early childhood predictors of the social competence of adults with autism. *Journal of Autism and Developmental Disorders, 42*, 161–174.

Gilman, S. E. (2012). The successes and challenges of life course Epidemiology: A commentary on Gibb, Fergusson and Horwood (2012). *Social Science & Medicine, 75*, 2124–2128.

Gilman, S. E., & Loucks, E. B. (2012). Invited commentary: Does the childhood environment influence the Association between every X and every Y in adulthood? *American Journal of Epidemiology, 176*, 684–688.

Gilmore, D. D. (1990). *Manhood in the making: Cultural concepts of masculinity*. New Haven: Yale University Press.

Greene, A., Wheatley, S. M., & Aldava, J. F. (1992). Stages on Life's way Adolescents' implicit theories of the life course. *Journal of Adolescent Research, 7*, 364–381.

Grotevant, H. D., & Cooper, C. R. (1986). Individuation in family relationships. *Human Development, 29*, 82–100.

Guerra, N. G., & Bradshaw, C. P. (2008). Linking the prevention of problem behaviors and positive youth development: Core competencies for positive youth development and risk prevention. *New Directions for Child and Adolescent Development, 2008*, 1–17.

Halfon, N., & Forrest, C. B. (2017). The emerging theoretical framework of life course health development. In N. Halfon, C. B. Forrest, R. M. Lerner, & E. Faustman (Eds.), *Handbook of life course health-development science*. Cham: Springer.

Helgeson, V. S., Snyder, P. R., Escobar, O., Siminerio, L., & Becker, D. (2007). Comparison of adolescents with and without diabetes on indices of psychosocial functioning for three years. *Journal of Pediatric Psychology, 32*, 794–806.

Hogg, R. J., Furth, S., Lemley, K. V., Portman, R., Schwartz, G. J., Coresh, J., Balk, E., Lau, J., Levin, A., & Kausz, A. T. (2003). National Kidney Foundation's kidney disease outcomes quality initiative clinical practice guidelines for chronic kidney disease in children and adolescents: Evaluation, classification, and stratification. *Pediatrics, 111*, 1416–1421.

Holmes-Walker, D., Llewellyn, A., & Farrell, K. (2007). A transition care Programme which improves diabetes control and reduces hospital admission rates in young adults with type 1 diabetes aged 15–25 years. *Diabetic Medicine, 24*, 764–769.

Howlin, P., Goode, S., Hutton, J., & Rutter, M. (2004). Adult outcome for children with autism. *Journal of Child Psychology and Psychiatry, 45*, 212–229.

Jacquet, S. E., & Surra, C. A. (2001). Parental divorce and premarital couples: Commitment and other relationship characteristics. *Journal of Marriage and Family, 63*, 627–638.

Kessler, R. C., Berglund, P., Demler, O., Jin, R., Merikangas, K. R., & Walters, E. E. (2005). Lifetime prevalence and age-of-onset distributions of Dsm-iv disorders in the National Comorbidity Survey Replication. *Archives of General Psychiatry, 62*, 593–602.

Kim, P., Neuendorf, C., Bianco, H., & Evans, G. W. (2015). Exposure to childhood poverty and mental health symptomatology in adolescence: A role of coping strategies. *Stress and Health, 32*, 494–502.

Koukourgianni, F., Harambat, J., Ranchin, B., Euvrard, S., Bouvier, R., Liutkus, A., & Cochat, P. (2010). Malignancy incidence after renal transplantation in children: A 20-year single-Centre experience. *Nephrology Dialysis Transplantation, 25*, 611–616.

Lerner, R. M. (2014). Developmental science, developmental systems, and contemporary theories of human development. In *Handbook of child psychology*. New York: Wiley and Sons.

Lotstein, D. S., Inkelas, M., Hays, R. D., Halfon, N., & Brook, R. (2008). Access to care for youth with special health care needs in the transition to adulthood. *Journal of Adolescent Health, 43*, 23–29.

Luciana, M., Conklin, H. M., Hooper, C. J., & Yarger, R. S. (2005). The development of nonverbal working memory and executive control processes in adolescents. *Child Development, 76*, 697–712.

Madsen, S. D., Roisman, G. I., & Collins, W. A. (2002). The intersection of adolescent development and intensive intervention: Age-related psychosocial correlates of treatment regimens in the diabetes control and complication trial. *Journal of Pediatric Psychology, 27*, 451–459.

Masten, A. S., & Coatsworth, J. D. (1998). The development of competence in favorable and unfavorable environments: Lessons from research on successful children. *American Psychologist, 53*, 205.

Masten, A. S., Coatsworth, J. D., Neemann, J., Gest, S. D., Tellegen, A., & Garmezy, N. (1995). The structure and coherence of competence from childhood through adolescence. *Child Development, 66*, 1635–1659.

Masten, A. S., Hubbard, J. J., Gest, S. D., Tellegen, A., Garmezy, N., & Ramirez, M. (1999). Competence in the context of adversity: Pathways to resilience and maladaptation from childhood to late adolescence. *Development and Psychopathology, 11*, 143–169.

Masten, A. S., Burt, K. B., Roisman, G. I., Obradovic, J., Long, J. D., & Tellegen, A. (2004). Resources and resilience in the transition to adulthood: Continuity and change. *Development and Psychopathology, 16*, 1071–1094.

Masten, A. S., Roisman, G. I., Long, J. D., Burt, K. B., Obradović, J., Riley, J. R., Boelcke-Stennes, K., & Tellegen, A. (2005). Developmental cascades: Linking academic achievement and externalizing and internalizing symptoms over 20 years. *Developmental Psychology, 41*, 733.

Masten, A. S., Burt, K. B., & Coatsworth, J. D. (2006). Competence and psychopathology in development. D. Cicchetti, C. Dante, & J. Donald (Eds). *Developmental psychopathology: Risk, disorder, and adaptation* (Vol. 3, 2nd ed., pp. 696–738). Hoboken: John Wiley & Sons Inc, xvi 944 pp.

Mawhood, L., & Howlin, P. (1999). The outcome of a supported employment scheme for high-functioning adults with autism or Asperger syndrome. *Autism, 3*, 229–254.

Mckenna, A. M., Keating, L. E., Vigneux, A., Stevens, S., Williams, A., & Geary, D. F. (2006). Quality of life in children with chronic kidney disease—Patient and caregiver assessments. *Nephrology Dialysis Transplantation, 21*, 1899–1905.

Mikulincer, M., & Shaver, P. R. (2009). The attachment and behavioral systems perspective on social support. *Journal of Social and Personal Relationships, 26*(1), 7–19.

Miller, G. E., Yu, T., Chen, E., & Brody, G. H. (2015 Aug 18). Self-control forecasts better psychosocial outcomes but faster epigenetic aging in low-Ses youth. *Proceedings Of The National Academy Of Sciences., 112*(33), 10325–10330.

Modell, J. (1991). *Into One's own: From youth to adulthood in the United States, 1920–1975.* Berkeley: University of California Press.

Moffitt, T. E., & Caspi, A. (2001). Childhood predictors differentiate life-course persistent and adolescence-limited antisocial pathways among males and females. *Devcelopment and Psychopathology, 13*, 355–375.

Nelson, C. A., Thomas, K. M., & De Haan, M. (2012). *Neuroscience of cognitive development: The role of experience and the developing brain.* Hoboken: John Wiley & Sons.

Newman, L., Wagner, M., Knokey, A.-M., Marder, C., Nagle, K., Shaver, D., & Wei, X. (2011). *The post-high school outcomes of young adults with disabilities up to 8 years after high school: A Report from the National Longitudinal Transition Study-2 (Nlts2). Ncser 2011–3005.* Washington, DC: National Center For Special Education Research.

Nurmi, J.-E. (1999). 15 self-definition and mental health during adolescence and young adulthood. In J. Schulenberg, J. L. Maggs, & K. Hurrelmann (Eds.), *Health risks and developmental transitions during adolescence* (p. 395). New York: Cambridge University Press.

Oeffinger, K. C., Mertens, A. C., Sklar, C. A., Kawashima, T., Hudson, M. M., Meadows, A. T., Friedman, D. L., Marina, N., Hobbie, W., & Kadan-Lottick, N. S. (2006). Chronic health conditions in adult survivors of childhood cancer. *New England Journal of Medicine, 355*, 1572–1582.

Osgood, D. W., Ruth, G., Eccles, J. S., Jacobs, J. E. & Barber, B. L. (2005). *Six paths to adulthood: Fast starters, parents without careers, educated partners, educated singles, working singles, and slow starters.* na.

Reiss, J. G., Gibson, R. W., & Walker, L. R. (2005). Health care transition: Youth, family, and provider perspectives. *Pediatrics, 115*, 112–120.

Rifkin, J. (2011). *The Thired industrial revolution.* New York: St. Martin's Press.

Roisman, G. I., Aguilar, B., & Egeland, B. (2004). Antisocial behavior in the transition to adulthood: The independent and interactive roles of developmental history and emerging developmental tasks. *Development and Psychopathology, 16*, 857–871.

Rotundo, E. A. (1994). *American manhood: Transformations in masculinity from the revolution to the modern era.* New York: Basic Books.

Roux, A. M., Shattuck, P. T., Rast, J. E., Rava, J. A., & Anderson, K.,. A. (2015). *National autism indicators report: Transition into young adulthood.* Philadelphia: Life Course Outcomes Research Program/A.J. Drexel Autism Institute/Drexel University.

Ryan, R. M., & Lynch, J. H. (1989). Emotional autonomy versus detachment: Revisiting the vicissitudes of adolescence and young adulthood. *Child Development, 60*(2), 340–356.

Saran, R., Li, Y., Robinson, B., Ayanian, J., Balkrishnan, R., Bragg-Gresham, J., Chen, J., Cope, E., Gipson, D., & He, K. (2015). US renal data system 2014 annual data Report: Epidemiology of kidney disease in the United States. *American Journal of Kidney Diseases: The Official Journal of the National Kidney Foundation, 65*, A7.

Sarnak, M. J. (2003). Cardiovascular complications in chronic kidney disease. *American Journal of Kidney Diseases, 41*, 11–17.

Scheer, S. D., Unger, D. G., & Brown, M. B. (1996). Adolescents becoming adults: Attributes for adulthood. *Adolescence, 31*, 127.

Schlegel, A., & Barry Iii, H. (1991). *Adolescence: An anthropological inquiry.* New York: Free Press.

Schulenberg, J. E., & Maggs, J. L. (2002). A developmental perspective on alcohol use and heavy drinking during adolescence and the transition to young adulthood. *Journal of Studies on Alcohol, Supplement No. 14*, 54–70.

Schulenberg, J. E., Sameroff, A. J., & Cicchetti, D. (2004). The transition to adulthood as a critical juncture in the course of psychopathology and mental health. *Development and Psychopathology, 16*, 799–806.

Shanahan, M. J. (2000). Pathways to adulthood in changing societies: Variability and mechanisms in life course perspective. *Annual Review of Sociology, 26*, 667–692.

Shroff, R., Weaver, D. J., & Mitsnefes, M. M. (2011). Cardiovascular complications in children with chronic kidney disease. *Nature Reviews Nephrology, 7*, 642–649.

Silbereisen, R. K., & Lerner, R. M. (2007). *Approaches to positive youth development.* Los Angeles/London: Sage.

Skokauskas, N., & Gallagher, L. (2010). Psychosis, affective disorders and anxiety in autistic Spectrum disorder: Prevalence and Nosological considerations. *Psychopathology, 43*, 8–16.

So, T.-Y., Bradley Layton, J., Bozik, K., Farrington, E., Gipson, P. E., Gibson, K., Primack, W., Conley Iii, W., Gipson, D. S., & Ferris, M. (2011). Cognitive pharmacy services at a pediatric nephrology and hypertension clinic. *Renal Failure, 33*, 19–25.

Spear, L. P. (2000). The adolescent brain and age-related behavioral manifestations. *Neuroscience & Biobehavioral Reviews, 24*(4), 417–463.

Steelman, L. C., & Powell, B. (1991). Sponsoring the next generation: Parental willingness to pay for higher education. *American Journal of Sociology, 96*(6), 1505–1529.

Steinberg, L., Dahl, R., Keating, D., Kupfer, D. J., Masten, A. S., & Pine, D. S. (2006). The study of developmental psychopathology in adolescence: Integrating affective neuroscience with the study of context. In D. Cicchetti & D. Cohen (Eds.), *Handbook of developmental psychopathology* (Vol. 2, pp. 710–741). New York: Wiley.

Taylor, J. L., & Seltzer, M. M. (2010). Changes in the autism behavioral phenotype during the transition to adulthood. *Journal of Autism and Developmental Disorders, 40*, 1431–1446.

Taylor, J. L., & Seltzer, M. M. (2011a). Changes in the mother–child relationship during the transition to adulthood for youth with autism Spectrum disorders. *Journal of Autism and Developmental Disorders, 41*, 1397–1410.

Taylor, J. L., & Seltzer, M. M. (2011b). Employment and post-secondary educational activities for young adults with autism Spectrum disorders during the transition to adulthood. *Journal of Autism and Developmental Disorders, 41*, 566–574.

Wadsworth, M. E., et al. (2016). Poverty and the development of psychopathology. In: M. E. Wadsworth, G. W. Evans, K. Grant, J. S. Carter, & S. Duffy (Eds.), *Development and psychopathology. Volume Four. Risk, resilience, and intervention*, Ch 8 (pp. 215–237). Hoboken: John Wiley & Sons.

Walker, J. S., & Gowen, L. K. (2011). *Community-based approaches for supporting positive development in youth and young adults with serious mental health conditions*. Portland: Research and Training Center for Pathways to Positive Futures, Portland State University.

Watson, A. R. (2000). Non-compliance and transfer from Paediatric to adult transplant unit. *Pediatric Nephrology, 14*, 469–472.

Watson, A. R. (2005). Problems and pitfalls of transition from Paediatric to adult renal care. *Pediatric Nephrology, 20*, 113–117.

Watson, A. R., Harden, P., Ferris, M., Kerr, P. G., Mahan, J., & Ramzy, M. F. (2011). Transition from pediatric to adult renal services: A consensus statement by the international society of nephrology (Isn) and the international pediatric nephrology Association (Ipna). *Pediatric Nephrology, 26*, 1753–1757.

Webster, B. H., Jr., & Bishaw, A. (2006). *U.S. Census Bureau, American Community Survey Reports, ACS-02, Income, Earnings, and Poverty Data From the 2005 American Community Survey*. Washington, DC: U.S. Government Printing Office.

Whitbeck, L., Hoyt, D. R., & Huck, S. M. (1994). Early family relationships, intergenerational solidarity, and support provided to parents by their adult children. *Journal of Gerontology, 49*, S85–S94.

White, S. W., Oswald, D., Ollendick, T., & Scahill, L. (2009). Anxiety in children and adolescents with autism Spectrum disorders. *Clinical Psychology Review, 29*, 216–229.

Yeager, D. S., & Dweck, C. S. (2012). Mindsets that promote resilience: When students believe that personal characteristics can be developed. *Educational Psychologist, 47*(4), 302–314.

Yeung, E., Kay, J., Roosevelt, G. E., Brandon, M., & Yetman, A. T. (2008). Lapse of care as a predictor for morbidity in adults with congenital heart disease. *International Journal of Cardiology, 125*, 62–65.

Pregnancy Characteristics and Women's Cardiovascular Health

Abigail Fraser, Janet M. Catov, Deborah A. Lawlor, and Janet W. Rich-Edwards

1 Introduction

Growing evidence suggests that pregnancy is a "critical period" in a woman's life when her health development is especially sensitive to certain internal and external stimuli. As a normal response to pregnancy and in order to support the developing fetus, women become more insulin resistant and hyperlipidemic and experience an increase in blood pressure (BP; after an initial drop) and upregulation of coagulation factors and the inflammatory cascade (Sattar 2004). This is perhaps the prime example of health as an emergent property as it is one that enables the bearing of offspring and thus the perpetuation of humanity. While for a majority of women, this adaptation to pregnancy remains "healthy," in some women it develops into a complication of pregnancy such as gestational diabetes mellitus (GDM), preeclampsia, fetal growth restriction (FGR), and preterm delivery.

It has long been understood that pregnancy complications are important for the life course health development of offspring, but much less appreciated that these complications also have key implications for the long-term health development of the mother. An accumulating body of research has shown that these common pregnancy

This chapter contains a modified version of a previously published review and analysis of existing research that appeared in *Epidemiologic Reviews*. Reprinted with permission from:
Janet W. Rich-Edwards, Abigail Fraser, Deborah A. Lawlor, Janet M. Catov; Pregnancy Characteristics and Women's Future Cardiovascular Health: An Underused Opportunity to Improve Women's Health?. Epidemiol Rev 2014;36(1):57–70. doi: 10.1093/epirev/mxt006

AF and DAL work in a unit that receives infrastructure funding from the United Kingdom Medical Research Council (MC_UU_12013), and AF is funded by a United Kingdom Medical Research Council fellowship (MR/M009351/1). A grant to DAL from the Wellcome Trust also supports this collaborative work (WT094529MA). JMC is funded by RO1HL103825 and K12HD43441. JRE is supported by an American Heart Association Founder's Grant (13GRNT17070022). The authors have no relevant disclosures, financial or otherwise.

A. Fraser (✉) • D.A. Lawlor
Medical Research Council Integrative Epidemiology Unit at the University of Bristol, University of Bristol, Bristol, UK BS8 2BN
e-mail: abigail.fraser@bristol.ac.uk

J.M. Catov
Department of Obestetrics and Gynecology, University of Pittsburgh, Pittsburgh, PA 15213, USA

University of Pittsburgh, Department of Epidemiology, Pittsburgh, PA 15261, USA

Magee-Womens Research Institute, Pittsburgh, PA 15213, USA

J.W. Rich-Edwards
Connors Center for Women's Health and Gender Biology, Brigham and Women's Hospital, Boston, MA 02120, USA

Harvard Medical School, Boston, MA 02115, USA

Harvard School of Public Health, Boston, MA 02120, USA

N. Halfon et al. (eds.), *Handbook of Life Course Health Development*,
DOI 10.1007/978-3-319-47143-3_8

complications predict the future risk of chronic diseases in women, including cardiovascular disease, diabetes, and breast cancer (Rich-Edwards 2009). In this chapter we use life course health development theoretical principles as a lens for an examination of the implications of pregnancy history for cardiovascular disease (CVD), a leading cause of female mortality (Oblast 1999; Yusuf et al. 2001).

Globally, one out of three women dies from CVD (Shah et al. 2009; Mathers et al. 2008). We do a worse job of recognizing and predicting CVD in women than in men, in part because CVD presents itself differently between the sexes (Mosca et al. 2011; Shaw et al. 2006). This has important implications for the prevention of CVD. Primary prevention, if applied to high risk populations early enough to avert the cumulative damage of chronic disease, can reduce CVD incidence (Scarborough and Weissberg 2011; Shay et al. 2012; MMWR 1989). In response to the growing appreciation that many preventive efforts start too late to be effective, there has been a call for "primordial prevention"—the prevention of the major CVD risk factors themselves (Labarthe 1999; Weintraub et al. 2011). In this context, pregnancy complications have the potential to be effective CVD risk "stress tests" to identify women who would most benefit from primordial or primary prevention efforts to reduce CVD risk (Sattar and Greer 2002). The concept of primordial prevention is consistent with the life course health development principle that health development is an emergent phenomenon and the best way to prevent future disease is to build health assets that have long-term salutary benefits.

On average, more than 80% of women in high-income countries bear at least one child (Martinez et al. 2012; OECD Family D 2014), as do upward of 90% of women in most lower- and middle-income nations (United Nations DoEaSA, Population Division 2009). A high proportion of women will, in the course of their reproductive career, have a pregnancy complicated by GDM, a hypertensive disorder of pregnancy, FGR macrosomia, or preterm delivery. The prevalence of any one of these conditions in any given pregnancy ranges from 2% to greater than 12%. In one UK study, 36% of singleton pregnancies were complicated by at least one of these factors (Fraser et al. 2012). In the U.S. national Nurses' Health Study 2, we estimated that 29% of parous study participants have had one of these pregnancy complications. As reviewed below, each of these complications has been associated with roughly a twofold increase in the risk of CVD events. If 80% of women are parous and 30% of them have had a pregnancy complication predictive of CVD, then about 25% of women are at heightened risk for future CVD risk.

We begin with a review of the evidence for associations of parity and common pregnancy complications (low birth weight, fetal growth restriction, preterm delivery, hypertensive disorders of pregnancy, and GDM) with future CVD risk. We conducted MEDLINE searches for English-language cohort and case-control studies published in the peer-reviewed literature through December 2012, as described in detail elsewhere (Rich-Edwards et al. 2014). Whether pregnancy is a sensitive period in terms of cardiovascular health development across the life course and complications per se contribute to long term CVD risk, whether they simply unmask women with an underlying propensity for CVD, or whether both pathways are in play remains unclear. As suggested by life course health development, longitudinal studies are needed to untangle these temporal effects. In the second part of the chapter, we further explore the physiologic mechanisms that might explain the associations between pregnancy complications and CVD. Finally, we discuss the implications of these findings for future research as well as for health care design and policy.

2 Associations of Parity and Pregnancy Complications with CVD Risk in Mothers

2.1 Parity and CVD

Most (Green and Moser 1988; Ness et al. 1993) but not all studies (Steenland et al. 1996) have found a positive association between parity (number of children) and later CVD. In the largest study to date, the association was examined in

1.3 million with a median follow-up time of 9.5 years (range 0–24) women using Swedish registry data (Parikh et al. 2010). Parity was associated with CVD in a J-shaped fashion, with two births representing the nadir of risk. Compared with women with two births, the multivariable-adjusted hazard ratios (95% confidence interval (CI)) for women with 0 and ≥5 births were 1.11 (1.09–1.14) and 1.57 (1.52–1.64), respectively.

Desired family size may affect the shape of the parity-CVD risk distribution in different societies and is an example of how societal norms and social structures may affect health development and its determinants. In Sweden, the modal family size (two children) coincides with the nadir of maternal cardiovascular risk (Parikh et al. 2010). This suggests that many women who bore only one child suffered from secondary infertility, first pregnancy complications that precluded further pregnancies, or severe neonatal outcomes that discouraged further childbearing. To the extent that subfertility and severe pregnancy complications predict future CVD risk, they may explain the low-parity "hook" of the J-shaped association of parity and maternal CVD. The increase in CVD risk with increasing parity after two children may be the result of different phenomena. These include rival, but not mutually exclusive, theories that (1) adverse physiologic change accumulates over pregnancies; (2) adverse lifestyle habits accrue with more children; and/or (3) selection bias in which women at higher CVD risk opt for larger families. Thus, it is unclear whether the association of higher parity with CVD risk is causal or correlational.

Some insight into the association of parity with maternal CVD risk may be gleaned by examining the association of number of children with paternal CVD risk. Similar associations for mothers and fathers would suggest that the association between parity and maternal CVD is not causal, but is more likely a result of confounding by socioeconomic position and/or behaviors related to child-rearing. Three reports examined associations of number of children with CVD in fathers. In general, men who have fathered the most children appear to have small increased CVD risk, though this association is not always statistically significant and is weaker than the associations observed among mothers (Dekker and Schouten 1993; Lawlor et al. 2003; Ness et al. 1995). Adjustment for lifestyle factors tends to reduce the associations in both mothers and fathers (Lawlor et al. 2003; Catov et al. 2007a). These results suggest that the association between high parity and CVD in later life may be largely the result of socioeconomic position and/or behavioral risk factors associated with child-rearing that are shared by both parents.

2.2 Common Pregnancy Complications and CVD in Mothers

Offspring birth weight predicts maternal lifespan (Catov et al. 2007a; Davey Smith et al. 1997, 2000a, b, 2007). Figure 1 presents the findings from studies that have examined associations of offspring birth weight or fetal growth—a function of birth weight and gestation length—with maternal CVD risk (Davey Smith et al. 1997, 2007, 2000a, b, 2005; Bellamy et al. 2007, 2011; Friedlander et al. 2007; Lykke et al. 2010a; Mongraw-Chaffin et al. 2010; Smith et al. 2001; Wikström et al. 2005; Fraser et al. 2012; Ness et al. 1993). One meta-analysis has calculated that, for every standard deviation (roughly 500 g) higher birth weight of the firstborn child, maternal CVD mortality is decreased by 25% (Davey Smith et al. 2007). It is unclear whether the inverse association of offspring birth weight with mortality is constant across the entire range of birth weight, as the association of high birth weight with maternal CVD risk varies by study. In some populations, the mothers of the largest infants (>4000 g or >4500 g) have the lowest risks of CVD (Davey Smith et al. 1997, 2000b), while in other populations there is an uptick in CVD risk for the mothers of macrosomic newborns (Davey Smith et al. 2007; Bonamy et al. 2011; Friedlander et al. 2007; Lykke et al. 2012). Given the strong associations of macrosomia with GDM and later type 2 diabetes (Metzger et al. 1993), the presence and magnitude of the association of large birth weight with future CVD risk may depend on the population prevalence of GDM and chronic diabetes during pregnancy (in other words,

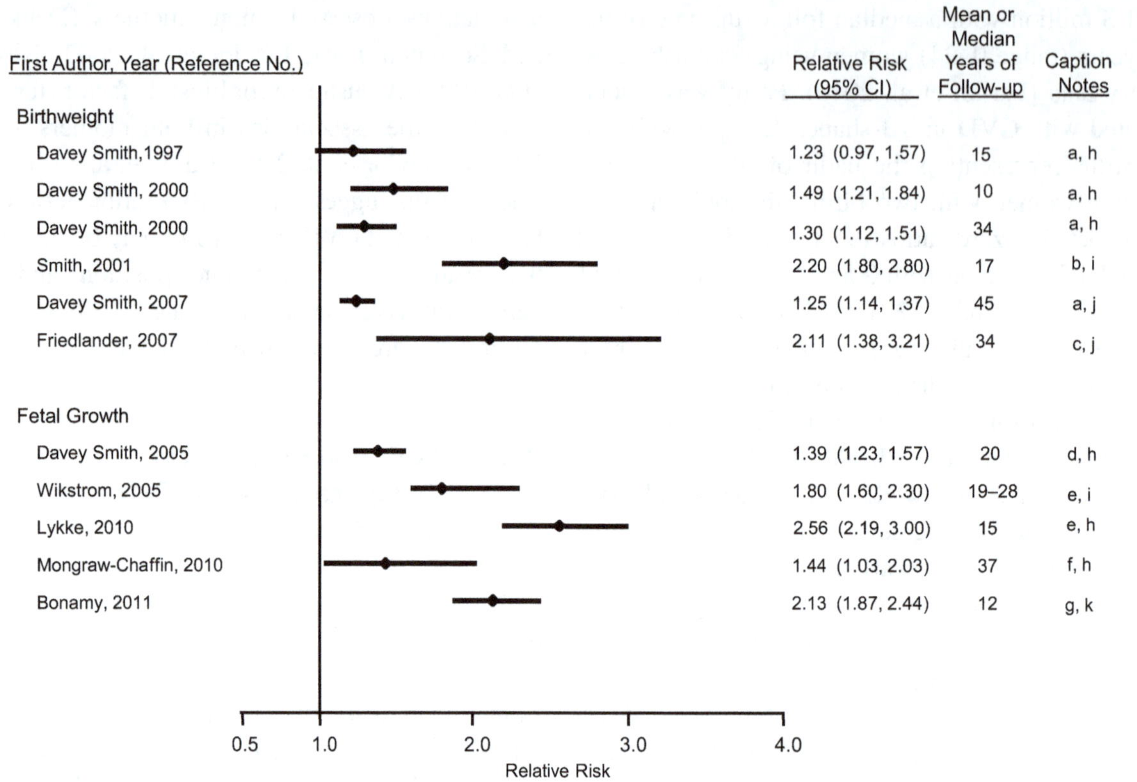

Fig. 1 Results from studies of offspring birth weight or fetal growth and relative risk of maternal cardiovascular disease (CVD). *a* Per 1 standard deviation (SD) lower birth weight; *b* lowest birth weight quintile compared to all others; *c* <2500 g compared to 1500–3999 g birth weight; *d* per 1 SD lower birth weight, adjusted for gestational age; *e* small for gestational age; *f* intrauterine growth retardation; *g* ~2 SD below mean birth weight adjusted for gestational age; *h* CVD mortality; *i* coronary heart disease (CHD) events ; *j* CHD mortality; *k* CVD events (*CI* confidence interval)

the extent to which large infant size is pathological). Indeed, the association of macrosomia with CVD risk is attenuated by adjustment for GDM(36) (Bonamy et al. 2011), indicating that a substantial portion of the association of macrosomia and CVD is explained by metabolic risk.

It is abundantly clear, however, that the 8% of deliveries that are low birth weight (<2500 g) are associated with twice the maternal CVD incidence and mortality of other deliveries (Davey Smith et al. 1997, 2000a, b, 2007). Associations of offspring birth weight with maternal CVD are only modestly diminished by adjustment for cigarette smoking and not affected by control for prepregnancy body mass index (Bonamy et al. 2011; Davey Smith et al. 2005).

Birth weight is the product of fetal growth rate and gestation length. Fetal growth, represented as birth weight corrected for gestation length, predicts maternal CVD risk (Bonamy et al. 2011; Lykke et al. 2012), as does gestation length (discussed below). In fact, the coincidence of restricted fetal growth and prematurity yields a more than threefold increased CVD risk (Bonamy et al. 2011). The curvilinear association of offspring birth weight with maternal CVD risk observed in many populations may be the product of competing pathological phenomena. At one end of the birth weight spectrum, the association of macrosomia with maternal CVD risk may be explained by underlying metabolic risk; at the other end of the spectrum, the association of low birth weight with maternal CVD risk may be driven by endothelial dysfunction and other pathologies associated with restricted fetal growth and preterm birth.

First offspring birth weight also predicts paternal CVD, although the magnitude of the positive association of offspring birth weight with paternal

CVD risk is less than a third of that for the infant's mother (Davey Smith et al. 2007). The fact that the birth weight of their first child predicts CVD events in both parents suggests that shared lifestyle or environmental factors, such as cigarette smoking, might influence both the growth of the fetus and CVD risk in the parents and/or that pleiotropic genetic variants affect both growth and CVD risk. Birth weight is passed down through maternal and paternal lines (Lie et al. 2006), opening the possibility that paternal CVD/fetal growth genes could affect both the pregnancy outcome and long-term chronic disease risk in the father (Freathy et al. 2007). However, the stronger association in mothers than in fathers suggests either parent-specific genomic imprinting or—as seems more parsimonious—that maternal health during pregnancy affects fetal growth and is a marker of her future CVD risk.

Preterm delivery (<37 weeks' gestation) accounts for 6–12% of deliveries in the developed world (Beck et al. 2010). The hazard ratios for CVD associated with total preterm delivery are depicted in Fig. 2 and are on the order of 1.3–2.6 for births <37 completed weeks compared with term births (Davey Smith et al. 2000b, 2005; Bonamy et al. 2011; Lykke et al. 2010a, b; Smith et al. 2001; Wikström et al. 2005; Catov et al. 2010a; Irgens et al. 2001; Nardi et al. 2006; Pell et al. 2004; Rich-Edwards et al. 2012). There is a greater range of relative risk when distinct preterm phenotypes are examined separately. While most preterm deliveries follow spontaneous labor or preterm premature rupture of membranes, a significant and growing fraction results from medically induced labor or Caesarean section without labor. The chief reasons for these medically indicated deliveries include preeclampsia and FGR, both of which have been associated with increased maternal CVD risk. In studies that have distinguished them, hypertensive preterm deliveries consistently have a stronger association with maternal CVD outcomes than do normotensive preterm deliveries, though the latter are still associated with a 1.2- to threefold increased risk compared with term deliveries (Catov et al. 2010a; Irgens et al. 2001). In the two studies that have contrasted CVD risk among mothers with spontaneous versus indicated preterm deliveries (Rich-Edwards et al. 2012; Hastie et al. 2011a), indicated delivery was associated with higher risks of CVD mortality than spontaneous preterm delivery. Nevertheless, spontaneous preterm delivery—compared with term delivery—was associated with doubling of CVD risk (Rich-Edwards et al. 2012; Hastie et al. 2011a).

Unlike the associations of parity or birth weight with paternal CVD risk, two studies (Davey Smith et al. 2005; Irgens et al. 2001) have reported that preterm delivery is not associated with paternal risk of CVD, implying that the association of preterm delivery with maternal CVD risk is not the product of a high-CVD risk lifestyle or genetic variants shared between both parents and their offspring. Of relevance, preterm birth risk appears to be passed only through the maternal line (Wilcox et al. 2008). These observations suggest that maternal intrauterine environment and health determine the risk of preterm delivery and explain its association with maternal CVD risk, rather than shared lifestyle or environment of the mother and father.

Gestational diabetes mellitus is a common and growing pregnancy complication that affects as many as 5% of pregnancies. It is well established that women with GDM are at increased risk of developing diabetes later in life (Bellamy et al. 2009); between 3% and 70% of women with a history of GDM will develop type 2 diabetes within three decades of the pregnancy (Kim et al. 2002), with a meta-analysis of 675,455 women finding a sevenfold increase in risk of later type 2 diabetes (Bellamy et al. 2009). Type 2 diabetes is an important CVD risk factor, having a markedly higher relative and absolute association with CVD in women than it does in men (Sarwar et al. 2010). Given these associations, it seems self-evident that a history of GDM would be associated with increased CVD risk. However, due largely to the fact that GDM screening during pregnancy was neither routine nor standardized until recent decades, there are few cohorts with long enough follow-up of screened populations to detect CVD incidence or mortality among women with a history of GDM (Shah et al. 2008; Carr et al. 2006). These are displayed in Fig. 3. The only large population-based study of this topic is a

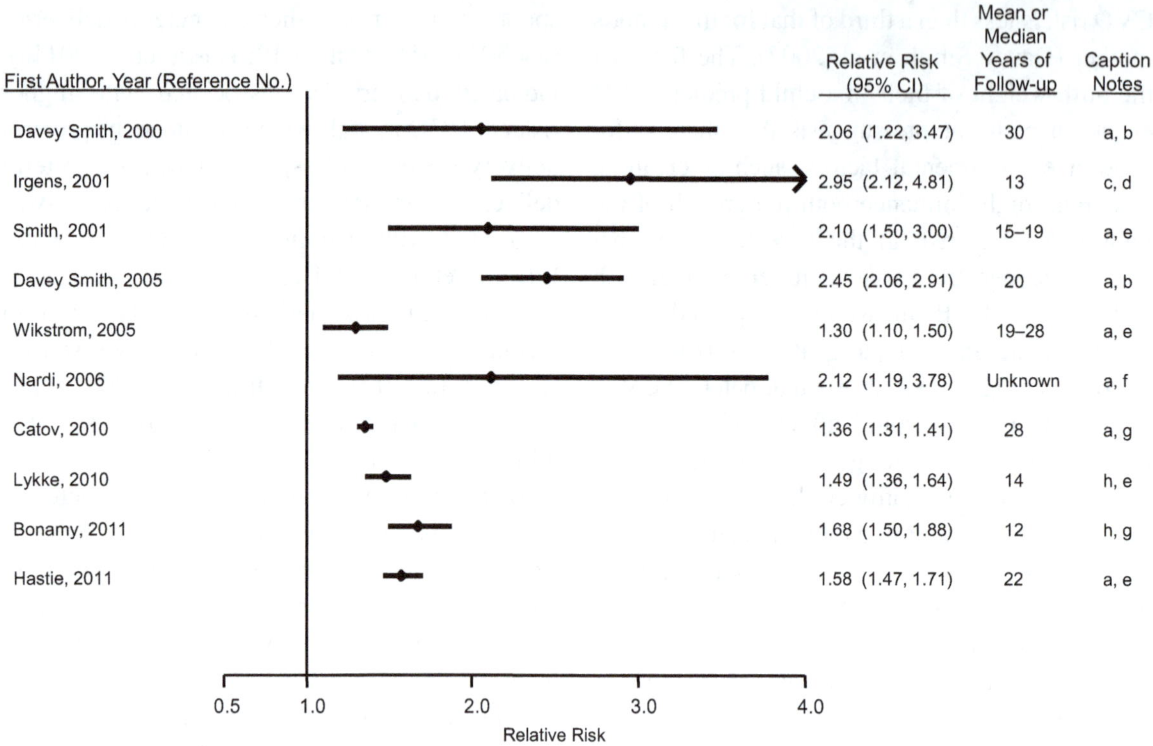

Fig. 2 Results from studies of preterm delivery and relative risk of maternal cardiovascular disease (CVD). *a* <37 weeks' gestation weeks compared with term; *b* CVD mortality; *c* <37 weeks' gestation length compared with term normotensive pregnancies; *d* CVD mortality, excluding stroke mortality; *e* coronary heart disease (CHD) events; *f* myocardial infarction; *g* CVD events; *h* 32–36 weeks' gestation length compared with term (*CI* confidence interval)

record linkage study conducted in Ontario, Canada, with a median follow-up of 11.5 years (Shah et al. 2008). In that study, a history of GDM was associated with a greater risk of hospital admission for acute myocardial infarction, coronary bypass, coronary angioplasty, stroke, or carotid endarterectomy (hazard ratio (HR) = 1.71; 95% CI, 1.08–2.69). Upon adjustment for diabetes after pregnancy, the association was attenuated toward the null (adjusted HR, 1.13; 0.67–1.89). A smaller, cross-sectional study found that women with a history of GDM had a higher CVD risk than women without a history of GDM (adjusted OR = 1.85, 1.21–2.82) and experienced CVD events 7 years earlier, on average (Carr et al. 2006).

Lesser degrees of antepartum hyperglycemia have also been associated with an elevated risk of subsequent diabetes and CVD. In the Ontario study, women with evidence of elevated glycemia short of GDM criteria were at an increased risk of diabetes (HR = 2.56, 2.28–2.87) (Retnakaran and Shah 2009a) and CVD (HR = 1.19, 1.02–1.39) (Retnakaran and Shah 2009b) compared to normoglycemic women.

Hypertensive disorders of pregnancy (HDPs) are common pregnancy complications that presage CVD. *Preeclampsia*, the combination of hypertension and proteinuria, affects approximately 2–5% of pregnancies, with a predominance among first pregnancies (Fraser et al. 2012; Wallis et al. 2008; North et al. 2011). Estimates of the prevalence of *gestational hypertension*, new-onset hypertension without proteinuria, vary from 3% to 14% (Fraser et al. 2012; Wallis et al. 2008; Roberts et al. 2005). Women with a history of preeclampsia have roughly fourfold higher incidence of hypertension and twofold elevated risks of heart disease, stroke, and venous thromboembolism (Bellamy et al. 2007; McDonald et al. 2008). Two systematic reviews, one of cohort studies (n = 25) and the other of both cohort (n = 10) and case-control (n = 5) studies,

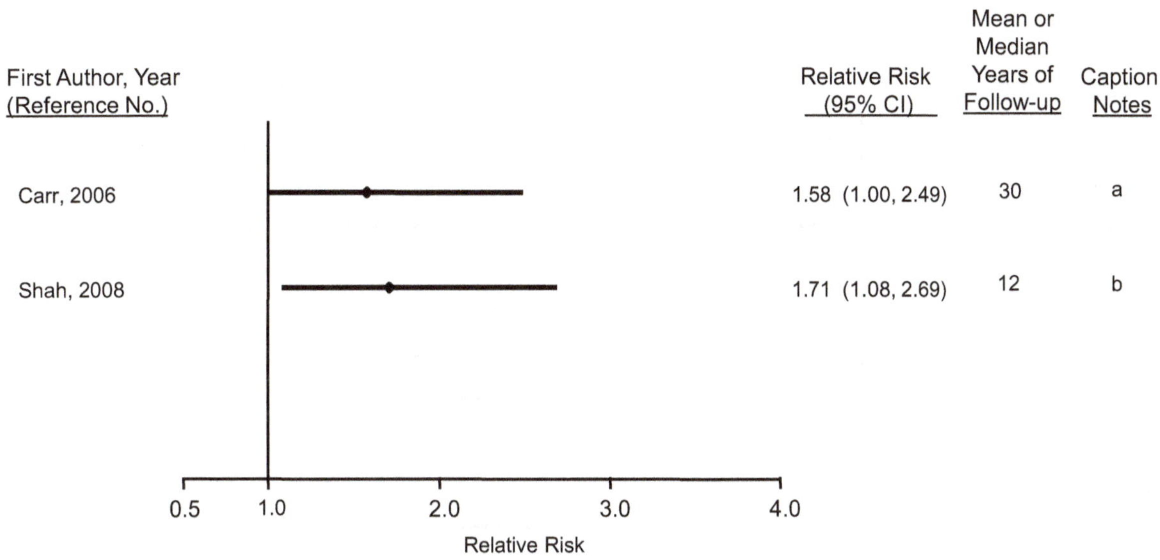

Fig. 3 Results from studies of gestational diabetes mellitus and relative risk of maternal cardiovascular disease (CVD). *a* Self-reported coronary artery disease, *b* CVD events (*CI* confidence interval)

have both reported a doubling of risk for different measures of CVD comparing women with preeclampsia to normotensive women over a median of 10–12-year follow-up (Bellamy et al. 2007; McDonald et al. 2008). Figure 4 depicts the relative risk of coronary heart disease (CHD) and CVD outcomes among mothers with a history of preeclampsia (Mongraw-Chaffin et al. 2010; Smith et al. 2001; Wikström et al. 2005; Irgens et al. 2001; Funai et al. 2005; Hannaford et al. 1997; Jónsdóttir et al. 1995; Kestenbaum et al. 2003; Lin et al. 2011; Lykke et al. 2009; Wilson et al. 2003).

Publications from three cohort studies published since those reviews give some insight into the onset and duration of CVD risk following HDP (Mongraw-Chaffin et al. 2010; Smith et al. 2001; Lin et al. 2011; Lykke et al. 2009). In a short-term follow-up of over 1,000,000 pregnancies in Taiwan, women with preeclampsia/eclampsia were at double the risk of major CVD from the third trimester of pregnancy up to three years postpartum, with particularly high relative risks for stroke (HR = 14.5, 1.3–165.1) and myocardial infarction (HR = 13.0, 4.6–6.3) (Lin et al. 2011). While these results suggest a high relative risk immediately following HDP, the confidence intervals are wide, and the absolute risk of CVD events is very small at this age, so that this immediate risk is unlikely to account for a large number of CVD events. The Child Health and Development Study in California has provided some of the longer follow-up; over 37 years after pregnancy, women with a history of preeclampsia in any pregnancy had double the risk of CVD death (HR = 2.14; 1.29–3.57) (Mongraw-Chaffin et al. 2010). This doubling of risk is consistent with studies with shorter duration of follow-up. Considering the exponential increase in the absolute numbers of CVD events with increasing age, this suggests that the elevated risk of CVD among women with a history of HDP is not limited to the early years postpartum.

Thus, studies repeatedly report a doubling of CVD risk among women with a history of preeclampsia and suggest lesser degrees of excess risk among women with a history of gestational hypertension, despite the strong association of gestational hypertension with development of chronic hypertension (Lykke et al. 2009). The combination of preterm delivery and preeclampsia—a likely marker of the severity of preeclampsia—is a particularly potent predictor of CVD risk. Compared to normotensive term pregnancies, women delivering preterm preeclamptic pregnancies have very high relative risks of future

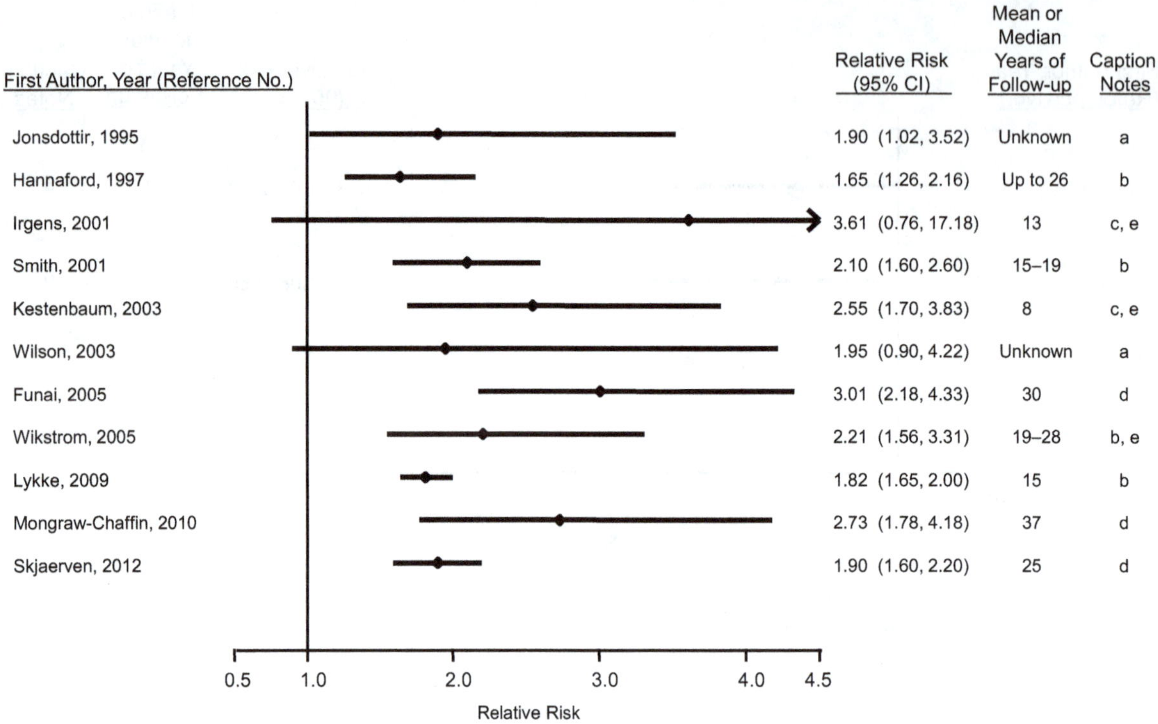

Fig. 4 Results from studies of hypertensive disorders of pregnancy and relative risk of maternal cardiovascular disease (CVD). *a* Coronary heart disease (CHD) mortality, *b* CHD events, *c* CVD events, *d* CVD mortality, *e* composite estimate provided by Bellamy review (18). A 2011 study by Lin (62) reported a relative risk of 23.0 (95% confidence interval (CI), 5.1–103.7) for CVD events (except stroke) during pregnancy and up to three years after delivery. We omitted that study from the figure so that we could keep the relative risk scale consistent across figures

CVD ranging from 2.5 to 9.5. (Mongraw-Chaffin et al. 2010; Smith et al. 2001; Lin et al. 2011; Skjaerven et al. 2012)

2.3 Recurrent Pregnancy Complications, Last Pregnancy Complications, and Maternal CVD Risk

Much of the literature is based on first pregnancies, precluding examination of the association of recurring pregnancy complications with CVD risk. There is evidence that recurrent preeclampsia (Lykke et al. 2009) and preterm delivery(Catov et al. 2010a; Lykke et al. 2010b) are associated with a greater risk of CVD than a single complicated pregnancy in multiparous women. Although the association of recurrent GDM with CVD risk has not been studied, after a first GDM pregnancy, each subsequent GDM pregnancy has been associated with a modestly increased risk of type 2 diabetes (adjusted HR = 1.16, 1.01–1.34) and each non-GDM pregnancy with a reduced risk of diabetes (HR = 0.34, 0.27–0.41) (Retnakaran et al. 2011). In fact, this highlights an intriguing pattern that is emerging with respect to last births: having preeclampsia (Skjaerven et al. 2012), preterm delivery (Rich-Edwards et al. 2012), or GDM (Retnakaran et al. 2011) in the last pregnancy appears to be associated with especially high risk of future CVD in mothers. Perhaps reflecting the same phenomenon, women who have one preterm delivery and one term delivery in their first two births appear to be at higher risk of CHD if the preterm delivery was the second birth (Catov et al. 2010a; Lykke et al. 2010b). This suggests that pregnancy complications severe enough to contraindicate or discourage a subsequent pregnancy may be particularly potent predictors of future CVD risk.

3 Physiological Mechanisms Linking Pregnancy Complications to Maternal CVD Risk

Pathways that link pregnancy exposures to later life CVD are not well understood. Considerable evidence supports the existence of common predisposing factors for both pregnancy complications and CVD risk suggesting that pregnancy complications can be thought of as a failed stress test, with pregnancy being the stressor. There have been almost no studies examining the alternative that pregnancy complications might *cause* increased CVD risk. To address this issue, we summarize evidence that compares CVD risk before, during, and after pregnancies with and without complications.

3.1 Cardiovascular Risk Factors Preceding Pregnancy Complications

Higher *prepregnancy blood pressure* is a risk factor for preeclampsia (Magnussen et al. 2007) and preterm delivery (Catov et al. 2013). Chronic hypertension has a well-established relation to increased risk of preeclampsia—known as "superimposed" preeclampsia. Even within the normotensive range, there is a positive dose-response association of prepregnancy systolic and/or diastolic blood pressure with preeclampsia, (Magnussen et al. 2007) and women who develop hypertensive disorders of pregnancy have higher blood pressure at 8 weeks' gestation than normotensive (Macdonald-Wallis et al. 2012). Preexisting hypertension has also been associated with FGR, especially in cases that were also preterm (Catov et al. 2008a). Risks for these complications also rise with increasing maternal age, suggesting that the aging endothelium may less successfully adapt to the profound vascular demands of pregnancy.

Prepregnancy lipid concentrations are also associated with pregnancy complications and offspring birth weight; the nature of the association varies with the pregnancy outcome in question. Lipid profiles consistent with elevated CVD risk, including higher prepregnancy triglyceride levels, total cholesterol, and lower HDL cholesterol, have been associated with preeclampsia and preterm delivery in the study in Norway (Magnussen et al. 2007, 2011). The US Coronary Artery Risk Development in Young Adults Study (CARDIA) found a curvilinear association of prepregnancy cholesterol levels with risk of delivering preterm (Catov et al. 2010b). With respect to fetal growth, women with a more atherogenic lipid profile may bear larger infants (Romundstad et al. 2007); this suggests that the association of low birth weight—at least the fetal growth component of low birth weight—with maternal CVD risk may not operate via dyslipidemia.

Prepregnancy adiposity and glucose/insulin dysregulation is strongly implicated in the etiology of GDM, based on the observation that women with GDM tend to have a family history of type 2 diabetes and higher body mass index (BMI) before pregnancy (Solomon et al. 1997), as well as higher levels of glucose and insulin and lower levels of adiponectin before the onset of the midpregnancy hyperglycemia that defines GDM (Nanda et al. 2011; Riskin-Mashiah et al. 2010; Sacks et al. 2003; Williams et al. 2004). Higher BMI and family history of diabetes are also associated with increased risk of preeclampsia (Qiu et al. 2003; O'Brien et al. 2003). The risk of preeclampsia doubles with every 5–7 kg/m^2 increase in body mass index before pregnancy (O'Brien et al. 2003).

Thus, subclinical elevations in the classic CVD risk factors of blood pressure, lipid levels, elevated BMI, and glucose/insulin dysregulation appear to predate both preeclampsia and GDM. Less clear is the extent to which CVD risk factors precede spontaneous preterm deliveries or FGR in normotensive pregnancies. Furthermore, the roles of prepregnancy inflammatory and coagulation factors with respect to pregnancy complications remain to be elucidated, despite the importance of these systems for both reproduction and CVD risk (Romero et al. 2007).

3.2 Cardiovascular Risk Factors During Pregnancy

3.2.1 Cardiovascular Adaptation in Normal Pregnancy

In normal gestation, maternal blood volume increases progressively from 6 to 8 weeks' gestation, peaking at an increase of 45% by 32 weeks (Monga and Creasy 1994). Cardiac output increases by 30–50%, with half of this increase occurring very early in gestation. Pulse rate increases 17%, and there are striking alterations in renal physiology. Although the insulin response to glucose is augmented in early pregnancy, insulin resistance emerges in the second half of pregnancy (Butte 2000). In addition, cholesterol and triglyceride profiles change after gestation week 9 to support steroid synthesis and fetal growth (Butte 2000). In uncomplicated pregnancy, there is a tendency for low-density lipoprotein (LDL) to shift across gestation from large, buoyant particles to smaller, denser, and more atherogenic particles (Hubel et al. 1998a). Fat is accumulated during the second trimester and then mobilized to support the dramatic fetal growth of the third trimester (Herrera 2000).

3.2.2 Cardiovascular Risk Factors During Pregnancy Complications

Vascular and endothelial dysfunction is characteristic of pregnancies complicated by preeclampsia or growth restriction. Placental underperfusion is common, and there are elevated markers of endothelial dysfunction in the maternal circulation. Women with hypertensive disorders of pregnancy demonstrate increased resistance in the uterine arteries (Ducey et al. 1987; Campbell and Griffin 1983), vascular stiffness, and impaired endothelial response (Savvidou et al. 2003, 2011). In addition, placental vascular lesions indicative of failed spiral artery remodeling, ischemia, or hemorrhage have also been reported in cases of both medically indicated and spontaneous preterm birth (Kelly et al. 2009).

During pregnancy, *lipid aberrations* accompany several pregnancy complications. Again, the direction of the associations appears to depend on the nature of the pregnancy complication. The dyslipidemias associated with atherosclerosis (hypertriglyceridemia, hypercholesterolemia, elevated free fatty acids, and excess oxidized LDL) are frequently seen during preeclampsia … (Clausen et al. 2001; Hubel et al. 1996, 1998b; Sattar et al. 1997). There is also emerging evidence to suggest that this atherogenic lipid profile is associated with both spontaneous and indicated preterm births (Edison et al. 2007; Catov et al. 2007b). Similarly, women with GDM exhibit elevations in triglycerides and, less consistently, total cholesterol and LDL during pregnancy (Enquobahrie et al. 2005). On the other hand, low maternal total and LDL-cholesterol concentrations appear in the third trimester in pregnancies complicated by FGR (Sattar et al. 1999). Placental studies are conflicting, with some suggesting reduced expression of lipoprotein receptors in placentas from FGR vs. appropriate weight for gestational age births (Wadsack et al. 2007) and others suggesting overexpression of these receptors (Stepan et al. 1999). FGR studies are hampered by nonstandard phenotyping, and thus findings may represent differing levels of severity. Despite these limitations, these data suggest that extremes of lipid concentrations are associated with adverse pregnancy outcomes. Longitudinal studies are needed to better understand how the relative contributions of low or high cholesterol are related to failed or compensatory lipid adaptation required to optimize fetal growth.

Metabolic dysregulation in pregnancy defines GDM and is a strong risk factor for preeclampsia; there is considerable overlap of the two conditions, with twice the rate of preeclampsia in diabetic versus nondiabetic pregnancies (Ostlund et al. 2004). However, GDM has only a modest association with spontaneous preterm birth (Hedderson et al. 2003). Higher early-pregnancy BMI is associated with increased risk of HDP and GDM (Solomon et al. 1997; O'Brien et al. 2003; Lawlor et al. 2012), but with reduced risk of SGA and spontaneous preterm birth in most studies (Smith et al. 2007).

Systemic inflammation during pregnancy may be important in the pathogenesis of several pregnancy complications. Elevated serum levels of C-reactive protein and/or leukocytes have been detected in women who experience GDM, FGR, and both spontaneous and indicated preterm deliveries (Catov et al. 2007c; Ernst et al. 2011; Freeman et al. 2004; Pitiphat et al. 2005; Wolf et al. 2001). However, neither mid-gestation circulating levels of C-reactive protein nor pro-inflammatory cytokines have proven to have prognostic value for specific pregnancy outcomes (Curry et al. 2007; Gammill et al. 2010).

Normal pregnancy is a state of *hypercoagulability*, and complications such as preeclampsia and preterm birth are characterized by particularly high biomarkers of an activated fibrinolytic cascade, as well as perhaps an impaired ability to mount this response appropriately (Catov et al. 2008b; Hackney et al. 2010; Heilmann et al. 2007). It has been hypothesized that aberrations in the cross talk between inflammation and the coagulation cascades could contribute to the pathophysiology of these pregnancy complications (Girardi 2011).

3.3 Cardiovascular Risk Factors After Pregnancy

3.3.1 Enduring Cardiovascular Impact of Normal Pregnancy

Most of the cardiovascular adaptations to normal pregnancy resolve in the postpartum period, although there are some detectable and lasting pregnancy effects. Blood pressure is modestly decreased in the postpartum period after a first uncomplicated pregnancy (Hackney et al. 2010). However, other lingering effects are not as salutary. Importantly, women retain, on average, 0.5–5.0 kg of weight following each pregnancy (Heilmann et al. 2007; Girardi 2011). Lactation may help resolve the cardiometabolic adaptations and fat accumulation associated with pregnancy (Agatisa et al. 2004; Berends et al. 2008; Catov et al. 2011).

The first birth may be a sentinel marker for complications in later pregnancies and future CVD risk (Lauenborg et al. 2005; Meyers-Seifer and Vohr 1996; Verma et al. 2002). Several factors distinguish first births. First, longitudinal studies suggest that the lasting blood pressure and lipid changes associated with pregnancy occur after first but not subsequent births (Hackney et al. 2010). In addition, first births are at higher risk for the major obstetric complications of preterm delivery, HDP, FGR, and stillbirth. Women with any of these complications are at higher risk in subsequent pregnancies for recurrence of the same complication as well as the onset of other complications. Importantly, complications during a first pregnancy impact the likelihood of having a subsequent pregnancy. As noted above, complications in a last pregnancy appear to be associated with especially high relative risks of CVD events. Thus, health status of the first and last pregnancies may be particularly telling of future maternal health.

The cumulative effect of these adaptations and resolutions and risks may contribute to the above-noted J-shaped association between parity and maternal CVD risk, with lowest risk for women who have delivered two infants. It is not clear whether pregnancies exert a cumulative cardiovascular burden with increasing parity, whether higher-order pregnancies at more advanced maternal age exert more cardiovascular risk, or whether women at high cardiovascular risk bear more children.

3.3.2 Cardiovascular Risk After Pregnancy Complications

The association of *vascular and endothelial dysfunction* with pregnancy complications continues after delivery. Women with preeclampsia have impaired endothelial function after pregnancy (Agatisa et al. 2004). This may also be true, although to a lesser extent, of women who deliver small babies due to FGR or preterm delivery. For example, lower offspring birth weight is associated with higher maternal blood pressure in the years after pregnancy (Davey Smith et al. 2005). Some (Catov et al. 2013; Berends et al. 2008) but not all (Catov et al. 2011) studies report higher blood pressure and atherosclerotic carotid vessel remodeling among women who have delivered an FGR neonate. Although studies are not unanimous (Macdonald-

Wallis et al. 2012; Lauenborg et al. 2005), women with a history of GDM are more likely to have hypertension (Meyers-Seifer and Vohr 1996; Verma et al. 2002), vascular dysfunction (Heitritter et al. 2005), impaired endothelium-dependent vasodilatation (Anastasiou et al. 1998), and higher carotid artery intima-media thickness (Tarim et al. 2006). These differences are not fully explained by the higher BMI typical of women with a history of GDM.

Studies of *lipid profiles after pregnancies* complicated by preeclampsia are consistent with increased atherogenesis risk, including consistently reported higher total cholesterol, LDL cholesterol, and triglycerides, although these differences are not always statistically significant (Fraser et al. 2012; Manten et al. 2007; Hubel et al. 2008; Laivuori et al. 1996; Magnussen et al. 2009; Romundstad et al. 2010; Sattar et al. 2003; Smith et al. 2009). Associations of reduced HDL cholesterol after preeclampsia have been reported by some (Fraser et al. 2012; Magnussen et al. 2009; Romundstad et al. 2010; Smith et al. 2009) but not all (Manten et al. 2007; Laivuori et al. 1996; Sattar et al. 2003) studies. One study has reported dyslipidemia among women with a history of spontaneous and indicated preterm births (Catov et al. 2011). Some (Lauenborg et al. 2005; Meyers-Seifer and Vohr 1996; Verma et al. 2002; Di Cianni et al. 2007) but not all (Schwarz et al. 2009) have reported elevated total cholesterol, LDL cholesterol, and/or triglycerides in women with a history of GDM. As with the studies of lipid concentrations before and during pregnancy, studies of lipid concentrations in women in the years after FGR are conflicting, with some reporting hyperlipidemia (Kanagalingam et al. 2009) and others reporting no differences compared to women with uncomplicated births (Catov et al. 2011).

It is now firmly established that women with a history of GDM have a manifold higher risk of developing *type 2 diabetes* than women with normoglycemic pregnancies (Bellamy et al. 2009). It is less widely appreciated that women with a history of preeclampsia are also at high risk of type 2 diabetes. After preeclampsia, mothers are three times more likely to develop diabetes within 16 years (Lykke et al. 2009), an observation bolstered by evidence of dysregulated glucose and insulin, as well as insulin resistance as early as 2 years after preeclamptic pregnancy (Fraser et al. 2012; Manten et al. 2007; Laivuori et al. 1996; Magnussen et al. 2009; Smith et al. 2009; Wolf et al. 2004). However, not all pregnancy complications are associated with risk of future metabolic disorder: in the Nurses' Health Study 2, although 2% of women who delivered a very preterm infant (<32 weeks' gestation) had a 35% higher risk of developing type 2 diabetes, moderate preterm delivery was not associated with increased diabetes risk (James-Todd et al. 2010).

After pregnancy, plasma C-reactive protein is elevated among women with prior eclampsia and indicated preterm births suggesting that systemic low-grade *inflammation* may link some adverse pregnancy outcomes and later CVD (Hastie et al. 2011b; Hubel et al. 2006). Several studies have documented higher C-reactive protein levels among women with a history of GDM (Heitritter et al. 2005; Di Cianni et al. 2007; Winzer et al. 2004). Although inflammation seems a likely culprit to explain the association of spontaneous preterm delivery with CVD risk, the only study to date that has examined this question has reported no differences in plasma C-reactive protein levels of women with a history of spontaneous preterm delivery compared to term delivery (Hastie et al. 2011b).

Women with a history of pregnancies complicated by preeclampsia may maintain a *procoagulation state* in the years after pregnancy, predisposing them to vascular and thrombotic events (Portelinha et al. 2009), although this pathway is less studied than others linking pregnancy complications to maternal CVD risk.

Thus, the associations of pregnancy complications with future CVD events in women are likely explained, at least in part, by their associations with classic CVD risk factors of hypertension, dyslipidemia, type 2 diabetes, and perhaps inflammation and thrombosis, which are evident before, during, and after such complicated pregnancies. Pregnancy provides a challenge to women's cardiovascular system, and pregnancy complications may serve as precursors, i.e., early indications that a woman is on a high-CVD risk trajectory, before these classic CVD risk factors are clinically detected. That said, this trajectory is complex and likely to be nonlinear. Given that most pregnancies occur in early adulthood, long before most CVD events occur, there is ample opportunity to influence that trajectory by recognizing that health develops continuously over the lifespan and that health development is a process resulting from the ongoing interactions between person and environment.

4 Recommendations for Future Research

4.1 Major Themes and Findings

The associations of pregnancy complications with CVD events are remarkably consistent.

Several pregnancy complications are more common among racial minority groups, who are also at higher risk of metabolic and cardiovascular disease. Although untested, the use of pregnancy complication history to screen women for targeted CVD prevention has potential to improve public health, given the magnitude of the associations, the prevalence of the pregnancy complications, and the importance of CVD in women. Pregnancy complications occur early enough in a woman's life course to offer a significant meaningful "runway" for primordial CVD prevention by lifestyle intervention and primary prevention by statins and antihypertensive drugs. In 2011, both the American Heart Association and the European Society of Cardiology included histories of preeclampsia and (in the case of the American Heart Association) GDM as part of CVD risk assessment that would trigger closer monitoring and control of CVD risk factors (Mosca et al. 2011; Regitz-Zagrosek et al. 2011). Pregnancy appears to be a critical transition period for a woman that stresses her cardiovascular system in ways that may shed light on future disease risk.

4.2 Research Priorities

(a) Epidemiologic research
- Establishing whether pregnancy complications per se contribute to CVD risk

We need to establish whether pregnancy complications act as stress tests to unmask women who are already at increased risk of CVD in later life and/or whether (and which) pregnancy complications have a causal, direct contribution to a woman's CVD risk. If pregnancy complications per se contribute to CVD risk independently of prepregnancy cardiovascular health, prevention strategies and treatment of pregnancy complications could be important not only for women and their offspring during the pregnancy but also later in life.

(b) Mechanism research
- Identifying mechanistic pathways to pregnancy complications and CVD

Should epidemiologic evidence suggest that pregnancy complications are causally associated with greater future CVD risk, it will be important to ascertain the underlying pathways responsible for these effects in order to identify potential treatment pathways. Gaining better understanding of the mechanisms underlying pregnancy complications themselves will also be important in informing prevention strategies.

(c) Translational research
- Improving risk stratification

Irrespective of whether pregnancy complications causally contribute to future CVD risk, a key question is the extent to which pregnancy history can be used to improve CVD risk scoring systems for women, such as the Framingham Risk Score. At present, these scoring systems are of debatable utility for women under age 70 (Greenland et al. 2010), and addition of pregnancy complications to prediction at these relatively younger ages may be particularly important. Several pregnancy complications are more common among racial minority groups, who are also at higher risk of metabolic and cardiovascular disease. Pregnancy history may be of particular importance in identifying risk in these groups.

- Establishing strategies to mitigate future CVD risk in women with pregnancy complications

If pregnancy complications are useful for early CVD risk prediction, the next question is whether earlier risk identification—as early as at the time of pregnancy—is a cost-effective way of reducing future risk. To do so it is important to examine whether women who experienced pregnancy complications should undergo more intense or earlier screening and monitoring in the postpartum years in order to determine whether they cross thresholds for treatment (e.g., with statins) earlier than women without pregnancy complications. We would also need to test the extent to which different lifestyle or pharmacologic preventions are effective at preventing future CVD in young or middle-aged women with a history of pregnancy complications. Key to this is identifying stages in the lifespan when women are (or are not) receptive to CVD prevention, including the postpartum year.

4.3 Data and Methods Development Priorities

(a) Importance of linking research across life stages: need for extended follow-up of women with known reproductive histories

The bulk of the research associating pregnancy history to CVD risk is derived from the linkage of large, often national, vital statistics registries for birth, hospitalization, and mortality statistics. These exercises have yielded consistent associations of pregnancy complications with CVD risk. However, as most registries were founded in the 1950s or 1960s, the longest-running has been able to follow women only into the early postmenopausal years. The data on GDM are further limited by the lack of consistent methods for screening and diagnosing GDM. Further follow-up will determine the extent to which the associations of pregnancy complications are maintained into the age range at which CVD events are most common in women. In the meantime, the stratification of risk by time since pregnancy is a helpful way to examine the extent to which risk associated with pregnancy complications changes over time (Hastie et al. 2011a). Although relative risk of CVD events may weaken with time, the absolute risks associated with a history of pregnancy complications is likely to grow with time since pregnancy, as women age. In addition, we should incorporate pregnancy history data into existing CVD cohorts with decades of follow-up. By illuminating the *timing* with which *particular CVD risk factors* emerge in the wake of specific pregnancy complications, we may be able to leverage the information contained by pregnancy history to predict CVD risk *earlier* than conventional risk screening protocols.

(b) Importance of linking research across life stages: need for studies with established CVD risk factors measured before, during, and after pregnancy

To understand the trajectory of CVD risk and the role of pregnancy complications in that trajectory, we need more studies to measure CVD risk factors prior to conception, particularly as evidence suggests that changes in blood pressure, augmentation index, and pulse wave velocity occur as early as 6 weeks' gestation, indicating that maternal adaptations occur very early in gestation (Mahendru et al. 2014). This raises the question of whether "booking" first trimester measures that are available in several birth cohorts is representative of prepregnancy values and emphasizes the importance of ascertaining cardiovascular health trajectories from pre- to postpartum.

(c) Need for innovative analytical approaches to improve causal inference

Methods for improving our understanding of whether pregnancy complications are causally related to later maternal health need to go beyond conventional multivariable approaches in prospective cohorts. For example, if it is found that genetic variants associated with high blood pressure and glucose intolerance/type 2 diabetes in general populations of men and nonpregnant women are also associated with HDP and GDM, this would lend some support to the hypothesis of a common etiology and pregnancy unmasking a preexisting (genetic) risk. There is some evidence that several type 2 diabetes mellitus variants from genome-wide association studies show robust associations with GDM (Karlsson et al. 2007; Lauenborg et al. 2009; Cho et al. 2009; Kwak et al. 2012).

Although it is not feasible to randomize women to pregnancy complications, long-term follow-up of women who have been in randomized controlled trials that have effectively prevented or treated the pregnancy complication will also address some of the research questions above. Lastly, experimental induction of pregnancy complications in animal models and following the mothers after delivery to examine whether vascular damage was sustained or metabolic risk increased are important for examining the question of a pregnancy causal effect (Bytautiene et al. 2010). However, the generalizability of the animal models depends on the fidelity with which the human pregnancy complications, such as preeclampsia, can be mimicked in other species, where they may not occur naturally.

4.4 Translational Priorities

We are just beginning to investigate the clinical implications of this growing body of research. First, we need to establish the role of pregnancy complications in determining maternal chronic disease risk. Independently of that, we also need to determine our ability to change the health trajectories of women with histories of complicated pregnancy. We will then have to consider the many issues of integrating the findings into clinical and public health systems. Some potential clinical implications include the need to link prenatal with primary care medical records, development of clinical screening strategies, prevention and treatment protocols after pregnancy complications, and increasing awareness among clinicians of these associations that span typical clinical silos between obstetrics and medicine (Rich-Edwards et al. 2010).

5 Conclusions

The stress test of pregnancy provides glimpses into the otherwise silent early adult years in which health development and chronic disease trajectories are set. Research to characterize the ways in which pregnancy complications inform us about subclinical and clinical vascular and metabolic risk in the mother is in its infancy. Future research will require large datasets that have prospectively collected accurate data on cardiovascular risk factors before, during, and after pregnancy, into middle age and beyond, when disease begins to emerge; data on pregnancy complications is also required. Only with such detailed information can we determine the extent to which specific pregnancy complications are related to future CVD, over and above prepregnancy risk factors, and whether they add to established risk factor scores calculated in middle age. With large birth cohorts increasingly recognizing the importance of long-term follow-up of the mother as well as their infant, the potential for this research is increasing. Ultimately, randomized controlled trials will be necessary to establish whether pregnancy advice and/or continued monitoring and early treatment of women identified as at risk during pregnancy is a cost-effective way of reducing CVD risk in women. Research in this area will require integration across such diverse specialties including obstetrics, primary care, pediatrics, endocrinology, and cardiology. This broader perspective may yield novel insights into the determinants of pregnancy outcomes and health development across the lifespan, perhaps creating a large shift in the ways in which we promote the health of women and children.

References

Agatisa, P. K., Ness, R. B., Roberts, J. M., Costantino, J. P., Kuller, L. H., & McLaughlin, M. K. (2004). Impairment of endothelial function in women with a history of preeclampsia: An indicator of cardiovascular risk. *American Journal of Physiology – Heart and Circulatory Physiology, 286*, H1389–H1393.

Anastasiou, E., Lekakis, J. P., Alevizaki, M., et al. (1998). Impaired endothelium-dependent vasodilatation in women with previous gestational diabetes. *Diabetes Care, 21*, 2111–2115.

Beck, S., Wojdyla, D., Say, L., et al. (2010). The worldwide incidence of preterm birth: A systematic review of maternal mortality and morbidity. *Bulletin of the World Health Organization, 88*, 31–38.

Bellamy, L., Casas, J. P., Hingorani, A. D., & Williams, D. J. (2007). Pre-eclampsia and risk of cardiovascular disease and cancer in later life: Systematic review and meta-analysis. *British Medical Journal, 335*, 974.

Bellamy, L., Casas, J. P., Hingorani, A. D., & Williams, D. (2009). Type 2 diabetes mellitus after gestational diabetes: A systematic review and meta-analysis. *Lancet, 373*, 1773–1779.

Berends, A. L., de Groot, C. J., Sijbrands, E. J., et al. (2008). Shared constitutional risks for maternal vascular-related pregnancy complications and future cardiovascular disease. *Hypertension, 51*, 1034–1041.

Bonamy, A. K., Parikh, N. I., Cnattingius, S., Ludvigsson, J. F., & Ingelsson, E. (2011). Birth characteristics and subsequent risks of maternal cardiovascular disease: Effects of gestational age and fetal growth. *Circulation, 124*, 2839–2846.

Butte, N. F. (2000). Carbohydrate and lipid metabolism in pregnancy: Normal compared with gestational diabetes mellitus. *The American Journal of Clinical Nutrition, 71*, 1256S–1261S.

Bytautiene, E., Lu, F., Tamayo, E. H., et al. (2010). Long-term maternal cardiovascular function in a mouse model of sFlt-1-induced preeclampsia. *American Journal of Physiology. Heart and Circulatory Physiology, 298*, H189–H193.

Campbell, S., Griffin, D. R., Pearce, J. M., et al. (1983). New doppler technique for assessing uteroplacental blood flow. *Lancet, 321*, 675–677.

Carr, D. B., Utzschneider, K. M., Hull, R. L., et al. (2006). Gestational diabetes mellitus increases the risk of cardiovascular disease in women with a family history of type 2 diabetes. *Diabetes Care, 29*, 2078–2083.

Catov, J., Newman, A., Roberts, J., et al. (2007a). Association between infant birth weight and maternal cardiovascular risk factors in the health, aging, and body composition study. *Annals of Epidemiology, 17*, 36–43.

Catov, J. M., Bodnar, L. M., Kip, K. E., et al. (2007b). Early pregnancy lipid concentrations and spontaneous preterm birth. *American Journal of Obstetrics and Gynecology, 197*, 610. e611–610. e617.

Catov, J. M., Bodnar, L. M., Ness, R. B., Barron, S. J., & Roberts, J. M. (2007c). Inflammation and dyslipidemia related to risk of spontaneous preterm birth. *American Journal of Epidemiology, 166*, 1312–1319.

Catov, J. M., Nohr, E. A., Olsen, J., & Ness, R. B. (2008a). Chronic hypertension related to risk for preterm and term small-for-gestational-age births. *Obstetrics and Gynecology, 112*, 290.

Catov, J., Bodnar, L., Hackney, D., Roberts, J., & Simhan, S. (2008b). Activation of the fibrinolytic cascade early in pregnancy among women with spontaneous preterm birth. *Obstetrics and Gynecology, 112*, 1116–1122.

Catov, J. M., Wu, C. S., Olsen, J., Sutton-Tyrrell, K., Li, J., & Nohr, E. A. (2010a). Early or recurrent preterm birth and maternal cardiovascular disease risk. *Annals of Epidemiology, 20*, 604–609.

Catov, J. M., Ness, R. B., Wellons, M. F., Jacobs, D. R., Roberts, J. M., & Gunderson, E. P. (2010b). Prepregnancy lipids related to preterm birth risk: The coronary artery risk development in young adults study. *Journal of Clinical Endocrinology and Metabolism, 95*, 2009–2028.

Catov, J. M., Dodge, R., Yamal, J. M., Roberts, J. M., Piller, L. B., & Ness, R. B. (2011). Prior preterm or small-for-gestational-age birth related to maternal metabolic syndrome. *Obstetrics and Gynecology, 117*, 225–232.

Catov, J. M., Dodge, R., Barinas-Mitchell, E., et al. (2013). Prior preterm birth and maternal subclinical cardiovascular disease 4 to 12 years after pregnancy. *Journal of Women's Health, 22*(2002), 835–843.

Cho, Y. M., Kim, T. H., Lim, S., et al. (2009). Type 2 diabetes-associated genetic variants discovered in the recent genome-wide association studies are related to gestational diabetes mellitus in the Korean population. *Diabetologia, 52*, 253–261.

Clausen, T., Djurovic, S., & Henriksen, T. (2001). Dyslipidemia in early second trimester is mainly a feature of women with early onset pre-eclampsia. *BJOG, 108*, 1081–1087.

Curry, A., Vogel, I., Drews, C., et al. (2007). Mid-pregnancy maternal plasma levels of interleukin 2, 6, and 12, tumor necrosis factor-alpha, interferon-gamma, and granulocyte-macrophage colony-stimulating factor and spontaneous preterm delivery. *Acta Obstetricia et Gynecologica Scandinavica, 86*, 1103–1110.

Davey Smith, G., Hart, C., Ferrell, C., et al. (1997). Birth weight of offspring and mortality in the Renfrew and Paisley study: Prospective observational study. *British Medical Journal, 315*, 1189–1193.

Davey Smith, G., Harding, S., & Rosato, M. (2000a). Relation between infants' birth weight and mothers' mortality: Prospective observational study. *British Medical Journal, 320*, 839–840.

Davey Smith, G., Whitley, E., Gissler, M., & Hemminki, E. (2000b). Birth dimensions of offspring, premature birth, and the mortality of mothers. *Lancet, 356*, 2066–2067.

Davey Smith, G., Sterne, J., Tynelius, P., Lawlor, D. A., & Rasmussen, F. (2005). Birth weight of offspring and subsequent cardiovascular mortality of the parents. *Epidemiology, 16*, 563–569.

Davey Smith, G., Hypponen, E., Power, C., & Lawlor, D. A. (2007). Offspring birth weight and parental mortality: Prospective observational study and meta-analysis. *American Journal of Epidemiology, 166*, 160–169.

Dekker, J. M., & Schouten, E. G. (1993). Number of pregnancies and risk of cardiovascular disease. *The New England Journal of Medicine, 329*, 1893–1894. author reply 1894–1895.

Di Cianni, G., Lencioni, C., Volpe, L., et al. (2007). C-reactive protein and metabolic syndrome in women with previous gestational diabetes. *Diabetes/Metabolism Research and Reviews, 23*, 135–140.

Ducey, J., Schulman, H., Farmakides, G., et al. (1987). A classification of hypertension in pregnancy based on Doppler velocimetry. *American Journal of Obstetrics and Gynecology, 157*, 680–685.

Edison, R. J., Berg, K., Remaley, A., et al. (2007). Adverse birth outcome among mothers with low serum cholesterol. *Pediatrics, 120*, 723–733.

Enquobahrie, D. A., Williams, M. A., Qiu, C., & Luthy, D. A. (2005). Early pregnancy lipid concentrations and the risk of gestational diabetes mellitus. *Diabetes Research and Clinical Practice, 70*, 134–142.

Ernst, G. D. S., de Jonge, L. L., Hofman, A., et al. (2011). C-reactive protein levels in early pregnancy, fetal growth patterns, and the risk for neonatal complications: The Generation R Study. *American Journal of Obstetrics and Gynecology, 205*, 132.e131–132.e112.

Fraser, A., Nelson, S. M., Macdonald-Wallis, C., et al. (2012). Associations of pregnancy complications with calculated cardiovascular disease risk and cardiovascular risk factors in middle age/clinical perspective. *Circulation, 125*, 1367–1380.

Freathy, R. M., Weedon, M. N., Bennett, A., et al. (2007). Type 2 diabetes TCF7L2 risk genotypes alter birth weight: A study of 24,053 individuals. *American Journal of Human Genetics, 80*, 1150–1161.

Freeman, D. J., McManus, F., Brown, E. A., et al. (2004). Short-and long-term changes in plasma inflammatory markers associated with preeclampsia. *Hypertension, 44*, 708–714.

Friedlander, Y., Paltiel, O., Manor, O., et al. (2007). Birthweight of offspring and mortality of parents: The Jerusalem perinatal study cohort. *Annals of Epidemiology, 17*, 914–922.

Funai, E. F., Friedlander, Y., Paltiel, O., et al. (2005). Long-term mortality after preeclampsia. *Epidemiology, 16*, 206–215.

Gammill, H. S., Powers, R. W., Clifton, R. G., et al. (2010). Does C-reactive protein predict recurrent preeclampsia? *Hypertension in Pregnancy, 29*, 399–409.

Girardi, G. (2011). Role of tissue factor in pregnancy complications: Crosstalk between coagulation and inflammation. *Thrombosis Research, 127*(Suppl 3), S43–S46.

Green, A. B. V., & Moser, K. (1988). Mortality in women in relation to their childbearing history. *BMJ (Clinical research ed), 297*, 391–395.

Greenland, P., Alpert, J. S., Beller, G. A., et al. (2010). 2010 ACCF/AHA guideline for assessment of cardiovascular risk in asymptomatic adults: A report of the American College of Cardiology Foundation/American Heart Association Task Force on Practice Guidelines. *Circulation, 122*, e584–e636.

Hackney, D. N., Catov, J. M., & Simhan, H. N. (2010). Low concentrations of thrombin-inhibitor complexes and the risk of preterm delivery. *American Journal of Obstetrics and Gynecology, 203*, 184.e181–184.e186.

Hannaford, P., Ferry, S., & Hirsch, S. (1997). Cardiovascular sequelae of toxaemia of pregnancy. *Heart, 77*, 154–158.

Hastie, C. E., Smith, G. C., MacKay, D. F., & Pell, J. P. (2011a). Maternal risk of ischaemic heart disease following elective and spontaneous pre-term delivery: Retrospective cohort study of 750 350 singleton pregnancies. *International Journal of Epidemiology, 40*, 914–919.

Hastie, C. E., Smith, G. C. S., Mackay, D. F., & Pell, J. P. (2011b). Association between preterm delivery and subsequent C-reactive protein: A retrospective cohort study. *American Journal of Obstetrics and Gynecology, 205*, 556.e551–556.e554.

Hedderson, M. M., Ferrara, A., & Sacks, D. A. (2003). Gestational diabetes mellitus and lesser degrees of pregnancy hyperglycemia: Association with increased risk of spontaneous preterm birth. *Obstetrics and Gynecology, 102*, 850–856.

Heilmann, L., Rath, W., & Pollow, K. (2007). Hemostatic abnormalities in patients with severe preeclampsia. *Clinical and Applied Thrombosis/Hemostasis, 13*, 285–291.

Heitritter, S. M., Solomon, C. G., Mitchell, G. F., Skali-Ounis, N., & Seely, E. W. (2005). Subclinical inflammation and vascular dysfunction in women with previous gestational diabetes mellitus. *Journal of Clinical Endocrinology and Metabolism, 90*, 3983–3988.

Herrera, E. (2000). Metabolic adaptations in pregnancy and their implications for the availability of substrates to the fetus. *European Journal of Clinical Nutrition, 54*, S47.

Hubel, C. A., McLaughlin, M. K., Evans, R. W., Hauth, B. A., Sims, C. J., & Roberts, J. M. (1996). Fasting serum triglycerides, free fatty acids, and malondialdehyde are increased in preeclampsia, are positively correlated, and decrease within 48 hours post partum. *American Journal of Obstetrics and Gynecology, 174*, 975–982.

Hubel, C., Shakir, Y., Gallaher, M., McLaughlin, M., & Roberts, J. (1998a). Low-density lipoprotein particle size decreases during normal pregnancy in association with triglyceride increases. *Journal of the Society for Gynecologic Investigation, 5*, 244–250.

Hubel, C. A., Lyall, F., Weissfeld, L., Gandley, R. E., & Roberts, J. M. (1998b). Small low-density lipoproteins and vascular cell adhesion molecule-1 are increased in association with hyperlipidemia in preeclampsia. *Metabolism, 47*, 1281–1288.

Hubel, C. A., Powers, R., Snaedal, S., et al. (2006). C-reactive protein is increased 30 years after eclamptic pregnancy. *J Soc Gynecol Invest, 13*(2 Suppl), 292A.

Hubel, C. A., Powers, R. W., Snaedal, S., et al. (2008). C-reactive protein is elevated 30 years after eclamptic pregnancy. *Hypertension, 51*, 1499–1505.

Irgens, H. U., Reisaeter, L., Irgens, L. M., & Lie, R. T. (2001). Long term mortality of mothers and fathers after pre-eclampsia: Population based cohort study. *BMJ (Clinical research ed), 323*, 1213–1217.

James-Todd, T. K. A., Hibert, E., Mason, S., Vadnais, M., Hu, F., & Rich-Edwards. J. (2010). Gestation length, birth weight and subsequent risk of type 2 diabetes in mothers. Oral presentation. *Presented at American Diabetes Association's 70th Scientific Sessions*, June 2010, Orlando, FL.

Jónsdóttir, L., Arngrimsson, R., Geirsson, R. T., Slgvaldason, H., & Slgfússon, N. (1995). Death rates from ischemic heart disease in women with a history of hypertension in pregnancy. *Acta Obstetricia et Gynecologica Scandinavica, 74*, 772–776.

Kanagalingam, M. G., Nelson, S. M., Freeman, D. J., et al. (2009). Vascular dysfunction and alteration of novel and classic cardiovascular risk factors in mothers of growth restricted offspring. *Atherosclerosis, 205*, 244–250.

Kelly, R., Holzman, C., Senagore, P., et al. (2009). Placental vascular pathology findings and pathways to preterm delivery. *American Journal of Epidemiology, 170*, 148–158.

Kestenbaum, B., Seliger, S. L., Easterling, T. R., et al. (2003). Cardiovascular and thromboembolic events following hypertensive pregnancy. *American Journal of Kidney Diseases, 42*, 982–989.

Kim, C., Newton, K. M., & Knopp, R. H. (2002). Gestational diabetes and the incidence of type 2 diabetes a systematic review. *Diabetes Care, 25*, 1862–1868.

Kwak, S. H., Kim, S. H., Cho, Y. M., et al. (2012). A genome-wide association study of gestational diabetes mellitus in Korean women. *Diabetes, 61*, 531–541.

Labarthe, D. R. (1999). Prevention of cardiovascular risk factors in the first place. *Preventive Medicine, 29*, S72–S78.

Laivuori, H., Tikkanen, M. J., & Ylikorkala, O. (1996). Hyperinsulinemia 17 years after preeclamptic first pregnancy. *The Journal of Clinical Endocrinology and Metabolism, 81*, 2908–2911.

Lauenborg, J., Mathiesen, E., Hansen, T., et al. (2005). The prevalence of the metabolic syndrome in a danish population of women with previous gestational diabetes mellitus is three-fold higher than in the general population. *The Journal of Clinical Endocrinology and Metabolism, 90*, 4004–4010.

Lauenborg, J., Grarup, N., Damm, P., et al. (2009). Common type 2 diabetes risk gene variants associate with gestational diabetes. *The Journal of Clinical Endocrinology and Metabolism, 94*, 145–150.

Lawlor, D. A., Emberson, J. R., Ebrahim, S., et al. (2003). Is the association between parity and coronary heart disease due to biological effects of pregnancy or adverse lifestyle risk factors associated with child-rearing? *Circulation, 107*, 1260–1264.

Lawlor, D. A., Relton, C., Sattar, N., & Nelson, S. M. (2012). Maternal adiposity—a determinant of perinatal and offspring outcomes? *Nature Reviews Endocrinology, 8*, 679–688.

Lie, R. T., Wilcox, A. J., & Skjaerven, R. (2006). Maternal and paternal influences on length of pregnancy. *Obstetrics and Gynecology, 107*, 880–885.

Lin, Y.-S., Tang, C.-H., Yang, C.-Y. C., et al. (2011). Effect of pre-eclampsia–eclampsia on major cardiovascular events among peripartum women in Taiwan. *The American Journal of Cardiology, 107*, 325–330.

Lykke, J. A., Langhoff-Roos, J., Sibai, B. M., Funai, E. F., Triche, E. W., & Paidas, M. J. (2009). Hypertensive pregnancy disorders and subsequent cardiovascular morbidity and type 2 diabetes mellitus in the mother. *Hypertension, 53*, 944–951.

Lykke, J. A., Langhoff-Roos, J., Lockwood, C. J., Triche, E. W., & Paidas, M. J. (2010a). Mortality of mothers from cardiovascular and non-cardiovascular causes following pregnancy complications in first delivery. *Paediatric and Perinatal Epidemiology, 24*, 323–330.

Lykke, J., Paidas, M., Damm, P., Triche, E., Kuczynski, E., & Langhoff-Roos, J. (2010b). Preterm delivery and risk of subsequent cardiovascular morbidity and type-II diabetes in the mother. *BJOG: An International Journal of Obstetrics & Gynaecology, 117*, 274–281.

Lykke, J. A., Paidas, M. J., Triche, E. W., & LANGHOFF-ROOS, J. (2012). Fetal growth and later maternal death, cardiovascular disease and diabetes. *Acta Obstetricia et Gynecologica Scandinavica, 91*, 503–510.

Macdonald-Wallis, C., Lawlor, D. A., Fraser, A., May, M., Nelson, S. M., & Tilling, K. (2012). Blood pressure change in normotensive, gestational hypertensive, preeclamptic, and essential hypertensive pregnancies. *Hypertension, 59*, 1241–1248.

Magnussen, E. B., Vatten, L. J., Lund-Nilsen, T. I., Salvesen, K. A., Smith, G. D., & Romundstad, P. R. (2007). Prepregnancy cardiovascular risk factors as predictors of pre-eclampsia: Population based cohort study. *BMJ (Clinical research ed), 335*, 978.

Magnussen, E. B., Vatten, L. J., Smith, G. D., & Romundstad, P. R. (2009). Hypertensive disorders in pregnancy and subsequently measured cardiovascular risk factors. *Obstetrics and Gynecology, 114*, 961–970.

Magnussen, E. B., Vatten, L. J., Myklestad, K., Salvesen, K. Å., & Romundstad, P. R. (2011). Cardiovascular risk factors prior to conception and the length of pregnancy: Population-based cohort study. *American Journal of Obstetrics and Gynecology, 204*, 526.e521–526.e528.

Mahendru, A. A., Everett, T. R., Wilkinson, I. B., Lees, C. C., & McEniery, C. M. (2014). A longitudinal study of maternal cardiovascular function from preconception to the postpartum period. *Journal of Hypertension, 32*, 849–856.

Manten, G. T., Sikkema, M. J., Voorbij, H. A., Visser, G. H., Bruinse, H. W., & Franx, A. (2007). Risk factors for cardiovascular disease in women with a history of pregnancy complicated by preeclampsia or intrauterine growth restriction. *Hypertension in Pregnancy, 26*, 39–50.

Martinez, G., Daniels, K., & Chandra, A. (2012). Fertility of men and women aged 15–44 years in the United States: National survey of family growth, 2006–2010. *Natl Health Stat Report, 12*, 1–28.

Mathers, C., Boerma, J. T., Fat, D. M., & World Health Organization. (2008). *The global burden of disease : 2004 update*. Geneva: World Health Organization.

McDonald, S. D., Malinowski, A., Zhou, Q., Yusuf, S., & Devereaux, P. J. (2008). Cardiovascular sequelae of preeclampsia/eclampsia: A systematic review and meta-analyses. *American Heart Journal, 156*, 918–930.

Metzger, B. E., Cho, N. H., Roston, S. M., & Radvany, R. (1993). Prepregnancy weight and antepartum insulin secretion predict glucose tolerance five years after gestational diabetes mellitus. *Diabetes Care, 16*(1wik), 42–1605.

Meyers-Seifer, C. H., & Vohr, B. R. (1996). Lipid levels in former gestational diabetic mothers. *Diabetes Care, 19*, 1351–1356.

MMWR. (1989). Chronic disease reports in the Morbidity and Mortality Weekly Report (MMWR). *MMWR Morb Mortal Wkly Rep, 38*, 1–8.

Monga, M., & Creasy, R. (1994). Cardiovascular and renal adaptation to pregnancy. In R. Creasy, R. Resnik, J. D. Iams, et al. (Eds.), *Maternal-fetal medicine: Principles and practice* (pp. 758–767). Philadelphia: WB Saunders.

Mongraw-Chaffin, M. L., Cirillo, P. M., & Cohn, B. A. (2010). Preeclampsia and cardiovascular disease death. *Hypertension, 56*, 166–171.

Mosca, L., Benjamin, E. J., Berra, K., et al. (2011). Effectiveness-based guidelines for the prevention of cardiovascular disease in women – 2011 update: A guideline from the american heart association. *Circulation, 123*, 1243–1262.

Nanda, S. S. M., Syngelaki, A., Akolekar, R., & Nicolaides, K. H. (2011). Prediction of gestational diabetes mellitus by maternal factors and biomarkers at 11 to 13 weeks. *Prenatal Diagnosis, 31*, 135–141.

Nardi, O., Zureik, M., Courbon, D., Ducimetière, P., & Clavel-Chapelon, F. (2006). Preterm delivery of a first child and subsequent mothers' risk of ischaemic heart disease: A nested case–control study. *European Journal of Cardiovascular Prevention & Rehabilitation, 13*, 281–283.

Ness, R. B., Harris, T., Cobb, J., et al. (1993). Number of pregnancies and the subsequent risk of cardiovascular disease. *The New England Journal of Medicine, 328*, 1528–1533.

Ness, R. B., Cobb, J., Harm, T., & D'Agostino, R. B. (1995). Does number of children increase the rate of coronary heart disease in men? *Epidemiology, 6*, 442–445.

North, R. A., McCowan, L. M., Dekker, G. A., et al. (2011). Clinical risk prediction for pre-eclampsia in nulliparous women: Development of model in international prospective cohort. *BMJ (Clinical research ed), 342*, d1875.

O'Brien, T. E., Ray, J. G., & Chan, W. S. (2003). Maternal body mass index and the risk of preeclampsia: A systematic overview. *Epidemiology, 14*, 368–374.

Oblast, T. I. (1999). Decline in deaths from heart disease and stroke—United States, 1900–1999. *Heart Disease and Stroke, 63*(1900), 593–597.

OECD Family D. (2014). Childlessness (SF 2.5) In: *Social Policy Division, Organisation for Economic Co-operation and Development.* Paris, France: 2010. SF2.5 report on childlessness. www.oecd.org/social/family/database. Accessed 24 June, 2013.

Ostlund, I., Haglund, B., & Hanson, U. (2004). Gestational diabetes and preeclampsia. *European Journal of Obstetrics, Gynecology, and Reproductive Biology, 113*, 12–16.

Parikh, N. I., Cnattingius, S., Dickman, P. W., Mittleman, M. A., Ludvigsson, J. F., & Ingelsson, E. (2010). Parity and risk of later-life maternal cardiovascular disease. *American Heart Journal, 159*, 215–221.e216.

Pell, J. P., Smith, G. C., & Walsh, D. (2004). Pregnancy complications and subsequent maternal cerebrovascular events: A retrospective cohort study of 119,668 births. *American Journal of Epidemiology, 159*, 336–342.

Pitiphat, W., Gillman, M. W., Joshipura, K. J., Williams, P. L., Douglass, C. W., & Rich-Edwards, J. W. (2005). Plasma C-reactive protein in early pregnancy and preterm delivery. *American Journal of Epidemiology, 162*, 1108–1113.

Portelinha, A., Cerdeira, A. S., Belo, L., et al. (2009). Haemostatic factors in women with history of Preeclampsia. *Thrombosis Research, 124*, 52–56.

Qiu, C., Williams, M. A., Leisenring, W. M., et al. (2003). Family history of hypertension and type 2 diabetes in relation to preeclampsia risk. *Hypertension, 41*, 408–413.

Regitz-Zagrosek, V., Lundqvist, C. B., Borghi, C., et al. (2011). ESC Guidelines on the management of cardiovascular diseases during pregnancy. The Task Force on the Management of Cardiovascular Diseases during Pregnancy of the European Society of Cardiology (ESC). *European Heart Journal, 32*, 3147–3197.

Retnakaran, R., & Shah, B. R. (2009a). Abnormal screening glucose challenge test in pregnancy and future risk of diabetes in young women. *Diabetic Medicine, 26*, 474–477.

Retnakaran, R., & Shah, B. R. (2009b). Mild glucose intolerance in pregnancy and risk of cardiovascular disease: A population-based cohort study. *Canadian Medical Association Journal, 181*, 371–376.

Retnakaran, R., Austin, P. C., & Shah, B. R. (2011). Effect of subsequent pregnancies on the risk of developing diabetes following a first pregnancy complicated by gestational diabetes: A population-based study. *Diabetic Medicine, 28*, 287–292.

Rich-Edwards, J. W. (2009). Reproductive health as a sentinel of chronic disease in women. *Women's Health (London, England), 5*, 101–105.

Rich-Edwards, J. W., McElrath, T. F., Karumanchi, S. A., & Seely, E. W. (2010). Breathing life into the lifecourse approach: Pregnancy history and cardiovascular disease in women. *Hypertension, 56*, 331–334.

Rich-Edwards, J. W. K. K., Wilcox, A., & Skjaerven, R. (2012). Duration of first pregnancy predicts maternal cardiovascular death, whether delivery was medically indicated or spontaneous. *American Journal of Epidemiology, 175*(Suppl 11), S64.

Rich-Edwards, J. W., Fraser, A., Lawlor, D. A., & Catov, J. M. (2014). Pregnancy characteristics and women's future cardiovascular health: An underused opportunity to improve women's health? *Epidemiologic Reviews, 36*, 57–70.

Riskin-Mashiah, S., Damti, A., Younes, G., & Auslender, R. (2010). First trimester fasting hyperglycemia as a predictor for the development of gestational diabetes mellitus. *European Journal of Obstetrics, Gynecology, and Reproductive Biology, 152*, 163–167.

Roberts, C. L., Algert, C. S., Morris, J. M., Ford, J. B., & Henderson-Smart, D. J. (2005). Hypertensive disorders in pregnancy: A population-based study. *The Medical Journal of Australia, 182*, 332–335.

Romero, R., Espinoza, J., Gonçalves, L. F., Kusanovic, J. P., Friel, L., & Hassan, S. (2007). The role of inflammation and infection in preterm birth. *Seminars in Reproductive Medicine, 25*, 021–039.

Romundstad, P. R., Davey Smith, G., Nilsen, T. I., & Vatten, L. J. (2007). Associations of prepregnancy cardiovascular risk factors with the offspring's birth weight. *American Journal of Epidemiology, 166*, 1359–1364.

Romundstad, P. R., Magnussen, E. B., Smith, G. D., & Vatten, L. J. (2010). Hypertension in pregnancy and later cardiovascular risk: Common antecedents? *Circulation, 122*, 579–584.

Sacks DA, C. W., Wolde-Tsadik, G., & Buchanan, T. A. (2003). Fasting plasma glucose test at the first prenatal visit as a screen for gestational diabetes. *Obstetrics and Gynecology, 101*, 1197–1203.

Sarwar, N., Gao, P., Seshasai, S. R., et al. (2010). Diabetes mellitus, fasting blood glucose concentration, and risk of vascular disease: A collaborative meta-analysis of 102 prospective studies. *Lancet, 375*, 2215–2222.

Sattar, N. (2004). Do pregnancy complications and CVD share common antecedents? *Atherosclerosis Supplements, 5*, 3–7.

Sattar, N., & Greer, I. A. (2002). Pregnancy complications and maternal cardiovascular risk: Opportunities for intervention and screening? *British Medical Journal, 325*, 157–160.

Sattar, N., Bendomir, A., Berry, C., Shepherd, J., Greer, I. A., & Packard, C. J. (1997). Lipoprotein subfraction concentrations in preeclampsia: Pathogenic parallels to atherosclerosis. *Obstetrics and Gynecology, 89*, 403–408.

Sattar, N., Greer, I., Galloway, P., et al. (1999). Lipid and lipoprotein concentrations in pregnancies complicated by intrauterine growth restriction. *Journal of Clinical Endocrinology and Metabolism, 84*, 128–130.

Sattar, N., Ramsay, J., Crawford, L., Cheyne, H., & Greer, I. A. (2003). Classic and novel risk factor parameters in women with a history of preeclampsia. *Hypertension, 42*, 39–42.

Savvidou, M. D., Hingorani, A. D., Tsikas, D., Frölich, J. C., Vallance, P., & Nicolaides, K. H. (2003). Endothelial dysfunction and raised plasma concentrations of asymmetric dimethylarginine in pregnant women who subsequently develop pre-eclampsia. *The Lancet, 361*, 1511–1517.

Savvidou, M. D., Kaihura, C., Anderson, J. M., & Nicolaides, K. H. (2011). Maternal arterial stiffness in women who subsequently develop pre-eclampsia. *PLoS ONE, 6*, e18703.

Scarborough, P., & Weissberg, P. (2011). *Trends in coronary heart disease, 1961–2011*. London: British Heart Foundation.

Schwarz, E. B., Ray, R. M., Stuebe, A. M., et al. (2009). Duration of lactation and risk factors for maternal cardiovascular disease. *Obstetrics and Gynecology, 113*, 974–982.

Shaat, N. L. A., Karlsson, E., Ivarsson, S., Parikh, H., Berntorp, K., & Groop, L. (2007). A variant in the transcription factor 7-like 2 (TCF7L2) gene is associated with an increased risk of gestational diabetes mellitus. *Diabetologia, 50*, 972–979.

Shah, B. R., Retnakaran, R., & Booth, G. L. (2008). Increased risk of cardiovascular disease in young women following gestational diabetes mellitus. *Diabetes Care, 31*, 1668–1669.

Shah, R. U., Klein, L., & Lloyd-Jones, D. M. (2009). Heart failure in women: Epidemiology, biology and treatment. *Women's Health (London, England), 5*, 517–527.

Shaw, L. J., Bairey Merz, C. N., Pepine, C. J., et al. (2006). Insights from the NHLBI-Sponsored Women's Ischemia Syndrome Evaluation (WISE) Study: Part I: Gender differences in traditional and novel risk factors, symptom evaluation, and gender-optimized diagnostic strategies. *Journal of the American College of Cardiology, 47*, S4–S20.

Shay, C. M., Ning, H., Allen, N. B., et al. (2012). Status of cardiovascular health in US adults clinical perspective prevalence estimates from the National Health and Nutrition Examination Surveys (NHANES) 2003–2008. *Circulation, 125*, 45–56.

Skjaerven, R., Wilcox, A. J., Klungsoyr, K., et al. (2012). Cardiovascular mortality after pre-eclampsia in one child mothers: Prospective, population based cohort study. *BMJ (Clinical research ed), 345*, e7677.

Smith, G. C., Pell, J. P., & Walsh, D. (2001). Pregnancy complications and maternal risk of ischaemic heart disease: A retrospective cohort study of 129,290 births. *Lancet, 357*, 2002–2006.

Smith, G. C. S., Shah, I., Pell, J. P., Crossley, J. A., & Dobbie, R. (2007). Maternal obesity in early pregnancy and risk of spontaneous and elective preterm deliveries: A retrospective cohort study. *American Journal of Public Health, 97*, 157–162.

Smith, G. N., Walker, M. C., Liu, A., et al. (2009). A history of preeclampsia identifies women who have underlying cardiovascular risk factors. *American Journal of Obstetrics and Gynecology, 200*(58), e51–e58.

Solomon, C. G., Willett, W. C., Carey, V. J., et al. (1997). A prospective study of pregravid determinants of gestational diabetes mellitus. *JAMA, 278*, 1078–1083.

Steenland, K., Lally, C., & Thun, M. (1996). Parity and coronary heart disease among women in the American Cancer Society CPS II population. *Epidemiology, 7*, 641–643.

Stepan, H., Faber, R., & Walther, T. (1999). Expression of low density lipoprotein receptor messenger ribonucleic acid in placentas from pregnancies with intrauterine growth retardation. *British Journal of Obstetrics and Gynaecology, 106*, 1221–1222.

Tarim, E., Yigit, F., Kilicdag, E., et al. (2006). Early onset of subclinical atherosclerosis in women with gestational diabetes mellitus. *Ultrasound in Obstetrics & Gynecology, 27*, 177–182.

United Nations DoEaSA, Population Division. (2009). *World fertility report*. New York: United Nations Publications.

Verma, A., Boney, C. M., Tucker, R., & Vohr, B. R. (2002). Insulin resistance syndrome in women with prior history of gestational diabetes mellitus. *The Journal of Clinical Endocrinology and Metabolism, 87*, 3227–3235.

Wadsack, C., Tabano, S., Maier, A., et al. (2007). Intrauterine growth restriction is associated with alterations in placental lipoprotein receptors and maternal lipoprotein composition. *American Journal of Physiology - Endocrinology and Metabolism, 292*, E476–E484.

Wallis, A. B., Saftlas, A. F., Hsia, J., & Atrash, H. K. (2008). Secular trends in the rates of preeclampsia, eclampsia, and gestational hypertension, United States, 1987–2004. *American Journal of Hypertension, 21*, 521–526.

Weintraub, W. S., Daniels, S. R., Burke, L. E., et al. (2011). Value of primordial and primary prevention for cardiovascular disease: A policy statement from the American Heart Association. *Circulation, 124*, 967–990.

Wikström, A. K., Haglund, B., Olovsson, M., & Lindeberg, S. N. (2005). The risk of maternal ischaemic heart disease after gestational hypertensive disease. *BJOG: An International Journal of Obstetrics & Gynaecology, 112*, 1486–1491.

Wilcox, A. J., Skjaerven, R., & Lie, R. T. (2008). Familial patterns of preterm delivery: Maternal and fetal contributions. *American Journal of Epidemiology, 167*, 474–479.

Williams, M. A., Qiu, C., Muy-Rivera, M., Vadachkoria, S., Song, T., & Luthy, D. A. (2004). Plasma adiponectin concentrations in early pregnancy and subsequent risk of gestational diabetes mellitus. *The Journal of Clinical Endocrinology and Metabolism, 89*, 2306–2311.

Wilson, B. J., Watson, M. S., Prescott, G. J., et al. (2003). Hypertensive diseases of pregnancy and risk of hypertension and stroke in later life: Results from cohort study. *British Medical Journal, 326*, 845.

Winzer, C., Wagner, O., Festa, A., et al. (2004). Plasma adiponectin, insulin sensitivity, and subclinical inflammation in women with prior gestational diabetes mellitus. *Diabetes Care, 27*, 1721–1727.

Wolf, M., Kettyle, E., Sandler, L., Ecker, J. L., Roberts, J., & Thadhani, R. (2001). Obesity and preeclampsia: The potential role of inflammation. *Obstetrics and Gynecology, 98*, 757–762.

Wolf, M., Hubel, C. A., Lam, C., et al. (2004). Preeclampsia and future cardiovascular disease: Potential role of altered angiogenesis and insulin resistance. *The Journal of Clinical Endocrinology and Metabolism, 89*, 6239–6243.

Yusuf, S., Reddy, S., Ôunpuu, S., & Anand, S. (2001). Global burden of cardiovascular diseases. *Circulation, 104*, 2746–2753.

Part III

The Life Course Origins and Consequences of Select Major Health Conditions and Issues

Early in the Life Course: Time for Obesity Prevention

Summer Sherburne Hawkins, Emily Oken, and Matthew W. Gillman

1 Introduction

Although the dramatic rise in obesity in the USA experienced in recent decades (Wang and Beydoun 2007) may have now stabilized (Ogden et al. 2014; Wen et al. 2012), the prevalence of obesity remains high. The most recent nationally representative data collected in 2012 showed that 17% of children ages 2–19 years were obese (Ogden et al. 2014). From 2003 through 2010, the prevalence of obesity in low-income children aged 2–4 years remained at approximately 15% (Pan et al. 2012), while one regional study suggested that from 2004 through 2008, obesity prevalence started to drop among 0 to 6-year-olds from non-low-income families (Wen et al. 2012). The reasons for this potential slowing or slight reversal of the trend among some subgroups in the USA remain unknown. However, obesity has not affected all segments of the population equally (Wang and Beydoun 2007; Wang et al. 2011), and racial/ethnic differences in obesity are already evident by the preschool years (Ogden et al. 2014).

The short- and long-term consequences of obesity include conditions involving nearly every organ system, such as asthma, type 2 diabetes, high blood pressure, cardiovascular disease, depression, and orthopedic problems, starting in childhood and escalating among adults (Han et al. 2010; Lobstein et al. 2004). Children who are obese are much more likely to be obese adults, and obesity at any age is very difficult to treat (Lobstein et al. 2004). Furthermore, the population-level effects of obesity are substantial. Nationwide, 9.1% of annual medical spending is attributable to adult obesity, representing a cost of $147 billion per year (Finkelstein et al. 2009). This combination of evidence on the epidemiology, health consequences, and public health impact of obesity suggests that prevention is essential.

2 Conceptual Framework

One of the reasons for the intractability of childhood obesity is the failure to take into account the complexity and interconnectedness of contributing factors ranging from the social, built, and economic environments to behavior, physiology, and epigenetics. These factors may also interact with each other creating a self-perpetuating cycle

S.S. Hawkins (✉)
Boston College, Chestnut Hill, MA, USA
e-mail: summer.hawkins@bc.edu

E. Oken • M.W. Gillman
Harvard Medical School and Harvard Pilgrim Health Care Institute, Boston, MA, USA
e-mail: emily_oken@harvardpilgrim.org; matthew.gillman@nih.gov

N. Halfon et al. (eds.), *Handbook of Life Course Health Development*,
DOI 10.1007/978-3-319-47143-3_9

of obesity, as we illustrate using gestational diabetes mellitus (Sect. 4.3; Gillman 2016). Based on the life course health development approach to chronic disease epidemiology, biological, behavioral, and psychosocial exposures that occur at particular stages in the life course may have differential and/or lasting effects on later outcomes (Ben-Shlomo and Kuh 2002; Halfon and Forrest 2017).

The effects of these exposures can be cumulative across an individual's life as well as operate across generations to influence future generation's risk for chronic disease. Factors can also interact with each other over the life course and be more or less important at particular stages. These periods of particular influence are often termed critical or sensitive (Ben-Shlomo and Kuh 2002). Throughout the chapter, we demonstrate that multiple critical and sensitive periods for obesity risk exist across the life course, although practically they may be hard to identify. Given the plasticity inherent in early human development, the pre- and perinatal periods may present the most important opportunity for critical or sensitive period effects. Added to the fact that treatment of obesity is impeded by cultural, behavioral, and physiological feedback loops, modifying environment, behaviors, and physiology early in life is likely an especially effective strategy for preventing obesity and its consequences.

Consistent with LCHD principles (see Halfon and Forrest 2017), Glass and McAtee (2006) propose that the multilevel approach shown in Fig. 1 places obesity prevention in a complex system with individual risk factors being influenced by multiple "above-water" levels (families, neighborhood, policies) as well as by the interaction with biology and "underwater" levels (genes, epigenetics, physiology) over time. This framework adds to a life course health development approach by emphasizing feedback loops and cross-level influences, such as gene-environment interactions, thus highlighting the need for methodology that takes into account these complex relationships to help identify the important and modifiable levers of change (Huang and Glass 2008).

We have organized this chapter to reflect the current thinking on periods in the life course that appear to be most important for the development of obesity. We focus primarily on the early portion of the life course, but also discuss later periods that may be key time points for intervening. These periods often represent times of active growth or turning points when the primary sources of influence change.

At each stage of the life course, we discuss specific macro-level factors if they are directly relevant to that time period. Most macro-level factors, however, either indirectly or directly influence all age groups, so we present them together after reviewing each life course stage individually. While this chapter does not represent a systematic review of the literature, we present key examples at each stage of the life course to illustrate important risk factors, mechanisms, and gaps in research. We conclude with recommendations for future work on methodology, research in emerging areas, and implications for practice and policy.

3 Measurement of Overweight and Obesity

Body mass index (BMI; weight/height^2) is the most commonly used indirect measure of adiposity, or fatness, at the population level. The US Centers for Disease Control and Prevention (CDC) recommends monitoring growth in children aged 0–2 years using the World Health Organization weight for recumbent length growth standards and defines excess weight as at or above the 97.7th percentile (Grummer-Strawn et al. 2010). The CDC defines obesity in children aged 2–19 years as a BMI at or above the 95th percentile for age and sex, with overweight between the 85th and 95th percentiles, using the CDC sex-specific BMI-for-age growth charts from 2000 (Kuczmarski et al. 2002; Ogden and Flegal 2010).

4 Prenatal Period

4.1 Birth Weight

Numerous studies have confirmed the associations of higher birth weight with risk of later obesity and type 2 diabetes mellitus; lower birth

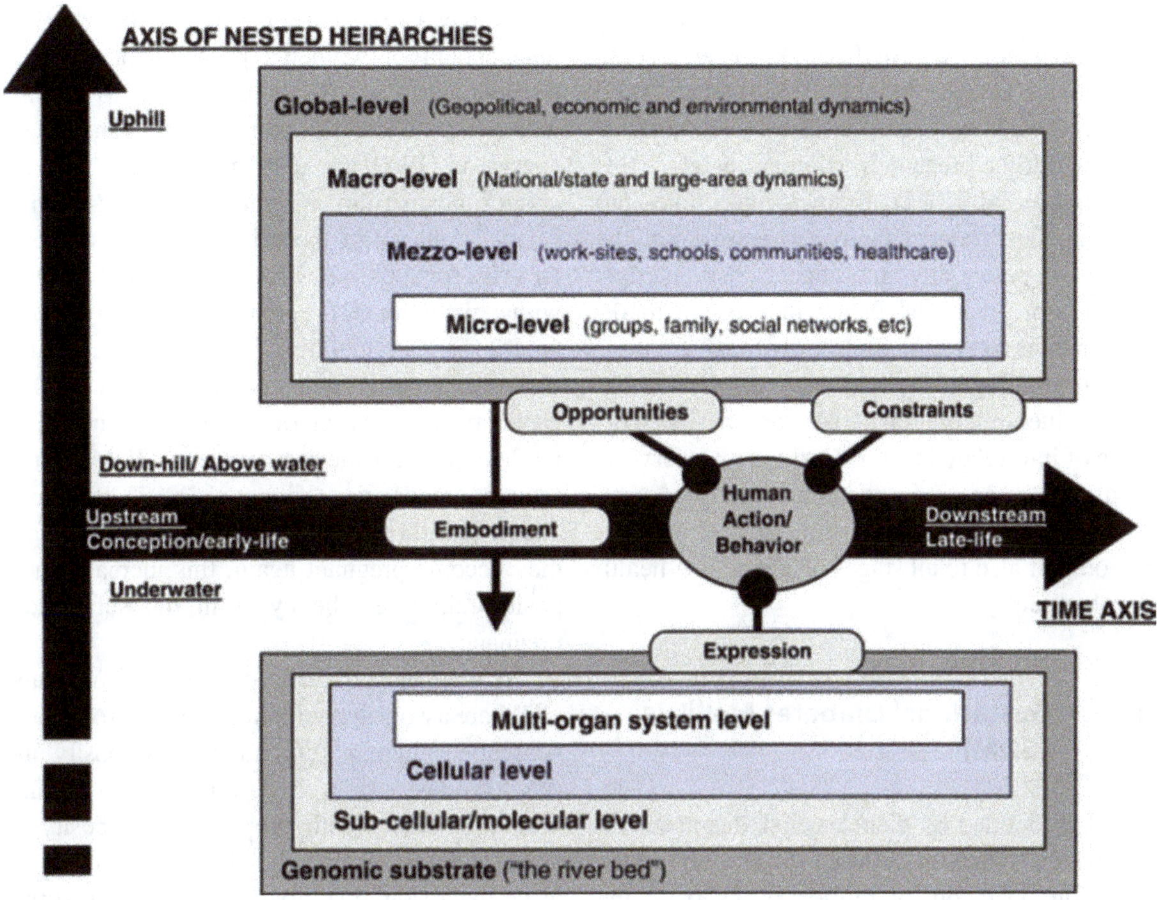

Fig. 1 Conceptual framework for etiology of childhood obesity (Reproduced from Glass and McAtee (2006))

weight is consistently associated with increased risk for central adiposity and its metabolic correlates, including type 2 diabetes mellitus and cardiovascular disease (Parsons et al. 1999; Yu et al. 2011). Birth weight, however, is not an etiologic factor in itself. Some have used birth weight as a marker of in utero programming during sensitive periods of development (Gillman 2005). However, many factors could explain the relationship between birth weight and later obesity. For example, maternal obesity, a risk factor for higher birth weight, is also highly related to childhood obesity (Perng et al. 2014). This association may be due to genomic inheritance and shared postnatal environment of eating habits and physical activity or inactivity in addition to in utero effects (Gillman and Poston 2012). However, even after controlling for maternal obesity, sociodemographic characteristics, and other risk factors, the birth weight-obesity association remains, raising the possibility of a lasting effect of fetal programming on later health (Gillman 2004; Oken and Gillman 2003).

4.2 Maternal Prepregnancy Obesity

Many women start their pregnancy already overweight or obese. In 2009, a representative survey from 20 states found that 21% of women were obese prepregnancy and an additional 25% were overweight (Fisher et al. 2013). Mothers who are overweight or obese prepregnancy are more likely to have infants with higher birth weight and an increased risk for being large-for-gestational age (LGA; >90th percentile of weight-for-gestational age) or macrosomic (birth weight > 4000 g) (Institute of Medicine 2009).

Women who are overweight or obese going into pregnancy are at higher risk for developing gestational diabetes mellitus (Torloni et al. 2009) and more likely to gain excessive amounts of weight during pregnancy (Battista et al. 2011; Dalenius et al. 2012). Studies must take into account these related factors to tease apart the roles of potentially modifiable risk factors. Furthermore, these risk factors may also be markers for shared genes and/or the postnatal environment (including lifestyle behaviors), which could also influence children's risk for obesity. This issue of interrelated factors—which may serve as mediators, moderators, or confounders of each other—is applicable not just to the prenatal period, but also to all stages of life course health development.

4.3 Gestational Diabetes Mellitus (GDM)

GDM is defined as diabetes first diagnosed in pregnancy, typically between 24 and 28 weeks gestation. Data on 59 million births from the National Hospital Discharge Survey showed that GDM increased from 1.9% to 4.2% from 1989 through 2004 (Getahun et al. 2008). Over this time period, the relative increase in GDM was 94% for white women (from 2.2% to 4.2%), but 260% for black women (from 0.6% to 2.1%) (Getahun et al. 2008).

GDM may be fueling the obesity epidemic (Battista et al. 2011; Herring and Oken 2011). Figure 2 shows the interrelationships of maternal, fetal, and child factors across the life course that may propagate the intergenerational transmission of obesity and diabetes (Gillman 2016). Both maternal prepregnancy obesity and excessive gestational weight gain (GWG) independently increase mothers' risk for developing GDM. A systematic review found that higher maternal prepregnancy BMI was associated with an increase in risk for GDM, such that overweight, moderately obese, and morbidly obese women were 2, 3, and 5.5 times more likely to develop GDM compared to women with normal BMI (Torloni et al. 2009). Excess GWG during pregnancy may also increase mothers' risk for GDM, independent of women's prepregnancy weight (Hedderson et al. 2010). Compared to women with adequate levels of weight gain, women with excessive GWG are also more likely to have greater postpartum weight retention (Nehring et al. 2011). All of these factors increase women's risk for subsequent health problems. Women with a history of GDM are more likely to develop type 2 diabetes mellitus, particularly within the first decade after delivery (Kim et al. 2002). Developing GDM in one pregnancy increases mothers' risk for the recurrence of GDM in subsequent pregnancies (Kim et al. 2007). If women do not lose the excess weight they gained before they become pregnant again, this increased adiposity reinforces the cycle in the subsequent pregnancy.

Prepregnancy obesity, excessive GWG, and GDM are associated with higher fetal growth and subsequent increases in children's adiposity and risk for obesity (Fig. 2) (Gillman 2016). Infants born to mothers with prepregnancy obesity or GDM are more likely to be of higher birth weight or be macrosomic (Battista et al. 2011; Institute of Medicine 2009), and trials of GDM treatment show reductions in macrosomia (Crowther et al. 2005; Gillman et al. 2010; Landon et al. 2009). A study found that children born to mothers with GDM had higher levels of adiposity and insulin secretion at age 5–10 years, independent of current BMI (Chandler-Laney et al. 2012). Boney et al. (2005) found that children who were LGA at birth and exposed to either GDM or maternal obesity in utero were at an increased risk for developing metabolic syndrome. The cycle continues when girls who are obese mature and have children of their own.

Plausible developmental mechanisms exist for the influence of GDM on childhood obesity. Pancreatic β-cells normally increase their insulin secretion to compensate for the insulin resistance during pregnancy. Glucose intolerance results when the β-cells are not able to respond to this increasing demand (Battista et al. 2011). Since glucose crosses the placenta but insulin does not, the fetus is exposed to greater levels of glucose (Freinkel 1980). The developing fetal pancreas

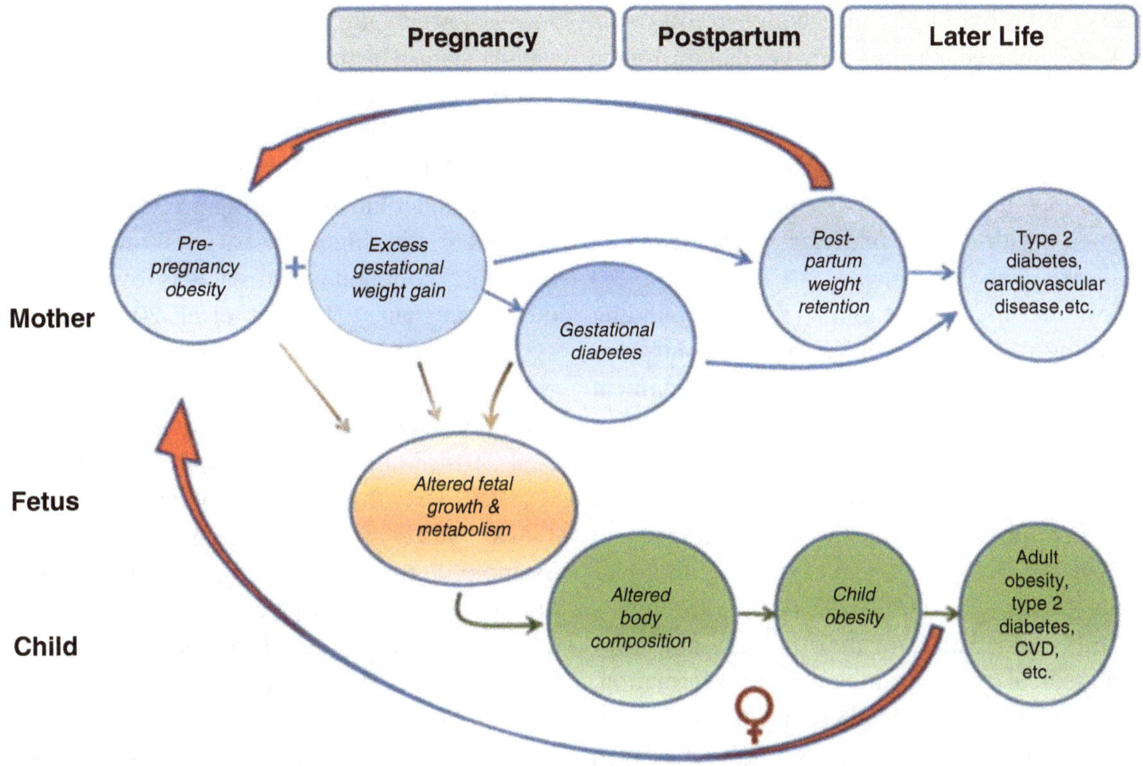

Fig. 2 Intergenerational transmission of obesity and gestational diabetes mellitus (Reproduced from Gillman (2016))

responds to the additional glucose by producing insulin, which can increase fetal adiposity (Freinkel 1980). Current research on the mechanisms of GDM is focusing on the areas of genetics, glucose, amino acid, lipid transport, and adipokines (Harlev and Wiznitzer 2010).

Methodological challenges abound in studying the association between GDM and later obesity. Kim et al. (2011) have argued that many studies combine pregestational diabetes mellitus and GDM into one category, examine only exposed or high-risk infants without an appropriate control group, and fail to control for potential confounding factors, most notably BMI. Their systematic review identified 12 studies of children exposed prenatally to GDM (excluding pregestational diabetes), with resulting crude odds ratios of 0.7–6.3 for offspring obesity. However, in many studies, it is not possible to distinguish women with GDM with true onset during pregnancy from undiagnosed pregestational diabetes (Herring and Oken 2011; Kim et al. 2011). In the two studies that adjusted for maternal prepregnancy BMI, results attenuated and were no longer significant after the covariate was included (Kim et al. 2011), which suggests that GDM may be a marker for preexisting maternal factors.

Randomized controlled trials (RCTs) of risk factor manipulation in pregnancy with childhood follow-up are especially valuable because they minimize the effect of confounding and thus are the most direct assessment of in utero programming in humans. In a US-based RCT of the treatment for mild GDM on pregnancy-related outcomes, Landon et al. (2009) found reduction in LGA and macrosomia; however, no childhood follow-up has been done. Gillman et al. (2010) followed up a subset of children who participated in an Australian-based multicenter RCT of treatment for mild GDM. Although the parent trial showed halving of macrosomia at birth, there were no differences in child BMI at age 4–5 years. One possible explanation for the null result is that offspring of mothers with GDM appear to lose their excess fat in the first year of life and do not again begin to diverge from their unexposed peers until school age; thus, continued follow-up of these children may be needed to demonstrate a longer-lasting effect of prenatal GDM treatment. Furthermore, as this study included women with mild GDM only, a more dramatic benefit of treatment may be experienced among offspring of women with more extreme hyperglycemia (Gillman et al. 2010).

Another method for minimizing confounding is sibling-pair designs, which partially control for differences in the pre- and postnatal environment (Brion 2010). This method relies on discrepant in utero exposure between siblings, such that the mother experienced GDM during her pregnancy with one sibling but not the other. Lawlor and colleagues (2011b) conducted a sibling-pair study of over 280,000 Swedish men through a record linkage study of their military conscription medical examination with birth information. They found that BMI at age 18 was higher in men whose mothers had GDM during pregnancy than those who did not; these differences were still evident in the within-sibling analyses and independent of maternal BMI. The authors concluded that GDM may influence later obesity risk through intrauterine mechanisms (Lawlor et al. 2011b).

4.4 Gestational Weight Gain (GWG)

In 1990, the Institute of Medicine (IOM) (1990) issued guidelines for the appropriate amount of weight women should gain during pregnancy. However, over the last two decades, excessive GWG has been common and increasing. In 2010, based on the Pregnancy Nutrition Surveillance System (PNSS) from 29 states and the District of Columbia, approximately 48% of low-income women gained more weight than recommended (Dalenius et al. 2012). Excessive weight gain is associated with adverse infant outcomes, including macrosomia and LGA infants, as well as postpartum weight retention in mothers (Siega-Riz et al. 2009). In 2009, the IOM published new guidelines, which for the first time include a weight gain range for obese women that recommends lower gains than for women with lower weight status (Institute of Medicine 2009).

GWG may also have a lasting effect on body size across the life course through in utero conditioning. Although some evidence suggests that extreme undernutrition during pregnancy may be associated with higher obesity risk in offspring, the more common occurrence is overnutrition during pregnancy (Herring et al. 2012). Recent systematic reviews found that excessive GWG was associated with an increased risk for offspring obesity compared to adequate GWG (Lau et al. 2014; Mamun Mamun et al. 2014; Nehring et al. 2013), with an overall pooled odds ratio of 1.4 (Mamun et al. 2014; Nehring et al. 2013). For example, Perng et al. (2014) found that every 5 kilograms of GWG was associated with greater adiposity (measured total fat and trunk fat) and higher leptin in children at ages 6–10 years, independent of maternal prepregnancy BMI.

GWG may influence childhood obesity through several potential developmental pathways. Mothers who are more prone to gain weight through genetic risk, poor diet, or other behavioral factors may have children who are also themselves exposed to these same risks. However, associations still remain after adjustment for maternal and paternal BMI, reducing some influence of shared genes and the postnatal environment. An alternative explanation may be through fetal conditioning (Gillman 2005), similar to that proposed for GDM. In animal models, overnutrition during pregnancy has resulted in insulin resistance, increased adiposity, and hypertension in offspring (Alfaradhi and Ozanne 2011).

One methodology to test causality is through an intervention aimed at influencing maternal weight gain during pregnancy through positive lifestyle changes. Three recent meta-analyses summarized the evidence on RCTs for prenatal dietary, physical activity, and behavioral or lifestyle interventions on maternal weight gain and infant outcomes (Agha et al. 2014; Oteng-Ntim et al. 2012; Thangaratinam et al. 2012). The reviews found that dietary and lifestyle interventions resulted in a small reduction in GWG (1.42–2.21 kg), but together the interventions did not appear to influence birth weight or LGA (Agha et al. 2014; Oteng-Ntim et al. 2012; Thangaratinam et al. 2012). However, none of the trials to date have looked at longer-term outcomes of child adiposity. Several ongoing RCTs targeted at changing GWG will follow offspring for development of obesity and its consequences (Dodd et al. 2011; Moholdt et al. 2011; Vesco et al. 2012). Vesco et al. (2014) found that obese women randomized to a dietary intervention gained less weight during pregnancy and had a lower proportion of babies born LGA, with further follow-up planned.

Two separate sibling-pair analyses have examined GWG and offspring obesity. Lawlor and colleagues (2011a) examined the association of maternal weight gain during pregnancy with obesity in men at age 18 years. They found that among mothers with a normal BMI, there was no relationship between GWG and later obesity. However, among mothers who were already overweight or obese, GWG was associated with an increased risk for later obesity, even in the within-sibling analyses, suggesting an influence of the intrauterine environment (Lawlor et al. 2011a). Although Branum et al. (2011) found that women with higher prepregnancy BMI and gestational weight gain had children with a higher BMI at age 4, differences were no longer significant in the sibling fixed-effects analysis. The interaction between maternal prepregnancy BMI and GWG on childhood obesity risk is an area of active investigation (Institute of Medicine 2009).

4.5 Maternal Smoking During Pregnancy

In 2010, approximately 9% of US women smoked during pregnancy, with white mothers and mothers with lower education more likely to smoke during pregnancy (Hawkins and Baum 2014). Many short- and long-term health effects of smoking during pregnancy on mothers and infants are well known, including lower fetal growth (U.S. Department of Health and Human Services 2004). It may seem paradoxical then that numerous studies, as summarized in recent meta-analyses, have shown that prenatal smoking exposure is associated with an increased risk for later obesity, even in studies that adjusted for potential confounding factors (Oken et al. 2008; Weng et al. 2012). Although mechanisms for the relationship between maternal smoking during pregnancy and childhood obesity are not fully understood, animal studies have shown an association between prenatal nicotine exposure and increased adiposity in offspring (Gao et al. 2005).

However, the extent to which this association, seen mainly in observational studies, is causal remains uncertain, especially since smoking is so strongly socially patterned. Several approaches have been used to minimize confounding, including accounting for paternal smoking, a proxy for sociodemographic risk that is likely to provide little direct exposure to the fetus. One study with information on both maternal smoking during pregnancy and paternal smoking status postpartum found that the association remained after adjustment for sociodemographic characteristics and paternal smoking (von Kries et al. 2008), while in another study the association was no longer evident after adjustment (Fleten et al. 2012).

Others have used alternative study designs to test whether the association may be causal. Although RCTs have demonstrated that smoking cessation during pregnancy reduces rates of low birth weight and preterm birth (Lumley et al. 2009), none have examined later child obesity risk. Two studies have used sibling-pair designs to examine smoking during pregnancy (Gilman et al. 2008; Iliadou et al. 2010). Although both found a relationship between smoking and later obesity, the association was no longer evident after including the sibling fixed-effect. These results raise the possibility that the association may be confounded by unmeasured factors that are shared within families rather than being causal.

4.6 Hormonal Influences: Leptin

In 1973, Douglas L. Coleman published his seminal work in two papers, discussing an unknown circulating factor responsible for the obese/diabetic state in the *ob/ob* mouse, later called leptin (Grayson and Seeley 2012). Leptin is a hormone primarily produced by adipose tissue known to be responsible for the regulation of appetite, energy expenditure, and neuroendocrine function (Hauguel-de Mouzon et al. 2006). It is sometimes called the satiety hormone because of its effects on inducing a sense of fullness.

The developmental role of leptin in the perinatal period may differ from that later in the life course. The placenta releases leptin into maternal and fetal circulation, which may influence appetite and weight regulation. Maternal plasma leptin concentrations during gestation are two times higher than during non-gravid periods (Hauguel-de Mouzon et al. 2006). Fetuses born to obese mothers and mothers with GDM have higher cord leptin levels than fetuses of lean mothers or mothers without GDM, respectively (Catalano et al. 2009; Okereke et al. 2002). Umbilical cord leptin levels are positively associated with fetal fat mass, percent body fat, and birth weight (Okereke et al. 2002).

Sensitive period(s) may exist for the role of leptin in later obesity risk. A series of studies from Project Viva, a US pre-birth cohort, has examined relationships of leptin with early growth. Lower cord blood leptin levels were associated with smaller size at birth, but higher weight gain from birth to 6 months and higher BMI at age 3 years (Mantzoros et al. 2009; Parker et al. 2011). In a follow-up study, Boeke et al. (2013) found that lower leptin levels during pregnancy and in cord blood were associated with more adiposity at age 3 years; however, higher leptin levels at age 3 were associated with greater weight gain and higher adiposity through age 7. These findings were independent of maternal BMI and birth weight. The authors concluded there may be a sensitive period of leptin influence during the prenatal period followed by accumulation of leptin tolerance during early childhood, with different effects of leptin exposure by timing (Boeke et al. 2013). These observations are consistent with animal studies showing conditioning impact of heightened leptin sensitivity on later obesity, with differences evident across the life course (Bouret et al. 2004). There is great interest in identifying the correct sensitive period(s) for leptin to influence fetal development and reduce later obesity risk. To date, however, little is known about modifiable factors influencing fetal leptin regulation in humans (Boeke et al. 2013).

5 Infancy

5.1 Rapid Weight Gain

Infants grow in both length and weight, and weight changes include growth in both fat-free mass and fat mass. Many studies have used change in weight as a proxy for gain in adiposity, which may or may not be a valid assumption. There are many different definitions of rapid growth, which are often based on country- or population-specific references (Monteiro and Victora 2005).

Several meta-analyses have demonstrated that infants who gain weight more quickly than average during the first 2 years of life are at higher risk for later obesity (Baird et al. 2005; Monteiro and Victora 2005; Weng et al. 2012). Taveras and colleagues (2011c) examined the number of major weight-for-length percentiles crossed on the CDC 2000 growth chart during each of the 6-month periods from birth to 2 years with outcomes of obesity at ages 5 and 10 years. They found that crossing upward 2 or more percentiles in the first 2 years was associated with an increased risk for obesity at both ages. The highest prevalence of later obesity was seen in children with the crossing upward of 2 or more weight-for-length percentiles within the first 6 months of life (Taveras et al. 2011c).

Debate continues as to the exact time frame that rapid weight gain matters the most for later obesity risk. A major limitation of current research is the lack of repeated measurements at small intervals during infancy. Studies with repeat detailed measurements often include small, homogeneous samples of children, and thus their generalizability is limited. An important area of future research is to more precisely define the critical window for rapid gain in adiposity (or length) as well as modifiable determinants of rapid weight gain.

Although based on the research we summarize here a potential conclusion might be to limit rapid weight gain in infants to prevent later obesity, an important consideration is the potential detrimental effects of restricting weight gain for other organ systems. For infants born preterm, more rapid postnatal weight gain has an important benefit for neurodevelopment and attained size (Ehrenkranz et al. 2006) Although no association was seen between slower infant weight gain and poorer neurodevelopmental outcomes in a study of healthy, term infants (Belfort et al. 2008), this area requires more study to help determine optimal length and BMI patterns to promote healthy neurodevelopment as well as reduce childhood obesity.

One important modifiable determinant of the rate of infant weight gain is infant feeding, both the type and the approach. Although exclusively breastfed infants gain weight more rapidly in the early postnatal period, infants who are formula fed or fed a combination of breast milk and formula gain BMI more rapidly during the latter half of the first year of life (Kramer et al. 2004). In an Australian RCT promoting positive feeding practices, Mihrshahi et al. (2011) found that formula feeding and feeding on a schedule were independently associated with rapid weight gain between birth and age 4–7 months. Although the association between breastfeeding and childhood obesity is discussed in the next section, infant gain in length or adiposity and nutrition are closely linked and, in fact, may be challenging to tease apart.

5.2 Breastfeeding

Despite the numerous demonstrated health benefits of breastfeeding (Section on Breastfeeding 2012), according to the CDC's 2014 Breastfeeding Report Card, only 79% of US mothers initiated breastfeeding and only 49% breastfed for at least 6 months (Centers for Disease Control and Prevention 2014). Moreover, racial/ethnic disparities in breastfeeding are substantial. Using national data from 2004 to 2008, there was a 20% point differential between black and white mothers for both breastfeeding initiation (54% versus 74%) and breastfeeding for at least 6 months (27% versus 43%) (Centers for Disease Control and Prevention 2010).

Systematic reviews and meta-analyses of observational studies have demonstrated an inverse association of breastfeeding initiation or duration with later obesity (Arenz et al. 2004; Harder et al. 2005; Owen et al. 2005b). Two reviews found that an inverse relationship still remained after adjusting for confounding factors, such as parental obesity or social class (Arenz et al. 2004; Owen et al. 2005b). However, a third showed attenuation of the association with BMI to null after such adjustment (Owen et al. 2005a). There was also evidence for a dose-response relationship, such that a longer duration of breastfeeding conferred a greater reduction in obesity risk (Harder et al. 2005; Owen et al. 2005b). As the majority of study samples were often homogeneous with children of mostly white European descent, there is debate about the extent to which these relationships apply to all racial/ethnic groups (Gillman 2011; Harder et al. 2005).

Plausible mechanisms abound for the relationship between breastfeeding and childhood obesity (Bartok and Ventura 2009). Breastfed infants may be better at self-regulation than bottle-fed infants because they come off the breast when they are full, which may help them learn to regulate energy intake (Li et al. 2010). Breast milk contains hormones, such as leptin, involved in regulating growth and development during infancy (Savino and Liguori 2008). After the first 3 months of life, breastfed infants have slower weight gain for the remainder of the year than formula-fed infants (Savino and Liguori 2008).

Nevertheless, evidence is mounting to question the extent to which this relationship is causal (Gillman 2011). The majority of research has been based on observational studies, and associations may still be due to unmeasured factors. The few studies using a sibling-pair design showed that breastfeeding duration reduced risk for later obesity, but because mothers often breastfeed similarly across siblings, there are a limited number of discordant pairs to detect effects (Gillman et al. 2006; Metzger and McDade 2010; Nelson et al.

2005; O'Tierney et al. 2009). Furthermore, these designs may not eliminate the role of infant growth and behavior as a predictor—rather than result—of breastfeeding intensity and duration.

Another methodological design to infer causality is to examine the association in a context with different social gradients for both the exposure and outcome measures (Brion 2010; Gillman 2011). Brion et al. (2011) compared the association between breastfeeding duration and BMI from two cohorts—in England where breastfeeding is associated with more advantaged social circumstances and in Brazil where there is little social patterning. There was an inverse association between breastfeeding duration and obesity risk for children in England, but no such association for children in Brazil, from which the authors concluded the effects are likely due to residual confounding (Brion et al. 2011). Similarly, a study in Hong Kong also found no association between breastfeeding and childhood obesity, where breastfeeding and obesity follow different social patterns (Kwok et al. 2010).

The Promotion of Breastfeeding Intervention Trial (PROBIT) in Belarus is a cluster-randomized trial of breastfeeding promotion (Kramer et al. 2001). Mothers who started breastfeeding were randomly assigned to an intervention group that provided additional breastfeeding support or a standard care control group. Although mothers in the breastfeeding promotion group showed increases in duration and exclusivity of breastfeeding, there was no evidence for a protective effect of breastfeeding on skinfold thickness or obesity in children at age 6.5 or 11 years (Kramer et al. 2007; Martin et al. 2013). Based on the existing evidence, breastfeeding may only confer modest protection against obesity rather than being a major determinant (Gillman 2011).

5.3 Disparities in Obesity Partially Explained by Early-Life Factors

Beyond breastfeeding, many other early-life obesogenic exposures may be socially patterned (Dixon et al. 2012). Several investigators have attempted to investigate whether observed racial/ethnic disparities in obesity rates (Ogden et al. 2014) are related to early-life factors. Taveras and colleagues (2010) have shown that compared to white children, black and Hispanic children were more likely to have risk factors for childhood obesity including excessive weight gain during infancy and early introduction of solid foods, while after 2 years, they were more likely to have a television in their bedrooms, shorter sleep duration, and higher intake of sugar-sweetened beverages and fast food (Taveras et al. 2010). In contrast, they were less likely to be exposed to factors associated with protection against obesity, including exclusive breastfeeding (Taveras et al. 2010). The same investigators more recently examined whether racial/ethnic differences in childhood obesity at age 7 were explained by these early risk factors (Taveras et al. 2013). Although black and Hispanic children had higher BMI z-scores than white children, there were no longer differences in BMI after adjustment for infancy- and childhood-related risk factors. The authors conclude that racial/ethnic disparities in obesity may be determined by modifiable factors in early life (Taveras et al. 2013).

6 Early to Mid-childhood

6.1 Family

Although family members have similar levels of adiposity, meaning that children are more likely to have a high BMI if their parents have a high BMI (Patel et al. 2011), the influence of parents on child adiposity almost certainly extends beyond shared genes. Parents (including caregivers) also share a similar family, neighborhood, and social environment. During the early years, parents are the primary influence on children's dietary and physical activity/inactivity choices. Parents not only physically provide children with food and opportunities for physical activity, but they also influence children's preferences through modeling or other experiences (Birch and Davison 2001; Van Der Horst et al. 2007). In the next two sections on early childhood to mid-childhood and adolescence, we focus on "above-water" macro-level factors where there is potential for population-level interventions and public health impact.

6.2 Diet, Physical Activity, and Inactivity

In the simplest terms, excessive weight gain occurs when there is more "energy in" than "energy out." The dietary and physical activity patterns of children and adolescents in the USA have changed substantially over the last few decades. Total energy intake and portion sizes from energy-dense, nutrient-poor foods have increased, and more meals are being eaten away from home (Duffey and Popkin 2013; Piernas and Popkin 2011). Among school-aged children, daily calories from sugar-sweetened beverages have increased from 130 to 212 kcal/day over the last 20 years (Lasater et al. 2011). Although children and adolescents are recommended to participate in 60 min or more of physical activity daily (U.S. Department of Health and Human Services 2008), many children are not achieving this goal. In 2013, nationwide, 15% of students did not engage in at least 60 min of physical activity on any of the prior 7 days (Kann et al. 2014). As children transition from childhood through adolescence, physical activity levels decrease (Kahn et al. 2008), and media exposure and sedentary behaviors increase (Kann et al. 2014; Rideout and Hamel 2006). In recent decades, screen time and media use have increased. Currently, 41% of students play video or computer games 3 or more hours per day, and an additional 33% watch television 3 or more hours per day (Kann et al. 2014). Even by age 1, children are using approximately 50 min of screen media daily, which increases to nearly 2 hours by age 4–6 years (Rideout and Hamel 2006).

As media use has increased, so has children's exposure to advertisements and food marketing. Food advertising has been linked to influencing children's food preferences, purchasing requests, and consumption patterns (McGinnis et al. 2006), suggesting a potential mechanism by which television and media use may increase children's risk for obesity. US guidelines for the responsible advertising to children are voluntary self-regulatory initiatives, and the Rudd Center for Food Policy and Obesity (2013) suggested that loopholes in industry pledges may provide for more public relations benefits than health benefits.

6.3 Food Insecurity

In 2013, 14% of US households with children were food insecure at least once during the year, meaning they were unable to provide adequate food for one or more household members due to insufficient means (Coleman-Jensen et al. 2014). Black and Hispanic households, low-income households, and single-parent households with children had rates of food insecurity higher than the national average (Coleman-Jensen et al. 2014). Since children from lower-income families are at higher risk for obesity, the challenge for many families is to dependably provide nutritious and high-quality food rather than obtaining enough food (Ludwig et al. 2012). The Supplemental Nutrition Assistance Program (SNAP) has no regulations on the quality of foods purchased (US Department of Agriculture, 2013b), and families may be spending their limited food budget on foods that are high in calories but with low nutrient quality such as sugar-sweetened beverages.

Three systematic reviews found that although food insecurity was associated with an increased risk for obesity in adults, particularly women, the evidence was mixed for children (Dinour et al. 2007; Eisenmann et al. 2011; Franklin et al. 2012). A challenge for studies is identifying whether the measure of food insecurity is at the family or child level as parents may protect children from being food insecure. Echoing the conclusion from a review by Eisenmann et al. (2011), even if the association is not causal, both food insecurity and obesity exist in low-income households. It is essential, therefore, to learn more about purchasing patterns, diet, and physical activity in these families to learn why food insecurity and obesity coexist and identify areas for intervention.

6.4 Child Care and School

Policies and programs in child care and school can influence children's dietary intake, physical activity patterns, and risk for obesity. Approximately 30% of children are in center-based programs by age 2 and 40% of children by age 3, spending nearly 30 hours in nonparental care each week (National Center for Education Statistics 2005). Thus, child care is a setting in which obesogenic behaviors can be allowed or prevented (Larson et al. 2011a). A review by Larson and colleagues (2011b) identified 18 obesity prevention interventions that take place in child care centers/preschools and 2 of the 5 interventions that used weight status as an outcome found evidence for reduced weight.

In 2007, Benjamin et al. (2008) reviewed state child care regulations for policies related to nutrition and physical activity that may contribute to childhood obesity. They found that 80% of states had regulations to ensure that water is freely available in child care centers, 33% regulated screen time, 18% had regulations for the provision of breast milk, 14% restricted sugar-sweetened beverages, and only three states required a specified number of minutes of physical activity. Four states had no policies related to obesogenic practices in child care. The proportion of states with these regulations for family child care homes—as opposed to centers—was either the same or less. As of 2013, up to one quarter of states did not comply with any of the five recommendations from the IOM to promote physical activity among infants in child care centers or family child care homes (Slining et al. 2014). Benjamin et al. (2009) showed that infants who attended home-based child care early in life had an increased weight for length at 1 year and BMI at 3 years, suggesting that more research is needed into the food and physical activity policies of family child care homes. Additional studies in Denmark (Neelon et al. 2015) and Finland (Lehto et al. 2015) have demonstrated an association between starting child care before age 1 and an increased risk for later obesity. In 2011, the White House Task Force on Childhood Obesity supported the development of new national standards for healthy eating, encouraging breastfeeding, promoting physical activity, and limiting screen time in early-care settings (American Academy of Pediatrics, American Public Health Association, and National Resource Center for Health and Safety in Child Care and Early Education 2012).

Since children spend most of their time in school and may eat two daily meals there, the school environment can play an important role in shaping health behaviors (Institute of Medicine 2007; Story et al. 2009). A systematic review and meta-analysis by Waters et al. (2011) identified 55 interventions for preventing obesity in children aged 0–18 years, with 5 of the 6 most promising strategies related to the school environment: school curricula that include healthy eating and physical activity, increases in opportunities for physical activity throughout the school week, improvements in the nutritional quality of the food served in schools, environments and cultural practices that support children eating healthier foods and being active throughout the day, and support for teachers and staff to implement health promotion strategies and activities. They also concluded that interventions did not increase disparities. There have been a number of reviews that examined the impact of school-based interventions overall or school food and physical activity, separately, on obesity risk (Gonzalez-Suarez et al. 2009; Katz et al. 2008; Kropski et al. 2008).

Food and beverages available in schools are either part of the federal school lunch and breakfast programs or are competitive foods sold outside the federal programs. Meals served in the National School Lunch Program and School Breakfast Program must adhere to federally defined nutrition standards in order for schools to be eligible for federal subsidies (Institute of Medicine 2007). In 2013, the US Department of Agriculture issued the new "Smart Snacks in Schools" nutrition standards for competitive foods and beverages, which limit calories, fat, sugar, and sodium (U.S. Department of Agriculture 2013a). A study by Masse et al. (2013) found that between 2003 and 2008, states significantly strengthened their school nutrition-related laws, particularly those related to the sale of competitive foods. Overall, laws for competitive food policies were stronger for elementary schools than for middle and high schools. As of 2008, 7 states had no school nutrition laws across the 16 categories they examined (Masse et al. 2013).

The National Association for Sport and Physical Education (NASPE) sets standards for physical education, including time allotment, curriculum, and staffing (National Association for Sport and Physical Education 2004). Perna et al. (2012) found that public schools in states with specific and stringent physical education laws reported more weekly time for physical education: specifically, elementary schools reported 40 more minutes and middle schools reported 60 more minutes than schools within states with no laws. There were no differences between high schools. However, overall, only 8.5% of schools fully met the NASPE guidelines for physical education time (Perna et al. 2012). Without federal legislation for physical education, policies vary widely by state and even by schools themselves.

7 Adolescence

7.1 Social Influences

Adolescence is a developmental period characterized by hormonal changes and a period of rapid growth both physically and psychologically (Viner et al. 2012). As children become more independent, their sphere of influence moves from parents to peers with increasing autonomy in making choices. Although influences of dietary and physical activity habits on obesity risk are similar to those described during the early- to mid-childhood periods, these habits are often influenced by peer norms. Strong peer relationships are an important developmental change during adolescence, and peer groups can influence health behaviors both positively and negatively (Viner et al. 2012).

Using social network theory and analysis, Christakis and colleagues (2007) found that weight gain in one person spread through social ties and influenced risk of obesity in a friend, sibling, or spouse among adults in the Framingham Study. Trogdon et al. (2008) used the National Longitudinal Study of Adolescent Health (Add Health) to examine the influence of peer effects on adolescents' own BMI by constructing a detailed definition of peer groups based on nominated friendship relationships. They found that mean peer BMI was associated with adolescent BMI, females were more sensitive to peer BMI and overweight status than males, and peer weight was more influential among adolescents with the highest BMI (Trogdon et al. 2008).

Ali et al. (2011) also used data from the Add Health study to understand potential mechanisms of peer effects on obesity-related health behaviors. They found evidence for the influence of peers on adolescents pursuing an active sport, regular exercise, and eating in fast-food restaurants, but no consistent relationships with television viewing, short sleep duration, or other dietary factors (Ali et al. 2011). Although additional research is needed to confirm these findings, the potential implications are that obesity prevention programs aimed at adolescents will need to consider the influence of peer groups.

8 Macro-level Factors

Although we have touched upon policies and social issues that have their strongest influence in particular age groups, this section presents macro-level factors that either indirectly or directly influence obesity risk across all stages in life course health development.

8.1 Environment

The term "obesogenic environment" often refers to features of the built and natural environments that limit healthful behaviors related to eating, sleeping, screen time, and physical activity. The definition used to study the built environment varies widely across studies (Dunton et al. 2009; Lovasi et al. 2009; Papas et al. 2007). The most common measures of access to food are distances to the nearest fast-food restaurants or grocery stores or density of food outlets within a defined area. The most common measures of access to physical activity resources are measured distance to facilities for physical activity such as parks, density of such facilities, walkability, or aspects of community design. Related measures included assessments of aesthetics or neighborhood safety. Papas et al. (2007) found that 17 of the 20 studies identified found a significant association between some aspect of the built environment and risk for obesity across the life course, with the majority of studies looking at features of the environment related to physical activity. Dunton et al. (2009) examined aspects of the built environment related to physical activity and childhood obesity. While they found few consistent findings in children, in adolescents obesity was associated with access to equipment and facilities, neighborhood type (urban/rural), and urban sprawl. Lovasi et al. (2009) examined how the built environment may be contributing to disparities in obesity and its risk factors. They focused on studies that included individuals who were poor or of low socioeconomic status, black, or Hispanic. The authors found that lack of access to supermarkets, exercise facilities or places to be active, and safety because of crime or traffic was all associated with BMI or related behaviors, and they concluded that prevention strategies should focus on these areas (Lovasi et al. 2009).

There are many methodological challenges to understanding the effects of the neighborhood environment on children because of the diversity of populations, measures, and outcomes across studies (Dunton et al. 2009; Lovasi et al. 2009; Papas et al. 2007). A further limitation is that nearly all of the studies have been cross-sectional, so the temporality of associations is not clear. Effects of the built environment on health vary across the life course because exposure to and interaction with the environment change by age. For example, distance to playgrounds matters more for children than adolescents, whereas walkability may have less impact on young children. While subjective measures of the built environment are often from parents or children themselves, more studies are using objective measures of the environment, such as geographic information system (GIS) mapping or even personal devices to determine time, place, and activity simultaneously. The most important aspect is the definition of the built environment. Studies that examine the same construct, such as walkability, may be using different definitions and measurements, which limit the ability to synthesize the evidence. As Dunton et al. (2009) conclude, it is imperative to identify "modifiable and specific" features of the built environment to inform the development of interventions.

Neighborhoods vary in many ways, most of which are unmeasured but likely interrelated; observed associations that remain after adjustment are still subject to residual confounding. RCTs, which balance both measured and unmeasured confounders, are uncommon in this area primarily due to the feasibility of manipulating aspects of the built environment. The Department of Housing and Urban Development conducted a unique social experiment from 1994 through 1998 to better understand the effects of neighborhood characteristics on health and social outcomes (Sanbonmatsu et al. 2011). Women with children living in public housing in high-poverty areas were randomly assigned to one of three groups: experimental housing vouchers redeemable only if they moved to a low-poverty area, unrestricted traditional vouchers, and a control group that offered neither opportunity (Ludwig et al. 2011). Ludwig et al. (2011) followed up the participants from 2008 to 2010 and found that women assigned to the experimental group had lower levels of extreme obesity and diabetes than women in the control group, although there were no baseline measures of these outcomes. However, among youth, there were no differences in physical health outcomes, including obesity (Sanbonmatsu et al. 2011). The authors concluded that although the mechanisms for these reductions were unknown, the intervention provides some causal evidence for the impact of the neighborhood environment on health (Ludwig et al. 2011).

A methodology for future research in this area is quasi-experimental designs that evaluate a clearly defined change—often a wide-ranging policy—that are referred to as natural experiments. Taking measurements of residents before and after this change, or using secondary measures such as data from electronic medical records, especially in comparison with an unexposed control group, can help assess the impact of neighborhood factors on obesity itself or related health behaviors. Such alternative study designs are needed to identify important levers of change to help inform the development of interventions conducted at the neighborhood or community levels.

8.2 Local and State

In recent years, city and state governments have taken bold actions to change the environment and encourage healthy choices. New York City (NYC) has been a pioneer in this effort by using a multiagency approach to tackle obesity and its risk factors (Mello 2009). In 2006, NYC passed the first regulation in the USA banning trans fat use in restaurants. An evaluation comparing food purchase data before and after the ban found a significant decrease in the trans fat content of purchases from fast-food chains after the law, with benefits for patrons from both high- and low-poverty neighborhoods (Angell et al. 2012). In 2008, NYC required chain restaurants to post calorie information prominently on menu boards and menus. Although children and adolescents' reported they noticed the posted information, there were no differences in calories purchased after versus before the introduction of calorie postings (Elbel et al. 2011). NYC initiatives have also extended to schools and the built environment (Office of the Mayor 2012). NYC established nutritional standards for every city agency that purchases or serves meals to clients, including the 1.1 million students that attend city schools, as well as standards for city vending machines. The most controversial proposal was to limit the size of sugar-sweetened beverages sold in food service establishments to 16 ounces, which caused much debate both for and against this measure and was ultimately blocked (Grynbaum 2012).

Although these policies in NYC provide assessable natural experiments to allow for evaluation of specific environmental factors that might promote weight gain (or loss), a challenge is learning what may be the critical lever(s) for change. When policies and programs are implemented simultaneously or within short time periods, it may not be possible to tease apart the individual effects of each policy. Furthermore, these efforts may not be generalizable; budgets are often limited, and other cities or states may not have the resources to implement the whole suite of policies that have been enacted in NYC. Nevertheless, these efforts provide valuable data to clinicians and policy makers to help elucidate what policies or programs will have the biggest effect on obesity levels.

A relatively new area is using legislation to financially penalize the purchase and consumption of obesogenic foods and beverages. One approach draws from the lessons of tobacco control and the success of cigarette taxes. Taxes on sugar-sweetened beverages are a prime example, although taxes have also been proposed to reduce the consumption of fast food (Powell et al. 2013). The consumption of sugar-sweetened beverages is strongly related to increased body weight (Te Morenga et al. 2012). As of January 2014, 34 states and DC had a sales tax on regular soda sold in food stores, with a mean tax rate of 5.2% (Chriqui et al. 2014). A systematic review by Powell et al. (2013) found that soda taxes had little impact on weight outcomes, but the authors argued that they were based on state-level sales taxes that were relatively low and therefore unlikely to effect substantial change in behavior.

Brownell et al. (2009) have proposed a national excise tax on sugar-sweetened beverages as a public health strategy to address the obesity epidemic. They recommended implementing an excise tax of 1 cent per ounce for beverages that have any added caloric sweetener, which would increase the cost of a 20-ounce soda by 15–20% (Brownell et al. 2009). This type of tax, which is similar to cigarette excise taxes, is preferable to a sales tax because it provides an incentive to reduce the amount of sugar per ounce of sugar-sweetened beverage (Brownell et al. 2009). Since the cost would be passed onto retailers, they would likely increase the retail price, and consumers would be aware of the cost when they are deciding to purchase the product. Andreyeva et al. (2011) estimated that a 1 cent per ounce tax on sugar-sweetened beverages could reduce consumption by 24% and daily per capita caloric intake from sugar-sweetened beverages from current levels of 190–200 calories to 145–150 calories. Brownell et al. (2009) suggest that the public health impact could be greater for groups at higher risk for obesity, such as children and low-income groups, who consume greater amounts of sugar-sweetened beverages.

An alternative approach to promoting a healthful diet is a subsidy to reduce price and encourage the consumption of healthful foods. Unfortunately, in recent decades, just the opposite situation has occurred. The real inflation-adjusted price of fruits and vegetables has increased, while soda prices have declined and fast-food prices have remained stable (Powell et al. 2013). In the USA, subsidies on food have been designed to alleviate food insecurity for low-income families rather than increasing consumption of healthful foods by everyone. Powell et al. (2013) found that lower fruit and vegetable prices were associated with lower body weight among low-income populations; however, cohort studies are mixed when it comes to the effects of fruits and vegetables on weight gain (Casazza et al. 2013). Based on the long history of tobacco control, the area of taxes and subsidies related to obesity is still in its infancy.

8.3 National

Reducing and preventing obesity is a federal priority. At a national level, the White House Task Force on Childhood Obesity and the accompanying *Let's Move!* campaign aim to reduce childhood obesity and raise a healthier generation through an intra-agency collaboration (White House Task Force on Childhood Obesity 2010). The 70 recommendations were summarized into five themes: getting children a healthy start on life; empowering parents and caregivers; providing healthy foods in schools; improving access to healthy, affordable food; and getting children more physically active. The strategy emphasized that changes are needed at many macro levels to promote healthy behaviors, including improvements to schools and the built environment. The White House Task Force reported some progress on many of these areas after just 1 year (White House Task Force on Childhood Obesity 2011). The IOM's Standing Committee on Childhood Obesity Prevention (Institute of Medicine 2011) and the US Department of Health and Human Services' National Prevention Strategy (National Prevention Council 2011) echo these priorities.

9 Recommendations

9.1 Major Themes

A multilevel approach for obesity prevention is needed, which takes into account individual risk factors that operate at multiple levels ("above-water" and "underwater" influences) and recognizes that these factors also interact across the life course (Fig. 1). We reviewed phases of life course health development, prenatal through adolescence, that appear to be most important for the development of obesity. We also presented alternative methodological approaches to observational studies that can help disentangle causal associations. The following sections outline research priorities and data/methods development priorities, and conclude with recommendations for practice and policy.

9.2 Research Priorities

Of the many emerging risk factors for obesity, we briefly highlight sleep duration, endocrine-disrupting chemicals, epigenetic markers, and microbial colonization.

- Sleep duration and quality: Disruption of sleep may have adverse health consequences, including childhood obesity. Biologically plausible mechanisms exist for why short sleep duration could increase children's risk for obesity: tiredness and fatigue lead to reduced physical activity; hormone changes associated with insufficient sleep, particularly lower leptin levels and higher ghrelin levels, result in increased hunger and eating; and with less sleep, there is more awake time to eat (Taheri 2006). Although most of the studies in this area have been cross-sectional, prospective cohort studies do provide some evidence for causality. Chen et al. (2008) identified 17 studies from 1980 to 2007 on sleep duration and adiposity in children, of which 3 were prospective cohort studies. Nielsen et al. (2011) reviewed the literature from 2007 to 2009 and identified an additional 13 studies in children. Of the eight prospective cohort studies, all found a significant inverse relationship between duration of sleep and adiposity (Nielsen et al. 2011). Recent studies from Project Viva have shown that chronic sleep curtailment from infancy was associated with an increase in adiposity and metabolic risk at age 7 (Cespedes et al. 2014; Taveras et al. 2014).

- Early relational environment: Two aspects of children's early relational environment—the quality of parental relationships and children's exposure to adverse experiences—have been identified as potential risk factors for child and adolescent obesity. The psychological and physiological consequences of insecure attachments and trauma are well established, including poor emotional regulation and heightened stress responses, which may directly lead to obesity through biological changes (Glaser and Kiecolt-Glaser 2005) or indirectly through emotional eating (Michopoulos et al. 2015; Torres and Nowson 2007) and sleep disturbances (Vgontzas et al. 2008). Studies in children and adolescents have found that those with poor-quality maternal-child relationships (Anderson et al. 2012) or insecure attachment (Anderson and Whitaker 2011) in early childhood were more likely to be obese compared to those with higher-quality relationships. Danese and Tan (2014) conducted a meta-analysis of 41 studies and found that childhood maltreatment was associated with an increased risk of obesity across the life course with an overall pooled odds ratio of 1.36 and associations remained after adjustment for socioeconomic status and health behaviors. An additional meta-analysis of 23 cohort studies found that adults who reported physical, emotional, sexual, or general abuse during childhood were more likely to be obese (pooled odds ratios of 1.28–1.45) and four studies reported dose-response relationships (Hemmingsson et al. 2014). While this evidence suggests a role of children's early relational environment in the development of obesity, further research is needed to better understand the mechanisms to help inform interventions.
- Endocrine-disrupting chemicals (EDCs): EDCs are compounds that mimic or interfere with the normal actions of endocrine hormones, including estrogens, androgens, and thyroid and pituitary hormones (Newbold et al. 2007). Although some EDCs are naturally occurring, man-made organic compounds pose greater risks to human health and include flame retardants, bisphenol A (BPA), pesticides, and polychlorinated biphenyls (PCBs). EDCs that are lipophilic, resistant to metabolism, and/or able to bioconcentrate up the food chain become stored in body fats and are of particular concern (Elobeid and Allison 2008). Thus, in utero exposure to environmental chemicals, including EDCs, during critical periods may play a role in the development of obesity through fetal programming (Newbold et al. 2007). Only recently has evidence been synthesized from animal models and epidemiologic studies in humans to suggest a possible link between EDCs and later obesity (Elobeid and Allison 2008). Trasande et al. (2012) found that urinary BPA concentrations were associated with obesity in children and adolescents, although alternative explanations cannot be ruled out because the study was cross-sectional.
- Epigenetics: The notion that early environmental influences, such as maternal diet, or toxic substances, like air pollution, alter offspring outcomes through epigenetic changes that influence gene regulation could unite several strands of human and animal observations about the origins of obesity. Proof of principle emanates from agouti mice (Waterland and Jirtle 2004). The epigenetic mechanism associated with dif-

ferences in body fat and cardiometabolic disease risk of the offspring involves switching off the agouti gene by methyl groups from a dietary supplement (Waterland and Jirtle 2004). These and similar findings show, in principle, how genetically identical individuals raised in similar postnatal environments can nonetheless develop widely differing phenotypes.

- Gut microbiota: Infants get their first priming dose of microbes in utero via the placenta, followed by a more thorough colonization as they pass through the birth canal and are exposed to the mother's skin, so that by the time they are a few days or weeks old, their gastrointestinal tracts are colonized by a population of microbes notable not only for their abundance but also variety. Gut microbiota are likely to affect many organs and systems, including the regulation of energy balance and weight gain. Although research on animal models suggests a role of gut microbiota in the development of obesity, studies in humans are limited (DiBaise et al. 2008). One model system for evaluating the role of gut microbiota is the route of delivery. Microbes from the mother and the environment colonize the infant's intestinal tract during delivery (Neu and Rushing 2011). During cesarean delivery, the direct contact with maternal vaginal and intestinal flora is absent. The intestinal microbial composition of infants via cesarean delivery resembles that of the mother's skin, whereas the intestinal flora of infants born vaginally resembles the mother's vaginal flora and intestinal tract (Dominguez-Bello et al. 2010). A systematic review by Li et al. (2013) found that delivery by cesarean section was associated with an increased risk for overweight/obesity across the life course compared to vaginal delivery, with an overall pooled odds ratio of 1.33.

9.3 Data/Methods Development Priorities

There are a number of major challenges to understanding causal influences on obesity risk throughout the life course. Here, we discuss some of these challenges as well as approaches to overcoming or minimizing them.

- One recurrent issue is the extent to which associations described in observational studies are causal. One notable example is breastfeeding (Gillman 2011). Mothers who choose to breastfeed often have substantially different social and economic circumstances from mothers who do not breastfeed their infants. Furthermore, factors that predict successful initiation and long-term maintenance of breastfeeding, such as maternal obesity and cesarean delivery, are themselves putative causes of child obesity. Also, it is possible that infant characteristics themselves predict breastfeeding duration, since mothers may be more likely to supplement faster growing infants, who appear hungrier.
- In cross-sectional studies, both confounding and reverse causation are important considerations. Longitudinal cohort studies with adjustment for multiple measured characteristics can go part of the way in minimizing confounding, but other approaches such as sibling-pair design, maternal versus paternal effects, cohorts with different confounding structures, and RCTs can help control for unmeasured confounding. Others have applied Mendelian randomization, a method that takes advantage of variation in genes of known function to examine the causal effect of a modifiable exposure on disease in nonexperimental studies (Smith and Ebrahim 2003). The genotype must affect the disease status only via its effect on the exposure of interest and should be randomly distributed with respect to other covariates (Ding and Hu 2008). This approach can produce unbiased estimates of the effects of a putative causal variable without a traditional RCT. One example is the study of the maternal and offspring FTO genotype and offspring obesity risk, which suggests that maternal obesity affects childhood obesity only through pathways other than the intrauterine environment (Lawlor et al. 2008). However, many times these approaches are not feasible. For example, data may not be readily available on

large numbers of siblings with discordant exposures; RCTs are costly and may not be ethical; and the few common genes that influence obesity risk do not have strong associations and also may influence multiple metabolic pathways.

- Another challenge is that of appropriate exposure assessment, which is relevant for multiple factors of great interest including diet, physical activity, and the toxic, built, and social environments. Multiple factors may interact among each other. For example, breastfeeding may particularly affect childhood obesity risk only in the presence of an obesogenic environment, whereas two important null studies of breastfeeding and obesity (Brion et al. 2011; Kramer et al. 2007; Martin et al. 2013) were both conducted in middle-income countries with relatively low population obesity rates (Belarus and Brazil).
- Current statistical techniques typically cannot take into account the multitude of factors both hierarchically and across the life course that impact obesity. Traditional longitudinal analyses, even those that account for multiple levels of influence, are often not powerful enough to account for the complexity and interconnectedness of obesity. Systems science approaches such as agent-based and system dynamics modeling can include not only longitudinal and multiple levels but also more complex features of relationships like nonlinearity, path dependence, loops, and tipping (Hammond 2009; Huang et al. 2009). These approaches have just recently been imported into public health from disciplines such as engineering (Mani et al. 2010) and evolutionary biology (Kitano 2002) and may very well contribute to understanding and ultimately solving childhood obesity.

9.4 Translational Priorities

The key to reducing childhood obesity is finding the right level and time in the life course to intervene for the maximal effectiveness and efficiency. Many intervention studies early in the life course are getting underway or are ongoing, and will be invaluable in informing not only what factors to change but how to change them. Such interventions may be complex and costly, but ultimately may be what is required to reverse the tide of obesity.

- Interventions to modify determinants of obesity through life course health development may invoke multiple settings, e.g., medical care, homes, child care, and school (Foster et al. 2010; Taveras et al. 2011a, b, 2012); involve multiple components, e.g., system redesign and individual behavior change strategies including e-technology (Lubans et al. 2010; Taveras et al. 2012); and target single or multiple factors (Dodd et al. 2011; Taveras et al. 2011b; Vesco et al. 2012). Interventions within medical care may be especially valuable during pregnancy and infancy, when individuals see their providers more often than any other time during the life course.
- Some recommendations are already clear. For prenatal factors, smoking avoidance has been a priority for decades (U.S. Department of Health and Human Services 2004). Guidelines exist for appropriate GWG (Institute of Medicine 2009). For mild-moderate GDM, treatment with lifestyle and insulin reduces neonatal complications (Crowther et al. 2005; Landon et al. 2009); the protocol and criteria for diagnosing GDM are undergoing new scrutiny.
- Among early childhood factors, "feeding up" small-for-gestational age infants should be abandoned for most because such infants who gain weight rapidly in infancy are at higher risk of chronic disease and derive no neurocognitive benefits (Belfort and Gillman 2011). The World Health Organization recommends exclusive breastfeeding for 6 months, but in the developed world, recommendations are moving toward 4–6 months (Section on Breastfeeding 2012); that interval appears to be appropriate for introducing solid foods for obesity prevention (Huh et al. 2011; Pearce et al. 2013).
- Among dietary factors, evidence is strongest for intake of sugary beverages at many ages. Avoiding introducing these into infant diets may be especially valuable, given most

humans'—especially children's—inherent "sweet tooth" (Ventura and Mennella 2011).

- The American Academy of Pediatrics recommends zero screen time under age 2 years and no more than 2 hours/day of screen time for child age 2 years and older (Strasburger 2011). Avoiding from the outset having a TV in the room where a child sleeps appears to be key to reducing screen time (Schmidt et al. 2012).
- Among the newer risk factors, improving sleep duration and quality may be an especially effective maneuver—and preliminary studies suggest it is feasible (Taveras et al. 2011a)—because all parents want more sleep!

Funding Funded by grants from NIH R00 HD068506 to Dr. Hawkins, K24 HD069408 and P30 DK092924 to Dr. Oken, and K24 HL060841 to Dr. Gillman. The content is solely the responsibility of the authors and does not necessarily represent the official views of the National Institutes of Health.

References

Agha, M., Agha, R. A., & Sandell, J. (2014). Interventions to reduce and prevent obesity in pre-conceptual and pregnant women: A systematic review and meta-analysis. *PloS One, 9*(5), e95132.

Alfaradhi, M. Z., & Ozanne, S. E. (2011). Developmental programming in response to maternal overnutrition. *Frontiers in Genetics, 2*, 27.

Ali, M. M., Amialchuk, A., & Heiland, F. W. (2011). Weight-related behavior among adolescents: The role of peer effects. *PloS One, 6*(6), e21179.

American Academy of Pediatrics, American Public Health Association, and National Resource Center for Health and Safety in Child Care and Early Education. (2012). *Preventing childhood obesity in early care and education: Selected standards from caring for our children; National health and safety performance standards; Guidelines for early care and education programs, 3rd edition.* http://nrckids.org/CFOC3/PDFVersion/preventing_obesity.pdf. Accessed 8 Feb 2013.

Anderson, S. E., Gooze, R. A., Lemeshow, S., & Whitaker, R. C. (2012). Quality of early maternal–child relationship and risk of adolescent obesity. *Pediatrics, 129*(1), 132–140.

Anderson, S. E., & Whitaker, R. C. (2011). Attachment security and obesity in US preschool-aged children. *Archives of Pediatrics & Adolescent Medicine, 165*(3), 235–242.

Andreyeva, T., Chaloupka, F. J., & Brownell, K. D. (2011). Estimating the potential of taxes on sugar-sweetened beverages to reduce consumption and generate revenue. *Preventive Medicine, 52*(6), 413–416.

Angell, S. Y., Cobb, L. K., Curtis, C. J., Konty, K. J., & Silver, L. D. (2012). Change in trans fatty acid content of fast-food purchases associated with New York City's restaurant regulation: A pre-post study. *Annals of Internal Medicine, 157*(2), 81–86.

Arenz, S., Ruckerl, R., Koletzko, B., & von Kries, R. (2004). Breast-feeding and childhood obesity–a systematic review. *International Journal of Obesity and Related Metabolic Disorders, 28*(10), 1247–1256.

Baird, J., Fisher, D., Lucas, P., Kleijnen, J., Roberts, H., & Law, C. (2005). Being big or growing fast: Systematic review of size and growth in infancy and later obesity. *BMJ, 331*(7522), 929.

Bartok, C. J., & Ventura, A. K. (2009). Mechanisms underlying the association between breastfeeding and obesity. *International Journal of Pediatric Obesity, 4*(4), 196–204.

Battista, M. C., Hivert, M. F., Duval, K., & Baillargeon, J. P. (2011). Intergenerational cycle of obesity and diabetes: How can we reduce the burdens of these conditions on the health of future generations? *Experimental Diabetes Research, 2011*, 596060.

Belfort, M. B., & Gillman, M. W. (2011). Healthy infant growth: What are the trade-offs in the developed world? In M. W. Gillman, P. D. Gluckman, & R. G. Rosenfeld (eds): *Recent Advances in Growth Research: Nutritional, Molecular and Endocrine Perspectives*. Nestlé Nutr Inst Workshop Ser, vol 71, pp 171–184

Belfort, M. B., Rifas-Shiman, S. L., Rich-Edwards, J. W., Kleinman, K. P., Oken, E., & Gillman, M. W. (2008). Infant growth and child cognition at 3 years of age. *Pediatrics, 122*(3), e689–e695.

Ben-Shlomo, Y., & Kuh, D. (2002). A life course approach to chronic disease epidemiology: Conceptual models, empirical challenges and interdisciplinary perspectives. *International Journal of Epidemiology, 31*(2), 285–293.

Benjamin, S. E., Cradock, A., Walker, E. M., Slining, M., & Gillman, M. W. (2008). Obesity prevention in child care: A review of U.S. state regulations. *BMC Public Health, 8*, 188.

Benjamin, S. E., Rifas-Shiman, S. L., Taveras, E. M., Haines, J., Finkelstein, J., Kleinman, K., & Gillman, M. W. (2009). Early child care and adiposity at ages 1 and 3 years. *Pediatrics, 124*(2), 555–562.

Birch, L. L., & Davison, K. K. (2001). Family environmental factors influencing the developing behavioral controls of food intake and childhood overweight. *Pediatric Clinics of North America, 48*(4), 893–907.

Boeke, C. E., Mantzoros, C. S., Hughes, M. D., L Rifas-Shiman, S., Villamor, E., Zera, C. A., & Gillman, M. W. (2013). Differential associations of leptin with adiposity across early childhood. *Obesity, 21*(7), 1430–1437.

Boney, C. M., Verma, A., Tucker, R., & Vohr, B. R. (2005). Metabolic syndrome in childhood: Association with birth weight, maternal obesity, and gestational diabetes mellitus. *Pediatrics, 115*(3), e290–e296.

Bouret, S. G., Draper, S. J., & Simerly, R. B. (2004). Trophic action of leptin on hypothalamic neurons that regulate feeding. *Science, 304*(5667), 108–110.

Branum, A. M., Parker, J. D., Keim, S. A., & Schempf, A. H. (2011). Prepregnancy body mass index and gestational weight gain in relation to child body mass index among siblings. *American Journal of Epidemiology, 174*(10), 1159–1165.

Brion, M. J. (2010). Commentary: Assessing the impact of breastfeeding on child health: Where conventional methods alone fall short for reliably establishing causal inference. *International Journal of Epidemiology, 39*(1), 306–307.

Brion, M. J., Lawlor, D. A., Matijasevich, A., Horta, B., Anselmi, L., Araujo, C. L., Menezes, A. M., Victora, C. G., & Smith, G. D. (2011). What are the causal effects of breastfeeding on IQ, obesity and blood pressure? Evidence from comparing high-income with middle-income cohorts. *International Journal of Epidemiology, 40*(3), 670–680.

Brownell, K. D., Farley, T., Willett, W. C., Popkin, B. M., Chaloupka, F. J., Thompson, J. W., & Ludwig, D. S. (2009). The public health and economic benefits of taxing sugar-sweetened beverages. *The New England Journal of Medicine, 361*(16), 1599–1605.

Casazza, K., Fontaine, K. R., Astrup, A., Birch, L. L., Brown, A. W., Bohan Brown, M. M., Durant, N., Dutton, G., Foster, E. M., Heymsfield, S. B., McIver, K., Mehta, T., Menachemi, N., Newby, P. K., Pate, R., Rolls, B. J., Sen, B., Smith, D. L., Jr., Thomas, D. M., & Allison, D. B. (2013). Myths, presumptions, and facts about obesity. *The New England Journal of Medicine, 368*(5), 446–454.

Catalano, P. M., Presley, L., Minium, J., & Hauguel-de Mouzon, S. (2009). Fetuses of obese mothers develop insulin resistance in utero. *Diabetes Care, 32*(6), 1076–1080.

Centers for Disease Control and Prevention. (2010). Racial and ethnic differences in breastfeeding initiation and duration, by state – National Immunization Survey, United States, 2004–2008. *MMWR. Morbidity and Mortality Weekly Report, 59*(11), 327–334.

Centers for Disease Control and Prevention. (2014). Breastfeeding report card: United States, 2014. http://www.cdc.gov/breastfeeding/pdf/2014breastfeedingreportcard.pdf. Accessed 2 Dec 2014.

Cespedes, E. M., Rifas-Shiman, S. L., Redline, S., Gillman, M. W., Pena, M. M., & Taveras, E. M. (2014). Longitudinal associations of sleep curtailment with metabolic risk in mid-childhood. *Obesity, 22*(12), 2586–2592.

Chandler-Laney, P. C., Bush, N. C., Granger, W. M., Rouse, D. J., Mancuso, M. S., & Gower, B. A. (2012). Overweight status and intrauterine exposure to gestational diabetes are associated with children's metabolic health. *Pediatr Obes, 7*(1), 44–52.

Chen, X., Beydoun, M. A., & Wang, Y. (2008). Is sleep duration associated with childhood obesity? A systematic review and meta-analysis. *Obesity, 16*(2), 265–274.

Chriqui, J. F., Eidson, S. S., & Chaloupka, F. J. (2014). State sales taxes on regular soda (as of January 2014) – BTG Fact Sheet. http://www.bridgingthegapresearch.org/_asset/s2b5pb/BTG_soda_tax_fact_sheet_April2014.pdf. Accessed 3 Dec 2014.

Christakis, N. A., & Fowler, J. H. (2007). The spread of obesity in a large social network over 32 years. *The New England Journal of Medicine, 357*(4), 370–379.

Coleman-Jensen, A., Gregory, C., & Singh, A. (September 2014). *Household food security in the United States in 2013, ERR-173*. Washington, DC: U.S. Department of Agriculture, Economic Research Service.

Crowther, C. A., Hiller, J. E., Moss, J. R., McPhee, A. J., Jeffries, W. S., & Robinson, J. S. (2005). Effect of treatment of gestational diabetes mellitus on pregnancy outcomes. *The New England Journal of Medicine, 352*(24), 2477–2486.

Dalenius, K., Brindley, P., Smith, B. L., Reinold, C. M., & Grummer-Strawn, L. (2012). *Pregnancy nutrition surveillance 2010 report*. Atlanta, GA: US Department of health and human services; Centers for Disease Control and Prevention.

Danese, A., & Tan, M. (2014). Childhood maltreatment and obesity: Systematic review and meta-analysis. *Molecular Psychiatry, 19*(5), 544–554.

DiBaise, J. K., Zhang, H., Crowell, M. D., Krajmalnik-Brown, R., Decker, G. A., & Rittmann, B. E. (2008). Gut microbiota and its possible relationship with obesity. *Mayo Clinic Proceedings, 83*(4), 460–469.

Ding, E. L., & Hu, F. B. (2008). Determining origins and causes of childhood obesity via Mendelian randomization analysis. *PLoS Medicine, 5*(3), e65.

Dinour, L. M., Bergen, D., & Yeh, M. C. (2007). The food insecurity-obesity paradox: A review of the literature and the role food stamps may play. *Journal of the American Dietetic Association, 107*(11), 1952–1961.

Dixon, B., Pena, M. M., & Taveras, E. M. (2012). Lifecourse approach to racial/ethnic disparities in childhood obesity. *Advances in Nutrition, 3*(1), 73–82.

Dodd, J. M., Turnbull, D. A., McPhee, A. J., Wittert, G., Crowther, C. A., & Robinson, J. S. (2011). Limiting weight gain in overweight and obese women during pregnancy to improve health outcomes: The LIMIT randomised controlled trial. *BMC Pregnancy and Childbirth, 11*, 79.

Dominguez-Bello, M. G., Costello, E. K., Contreras, M., Magris, M., Hidalgo, G., Fierer, N., & Knight, R. (2010). Delivery mode shapes the acquisition and structure of the initial microbiota across multiple body habitats in newborns. *Proceedings of the National Academy of Sciences of the United States of America, 107*(26), 11971–11975.

Duffey, K. J., & Popkin, B. M. (2013). Causes of increased energy intake among children in the U.S., 1977–2010.

American Journal of Preventive Medicine, 44(2), e1–e8.

Dunton, G. F., Kaplan, J., Wolch, J., Jerrett, M., & Reynolds, K. D. (2009). Physical environmental correlates of childhood obesity: A systematic review. *Obesity Reviews, 10*(4), 393–402.

Ehrenkranz, R. A., Dusick, A. M., Vohr, B. R., Wright, L. L., Wrage, L. A., & Poole, W. K. (2006). Growth in the neonatal intensive care unit influences neurodevelopmental and growth outcomes of extremely low birth weight infants. *Pediatrics, 117*(4), 1253–1261.

Eisenmann, J. C., Gundersen, C., Lohman, B. J., Garasky, S., & Stewart, S. D. (2011). Is food insecurity related to overweight and obesity in children and adolescents? A summary of studies, 1995–2009. *Obesity Reviews, 12*(5), e73–e83.

Elbel, B., Gyamfi, J., & Kersh, R. (2011). Child and adolescent fast-food choice and the influence of calorie labeling: A natural experiment. *International Journal of Obesity, 35*(4), 493–500.

Elobeid, M. A., & Allison, D. B. (2008). Putative environmental-endocrine disruptors and obesity: A review. *Current Opinion in Endocrinology, Diabetes, and Obesity, 15*(5), 403–408.

Finkelstein, E. A., Trogdon, J. G., Cohen, J. W., & Dietz, W. (2009). Annual medical spending attributable to obesity: Payer-and service-specific estimates. *Health Affairs, 28*(5), 822–831.

Fisher, S. C., Kim, S. Y., Sharma, A. J., Rochat, R., & Morrow, B. (2013). Is obesity still increasing among pregnant women? Prepregnancy obesity trends in 20 states, 2003–2009. *Preventive Medicine, 56*(6), 372–378.

Fleten, C., Nystad, W., Stigum, H., Skjaerven, R., Lawlor, D. A., Davey Smith, G., & Naess, O. (2012). Parent-offspring body mass index associations in the Norwegian Mother and Child Cohort Study: A family-based approach to studying the role of the intrauterine environment in childhood adiposity. *American Journal of Epidemiology, 176*(2), 83–92.

Foster, G. D., Linder, B., Baranowski, T., Cooper, D. M., Goldberg, L., Harrell, J. S., Kaufman, F., Marcus, M. D., Treviño, R. P., & Hirst, K. (2010). A school-based intervention for diabetes risk reduction. *The New England Journal of Medicine, 363*(5), 443–453.

Franklin, B., Jones, A., Love, D., Puckett, S., Macklin, J., & White-Means, S. (2012). Exploring mediators of food insecurity and obesity: A review of recent literature. *Journal of Community Health, 37*(1), 253–264.

Freinkel, N. (1980). Banting lecture 1980. Of pregnancy and progeny. *Diabetes, 29*(12), 1023–1035.

Gao, Y. J., Holloway, A. C., Zeng, Z. H., Lim, G. E., Petrik, J. J., Foster, W. G., & Lee, R. M. (2005). Prenatal exposure to nicotine causes postnatal obesity and altered perivascular adipose tissue function. *Obesity Research, 13*(4), 687–692.

Getahun, D., Nath, C., Ananth, C. V., Chavez, M. R., & Smulian, J. C. (2008). Gestational diabetes in the United States: Temporal trends 1989 through 2004. *American Journal of Obstetrics and Gynecology, 198*(5), e521–e525.

Gillman, M. W. (2004). A life course approach to obesity. In D. Kuh (Ed.), *A life course approach to chronic disease epidemiology*. Oxford: Oxford University Press.

Gillman, M. W. (2005). Developmental origins of health and disease. *The New England Journal of Medicine, 353*(17), 1848–1850.

Gillman, M. W. (2011). Commentary: Breastfeeding and obesity–the 2011 Scorecard. *International Journal of Epidemiology, 40*(3), 681–684.

Gillman, M. W. (2016). Interrupting intergenerational cycles of maternal obesity. In M. S. Fewtrell, F. Haschke, & S. L. Prescott (eds): Preventive Aspects of Early Nutrition. Nestlé Nutr Inst Workshop Ser, vol 85, pp 59–69.

Gillman, M. W., Oakey, H., Baghurst, P. A., Volkmer, R. E., Robinson, J. S., & Crowther, C. A. (2010). Effect of treatment of gestational diabetes mellitus on obesity in the next generation. *Diabetes Care, 33*(5), 964–968.

Gillman, M. W., & Poston, L. (2012). *Maternal obesity*. Cambridge, UK: Cambridge University Press.

Gillman, M. W., Rifas-Shiman, S. L., Berkey, C. S., Frazier, A. L., Rockett, H. R., Camargo, C. A., Jr., Field, A. E., & Colditz, G. A. (2006). Breast-feeding and overweight in adolescence: Within-family analysis [corrected]. *Epidemiology, 17*(1), 112–114.

Gilman, S. E., Gardener, H., & Buka, S. L. (2008). Maternal smoking during pregnancy and children's cognitive and physical development: A causal risk factor? *American Journal of Epidemiology, 168*(5), 522–531.

Glaser, R., & Kiecolt-Glaser, J. K. (2005). Stress-induced immune dysfunction: Implications for health. *Nature Reviews Immunology, 5*(3), 243–251.

Glass, T. A., & McAtee, M. J. (2006). Behavioral science at the crossroads in public health: Extending horizons, envisioning the future. *Social Science & Medicine, 62*(7), 1650–1671.

Gonzalez-Suarez, C., Worley, A., Grimmer-Somers, K., & Dones, V. (2009). School-based interventions on childhood obesity: A meta-analysis. *American Journal of Preventive Medicine, 37*(5), 418–427.

Grayson, B. E., & Seeley, R. J. (2012). Deconstructing obesity: The face of fatness before and after the discovery of leptin. *Diabetologia, 55*(1), 3–6.

Grummer-Strawn, L. M., Reinold, C., & Krebs, N. F. (2010). Use of World Health Organization and CDC growth charts for children aged 0–59 months in the United States. *MMWR – Recommendations and Reports, 59*(RR-9), 1–15.

Grynbaum, M. M. (2012). Will soda restrictions help New York win the war on obesity? *BMJ, 345*, e6768.

Halfon, N., & Forrest, C. B. (2017). The emerging theoretical framework of life course health development. In N. Halfon, C. B. Forrest, R. M. Lerner, & E. Faustman (Eds.), *Handbook of life course health-development science*. Cham: Springer.

Hammond, R. A. (2009). Complex systems modeling for obesity research. *Preventing Chronic Disease, 6*(3), A97.

Han, J. C., Lawlor, D. A., & Kimm, S. Y. (2010). Childhood obesity. *Lancet, 375*(9727), 1737–1748.

Harder, T., Bergmann, R., Kallischnigg, G., & Plagemann, A. (2005). Duration of breastfeeding and risk of overweight: A meta-analysis. *American Journal of Epidemiology, 162*(5), 397–403.

Harlev, A., & Wiznitzer, A. (2010). New insights on glucose pathophysiology in gestational diabetes and insulin resistance. *Current Diabetes Reports, 10*(3), 242–247.

Hauguel-de Mouzon, S., Lepercq, J., & Catalano, P. (2006). The known and unknown of leptin in pregnancy. *American Journal of Obstetrics and Gynecology, 194*(6), 1537–1545.

Hawkins, S. S., & Baum, C. F. (2014). Impact of state cigarette taxes on disparities in maternal smoking during pregnancy. *American Journal of Public Health, 104*(8), 1464–1470.

Hedderson, M. M., Gunderson, E. P., & Ferrara, A. (2010). Gestational weight gain and risk of gestational diabetes mellitus. *Obstetrics and Gynecology, 115*(3), 597–604.

Hemmingsson, E., Johansson, K., & Reynisdottir, S. (2014). Effects of childhood abuse on adult obesity: A systematic review and meta-analysis. *Obesity Reviews, 15*(11), 882–893.

Herring, S. J., & Oken, E. (2011). Obesity and diabetes in mothers and their children: Can we stop the intergenerational cycle? *Current Diabetes Reports, 11*(1), 20–27.

Herring, S. J., Rose, M. Z., Skouteris, H., & Oken, E. (2012). Optimizing weight gain in pregnancy to prevent obesity in women and children. *Diabetes, Obesity & Metabolism, 14*(3), 195–203.

Huang, T. T., Drewnosksi, A., Kumanyika, S., & Glass, T. A. (2009). A systems-oriented multilevel framework for addressing obesity in the 21st century. *Preventing Chronic Disease, 6*(3), A82.

Huang, T. T., & Glass, T. A. (2008). Transforming research strategies for understanding and preventing obesity. *JAMA, 300*(15), 1811–1813.

Huh, S. Y., Rifas-Shiman, S. L., Taveras, E. M., Oken, E., & Gillman, M. W. (2011). Timing of solid food introduction and risk of obesity in preschool-aged children. *Pediatrics, 127*(3), e544–e551.

Iliadou, A. N., Koupil, I., Villamor, E., Altman, D., Hultman, C., Langstrom, N., & Cnattingius, S. (2010). Familial factors confound the association between maternal smoking during pregnancy and young adult offspring overweight. *International Journal of Epidemiology, 39*(5), 1193–1202.

Institute of Medicine. (1990). *Nutrition during pregnancy. Part I, weight gain.* Washington, DC: National Academies Press.

Institute of Medicine. (2007). *Nutrition standards for foods in schools: Leading the way toward healtheir youth.* Washington, DC: National Academies Press.

Institute of Medicine. (2009). *Weight gain during pregnancy: Reexamining the guidelines.* Washington, DC: National Academies Press.

Institute of Medicine. (2011). *Early childhood obesity prevention policies.* Washington DC: National Academies Press.

Kahn, J. A., Huang, B., Gillman, M. W., Field, A. E., Austin, S. B., Colditz, G. A., & Frazier, A. L. (2008). Patterns and determinants of physical activity in U.S. adolescents. *The Journal of Adolescent Health, 42*(4), 369–377.

Kann, L., Kinchen, S., Shanklin, S. L., Flint, K. H., Kawkins, J., Harris, W. A., Lowry, R., Olsen, E. O., McManus, T., Chyen, D., Whittle, L., Taylor, E., Demissie, Z., Brener, N., Thornton, J., Moore, J., Zaza, S., & Centers for Disease Control and Prevention (CDC). (2014). Youth risk behavior surveillance–United States, 2013. *MMWR Surveillance Summaries, 63*(4), 1–168.

Katz, D. L., O'Connell, M., Njike, V. Y., Yeh, M. C., & Nawaz, H. (2008). Strategies for the prevention and control of obesity in the school setting: Systematic review and meta-analysis. *International Journal of Obesity, 32*(12), 1780–1789.

Kim, C., Berger, D. K., & Chamany, S. (2007). Recurrence of gestational diabetes mellitus: A systematic review. *Diabetes Care, 30*(5), 1314–1319.

Kim, C., Newton, K. M., & Knopp, R. H. (2002). Gestational diabetes and the incidence of type 2 diabetes: A systematic review. *Diabetes Care, 25*(10), 1862–1868.

Kim, S. Y., England, J. L., Sharma, J. A., & Njoroge, T. (2011). Gestational diabetes mellitus and risk of childhood overweight and obesity in offspring: A systematic review. *Experimental Diabetes Research, 2011*, 541308.

Kitano, H. (2002). Systems biology: A brief overview. *Science, 295*(5560), 1662–1664.

Kramer, M. S., Chalmers, B., Hodnett, E. D., Sevkovskaya, Z., Dzikovich, I., Shapiro, S., Collet, J. P., Vanilovich, I., Mezen, I., Ducruet, T., Shishko, G., Zubovich, V., Mknuik, D., Gluchanina, E., Dombrovsky, V., Ustinovitch, A., Ko, T., Bogdanovich, N., Ovchinikova, L., & Helsing, E. (2001). Promotion of Breastfeeding Intervention Trial (PROBIT): A randomized trial in the Republic of Belarus. *JAMA, 285*(4), 413–420.

Kramer, M. S., Guo, T., Platt, R. W., Vanilovich, I., Sevkovskaya, Z., Dzikovich, I., Michaelsen, K. F., Dewey, K., & Promotion of Breastfeeding Interven tion Trials Study Group. (2004). Feeding effects on growth during infancy. *The Journal of Pediatrics, 145*(5), 600–605.

Kramer, M. S., Matush, L., Vanilovich, I., Platt, R. W., Bogdanovich, N., Sevkovskaya, Z., Dzikovich, I., Shishko, G., Collet, J. P., Martin, R. M., Davey Smith, G., Gillman, M. W., Chalmers, B., Hodnett, E., Shapiro, S., & PROBIT Study Group. (2007). Effects of prolonged and exclusive breastfeeding on child height, weight, adiposity, and blood pressure at age 6.5 y: Evidence from a large randomized trial. *The American Journal of Clinical Nutrition, 86*(6), 1717–1721.

Kropski, J. A., Keckley, P. H., & Jensen, G. L. (2008). School-based obesity prevention programs: An evidence-based review. *Obesity, 16*(5), 1009–1018.

Kuczmarski, R. J., Ogden, C. L., Guo, S. S., Grummer-Strawn, L. M., Flegal, K. M., Mei, Z., Curtin, L. R., Roche, A. F., & Johnson, C. L. (2002). 2000 CDC growth charts for the United States: Methods and development. *Vital and Health Statistics, 11*(246), 1–190.

Kwok, M. K., Schooling, C. M., Lam, T. H., & Leung, G. M. (2010). Does breastfeeding protect against childhood overweight? Hong Kong's 'Children of 1997' birth cohort. *International Journal of Epidemiology, 39*(1), 297–305.

Landon, M. B., Spong, C. Y., Thom, E., Carpenter, M. W., Ramin, S. M., Casey, B., Wapner, R. J., Varner, M. W., Rouse, D. J., Thorp, J. M., Jr., Sciscione, A., Catalano, P., Harper, M., Saade, G., Lain, K. Y., Sorokin, Y., Peaceman, A. M., Tolosa, J. E., Anderson, G. B., & Eunice Kennedy Shriver National Institute of Child Health and Human Development Maternal-Fetal Medicine Units Network. (2009). A multicenter, randomized trial of treatment for mild gestational diabetes. *The New England Journal of Medicine, 361*(14), 1339–1348.

Larson, N., Ward, D., Neelon, S. B., & Story, M. (2011a). *Preventing obesity among preschool children: How can child-care settings promote healthy eating and physical activity? Research synthesis*. Princeton, NJ: Robert Wood Johnson Foundation.

Larson, N., Ward, D. S., Neelon, S. B., & Story, M. (2011b). What role can child-care settings play in obesity prevention? A review of the evidence and call for research efforts. *Journal of the American Dietetic Association, 111*(9), 1343–1362.

Lasater, G., Piernas, C., & Popkin, B. M. (2011). Beverage patterns and trends among school-aged children in the US, 1989–2008. *Nutrition Journal, 10*, 103.

Lau, E. Y., Liu, J., Archer, E., McDonald, S. M., & Liu, J. (2014). Maternal weight gain in pregnancy and risk of obesity among offspring: A systematic review. *Journal of Obesity, 2014*, 524939.

Lawlor, D. A., Lichtenstein, P., Fraser, A., & Langstrom, N. (2011a). Does maternal weight gain in pregnancy have long-term effects on offspring adiposity? A sibling study in a prospective cohort of 146,894 men from 136,050 families. *The American Journal of Clinical Nutrition, 94*(1), 142–148.

Lawlor, D. A., Lichtenstein, P., & Langstrom, N. (2011b). Association of maternal diabetes mellitus in pregnancy with offspring adiposity into early adulthood: Sibling study in a prospective cohort of 280,866 men from 248,293 families. *Circulation, 123*(3), 258–265.

Lawlor, D. A., Timpson, N. J., Harbord, R. M., Leary, S., Ness, A., McCarthy, M. I., Frayling, T. M., Hattersley, A. T., & Smith, G. D. (2008). Exploring the developmental overnutrition hypothesis using parental-offspring associations and FTO as an instrumental variable. *PLoS Medicine, 5*(3), e33.

Lehto, R., Mäki, P., Ray, C., Laatikainen, T., & Roos, E. (2015). Childcare use and overweight in Finland: Cross-sectional and retrospective associations among 3- and 5-year-old children. *Pediatric Obesity, 11*(2), 136–143. doi:10.1111/ijpo.12036.

Li, H. T., Zhou, Y. B., & Liu, J. M. (2013). The impact of cesarean section on offspring overweight and obesity: A systematic review and meta-analysis. *International Journal of Obesity, 37*(7), 893–899.

Li, R., Fein, S. B., & Grummer-Strawn, L. M. (2010). Do infants fed from bottles lack self-regulation of milk intake compared with directly breastfed infants? *Pediatrics, 125*(6), e1386–e1393.

Lobstein, T., Baur, L., & Uauy, R. (2004). Obesity in children and young people: A crisis in public health. *Obesity Reviews, 5*(1), 4–104.

Lovasi, G. S., Hutson, M. A., Guerra, M., & Neckerman, K. M. (2009). Built environments and obesity in disadvantaged populations. *Epidemiologic Reviews, 31*, 7–20.

Lubans, D. R., Morgan, P. J., Dewar, D., Collins, C. E., Plotnikoff, R. C., Okely, A. D., Batterham, M. J., Finn, T., & Callister, R. (2010). The Nutrition and Enjoyable Activity for Teen Girls (NEAT girls) randomized controlled trial for adolescent girls from disadvantaged secondary schools: Rationale, study protocol, and baseline results. *BMC Public Health, 10*, 652.

Ludwig, D. S., Blumenthal, S. J., & Willett, W. C. (2012). Opportunities to reduce childhood hunger and obesity: Restructuring the supplemental nutrition assistance program (the food stamp program). *JAMA, 308*(24), 2567–2568.

Ludwig, J., Sanbonmatsu, L., Gennetian, L., Adam, E., Duncan, G. J., Katz, L. F., Kessler, R. C., Kling, J. R., Lindau, S. T., Whitaker, R. C., & McDade, T. W. (2011). Neighborhoods, obesity, and diabetes–a randomized social experiment. *The New England Journal of Medicine, 365*(16), 1509–1519.

Lumley, J., Chamberlain, C., Dowswell, T., Oliver, S., Oakley, L., & Watson, L. (2009). Interventions for promoting smoking cessation during pregnancy. *Cochrane Database of Systematic Reviews, 3*, CD001055.

Mamun, A. A., Mannan, M., & Doi, S. A. (2014). Gestational weight gain in relation to offspring obesity over the life course: A systematic review and bias-adjusted meta-analysis. *Obesity Reviews, 15*(4), 338–347.

Mani, M., Mandre, S. B., & M. (2010). Events before droplet splashing on a solid surface. *Journal of Fluid Mechanics, 647*, 163.

Mantzoros, C. S., Rifas-Shiman, S. L., Williams, C. J., Fargnoli, J. L., Kelesidis, T., & Gillman, M. W. (2009). Cord blood leptin and adiponectin as predictors of adiposity in children at 3 years of age: A prospective cohort study. *Pediatrics, 123*(2), 682–689.

Martin, R. M., Patel, R., Kramer, M. S., Guthrie, L., Vilchuck, K., Bogdanovich, N., Sergeichick, N., Gusina, N., Foo, Y., Palmer, T., Rifas-Shiman, S. L., Gillman, M. W., Smith, G. D., & Oken, E. (2013). Effects of promoting longer-term and exclusive breastfeeding on adiposity and insulin-like growth factor-I at age 11.5 years: A randomized trial. *JAMA, 309*(10), 1005–1013.

Masse, L. C., Perna, F., Agurs-Collins, T., & Chriqui, J. F. (2013). Change in school nutrition-related laws from 2003 to 2008: Evidence from the school nutrition-environment state policy classification system. *American Journal of Public Health, 103*(9), 1597–1603.

McGinnis, J. M., Gootman, J. A., & Kraak, V. I. (2006). *Food marketing to children and youth: Threat or opportunity?* Washington, DC: National Academies Press.

Mello, M. M. (2009). New York City's war on fat. *The New England Journal of Medicine, 360*(19), 2015–2020.

Metzger, M. W., & McDade, T. W. (2010). Breastfeeding as obesity prevention in the United States: A sibling difference model. *American Journal of Human Biology, 22*(3), 291–296.

Michopoulos, V., Powers, A., Moore, C., Villarreal, S., Ressler, K. J., & Bradley, B. (2015). The mediating role of emotion dysregulation and depression on the relationship between childhood trauma exposure and emotional eating. *Appetite, 91*, 129–136.

Mihrshahi, S., Battistutta, D., Magarey, A., & Daniels, L. A. (2011). Determinants of rapid weight gain during infancy: Baseline results from the NOURISH randomised controlled trial. *BMC Pediatrics, 11*, 99.

Moholdt, T. T., Salvesen, K., Ingul, C. B., Vik, T., Oken, E., & Morkved, S. (2011). Exercise Training in Pregnancy for obese women (ETIP): Study protocol for a randomised controlled trial. *Trials, 12*, 154.

Monteiro, P. O., & Victora, C. G. (2005). Rapid growth in infancy and childhood and obesity in later life–a systematic review. *Obesity Reviews, 6*(2), 143–154.

National Association for Sport and Physical Education. (2004). *Moving into the future: National standards for physical education* (2nd ed.). Reston, VA: McGraw-Hill.

National Prevention Council. (2011). *National prevention strategy*. Washington, DC: U.S. Department of Health and Human Services, Office of the Surgeon General.

Neelon, S. B., Andersen, C. S., Morgen, C. S., Kamper-Jørgensen, M., Oken, E., Gillman, M. W., & Sørensen, T. I. A. (2015). Early child care and obesity at 12 months of age in the Danish National Birth Cohort. *International Journal of Obesity, 39*(1), 33–38.

Nehring, I., Lehmann, S., & von Kries, R. (2013). Gestational weight gain in accordance to the IOM/NRC criteria and the risk for childhood overweight: A meta-analysis. *Pediatric Obesity, 8*(3), 218–224.

Nehring, I., Schmoll, S., Beyerlein, A., Hauner, H., & von Kries, R. (2011). Gestational weight gain and long-term postpartum weight retention: A meta-analysis. *The American Journal of Clinical Nutrition, 94*(5), 1225–1231.

Nelson, M. C., Gordon-Larsen, P., & Adair, L. S. (2005). Are adolescents who were breast-fed less likely to be overweight? Analyses of sibling pairs to reduce confounding. *Epidemiology, 16*(2), 247–253.

Neu, J., & Rushing, J. (2011). Cesarean versus vaginal delivery: Long-term infant outcomes and the hygiene hypothesis. *Clinics in Perinatology, 38*(2), 321–331.

Newbold, R. R., Padilla-Banks, E., Snyder, R. J., Phillips, T. M., & Jefferson, W. N. (2007). Developmental exposure to endocrine disruptors and the obesity epidemic. *Reproductive Toxicology, 23*(3), 290–296.

Nielsen, L. S., Danielsen, K. V., & Sorensen, T. I. (2011). Short sleep duration as a possible cause of obesity: Critical analysis of the epidemiological evidence. *Obesity Reviews, 12*(2), 78–92.

Office of the Mayor. (2012). Reversing the epidemic: The New York City obesity task force plan to prevent and control obesity. http://www.nyc.gov/html/om/pdf/2012/otf_report.pdf. Accessed 5 Feb 2013.

O'Tierney, P. F., Barker, D. J., Osmond, C., Kajantie, E., & Eriksson, J. G. (2009). Duration of breast-feeding and adiposity in adult life. *The Journal of Nutrition, 139*(2), 422S–425S.

Ogden, C. L., Carroll, M. D., Kit, B. K., & Flegal, K. M. (2014). Prevalence of childhood and adult obesity in the United States, 2011–2012. *JAMA, 311*(8), 806–814.

Ogden, C. L., & Flegal, K. M. (2010). Changes in terminology for childhood overweight and obesity. *National Health Statistics Reports, 25*, 1–5.

Oken, E., & Gillman, M. W. (2003). Fetal origins of obesity. *Obesity Research, 11*(4), 496–506.

Oken, E., Levitan, E. B., & Gillman, M. W. (2008). Maternal smoking during pregnancy and child overweight: Systematic review and meta-analysis. *International Journal of Obesity, 32*(2), 201–210.

Okereke, N. C., Uvena-Celebrezze, J., Hutson-Presley, L., Amini, S. B., & Catalano, P. M. (2002). The effect of gender and gestational diabetes mellitus on cord leptin concentration. *American Journal of Obstetrics and Gynecology, 187*(3), 798–803.

Oteng-Ntim, E., Varma, R., Croker, H., Poston, L., & Doyle, P. (2012). Lifestyle interventions for overweight and obese pregnant women to improve pregnancy outcome: Systematic review and meta-analysis. *BMC Medicine, 10*, 47.

Owen, C. G., Martin, R. M., Whincup, P. H., Davey-Smith, G., Gillman, M. W., & Cook, D. G. (2005a). The effect of breastfeeding on mean body mass index throughout life: A quantitative review of published and unpublished observational evidence. *The American Journal of Clinical Nutrition, 82*(6), 1298–1307.

Owen, C. G., Martin, R. M., Whincup, P. H., Smith, G. D., & Cook, D. G. (2005b). Effect of infant feeding on the risk of obesity across the life course: A quantitative review of published evidence. *Pediatrics, 115*(5), 1367–1377.

Pan, L., Blanck, H. M., Sherry, B., Dalenius, K., & Grummer-Strawn, L. M. (2012). Trends in the prevalence of extreme obesity among US preschool-aged children living in low-income families, 1998–2010. *JAMA, 308*(24), 2563–2565.

Papas, M. A., Alberg, A. J., Ewing, R., Helzlsouer, K. J., Gary, T. L., & Klassen, A. C. (2007). The built environment and obesity. *Epidemiologic Reviews, 29*, 129–143.

Parker, M., Rifas-Shiman, S. L., Belfort, M. B., Taveras, E. M., Oken, E., Mantzoros, C., & Gillman, M. W. (2011). Gestational glucose tolerance and cord blood leptin levels predict slower weight gain in early infancy. *The Journal of Pediatrics, 158*(2), 227–233.

Parsons, T. J., Power, C., Logan, S., & Summerbell, C. D. (1999). Childhood predictors of adult obesity: A systematic review. *International Journal of Obesity and Related Metabolic Disorders, 23*(8), S1–107.

Patel, R., Martin, R. M., Kramer, M. S., Oken, E., Bogdanovich, N., Matush, L., Smith, G. D., & Lawlor, D. A. (2011). Familial associations of adiposity: Findings from a cross-sectional study of 12,181 parental-offspring trios from Belarus. *PloS One, 6*(1), e14607.

Pearce, J., Taylor, M. A., & Langley-Evans, S. C. (2013). Timing of the introduction of complementary feeding and risk of childhood obesity: A systematic review. *International Journal of Obesity, 37*(10), 1295–1306.

Perna, F. M., Oh, A., Chriqui, J. F., Masse, L. C., Atienza, A. A., Nebeling, L., Agurs-Collins, T., Moser, R. P., & Dodd, K. W. (2012). The association of state law to physical education time allocation in US public schools. *American Journal of Public Health, 102*(8), 1594–1599.

Perng, W., Gillman, M. W., Mantzoros, C. S., & Oken, E. (2014). A prospective study of maternal prenatal weight and offspring cardiometabolic health in midchildhood. *Annals of Epidemiology, 24*(11), 793–800 e791.

Piernas, C., & Popkin, B. M. (2011). Increased portion sizes from energy-dense foods affect total energy intake at eating occasions in US children and adolescents: Patterns and trends by age group and sociodemographic characteristics, 1977–2006. *The American Journal of Clinical Nutrition, 94*(5), 1324–1332.

Powell, L. M., Chriqui, J. F., Khan, T., Wada, R., & Chaloupka, F. J. (2013). Assessing the potential effectiveness of food and beverage taxes and subsidies for improving public health: A systematic review of prices, demand and body weight outcomes. *Obesity Reviews, 14*(2), 110–128.

Rideout, V. J., & Hamel, E. (2006). *The media family: Electronic media in the lives of infants, toddlers, preschoolers, and their parents*. Menlo Park, CA: Kaiser Family Foundation.

Rudd Center for Food Policy & Obesity. (2013). *Industry self-regulation of food marketing.*. http://www.yaleruddcenter.org/what_we_do.aspx?id=25. Accessed 5 Feb 2013.

Sanbonmatsu, L., Ludwig, J., Katz, L. F., Gennetian, L. A., Duncan, G. J., Kessler, R. C., Adam, E., TW, M. D., & Lindau, S. T. (2011). *Moving to opportunity for fair housing demonstration program – Final impacts evaluation*. Washington, DC: U.S. Department of Housing and Urban Development.

Savino, F., & Liguori, S. A. (2008). Update on breast milk hormones: Leptin, ghrelin and adiponectin. *Clinical Nutrition, 27*(1), 42–47.

Schmidt, M. E., Haines, J., O'Brien, A., McDonald, J., Price, S., Sherry, B., & Taveras, E. M. (2012). Systematic review of effective strategies for reducing screen time among young children. *Obesity, 20*(7), 1338–1354.

Section on Breastfeeding. (2012). Breastfeeding and the use of human milk. *Pediatrics, 129*(3), e827–e841.

Siega-Riz, A. M., Viswanathan, M., Moos, M. K., Deierlein, A., Mumford, S., Knaack, J., Thieda, P., Lux, L. J., & Lohr, K. N. (2009). A systematic review of outcomes of maternal weight gain according to the Institute of Medicine recommendations: Birthweight, fetal growth, and postpartum weight retention. *American Journal of Obstetrics and Gynecology, 201*(4), 339.e331–339.e314.

Slining, M. M., Benjamin Neelon, S. E., & Duffey, K. J. (2014). A review of state regulations to promote infant physical activity in child care. *International Journal of Behavioral Nutrition and Physical Activity, 11*(1), 139.

Smith, G. D., & Ebrahim, S. (2003). 'Mendelian randomization': Can genetic epidemiology contribute to understanding environmental determinants of disease? *International Journal of Epidemiology, 32*(1), 1–22.

National Center for Education Statistics. (2005). *Number of children under 6 years old and not yet enrolled in kindergarten, percentage in center-based programs, average weekly hours in nonparental care, and percentage in various types of primary care arrangements, by selected child and family characteristics: 2005*. http://nces.ed.gov/programs/digest/d09/tables/dt09_044.asp. Accessed 5 Feb 2013.

Story, M., Nanney, M. S., & Schwartz, M. B. (2009). Schools and obesity prevention: Creating school environments and policies to promote healthy eating and physical activity. *The Milbank Quarterly, 87*(1), 71–100.

Strasburger, V. C. (2011). Children, adolescents, obesity, and the media. *Pediatrics, 128*(1), 201–208.

Taheri, S. (2006). The link between short sleep duration and obesity: We should recommend more sleep to prevent obesity. *Archives of Disease in Childhood, 91*(11), 881–884.

Taveras, E. M., Blackburn, K., Gillman, M. W., Haines, J., McDonald, J., Price, S., & Oken, E. (2011a). First steps for mommy and me: A pilot intervention to improve nutrition and physical activity behaviors of postpartum mothers and their infants. *Maternal and Child Health Journal, 15*(8), 1217–1227.

Taveras, E. M., Gillman, M. W., Kleinman, K., Rich-Edwards, J. W., & Rifas-Shiman, S. L. (2010). Racial/ethnic differences in early-life risk factors for childhood obesity. *Pediatrics, 125*(4), 686–695.

Taveras, E. M., Gillman, M. W., Kleinman, K. P., Rich-Edwards, J. W., & Rifas-Shiman, S. L. (2013). Reducing racial/ethnic disparities in childhood obesity: The role of early life risk factors. *JAMA Pediatrics, 167*(8), 731–738.

Taveras, E. M., Gillman, M. W., Pena, M. M., Redline, S., & Rifas-Shiman, S. L. (2014). Chronic sleep curtailment and adiposity. *Pediatrics, 133*(6), 1013–1022.

Taveras, E. M., Gortmaker, S. L., Hohman, K. H., Horan, C. M., Kleinman, K. P., Mitchell, K., Price, S., Prosser, L. A., Rifas-Shiman, S. L., & Gillman, M. W. (2011b). Randomized controlled trial to improve primary care to prevent and manage childhood obesity: The high five for kids study. *Archives of Pediatrics & Adolescent Medicine, 165*(8), 714–722.

Taveras, E. M., McDonald, J., O'Brien, A., Haines, J., Sherry, B., Bottino, C. J., Troncoso, K., Schmidt, M. E., & Koziol, R. (2012). Healthy habits, happy homes: Methods and baseline data of a randomized controlled trial to improve household routines for obesity prevention. *Preventive Medicine, 55*(5), 418–426.

Taveras, E. M., Rifas-Shiman, S. L., Sherry, B., Oken, E., Haines, J., Kleinman, K., Rich-Edwards, J. W., & Gillman, M. W. (2011c). Crossing growth percentiles in infancy and risk of obesity in childhood. *Archives of Pediatrics & Adolescent Medicine, 165*(11), 993–998.

Te Morenga, L., Mallard, S., & Mann, J. (2012). Dietary sugars and body weight: Systematic review and meta-analyses of randomised controlled trials and cohort studies. *BMJ, 346*, e7492.

Thangaratinam, S., Rogozinska, E., Jolly, K., Glinkowski, S., Roseboom, T., Tomlinson, J. W., Kunz, R., Mol, B. W., Coomarasamy, A., & Khan, K. S. (2012). Effects of interventions in pregnancy on maternal weight and obstetric outcomes: Meta-analysis of randomised evidence. *BMJ, 344*, e2088.

Torloni, M. R., Betran, A. P., Horta, B. L., Nakamura, M. U., Atallah, A. N., Moron, A. F., & Valente, O. (2009). Prepregnancy BMI and the risk of gestational diabetes: A systematic review of the literature with meta-analysis. *Obesity Reviews, 10*(2), 194–203.

Torres, S. J., & Nowson, C. A. (2007). Relationship between stress, eating behavior, and obesity. *Nutrition, 23*(11–12), 887–894.

Trasande, L., Attina, T. M., & Blustein, J. (2012). Association between urinary bisphenol a concentration and obesity prevalence in children and adolescents. *JAMA, 308*(11), 1113–1121.

Trogdon, J. G., Nonnemaker, J., & Pais, J. (2008). Peer effects in adolescent overweight. *Journal of Health Economics, 27*(5), 1388–1399.

U.S. Department of Agriculture. (2013a). National school lunch program and school breakfast program: Nutrition standards for all foods sold in school as required by the Healthy, Hunger-Free Kids Act of 2010; Interim Final Rule. *Federal Register, 78*(125), 39067–39120.

U.S. Department of Agriculture. (2013b). *Supplemental Nutrition Assistance Program (SNAP)*. http://www.fns.usda.gov/snap. Accessed 5 Feb 2013.

U.S. Department of Health and Human Services. (2004). *The health consequences of smoking: A report of the surgeon general*. Atlanta, GA: U.S. Department of Health and Human Services; Centers for Disease Control and Prevention; National Center for Chronic Disease Prevention and Health Promotion; Office on Smoking and Health.

U.S. Department of Health and Human Services. (2008). *2008 physical activity guidelines for Americans*. Washington, DC: U.S. Department of Health and Human Services.

Van Der Horst, K., Paw, M. J., Twisk, J. W., & Van Mechelen, W. (2007). A brief review on correlates of physical activity and sedentariness in youth. *Medicine and Science in Sports and Exercise, 39*(8), 1241–1250.

Ventura, A. K., & Mennella, J. A. (2011). Innate and learned preferences for sweet taste during childhood. *Current Opinion in Clinical Nutrition and Metabolic Care, 14*(4), 379–384.

Vesco, K. K., Karanja, N., King, J. C., Gillman, M. W., Leo, M. C., Perrin, N., CT, M. E., Eckhardt, C. L., Smith, K. S., & Stevens, V. J. (2014). Efficacy of a group-based dietary intervention for limiting gestational weight gain among obese women: A randomized trial. *Obesity, 22*(9), 1989–1996.

Vesco, K. K., Karanja, N., King, J. C., Gillman, M. W., Perrin, N., McEvoy, C., Eckhardt, C., Smith, K. S., & Stevens, V. J. (2012). Healthy moms, a randomized trial to promote and evaluate weight maintenance among obese pregnant women: Study design and rationale. *Contemporary Clinical Trials, 33*(4), 777–785.

Vgontzas, A. N., Lin, H. M., Papaliaga, M., Calhoun, S., Vela-Bueno, A., Chrousos, G. P., & Bixler, E. O. (2008). Short sleep duration and obesity: The role of emotional stress and sleep disturbances. *International Journal of Obesity, 32*(5), 801–809.

Viner, R. M., Ozer, E. M., Denny, S., Marmot, M., Resnick, M., Fatusi, A., & Currie, C. (2012). Adolescence and the social determinants of health. *Lancet, 379*(9826), 1641–1652.

von Kries, R., Bolte, G., Baghi, L., & Toschke, A. M. (2008). Parental smoking and childhood obesity–is maternal smoking in pregnancy the critical exposure? *International Journal of Epidemiology, 37*(1), 210–216.

Wang, Y., & Beydoun, M. A. (2007). The obesity epidemic in the United States–gender, age, socioeconomic, racial/ethnic, and geographic characteristics: A systematic review and meta-regression analysis. *Epidemiologic Reviews, 29*, 6–28.

Wang, Y. C., Gortmaker, S. L., & Taveras, E. M. (2011). Trends and racial/ethnic disparities in severe obesity among US children and adolescents, 1976–2006. *International Journal of Pediatric Obesity, 6*(1), 12–20.

Waterland, R. A., & Jirtle, R. L. (2004). Early nutrition, epigenetic changes at transposons and imprinted genes, and enhanced susceptibility to adult chronic diseases. *Nutrition, 20*(1), 63–68.

Waters, E., de Silva-Sanigorski, A., Hall, B. J., Brown, T., Campbell, K. J., Gao, Y., Armstrong, R., Prosser, L., & Summerbell, C. D. (2011). Interventions for preventing obesity in children. *Cochrane Database of Systematic Reviews, 12*, CD001871.

Wen, X., Gillman, M. W., Rifas-Shiman, S. L., Sherry, B., Kleinman, K., & Taveras, E. M. (2012). Decreasing prevalence of obesity among young children in Massachusetts from 2004 to 2008. *Pediatrics, 129*(5), 823–831.

Weng, S. F., Redsell, S. A., Swift, J. A., Yang, M., & Glazebrook, C. P. (2012). Systematic review and meta-analyses of risk factors for childhood overweight identifiable during infancy. *Archives of Disease in Childhood, 97*(12), 1019–1026.

White House Task Force on Childhood Obesity. (2011). *One year progress report*. http://www.letsmove.gov/sites/letsmove.gov/files/Obesity_update_report.pdf. Accessed 8 Feb 2013.

White House Task Force on Childhood Obesity. (2010). *Solving the problem of childhood obesity within a generation: The White House task force on childhood obesity report to the president* http://www.letsmove.gov/sites/letsmove.gov/files/TaskForce_on_Childhood_Obesity_May2010_FullReport.pdf. Accessed 19 July 2012.

Yu, Z. B., Han, S. P., Zhu, G. Z., Zhu, C., Wang, X. J., Cao, X. G., & Guo, X. R. (2011). Birth weight and subsequent risk of obesity: A systematic review and meta-analysis. *Obesity Reviews, 12*(7), 525–542.

Pediatric Type 2 Diabetes: Prevention and Treatment Through a Life Course Health Development Framework

Pamela Salsberry, Rika Tanda, Sarah E. Anderson, and Manmohan K. Kamboj

1 Introduction

Estimates project that one in three US adults may have diabetes in 2050 (Boyle et al. 2010). The rates are even higher in some subgroups; for example, in Hispanic females it is 1 in 2 (Venkat Narayan et al. 2003). This problem is not limited to the USA. Shaw et al. 2010 estimate that 7.7% or 434 million adults will have diabetes by 2030 worldwide (Shaw et al. 2010). Until very recently, type 2 diabetes mellitus (T2DM) was a disease diagnosed in adults, but as the childhood obesity epidemic has spread in both magnitude and severity, the diagnosis of T2DM in adolescents and young adults has become more common. The prevalence of prediabetes in 12–19 years, estimated using National Health and Nutrition Examination Survey (NHANES) data, increased from 9% in 1999–2000 to 23% in 2007–2008 (May et al. 2012). Analyses using data from the SEARCH for Diabetes in Youth Study (SEARCH) indicate a 30.5% overall increase in the prevalence of T2DM in children/adolescents from 2001 to 2009 (Dabelea et al. 2014). Because of the newness of this diagnosis in children and adolescents, very little is known about the natural history of the disease, and it will likely take decades to fully understand the determinants and consequences of this new epidemic. Early indicators suggest that the disease may be more severe (Elder et al. 2012) and more difficult to manage when diagnosed in adolescents (Zeitler et al. 2012).

A recent analysis estimates that adolescents with T2DM will lose approximately 15 years of life and will experience severe and chronic complications by their 40s as a result of the disease (Rhodes et al. 2012). The mean direct cost for medical care for a man diagnosed with T2DM for less than 15 years is estimated at $2465. The economic burden of T2DM rises significantly as the

P. Salsberry, PhD, RN, FAAN (✉)
College of Public Health, Division of Health Behavior, Health Promotion, Institute for Population Health, The Ohio State University, 1841 Neil Avenue, 353 Cunz Hall, Columbus, OH 43210, USA
e-mail: Salsberry.1@osu.edu

R. Tanda, PhD, RN
College of Health Science and Professions, Ohio University, Grover Center W133B, Athens, OH 45701, USA
e-mail: tandar@ohio.edu

S.E. Anderson, PhD
The Ohio State University, College of Public Health, 336 Cunz Hall, 1841 Neil Avenue, Columbus, OH 43210, USA
e-mail: sanderson@cph.osu.edu

M.K. Kamboj, MD
The Ohio State University, College of Medicine, Endocrinology, Metabolism and Diabetes, Nationwide Children's Hospital, 700 Children's Drive (ED425), Columbus, OH 43205, USA
e-mail: Manmohan.Kamboj@Nationwidechildrens.org

N. Halfon et al. (eds.), *Handbook of Life Course Health Development*,
DOI 10.1007/978-3-319-47143-3_10

years with disease increase. For those with disease 15 years or more, the costs are estimated to be 10–50% higher. This grim forecast highlights that not only will the disease burden be significant but the economic burden will be high in youth diagnosed with T2DM (Li et al. 2013). Metabolic comorbidities occur with alarming frequency (West et al. 2009). Within the SEARCH study, a significant portion of adolescents with T2DM had hypertension, high LDL cholesterol, or high triglycerides (Lawrence et al. 2009a; Mayer-Davis et al. 2009). It is clear that there is much to do to understand the epidemic, to determine effective prevention strategies, and to develop interventions for those diagnosed with the disease. It is also clear from what we are learning that preventive and treatment strategies need to begin early.

The risk for a child developing T2DM begins in utero. Individual health development trajectories emerge from this starting point and are the result of factors that accumulate across time and/or are the result of biological conditioning during sensitive periods of development. Understanding how these trajectories emerge, and which factors and events result in disease-causing pathways, is key to not only understanding the onset and variable natural history of the disease but in determining ways to prevent and treat it. There is an extensive and emergent body of literature that examines the mechanisms, pathways, and determinants of T2DM in children and adolescents. Genetic and epigenetic mechanisms are clearly a part of the story, but several studies also demonstrate the influence and importance of the social context on developing biological processes (Kempf et al. 2008). These include behaviors and psychological stressors nested within families, neighborhoods, and communities. Consistent with the principles of life course health development that are presented by Halfon and Forrest (2017), there is a growing consensus that T2DM is the result of the multilevel interaction of genetic, behavioral, social, and economic factors with the timing, sequence, and dose of exposure central to long-term outcomes.

A life course health development approach that details risks and protective factors, as well as preventive and treatment strategies, contextualized within the developmental stage of the child, is required. While one's genetic code may establish susceptibility toward T2DM development, its development is the result of a complex process of person-environment interactions that are multidimensional, multidirectional, and multilevel. A major aim of this chapter is to demonstrate that a life course health development approach to pediatric T2DM is critical to the development of a sound national strategy to prevent and treat T2DM in children. We review major factors known to influence the development of pediatric T2DM and track these across childhood. This set of factors will likely change over the next decade as our understanding of disease mechanisms deepens, but what will not change is the importance of placing these factors into context and recognizing that T2DM development is highly sensitive to the timing and social structuring of multiple environmental exposures. Research recommendations relevant to the field of maternal and child health regarding T2DM will be discussed through a life course lens. This chapter is organized around four key developmental stages: preconception and intrauterine life, infancy, childhood (early and middle), and adolescence. These health development stages unfold against the "backdrop" of each child's genetics, race/ethnicity, and family economic status.

2 The Backdrop

2.1 Genetics

Having a relative with T2DM is an established risk factor for the disease (Rosenbloom et al. 1999). Through a series of twin studies, heritability of fasting glucose levels has been estimated to range from 38% to 51% (Katoh et al. 2005; Snieder et al. 1999). Heritability is a population parameter that measures the fraction of variation, i.e., fasting glucose levels, among individuals in a population that is attributable to their genotypes (Visscher et al. 2008). At the individual level, a positive family history of T2DM has been associated with reduced insulin sensitivity at younger ages in children and adolescents when compared with children with no family history (Arslanian et al. 2005). There is a 40% increased lifetime risk for T2DM for children if one parent has T2DM; this increases to 70% if both parents have T2DM (Groop and Tuomi 1997). Studies have found that as many as 80% of youth with T2DM have a close relative with diabetes (Arslanian et al. 2005; Copeland et al. 2011).

Most of the genetic studies of T2DM have been carried out with adults; genetic studies of T2DM in children and youth are limited because of low number of subjects (Morgan 2012). An exception to this is a large meta-analysis that combined data from 6 European cohorts to test whether associations of common genetic variants identified for fasting glucose or insulin levels in nondiabetic adults were detectable in healthy children and adolescents. They found that the majority of novel fasting glucose loci identified in genome-wide associations studies (GWAS) in adults were detectable in childhood and at similar effect sizes (Barker et al. 2011). Work is progressing to examine whether associations between adult-identified susceptibility genes with T2DM hold in pediatric T2DM. For example, transcription factor 7-like 2 (TCF7L2) has been found to be associated with an increased risk of T2DM in African-American youth but not in non-Hispanic whites (Dabelea et al. 2011).

There is clear evidence that genetics plays a role in childhood susceptibility to T2DM, but significant research is needed. This research will require substantial collaboration across sites to achieve sample sizes large enough to test hypotheses. While progress is being made in elucidating underlying gene variants in adults, testing to determine if the same variants are operating in children and adolescents is required (Morgan 2012).

2.2 Prevalence and Incidence of T2DM Related to Age, Race, and Ethnicity

The prevalence of T2DM among children has risen with population increases in obesity, but compared to adolescents, T2DM in preadolescent children occurs less frequently. The highest rates are noted for adolescents aged 15–19 years, while incidence in children below 10 years in age is low. These results come from the SEARCH study, a multiethnic, population-based study designed to estimate rates of diabetes (both type 1 and type 2) based upon health-care provider assessment and in a subpopulation with further blood analyses. Data from SEARCH indicated a prevalence of diagnosed T2DM among 10–14-year-olds of 0.23 cases per 1000 children in 2009, up from 0.15 per 1000 in 2001 (Dabelea et al. 2014). Comparable prevalence estimates for adolescents (15–19 years) in 2001 and 2009 were respectively 0.54 and 0.68 per 1000 (Dabelea et al. 2014). Data from 1999 to 2010 NHANES, representative of US youth 12–19 years, indicated a total prevalence of T2DM of 0.36 per 1000 (Demmer et al. 2013). This estimate combines diagnosed and undiagnosed cases of T2DM, with approximately 1/3 of the total being undiagnosed but having a fasting glucose level of ≥126 mg/dL (Demmer et al. 2013). The prevalence of pediatric T2DM is higher for females and among minorities in the USA (Dabelea et al. 2014). SEARCH researchers modeling T2DM incidence by age and race/ethnicity report increasing incidence during the elementary school years with a peak in incidence at approximately age 14 years for all racial-ethnic groups (Imperatore et al. 2012). At any age, the incidence of T2DM for African-American, Hispanic, and Asian/Pacific Islander youth is higher than for non-Hispanic whites (Imperatore et al. 2012; Dabelea et al. 2007), and the incidence for children under 10 years old is very low (annual incidence <1 per 100,000) (Dabelea et al. 2007). However, because T2DM develops gradually, can be asymptomatic, and may be misdiagnosed as type 1 diabetes mellitus (T1DM) in children, population estimates of prevalence and incidence must be interpreted cautiously (Amed et al. 2010a).

2.3 Economic Status

Data on the relationship between economic status (of parents) and children and adolescents diagnosed with T2DM are limited, but there are indications of a positive correlation. The treatment options for T2DM in adolescents and youth study (TODAY Study) found that 41.5% of their subjects came from households with an annual income of less than $25,000, and 26.3% were in families in which the highest education level of the parent/guardian was less than a high school degree (Copeland et al. 2011). The association of economic status measured by educational level, occupation, and income with T2DM in adults has been studied extensively and likely offers clues to risk in children and adolescents. A systematic review and meta-analysis that was global in scope found associations with low levels of education (relative risk (RR) = 1.41, 95% CI: 1.28–1.51), with occupation (RR = 1.31, 95% CI: 1.09–1.57), and with low income (RR = 1.31, 95% CI: 1.09–1.57). While the data were limited from middle- and low-income countries in this study, the increased risks were independent of the income levels of countries (Agardh et al. 2011). Another systematic review examining childhood socioeconomic status (SES) as a risk for T2DM found a strong relationship; although this relationship was attenuated by adult SES, a significant relationship remained (Tamayo et al. 2010). Parental education has been found to be associated with insulin resistance in the CARDIA study participants, and the association differed by race and gender. Low parental education was associated with greater insulin resistance in African-American and white females and in African-American males, but not in white males (Tamayo et al. 2012). Smith et al. 2011 found similar results in the Framingham Offspring Study where an inverse relation between cumulative economic status and T2DM in women, but not men, was noted (Smith et al. 2011). These results highlight why untangling the pathways for risk will be difficult.

2.4 Social (Psychological) Stressors

There is strong evidence that acute or chronic stress during critical periods in early life, childhood, and/or adolescence has long-term risks for altered metabolic function including the development of T2DM (Pervanidou and Chrousos 2012). Obesity likely mediates this relation brought on by unhealthy behaviors related to eating and activity patterns as coping mechanisms for chronic stress. Furthermore, chronic stress leads to the dysregulation of the hypothalamic-pituitary-adrenal (HPA) axis, with increased cortisol, catecholamine, and elevated insulin concentrations (Pervanidou and Chrousos 2011). Key stressors in children are recognized as those related to the creation of a safe, stable, and nurturing environment, and when these are disrupted, the child's long-term health suffers (Shonkoff and Garner 2012).

2.5 Summary

These "backdrop" factors are the platform upon which health develops and emerges over time, influenced by dynamic interactions at multiple levels (biological, behavioral, social/cultural) at sensitive periods transacting simultaneously. The next sections illustrate this principle by highlighting key factors within developmental stage that have been linked to pediatric T2DM.

3 Preconception and Intrauterine Life

Over the last 20 years, a significant body of evidence from epidemiological and animal studies has established a strong link between the intrauterine environment and long-term health (Dyer and Rosenfeld 2011; Gluckman et al. 2008; McMillen and Robinson 2005; Sebert et al. 2011; Sinclair et al. 2007). The notion of biological embedding is now widely accepted, even though the mechanisms are not completely understood (Tarry-Adkins and Ozanne 2011). Maternal nutritional status, gestational diabetes, high levels of maternal stress, hypoxia/placental insufficiency, and environmental toxins have been associated with the development of T2DM in children and adolescents (Warner and Ozanne 2010; Boekelheide et al. 2012). Furthermore, the relationship of these high-risk maternal factors to intrauterine growth restriction (IUGR) and small-for-gestational-age (SGA) newborns with their predisposition for obesity, insulin resistance, and T2DM later in life has been established as well. These factors are briefly reviewed below. Several excellent papers review the underlying mechanisms of these relationships in greater depth (Dyer and Rosenfeld 2011; Armitage et al. 2004; Berends and Ozanne 2012; Martin-Gronert and Ozanne 2012; Thayer et al. 2012; Prince et al. 2014).

3.1 Maternal Nutrition: Prior to and During Pregnancy

3.1.1 Maternal Under Nutrition

A series of studies linking low birth weight, maternal undernutrition, and the development of cardiovascular disease has fueled much work on the impact of caloric restriction on the developing fetus (Hales and Barker 2001; Barker et al. 1993). Animal studies have found endocrine and metabolic abnormalities associated with food restrictions (Warner and Ozanne 2010). Data suggest that undernutrition alters the structure and/or function of the developing endocrine-metabolic axis, leading to an insulin resistance and energy conservation in light of reduced calories. An overactivation of the HPA axis leads to increased cortisol levels in growth-restricted fetuses, a situation that mimics chronic stress (Kanaka-Gantenbein 2010; Kapoor et al. 2006). The effects of the undernutrition seem to depend on the timing and extent of the deprivation. In a rodent study, a 50% caloric restriction at the end of the fetal period resulted in reduced β-cell mass (Bertin et al. 2002), and if the caloric restriction continued through early life, the reduction in β-cell mass was permanent (Garofano et al. 1998). Furthermore, the type of diet seems to be important as well. Because of the importance of amino acids in fetal development, studies on the effects of low-protein diets on fetal growth have been pursued with high interest (Fernandez-Twinn et al. 2005). Studies have shown that when dams were fed a low-protein diet, the results were growth-restricted pups, and if the maternal diets remained low protein during suckling, the growth restriction was permanent. Most importantly, these offspring then went on to develop glucose intolerance and T2DM (Hoet et al. 1992).

3.1.2 Maternal Overnutrition

Maternal obesity at the time of pregnancy is known to be associated with a greater risk for child obesity (Salsberry and Reagan 2005), placing them at increased risk for the development of T2DM. Fetal overnutrition has also been associated with insulin resistance and adult diabetes (Armitage et al. 2008). In animal studies, offspring born to obese maternal rats had higher fat-to-lean ratios at birth, and by 3 months of age, these pups were insulin resistant (Samuelsson et al. 2008). When pregnant dams are fed a high-fat content, the offspring are noted to develop a phenotype resembling the human metabolic syndrome (Armitage et al. 2008).

3.2 Maternal Stress

Increased maternal stress is associated with adverse birth outcomes, in particular low birth weight and preterm birth (Christian 2012). Studies demonstrate that maternal exposure to glucocorticoids reduces birth weight in sheep and rats (Tarry-Adkins and Ozanne 2011). Meaney et al. (2007) have suggested that these birth outcomes are mediated by effects on the HPA axis. Stressors in the environment alter maternal physiology and behavior, which then programs HPA activity in the offspring (Meaney et al. 2007). These changes have been linked to the development of T2DM and other components of the metabolic syndrome in the offspring (Brunton 2010).

3.3 Maternal Hypoxia/Placental Insufficiency

Fetal oxygenation is also an independent risk factor for fetal growth abnormalities and long-term development of T2DM. Reduction in fetal oxygenation has also been associated with IUGR, a known risk factor for metabolic syndrome.

Multiple underlying pathophysiological reasons for fetal hypoxia include placental insufficiency, uterine placental ligation, and smoking. These effects all result in IUGR (Tarry-Adkins and Ozanne 2011).

3.4 Environmental Exposures

Exposures to environmental toxins during pregnancy are under increased scrutiny as the evidence builds suggesting significant life course health affects with early-life exposures to a range of chemicals (Thayer et al. 2012). In particular, nicotine, arsenic, and endocrine disrupting chemicals (EDC) are tied to metabolic outcomes. For example, high levels of arsenic exposure have been linked to T2DM in adults, and there is some suggestion that even low doses may also confer an increased T2DM risk (Navas-Acien et al. 2008; Maull et al. 2012). The causal mechanisms include altered glucose metabolism, insulin resistance, and obesity as a result of exposure (Seki et al. 2012). Exposure to EDC, particularly bisphenol A (BPA), is thought to lead to functional changes in gene expression and increased risk for development of obesity and T2DM (Barouki et al. 2012; Liu et al. 2013). This is an area of intense activity that will likely result in significant new knowledge over the next decade.

3.5 Microbiome

There is growing recognition of the importance of the human microbiome in pediatrics (Johnson and Versalovic 2012). During pregnancy a woman's microbiome undergoes significant change from the first to third trimester, changes thought to be beneficial to the mother and the establishment of the neonatal microbiome (Prince et al. 2014; Koren et al. 2012). The infant's microbiota is influenced by the mode of delivery, with colonization in vaginally delivered newborns a function of maternal vaginal and intestinal microbiota, while cesarean delivered newborns exhibit the microbiome of the maternal skin microbiota. The infant's environment and nutrition further influence the infant's developing microbiome (Johnson and Versalovic 2012). These environmental influences on the developing microbiome are critical, as the microbiome is thought to play a role in health and disease (Cenit et al. 2014; Devaraj et al. 2013). Evidence from research in adults suggests that the microbiome plays a critical role in T2DM. Ongoing research is beginning to demonstrate implications for prevention and treatment of metabolic conditions based upon knowledge of the microbiome; extending this work to children is of high importance (Szajewska 2013; Versalovic 2013).

3.6 Gestational Diabetes (GDM)

GDM represents a form of impaired glucose tolerance that is first recognized during pregnancy. Insulin resistance normally occurs in pregnancy. This allows the metabolic needs of the fetus to be met, while an increased maternal insulin secretion compensates for the insulin resistance. But in GDM, this increased resistance is coupled with a failure of increased insulin secretion, resulting in hyperglycemia (Battista et al. 2011). GDM is harmful to the mother and to the fetus. GDM has been shown to alter pancreatic development and insulin sensitivity in the fetus (Warner and Ozanne 2010). Fetal growth is often affected, resulting in macrosomia or large-for-gestational-age infants (Dyer and Rosenfeld 2011). The Hyperglycemia and Adverse Pregnancy Outcome (HAPO) study found a strong linear relation between fasting glucose and post challenge glucose with macrosomia and neonatal adiposity (Metzger et al. 2008). Macrosomic infants born to diabetic mothers have been found to be more glucose intolerant between the ages of 10–16 years, are more likely to be obese, and are at a greater risk for T2DM (Silverman et al. 1998). Because of methodological differences in current studies, the long-term effect of GDM on child outcomes is not fully understood, but studies do suggest that increased rates of obesity, T2DM, and other cardiovascular conditions may result (Kim et al. 2011; Simeoni and Barker 2009).

Screening and Diagnosis Given the convincing evidence that diabetes and gestational diabetes are harmful to both the mother and fetus, considerable effort has been directed toward establishing consensus criteria for the diagnosis of diabetes in pregnancy. There is controversy over the "correct" diabetes threshold, that is, the level at which maternal blood glucose conveys a significant risk to the fetus. The HAPO study, a multisite and multinational study, was designed to address some of these questions. HAPO study results showed a linear relation between increasing levels of fasting and 1 and 2 hour plasma glucose levels post a 75 g oral glucose tolerance test (OGTT) on the primary study outcomes, including birth weight above 90th percentile, cord blood C-peptide level above the 90th percentile, primary cesarean delivery, and neonatal hypoglycemia (Hadar and Hod 2010). These results have led to guidelines issued in 2010 by the International Association of Diabetes and Pregnancy Study Groups (IADPSG) for the detection and diagnosis of hyperglycemic disorders in pregnancy. These guidelines include the determination of the diabetes status of the pregnant woman at the first prenatal visit. Following these guidelines is expected to increase the number of all women with diabetes during pregnancy. These guidelines, however, remain controversial (Moses 2010). There are concerns over increasing costs associated with the identification of a greater number of women with diabetes resulting in an increased number of women receiving treatment.

The American College of Obstetricians and Gynecologists and the National Diabetes Education program have joined together in a call for action, specifically recommending follow-up testing during the postpartum period in women who experienced GDM. Currently only approximately one-half of these women are tested. Recommendations include the following: If the postpartum test is normal, retest every 3 years and at the first prenatal visit for subsequent pregnancies. If prediabetes is diagnosed at the postpartum check, then the recommendation is to test annually (Gabbe et al. 2012).

Treatment Intrauterine conditions are being targeted in the HAPO study. The initial results showed that close control of glucose improved birth outcomes, leading to the new recommendations for the diagnosis and classification of hyperglycemia during pregnancy (Metzger et al. 2010). The HAPO study is also following the outcomes in children born to women with GDM; this longitudinal follow-up may yield important insights for the health of the offspring as well. Early results, however, on offspring at ages 4 and 5 show no difference in body mass index (BMI) in the treatment group (Gillman et al. 2010). Further work with longer follow-up is required to determine if there are latent effects of treatment that will potentially influence outcomes at a later age.

3.7 Summary

Intrauterine life is a sensitive period for T2DM risk development. Building upon the backdrop of genetic susceptibility and within the social and economic context of the mother, the fetus develops an underlying propensity toward T2DM development. Much of this comes through epigenetic changes influenced by maternal nutrition, life stressors, chemical exposures, and maternal behaviors. The occurrence of higher levels of risk is strongly correlated with maternal economic disadvantage and the result of molecular, physiological, behavioral, cultural, and evolutionary processes that interact across time and space. Consistent with the principles of life course health development (LCHD), development of a phenotype at high risk for T2DM development is thus the result of person-environment interactions that are multidimensional, multidirectional, and multilevel, which are highly sensitive to the timing and social structure of environmental exposures.

4 Infancy

4.1 Feeding

Multiple advantages of breastfeeding are well accepted (American Academy of Pedicatrics 2012; James and Lessen 2009), but clarifying the relationship between breastfeeding and future metabolic function is not simple and requires consideration of multiple factors that have effects over one's life course. Controlling social and environmental factors between infancy and some later age is difficult because information for such a long interval is often missing. Despite the limitations, there are several studies that have examined infant feeding type or breastfeeding duration and their relation to dietary habits or cardiometabolic risks. For example, a study that used the Hertfordshire cohort has found an independent association between exclusive breastfeeding (vs. mixed or bottle-feeding) and adherence to healthy dietary recommendations and less intake of processed meat in middle to late adulthood (Robinson et al. 2013). Socioeconomic factors were not associated with the dietary recommendation adherence. The authors speculate breast milk may have provided significant impact on dietary flavor learning during infancy.

In a recent study by Martin et al. (2014), the relationship between cardiometabolic risks and long-term exclusive breastfeeding was examined. This study was a follow-up study of a randomized control study where one group of new mothers was encouraged to undertake exclusive breastfeeding and the other nonexclusive breastfeeding. While the original intervention significantly prolonged breastfeeding duration and exclusiveness, the intervention effect did not influence cardiometabolic factors, such as blood pressure, fasting glucose, insulin, insulin resistance, and adiponectin, when children were at age 11.5 years. A previous follow-up study of this cohort also failed to show intervention effects on anthropometry (height, weight, BMI, and skinfold) and blood pressure at age 6.5 years (Kramer et al. 2009).

Investigating the effects of breastfeeding is complex as there are likely multiple biological and behavioral ways that breastfeeding may influence the infant's health development. Nutrition-focused research studies that examine the importance of the nutrients within breast milk are ongoing. But there are also suggestions that breastfeeding may impact an infant's ability to self-regulate behavior. For example, Taveras et al. (2004), using the US mixed-race cohort, have found that restrictive feeding style is associated with bottle-feeding and shorter breastfeeding duration, which could disrupt the infant's ability to self-regulate feeding behavior. Maternal restrictive feeding style was also found to be associated with increased child's weight for age at 18 months among an African-American sample (Thompson and Bentley 2013).

There has been particular interest in the effects of breastfeeding on children who are exposed to maternal diabetes in utero. The evidence is mixed regarding the effects of breastfeeding among offspring of diabetic mothers (ODM) and development of obesity and T2DM during childhood. A study from Germany found that high consumption of breastmilk during the first 7 days of life among ODM may pose deleterious effects on body weight and glucose tolerance measured at age 2 years (Plagemann et al. 2002). These authors suggest that certain substances contained in early milk of mother's with diabetes may program for metabolic dysregulation in their offspring.

In the Nurses' Health Study II (Mayer-Davis et al. 2006), researchers found that exclusive breastfeeding compared to exclusive formula feeding, or longer duration of breastfeeding (>9 months) compared to never breastfed, was associated with lower odds of being overweight at ages 9–14 years, controlling for child's age, gender, and pubertal development. However, further controlling for other maternal and child factors resulted in null association, and a separate analysis for ODM did not reach statistical significance. A case control study using the SEARCH participants found that longer duration of breastfeeding resulted in a reduction in T2DM, controlling for maternal, child's, and social factors. When the child's weight (measured using BMIz) was included in the analysis, the association was attenuated to null, suggesting that the child's BMIz may mediate the pathway to a diagnosis of T2DM (Mayer-Davis et al. 2008).

The mechanisms involved in the effects of breastfeeding on child's future weight status or risks for T2DM are unclear. However, insulin and other metabolic hormones that are present in breast milk likely play some role. Insulin is present at more than threefold concentration in early milk collected within the first weeks of the postpartum period than in mature milk collected 3 months postpartum (Ley et al. 2012). The insulin concentration in early milk does not appear to be affected by the mother's gestational diabetes status. While the insulin concentration in mature milk of nondiabetic women is not different from that of women with GDM (Ley et al. 2012), maternal prenatal metabolic indicators, such as BMI, fasting glucose, insulin resistance, insulin sensitivity, and adiponectin levels, can predict insulin concentration in mature milk (Ley et al. 2012; Whitmore et al. 2012).

Other research efforts have been focused on infant feeding practices, such as timing of solid food introduction and amount of sugar-sweetened drink during infancy and early childhood, and their effects on childhood obesity development (Gaffney et al. 2012). Another area is investigation of micro- and macronutrient constituents of breast milk. A randomized clinical trial demonstrated that health modifications made to the diets of pregnant and lactating women improved infant metabolic health (Aaltonen et al. 2011). More research is needed to investigate how infant feeding may influence metabolic health development over the life course. An excellent review article summarizes the critical next questions in lactation and neonatal nutrition, providing a road map for this necessary research (Neville et al. 2012).

4.2 Infant Growth Patterns

Several studies (Fabricius-Bjerre et al. 2011; Ekelund et al. 2007; Eriksson et al. 2006) highlight significant associations between infant/childhood growth patterns and development of T2DM and later cardiovascular disease. Because growth is orchestrated by a complex series of interactions between growth hormone, sex steroids, and insulin, tracking growth over time is an important global health measure. Understanding high-risk growth patterns may assist in earlier identification of high-risk children with the potential to begin interventions at an earlier age. The Helsinki Birth Cohort Study (HBCS) 1934–1944 has shown that a small body size at birth with thinness during the first year followed by higher BMIs later in childhood is associated with the development of T2DM (Eriksson 2006). Also, this study found that an early age at adiposity rebound was associated with a markedly increased risk of T2DM in adulthood (Eriksson 2011). An important recent finding suggests that breastfeeding may alter childhood growth even in children exposed to overnutrition during the pregnancy. In the Exploring Perinatal Outcomes among Children (EPOCH) study, breastfeeding was associated with long-term effects on childhood BMI growth extending into late childhood. Slower BMI growth velocity was seen among adequately breastfed (breastfeeding >6 months) children compared with infants who had low breastfeeding status, and these benefits lasted through age 9 years (Crume et al. 2012).

4.3 Sleep Duration

Shortened sleep duration is suggested as a risk factor for obesity, insulin resistance, and Type 2 diabetes among adults. Long-term effects of shortened sleep during infancy on metabolic function are unknown. A limited number of studies that examined the relationship between sleep duration during infancy and subsequent obesity in early childhood have produced conflicting results. For example, studies of US children (Taveras et al. 2008, 2014) have found chronic sleep curtailment from infancy to age 7 years was associated with increased BMI z-scores. Because short sleep hours were associated with longer TV viewing time, the investigators suggested the screen time as one of the potential pathways for the association. Similarly, Bell and Zimmerman (2010) using sample from the Panel Survey of Income Dynamics-Child Development Supplement, reported that shortened night time sleep (less than 9 hours) during early childhood (ages 0–59 months) but not during school age was associated with increased likelihood of being overweight or obese at follow-up at age 5–10 years. Both US studies include relatively large number of minority population (30–50%) whose nighttime sleep is on average shorter than white children. However, studies of Dutch children and Australian children have shown no such association (Hiscock et al. 2011; Klingenberg et al. 2013). The latter two studies utilized objective measures of sleep duration such as actinography, while the US studies have relied on parental report. Improvement in measurement of child's sleep duration and other behavioral markers in longitudinal studies are needed to advance the knowledge in this area.

4.4 Parenting and Postpartum Depression

The impact of maternal postpartum depression on parenting is significant during the first year of life. Mothers who suffer from postpartum depression may lack responsiveness to infant cues for hunger or satiety. However, the studies examining the association between maternal depressive symptoms and child weight status have produced mixed results. Several studies conducted in the USA have shown the association between maternal postpartum depressive symptoms and inappropriate parenting practices such as shorter or less intense breastfeeding (McLearn et al. 2006; Gaffney et al. 2014), inappropriate early feeding practices (Gaffney et al. 2014), and fewer healthy interactions with infants (McLearn et al. 2006). Exposure to chronic maternal depressive symptoms has also been associated with increased risk of childhood overweight (Wang et al. 2013). Cumulative exposure to maternal depressive symptoms in early infancy can lead to disruption of behavioral and metabolic cues for sensation of hunger and satiety. A study involving five European countries, however, has shown no relationship between maternal depressive symptoms and adiposity measures at age 24 months (Grote et al. 2010). The investigators of the latter study noted that prevalence of high depressive symptom scores differed significantly by the participating countries, and therefore, the instrument to measure depressive symptoms used in this study may not be comparably used by the participants across different study sites. More prospective cohort studies focused on the relationship between infant/child development and maternal lifestyles as well as infant's surrounding environment are needed. Cohort studies such as the Amsterdam Born Children and their Development (ABCD) study (van Eijsden et al. 2011) may provide further knowledge on this area.

4.5 Summary

Infant development occurs within a context of "backdrop" factors and as an extension of what has happened during the prior period (fetal life). Because evolutionary life-history theory suggests that development during fetal life prepares the neonate for a particular external environment, when conditions in utero match the conditions in infancy, development unfolds as an extension of pathways begun in utero. When a mismatch occurs between these environments, aspects of development may be compromised. This may be the case when undernutrition in fetal life is followed by an abundance of nutrients postnatally, a particularly risky circumstance for metabolic health. The important point is that infant health development must be seen as conditioned by the interaction of processes and conditions during intrauterine life, and that this wider lens brings into sharper focus the multiple interacting risks contributing to the development of T2DM. Our examinations of how experiences in infancy feed forward into this continuously evolving health developmental process suggest that long-term health behaviors are beginning to be set through complex transactions between maternal behaviors and preferences regarding feeding and sleep (both of which are influenced by the mother's own environment and psychological state) and the infant's developing behavioral response patterns.

5 Childhood

5.1 Childhood Overweight and Obesity

Almost all children and adolescents with T2DM are also overweight or obese, and excess adiposity, particularly visceral adiposity, is associated with insulin resistance (Dabelea et al. 2007; Haines et al. 2007; Amed et al. 2010b). Studies with US and Canadian youth have found that 75–95% of those with T2DM are obese (BMI percentile > 95th for age and sex) (Mayer-Davis et al. 2009; Amed et al. 2010b; Liu et al. 2009; Lawrence et al. 2009b; Bell et al. 2009). Another study in obese children found that 25% of obese children 4–10 years of age and 21% of 11–18 years of age were found to have an impaired glucose tolerance. Silent T2DM was identified in 4% of the obese adolescents (Sinha et al. 2002). Researchers in the UK using the International Obesity Task Force (IOTF) cut point for defining obesity (which is higher than the US reference (Rolland-Cachera 2011)) found that 83% of youth with T2DM were obese (Haines et al. 2007). These results clearly point to the importance of understanding the underlying factors that contribute to childhood obesity, and also point toward the complex path that underlies the development of T2DM. Further understanding of how multiple factors interact, with a key emphasis toward the timing of these factors in reference to the life course is needed (Ong 2010; Tounian 2011).

5.2 Impaired Glucose Tolerance and Progression to T2DM

Obese children may have deficits in glucose regulation that predict future T2DM, as well as less favorable risk factor profiles for cardiovascular disease (West et al. 2009; Burns et al. 2014). Evidence of impaired glucose tolerance, elevated fasting glucose, insulin resistance, and/or previously undiagnosed "silent" T2DM has been documented in multiple samples of obese youth (Wabitsch et al. 2004; Sinha et al. 2002; Morrison et al. 2012). Morrison et al. (2012) studied 259 overweight and obese children and adolescents (aged 5–17 years) who were seeking weight-loss treatment and found that >20% had prediabetes—impaired glucose tolerance as measured by an oral glucose tolerance test or elevated fasting glucose (Morrison et al. 2012). Among these youth with prediabetes, a majority with impaired glucose tolerance did not have elevated fasting glucose levels (Morrison et al. 2012), which is consistent with findings from an Italian study (Morandi et al. 2014). The current American Diabetes Association (ADA) guidelines (American Diabetes Association 2010) recommend that overweight children ≥10 years or pubertal with two or more additional risk factors for T2DM have their fasting glucose measured (see Table 1). ADA guidelines do not recommend screening youth with an oral glucose tolerance test. Morrison et al. found that the sensitivity and specificity of the ADA criteria to identify youth with prediabetes were respectively 39% and 70%. Furthermore, in their sample the prevalence of prediabetes in children 5–9 years old was not significantly different from that of youth ≥10 years old (Morrison et al. 2012). Some evidence indicates that elevated fasting triglycerides may help to identify obese children and adolescents who would benefit from an oral glucose tolerance test (Morrison et al. 2012; Morandi et al. 2014). More longitudinal studies of children at risk for T2DM are needed to elucidate the natural history and progression of the disorder. In a sample of 117 obese children and adolescents (4–18 years) in which two oral glucose tolerance tests were administered between 18 and 24 months apart, Weiss et al. 2005 found that of 38 youth with impaired glucose tolerance at the first time point, 8 developed T2DM, 10 still had impaired glucose tolerance, and 15 (46%) had normal glucose tolerance at the second time point (Weiss et al. 2005). Among the 84 youth with normal glucose tolerance initially, 8 had impaired glucose tolerance at the follow-up assessment (Weiss et al. 2005). Progression from prediabetes to T2DM has been studied among adults (Morris

Table 1 Summary of screening guidelines for T2DM: Childhood overweight and obesity

	Year	Recommendations	Other risk factors
Diabetes screening			
Expert Committee (Barlow 2007)	2007	BMI > 85th% and aged ≥ 10 years with ≥2 other risk factors FGT or 2 h. GTT; BMI ≥ 95th% and aged ≥ 10 years FGT every 2 years	Parental obesity Family history Current lifestyle BMI trajectory CVD risk factors (HBP, cholesterol)
ADA (Amercian Diabetes Association 2000)	2012	BMI > 85th% or weight > % of ideal for height with ≥2 other risk factors screened every 3 years beginning at age 10 years or onset of puberty, whichever is earlier. Testing done every 2 years	Family history of T2DM in first or second-degree relatives Certain race/ethnic groups[b] Signs of insulin resistance or conditions associated with insulin resistance (AN, HTN, dyslipidemia, PCOS, SGA) Maternal diabetes or GDM
ISPAD[a] (International Society for Pediatric and Adolescent Diabetes)	2011	BMI > 85th% with other risk factors. In Asian children, screen with low or high birth weight with 1 risk factor, regardless of BMI	Immediate family history of T2DM, early family history of CVD, or Signs of insulin resistance (AN, dyslipidemia, HBP, PCOS)
Overweight/Obesity screening			
USPSTF (Barton 2010)	2010	Screen at 6 year and older for obesity	
Expert Committee (Barlow 2007)	2007	Every well child visit: height and weight, calculate and plot BMI	

[a]The ISPAD guidelines are also sensitive to country resources, so that screening decisions will likely be tied directly to the health-care resources with a country
[b]Native American, African-American, Latino, Asian American, Pacific Islander

et al. 2013), and although less is currently known about how the disease develops in children and adolescents, this is an area of active investigation.

5.3 Diabetes Prevention

A number of lifestyle interventions to prevent T2DM in youth at high risk have been evaluated in randomized trials. The Yale Bright Bodies Healthy Lifestyle program is an intensive 6-month behavioral intervention for obese youth and their families that has been evaluated in multiple randomized controlled trials (Savoye et al. 2007, 2011, 2014). Among 174 ethnically diverse children and adolescents aged 8–16 years—69 assigned to the control condition—the youth in the intervention group showed reductions in adiposity at 6 months that were maintained at 1 year as well as reductions in fasting insulin levels, which were seen at 6 months and also maintained for 1 year (Savoye et al. 2007). These youth were also assessed 24 months after the start of the trial and the favorable changes in body composition and insulin sensitivity seen at 6 and 12 months were sustained at similar levels at 24 months (Savoye et al. 2011). A subsequent trial among 10–16-year-olds with prediabetes ($n = 38$ receiving the Bright Bodies intervention and $n = 37$ standard clinical care) also demonstrated improvements in glucose metabolism and insulin sensitivity as well as reductions in adiposity and improved fitness (Savoye et al. 2014). Such results are encouraging, and although the intervention is intensive, it uses a standardized curriculum and is likely to be cost-effective long term (Savoye et al. 2014).

The HEALTHY Study was a national 3-year middle-school intervention program designed to reduce risk factors for type 2 diabetes. It used a randomized trial designed to determine whether changes to the school environment of middle-school students over a 3-year period could impact their risk for T2DM (Foster et al. 2010; Hirst et al. 2009). Prevention of T2DM in youth involves encouraging changes in eating and activity behaviors that should also reduce risk for obesity. Although many large and well-conducted randomized trials of school-based interventions to prevent obesity have had limited impact on obesity prevalence (Luepker et al. 1996; Caballero et al. 2003; Brown and Summerbell 2009), such interventions may improve glucose homeostasis and other risk factors for T2DM (Trevino et al. 2004; Rosenbaum et al. 2007). The Healthy Study was a group randomized trial conducted in 42 middle schools (21 intervention, 21 control) in 7 areas of the USA between fall 2006 and spring 2009 (Hirst et al. 2009). Students were in 6th grade when enrolled and in 8th grade when outcomes were assessed. The interventions in the Healthy Study included changes to the school environment with regard to nutrition (Gillis et al. 2009), physical activity (McMurray et al. 2009), and health messaging (Venditti et al. 2009). The primary outcome was prevalence of BMI ≥85th percentile (overweight and obesity), and at baseline about 50% of students in intervention and control schools were overweight or obese (Kaufman et al. 2009). Over the course of the study, this prevalence decreased in intervention schools to 45.8% and in control schools to 45.2%, and thus there was not an effect of the intervention on the prevalence of overweight and obesity (Foster et al. 2010). However, the intervention did have a modest and statistically impact on the secondary outcomes of obesity, mean BMI z-score, high waist circumference, and fasting insulin levels (Foster et al. 2010). These results suggest that changes to the school environment regarding nutrition, physical activity, and health messaging may reduce the risk of childhood onset of T2DM (Foster et al. 2010)

Some evidence suggests that interventions targeting physical fitness may be as effective in reducing risk for T2DM in youth as multicomponent interventions. Among obese 7–11-year-old children, a program of 40 min of aerobic exercise 5 days per week for 4 months reduced adiposity and insulin levels, but these effects were not sustained in the absence of the program (Ferguson et al. 1999). A dose-response effect for the benefit of time spent in exercise on fitness and cardiometabolic measures of T2DM risk was demonstrated in a subsequent study of overweight and obese 7–11-year-olds randomized to a 10–15-week program of 20 or 40 min per school day of aerobic activity or to a control group (Davis et al. 2012). Similar findings were noted in a pilot randomized study in which physical activity was added to a family-based weight control treatment. The exercise group had lower visceral abdominal fat posttreatment, a result that may be key in future work to reduce diabetes risk (Saelens et al. 2011). In a YMCA-based program targeted to prevent the development of T2DM in high-risk inner-city African-American children (TAT: Taking Action Together), initial results were encouraging with improvement in glucoregulation in boys (but not girls) and a decrease in BMI z-scores in the treatment group (Ritchie et al. 2010; Raman et al. 2010).

5.4 Obesity Prevention

Because of the strong association between obesity and T2DM, much of the literature that discusses prevention of T2DM focuses on weight reduction or healthy weight maintenance throughout childhood. In a systematic review of the effectiveness of weight management interventions in children, the US Preventative Services Task Force (USPSTF) results support at least in the short term benefits of comprehensive medium-to-high intensity behavioral interventions in children 6 years and older (Whitlock et al. 2010). The outcomes studied in the USPSTF review were limited to childhood weight and not the progression to T2DM (see Table 1).

Recent evidence points to the importance and benefit of intervening early in children's lives to reduce obesity (Knowlden and Sharma 2012), and a number of randomized controlled treatment trials in preschool-aged children have demonstrated success. An intensive 16-week multidisciplinary program for overweight or obese Dutch children aged 3–5 years and their parent was compared to a "usual-maintained care" control, and results showed reductions in BMI and waist circumference that were for 12 months (Bocca et al. 2012a). Among 33 obese preschool-aged (2–5 years) children in the Midwest USA, a pilot randomized trial compared two 6-month multidisciplinary treatment programs (one in which all sessions were held at a clinic and another program that alternated between clinic sessions and individual home-based visits by a pediatric psychology fellow); both interventions were consistent with Expert Committee (Barlow 2007) stage 3 recommendations and were compared to a control condition of pediatrician counseling as recommended by the Expert Committee as stage 1 treatment (Stark et al. 2014). Compared to pediatrician counseling, children in the intervention with home visits group had greater reductions in BMI z-score at 6 months (end of intervention) and at 12 months than did children in the clinic only intervention (Stark et al. 2014). These results suggest that parents of obese preschool-aged children may benefit from in-home guidance regarding implementation and maintenance of parenting behaviors related to weight reduction. In an observational study of children aged 6–16 years seeking treatment for obesity in Sweden, researchers evaluated whether age and severity of obesity impacted the likelihood of treatment success over a 3-year period (Danielsson et al. 2012). They found that younger children (6–9 years) were more likely to have clinically meaningful reductions in weight status than older children and adolescents, and that treatment success was rare for adolescents particularly if they were severely obese (Danielsson et al. 2012). The difficulties associated with treating obesity once it is established underscore the need to prevent excess weight gain in young children before they become obese.

It is well established that parents play a key role in obesity treatment efforts directed at youth (Kitzmann et al. 2010), and for obvious reasons parents are the main audience for obesity prevention efforts in early childhood (Skouteris et al. 2011, 2012; Hesketh and Campbell 2010). Interventions directed at parents of infants have shown promise in reducing children's risk for obesity (Campbell et al. 2013; Wen et al. 2012), and parents of infants may be receptive to messaging aimed at increasing adoption of healthy eating and activity behaviors. Emerging evidence also suggests that interventions to promote positive parenting in general may help to reduce risk for childhood obesity (Harvey-Berino and Rourke 2003; Brotman et al. 2012). Maternal warmth and sensitivity are associated in prospective cohort studies with lower risk for obesity (Anderson et al. 2012, 2014). An explanatory mechanism may involve the impact of responsive parenting on the child's developing stress response system and regulatory pathways in the limbic areas of the brain (McEwen 2008; Schore 2005). In a national sample of preschool-aged children, the household routines of having family meals, ensuring that children get adequate sleep, and limiting time spent watching television were associated with lower prevalence of obesity (Anderson and Whitaker 2010). A randomized trial of a 6-month home-based intervention to promote these household routines in a sample of low-income families of 2–5-year-old children reduced children's BMI (Haines et al. 2013).

Recent evidence points to the importance of intervening early. In a randomized clinical trial targeting 3–5-year-old overweight or obese children, a multidisciplinary program reduced BMI, BMI z-scores, waist circumference, and waist circumference z-scores compared to a usual treatment control group. The treatment results were still present 12 months after the start of the intervention (Bocca et al. 2012b). A 6-month intensive home-based behavioral intervention program aimed at obese preschoolers (ages 2–5 years) has also shown promise in reducing BMI z-scores, both during the treatment period and at 12 months follow-up (Saelens et al. 2011). In an observational study of obese children ages 6–16 years, all were exposed to a behavioral treatment; changes in BMIs across a 3-year treatment window showed that younger aged children (6–9 compared with 14–16 years) were more successful in improving outcomes (Danielsson et al. 2012).

5.5 Screening Guidelines

Given what we know about factors associated with diabetes, screening for T2DM in children and adolescents is linked to weight status of the child, age of the child, and pubertal status. Several groups have published guidelines for T2DM screening in children. These guidelines are summarized in Table 1.

5.5.1 Growth in Childhood

Birth weight and growth trajectories have both been recognized as factors that are associated with the life course risk of T2DM. Given this, it seems key that individuals from the start understand their risk and that primary-care providers collect these data for all children. Surprisingly few guidelines currently recommend including birth weight as a component of a child's risk assessment for T2DM. An exception to this is the ISPAD screening guidelines that include birth size in their guidelines for Asian children. No recommendations were found that considered the actual growth of the child with respect to possible high-risk trajectories. Including birth size and growth as screeners for high-risk children has yet to be fully examined. A better understanding of the growth trajectory may be useful in identifying high-risk children earlier, but further work is needed in this area.

5.6 Summary

Childhood is the period where health behaviors are formed. While there is evidence that these behaviors are influenced by experience in the prior developmental periods, there is also evidence that significant change is still possible, especially in children under 5 years. Increasing evidence from both observational and intervention studies suggests that behavioral change is possible early on, but by middle childhood it becomes increasingly more difficult to affect real behavior change. These findings are pushing the research community to design studies that include young children, and the evidence is accumulating that interventions at the youngest ages achieve the best outcomes. During this period the child's world widens as he/she transitions into preschool and kindergarten, raising further the need to widen the focus of intervention beyond the family.

6 Adolescence

6.1 Transition into Adolescence

Puberty is an important phase in the life course that needs to be considered in studying the risks for T2DM. During puberty there is a known physiological insulin resistance and hyperinsulinemia that is thought to facilitate pubertal weight gain and growth (Burt Solorzano and McCartney 2010). The timing of the start of this insulin resistance has been reported to begin in mid-childhood, some years before puberty (Jeffery et al. 2012). Understanding this insulin resistance as it relates to the pubertal process is of high importance, as the rates of childhood diabetes continue to rise. Obesity exaggerates this pubertal insulin resistance, especially in girls, and may partially explain advanced maturation in obese females (Burt Solorzano and McCartney 2010).

6.2 Diagnosis of T2DM

The rising prevalence of both type 1 and type 2 among children and adolescents, in conjunction with increasing obesity throughout the population, has complicated the diagnosis of diabetes type. Past reliance on phenotype to distinguish and diagnose type of diabetes is not reliable (Amed et al. 2010a; Rosenbloom et al. 2008). In obese adolescents who present with new-onset diabetes, measurement of pancreatic autoantibodies is recommended as necessary to differentiate the type of diabetes (Zeitler 2010).

6.3 Treatment

Overall, there are few published evidence-based treatment studies for pediatric T2DM. The ADA and the ISPAD have published treatment recommendations, but these are primarily consensus based and built on current guidelines for adult T2DM (Amed et al. 2010a; Herbst et al. 2014). There are a handful of studies that have either been conducted or are ongoing specifically to address pediatric T2DM, studies which address both questions of prevention and treatment.

Treatment for T2DM has been addressed in a large multicenter randomized clinical trial, the Treatment Options for T2DM in Adolescents and Youth (known as the TODAY Study) (Copeland et al. 2011). Subjects were between the ages of 10 and 17, diagnosed with T2DM for less than 2 years, and had a BMI percentile at or above the 85th percentile for age and sex. Subjects were randomized into one of 3 comparison groups: metformin monotherapy, metformin plus rosiglitazone, or metformin plus an intensive family lifestyle program. Rates of failure (defined as poor glycemic control) were 52% in metformin alone, 39% in metformin plus rosiglitazone, and 47% in metformin plus the lifestyle program. Greatest weight loss was seen in the metformin plus the lifestyle program (Zeitler et al. 2012). These results highlight the difficulty that the majority of adolescents have in maintaining good glycemic control and suggest that many will require insulin within a few years of diagnosis. Ongoing research is needed to determine optimal management strategies in adolescents with T2DM.

The goal of therapy is to achieve euglycemia. The blood glucose levels should be monitored based on individual needs. Self- monitored blood glucose testing may be done at premeal times, or limited to before breakfast and before dinner only. Postprandial blood glucose levels, obtained 2 h after dinner, also offer helpful data for dose titration. The hemoglobin A1c is monitored at the time of clinic follow-up every 3 months. This reflects the average blood glucose over the past 3-month period. The aim of treatment is to achieve a hemoglobin A1c of less than 6.5% and the target blood glucose range = 70–120 mg/dl.

The first intervention for treatment of T2DM remains healthy lifestyle modifications including dietary modifications (including decreasing caloric intake) and increasing physical activity and exercise regimens to achieve weight stabilization and ultimately weight loss. Data from a recent study suggests that regular exercise was associated with lowering of the hemoglobin A1c (Herbst et al. 2014). Initiating changes in portion control as well as food choices and implementing modest amounts of exercise often prove difficult. Often adolescents have long-standing overweight and obesity concerns. Lifestyle changes tend to be more successful if initiated by the whole family instead of the particular individual being targeted.

If the diagnostic parameters are consistent with T2DM, pharmacologic treatment will need to be initiated. The particular therapeutic regimen initiated is determined by the initial presentation of T2 DM. If the adolescent presents in diabetic ketoacidosis, insulin therapy is instituted, initially intravenously, with subsequent transition to subcutaneous insulin therapy after the resolution of the acute diabetes ketoacidosis phase. Oral medication, specifically metformin, is initiated as well once the ketosis has resolved. If the presentation of T2DM is less acute, with the diagnosis being made on routine office testing, and hemoglobin A1c is less than 9%, medication therapy may be initiated first with metformin. In patients with symptomatology in between these 2 scenarios, where hemoglobin A1c is more than 9% in the presence of typical symptomatology, but no diabetes ketoacidosis, therapy may be initiated with metformin along with basal insulin (Zeitler et al. 2014). Other medications used for treatment of T2DM in adults are not approved for adolescents below 16 years of age.

Adherence to therapeutic interventions is key for achieving adequate diabetes control and is strongly emphasized. Modifications to regimen are based on hemoglobin A1c and review of blood glucose data. Adolescents who are on metformin therapy as well as basal insulin may need additional rapid acting insulin to cover their meals. Adolescents who were initiated on insulin and metformin, and achieve goal A1c, are feasible to gradually decrease the insulin dose, after they are on maximal metformin dosing. If adolescents are able to modify lifestyle factors as well as manage medication therapy adequately, it may be feasible to discontinue insulin altogether, while continuing on metformin therapy, albeit done very gradually with close monitoring.

6.3.1 Bariatric Surgery

Bariatric surgery for weight loss or uncontrolled T2DM is not commonly undertaken in the adolescent population. Results obtained in studies with adults that report weight loss and improvement in T2DM after bariatric surgery procedures (Courcoulas et al. 2014) has caused increased interest in its use in adolescents with morbid obesity. When bariatric surgery has been used as a treatment strategy for extreme obesity in adolescents, it has been found to be effective in improving or reversing abnormal glucose metabolism, but long-term outcome data in this age group is not yet available. This treatment option is limited to a very specific population because of potential complications (Brandt et al. 2010).

6.4 Surveillance

Comorbidities associated with T2DM should be investigated and treated as needed based on individual clinical presentation. The ADA and the ISPAD have published guidelines for comorbidity screening in youth diagnosed with T2DM. These guidelines are summarized in Table 2.

In a study examining adherence to ADA recommendations for lipid levels, blood pressure, hemoglobin A1c, microalbuminuria, and eye examinations, 95% of the participants reported having their blood pressure checked at all or most visits, 88% had lipid levels measured, 83% had kidney function tested, 68% underwent HbA1c testing, and 66% underwent an eye examination (Waitzfelder et al. 2011). Participants aged 18 years or older, particularly those with T2DM, tended to have fewer tests of all kinds performed. Age and family income emerged as important correlates of overall quality of care in multivariate models: older age and lower income were associated with not meeting the guidelines. Overall, while there was good compliance with the ADA-recommended guidelines, efforts to improve HbA1c testing and eye examinations were needed, especially among older adolescents and young adults (Waitzfelder et al. 2011).

6.5 Comorbidities

The TODAY study has demonstrated that a significant portion of adolescents with T2DM develop comorbidities. Careful attention to these

Table 2 Summary of surveillance guidelines for comorbidities

	Year	Recommendations
ADA (American Diabetes Association 2000)	2012	Blood pressure measurement annually Fasting lipid profile Microalbuminuria assessment Dilated eye examination performed at the time of diagnosis Evaluation of polycystic ovarian disease and other comorbidities such as sleep apnea, hepatic steatosis, orthopedic complications, and psychosocial concerns
ISPAD (ISPAD 2011)	2011	Blood pressure measured at least annually Initial eye examination within 3 months of diagnosis and then annually from 11 years on after 2 years of diabetes duration Annual screening for microalbuminuria from age 11 and after 2 years of diabetes duration Fasting blood lipids after initial diagnosis and stabilization of diabetes ≥12 years; if family history of hypercholesterolemia, early CVD, or family history is unknown, screening should start at 2 years Peripheral and autonomic neuropathy assessed by history and physical exam from age 11 years with 2 years of diabetes duration

must be part of any management plan for these youths. Common comorbidities include hypertension and other metabolic conditions. Table 2 summarizes guidelines for monitoring the development of comorbidities in children/adolescents with T2DM.

6.6 Care Transition into Adult Practice

The emerging adult period (ages 18–30 years) is a high-risk time for youth with T2DM. These transitions from the pediatric to adult care setting often result in loss to follow-up at a time when the emergence of complications is occurring and the youth are engaging in high-risk health behaviors (Peters and Laffel 2011). In the majority of health-care institutions, there are no well-structured, seamless processes in place to ensure smooth transitions of care for any chronic care condition. Furthermore, there is little evidence-based research to guide practice on the management of this care transition in youth with T2DM. In the absence of evidenced-based programs and because of concerns about this transition, many programs are in the process of designing and/or implementing transition of care initiatives (Lee 2013). In 2011, a consensus-based document outlining recommendations for transition from pediatric and to adult diabetes care systems was published. Part of this document specifically highlighted the need for research to determine the best strategies for transition to diabetic adult care to assure optimal outcomes for the youth (Peters and Laffel 2011).

6.7 Summary

Because T2DM is most likely diagnosed during or shortly after puberty, the emphasis in adolescence is focused on understanding the components of care for the disease, including the surveillance for and management of comorbidities. In adolescence the consequences of the child's early environments are becoming clear and the window for prevention has narrowed.

7 Summary and Recommendations

7.1 Summary

- Pediatric T2DM is a life course problem—this chapter demonstrates that no one factor and no one time period provides the explanation; prevention and treatment is not simple. To optimize childhood metabolic health, we must begin prior to conception and at every age seize the opportunities to shape the child's environment to enhance metabolic health development.
- Significant progress has been made in describing the growing pediatric T2DM epidemic and in identifying individual risk factors that contribute to its development. Work is ongoing to understand the underlying mechanisms of pediatric T2DM. This knowledge base will likely grow rapidly over the next decade.
- A major limitation of much of this work is that the studies tend to be singularly focused on exploring and understanding a particular risk, and are completed using a specific disciplinary approach. What is missing from most of this literature is the recognition that these risks exist within a dynamic developmental context with implications from micro- to macrosystems. The next generation of studies needs to consider how risks play out differently depending upon prior or current exposures and environments. What are the risk modifiers and mediators?
- Accounting for the influence of time-specific exposures during sensitive developmental periods in conjunction with exposures across time is limited in the current research, and must be addressed more thoroughly in future studies.
- Another major task facing pediatric T2DM researchers is to understand the developmental similarities and differences in T2DM between children and adults. When T2DM "threatens" or occurs in children/adolescents, the challenges of understanding and intervening are different from those in the adult population, both biologically and behaviorally.

- Pediatric T2DM must be understood within the dynamic context of the child's overall health development. Research on the factors and developmental processes occurring early in life has shown how the emergence of T2DM children and adolescents is conditioned by prior experiences, exposures, and response patterns earlier in the life course.
- Translating the current knowledge into practice-relevant evidence is lagging and must be accelerated.

7.2 Recommendations

7.2.1 Recommendation 1: To Continue to Elucidate Mechanisms that Contributes to Pediatric T2DM by Focusing the Research in Key Areas

There are several parts to this recommendation including the identification of substantive research areas to guide further work, as well as recommendations about the process for doing the work. Life course health development research will require transdisciplinary teams of scientists that examine phenomenon across different levels (genetic, cellular, biological systems, families, neighborhoods, and large and complex macrosystems) at different developmental stage of the child. No one individual, and no one discipline, can achieve this knowledge by working in a disciplinary silo.

There are several areas that will require further investigation, and in particular we need to increase our understanding of factors that may mitigate the effects of adverse early-life programming. Childhood adversity, including the type of adversity (e.g., resource lack compared with family chaos), and chronic stress are noted as likely to be involved in the biological programming of several chronic health conditions including pediatric T2DM, but this is poorly accounted for in most of the current studies. Inclusion of poverty and family stress get at some of these factors, but better conceptual and empirical models are needed. Furthermore, the timing of the exposure for these risks is also not well documented, and their time-specific impacts are not well understood (i.e., is it poverty during pregnancy, during early childhood, or both?). On the positive side, there is a small but growing literature on the importance of parenting style, particularly nurturing behaviors, as possibly ways of mitigating the negative effects of various types of adverse environmental contexts.

Research priorities include:

- Understanding the health capital and health development capacity that mothers (and fathers) bring to conception and determine which of these factors are most important for child health development
- Determining how adult-recognized T2DM genetic susceptibility applies in pediatric T2DM
- Increased work to identify the epigenetic changes that occur in response to risk exposures (e.g., environmental toxins, stressors)
- Nutrition research, at every stage of childhood
- Understanding how health behaviors develop across time

But none of these are factors will provide a satisfactory explanation in isolation; each must be conditioned on prior and co-occurring factors. A life course health development perspective suggests that research must be embedded within the life stage of the child, taking into account the child's full developmental history, including the intrauterine period. Exploring contemporaneous factors, e.g., physical activity, and their association with T2DM should be done conditional on prior life course exposures, not simply on current factors; for example, knowing that the child was exposed to diabetes in utero and the birth size of the infant may be key markers for understanding differential effects of contemporaneous factors. Figure 1 integrates these ideas to display the life stages along the horizontal axis and prevention, screening, and treatment/surveillance along the y axis. Embedded within this figure but not displayed because of the complexity is that at each point multiple factors from multiple levels are transacting simultaneously to bring about an outcome.

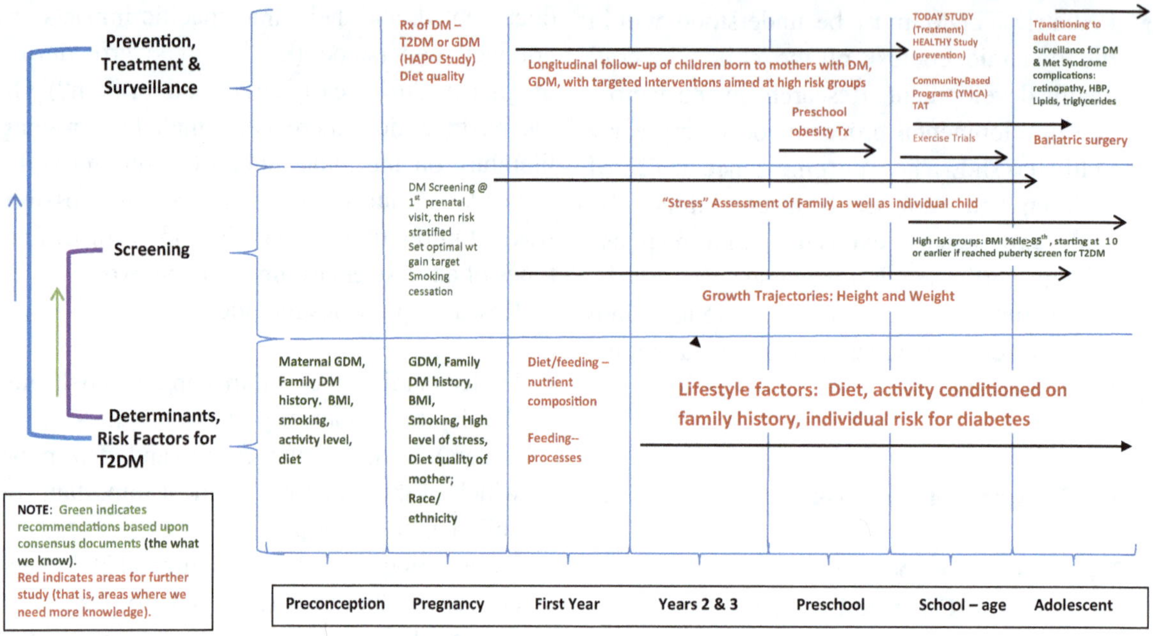

Fig. 1 A life course approach for understanding the risks, prevention and treatment of type 2 diabetes

7.2.2 Recommendation 2: To Strengthen Data and Methods Used to Address Identified Research Priorities and Explore the Feasibility of an International Effort to Harmonize Ongoing Birth Cohorts for the Purpose of Developing a Better Understanding of the Timing, Dose, and Interaction of Factors that Contribute to Pediatric T2DM Worldwide

Few data sets used to study the onset and impacts of T2DM include significant information on the broader context of the family, school, or neighborhood. In studies with good social data, biological data are often not included. A wider (micro to macro contexts) and longer (birth through adolescence) lens is needed to study T2DM. The need for longitudinal studies that can provide this lens is widely noted in the research literature, but because of the costs and subject burden, these long-term studies are difficult to carry out. However, there are a large number of longitudinal birth cohort studies ongoing worldwide that may have the potential for improving the understanding of pediatric T2DM. The recommendation here is to explore the feasibility of an international effort to harmonize ongoing birth cohorts to develop a better understanding of the timing, dose, and interactions of factors that contribute to T2DM worldwide. An added benefit of the development of such a data set is that it would provide the data to generate and test hypotheses, not just about T2DM but data directly relevant to the testing of the life course health development theoretical framework.

Table 3 presents an overview of international birth cohort studies. Of these studies, one dates to the 1950s, one to the 1960s, two during the 1970s, and another two in the 1980s. Twelve of the birth cohorts began data collection in the 1990s and 21 began data collection between 2000 and 2011. From this list, there are a handful of studies with data elements (birth data, multiple data collection points throughout childhood, including adolescent health and height and weight) pertinent to informing a life course picture of key pathways in this epidemic. Six birth cohorts were identified as having collected data beyond 1995 and included at least one data collection point in adolescence (defined as data

Table 3 Birth cohort longitudinal studies

Cohort/country	Years	Ages/data collection points	Sample characteristics	Measures	Comments: PI/Managing entity// website
Early Childhood Longitudinal Study—Birth cohort/US (ECLS)	Births in 2001	Birth through kindergarten entry: 9 months, 2 years, 4 years, and kindergarten	14,000 diverse nationally rep. sample; oversampling of API, AI, and Alaskan natives, twins, LBW	Cognitive, social, emotional, physical development—assessments, parents, child care settings, and KGT	National Center for Education Statistics http://nces.ed.gov/ecls
National Child Development Study (NCDS): UK 1958 Cohort	Births in 1958	1958, 7, 11, 16, 23, 33, 42, 46, 50; in 2003 @45, 9000 in biomedical screens	17,000 born during 1 week in 1958 in England, Scotland, Wales	Physical, educational, economic, employment, family life, health behaviors, well-being, social participation, attitudes	Centre for Longitudinal Studies, Institute of Education: Jane Elliot, PI http://www.cls.ioe.ac.uk/
1970 British Cohort Study	Births in 1970	1970, 5, 10, 16, 30, 34, and 42 (in 2012)	17,000 people born in England, Scotland, Wales in single week in 1970	Health, physical educational and social development, economic circumstances	Managed by Centre for Longitudinal Studies, Institute of Education; Alice Sullivan, PI http://www.cls.ioe.ac.uk/
Millennium Cohort Study	Births in 2000–2001	9 months, 3, 5, 7, 11 (in 2012) plus health visitor survey report and fertility survey report	19,000 people in the UK	Sibling and parent info; parenting, childcare, school choice, child behavior and cognitive development, child and parent health, parent's employment and education, income, poverty, neighborhood, and residential mobility; social capital and ethnicity	Managed by Centre for Longitudinal Studies, Institute of Education Lucinda Platt, PI http://www.cls.ioe.ac.uk/
Growing up in Scotland (GUS)	Births in Scotland: 2003/2004 birth cohort 1 and 2010/2011 birth cohort 2	Data collection yearly on the early cohorts; for the 2010 cohorts—only at key transitions	8000 children were enrolled into the study in 2005–20065000 were babies (~10 months) born between 6/ 2004 and 5/ 20053000 were toddlers (~34 months) born between 6/2002 and 5/ 2003. 6000 children born between 3/2010 and 2/ 2011 will be enrolled during 2010–2011; data collection at 10 months old.	Education, social work/support for parents, health, childcare, social inclusion	*Centre for Research onFamilies and Relationships*—University of Edinburghhttp://growingupinscotland.org.uk/
Growing up in Ireland	Births in 1999/2000 for older cohort; 2007/2008 for infant cohort	Two rounds of data collections with each group	8500 9-year-olds and 11,000 9-month-olds interviewed during September 2008 to April 2009. Second round data collection took place between January and August 2011.	The main aim of the study is to paint a full picture of children in Ireland and how they are developing in the current social, economic, and cultural environment	PI: Professor James Williams at Trinity College Dublin. http://www.growingup.ie/

(continued)

Table 3 (continued)

Cohort/country	Years	Ages/data collection points	Sample characteristics	Measures	Comments: PI/Managing entity// website
NLSY: Children of the '79	US	The NLSY child sample is comprised of all children born to the NLSY79 mothers; mothers have been interviewed biennially; data on child begins at birth through adulthood	More than 11,000 children have been identified; birth years range from 1979 through 2010	Cognitive, behavioral, health status, home environment, psychosocial, parental involvement, economic conditions of the family, risky behaviors	Access to in data available at Bureau of Labor Statistics web site www.bls.gov/nls/nlsy79.htm
Panel study of income dynamics (PSID)	US Birth 1968 and ongoing	Birth through adulthood. Annually from 1968 to 1997, biennially 1998. Child development supplement 1n 1997 from birth –12 and 2002/2003 for 5–18 years. 2007/2008 at 10–18 years. 18 years transition to adulthood at '05,'07, '09, '11	70,000 individuals over four decades. Includes initial participants from 1968 and their biological/adopted descendants. 1997 and 1999 included 511 immigrants to the USA	Cognitive, behavioral and health status. Afterschool physical activities, home environment, psychosocial, parental involvement, schooling and school environment	http://psidonline.isr.umich.edu/Guide/default.aspx
National Longitudinal Survey of Children and Youth	Canada 1994 and ongoing	Birth to early adulthood—eight cycles with varying age ranges (0–25 years)	Cycle 8: 35,795 children	Child health, family psychosocial, emotional, development, teenage risk behaviors	http://www.statcan.gc.ca/start-debut-eng.html

Danish Longitudinal Survey of Children	Denmark 1995 and 2003	Birth to adulthood: Birth 1995, 1996, 1999, 2003, 2007 (11 years old)	6011 children (born Sept 15-Oct 31, 1995 and mothers are Danish citizens); 611 children (born April 1-Dec 31, 1995 and mothers had been residing in Demark for 3 years); 6000 children born in 1995 who were placed in group homes/foster care—data collection began in 2003	Effect of differences in the socioeconomic situation, way of life, ethnicity, upbringing, and organization of home life within the family and its effects on childhood development. Consequences of the institutionalized childhood. Effectiveness of societal support of families and children. Effect of leave-of-absence schemes on the parents' perception of the father/mother role, or their perception of the role of the family/"the public sector." Effect of parents' mutual relations (conflict/harmony) on their children's daily life. Effect of parental education, way of life, cultural background and working conditions of the parents on the way they prioritize family life. Conditions in childhood/adolescence that effect social integrate. What social mechanisms influence child resiliency	http://www.sfi.dk/the_danish_longitudinal_survey_of_children-3214.aspx
Growing up in France (ELFE)	France 2011 (children born on specific days of year 2009 [4 days in each of the four different quarters])	Birth to adulthood: birth, 2 months, 3, 6, 11	1000 children (goal is 20,000)	To study the various factors interacting all over the life course up to adulthood (family structure, social and physical environment, schooling, health, and nutritional behavior) and to clarify the impact of the experience lived during infancy on the individual's physical, psychological, social, and professional development. Measure the cumulative exposures to specific environmental conditions or behaviors year after year and to analyze their consequences on social and health inequalities	http://www.cls.ioe.ac.uk/page.aspx?&sitesectionid=326&sitesectiontitle=ELFE+%28Growin%20g+up+in+France

(continued)

Table 3 (continued)

Cohort/country	Years	Ages/data collection points	Sample characteristics	Measures	Comments: PI/Managing entity// website
European Longitudinal Study of Pregnancy and Childhood (ELSPAC)	Europe born 1991 to 1995: Great Britain, Isle of Man, Czech Republic, Slovakia, Russia, Ukraine, Croatia and Estonia; recently added: Spain and Greece.	Pregnancy, birth to 19 years: 6 and 18 months; 3, 5, 7, 11, 15, 18 and 19 years	7589 children	Detect biological, psychological, and social factors as well as factors of external environment associated with survival and health of the fetus, infant and a child. Biopsychosocial determinants of the child's development from conception until the end of school age, while taking into consideration a lifestyle of the family, environment, care, or relationships among family members as well as personalities of the mother and the father. Furthermore, we are aiming to find the links between biopsychosocial determinants as well as origin and development of health disorders of a fetus, newborn, and a child. Medical issues during pregnancy—bleeding, eclampsia, infections, adolescent mothers. Specific termination of pregnancy—preterm delivery, intrauterine growth retardation of the fetus, abortions, child of diabetic mother. Growth— weight; height; length of long bones; circumference of head, waist, and arm; skin folders; and other anthropometric data. Development—developmental landmarks, motoric coordination, intellectual abilities	Research Institute of Preventive and Social Paediatrics at the Faculty of Medicine, Masaryk University Brno, Czech Republic: Lubomír Kukla, PI; Website: http://www.aloe-app.com/index-en.php
Growing up in Australia	Australia 2004	Two cohorts—families with 4–5-year-old children (4–19 years) and families with 0–1-year-old infants (birth to 16 years) Interviewed biennially	10,000 children – infant cohort (Dabelea et al. 2014; Grote et al. 2010) and child cohort (4991)	Children's social, economic, and cultural environments to their adjustment and well-being	Daryl Higgins, PI Website: http://www.aifs.gov.au/growingup/index.html

Birth to twenty	South Africa 1990	Birth through adulthood Birth to 14 years annually and 14 through adulthood biennially; multigenerational	3273 children (1594 recruited antenatal); 3273 women (singleton births)	Lifecycle approach and attempts to integrate historical, personal, social, and economic information with data collected during all major developmental stages. In the early years, the emphasis was on physical growth, health and health service usage; in the preschool years attention turned to social behavior, and home and center support for learning; during primary school, data has been collected on educational progress; in the teen years the study is concentrating on precursors to adult health and adjustment, including sexual behavior, school achievement, substance use, diet, activity, and conflict with the law. Regularly assessments are made of children's residential circumstances, household composition, and socioeconomic conditions. Growth measurements are taken and blood and urine samples subjected to a number of biochemical tests. Body composition, blood pressure and physical activity are also assessed	Child Youth Family and Social Development, Human Sciences Research Council: Linda Richter, PI http://www.wits.ac.za/academic/health/research/birthto20/10274/home.html
The Avon Longitudinal Study of Parents and Children 1992 (ALSPAC)—Children of the '90s study	UK	Birth to early adulthood	14,000 mothers in the former county of Avon enrolled during pregnancy in 1991 and 1992. The health and development of their children has been followed in great detail ever since	During pregnancy: medical history and physical health of mother and grandparents, exposure to environmental pollutants, sleeping patterns, diet, caffeine and alcohol consumption, smoking, illegal drug taking, psychological well-being of parents, their expectations and attitudes, social support networks. Early childhood: health, lifestyle, and development. At focus clinics, physical measurements and psychological tests, regular biological samples, DNA extraction, school performance on SATS and GCSEs. ALSPAC links to additional sources of data on participants include national pupil database and school census data, and information on death and cancer	http://www.bristol.ac.uk/alspac/

(continued)

Table 3 (continued)

Cohort/country	Years	Ages/data collection points	Sample characteristics	Measures	Comments: PI/Managing entity// website
Childhood Obesity – Early Programming by Infant Nutrition (CHOPIN)	Germany: 2002 to 2004 enrollment	Follow through to age 11; data collection yearly through 8 and then again at 11	1678 infants in Belgium, Germany, Italy, Poland, Spain	Birth outcomes (wt, length, gestational age, Apgar, sex); child exposures infancy through age 11; development; child health, biological samples. Also included a 1 year multicenter intervention trial on newborn infants, to test whether feeding infant formulae (differing in protein content), can influence growth trajectories during the first year of life	PI: Berthold Koletzko, Div. Metabolic and Nutritional Medicine, Dr. von Hauner Children's Hospital, Ludwig-Maximilians-University of Munich Medical http://www.ist-world.org/ProjectDetails.aspx?ProjectId=c63efc2bdd954069bed34a6d65d33dd4&SourceDatabaseId=e4fcfde0182a45898e8741a1abae3984
All Babies in Southeast Sweden	Sweden: Oct 1st 1997 to Oct 1st 1999	Multiple—beginning during fetal life, including bio-samples during pregnancy through age 14 years	17,000 infants	Main exposure: nutrition, physical activity, sleep pattern, infections, psychosocial factors, child care, stress, drugs, vaccinations, genetics, Outcomes: autoimmunity (Type 1 DM, celiac disease, RA), allergy, obesity, Type 2 DM	PI Johnny Ludvigsson; Dept of Clin Exp Medicine, Linköping university, Sweden http://www.researchweb.org/is/lio/ansokan/56531
Aarhus Birth Cohort	Births beginning in 1990 Denmark	Pre-pregnancy, second and third trimester	100,000 children and 100,000 mothers who gave birth at the Dept of Obst and Gyn, Aarhus Univ Hospital, Skejby	Fetal programming hypothesis and on various aspects of pregnancy, birth, and neonatal care. Birth outcomes (wt, lt, GA at birth, Apgar, congenital malformations, stillbirth, sex)	Dept. of Pediatrics and Perinatal Epidemiology Research Unit, Aarhus University Hospital, Skejby, Denmark:Tine Brink Henriksen, PI http://fetotox.au.dk/the-fetotox-birth-cohorts/aarhus-birth-cohort-biobank-abcb/
Amsterdam Born Children and their Development (ABCD study)	2003–2004	Pre-pregnancy, pregnancy (1st, 2nd, 3rd trimester), birth, 5 and 6 years to adulthood	6161 infants and 8266 mothers	Association between lifestyle, psychosocial conditions and nutritional status during pregnancy, and the child's health at birth (birth weight, pregnancy duration, perinatal mortality) and in later life (growth, physical development, behavior and cognitive functioning)	Academic Medical Centre/ University of Amsterdam: Manon van Eijsden; Tanja G.M. Vrijkotte, PI http://www.abcd-study.nl/
Babies After SCOPE: Evaluating the Longitudinal Impact using Neurological and Nutritional Endpoints	Ireland: Aug 1st 2008 to Oct 31 2011	Birth to 5 years, birth to 1, 2, and 5 years	2185 children born in Ireland	Maternal health, fetal growth, and childhood nutrition, growth and development in the first 2 years of life. Birth outcomes (wt, lt, GA at birth, sex)	University College Cork: PI Deirdre Murray, PI http://www.nationalchildrensresearchcentre.ie/research/baseline-study-babies-after-scope-evaluating-longitundinal-impact-using-neurological-and-nutritional-endpoints/

Bologna Birth Cohort	Italy 2004–2005	Birth to adulthood: birth, 1, 2, 3, and 7 years	654 children, 651 mothers, 593 fathers delivering at the University Hospital of Bolonga	Exposure: passive smoking, breastfeeding, nutrition, allergens, indoor pollution, motor vehicles pollution Outcome: wheezing, asthma, eczema, atopic dermatitis, sleep, cognitive development. Birth outcomes (wt, lt, GA at birth, Apgar, stillbirth, sex)	Maria Pia Fantini, PI
Born in Bradford	UK Jan 1st 2007 to Dec 24th 2010	Birth to adulthood: 1, 2, and 3 years	14,000 children, 14,000 mothers, and 3000 fathers	Describe health and ill-health within a largely bi-ethnic population; identify modifiable causal pathways that promote well-being, or contribute to ill-health; develop, design and evaluate interventions to promote health and well-being; Develop a model for integrating operational, epidemiological, and evaluative research into practice within the NHS and other health-related systems; build and strengthen the local research capacity	Bradford Institute for Health Research: John Wright, PI http://www.borninbradford.nhs.uk/
Copenhagen Child Cohort 2000 (CCC2000)	Denmark Births in 2000	Pregnancy, birth to adulthood: birth, 1, 6, and 11 years	6090 children, 6090 mothers	Developmental trajectories of psychopathology and mental disorders from birth in a general population birth cohort and to determine at risk states of mental illness in childhood and adolescence. Birth outcomes (wt, lt, GA at birth, Apgar, congenital malformations, stillbirth, sex)	Child and Adolescent psychiatric Centre, University Hospital of Copenhagen: Anne Mette Skovgaard, PI
Danish National Birth Cohort (DNBC)	Denmark Births 1996–2002	Pregnancy, birth to adulthood: birth—7 years, 11 years	95,000 children, 100,418 mothers	Pregnancy complications and diseases in offspring as a function of factors operating in pregnancy/fetal and early life. Fetal growth as an outcome and as a determinant of later health. Main exposures: infection, alcohol, tobacco, environments, medication, psychosocial factors. Nutrition in pregnancy, in general but with focus upon fish intake Outcome measures: life-long follow-up of children—mortality and morbidity. Birth outcomes (wt, lt, GA at birth, Apgar, congenital malformations, stillbirth, sex)	Statens Serum Institut, Copenhagen: Jørn Olsen, PI http://www.ssi.dk/English/RandD/Research%20areas/Epidemiology/DNBC/
Dortmund Nutritional and Anthropometric Longitudinally Designed Study (DONALD)	Germany Births from 1985 and ongoing	Infants 3–6 months old to adulthood: birth—18 years	1300 each children, mothers, and fathers; open cohort study. Annual recruitment of 30–40 infants	Environmental exposure is not the main focus of the birth outcomes (wt, lt, GA at birth, apgar, sex). Child exposures: child care, second hand smoke, smoking, alcohol, breastfeeding, diet, PA, medications, head circumference, sexual maturation, allergies, infections, cardiac, cancer, DM, BP, sleep, urine samples	Research Insitute of Child Nutrition: Anette Buyken, Thomas Remer, Ute Alexy, Mathilde Kersting – Pis

(continued)

Table 3 (continued)

Cohort/country	Years	Ages/data collection points	Sample characteristics	Measures	Comments: PI/Managing entity// website
Gateshead Millennium Study	UK births from June 1st 1999 to May 31st 2000	Birth to adulthood: birth, 1, 7, 9, and 12 years	1029 children and 1011 mothers	Feeding, weaning, and growth, including characteristics of maternal feeding style, eating attitudes, and depression. Childhood aspects of developmental psychopathology, behavioral and emotional development, and repetitive behaviors. Origins of childhood obesity, with particular reference to food intake, physical activity and sedentary behavior. Original purpose was investigation of weight faltering	Newcastle University: Ashley Adamson, PI http://www.cls.ioe.ac.uk/page.aspx?&sitesectionid=332&sitesectiontitle=Gateshead+Millennium+Study
GECKO Drenthe cohort	Netherlands born April 1st 2006 to April 1st 2007	Pregnancy, birth to adulthood: birth—5 years	2997 children born in Drenthe, Netherlands. Pregnant mothers recruited in the third trimester	The overall aim of the GECKO Drenthe cohort is to study the prevalence and early risk factors for the development of childhood overweight and fat distribution at very young age. Within this birth cohort the growth of the children is closely followed, starting at birth until adulthood. The children are followed using questionnaires that the parents have to answer and the regular visits to the Well Baby Clinics, where length, weight, head circumference, and hip and waist circumference are measured. Furthermore, physical activity is measured using accelerometers. At birth, cord blood was sampled and stored for (epi)genetic analysis and biomarkers. During the first 9 months of life, the children were measured every month (incl. questionnaire); thereafter this frequency decreased until once every 2 years from 3 years onward. The children are now 5 years old	University Medical Center Groningen: E. Corpeleijn, PI
Generation R	Netherlands birth Jan 21st 2002 to Feb 1st 2006	Pregnancy, birth to adulthood: birth—5, 7, and 9 years	10,000 children, 97,780 mothers, and 6500 fathers	Identification of early critical periods and causal pathways for growth, development, and health. Birth outcomes (wt, length, GA at birth, Apgar, congenital malformation, still birth, sex)	Erasmus Medical Center Rotterdam: Vincent Jaddoe, PI http://research.lunenfeld.ca/eagle/?page=841

Genetic and Environment: Prospective Study on Infancy in Italy (GASPII)	Italy June 1st 2003 to Oct 31st 2004	Birth to 20 years: birth, 1, 3, and 8 years	708 children, 693 mothers (>18 years), and 63 fathers	Environmental exposures, diet, air pollution asthma and allergies, accidents and injuries, obesity, minor birth defects, neurodevelopment. Birth outcomes (wt, length, GA at birth, Apgar, congenital malformation, still birth, sex)	Department of Epidemiology Regional Health Service lazio Region: Daniela Porta, PI
German Infant Study on the influence of Nutrition Intervention (GINIplus)	Germany births Jan 1st 1995 to Jan 1st 1998	Birth to adulthood: birth—4, 6, 10, and15 years	5991 children, maternal pregnancy outcomes	Intervention substudy; double -blinded randomized trial for hypoallergenic formulae, observational substudy: natural course of atopic diseases and metabolic disorders; mental health, nutrition, body weight and physical activity; Birth outcomes (wt, lt, GA at birth)	HelmholtzZentrum München: D. Berdel; A.v. Berg; C.P. Bauer; U. Krämer; S. Koletzko; J. Heinrich – PIs
Healthy Habits for two (HHf2)	Denmark births April 1st 1984 to April 1st 1987	Pregnancy, birth annually through 18 to 20 years	11,144 children of live birth singleton pregnancy, 11,980 mothers who attended 2 midwife in Aalborg or Odense during week 35 to 38 of pregnancy	Birth outcomes (wt, lt, GA at birth, Apgar, congenital malformations, sex). Converted from a trial to a birth cohort	The Danish Epidemiology Science Centre: Jørn Olsen, PI
KOALA Birth Cohort Study (KOALA)	Netherlands Birth Jan 1st 2000 to Oct 1st 2002	Pregnancy, Birth to adulthood: birth—2, 5–9 years	2843 children, 2900 mothers >14 weeks in a pregnancy pelvic pain or from an alternate lifestyle practices, 2900 fathers	Main outcomes: 1. allergy and asthma development, 2. growth and overweight development (inflammatory, immunological, metabolic, cardiorespiratory and cardiovascular aspects) Main exposures: microbial (infections, gut microbiota), breastfeeding and breast milk composition, nutrition, physical activity, parenting practices and parenting styles; home, neighborhood, and childcare environment. Birth outcomes (wt, lt, GA at birth, Apgar, congenital malformations, sex)	Maastricht University: Carel Thijs, PI http://www.koala-study.nl/
Lifeways Cross-Generation Cohort Study	Ireland 2001 to 2003	Pregnancy, birth: birth—3, 5, and 10 years	1074 children, 1061 mothers, 325 fathers	Physical and psychological health status, socioeconomic circumstances, birth, childhood, early adulthood and early middle age. Birth outcomes (wt, GA at birth, Apgar, congenital malformations, stillbirth, sex)	University College Dublin: Cecily Kelleher, PI http://www.ucd.ie/phpps/research/clinicalepidemiologygroup/lifewayscross-generationcohortstudy/

(continued)

Table 3 (continued)

Cohort/country	Years	Ages/data collection points	Sample characteristics	Measures	Comments: PI/Managing entity// website
Mother Child Cohort in Crete (RHEA)	Greece Feb 1st 2007 to Feb 29th 2008	Pregnancy, birth to 16 years: birth—4 years	1590 children; 1610 mothers >16 years and 9–13 wks gestation; 37 fathers	1. The evaluation of nutritional, environmental, biological, and psychosocial exposures in the prenatal period and in early childhood. 2. The evaluation of the association of these exposures with the development of the fetus and the child, reproductive outcomes, endocrine-related outcomes, neurodevelopment, obesity, and the occurrence of chronic diseases including asthma and allergies, metabolic syndrome, and endocrine disorders that appear first in childhood but that may perpetuate to adulthood. 3. The evaluation of mother's health during and after pregnancy. 4. The evaluation of genetic susceptibility and the interactions between genetic and environmental factors affecting child health. Birth outcomes (wt, lt, GA at birth, Apgar, stillbirth, sex)	Dept of Social Medicine, Medical School, Heraklion, University of Crete, Greece and CREAL, Barcelona, Spain: Manolis Kogevinas and Leda Chatzi – PIs
Norwegian Human Milk Study (HUMIS)	Norway 2003 to 2009	Birth to adulthood: Birth −2 years, 8 years	2500 children breastfeeding at 2 wks of age, 2500 mothers, 2400 fathers	Exposures: environmental toxicants, gut microbiota, pops, Pfos, organotins, gut microbiota, *Bifidobacterium*, *Lactobacillus*, early nutrition, human milk composition, duration of breastfeeding. Main outcomes: child health, reproductive health, asthma and allergy, ADHD, neuropsychological development, depression, overweight. Birth outcomes (wt, lt, GA at birth, Apgar, congenital malformations, sex)	Norwegian Institute of Public Health: Merete Eggesbø, PI
Norwegian Mother and Child Cohort Study (MoBa)	Norway Jan 1st 1999 to Dec 31 2008	Pregnancy, birth to adulthood: birth, 1, 3, 5, 7, 8 years	10,500 children, 90,700 mothers 17–20 wks pregnant, 72,100 fathers	Causes of diseases. Additional aims are to detect early signs of disease and to describe the development of diseases. Birth outcomes (wt, lt, GA at birth, apgar, congenital malformations, stillbirth)	Norwegian Institute of Public Health: Per Magnus, PI http://www.fhi.no/eway/default.aspx?pid=240&trg=Main_6664&Main_6664=6894:0:25,7372:1:0:0:::0:0&MainContent_6898=6671:0:25,7899:1:0:0:::0:0&List_6673=6674:0:25,7905:1:0:0:::0:0

Odense Child Cohort	Denmark Births beginning in 2010	Infants 0–5 months to 18 years	1650 children, 2249 mothers, 2102 fathers—living in Odense, Denmark	Interaction between the fetus/infant/child during pregnancy, birth, and childhood and the social and environmental determinants for health and disease. Birth outcomes (wt, lt, GA at birth, Apgar, stillbirth, sex)	Odense University Hospital, Hans Christian Andersen Children's Hospital, Paediatric Research Unit: Steffen Husby, PI http://www.sdu.dk/en/Om_SDU/Institutter_centre/Klinisk_institut/Forskning/Forskningsenheder/Paediatri/Odense+Børnekohorte
Study on the pre- and early postnatal determinants of child health and development (EDEN – France)	France Births 2003 to 2005	Pregnancy, birth to 8 years: birth to 5 years and 8 years	1900 children, 2000 mothers >18 years and <24 wks pregnant, 1800 fathers	Pre- and postnatal determinant of the child's development and health. Birth outcomes (wt, lt, GA at birth, Apgar, congenital malformations, stillbirth, sex)	CESP INSERM: Heude Barbara, PI

The cohorts outlined here met the following criteria: Enrollment of the mother/child into the cohort was either prior to the pregnancy, during the pregnancy, or at birth; there was data collected with some frequency in childhood; the studies were not single/narrow focused)

Key source is http://www.birthcohorts.net; this site is an inventory of birth cohort longitudinal studies maintained by Department of Public Health, University of Copenhagen, Professor Anne-Marie Nybo Andersen collection at 15 years or beyond). These cohorts also gathered data for childhood weight, height, health assessment, and various social parameters. The cohorts were the Canadian National Longitudinal Survey of Children and Youth (NLSCY, data collected at various age points from birth through age 25 over the course of 8 cycles), the European Longitudinal Study of Pregnancy and Childhood (ELSPAC, data collected at nine points from birth through 19 years and includes the countries of Great Britain, Isle of Man, Czech Republic, Slovakia, Russia, Ukraine, Croatia, Estonia, Spain and Greece), the Growing Up in Australia survey (data collected through two separate cohorts with one beginning at birth to 1 year and the second at 4/5 years with follow-up to age 19 years), the South Africa's Birth to 20 longitudinal study (data collected through two separate cohorts that followed children ages birth to 14 years and age 14 years through adulthood), the UK's Avon Longitudinal Study of Parents and Children (ALSPAC) (data collected on children born between 1990 and 1992 from birth through adulthood), and finally, the German Infant Study on the Influence of Nutrition Intervention (GINIplus), collected data on children born between 1995 and 1998 annually from birth through 4 years and then at 6, 10, and 15 years of age.

In addition to the data limitations currently facing the pediatric T2DM research community, there are also methodological/analytical challenges. To make progress in all of these research priorities, large amounts of data will be needed. These data will be diverse ranging from genetic and other biologicals to social structure factors. Management and analyses of such diverse data will require new methods and collaborations that will include basic scientists, mathematicians, data engineers, practitioners, and translational scientists. Researchers will need to employ big data analytics and a complex system perspective that can address multiple causes and outcomes. The challenges are significant, but the opportunities vast to make a real difference to the health development of all children

7.2.3 Recommendation 3: To Translate the Growing Body of Knowledge into Evidenced-Based Prevention and Treatment Strategies

There are clear needs for both prevention and treatment trials in children and adolescents. There is a dearth of evidence-based studies and guidelines available to pediatric practitioners and pediatric endocrinologist to address the multiple management issues faced when treating patients with T2DM. Areas of clear need include prevention strategies for children born at high risk. For example, low birth weight newborns, offspring of diabetic mothers, could be placed in programs to test interventions to modify risk. This is a very important area of pediatric and diabetes research with implications on health status and care for large number of children into adulthood and should be of high priority for funding agencies.

Prevention trials are needed that can identify strategies to reduce the risk for developing T2DM, and as recent work demonstrates, understanding the age at intervention is key. Prevention strategies may be gleaned from longitudinal data collected for other reasons. While not a prospective trial, the primary data elements could be supplemented either through new data collection efforts (e.g., during adolescence collecting insulin, glucose, etc.), or by combining the primary data with other administrative data—child electronic health records of heights and weights throughout childhood—or both. With home address information, child contexts could be tracked over time and neighborhoods accounted for in the analyses.

Finally, there is much work to be done to translate the knowledge into policy at every level. Pediatric practitioners need up-to-date guidelines to identify children at high risk for T2DM at young ages. Families must be given the information about the possible long-term consequences of decisions made in early life. Local, state, and national governments also need policies in place that enhance child health development throughout childhood. Only then will we be able to achieve the goal of optimal health development for every child.

References

Aaltonen, J., Ojala, T., Laitinen, K., Poussa, T., Ozanne, S., & Isolauri, E. (2011). Impact of maternal diet during pregnancy and breastfeeding on infant metabolic programming: A prospective randomized controlled study. *European Journal of Clinical Nutrition, 65*(1), 10–19.

Agardh, E., Allebeck, P., Hallqvist, J., Moradi, T., & Sidorchuk, A. (2011). Type 2 diabetes incidence and socio-economic position: A systematic review and meta-analysis. *International Journal of Epidemiology, 40*(3), 804–818.

Amed, S., Daneman, D., Mahmud, F. H., & Hamilton, J. (2010a). Type 2 diabetes in children and adolescents. *Expert Review of Cardiovascular Therapy, 8*(3), 393–406.

Amed, S., Dean, H. J., Panagiotopoulos, C., Sellers, E. A., Hadjiyannakis, S., Laubscher, T. A., et al. (2010b). Type 2 diabetes, medication-induced diabetes, and monogenic diabetes in Canadian children: A prospective national surveillance study. *Diabetes Care, 33*(4), 786–791.

Amercian Diabetes Association. (2000). Type 2 diabetes in children and adolescents. *Pediatrics, 105*(3 Pt 1), 671–680.

American Academy of Pedicatrics. (2012). Breastfeeding and the use of human milk. *Pediatrics, 129*(3), e827–e841.

American Diabetes Association. (2010). Diagnosis and classification of diabetes mellitus. *Diabetes Care, 33*(Suppl 1), S62–S69.

Anderson, S. E., & Whitaker, R. C. (2010). Household routines and obesity in US preschool-aged children. *Pediatrics, 125*(1), 420–428.

Anderson, S. E., Gooze, R. A., Lemeshow, S., & Whitaker, R. C. (2012). Quality of early maternal-child relationship and risk of adolescent obesity. *Pediatrics, 129*(1), 132–140.

Anderson, S. E., Lemeshow, S., & Whitaker, R. C. (2014). Maternal-infant relationship quality and risk of obesity at age 5.5 years in a national US cohort. *BMC Pediatrics, 14*(1), 54.

Armitage, J. A., Khan, I. Y., Taylor, P. D., Nathanielsz, P. W., & Poston, L. (2004). Developmental programming of the metabolic syndrome by maternal nutritional imbalance: How strong is the evidence from experimental models in mammals? *The Journal of Physiology, 561*(Pt 2), 355–377.

Armitage, J. A., Poston, L., Taylor, P., & D. (2008). Developmental origins of obesity and the metabolic syndrome: The role of maternal obesity. *Frontiers of Hormone Research, 36*, 73–84.

Arslanian, S. A., Bacha, F., Saad, R., & Gungor, N. (2005). Family history of type 2 diabetes is associated with decreased insulin sensitivity and an impaired balance between insulin sensitivity and insulin secretion in white youth. *Diabetes Care, 28910*, 115–119.

Barker, D. J., Hales, C. N., Fall, C. H., Osmond, C., Phipps, K., & Clark, P. M. (1993). Type 2 (non-insulin-dependent) diabetes mellitus, hypertension and hyperlipidaemia (syndrome X): Relation to reduced fetal growth. *Diabetologia, 36*(1), 62–67.

Barker, A., Sharp, S. J., Timpson, N. J., Bouatia-Naji, N., Warrington, N. M., Kanoni, S., et al. (2011). Association of genetic loci with glucose levels in childhood and adolescence: A meta-analysis of over 6,000 children. *Diabetes, 60*(6), 1805–1812.

Barlow, S. E. (2007). Expert committee recommendations regarding the prevention, assessment, and treatment of child and adolescent overweight and obesity: Summary report. *Pediatrics, 120*(Suppl 4), S164–S192.

Barouki, R., Gluckman, P. D., Grandjean, P., Hanson, M., & Heindel, J. J. (2012). Developmental origins of non-communicable disease: Implications for research and public health. *Environmental Health : A Global Access Science Source, 11*, 42.

Barton, M. (2010). Screening for obesity in children and adolescents: US preventive services task Force recommendation statement. *Pediatrics, 125*(2), 361–367.

Battista, M. C., Hivert, M. F., Duval, K., & Baillargeon, J. P. (2011). Intergenerational cycle of obesity and diabetes: How can we reduce the burdens of these conditions on the health of future generations? *Experimental Diabetes Research, 2011*, 596060. doi:10.1155/2011/596060.

Bell, J. F., & Zimmerman, F. J. (2010). Shortened nighttime sleep duration in early life and subsequent childhood obesity. *Archives of Pediatrics & Adolescent Medicine, 164*(9), 840–845.

Bell, R. A., Mayer-Davis, E. J., Beyer, J. W., D'Agostino, R. B., Jr., Lawrence, J. M., Linder, B., et al. (2009). Diabetes in non-Hispanic white youth: Prevalence, incidence, and clinical characteristics: The SEARCH for diabetes in youth study. *Diabetes Care, 32*(Suppl 2), S102–S111.

Berends, L. M., & Ozanne, S. E. (2012). Early determinants of type-2 diabetes. *Best Practice & Research. Clinical Endocrinology & Metabolism, 26*(5), 569–580.

Bertin, E., Gangnerau, M. N., Bellon, G., Bailbe, D., Arbelot De Vacqueur, A., & Portha, B. (2002). Development of beta-cell mass in fetuses of rats deprived of protein and/or energy in last trimester of pregnancy. *American Journal of Physiology. Regulatory, Integrative and Comparative Physiology, 283*(3), R623–R630.

Bocca, G., Corpeleijn, E., Stolk, R. P., & Sauer, P. J. J. (2012a). Results of a multidisciplinary treatment program in 3-year-old to 5-year-old overweight or obese children: A randomized controlled clinical trial. *Archives of Pediatrics & Adolescent Medicine, 166*(12), 1109–1115.

Bocca, G., Corpeleijn, E., Stolk, R. P., & Sauer, P. J. (2012b). Results of a multidisciplinary treatment program in 3-year-old to 5-year-old overweight or obese children: A randomized controlled clinical trial. *Archives of Pediatrics & Adolescent Medicine, 166*(12), 1109–1115.

Boekelheide, K., Blumberg, B., Chapin, R. E., Cote, I., Graziano, J. H., Janesick, A., et al. (2012). Predicting later-life outcomes of early-life exposures. *Environmental Health Perspectives, 120*(10), 1353–1361.

Boyle, J. P., Thompson, T. J., Gregg, E. W., Barker, L. E., & Williamson, D. F. (2010). Projection of the year 2050 burden of diabetes in the US adult population: Dynamic modeling of incidence, mortality, and pre-diabetes prevalence. *Population Health Metrics, 8*, 29. doi:10.1186/1478-7954-8-29.

Brandt, M. L., Harmon, C. M., Helmrath, M. A., Inge, T. H., McKay, S. V., & Michalsky, M. P. (2010). Morbid obesity in pediatric diabetes mellitus: Surgical options and outcomes. *Nature reviews. Endocrinology, 6*(11), 637–645.

Brotman, L. M., Dawson-McClure, S., Huang, K. Y., Theise, R., Kamboukos, D., Wang, J., et al. (2012). Early childhood family intervention and long-term obesity prevention among high-risk minority youth. *Pediatrics, 129*(3), e621–e628.

Brown, T., & Summerbell, C. (2009). Systematic review of school-based interventions that focus on changing dietary intake and physical activity levels to prevent childhood obesity: An update to the obesity guidance produced by the National Institute for health and clinical excellence. *Obesity Reviews, 10*(1), 110–141.

Brunton, P. J. (2010). Resetting the dynamic range of hypothalamic-pituitary-adrenal axis stress responses through pregnancy. *Journal of Neuroendocrinology, 22*(11), 1198–1213.

Burns, S. F., Lee, S., Bacha, F., Tfayli, H., Hannon, T. S., & Arslanian, S. A. (2014). Pre-diabetes in overweight youth and early atherogenic risk. *Metabolism, 63*(12), 1528–1235.

Burt Solorzano, C. M., & McCartney, C. R. (2010). Obesity and the pubertal transition in girls and boys. *Reproduction, 140*(3), 399–410.

Caballero, B., Clay, T., Davis, S. M., Ethelbah, B., Rock, B. H., Lohman, T., et al. (2003). Pathways: A school-based, randomized controlled trial for the prevention of obesity in American Indian schoolchildren. *American Journal of Clinical Nutrition, 78*(5), 1030–1038.

Campbell, K. J., Lioret, S., McNaughton, S. A., Crawford, D. A., Salmon, J., Ball, K., et al. (2013). A parent-focused intervention to reduce infant obesity risk behaviors: A randomized trial. *Pediatrics, 131*(4), 652–660. doi:10.1542/peds.2012-2576.

Cenit, M. C., Matzaraki, V., Tigchelaar, E. F., & Zhernakova, A. (2014). Rapidly expanding knowledge on the role of the gut microbiome in health and disease. *Biochimica et Biophysica Acta, 1842*(10), 1981–1992.

Christian, L. M. (2012). Physiological reactivity to psychological stress in human pregnancy: Current knowledge and future directions. *Progress in Neurobiology, 99*(2), 106–116. doi:10.1016/j.pneurobio.2012.07.003.

Copeland, K. C., Zeitler, P., Geffner, M., Guandalini, C., Higgins, J., Hirst, K., et al. (2011). Characteristics of adolescents and youth with recent-onset type 2 diabetes: The TODAY cohort at baseline. *Journal of Clinical Endocrinology and Metabolism, 96*(1), 159–167.

Courcoulas, A., Goodpaster, B., Eagleton, J., Belle, S., Kalarchian, M., Lang, W., et al. (2014). Surgical vs medical treatments for type 2 diabetes mellitus: A randomized clinical trial. *JAMA Surgery, 7*(149), 707–715.

Crume, T. L., Ogden, L. G., Mayer-Davis, E. J., Hamman, R. F., Norris, J. M., Bischoff, K. J., et al. (2012). The impact of neonatal breast-feeding on growth trajectories of youth exposed and unexposed to diabetes in utero: The EPOCH study. *International Journal of Obesity, 36*(4), 529–534.

Dabelea, D., Bell, R. A., D'Agostino, R. B., Jr., Imperatore, G., Johansen, J. M., Linder, B., et al. (2007). Incidence of diabetes in youth in the United States. *JAMA, 297*(24), 2716–2724.

Dabelea, D., Dolan, L. M., D'Agostino, R., Jr., Hernandez, A. M., McAteer, J. B., Hammon, R. F., et al. (2011). Association testing of TCF7L2 polymorphisms with type 2 diabetes in multi-ethnic youth. *Diabetologia, 54*(3), 535–539.

Dabelea, D., Mayer-Davis, E. J., Saydah, S., Imperatore, G., Linder, B., et al. (2014). Prevalence of type 1 and type 2 diabetes among children and adolescents from 2001 to 2009. *JAMA, 311*(17), 1778–1786.

Danielsson, P., Kowalski, J., Ekblom, O., & Marcus, C. (2012a). Response of severely obese children and adolescents to behavioral treatment. *Archives of Pediatrics & Adolescent Medicine, 166*(12), 1103–1108.

Danielsson, P., Kowalski, J., Ekblom, O., & Marcus, C. (2012b). Response of severely obese children and adolescents to behavioral treatment. *Archives of Pediatrics & Adolescent Medicine, 166*(12), 1103–1108.

Davis, C. L., Pollock, N. K., Waller, J. L., Allison, J. D., Dennis, B. A., Bassali, R., et al. (2012). Exercise dose and diabetes risk in overweight and obese children: A randomized controlled trial. *JAMA, 308*(11), 1103–1112.

Demmer, R. T., Zuk, A. M., Rosenbaum, M., & Desvarieux, M. (2013). Prevalence of diagnosed and undiagnosed type 2 diabetes mellitus among US adolescents: Results from the continuous NHANES, 1999-2010. *American Journal of Epidemiology, 178*(7), 1106–1113.

Devaraj, S., Hemarajata, P., & Versalovic, J. (2013). The human gut microbiome and body metabolism: Implications for obesity and diabetes. *Clinical Chemistry, 59*(4), 617–628.

Dyer, J. S., & Rosenfeld, C. R. (2011). Metabolic imprinting by prenatal, perinatal, and postnatal overnutrition: A review. *Seminars in Reproductive Medicine, 29*(3), 266–276.

van Eijsden, M., Vrijkotte, T. G., Gemke, R. J., & van der Wal, M. F. (2011). Cohort profile: The Amsterdam born children and their development (ABCD) study. *International Journal of Epidemiology, 40*(5), 1176–1186.

Ekelund, U., Ong, K. K., Linne, Y., Neovius, M., Brage, S., Dunger, D. B., et al. (2007). Association of weight gain in infancy and early childhood with metabolic risk in young adults. *The Journal of Clinical Endocrinology and Metabolism, 92*(1), 98–103.

Elder, D. A., Herbers, P. M., Weis, T., Standiford, D., Woo, J. G., & D'Alessio, D. A. (2012). Beta-cell dysfunction in adolescents and adults with newly diagnosed type 2 diabetes mellitus. *Journal of Pediatrics, 160*(6), 904–910.

Eriksson, J. G. (2006). Early growth, and coronary heart disease and type 2 diabetes: Experiences from the Helsinki birth cohort studies. *International Journal of Obesity, 30*(Suppl 4), S18–S22.

Eriksson, J. G. (2011). Early growth and coronary heart disease and type 2 diabetes: Findings from the Helsinki birth cohort study (HBCS). *The American Journal of Clinical Nutrition, 94*(6 Supplement), 1799S–1802S.

Eriksson, J. G., Osmond, C., Kajantie, E., Forsen, T. J., & Barker, D. J. (2006). Patterns of growth among children who later develop type 2 diabetes or its risk factors. *Diabetologia, 49*(12), 2853–2858.

Fabricius-Bjerre, S., Jensen, R. B., Faerch, K., Larsen, T., Molgaard, C., Michaelsen, K. F., et al. (2011). Impact of birth weight and early infant weight gain on insulin resistance and associated cardiovascular risk factors in adolescence. *PloS One, 6*(6), e20595. doi:10.1371/journal.pone.0020595.

Ferguson, M. A., Gutin, B., Le, N. A., Karp, W., Litaker, M., Humphries, M., et al. (1999). Effects of exercise training and its cessation on components of the insulin resistance syndrome in obese children. *International Journal of Obesity and Related Metabolic Disorders, 23*(8), 889–895.

Fernandez-Twinn, D. S., Wayman, A., Ekizoglou, S., Martin, M. S., Hales, C. N., & Ozanne, S. E. (2005). Maternal protein restriction leads to hyperinsulinemia and reduced insulin-signaling protein expression in 21-mo-old female rat offspring. *American Journal of Physiology. Regulatory, Integrative and Comparative Physiology, 288*(2), R368–R373.

Foster, G. D., Linder, B., Baranowski, T., Cooper, D. M., Goldberg, L., Harrell, J. S., et al. (2010). A school-based intervention for diabetes risk reduction. *New England Journal of Medicine, 363*(5), 443–453.

Gabbe, S. G., Landon, M. B., Warren-Boulton, E., & Fradkin, J. (2012). Promoting health after gestational diabetes: A National Diabetes Education Program call to action. *Obstetrics and Gynecology, 119*(1), 171–176.

Gaffney, K. F., Kitsantas, P., & Cheema, J. (2012). Clinical practice guidelines for feeding behaviors and weight-for-age at 12 months: A secondary analysis of the infant feeding practices study II. *Worldviews on Evidence- Based Nursing, 9*(4), 234–242.

Gaffney, K. F., Kitsantas, P., Brito, A., & Swamidoss, C. S. (2014). Postpartum depression, infant feeding practices, and infant weight gain at six months of age. *Journal of Pediatric Health Care, 28*(1), 43–50.

Garofano, A., Czernichow, P., & Breant, B. (1998). Beta-cell mass and proliferation following late fetal and early postnatal malnutrition in the rat. *Diabetologia, 41*(9), 1114–1120.

Gillis, B., Mobley, C., Stadler, D. D., Hartstein, J., Virus, A., Volpe, S. L., et al. (2009). Rationale, design and methods of the HEALTHY study nutrition intervention component. *International Journal of Obesity, 33*(Suppl 4), S29–S36.

Gillman, M. W., Oakey, H., Baghurst, P. A., Volkmer, R. E., Robinson, J. S., & Crowther, C. A. (2010). Effect of treatment of gestational diabetes mellitus on obesity in the next generation. *Diabetes Care, 33*(5), 964–968.

Gluckman, P. D., Hanson, M. A., Cooper, C., & Thornburg, K. L. (2008). Effect of in utero and early-life conditions on adult health and disease. *New England Journal of Medicine, 359*(1), 61–73.

Groop, L. C., & Tuomi, T. (1997). Non-insulin-dependent diabetes mellitus–a collision between thrifty genes and an affluent society. *Annals of Medicine, 29*, 37–53.

Grote, V., Vik, T., von Kries, R., Luque, V., Socha, J., Verducci, E., et al. (2010). Maternal postnatal depression and child growth: A European cohort study. *BMC Pediatrics, 10*, 14. doi:10.1186/1471-2431-10-14.

Hadar, E., & Hod, M. (2010). Establishing consensus criteria for the diagnosis of diabetes in pregnancy following the HAPO study. *Annals of the New York Academy of Sciences, 1205*, 88–93.

Haines, L., Wan, K. C., Lynn, R., Barrett, T. G., & Shield, J. P. (2007). Rising incidence of type 2 diabetes in children in the U.K. *Diabetes Care, 30*(5), 1097–1101.

Haines, J., McDonald, J., O'Brien, A., Sherry, B., Bottino, C. J., Schmidt, M. E., et al. (2013). Healthy habits, happy homes: Randomized trial to improve household routines for obesity prevention among preschool aged children. *JAMA Pediatrics, 167*(11), 1072–1079.

Hales, C. N., & Barker, D. J. (2001). The thrifty phenotype hypothesis. *British Medical Bulletin, 60*, 5–20.

Halfon, N., & Forrest, C. B. (2017). The emerging theoretical framework of life course health development. In N. Halfon, C. B. Forrest, R. M. Lerner, & E. Faustman (Eds.), *Handbook of life course health-development science*. Cham: Springer.

Harvey-Berino, J., & Rourke, J. (2003). Obesity prevention in preschool native-American children: A pilot study using home visiting. *Obesity Research, 11*(5), 606–611.

Herbst, A., Kapellen, T., Schober, E., Graf, C., Meissner, T., & Holl, R. (2014). Impact of regular physical activity on blood glucose control and cardiovascular risk factors in adolescents with type 2 diabetes mellitus – a multicenter study of 578 patients from 225 centres. *Pediatric Diabetes, 16*(3), 204–210.

Hesketh, K. D., & Campbell, K. J. (2010). Interventions to prevent obesity in 0-5 year olds: An updated systematic review of the literature. *Obesity, 18*(Supple 1), S27–S35.

Hirst, K., Baranowski, T., DeBar, L., Foster, G. D., Kaufman, F., Kennel, P., et al. (2009). HEALTHY study rationale, design and methods: Moderating risk of type 2 diabetes in multi-ethnic middle school students. *International Journal of Obesity, 33*(Suppl 4), S4–20.

Hiscock, H., Scalzo, K., Canterford, L., & Wake, M. (2011). Sleep duration and body mass index in 0-7-year olds. *Archives of Disease in Childhood, 96*(8), 735–739.

Hoet, J. J., Dahri, S., Snoeck, A., Reusens-Billen, B., & Remacle, C. (1992). Importance of diets and their effect on fetal development: Function and structure of the endocrine pancreas following protein deficiency during intrauterine life. *Bulletin et Mémoires de l'Académie Royale de Médecine de Belgique, 147* (3–5), 174–181. discussion 81–83.

Imperatore, G., Boyle, J. P., Thompson, T. J., Case, D., Dabelea, D., Hamman, R. F., et al. (2012). Projections of type 1 and type 2 diabetes burden in the U.S. population aged <20 years through 2050: Dynamic modeling of incidence, mortality, and population growth. *Diabetes Care, 35*(12), 2515–2520.

ISPAD. (2011). *Global IDF/ISPAD guideline for childhood and Pediatric diabetes.* Brussels, Belgium: International Diabetes Foundation.

James, D. C., & Lessen, R. (2009). Position of the American dietetic association: Promoting and supporting breastfeeding. *Journal of the American Dietetic Association, 109*(11), 1926–1942.

Jeffery, A. N., Metcalf, B. S., Hosking, J., Streeter, A. J., Voss, L. D., & Wilkin, T. J. (2012). Age before stage: Insulin resistance rises before the onset of puberty: A 9-year longitudinal study (EarlyBird 26). *Diabetes Care, 35*(3), 536–541.

Johnson, C. L., & Versalovic, J. (2012). The human microbiome and its potential importance to pediatrics. *Pediatrics, 129*(5), 950–960.

Kanaka-Gantenbein, C. (2010). Fetal origins of adult diabetes. *Annals of the New York Academy of Sciences, 1205*, 99–105.

Kapoor, A., Dunn, E., Kostaki, A., Andrews, M. H., & Matthews, S. G. (2006). Fetal programming of hypothalamo-pituitary-adrenal function: Prenatal stress and glucocorticoids. *The Journal of Physiology, 572*(Pt 2), 31–44.

Katoh, S., Lehtovirta, M., Kaprio, J., Harjutsalo, V., Koskenvuo, M., Eriksson, J., et al. (2005). Genetic and environmental effects on fasting and postchallenge plasma glucose and serum insulin values in Finnish twins. *Journal of Clinical Endocrinology and Metabolism, 90*(5), 2642–2647.

Kaufman, F. R., Hirst, K., Linder, B., Baranowski, T., Cooper, D. M., Foster, G. D., et al. (2009). Risk factors for type 2 diabetes in a sixth-grade multiracial cohort: The HEALTHY study. *Diabetes Care, 32*(5), 953–955.

Kempf, K., Rathmann, W., & Herder, C. (2008). Impaired glucose regulation and type 2 diabetes in children and adolescents. *Diabetes/Metabolism Research and Reviews, 24*, 427–437.

Kim, S. Y., England, J. L., Sharma, J. A., & Njoroge, T. (2011). Gestational diabetes mellitus and risk of childhood overweight and obesity in offspring: A systematic review. *Experimental Diabetes Research, 2011*, 541308.

Kitzmann, K. M., Dalton, W. T., 3rd, Stanley, C. M., Beech, B. M., Reeves, T. P., et al. (2010). Lifestyle interventions for youth who are overweight: A meta-analytic review. *Health Psychology, 29*(1), 91–101.

Klingenberg, L., Christensen, L. B., Hjorth, M. F., Zangenberg, S., Chaput, J. P., Sjodin, A., et al. (2013). No relation between sleep duration and adiposity indicators in 9-36 months old children: The SKOT cohort. *Pediatric Obesity, 8*(1), e14–e18.

Knowlden, A. P., & Sharma, M. (2012). Systematic review of family and home-based interventions targeting paediatric overweight and obesity. *Obesity Reviews, 13*(6), 499–508.

Koren, O., Goodrich, J. K., Cullender, T. C., Spor, A., Laitinen, K., Backhed, H. K., et al. (2012). Host remodeling of the gut microbiome and metabolic changes during pregnancy. *Cell, 150*(3), 470–480.

Kramer, M. S., Matush, L., Vanilovich, I., Platt, R. W., Bogdanovich, N., Sevkovskaya, Z., et al. (2009). A randomized breast-feeding promotion intervention did not reduce child obesity in Belarus. *The Journal of Nutrition, 139*(2), 417S–421S.

Lawrence, J., Mayer-Davis, E., Ryeynolds, K., Beyer, J., Pettitt, D., D'Agostino, R. B., et al. (2009a). Diabetes in Hispanic American youths. *Diabetes Care, 32*(Supplement 2), S123–S132.

Lawrence, J. M., Mayer-Davis, E. J., Reynolds, K., Beyer, J., Pettitt, D. J., D'Agostino, R. B., et al. (2009b). Diabetes in Hispanic American youth: Prevalence, incidence, demographics, and clinical characteristics: The SEARCH for diabetes in youth study. *Diabetes Care, 32*(Suppl 2), S123–S132.

Lee, Y. (2013). Diabetes care for emerging adults: Transition from pediatric to adult diabetes care systems. *Annals of Pediatric Endocrinology & Metabolism, 18*, 106–110.

Ley, S. H., Hanley, A. J., Sermer, M., Zinman, B., & O'Connor, D. L. (2012). Associations of prenatal metabolic abnormalities with insulin and adiponectin concentrations in human milk. *The American Journal of Clinical Nutrition, 95*(4), 867–874.

Li, R., Bilik, D., Brown, M. B., Zhang, P., Ettner, S. L., Ackerman, R. T., et al. (2013). Medical costs associated with type 2 diabetes complications and comorbidities. *The American Journal of Managed Care, 19*(5), 421–430.

Liu, L. L., Yi, J. P., Beyer, J., Mayer-Davis, E. J., Dolan, L. M., Dabelea, D. M., et al. (2009). Type 1 and type 2 diabetes in Asian and Pacific Islander U.S. youth: The SEARCH for diabetes in youth study. *Diabetes Care, 32*(Suppl 2), S133–S140.

Liu, J., Yu, P., Qian, W., Li, Y., Zhao, J., Huan, F., et al. (2013). Perinatal bisphenol a exposure and adult glucose homeostasis: Identifying critical windows of exposure. *PloS One, 8*(5), e64143.

Luepker, R. V., Perry, C. L., McKinlay, S. M., Nader, P. R., Parcel, G. S., Stone, E. J., et al. (1996). Outcomes of a field trial to improve children's dietary patterns and physical activity. The child and adolescent trial for cardiovascular health. CATCH collaborative group. *The Journal of the American Medical Association, 275*(10), 768–776.

Martin, R. M., Patel, R., Kramer, M. S., Vilchuck, K., Bogdanovich, N., Sergeichick, N., et al. (2014). Effects of promoting longer-term and exclusive breastfeeding on cardiometabolic risk factors at age 11.5 years: A cluster-randomized, controlled trial. *Circulation, 129*(3), 321–329.

Martin-Gronert, M. S., & Ozanne, S. E. (2012). Mechanisms underlying the developmental origins of disease. *Reviews in Endocrine & Metabolic Disorders, 13*(2), 85–92.

Maull, E. A., Ahsan, H., Edwards, J., Longnecker, M. P., Navas-Acien, A., Pi, J., et al. (2012). Evaluation of the association between arsenic and diabetes: A National Toxicology Program workshop review. *Environmental Health Perspectives, 120*(12), 1658–1670.

May, A. L., Kuklina, E. V., & Yoon, P. W. (2012). Prevalence of cardiovascular disease risk factors among US adolescents, 1999–2008. *Pediatrics, 129*(6), 1035–1041.

Mayer-Davis, E. J., Rifas-Shiman, S. L., Zhou, L., Hu, F. B., Colditz, G. A., & Gillman, M. W. (2006). Breastfeeding and risk for childhood obesity: Does maternal diabetes or obesity status matter? *Diabetes Care, 29*(10), 2231–2237.

Mayer-Davis, E. J., Dabelea, D., Lamichhane, A. P., D'Agostino, R. B., Jr., Liese, A. D., et al. (2008). Breast-feeding and type 2 diabetes in the youth of three ethnic groups: The SEARCh for diabetes in youth case-control study. *Diabetes Care, 31*(3), 470–475.

Mayer-Davis, E. J., Beyer, J., Bell, R. A., Dabelea, D., D'Agostino, R., Jr., Imperatorek, G., et al. (2009). Diabetes in African American youth: Prevalence, incidence, and clinical characteristics: The SEARCH for diabetes in youth study. *Diabetes Care, 32*(Supplement 2), S112–S122.

McEwen, B. S. (2008). Understanding the potency of stressful early life experiences on brain and body function. *Metabolism Clinical and Experimental, 57*(Suppl 2), S11–S15.

McLearn, K. T., Minkovitz, C. S., Strobino, D. M., Marks, E., & Hou, W. (2006). Maternal depressive symptoms at 2 to 4 months post partum and early parenting practices. *Archives of Pediatrics & Adolescent Medicine, 160*(3), 279–284.

McMillen, I. C., & Robinson, J. S. (2005). Developmental origins of the metabolic syndrome: Prediction, plasticity, and programming. *Physiological Reviews, 85*(2), 571–633.

McMurray, R. G., Bassin, S., Jago, R., Bruecker, S., Moe, E. L., Murray, T., et al. (2009). Rationale, design and methods of the HEALTHY study physical education intervention component. *International Journal of Obesity, 33*(Suppl 4), S37–S43.

Meaney, M. J., Szyf, M., & Seckl, J. R. (2007). Epigenetic mechanisms of perinatal programming of hypothalamic-pituitary-adrenal function and health. *Trends in Molecular Medicine, 13*(7), 269–277.

Metzger, B. E., Lowe, L. P., Dyer, A. R., Trimble, E. R., Chaovarindr, U., Coustan, D. R., et al. (2008). Hyperglycemia and adverse pregnancy outcomes. *The New England Journal of Medicine, 358*(19), 1991–2002.

Metzger, B. E., Gabbe, S. G., Persson, B., Buchanan, T. A., Catalano, P. A., Damm, P., et al. (2010). International association of diabetes and pregnancy study groups recommendations on the diagnosis and classification of hyperglycemia in pregnancy. *Diabetes Care, 33*(3), 676–682.

Morandi, A., Maschio, M., Marigliano, M., Miraglia Del Giudice, E., Moro, B., Peverelli, P., et al. (2014). Screening for impaired glucose tolerance in obese children and adolescents: A validation and implementation study. *Pediatric Obesity, 9*(1), 17–25.

Morgan, A. R. (2012). Determining genetic risk factors for pediatric type 2 diabetes. *Current Diabetes Reports, 12*(1), 88–92.

Morris, D. H., Khunti, K., Achana, F., Srinivasan, B., Gray, L. J., Davies, M. J., et al. (2013). Progression rates from HbA(1c) 6.0-6.4% and other prediabetes definitions to type 2 diabetes: A meta-analysis. *Diabetologia, 56*(7), 1489–1493.

Morrison, K. M., Xu, L., Tarnopolsky, M., Yusuf, Z., Atkinson, S. A., & Yusuf, S. (2012). Screening for dysglycemia in overweight youth presenting for weight management. *Diabetes Care, 35*(4), 711–716.

Moses, R. G. (2010). New consensus criteria for GDM: Problem solved or a pandora's box? *Diabetes Care, 33*(3), 690–691.

Navas-Acien, A., Silbergeld, E. K., Pastor-Barriuso, R., & Guallar, E. (2008). Arsenic exposure and prevalence of type 2 diabetes in US adults. *JAMA, 300*(7), 814–822.

Neville, M. C., Anderson, S. M., McManaman, J. L., Badger, T. M., Bunik, M., Contractor, N., et al. (2012). Lactation and neonatal nutrition: Defining and refining the critical questions. *Journal of Mammary Gland Biology and Neoplasia, 17*(2), 167–188. doi:10.1007/s10911-012-9261-5.

Ong, K. K. (2010). Early determinants of obesity. *Endocrine Development, 19*, 53–61.

Pervanidou, P., & Chrousos, G. P. (2011). Stress and obesity/metabolic syndrome in childhood and adolescence. *International Journal of Pediatric Obesity, 6*(Supplement 1), 21–28.

Pervanidou, P., & Chrousos, G. P. (2012). Metabolic consequences of stress during childhood and adolescence. *Metabolism, 61*(5), 611–619.

Peters, A., & Laffel, L. (2011). Diabetes care for emerging adults: Recommendations for transition from pediatric to adult diabetes care systems: A position statement of the American Diabetes Association. *Diabetes Care, 34*(11), 2477–2485.

Plagemann, A., Harder, T., Franke, K., & Kohlhoff, R. (2002). Long-term impact of neonatal breast-feeding on body weight and glucose tolerance in children of diabetic mothers. *Diabetes Care, 25*(1), 16–22.

Prince, A. L., Antony, K. M., Ma, J., & Aagaard, K. M. (2014). The microbiome and development: A mother's perspective. *Seminars in Reproductive Medicine, 32*(1), 14–22.

Raman, A., Ritchie, L. D., Lustig, R. H., Fitch, M. D., Hudes, M. L., & Fleming, S. E. (2010). Insulin resistance is improved in overweight African American boys but not in girls following a one-year multidisciplinary community intervention program. *Journal of Pediatric Endocrinology & Metabolism, 23*(1–2), 109–120.

Rhodes, E. T., Prosser, L. A., Hoerger, T. J., Lieu, T., Ludwig, D. S., & Laffel, L. M. (2012). Estimated morbidity and mortality in adolescents and young adults diagnosed with type 2 diabetes mellitus. *Diabetic Medicine, 29*(4), 453–463.

Ritchie, L. D., Sharma, S., Ikeda, J. P., Mitchell, R. A., Raman, A., Green, B. S., et al. (2010). Taking action together: A YMCA-based protocol to prevent type-2 diabetes in high-BMI inner-city African American children. *Trials, 11*, 60.

Robinson, S., Ntani, G., Simmonds, S., Syddall, H., Dennison, E., Sayer, A. A., et al. (2013). Type of milk feeding in infancy and health behaviours in adult life: Findings from the Hertfordshire cohort study. *The British Journal of Nutrition, 109*(6), 1114–1122.

Rolland-Cachera, M. F. (2011). Childhood obesity: Current definitions and recommendations for their use. *International Journal of Pediatric Obesity, 6*(5–6), 325–331.

Rosenbaum, M., Nonas, C., Weil, R., Horlick, M., Fennoy, I., Vargas, I., et al. (2007). School-based intervention acutely improves insulin sensitivity and decreases inflammatory markers and body fatness in junior high school students. *The Journal of Clinical Endocrinology and Metabolism, 92*(2), 504–508.

Rosenbloom, A. L., Joe, J. R., Young, R. S., & Winter, W. E. (1999). Emerging epidemic of type 2 diabetes in youth. *Diabetes Care, 22*(2), 345–354.

Rosenbloom, A. L., Silverstein, J. H., Amemiya, S., Zeitler, P., & Klingensmith, G. J. (2008). ISPAD clinical practice consensus guidelines 2006-2007. Type 2 diabetes mellitus in the child and adolescent. *Pediatric Diabetes, 9*(5), 512–526.

Saelens, B. E., Grow, H. M., Stark, L. J., Seeley, R. J., & Roehrig, H. (2011). Efficacy of increasing physical activity to reduce children's visceral fat: A pilot randomized controlled trial. *International Journal of Pediatric Obesity, 6*(2), 102–112.

Salsberry, P. J., & Reagan, P. B. (2005). Dynamics of early childhood overweight. *Pediatrics, 116*(6), 1329–1338.

Samuelsson, A. M., Matthews, P. A., Argenton, M., Christie, M. R., McConnell, J. M., et al. (2008). Diet-induced obesity in female mice leads to offspring hyperphagia, adiposity, hypertension, and insulin resistance: A novel murine model of developmental programming. *Hypertension, 51*(2), 383–392.

Savoye, M., Shaw, M., Dziura, J., Tamborlane, W. V., Rose, P., Guandalini, C., et al. (2007). Effects of a weight management program on body composition and metabolic parameters in overweight children: A randomized controlled trial. *JAMA, 297*(24), 2697–2704.

Savoye, M., Nowicka, P., Shaw, M., Yu, S., Dziura, J., Chavent, G., et al. (2011). Long-term results of an obesity program in an ethnically diverse pediatric population. *Pediatrics, 127*(3), 402–410.

Savoye, M., Caprio, S., Dziura, J., Camp, A., Germain, G., Summers, C., et al. (2014). Reversal of early abnormalities in glucose metabolism in obese youth: Results of an intensive lifestyle randomized controlled trial. *Diabetes Care, 37*(2), 317–324.

Schore, A. N. (2005). Back to basics: Attachment, affect regulation, and the developing right brain: Linking developmental neuroscience to pediatrics. *Pediatrics in Review, 26*(6), 204–217.

Sebert, S., Sharkey, D., Budge, H., & Symonds, M. E. (2011). The early programming of metabolic health: Is epigenetic setting the missing link? *The American Journal of Clinical Nutrition, 94*(6 Supplement), 1953S–1958S.

Seki, Y., Williams, L., Vuguin, P. M., & Charron, M. J. (2012). Minireview: Epigenetic programming of diabetes and obesity: Animal models. *Endocrinology, 153*(3), 1031–1038.

Shaw, J. E., Socree, R. A., & Zimmet, P. Z. (2010). Global estimates of the prevalence of diabetes for 2010 and 2030. *Diabetes Research and Clinical Practice, 87*, 4–14.

Shonkoff, J. P., & Garner, A. S. (2012). The lifelong effects of early childhood adversity and toxic stress. *Pediatrics, 129*(1), e232–e246.

Silverman, B. L., Rizzo, T. A., Cho, N. H., & Metzger, B. E. (1998). Long-term effects of the intrauterine environment. The Northwestern University diabetes in pregnancy Center. *Diabetes Care, 21*(Suppl 2), B142–B149.

Simeoni, U., & Barker, D. J. (2009). Offspring of diabetic pregnancy: Long-term outcomes. *Seminars in Fetal & Neonatal Medicine, 14*(2), 119–124.

Sinclair, K. D., Lea, R. G., Rees, W. D., & Young, L. E. (2007). The developmental origins of health and disease: Current theories and epigenetic mechanisms. *Society of Reproduction and Fertility Supplement, 64*, 425–443.

Sinha, R., Fisch, G., Teague, B., Tamborlane, W. V., Banyas, B., Allen, K., et al. (2002). Prevalence of impaired glucose tolerance among children and adolescents with marked obesity. *The New England Journal of Medicine, 346*(11), 802–810.

Skouteris, H., McCabe, M., Swinburn, B., Newgreen, V., Sacher, P., & Chadwick, P. (2011). Parental influence and obesity prevention in pre-schoolers: A systematic review of interventions. *Obesity Reviews, 12*(5), 315–328.

Skouteris, H., McCabe, M., Ricciardelli, L., Milgrom, J., Baur, L., Aksan, N., et al. (2012). Parent–child interactions and obesity prevention: A systematic review of the literature. *Early Child Development and Care, 182*(2), 153–174.

Smith, B. T., Lynch, J. W., Fox, C. S., Harper, S., Abrahamowicz, M., Almeida, N. D., et al. (2011). Life-course socioeconomic position and type 2 diabetes mellitus: The Framingham offspring study. *American Journal of Epidemiology, 173*(4), 438–447.

Snieder, H., Boomsma, D. I., van Doornen, L. J., & Neale, M. C. (1999). Bivariate genetic analysis of fasting insulin and glucose levels. *Genetic Epidemiology, 16*(4), 426–446.

Stark, L. J., Clifford, L. M., Towner, E. K., Filigno, S. S., Zion, C., Bolling, C., et al. (2014). A pilot randomized controlled trial of a behavioral family-based intervention with and without home visits to decrease obesity in preschoolers. *Journal of Pediatric Psychology, 39*(9), 1001–1012. doi:10.1093/jpepsy/jsu059.

Szajewska, H. (2013). Microbiota modulation: Can probiotics prevent/treat disease in pediatrics? *Nestle Nutrition Institute Workshop Series, 77*, 99–110.

Tamayo, T., Christian, H., & Rathmann, W. (2010). Impact of early psychosocial factors (childhood socioeconomic factors and adversities) on future risk of type 2 diabetes, metabolic disturbances and obesity: A systematic review. *BMC Public Health, 10*, 525. doi:10.1186/1471-2458-10-525.

Tamayo, T., Jacobs, D. R., Jr., Strassburger, K., Giani, G., Seeman, T. E., Matthews, K., et al. (2012). Race- and sex-specific associations of parental education with insulin resistance in middle-aged participants: The CARDIA study. *European Journal of Epidemiology, 27*(5), 349–355.

Tarry-Adkins, J. L., & Ozanne, S. E. (2011). Mechanisms of early life programming: Current knowledge and future directions. *The American Journal of Clinical Nutrition, 94*(6 Supplement), 1765S–1771S.

Taveras, E. M., Scanlon, K. S., Birch, L., Rifas-Shiman, S. L., Rich-Edwards, J. W., & Gillman, M. W. (2004). Association of breastfeeding with maternal control of infant feeding at age 1 year. *Pediatrics, 114*(5), e577–e583.

Taveras, E. M., Rifas-Shiman, S. L., Oken, E., Gunderson, E. P., & Gillman, M. W. (2008). Short sleep duration in infancy and risk of childhood overweight. *Archives of Pediatrics & Adolescent Medicine, 162*(4), 305–311.

Taveras, E. M., Gillman, M. W., Pena, M. M., Redline, S., & Rifas-Shiman, S. L. (2014). Chronic sleep curtailment and adiposity. *Pediatrics, 133*(6), 1013–1022.

Thayer, K. A., Heindel, J. J., Bucher, J. R., & Gallo, M. A. (2012). Role of environmental chemicals in diabetes and obesity: A National Toxicology Program workshop review. *Environmental Health Perspectives, 120*(6), 779–789.

Thompson, A. L., & Bentley, M. E. (2013). The critical period of infant feeding for the development of early disparities in obesity. *Social Science & Medicine, 97*, 288–296.

Tounian, P. (2011). Programming towards childhood obesity. *Annals of Nutrition & Metabolism, 58*(Suppl 2), 30–41.

Trevino, R. P., Yin, Z., Hernandez, A., Hale, D. E., Garcia, O. A., & Mobley, C. (2004). Impact of the Bienestar school-based diabetes mellitus prevention program on fasting capillary glucose levels: A randomized controlled trial. *Archives of Pediatrics & Adolescent Medicine, 158*(9), 911–917.

Venditti, E. M., Elliot, D. L., Faith, M. S., Firrell, L. S., Giles, C. M., Goldberg, L., et al. (2009). Rationale, design and methods of the HEALTHY study behavior intervention component. *International Journal of Obesity, 33*(Suppl 4), S44–S51.

Venkat Narayan, K. M., Boyle, J. P., Thompson, T. J., Sorensen, S. W., & Willimason, D. F. (2003). Lifetime risk for riabetes mellitus in the United States. *JAMA, 290*(14), 1884–1889.

Versalovic, J. (2013). The human microbiome and probiotics: Implications for pediatrics. *Annals of Nutrition & Metabolism, 63*(Suppl 2), 42–52.

Visscher, P. M., Hill, W. G., & Wray, N. R. (2008). Heritability in the genomics era–concepts and misconceptions. *Nat Rev Genet, 9*(4), 255–266.

Wabitsch, M., Hauner, H., Hertrampf, M., Muche, R., Hay, B., Mayer, H., et al. (2004). Type II diabetes mellitus and impaired glucose regulation in Caucasian children and adolescents with obesity living in Germany. *International Journal of Obesity and Related Metabolic Disorders, 28*(2), 307–313.

Waitzfelder, B., Pihoker, C., Klingensmith, G., Case, D., Anderson, A., Bell, R. A., et al. (2011). Adherence to guidelines for youths with diabetes mellitus. *Pediatrics, 128*(3), 531–538.

Wang, L., Anderson, J. L., Dalton, W. T., Wu, T., Liu, X., & Zheng, S. (2013). Maternal depressive symptoms and the risk of overweight in their children. *Maternal and Child Health Journal, 17*(5), 940–948.

Warner, M. J., & Ozanne, S. E. (2010). Mechanisms involved in the developmental programming of adulthood disease. *The Biochemical Journal, 427*(3), 333–347.

Weiss, R., Taksali, S. E., Tamborlane, W. V., Burgert, T. S., Savoye, M., & Caprio, S. (2005). Predictors of changes in glucose tolerance status in obese youth. *Diabetes Care, 28*(4), 902–909.

Wen, L. M., Baur, L. A., Simpson, J. M., Rissel, C., Wardle, K., & Flood, V. M. (2012). Effectiveness of home based early intervention on children's BMI at age 2: Randomised controlled trial. *BMJ, 344*, e3732. doi:10.1136/bmj.e3732.

West, N. A., Hamman, R. F., Mayer-Davis, E. J., D'Agostino, R. B., Jr., Marcovina, S. M., Liese, A. S., et al. (2009). Cardiovascular risk factors among youth with and without type 2 diabetes: Differences and possible mechanisms. *Diabetes Care, 32*(1), 175–180.

Whitlock, E. P., O'Connor, E. A., Williams, S. B., Beil, T. L., & Lutz, K. W. (2010). Effectiveness of weight management interventions in children: A targeted systematic review for the US preventive service task Force. *Pediatrics, 125*(2), e396–e418.

Whitmore, T. J., Trengove, N. J., Graham, D. F., & Hartmann, P. E. (2012). Analysis of insulin in human breast milk in mothers with type 1 and type 2 diabetes mellitus. *International Journal of Endocrinology, 2012*, 296368. doi:10.1155/2012/296368.

Zeitler, P. (2010). Approach to the obese adolescent with new-onset diabetes. *The Journal of Clinical Endocrinology and Metabolism, 95*(12), 5163–5170.

Zeitler, P., Hirst, K., Pyle, L., Linder, B., Copeland, K., Arslanian, S., et al. (2012). A clinical trial to maintain glycemic control in youth with type 2 diabetes. *New England Journal of Medicine, 366*(24), 2247–2256.

Zeitler, P., Tandon, N., Nadeau, K., Urakami, T., Barrett, T., & Maahs, D. (2014). Type 2 diabetes in the child and adolescent. *Pediatric Diabetes, 20*(Supplement), 20–26.

Life Course Health Development in Autism Spectrum Disorders

Irene E. Drmic, Peter Szatmari, and Fred Volkmar

1 Introduction

Health development results from dynamic person-environment interactions that begin before conception and continue throughout the lifespan (Halfon et al. 2014; Russ et al. 2014). Life course health development (LCHD) incorporates theories and empirical evidence from the biological, physical, and social sciences to formulate a framework that explains how health develops over the life course. The principles of life course health development (see Halfon and Forrest 2017) describe health as an emergent set of capacities that develop continuously over the lifespan in complex, nonlinear processes that result from multilevel interactions of individuals and their environments. Furthermore, health is sensitive to the timing and social structuring of environmental exposures, as well as to timing and synchronization of molecular, physiological, behavioral, social, and cultural functions. Finally, evolution enables and constrains the range of adaptive plastic responses and health developmental pathways associated with these phenotypes.

The life course health development conceptual framework can be applied to autism spectrum disorders (ASD) to help prioritize a research agenda and improve health development across the lifespan for individuals with ASD, their families, and communities. Novel approaches to understanding ASD are welcome given that ASD represents a major public health challenge. The estimated annual cost of caring for individuals with ASD in the USA is \$137 billion, with a lifetime cost per individual estimated to be \$2.4 million for those with co-occurring intellectual disability and \$1.4 million for those without intellectual disability (Dawson and Bernier 2013). The following chapter is not an exhaustive review of the literature in ASD; rather, we highlight some issues and findings that are pertinent to an understanding of ASD using the lens of the life course health development principles.

I.E. Drmic (✉)
Hospital for Sick Children, Toronto, ON, Canada
e-mail: Irene.drmic@sickkids.ca

P. Szatmari
Centre for Addiction and Mental Health,
Hospital for Sick Children, University of Toronto,
Toronto, ON, Canada
e-mail: Peter.Szatmari@utoronto.ca

F. Volkmar
Child Study Center, Yale University School
of Medicine, New Haven, CT, USA
e-mail: Fred.Volkmar@yale.edu

1.1 What Is Autism Spectrum Disorder (ASD): The Clinical Phenotype

Autism spectrum disorders are a group of neuropsychiatric conditions all of which share

N. Halfon et al. (eds.), *Handbook of Life Course Health Development*,
DOI 10.1007/978-3-319-47143-3_11

difficulties in social engagement and social interaction as their major diagnostic feature. As a result of this basic problem, difficulties arise in learning, cognitive organization, attention, and adaptive skills. Autism, the prototypic disorder, was described by Kanner in 1943 as an "inborn disturbance" of social contact. Autism was first included in a new category of pervasive developmental disorders when first recognized officially in the third edition of *Diagnostic and Statistical Manual of Mental Disorders* (DSM;APA 1980).

Autism is a condition of early onset and poses multiple problems in health development. Many parents are concerned about affected children's development by age 1 with the vast majority of parents worried by age 2 (Chawarska et al. 2008). An increasing body of work has focused on autism as it first develops in infancy (Rogers 2009). In a minority of cases (about 20%), parents report some period of normal development followed by loss of skills; the clinical significance of regression continues to be debated (Parr et al. 2011; Shattuck et al. 2009).

Problems in social interaction are a hallmark of autism and related conditions. Social difficulties are distinctive even considering any associated developmental delays. Similarly, communication problems are present and persistent even in the more cognitively able children who lack verbal and nonverbal social communication skills such as gestures, facial expression, and eye contact. Even when children do speak, they exhibit a number of difficulties including echolalia, pronoun use difficulties, abnormal prosody, and in the social use of language (Paul 2008). Kanner noted the range of unusual behaviors frequent in autism including motor mannerisms (stereotyped movement), difficulties with change, and insistence on routines. The apparent over-engagement with the nonsocial world arises in the general lack of social engagement. This suggests a potential route both as a mechanism for learning difficulties and for intervention.

The original impression that autism was not associated with cognitive problems rested, in large part, on the unusual abilities of children in some areas; in some cases, these skills are highly circumscribed and may arise even in association with overall intellectual delay (Hermelin 2001). Even for the most able individuals, scatter in abilities is often present with a relative deficit in verbal as opposed to perceptual abilities. It is also the case that there is frequently a gap between abilities in a formal testing situation and "real-world" or adaptive skills – the latter reflecting the significant difficulties individuals have in generalization and in tasks that involved fast-paced decision making, executive functioning, and social interaction (Robinson et al. 2009). In more classical autism, nonverbal skills tend to be much stronger than verbal abilities; the opposite profile may hold true for Asperger's disorder although this has been debated (Klin et al. 1996; Meyer and Minshew 2002; Noterdaeme et al. 2010).

As noted above in addition to classic autism of the type described by Kanner, a number of other conditions with some apparent similarity to autism have been recognized, although their validity apart from autism continues to be hotly debated. Asperger's disorder was described (Asperger 1944) the year after Kanner's report first appeared. Although the children (all boys) had major problems in social interaction, in contrast to Kanner's (1943) cases, they demonstrated good language abilities and were more likely to exhibit motor difficulties, unusual and all-consuming esoteric special interests, and their problems seemed to come to clinical attention rather later (Woodbury-Smith and Volkmar 2009). Although included in DSM-IV and *International Statistical Classification of Diseases and Related Health Problems* (ICD)-10 as a distinctive disorder, Asperger's disorder has been the focus of much debate and is not considered a diagnosable disorder in DSM-V.

A subthreshold pervasive developmental disorder category was included in DSM since 1980 to encompass individuals whose difficulties appear to fall close to autism but do not achieve thresholds for diagnosis of that, or related, conditions. Interestingly this concept also was described in the 1940s although not with great precision. It has as always been recognized to significantly outnumber more classical autism (Fombonne 2005a, b) by probably four or five times although research in this area has, paradoxically, been limited. In recent years, the tendency to equate pervasive developmental disorder not otherwise specified with more classic autism has led to a broader autism spectrum concept although it must be emphasized that the DSM-5 autism spectrum disorder concept would likely exclude many cases that in the past had been said to have pervasive developmental disorder not otherwise specified (Volkmar and McPartland 2014).

1.2 Epidemiology

It is clear that ASD has a strong genetic component and is likely related to the interaction of multiple genes (Devlin and Scherer 2012); ASD invariably originates in the first years of life. Poverty and lack of access to adequate resources and intervention clearly impact identification, service provision, and likely outcome (Liptak et al. 2008; Thomas et al. 2007), but this area of work remains one that is relatively little studied. Various factors complicate the study of prevalence rates in ASD. There has been a concern that rates have risen over time although in his review of the topic Fombonne (2005a, b) suggests that a median rate of strictly defined autism would be about 1 per 800 to 1000 people with the much broader pervasive developmental disorder category being much more common. Several recent studies have reported higher rates (e.g., Brugha et al. 2011; Elsabbagh et al. 2012), but studies of adults in community settings report similar rates to those estimated by Fombonne and others (Brugha et al. 2011; Elsabbagh et al. 2012; Rutter 1973) and various factors which might account for apparent increases in rates have been identified (King and Bearman 2009; Rutter 1982) with potential overestimation due to methodology (i.e., case-confirmation strategies) and small sample sizes resulting in high estimates (Levy et al. 2009). Such factors include increased public awareness and increased recognition of more cognitively able individuals, applying the diagnosis to individuals with specific syndromes such as Down syndrome and widening of diagnostic criteria, sundry methodological problems, and "diagnostic substitution" – the latter referring to an issue, particularly in the USA, where an educational label of autism may be used to obtain services in preference to other labels such as mental retardation (Fombonne 2005a, b).

Most studies have reported significantly higher rates of ASD in boys than in girls although girls with more strictly defined autism are also more likely to have intellectual disability (Fombonne 2005a, b). The three- to fivefold increase in boys is similar to other neurodevelopmental disorders such as language disorders and attention deficit hyperactivity disorder (ADHD). It is possible that milder expression in some girls is underdiagnosed (Landa et al. 2007). There has been speculation that greater severity sometimes observed in girls is a function of a greater genetic risk for the condition (Fombonne 2005a, b) and that observed sex differences might relate to fundamental cognitive mechanisms (Baron-Cohen 2011). In reality, sex differences have been remarkably little studied and our understanding of this phenomenon remains very limited.

Potential social class correlates of autism first noted by Kanner (1943) in his original sample have not generally held up in subsequent research, presumably reflecting a referral bias in Kanner's original cases (Fombonne 2005a, b; Wing 1980). However, disparities in diagnosis rates are observed with children from backgrounds of poverty or minority status often going undiagnosed (LaFramboise et al. 2009). Although diagnostic presentation is rather similar around the world, cultural factors may impact both diagnosis and treatment (Brown and Rogers 2003).

1.3 Classification and Diagnosis

Several approaches were undertaken in the late 1970s to provide more operational definitions of autism. Rutter's approach (1978) emphasized difficulties in social interaction, communication, and unusual behaviors of early onset that were not solely attributable to mental retardation. Both family genetic and longitudinal studies provided important information on the stability and validity of the diagnosis apart from other conditions and led to the inclusion of autism in DSM-III (APA 1980). The DSM-III approach was modified in 1987 when DSM-III-R appeared and yet again with DSM-IV which appeared in 1994. The DSM-IV definition was based on results of a large international field trial and became consistent with the tenth revision of the ICD leading to two decades of diagnostic stability (Volkmar and McPartland 2014). For DSM-5, a number of changes were made and have proven controversial. The adoption of the term autism spectrum disorder seems well justified; however, the criteria proposed appear to really be more relevant to classic "Kanner's autism," and many individuals, particularly the more cognitively able, would likely lose their diagnosis (Volkmar and McPartland 2014). As a result, cases with "well-established" diagnosis of Asperger's or pervasive developmental disorder not otherwise specified (PDD-NOS; in DSM-IV terms) could retain an ASD diagnosis – thus effectively creating two diagnostic systems in current use; the advent of ICD-11 and the Research Domain Criteria (RDoC) approach suggest that for some time there may be considerable controversy about definitional issues (see Baker et al. 2012; Brand et al. 2012; Mattilla et al. 2011; McGrew et al. 2012; Watts 2012; Huerta et al. 2012).

2 Pathogenesis

2.1 Hereditability

ASD is now considered a disorder caused at least in part by genetic factors (Szatmari et al. 1998). The evidence for this comes from studies showing that ASD runs within families, from twin studies that show that this familial aggregation is due to genetic and possibly to shared environmental risk factors (Sullivan et al. 2012) and to the recent identification of several different networks of genes responsible for synaptic and axonal development and neuronal migration (Malhotra and Sebat 2012).

Early family studies looked at the recurrence risk to a sibling if one child in the family had ASD. Those sibling risks were around 2% which were considered to be very much higher than the general population rate estimated at that time to be 4 per 10,000 (Szatmari et al. 1998). With better study designs and with a better appreciation of the breadth of the ASD phenotype, these family studies now suggest that the risk to sibling is closer to 9% (Ritvo et al. 1989). This needs to be seen in the context thought of more recent prevalence estimates of ASD of around 1%. Thus, it seems the sibling recurrence risk is roughly ten times the population base rate (Constantino et al. 2010).

The baby sibs paradigm provides a more valid estimate of sibling recurrence risk. In these studies, the infant sibling of an older child with ASD is followed from birth to 3 years of age. In this context, the emergence of autistic signs and symptoms can be carefully documented prospectively, and the presence or absence of an ASD diagnosis is determined by 3 years of age. These studies have shown that signs and symptoms of the ASD phenotype begin to emerge around 6–12 months of age, and upward of 20% of siblings will have a diagnosis of ASD at 3 years of age (Chawarska et al. 2008; Zwaigenbaum et al. 2012). Interestingly, despite the fact that these studies have demonstrated that ASD can be diagnosed as early as 3 years and that best practice in ASD, such as the 2007 American Academy of Pediatrics guideline that all children should be screened for ASD at 18 and 24 months, the average age of diagnosis in the USA is still close to 5 years and higher in those with milder forms of ASD (CDC 2014).

Twin studies are used to determine the mechanism of familial aggregation. Earlier studies suggested very sharp discrepancies between monozygous and dizygous concordance rates suggesting not only that the mechanism of heritability was genetic but that there was little room for environmental risk factors in playing an important role in causation. The twin study with the largest sample size and the one carried out with the most methodological rigor was recently published (Hallmayer et al. 2011). In that study, monozygous concordance rates were closer to 60%, and dizygous rates were 20% rate seen in the recent infant sibling studies. While the Hallmayer et al. twin study also provides support for the importance of genetic factors in the etiology of the disorder, the higher than expected dizygous concordance rate also suggests a significant role for shared environmental risk factors.

2.2 Genetic Contribution

Hundreds of different genes have been described in ASD that have been disrupted by either deletions or duplications of copy number. These genes all appear to be related to different aspects of neuronal development (largely synaptic functioning) or neuronal migration (Li et al. 2012). This is an important finding as it steers mechanisms of etiology away from neurotransmitters and monoamines, a theory which had dominated the field for several decades (McDougle et al. 2005).

With the discovery of copy number variants as important structural genomic risk factors for a variety of human diseases has come the realization that these variants might play an important role in the etiology of ASD (Marshall et al. 2008). Copy number variants represent deletions or duplications covering more than 1000 kbs of DNA. In general, copy number variants can be common or rare, and they can be either de novo or inherited from parents. The first copy number variant identified in ASD in a genome-wide study was a rare deletion in the neurexin gene (Szatmari et al. 2007), and this has been followed up with many reports of other copy number variants affecting important brain-expressed genes (for a review see Malhotra and Sebat 2012). These copy number variants tend to be extremely rare, found in less than 1% of the ASD samples, and tend to rise de novo. This would explain the frequent lack of family history in ASD families and would provide a mechanism whereby the prevalence of the disorder remains stable in the context of a condition associated with reduced fertility (Power et al. 2012). Common genetic variants (either polymorphisms or copy number variants) have not been reliably identified in ASD, although such variants likely do exist and will require very large sample sizes for their identification (Devlin et al. 2011). If they do exist, their effect size must be very small or else they operate as modifying factors as opposed to susceptibility genes. Currently, copy number variants explain less than 10% of cases in ASD, and the population attributable risk is less than 5% (Pinto et al. 2010). The etiology of the vast majority of cases of ASD remains to be explained. The next generation of genetic studies will focus on much smaller copy number variants or DNA sequence variants identified either in exomes or in whole genome sequencing.

2.3 Nongenetic Contributions

The search for environmental risk factors has been underway for many decades. There seems reasonably good evidence that certain maternal anticonvulsants such as carbamazepine, valproic acid, and perhaps other anticonvulsants increase risk for ASD (Palac and Meador 2011). Other putative environmental risk factors that may have been more common in earlier decades such as congenital rubella have now virtually disappeared. A complication in all this work is disentangling the sometimes complex issues of severe mental handicap and “autistic-like” behaviors, particularly since stereotyped mannerisms become much more common with severe intellectual deficiency, but characteristic social-communicative features may be either difficult to judge or not clearly present (Volkmar et al. 2005). Pregnancy and birth complications have been studied extensively, and other than low birth weight or being small for gestational age, it is difficult to identify a risk factor (see Gardener et al. 2009 for a recent meta-analysis). It should be noted, however, that low birth weight may in fact represent a *consequence* of genetic vulnerability rather than an environmental risk factor interacting with genetic susceptibility (Rutter 2005). Other potential environmental markers signaled by inflammatory indices are of interest but remain highly speculative at this point (Muller et al. 2015). Perhaps the most convincing evidence for an environmental risk factor is that of advanced parental age (Shelton et al. 2010). Since paternal and maternal age is so highly correlated, it is difficult to determine if both are risk factors or if only one. This is important as the mechanism by which the risk factor might operate will be quite different based on the maternal/paternal risk factor (Veltman and Brunner 2012). De novo copy number variants are more common with advanced paternal age, while chromosomal abnormalities (like trisomies) are more common with advanced maternal age.

2.4 Epigenetic Contributions

Epigenetic studies of non-syndromic ASD are in their infancy but do hold promise once technological and methodical issues associated with this area of study are resolved. Genes that regulate DNA methylation have been implicated in the etiology of ASD, and single gene disorders associated with ASD have implicated epigenetic mechanisms (Loke et al. 2015). It is anticipated that this will be an active field in the future and will yield novel insights in how person-environment interactions lead to the development of ASD.

2.5 Physical Biomarkers

Magnetic resonance imaging and diffusion tensor imaging studies have provided some insight into brain structure, circuitry, and connectivity in ASD. Courchesne and colleagues followed toddlers from 12 months to 48 months and found an abnormal brain growth trajectory in autism (Schumann et al. 2010). Toddlers, who were ultimately diagnosed with ASD, showed enlargement of cerebral gray and white matter, which was most pronounced in the frontal, temporal, and cingulate cortices, and some gray matter regions showed an abnormal growth rate. In addition, in those infants who later developed ASD, there was a difference in the development of white matter tracks between 6 and 12 months of age (i.e., increases in fractional anisotropy), with a slowing in development by 24 months (Wolff et al. 2012). Thus, abnormal neurodevelopmental connectivity early in life could potentially serve as an important biomarker for ASD.

2.6 Genotype-Phenotype Contributions

In addition, genotype-phenotype correlations have been virtually impossible to establish, and the fact that the genetic variants identified in ASD also appear to be playing a role in intellectual disability, epilepsy, schizophrenia, and ADHD has emphasized the nonspecificity of these susceptibility risk factors (State 2010). These genetic findings in ASD have influenced healthcare recommendation and practice, such that microarray testing is part of the standard of care for diagnosis of ASD (McGrew et al. 2012). It is likely that in the future, whole exome sequencing will also become standard clinical practice. However, to date, no studies have directly assessed the impact of genetic testing on health outcomes such as earlier age of diagnosis or reduced use of other diagnostic tools such as MRI (Sun et al. 2015). In the future, we anticipate that there will be an increased application of genetics and neuroimaging to the early identification of ASD (Dawson and Bernier 2013). It is also likely that the discovery of genetic variants that impact the development of the synapse will lead to clinical trials of new (or "repurposed") drugs targeting those mechanisms. Such trials are already underway in fragile X and tuberous sclerosis but so far with disappointing results (Geschwind and State 2015).

3 Outcome Studies

3.1 An Overview of Developmental Course

Before reviewing approaches to assessing outcome, an overview of what is known, and what is not known, about the course of autism spectrum disorders may be helpful. It must be emphasized that outcome is usually very specifically defined as adult independence and that little information is available on health-related outcomes and vanishingly little relates to older individuals with ASD. Variations in life course are, in part, one of the rationales used to support previous diagnostic distinctions between subtypes. In more "classical" autism, it is clear that diagnosis in infancy is of great interest but also somewhat problematic until about age 3 when reasonable stability in clinical manifestations occurs. Before that time, the issue usually is between change from (or to) a more classic picture to a more "subthreshold" condition (an issue that may be mitigated by the broad approach adopted in DSM-5). Often the difficulty, using the DSM-IV, was that social and communication problems are present but the "restricted interests" criteria were not fully met (even though some likely precursor behaviors are present). Rarely a child moves off the autism spectrum entirely. There is good evidence (NRC 2001) that treatments are most effective when started early in life; although for reasons not well understood, some children do not improve as dramatically as others. It is important to emphasize that apart from a reasonably robust literature on adult outcome (i.e., early in adult life), the literature on adults with autism is very limited both in terms of actual numbers of studies and individuals studied and an absence of literature on the topic of aging in autism (Howlin 2013; Perkins and Berkman 2012). For example, few studies address the issue of rates of employment among adults with autism/ASD and rates of suicide or suicide attempts (even though depression is thought to be a frequent co-occurring condition), and no studies are available on the life course changes for individuals with autism/ASD. Put another way (and viewed in the starkest possible light), it is as if adults with autism/ASD vanish from the scene once they've become adult and "had their outcome," such as capacities in young adulthood for personal independence and self-sufficiency.

School-age children with more "classic" autism often become more sociable as they get older, and gains in cognitive and communication skills also typically are made – sometimes dramatic ones and other times not. Social language use and peer relationships often remain areas of difficulties, and problems with agitation and self-stimulatory behavior may require behavioral or pharmacologic intervention. As first observed by Leo Kanner (Kanner 1971), in adolescence, some children make major gains, while another group unfortunately exhibits some degree of deterioration in functioning. A number of outcome studies now suggest a gradual change in overall prognosis presumably reflecting both earlier and better intervention as well as some changes in diagnostic practice over the time (i.e., including recognizing autism in more cognitively able individuals) (Howlin 2005). An increasing number of individuals are able to live independently and self-sufficiently as adults, and many now go to college or pursue technical/vocational training. Major predictors of adult outcome include level of intellectual functioning and communication competence. Some adults require intermediate levels of support, and in many cases, affected individuals never attain independence and must live in highly structured residential settings. Age-related vulnerabilities have been noted, e.g., the risk of seizure disorder is substantially increased both in early childhood and again in adolescence and possibly well into adulthood. More able adults with autism and related conditions also are apparently more vulnerable to anxiety and depression which can require specific treatments (Howlin 2013; Skokauskas and Gallagher 2010; Szatmari and McConnell 2011; White et al. 2009).

Data on outcome in Asperger's disorder are, expectedly, less extensive but suggest (also as might be expected) overall better outcomes in terms of independence, educational attainment, employment, and social independence. However, comorbid conditions, such as anxiety and depression, can be a complicating factors and negatively impact outcomes (Skokauskas and Gallagher 2010; Szatmari and McConnell 2011; White et al. 2009; Volkmar et al. 2014). There is some suggestion of increased risk for both psychosis and legal difficulties in adolescence and adulthood, but the evidence for this consists largely of case reports (Skokauskas and Gallagher 2010; Szatmari and McConnell 2011; White et al. 2009).

Studies of children with "subthreshold" pervasive developmental disorder are very uncommon although, on balance, these individuals appear to have a better outcome than those with more classical autism (Towbin 2005). The outcome in childhood disintegrative disorder and Rett's does appear, unfortunately, to be poor (Volkmar et al. 2005; Van Acker et al. 2005). In childhood disintegrative disorder, children lose skills but then plateau and make relatively minimal gains. In Rett's, the course is well known with children becoming somewhat more sociable over time but also more incapacitated due to neurological and movement problems.

3.2 Adult Independence

Information on long-term prognosis is limited and difficult to interpret. This review will focus primarily on long-term follow-up outcome studies that have been published over the past decade (for reviews of earlier outcome studies see Gillberg 1991; Henninger and Taylor 2012; Howlin 2000; Howlin and Moss 2012; Levy and Perry 2011; Nordin and Gillberg 1998). The majority of studies that report on "outcomes" for people with ASD have focused on a few domains (e.g., work status, residential situation, friendships; see more detailed discussion below). Predicting outcome has been difficult due to the wide variability in cognitive, linguistic, social, and behavioral abilities in this group of individuals. Consistent interpretation of different findings has also been difficult due to varied sample size (generally small), sampling procedures (clinical versus population based), differences in diagnostic criteria over time, wide range of age at diagnosis, differences in amount of time between initial and follow-up assessments, differences in measures used, imprecise and/or poor quality data on early intellectual functioning, and the lack of information about early intervention services. These factors may account, in part, for the substantial variability reported in adult outcomes for people with ASD.

As noted previously, although psychosocial outcomes have generally been poor, there is a trend over time for higher rates of improvement (see Table 1 – description of how the outcome categories were defined is provided below; Beadle-Brown et al. 2002; Billstedt et al. 2005, 2007, 2011; Eaves and Ho 2008; Farley et al. 2009; Gillberg 1991; Hofvander et al. 2009; Howlin 1998; Howlin et al. 2004; Kobayashi et al. 1992; Lockyer and Rutter 1969, 1970; Lotter 1978; Lovaas 1987; Nordin and Gillberg 1998; Rutter et al. 1967; Rutter and Lockyer 1967; Szatmari et al. 1989). Studies conducted from the 1950s to 1970s reported that less than 15% of individuals had good/very good outcomes and the majority had poor/very poor outcomes (Eisenberg 1956; Rutter et al. 1967; Lotter 1974). Over the past three decades, outcomes have improved but remain variable; the proportion of good to very good outcomes ranges from 4% to 62% and poor to very poor outcome ranges from 3% to 78% (see Table 1). Outcomes have been classified into different outcome categories ranging from "very poor to very good" by various studies over the years. Of note, these ratings were more subjective in earlier studies (pre-2000), whereas more objective criteria have been used in recent studies (for a detailed discussion, see Henniger and Taylor 2012).

The group of studies published within the last decade used quantifiable outcome criteria to classify individuals with ASD into these different outcome categories ranging from very poor to very good (see Howlin et al. 2004, Appendix 2, for detailed criteria). In general, the criteria used to determine outcome were based on a 5-point composite rating of overall social and independent living functioning that was derived by summing individual scores for work status (ranging from 0 = employed or self-employed to 3 = no occupation), residential situation (ranging from 0 = living independently to 5 = being in hospital care or at home because nowhere else would accept the individual), and number and quality of meaningful friendships (ranging from 0 = more than one friendship to 3 = no friendships or joint activities) . Based on the 5-point composite rating, a score of 0 indicated a "very good" outcome (i.e., total for all three areas between 0 and 2); 1 = "good" outcome (total 3–4); 2 = "fair" outcome (total 5–7); 3 = "poor" outcome (total 8–10); and 4 = "very poor" outcome (total 11). Thus, the concept of "outcome" is related to practical independence and autonomy achieved in adult life.

Howlin and her colleagues (2004) surveyed 68 adults (average age of 29 years) with autism who had a performance IQ of 50 or above in childhood and found that the majority (58%) had

Table 1 Review of adult outcome studies

Authors	*N*	Mean age at intake (IN) and follow-up (FU) (years)	Functioning level at intake (IN) and follow-up (FU)	Mean follow-up time (years)	Method of initial assessment	*Dx*	Very poor to poor	Restricted to fair	Good to very good
Gillespie-Lynch et al. (2012)	AUT = 20	IN: 3.9 FU: 26.6	IN: 54.7[a] FU: n/a	–	DSM-III	AUT	50	20	30
Billstedt et al. (2011)[b]	TOT = 108 (AUT = 73 ATY = 35)	IN: <10 years FU: 25.5 (17–40)	AUT IN: 21% IQ > 70 FU: 7% IQ > 70 ATY IN: 14% IQ > 70 FU: 3% IQ > 70	17.8	DSM-III-R	AUT& ATY	12	26	62
Farley et al. (2009)	AUT = 48	IN: 7.2 (3–25) FU: 32.5 (22–46)	IN: IQ > 70 (IQ Estimate = 86.66) FU: FSIQ = 88.93	24.4	DSM-III	AUT	17	34	48
Eaves and Ho (2008)	AUT = 48 ASD = 40	IN: 6.8 (3–12) FU: 24.0 (19–31)	IN: 17% IQ ≥ 70 FU: n/a	–	DSM I–III; Rutter	AUT	46	32	21
Cederlund et al. (2008)	ASP = 70 AUT = 70 (includes AUT & ATY)	ASP IN: 11.3 (5–24) FU: 21.5 (16–33) AUT IN: <10.0 FU: 24.5 (16–36)	ASP: IN: 100% IQ ≥ 70 (FSIQ =101.4) FU: 98% IQ ≥ 70 (FSIQ = 103.0) AUT: IN: 19% IQ ≥ 70 FU: 7% IQ ≥ 70	–	Gillberg's criteria, DSM-III, DSM-III-R	ASP AUT	3 76	70 24	27 0
Billstedt et al. (2005)	TOT = 108 (AUT = 73 ATY = 35)	IN: <10.0 FU: 25.5 (17–40)	AUT: IN: 21% IQ > 70 FU: 7% IQ > 70 ATY IN: 14% IQ > 70 FU: 3% IQ > 70	17.8	Rutter, DSM-III	AUT& ATY	78	21	0
Howlin et al. 2004	AUT = 68	IN 7.24 (3–15) FU 29.3 (21–48)	IN: PIQ = 80.21 VIQ = 61.49 FU: PIQ = 75.00 VIQ = 79.78	–	Criteria applicable at time of diagnosis (1950–1979)	AUT	58	19	22

(continued)

Table 1 (continued)

Authors	*N*	Mean age at intake (IN) and follow-up (FU) (years)	Functioning level at intake (IN) and follow-up (FU)	Mean follow-up time (years)	Method of initial assessment	*Dx*	Very poor to poor	Restricted to fair	Good to very good
Engstrom et al. (2003)	ASP = 32 HFA = 10	IN: HFA 13.5 (4–20); ASP 28.0 (15–41) FU: 30.8 (18–49)	IN: n/a FU: 100% IQ > 70	–	DSM-IV	ASP& HFA	12	75	12
Howlin (2000) and Mawhood et al. (2000)	AUT = 19	IN: (7–8) FU: 23.8 (21–26)	IN: NVIQ ≥ 70 NVIQ = 94.28 VIQ = 66.56 FU: NVIQ = 82.78 VIQ = 82.33	–	Rutter	AUT	74	10	16
Larsen and Mouridsen (1997)	AUT = 9 ASP = 9	IN: ASP = 9.2; AUT = 5.9 FU: ASP 39.1 (33–44); AUT 36.5 (32–39)	IN: ASP: 100% IQ > 70 AUT: 56% IQ > 70 FU: N/A	30	ICD-10	ASP AUT	22 67	44 11	33 22
Ruble and Dalrymple (1996)	AUT = 46	IN: 5.2 FU: 17.1	IN: 26.7% IQ >70 FU: 15.2% IQ > 70	8.6	DSM-III-R	AUT	100	0	0
Kobayashi et al. (1992)	AUT = 201	IN: 6.4 FU: 21.5	IN: 23.4% IQ ≥ 70 FU: n/a	15.4	DSM-III-R	AUT	46	27	27
Gillberg and Steffenburg (1987)	AUT = 23	IN: <6 FU: (16–23)	IN: 26% IQ > 70 FU: n/a	6–11	DSM-III; Kanner & Eisenberg; Rutter	AUT	44	48	4
Lotter 1974	AUT = 32	IN: (8–10) FU: (16–18)	IN: 66.7% IQ < 55 FU: n/a	8	Creak (1961)	AUT	63	24	13
Rutter et al. (1967) and Rutter and Lockyer (1967)	IP = 57	IN: 5.9 (2–10) FU: 15.6	IN: 29% IQ > 70 (mean IQ 62) FU: n/a	9.7	Agreement among psychiatrists	IP	61	25	14
Eisenberg (1956)	AUT = 63	IN: 6 FU: 15	n/a	9	Unclear	AUT	73	22	5

ASP Asperger syndrome, *ATY* atypical autism, *AUT* autism, *HFA* high-functioning autism, *IP* infantile psychosis

[a]Developmental quotient (mental age divided by chronological age)

[b]QOL scale

poor or very poor outcomes, 19% had fair outcome, and 22% had good or very good outcome. Those individuals with a performance IQ of at least 70 in childhood had significantly better outcome than those with an IQ below 70. More specifically, of those individuals with a performance IQ between 50 and 69 (n = 23), only one individual had very good outcome, three were rated as fair, and the remaining had poor or very poor outcome. Individuals in this IQ category had much poorer prognosis with few having jobs, friends, or achieving independence as adults. In the group of individuals with near average to average IQ, outcome was generally better, although still quite variable. Of those individuals with an IQ of 70 or above (n = 45; parental data missing on one individual), 14 individuals were rated as good or very good, 10 as fair, and 20 as poor or very poor. Furthermore, there was no difference in outcome in those individuals with an IQ over 100 and those with and initial IQ between 70 and 99. Interestingly, many individuals with an IQ between 70 and 99 made better progress in terms of academics, jobs, and general level of functioning, than those with an IQ above 100. Thus, having an IQ of about 70 seemed to be a critical cutoff point for better outcome (e.g., level of independence); however, outcome in these individuals was still quite variable.

Other studies found a similar pattern of results. Billstedt et al. (2005) examined a group of low- to middle-functioning individuals (82% had an IQ below 70) with autism or atypical autism and found that 91% had poor or very poor outcome and none were reported to have good outcome. Eaves and Ho (2008) reported somewhat better outcomes in a group of low- to middle-functioning individuals (majority had IQ < 70) with approximately half having fair to good outcome and half poor (but none very poor). Similar outcomes were reported by Gillespie-Lynch et al. (2012), with 50% reporting poor outcome and 50% fair to very good outcome. Engstrom, Ekstrom, and Emilsson (2003) reported on the psychosocial functioning of a systematically selected sample of patients with Asperger syndrome (AS) and high-functioning autism (HFA) all of whom had an IQ above 70. The majority were rated as having a fair outcome (75%), with few being rated as good or poor (12% each) and none being rated as very poor. Farley et al. (2009) also examined adult outcomes for 41 individuals with average or near average cognitive abilities and found better outcomes compared to the other studies with 48% showing good or very good outcome, 34% with fair outcome, and only 17% with poor outcome (none with very poor outcome). Taken together, these studies suggest that outcomes for adults may be improving and that this is likely related to availability of services for individuals with ASD (Gillespie-Lynch et al. 2012; Kobayashi et al. 1992). However, it is important to also take into consideration the pattern of attrition in longitudinal studies. For instance, selective attrition of lower functioning individuals may account for the more positive outcomes in some studies (Eaves and Ho 2008; Gillespie-Lynch et al. 2012).

3.3 Quality of Life

Although the vast majority of studies have based outcomes on level of independence achieved in adulthood and IQ, symptom severity and language development are thought to be important factors in these outcomes; there is increasing interest in examining outcomes based on quality of life (QOL) indictors. QOL is a more comprehensive and multidimensional concept that also encompasses one's subjective evaluations of their experiences (Burgess and Gutstein 2007). According to the World Health Organization (WHO), the concept of QOL not only includes level of independence and social relationships but also is composed of the person's health, personal beliefs, and their relationship to salient features of their environment (Saxena and Orley 1997).

Generally, studies show that overall QOL and health-related QOL is relatively low for people with ASD (Kamp-Becker et al. 2011; van Heijst and Geurts 2015; Potvin et al. 2015). van Heijst and Geurts (2015) conducted a meta-analysis on QOL studies that included children, adolescents, and adults with ASD and found that QOL is lower in people with ASD compared to people without ASD and age did not have an effect. The lack of association with age has previously been reported (Kamino et al. 2012; Kamp-Becker et al. 2011), although it had also been reported that increasing age is associated with decreasing quality of life (Bennett et al. 2005). Characteristics that were relevant predictors in the traditional adult outcome studies, including symptom severity, IQ, and early language, were not examined because information was too sparse. Given the dearth of information about the elderly, the authors also conducted an empirical study examining QOL in intellectually able elderly individuals with ASD and again found large difference in QOL in people with versus without ASD with lower QOL in individuals with ASD. Interestingly, age, IQ, and symptom severity did not predict QOL in the elderly.

Billstedt et al. (2011) examined aspects of quality of life (QOL) in adults diagnosed with autism or atypical autism in childhood and found that the majority of the ASD group remained dependent on parents for support in education, recreation, and occupational situations in late adolescents and early adulthood, but QOL was quite positive (independent of intellectual functioning). The QOL scale used in this study measured both objective and subjective (although by proxy) indicators of well-being. The authors who evaluated the participants completed a QOL scale assessing "autism-friendly environment" using a five-item scale (QOL-1). The item categories were (1) staff and caregivers have specific "autism knowledge," (2) applied structured education implemented, (3) individual specific treatment/training plan for the person with autism implemented, (4) occupation or everyday life activity corresponding to his/her level of capacity, and (5) overall quality of life. Each item was rated on a 1 (very good) to 5 (very poor). A second QOL scale assessing "parent/care rating of individual's well-being" was obtained to estimate how the individual with autism enjoyed or liked his/her residential conditions (QOL-2). Sixty-two percent of individuals were rated as having a very good or good QOL by the authors (QOL-1), and 91% of families reported high or very high residential well-being (QOL-2). This is consistent with reports among young adults with intellectual disabilities who reported satisfaction with their lives even though they remained quite dependent on caregivers (Keogh et al. 2004) and a greater sense of empowerment than those individuals who were still in the school system (Kraemer et al. 2003). Howlin (2013) emphasized that traditional definitions of "good outcome" or "independent living" may not be the most suitable goal to strive for individuals with ASD, because it may lead to a life with little support that is isolated and lacking in stimulation. More research examining QOL is needed in ASD. Raphael et al. (1996) conceptualize a QOL model, which is relevant to persons with developmental disabilities, as containing three domains that include "being, belonging, and becoming" (p. 28). The "being" domain includes being who one is or wants to become, "belonging" includes how one fits within their environment, and "becoming" involves pursuit of personal goals and wants. They also noted that within each domain, it is important to consider the perceived importance, enjoyment experienced, perceived control, and opportunities for change and enhancement. Thus, it is important to also examine and understand the subjective experience of the individuals with ASD and their families when assessing outcome. As with any chronic disability, having a condition like ASD may predispose to other problems – particularly difficulties with depression and anxiety disorder; the relative dearth of work on adult outcome and complexities of the problems of comorbidity and diagnosis limit our understanding of the developmental pathways that result in these outcomes. Similarly, even for the most cognitively able adults (e.g., those who attend college), challenges remain in various areas including adaptive (real-world) skills and generalization, social interaction, organization abilities, and so forth (Farley et al. 2009). As noted previously, the significant limitations of the available literature must be emphasized – issues of QOL have not frequently been assessed, even more cognitively able individuals may lead lives of social isolation with comorbid mental health conditions, medication use is quite high, limitations in daily life can result from poor adaptive skills, and essentially no information is available on aging (Howlin 2013). Thus, given the large differences between quality of life in people with and without ASD, a great deal of work needs to be done to understand how to support optimal health development in individuals with ASD and provide their families with the kinds of interventions that will enable them to achieve a higher QOL and promote well-being. A shift in research focus is needed to understand factors that lead to a better QOL across the life course. There is some evidence indicating that a higher QOL is related to earlier diagnosis (Kamino et al. 2012), greater perceived support (Renty and Roeyers 2006), and supported employment, residential, and leisure programs (Garcia-Villamisar et al. 2002, García-Villamisar and Dattilo 2010; Gerber et al. 2011). Thus, considerable work is needed to improve QOL in people with ASD, and a better understanding of the developmental trajectory across the lifespan may help to better understand the need and interventions required to support these individuals.

3.4 Predictors of Adult Independence

Intellectual functioning (IQ) and language have been most consistently identified as the best predictor of adult personal independence as outcome in ASD (Billstedt et al. 2005, 2007; Gillberg and Steffenburg 1987; Gillespie-Lynch et al. 2012; Howlin et al. 2004; Kobayashi et al. 1992; Lotter 1974; Nordin and Gillberg 1998; Rumsey et al. 1985), although reports have been variable (Farley et al. 2009; Gillespie-Lynch et al. 2012). Farley et al. (2009) reported that early childhood variables were weakly associated with adult outcomes, but the participants in their study all had communicative phrase speech or better language by age 6 and near average to average IQ. Gillespie-Lynch et al. (2012) also found that early intellectual functioning did not predict adult outcomes but suggested that this may be because the average age of the first assessment was quite young (mean age of 3.9 years). Cognitive testing of children with autism older than 4–5 years of age is reported to give more stable measures than in those children who are tested at younger ages (Lord and Schopler 1989; Howlin et al. 2004). In general, however, the presence of an intellectual disability (ID) is associated with poorer outcome in people with ASD in adult life (Cederlund et al. 2008; Gillberg and Steffenberg 1987; Howlin et al. 2004; Rumsey et al. 1985; Shattuck et al. 2007), with the poorest outcomes for those individuals with an IQ below 50 (Lord and Bailey 2002). Few people with this level of cognitive impairment (IQ < 50), regardless of an ASD diagnosis, achieve a high level of independence as adults (Keogh et al. 2004; Kraemer and Blacher 2001). Conversely, higher levels of intellectual functioning (IQ > 70) are associated with better outcome (Billstedt et al. 2007; Eaves and Ho 2008; Gillberg and Steffenberg 1987; Howlin et al. 2004; Rumsey et al. 1985; Szatmari et al. 1989), but outcome can still be quite variable in these individuals (Billstedt et al. 2005; Howlin et al. 2004). These data further underscore the importance of focusing on early language development and learning (IQ) in early intervention programs for children with ASD.

With regard to verbal and performance (nonverbal) IQ, the results are more inconsistent. Some have reported that childhood verbal IQ is a better predictor of later functioning than performance IQ (Billstedt et al. 2005; Lord and Bailey 2002), whereas another study found neither to be a consistent prognostic indicator (Howlin et al. 2004). In addition, the presence of good early language skills before age 5–6 is crucial for positive outcome in ASD (Billstedt et al. 2007; Gillberg and Steffenberg 1987; Gillespie-Lynch et al. 2012; Lockyer and Rutter 1969; Lotter 1978; Szatmari et al. 2003). Mawhood et al. (2000) have shown that individuals who tended to have better linguistic outcome in adulthood were functioning at a higher cognitive level more generally.

Other factors have also been suggested to be related to outcome, including symptom severity, repetitive/stereotyped behaviors in childhood, adaptive behavior, education, gender, the presence of a diagnosed medical disorder, onset of epilepsy before age 5 years, and joint attention skills (Billstedt et al. 2007; De Meyer et al. 1973; Farley et al. 2009; Gillespie-Lynch et al. 2012; Howlin and Goode 1998; Totsika et al. 2010; Venter et al. 1992). For instance, Farley et al. (2009) reported that adaptive behavior measures (in particular the Daily Living Skills domain) evaluated at follow-up were most closely correlated to better outcomes. They described a group of individuals with a high IQ but poor practical living skills who felt frustrated by these limitations. Furthermore, they also described individuals who had a low IQ but who were able to manage with little assistance and obtained good or very good outcome rating despite poor cognitive skills. These results have important implications for intervention programs that foster these practical living skills in adulthood.

The development of joint attention skills may be another important area to target in early intervention programs because of the relationship of this developmental skill set with later health development outcomes. Joint attention skills typically develop between 6 and 18 months of age and refer to ability of the infant to coordinate their attention with another individual during a social interaction. Joint attention skills are important because they are considered early markers of social cognitive development; that is, they reflect the early development of the infant's ability to think about the perspective of another individual (Tomasello 1995). These skills are critical to social learning and social information processing (Mundy and Jarrold 2010), language development (Sigman and Kasari 1995), and the emergence of social and behavioral competence in childhood (Vaughan Van Hecke et al. 2007). Children with ASD present with deficits in joint attention regardless of their developmental or intellectual level, and these deficits are neither absolute nor uniform (Mundy et al. 2009).

In a recent longitudinal study into adult outcomes, responsiveness to joint attention, but not initiation of joint attention (IJA), was found to predict later outcomes. Responsiveness to joint attention was found to predict gains in IQ from early childhood (M = 3.9 years) to later childhood (M = 11.7 years) and receptive language in late adolescents/early adulthood (M = 18.3 years) (Sigman and McGovern 2005; Sigman and Ruskin 1999). In terms of adult outcomes, responsiveness to joint attention predicted adult nonverbal communication, social skills, and symptoms (Gillespie-Lynch et al. 2012). In addition, responsiveness to joint attention and early language both predicted a composite measure of adult social functioning and independence. Taken together, responsiveness to joint attention measured in early childhood may reflect early emerging social cognition, and preliminary evidence suggests that it may be a good predictor of social behaviors in adulthood. Gillespie-Lynch and colleagues also suggested examining the relationship with responsiveness to joint attention and early executive functioning in childhood on later outcomes given that executive functioning is related to adaptive functioning in children with autism (Gilotty et al. 2012).

Gulsrud et al. (2014) examined the developmental trajectories of specific joint attention gestures (i.e., pointing, showing, coordinated joint looking) and expressive language over a 6-year period and found that coordinated joint looking and showing increased over time and pointing to share interest increased over the preschool years (3–5 years of age) and then decreased. They also reported a causal relationship between early pointing and later language development; that is, those children with high rates of pointing in the preschool years had better expressive language skills later. Hence, an understanding of the developmental course of joint attention skills allows for better consideration deciding "when" to intervene. Based on the data, the authors suggested that it may be useful to focus on pointing in early childhood when the child is preverbal and less useful when the child begins to use spoken language. Thus, the interval when early joint attention skills develop may represent a critical or sensitive period to intervene and potentially impact the developmental trajectory and outcomes for individuals with ASD. In addition, the children who received the joint attention intervention showed the fastest improvement compared to the control condition or child who received a different intervention. Participation in the joint attention treatment placed these children on a different developmental trajectory. This highlights that "what" you target and "when" you intervene are important (Gulsrud et al. 2014).

3.5 Diagnostic Stability and Symptom Severity

There is considerable debate in the literature regarding the stability of a diagnosis of autism and other forms of ASD over time. Some studies report that individuals diagnosed in childhood continue to meet criteria for the disorder at follow-up (Billstedt et al. 2005; Cederlund et al. 2008; Howlin et al. 2004; Lotter 1978); whereas others report a change in diagnosis or movement "off" the spectrum in some individuals (Daniels et al. 2011; Kleinman et al. 2008; Turner and Stone 2007). Two recent studies reported that a diagnosis of autism was reasonably stable, whereas for other forms of ASD such as pervasive developmental disorder, the results were more variable (Rondeau et al. 2011; Woolfenden et al. 2012). Rondeau et al. (2011) did a meta-analysis on eight longitudinal studies, published between 1996 and 2009, examining autism and pervasive developmental disorder. All diagnoses were made before 36 months of age, and the interval between the initial and follow-up assessment was short, ranging from 12 to 84 months. They reported that an autism diagnosis tended to be a more stable than pervasive developmental disorder. Of those with pervasive developmental disorder, only 35% retained the same diagnosis (versus the 76% reported for autism), 39% moved to autism, and 25% moved off the spectrum. The authors concluded that those children diagnosed with pervasive developmental disorder at a young age should be reassessed at an older age.

The diagnosis of autism is relatively reliable and stable over time. Issues arise for very young children (the full syndrome picture sufficient for diagnosis may not be observed until age 3 years) and for individuals with "autistic-like" or "spectrum" conditions not so clearly satisfying strict diagnostic criteria. For example, Woolfenden et al. (2012) conducted a systematic review of 23 longitudinal studies (many overlapping with Rondeau et al. 2011) examining the stability of the diagnosis of children initially diagnosed with autism and other forms of ASD. The mean age of children at baseline ranged from 1.8 to 11.3 years, and mean duration at follow-up ranged from 2.1 to 32.5 years. Overall, autism was found to be a stable diagnosis although lower estimates (as low as 53%) were reported for children diagnosed in the preschool years (below 3 years of age). A small percentage of individuals diagnosed with autism, between 12% and 15%, move off the spectrum altogether. For other ASD's (including pervasive developmental disorder, Asperger's disorder, but not autism), based on the highest quality studies, the pattern of stability was more variable with 14–61% retaining their initial diagnosis at follow-up. A few studies reported on optimal outcome in autism (Fein group), and while these adults are indeed quite independent and functional, it appears that some autistic traits remain.

Taken together, a diagnosis of autism is more stable than the other ASD subtypes such as pervasive developmental disorder (Rondeau et al. 2011; Woolfenden et al. 2012), which is consistent with the rationale for the DSM-5 (Szatmari 2011). Given that the ASD category is less stable due to the inclusion of pervasive developmental disorder individuals, this presents challenges to clinicians when sharing a diagnosis of ASD with parents in terms of making appropriate intervention recommendations (Woolfenden et al. 2012).

Impairments in the core ASD symptoms (impairment in communication, reciprocal social interaction, and repetitive or stereotyped behaviors and interests) also tend to persist into adulthood (Billstedt et al. 2007; Howlin 2003; Matson et al. 2008), although symptom severity is reported to decrease in some individuals over time (Seltzer et al. 2003; Shattuck et al. 2007). Totsika et al. (2010) found that an older (50 years or older) group of adults with ASD and ID presented with fewer behavioral problems than the younger (<50 years) group, which is consistent with reports of decreases in behavior problems in the general adult intellectual disability population (Holden and Gitlesen 2006). Billstedt et al.

(2007) found that social interaction problems were still present in the vast majority of adults with ASD, but the occurrence of behavioral impairments (maladaptive and stereotyped behaviors) was much more variable with only a few symptoms in each category affecting half or more of the study sample. Others have reported that behavioral problems continue into the adult years (Ballaban-Gil et al. 1996) and that unusual responses to sensory (e.g., touch, pain, auditory, and visual) stimuli also remain common in adulthood (Billstedt et al. 2007; Leekam et al. 2006).

3.6 Cognitive Stability

There is considerable variability in measures of cognitive ability over time. Some have reported that IQ is relatively stable in ASD (e.g., Ballaban-Gil et al. 1996; Begovac et al. 2009; Howlin et al. 2004; Lockyer and Rutter 1970; Venter et al. 1992), whereas others have reported gains and/or losses over time (Billstedt et al. 2005; Farley et al. 2009; Mawhood et al. 2000). Howlin and colleagues reported that IQ remained remarkably stable over the life course; however, stability tended to be greatest among individuals with an initial IQ of at least 70. On the other hand, Billstedt et al. (2005) found that many individuals who initially had near average intelligence (IQ between 71 and 85) were later diagnosed with a mild (IQ 50–70) or severe (IQ < 50) intellectual disability, and those individuals with a severe intellectual disability (IQ < 50) in the original diagnostic study were all still in this category at follow-up. Overall, they found a downward shift of IQ level from the diagnostic study to the follow-up evaluation. A decrease in IQ may be an important biological marker in a subset of individuals with ASD (Farley et al. 2009). Farley et al. (2009) reported that over half of the sample had either large gains or losses in cognitive ability of greater than 1 standard deviation. Cognitive gain was associated with better outcome, as was better adaptive functioning. Some of the variability in results may be, in part, accounted for by the way IQ was measured or assessed, the age of initial assessment (IQ less stable in young children), and level of functioning of the participant, and the sometimes highly varied cognitive profiles of individuals which may evolve over time. This variability in IQ trajectory may also be due to the cumulative or time-specific impact of other risk or protective factors on the plasticity of IQ development.

4 Transitions Over the Life Course

4.1 Childhood

Children with ASD, like all other children, undergo several transitions throughout their school years. For instance, this may include the transition from early intervention to preschool, changing grades each year and moving into adolescence and then into adult life. Individuals with ASD also struggle with smaller transitions that are required on a daily basis, such as transitioning from one context to another. For example, this may include a transition between classes or transitions to unfamiliar settings (e.g., doctor's office). It is important to plan for these transitions because ineffective transition planning can have a negative impact on social and academic progress (Adreon and Stella 2001). Thus, numerous studies have emphasized the importance of transition planning for all children with special needs (Polloway et al. 2001), and this is particularly significant for children with ASD who frequently struggle with transitions. The ease with which a child transitions depends on the strategies adopted by educators when working with the child with ASD and their family (Harris and Handelman 2000). Parents of young children with ASD identified a number of factors that support successful and effective transitions, such as good communication between the school and home, transition plans that are child-centered, and inclusion of parents (Stoner et al. 2007).

Longitudinal studies of ASD have emphasized documenting the prevalence of certain outcomes (such as the stability of the diagnosis) rather than a more detailed look at developmentally related changes over time. Some studies are now taking a life course health development perspective by focusing on trajectories (Kim et al. 2015). The Pathways in ASD study, for example, followed roughly 400 children from the point of diagnosis at 2–4 years of age to the transition into primary school at 6 years of age allowing for the possibility of heterogeneous trajectories of autism symptoms and adaptive functioning. The results suggested (Szatmari et al. 2015) that heterogeneity in the rate of change of both phenotypes occurred, with some children doing remarkably well in adaptive function, but autism symptom severity remained more stable. There was little overlap of the autistic symptom severity and adaptive functioning developmental trajectories so that the course of the two seemed relatively independent, thereby highlighting the importance of close surveillance and treatment of these two domains independently over time because improvement in one area does not ensure improvement in the other area. These data also suggested that at least for the transition into primary school, continued improvement is possible for the majority of children with ASD.

A growing evidence base suggests that behavioral interventions can be associated with positive outcomes for children with ASD, with little evidence and generally poor quality studies available in adolescents and adults (Lounds Taylor et al. 2012; Weitlauf et al. 2014; National ASD Center National Standards Project 2009, 2015). Early interventions that were based on high-intensity applied behavior analysis over extended periods of time were associated with improvements in cognitive functioning and language skills, although the magnitude of effects varied across studies (Weitlauf et al. 2014). This variability may be related to the scarcity of information about modifying factors related to subgroups (Weitlauf et al. 2014). For instance, the majority of evidence supports the efficacy of comprehensive early intensive behavioral interventions (EIBI), which is currently the standard of care in many clinics and schools (Peters-Scheffer et al. 2011; Reichow 2012). Meaningful gains have been shown in IQ, language skills, and adaptive outcomes with medium to large effects (Reichow 2012; Strauss et al. 2013) and a decrease in autism severity over time (Zachor and Itzchak 2010). Gains are not universal, some making rapid progress and others only modest or no progress (Peters-Scheffer et al. 2011; Reichow and Wolery 2009). Inclusion of parents in skill generalization has led to overall higher effect sizes (Strauss et al. 2013). Early intensive parent programs have been shown to modify parent behavior during interactions, but there is less data about their ability to improve developmental skills beyond language gains for some children (Weitlauf et al. 2014). Predictors of positive outcome and/or changes in trajectory include younger age at entry into EIBI programs (between 18 months and 5 years), higher IQ or adaptive functioning or language (mild to moderate range of functioning), and less severe autism symptoms (Strauss et al. 2013). With regard to program characteristics, intensity of EIBI programs was related to gains in IQ, adaptive functioning, and language ability, whereas duration of the program was generally not related to gains with the exception of some evidence that it was related to language and adaptive behavior gains (Strauss et al. 2013). Contemporary early intervention ABA approaches are more naturalistic, child-directed, and guided by developmental theory and are currently referred to as naturalistic developmental behavioral interventions (NDBI's) (for detailed discussion see Schreibman et al. 2015). Other behavioral interventions that have shown some positive effects include, but are not limited to, social skills, treatment targeting joint attention, and cognitive behavior therapy (Weitlauf et al. 2014). Research is beginning to show that behaviorally based interventions have an effect on patterns of brain activity, particularly in regions involved in social processing (Dawson et al. 2012), and that neural plasticity in response to intervention may exist throughout the lifespan (Faja et al. 2012).

Thus, the evidence supports that early interventions are effective in ASD; however, less is known about how sustainable these intervention effects are after transitions from early intervention into preschool and elementary school. There is emerging evidence that young children with ASD who received early intervention sustained social, language, and/or nonverbal cognitive gains through a 6–37-month follow-up period (e.g., Kasari et al. 2010; Landa et al. 2011; Landa and Kalb 2012). For instance, Landa and Kalb (2012) examined outcomes in 2-year-old toddlers enrolled in a 6-month nursery school-based intervention immediately following intervention (M age = 35 months), at short-term (M age = 41 months) and long-term follow-up (M age = 72 months; 37 months after children completed intervention). At long-term follow-up, they found gains in IQ and communication; however, increases were not evenly distributed across the different time points. Gains in IQ and communication were robust initially from pre- to post-intervention, followed by a period of stabilization, which was then followed by another developmental burst. In contrast, the trajectory of autism severity was different with an initial decrease in severity form pre- to post-intervention, followed by an increase in severity to pre-intervention levels by the final time point. Magiati et al. (2011) reassessed outcomes even later at 5 years after departing preschool and found that children maintained standardized IQ scores, but adaptive functioning scores decreased. Longer-term outcome studies are needed to determine the sustainability of gains, as well as to determine whether there are sensitive periods in development as well as the developmental scaffolding that is necessary, especially during key life course transitions that are likely to promote optimal health development outcomes (e.g., age, type of intervention, duration, intensity, content, etc.) (Landa and Kalb 2012).

4.2 Transition from Adolescence into Adulthood

For youth with ASD and their families, the transition into adulthood is a time of uncertainty and loss of entitlement to many services that were available while in the school system. In comparison to early childhood, there often is a dearth of appropriate supports and opportunities for adults with ASD. Leaving high school can have a disruptive effect on youth and young adults with ASD in a number of areas, including ASD symptom presentation, maladaptive behaviors, and family functioning (Taylor and Seltzer 2010, 2011a, b). Taylor and Seltzer (2010) examined the impact of exiting high school and observed that in general, autism symptoms and maladaptive behaviors continued to improve while adolescents were part of the secondary school system, but improvement significantly slowed (by over half) after exiting high school for internalizing behavior and all but one of the autism symptom domains (i.e., verbal communication impairments). The authors suggested that this change was likely related to the lack of disability-related services or that occupational or day program services were less stimulating than those in the school system. Interestingly, youth without comorbid intellectual disability improved more in both autism symptoms and maladaptive behaviors while in high school compared to those with intellectual disability (Shattuck et al. 2007), but after exiting high school, improvement slowed more for those individuals without an ID (Taylor and Seltzer 2010). Indeed, only 6% of individuals with ASD without comorbid ID were receiving day services immediately after high school, compared to 74% with ASD and ID, and over one-quarter had no occupational, educational, or day activities. In addition, the improvement in the mother-youth relationship seen in high school slowed or stopped after high school (i.e., decreasing maternal warmth), with the greatest impact on relationships for youth with ASD and no ID (Taylor and Seltzer 2011a). Thus, leaving high school had a negative impact on individuals with ASD, with the most pronounced effect on those youth with ASD without an ID, suggesting a particular lack of adequate educational and occupational activities for this group of individuals in adulthood. It also highlights that individuals with ASD and no ID are often impaired in their adaptive skills and encounter difficulty generalizing these skills in daily life. When services are inadequate, parents will often take on this responsibility, leading some families to experience this transition period as a time of stress and anxiety (Howlin 2005). Other families view this period as an opportunity for new and more positive possibilities, such as finding more appropriate occupational placements and leaving high school, which for some youth, was a negative experience (Taylor 2009).

Access to autism-related services is also related to family income. Families with lower incomes and less parental education may have less access to autism-related services in childhood compared to families with higher incomes (Liptak et al. 2008; Thomas et al. 2007). Improvement in maladaptive behaviors slows after high school more so for those families with a lower income (Taylor and Seltzer 2011b). Thus, it is important to better understand the factors that promote optimal transition for individuals with ASD, as well as the impact on families. Taylor (2009) underscores the importance of examining contextual and environmental factors that are amenable to change or can be targeted in intervention in order to improve success with transition and suggests that exclusively focusing on characteristics such as IQ and early language that although are predictive of later outcome is more difficult to intervene once the individual with ASD becomes an adolescent or adult. For instance, the implementation of transition planning has been associated with more successful achievement of adult milestones (Frank and Siltington 2000). Indeed, factors such as the post-high school goals for the student and parental expectations were predictive of participation in postsecondary education (Chiang et al. 2012). In addition, the development of appropriate educational, occupational, and day programs for individuals with ASD of all ability levels is important as is a lifelong emphasis on generalization of skills.

4.2.1 Educational Attainment

With regard to education, many individuals in the follow-up studies published in the last decade attended specialized schools or classrooms (Billstedt et al. 2011; Farley et al. 2009, Howlin et al. 2004). Only a few individuals with ASD obtained formal qualifications (Eaves and Ho 2008; Howlin et al. 2004), although results of recent studies have been more promising (Hofvander et al. 2009; Farley 2009). For example, Farley and colleagues reported that 44% completed high school at grade 12 with a diploma, and 39% went on to postsecondary education. With regard to those students who are capable of entry into college or university, many do not seek or gain entry or drop out prematurely (Glennon 2001; VanBergeijk et al. 2008) due to a number of factors including social isolation and loneliness, difficulty managing changing routines and schedules, difficulty with independent living, and the absence of monitoring and guidance (Howlin et al. 2004; Jobe and White 2007; White et al. 2011).

Students with ASD are able to succeed both academically and socially in postsecondary education when the transition is carefully planned, appropriate accommodations are obtained, and supports are available (for detailed discussion, see VanBergeijk et al. 2008). Preparing students for the transition to postsecondary education is important for many adolescents but is particularly important for individuals with ASD, most of whom have difficulty with transitions. VanBergeijk and colleagues stress the importance of a good fit between the student and the prospective academic institution. For instance, this may include careful consideration of the size of the school and classes, level of supports, and receptiveness to serving students with disabilities – specifically ASD, access to mental health services, and availability of supports to address both academic concerns (e.g., organizational help, accommodations related to evaluation and test taking, support with complex assignments, etc.), as well as nonacademic concerns including life skills, issues of daily living (e.g., laundry, budgeting), organizational difficulties, communication limitations, and social skills (e.g., socializing with peers, getting along with roommates, romantic relationships). Indeed, adolescents with ASD reported greater concern about social acceptance and being able to function independently than about accessing academic accommodations and resources in postsecondary educational settings, and thereby identified a need for built in social supports and access to trained staff members as a resource (Camarena and Sarigiani 2009). Many individuals with ASD also have difficulty with issues related to sexuality and may require support or direct instruction (see Volkmar 2004). Furthermore, postsecondary educational programs must also include planning and preparation for the transition to work and independent living that includes vocational training and life coaching (VanBergeijk et al. 2008). Families and educators are also encouraged to support the development of self-advocacy skills which are important to the transition process so that adolescent and young adults are able to navigate the journey through higher education, work, and independent living (Camarena and Sarigiani 2009). Thus, for students with aspirations for postsecondary education, careful planning and supports are required to help students with ASD achieve academic success.

4.2.2 Employment, Independent Living, and Social Life

The research on transition into adulthood in individuals with ASD has primarily focused on the traditional view of transition which describes the degree of independence in living arrangements, ability to gain and maintain employment, and the presence of intimate relationships outside of the family unit (Fussell and Furstenberg 2005). The majority of individuals with ASD have difficulty achieving the developmental tasks of adulthood and remain dependent on parents/caregivers for support in employment and accommodation, and most do not have intimate relationships (friendship or romantic).

Many persons with ASD are able to work successfully within the community (Garcia-Villamisar et al. 2000; Mawhood and Howlin 1999); however, the majority experience difficulty securing meaningful employment (Billstedt et al. 2011; Eaves and Ho 2008; Howlin et al. 2004; Newman et al. 2011). Findings from the National Longitudinal Transition Study-2 (NLTS2) examined a nationally representative sample of youth and young adults with disabilities in the USA and found that up to 8 years post-high school, only 63% of adults with autism had worked at some point after high school and only 37% were employed at the time of the survey (Newman et al. 2011). In a group of individuals with near average to average intelligence, the outcomes were somewhat more promising with 54% in full-time or part-time independent paid jobs, 12% in supported employment or part-time volunteer positions, 24% in day programs, and 10% unemployed (Farley et al. 2009). Even among those who are employed, many worked few hours, and most jobs tended to be low level, were found by parental contacts (versus open job market), and were poorly paid such that individuals did not have adequate financial support to live independently (Cimera and Cowan 2009; Eaves and Ho 2008; Howlin et al. 2004). Furthermore, many individuals were in part-time, volunteer, supported, or sheltered employment; few worked independently with little or no support, and some had no daytime occupation at all. Jobs often ended prematurely because of social or behavioral difficulties or other work-related difficulties (Mawhood and Howlin 1999). Cimera and Cowan (2009) examined cost of services and employment outcomes achieved by adults with ASD in the vocational rehabilitation system. The study found that adults with autism were employed at higher rates than other disability groups; however, the rate of employment was only 41% (60% do not obtain employment), and as noted earlier, they worked fewer hours and earned lower wages. Adults with autism were also the most costly group of individual to serve, and services were difficult to implement. Howlin (2013) underscores that generic employment services do not meet the needs of individuals with ASD, and there is a need for more programs and research specific to individuals with ASD. Although limited, research is beginning to emerge showing that supported employment models for individuals with ASD are effective (Howlin et al. 2005; Keel et al. 1997; Shattuck et al. 2012; Taylor et al. 2012).

Critical factors in finding and maintaining a long-term placement include a thorough assessment to appropriately match the skills and abilities of the person with ASD to the requirements of the job, as well as having the appropriate level and type of employment support (Mawhood and Howlin 1999; Smith and Paulippen 1999).

Hagner and Cooney (2005) found that a set of supervisory accommodation strategies were commonly associated with successful supervision, including maintaining a consistent schedule and set of job responsibilities, using organizers to structure the job, minimizing unstructured or idle time, being direct with communication, and providing reminders and reassurances. Longer job retention has been correlated with higher levels of social inclusion and acceptance on the job (Belcher and Smith 1994). Furthermore, engaging in work is often related to other meaningful outcomes, such as contributing to one's self-worth and confidence, providing opportunities to shares one's strengths that are valued by others, opportunities to develop friendships or other supportive relationships, as well as engagement in the larger community (Lee and Carter 2012). On the other hand, failure to find suitable work resulted in frustration and in some serious problems with depression and/or anxiety (Mawhood and Howlin 1999). With supported employment, individuals with ASD are able to find and maintain suitable employment (Mawhood and Howlin 1999).

Most individuals with ASD live with their parents or in other supported arrangements (e.g., community-based group home), and few live independently either with or without some level of support (Billstedt et al. 2011; Farley et al. 2009). Eaves and Ho (2008) reported that 56% lived with their parents, 35% were in supported arrangements such as group homes or foster care, and the remainder lived more or less independently. With regard to friendship, it has been reported that up to approximately 30% of individuals have one or more friends (Eaves and Ho 2008; Howlin et al. 2004). Social contacts often result from special interests and skills rather than close friendships (Howlin 2000). Some individuals have been reported to want friendships but were unable to form these relationships, whereas others had no interest or did not understand the concept of friendship (Billstedt et al. 2011). Few individuals had close intimate relationships or were married at some point (Eaves and Ho 2008; Farley et al. 2009; Hofvander et al. 2009; Howlin et al. 2004). In a group of higher functioning individuals with ASD, Farley and colleagues reported that 7% were married, 5% divorced, 7% were in long-term relationships, 44% never dated, 32% dated in both group and couple situations, and 22% dated only in group settings. When parents were asked whether they felt their adult child wished to have a romantic relationship, of those participants not already in relationships, 44% felt their son or daughter would like to be in a relationship. On the other hand, 41% did not want a romantic partner because parents thought their children were concerned about passing on autism to a child or themselves being too difficult for a partner to manage.

4.2.3 Summary

Taken together, the research to date focuses primarily on the attainment of traditional skills that are indicative of successful transition into adulthood and less on more subjective or quality of life indicators. Although outcomes are quite variable, in general, outcomes related to level of independence, employment status, and intimate relationships are poor, suggesting that the transition to adulthood is fraught with many challenges. Evidence suggests that better outcomes are related to better cognitive abilities and earlier language skills, although even these individuals struggle with attaining the developmental tasks of adulthood. Furthermore, availability of appropriate resources, services, and supports for the individuals with ASD and their families are key ingredients for successful transition into adulthood and better outcomes throughout adult life. Lee and Carter (2012) identified seven elements that are important for high-quality transition services, which include individualized services that reflect the strengths of the individual, positive career development and early work experiences, collaboration and interagency involvement, family supports and expectations, fostering self-determination and independence, social- and employment-related skill instruction, and establishment of job-related supports. Thus, the impetus of future research is to examine factors that will support successful transition (e.g., environmental and contextual factors) and find other ways to define transition such as from a psychosocial or attachment perspective (for review, see Taylor 2009), especially as the epidemiology of ASD changes from autism with ID to a preponderance of ASD without ID.

4.3 Aging and ASD

Autism is a lifelong condition; however, little is known about older adults with ASD. Indeed, much of the research to date has examined the aging ASD population but not the aged (65 plus) (Perkins and Berkman 2012). Although information is quite limited, research suggests that life expectancy is shortened compared to the general population and causes of death include high rates of seizures and accidental deaths (e.g., drowning) (Mouridsen et al. 2008; Piven and Rabins 2011). It is unclear whether deaths that are related to diseases (e.g., nervous and sensory disease) in ASD are due to a predisposition to certain health concerns or due to poor health surveillance leading to poor diagnosis and management (Perkins and Berkman 2012). A number of medical and psychiatric concerns have been reported in children and adolescents with ASD, such as sleep disorders, psychiatric symptoms, gastrointestinal disorders, feeding selectivity and aversions, metabolic conditions, and epilepsy; however, there is little information about these concerns as individuals age (Piven and Rabins 2011). Similarly, it is unclear whether treatments that are effective in children and adolescents would also benefit adults. Given the dearth of information of older adults with ASD, a group of experts were convened to characterize the gaps in knowledge and define a research agenda to bridge this gap (see Piven and Rabins 2011). Research priorities included developing diagnostic criteria and tools to diagnose older adults, conducting cross-sectional descriptive studies in adults of phenomenology and associated features, longitudinal studies of lifespan trajectories, neurobiological studies examining underlying changes over time, intervention studies, and mechanism to support clinical and research training in aging. This research is needed to improve the lives of individuals with ASD and to inform clinical practice and policies that can address these healthcare disparities (Piven and Rabins 2011).

5 Mental Health Issues in ASD

5.1 Prevalence Rates

In terms of quality of adult life, there is increasing evidence suggesting that comorbid psychiatric symptoms and disorders are common in individuals with ASD, with estimated rates ranging from 30% to 70% (e.g., Bradley et al. 2004; Gjevik et al. 2011; Leyfer et al. 2006; Moseley et al. 2011; Simonoff et al. 2008; Skokauskas and Gallagher 2010). Understanding comorbid mental health problems is important not only because of the high prevalence but also because of the impact on daily functioning, long-term prognosis, and the added burden and challenges faced by individuals and their families. Individuals with ASD have higher rates of comorbidity compared to the general population (Ghaziuddin et al. 1998; Moseley et al. 2011), a psychiatrically referred population of youth without ASD (Joshi et al. 2010), as well as individuals with ID alone (Bradley et al. 2004; Brereton et al. 2006; LoVullo and Matson 2009), although the latter has not been consistently found (Tsakanikos et al. 2006). The most commonly reported psychiatric disorders include anxiety and depression (MacNeil et al. 2009; Sterling et al. 2008; White et al. 2009). ASD has also been found to co-occur with obsessive compulsive disorder (OCD), disruptive behavioral disorders, attention deficit hyperactivity disorder (ADHD), bipolar disorder, Tourette's disorder, tic disorder, and eating disorders (Drmic amd Szatmari 2014; Skokauskas and Gallagher 2010; Szatmari and McConnell 2011; Volkmar et al. 2014; White et al. 2009). Studies examining schizophrenia have been mixed; some studies report high rates (Chang et al. 2003), whereas others have not found an increased rate (Seltzer et al. 2004; Volkmar and Cohen 1991). Although the two disorders are quite different, misclassification of ASD as schizophrenia may also contribute to the variability in reported rates (Perlman 2000;

Palucka, Bradley, Lunsky 2008). Furthermore, ASD often co-occurs with multiple psychiatric disorders (Leyfer et al. 2006; Simonoff et al. 2008). For instance, Simonoff et al. (2008), using a population-based cohort, conducted a structured psychiatric interview (not modified for ASD) with 112 10–14-year olds and found that 70% of ASD participants had at least one comorbid disorder and 41% had two or more. It is important to better understand this comorbidity given that many individuals with ASD are likely to struggle with mental health concerns, and more importantly, psychiatric problems may cause considerable distress and interference with daily functioning and significantly impact long-term prognosis and outcome (Kim et al. 2000; Mattila et al. 2010; Muris et al. 1998; Russell and Sofronoff 2005; White et al. 2009).

To date, the majority of research on psychiatric comorbidity has been conducted in children and adolescents (Amr et al. 2012; Gjevik et al. 2011; Leyfer et al. 2006; Mattila et al. 2010; Skokauskas and Gallagher 2010). In a review conducted by Skokauskas and Gallagher (2010) examining comorbid disorders in children with autism and Asperger syndrome, wide ranges in rates of co-occurring symptoms or diagnoses were found: 0–6% for schizophrenia, 5–35% for generalized anxiety, 10–64% for simple phobias, 1–37% for OCD, and 0–50% for affective disorders or symptoms. Fewer studies have examined this issue in adults, although research in this area is beginning to emerge (Cederlund et al. 2010; Ghaziuddin and Zafar 2008; Hofvander et al. 2009; La Malfa et al. 2007; Lugnegard et al. 2011; Moseley et al. 2011), and a number of follow-up studies have reported on psychiatric outcomes (Billstedt et al. 2005; Eaves and Ho 2008; Farley et al. 2009). A study that examined young adults with Asperger syndrome found high rates of depression and anxiety, consistent with the literature in children and adolescents with ASD, whereas psychotic and substance-induced disorders were uncommon (Lugnegard et al. 2011). Hofvander et al. (2009) assessed 122 consecutively referred adults with ASD and normal intelligence ranging in age from 16 to 60 years. Lifetime axis I comorbidity was common, and they also found that mood (53%) and anxiety disorders (50%) were most common, followed by ADHD (43%), OCD (34%), and chronic tic disorders (20%). With regard to the rate of lifetime axis II disorders, 62% met criteria for at least one personality disorder. Other studies have reported somewhat lower rates of anxiety (Farley et al. 2009; Moseley et al. 2011) and depression (Billstedt et al. 2005; Eaves and Ho 2008; Farley et al. 2009; Moseley et al. 2011). A study examining adolescents and young adults with autism (over three-quarters had an intellectual disability) found that 42% had an additional mental health disorder, a rate that is two to four times seen in typically developing young people (Moseley et al. 2011). There is some evidence that the rates of mood and anxiety disorders in parents of children with autism is higher than that in the general population and when compared to Down syndrome (Bolton et al. 1998; Mazefsky et al. 2008). This may reflect an effect of stress on family members. A more thorough examination of genetic variable expressivity would involve a study of mood disorders in second- and third-degree relatives.

5.2 Mental Health Services

Given the high rate of psychiatric comorbidity, there is a need for appropriate mental health services for individuals with ASD of all ages. This includes preventive interventions designed to optimize mental functioning and life course trajectories. In a study investigating the healthcare experiences of children with ASD and their families, it was found that 15% of families reported unmet mental health services, and provider lack of skills was a barrier to obtaining these services (Chiri and Warfield 2012). With regard to the utilization of mental health services by individuals with ASD, the reports are mixed, with some reporting underutilization of services (Bryson et al. 2008) and others reporting relatively high rates of service use (Narendorf et al. 2011). Narendorf et al. (2011) reported that of those youth who received mental health services (i.e., 46%), 49% received it through the school.

African-American youth and youth from lower-income families were more likely to use school-based services than accessing community-based services, underscoring the importance of schools in providing these services for underserved group and the importance of ensuring the continuation of services after high school. For students with ASD, there is emerging research examining the delivery of mental health services in schools for anxiety (Drmic, Aljunied, Reaven 2017; Luxford, Hadwin, Kovshoff 2016). Bryson et al. (2008) found that short-term crisis-oriented mental health services were effective at stabilizing children with ASD but that many remained highly symptomatic at discharge, suggesting that changes are needed to the current system in order to serve those individuals with chronic and long-term needs.

Many individuals with ASD may be at risk for psychiatric hospitalization. Indeed, approximately 11% of children and youth aged 5–21 years experienced at least one psychiatric hospital inpatient admission (Mandell 2008), and 48% used psychiatric hospital services by age 40 (Mouridsen et al. 2008). Children with a diagnosis of Asperger's disorder and pervasive developmental disorder, compared to children with autism, were more likely to experience inpatient hospitalization (Bryson et al. 2008). Lunsky et al. (2009) compared patients with ASD and ID to other individuals accessing tertiary level mental healthcare in Ontario and found that individuals with ASD and ID were younger, spent more days in hospitals, and were less likely to have a psychotic disorder diagnosis than both patients with and without ID. Interestingly, fewer than half of the individuals with ASD and ID had an additional psychiatric diagnosis, although almost all (91%) were prescribed psychotropic medication, which is consistent with previous studies (Tsakanikos et al. 2006, 2007a). Tsakanikos et al. (2007b) reported that behavioral management problems predicted psychotropic medication and use of psychiatric services in adults with pervasive developmental disorder and ID. A study examining referral trends to specialist mental health services in south London from 1983 to 2000 for individuals with ASD and ID reported an increase in diagnosable psychiatric disorders over time and a significant reduction of medication at time of referral, but no change in the use of other therapeutic interventions, which is in contrast to services received by younger children with ASD. Thus, there continues to be a need for specialized inpatient and outpatient mental health services for individuals with ASD, as well as more training for service providers.

6 Summary

ASD is a neurodevelopmental disorder that represents a chronic, lifelong condition based on atypicalities in brain development. While there are changes in syndrome expression over time, new challenges often emerge. Much of the current research has focused on static or crosssectional outcomes as opposed to developmental trajectories and changes in those trajectories. This can include looking at the developmental course of the disorder, the developmental course of specific skills that are important to later outcomes such as joint attention skills, as well as trajectories, related to the effects of early intervention. Longer-term studies are critical to treatment research in order to determine the sustainability of early intervention treatment gains, to explore whether there are sensitive periods of child development when treatments are most effective, and to determine factors that promote treatment outcome. Research needs to include enough information about factors that might be important to outcome so that predictors can be better elucidated, as well as a shift to focus on mediators and moderators of outcome. There is a need for more longitudinal studies and some consensus about the type of information that should be gathered by all research groups so that findings are comparable among different studies and can be combined into meta-analyses. For instance, standardized IQ measures could be used to document intellectual abilities. It may be beneficial to convene a group of experts as well as parents and individuals with ASD to determine what basic set of factors are important.

The current review highlights that outcomes for people with ASD have been improving over time; although relative to typically developing children and adolescents, outcomes are still generally poor. Much of the work to date has focused on achieving the traditional developmental tasks of adulthood, including independence in living arrangements, gaining and maintaining employment, and developing intimate relationships outside of the family unit. Research examining quality of life is beginning to emerge, which is an important next step to further our understanding of how to help improve the lived experiences of individuals with ASD. QOL studies need to shift focus and include information about factors and developmental processes that are thought to be important to achieving better life course health development outcomes, such as IQ, symptom severity, and language development. In addition, examining other factors that promote thriving in individuals with ASD is needed. Understanding what those factors are is critical so that better programs and interventions can be developed, which include the developmental scaffolding that children and families need to optimize long-term health development outcomes. It is also important to understand what impact access to adequate resources and intervention has on the identification, service provision, and likely outcomes on people with ASD. Another key theme is the development and emergence of mental health comorbidities which often represent an enormous challenge for young adults with ASD and their families. Research needs to include information about the developmental pathways that lead to these outcomes so that risk and protective factors can be targeted early, with the intent of optimizing the trajectory of mental health outcomes. There is also a need for more basic research such as epigenetic studies of non-syndromic ASD, genetic studies that focus on much smaller copy number variants or DNA sequence variants identified either in exomes or in whole genome sequencing, and continued research examining environmental risk factors.

A number of recommendations to facilitate the transition periods and support individual with ASD and their families can be gleaned from the existing literature. Implementation of a transition plan is crucial since it is associated with more successful transition from early intervention into preschool (Stoner et al. 2007) and attainment of adult milestones (Frank and Siltington 2000) and may help temper the disruptive effect of leaving high school (Taylor and Seltzer 2010, 2011a, b). Parents, clinicians, and educators are encouraged to begin the transition planning process for the transition to adulthood early and include planning for treatment, independence (i.e., daily living skills, skills for independent living), education, employment, living arrangements, mental health, and medical care. For instance, good practical living skills, even in those individuals who have a cognitive disability, led to better outcomes and quality of life (Farley et al. 2009). Therefore, focusing on developing independence in daily living skills starting from a young age is an important target for intervention programs and transition planning. This highlights the importance of planning early so that skills can be integrated into treatment and educational programs at younger ages, allowing for ample practice and supervision of these skills well before the individual is expected to be able to manage on their own.

For many individuals and families, the transition to adulthood is a time of worry and uncertainty because many services that were available through the educational system are no longer available and there are few appropriate supports or services for adults with ASD. Taylor and Seltzer (2010) showed that the improvement slowed significantly after exiting high school, particularly for those youth with ASD and no ID. This change was likely related to a lack of services or that available services were less stimulating than those provided in the educational system. Thus, the development of new models of care that incorporate appropriate educational, occupational and day programs for adults with ASD of all ability levels is essential. However, simply having a program is not enough; it is also important to ensure that the appropriate training and support is provided on an ongoing basis to the individual with ASD and that service providers are adequately trained to work with this group of individuals. For instance, given the prevalence and impact of mental health issues in individuals with ASD and their families, there is a need for ongoing mental health services and staff who are trained in this area and able to support families. A worrying trend is the increased use of psychopharmacology in adults with ASD often as a result of lack of psychosocial services that might better meet those needs in a way that improves life course outcomes and promotes thriving. Another example relates to successfully obtaining and maintaining long-term employment, which may involve supportive employment programs that include training related to general job skills (e.g., resume writing, interviewing skills, proper social behavior), specific skills needed for a particular job (e.g., learning job requirements and skills, learning about the culture and expectations for that job), and ongoing support (e.g., job coach). Training and support should also be provided to the employers in order to educate them about ASD in general, help them understand the needs of a particular individual, as well as highlight their unique skills and abilities that can positively contribute to workplace. Indeed, parents, educators, employers, and other professionals are encouraged to appreciate the many strengths, skills, and unique talents of individuals with ASD and approach current programs and future planning from a strength-based approach, leveraging each individual's unique set of assets, versus a deficits-based approach that focuses on what needs to be fixed.

There is a stark lack of information about ASD in the aging and elderly population. Given this gap in knowledge, a group of experts were convened to identify and describe these gaps and define a research agenda (see Piven and Rabins 2011). The research proprieties included developing diagnostic criteria and tools to diagnose older adults, conducting cross-sectional descriptive studies in adults of phenomenology and associated features, longitudinal studies of lifespan trajectories, neurobiological studies examining underlying changes over time, and intervention studies and mechanism to support clinical and research training in aging.

This change in perspective might be part of a shift from treatment of deficits to accommodation of unique characteristics of the adult with ASD. There comes a time when the relentless pursuit of treatment to "make things better" will have a negative impact on the person with ASD and their family. People with ASD should not always be considered "disabled," and taking a lifespan perspective to developmental trajectories should be part of this switch for service providers as well as parents.

7 Research Priorities

There has been a marked increase in ASD-related research over the past decades. Considerable advances have been made in key areas, including: the genetic basis of ASD and its diagnosis; studies of the social brain; the connections between timing of diagnosis and long-term outcomes; new treatment models, some pharmacological and behavioral treatments can now be viewed as evidence based; psychiatric co-morbidities with particular emphasis on anxiety and depression; and, research on basic issues like employment, living arrangements, medical survelillance, etc. Thus, a number of gaps remain that need to be addressed. The following summarizes a number of recommendations for research, some of which were noted earlier in the paper, to better understand life course health development in ASD.

7.1 Research Priorities

(i) Basic mechanism research:
  (a) Better understanding of epigenetic mechanisms in non-syndromic ASD.
  (b) Continued research in the area of genetics and neuroimaging. For example, this could include:
  - Genetic studies that focus on much smaller copy number variants or DNA sequence variants identified either in exomes or in whole genome sequencing
  - Studies that assess the impact of genetic testing (e.g., microarrays) on health outcomes
  - Studies combining genetics and neuroimaging work

- Neuroimaging studies examining the trajectories of brain development
- Neuroimaging studies examining the impact of behavioral treatments on the brain

(c) Continued research examining environmental risk factors, as well as gene-environment interactions.

(d) Identification of biomarkers (e.g., genetics, neural circuitry) is a high priority. For instance, the National Institutes of Health Interagency Coordinating Committee Strategic Plan called for the identification of biological markers, which separately or in combination with behavioral markers accurately identified ASD before age 2 (Dawson and Bernier 2013).

(e) Development of novel therapeutics, e.g., creating medicine that can target core ASD symptoms.

(f) Focus on early developmental skills or early markers of development that may impact the developmental trajectory. For instance, there is evidence that early joint attention skills are important for social cognitive development and later language and adaptive skills. Further, interventions targeting joint attention have been shown to be effective. Thus, research further examining the role of joint attention skills in ASD would be beneficial. It is also important to identify other potential early developing skills that may provide early targets for intervention.

(ii) Clinical Research:

(a) Early diagnosis remains a treatment priority. The recent advances in technology (e.g., neuroimaging) and genetics suggest the next wave of advances in our ability to detect autism through the use of biomarkers and new screening tools. Thus, research examining the utility of these biomarkers in clinical contexts will be needed. The availability of predictive biomarkers could index risk for ASD before or at the onset of symptoms, thereby preventing the symptoms from developing or alleviating symptoms and improving the trajectory of outcomes.

(b) Development of more evidence-based treatment research throughout the lifespan is needed.

- A growing body of literature has shown that interventions can be associated with positive outcomes in children; however, there is still a need for studies across setting and improvements in methodological rigor.
- Little evidence is available about treatment in adolescents and adults. There is a need to develop treatment across the lifespan and determine "which" treatments are most needed and effective at the different life stages and "when" these treatments are most effective.
- Substantial scientific advances are needed to improve our understanding of which interventions are most effective for specific children with ASD and to elucidate the factors or components of interventions most associated with positive outcomes.
- Exciting potential to bring together basic science and treatment in development of new metrics/measures (e.g., predicting response to treatments – recent work on EEG/fMRI and treatment change).

(c) Very little evidence is available for specific treatment approaches in adolescents and adults; this is especially the case for evidence-based approaches to support the transition of youth with autism to adulthood. (Lounds et al. 2012). Thus, more research is needed to focus transition period.

(d) Little information exists about the aging population in ASD with virtually no information about the aged (65+). More research is needed in various areas from basic and clinical research to data/method development and translational research. A research agenda spanning all these areas for the aging population was described in Piven and Rabins (2011). As noted earlier, the research

priorities included developing diagnostic criteria and tools to diagnose older adults, conducting cross-sectional descriptive studies in adults of phenomenology and associated features, longitudinal studies of lifespan trajectories, neurobiological studies examining underlying changes over time, and intervention studies and mechanism to support clinical and research training in aging.
   (e) Studies examining quality of life and the person, environmental, and person-environmental interactions that lead to a thriving life.

(iii) Translational research:
   (a) Need innovative solutions for training physicians, clinicians, and other professionals working with individuals with ASD throughout the lifespan. In particular, there is a serious lack of well-trained healthcare professional to serve the large number of adults with ASD. This includes multiple areas, including diagnosis and assessment of adult, mental health and medical supports, and supports for daily life.
   (b) Research related to transition planning as it relates to treatment, independence, education, employment, living arrangements, mental health, and medical care.

7.2 Data/Method Development Priorities

(a) A shift toward longitudinal studies to better understand developmental trajectories (with attention to child and family characteristics – e.g., SES, parental education)
(b) Inclusion of characteristics that might be important to outcome (e.g., IQ, language ability, etc.) so that predictors of outcome can be better elucidated, as well as a shift to focus on mediators and moderators of outcome.
(c) A shift in focus examining not only risk factors but also on factors that are protective and promote thriving.
(d) Better metrics throughout the lifespan. There is an exciting potential to bring together basic science and treatment in development of new metrics/measures (e.g., predicting response to treatments as was seen in recent work on fMRI and treatment change).
(e) Development of better measures to look at outcome determination and more focus on quality of life (QOL) measures for the individual and family.
(f) Greater focus in critical or sensitive periods of development when environemntal exposures can have long-lasting effects on outcomes.

7.3 Translational Priorities

(a) Early diagnosis. A wide gap remains between our knowledge about best practices in ASD (e.g., screening for ASD at 18 and 24 months) and Centers for Disease Control and Prevention (CDC) data showing that the average age of diagnosis in the USA is 5 years and higher for individuals with milder forms of ASD. This is a problem given that much of the literature on early intervention shows best outcomes when intervention is initiated early (between 18 months and 5 years). This is a major challenge and will require innovative solutions and a focus on dissemination and implementation science.
(b) Better coordination of different systems related to children's health development (e.g., school and health systems).
(c) Development of physician guidelines for healthcare.
(d) Challenge in providing access to behavioral, mental health, and medical healthcare and, thus, the need for improved and expanded healthcare services with care providers who are well trained in working with individuals with ASD and their families.
(e) Innovative solutions to better serve those in remote regions or underserved population (e.g., individuals living in poverty).

(f) Incorporating independent living skills into treatment/educational programs starting at a young age.
(g) Although our understanding of autism has increased, there is a major gap in translating this to public school settings.
(h) Development of new models/systems of care that incorporate appropriate educational, occupational and day programs for adults with ASD of all ability levels is essential.
(i) Vocational system for adults.
(j) Generic employment services do not meet the needs of individuals with ASD, therefore the need for more programs and research specific to individuals with ASD (e.g., supported employment models). Supportive employment programs – training related to general job skills, specific skills needed for a particular job, and ongoing support (e.g., job coach).
(k) Training and support for employers.

8 Conclusions

Taken together, there has been a tremendous growth in research in the ASD field. However, there remain a number of gaps that need to be addressed, with a particular focus on optimizing life course trajectories for individuals and populations with ASD. The principles of the life course health development framework describe health as an emergent set of developmental capacities that develop continuously over the lifespan in a complex, nonlinear process occurring in multiple dimensions, levels, and phases and are sensitive to timing. This is a valuable framework to direct the research agenda to continue to move the field forward and to improve the lives of individuals with ASD, their families, and their communities.

References

Adreon, D., & Stella, J. (2001). Transition to middle and high school: Increasing the success of students with Asperger syndrome. *Intervention in School and Clinic, 36*, 266–271.

American Psychiatric Association. (1980). *Diagnostic and statistical manual*. Washington, DC: APA Press.

Amr, M., Raddad, D., El-Mehesh, F., Bakr, A., Sallam, K., & Amin, T. (2012). Comorbid psychiatric disorders in Arab children with autism spectrum disorders. *Research in Autism Spectrum Disorders, 6*, 240–248.

Asperger, H. (1944). Die "autistichen Psychopathen" im Kindersalter. *Archive fur psychiatrie und Nervenkrankheiten, 117*, 76–136.

Baker, T. B., Breslau, N., Covey, L., & Shiffman, S. (2012). DSM criteria for tobacco use disorder and tobacco withdrawal: A critique and proposed revisions for DSM-5. *Addiction, 107*(2), 263–275. doi:10.1111/j.1360-0443.2011.03657.x.

Ballaban-Gil, K., Rapin, I., Tuchman, R., & Shinner, S. (1996). Longitudinal examination of the behavioral, language and social changes in a population of adolescents and young adults with autistic disorder. *Pediatric Neurology, 15*, 217–223.

Baron-Cohen, S. (2011). *The science of evil: On empathy and the origins of cruelty*. New York: Basic Books.

Beadle-Brown, J., Murphy, G., Wing, L., Gould, J., Shah, A., & Holmes, N. (2002). Changes in social impairment for people with intellectual disabilities: A follow-up of the Camberwell cohort. *Journal of Autism and Developmental Disorders, 32*, 195–206.

Begovac, I., Begovac, B., Majic, G., & Vidovic, V. (2009). Longitudinal studies of IQ stability with childhood autism-literature survey. *Psychiatria Danubina, 21*(3), 310–319.

Belcher, R., & Smith, M. D. (1994). Coworker attitudes towards employees with autism. *Journal of Vocational Rehabilitation, 4*, 29–36.

Bennet, H. E., Wood, C. L., & Hare, D. J. (2005). Providing care for adults with autistic spectrum disorders in learning disability services: Needs-based or diagnosis-driven? *Journal of Applied Research in Intellectual Disabilities, 18*, 57–64.

Billstedt, E., Gillberg, C., & Gillberg, C. (2005). Autism after adolescents: Population-based 13- to 22-year follow-up study of 120 individuals with autism diagnosed in childhood. *Journal of Autism and Developmental Disorders, 35*(3), 351–360.

Billstedt, E., Gillberg, C., & Gillberg, C. (2007). Autism in adults: Symptom patterns and early childhood predictors. Use of the DISCO in a community sample followed from childhood. *Journal of Child Psychology and Psychiatry, 48*(11), 1102–1110.

Billstedt, E., Gillberg, I. C., & Gillberg, C. (2011). Aspects of quality of life in adults diagnosed with autism in childhood: A population-based study. *Autism, 15*(1), 7–20.

Bolton, P. F., Pickles, A., Murphy, M., & Rutter, M. (1998). Autism, affective, and other psychiatric disorders: Patterns of familial aggregation. *Psychological Medicine, 28*, 385–395.

Bradley, E. A., Summers, J. A., Wood, H. L., & Bryson, S. E. (2004). Comparing rates of psychiatric and behavior disorders in adolescents and young adults with severe intellectual disability with and without autism. *Journal of Autism and Developmental Disorders, 34*, 151–161.

Brand, B. L., Lanius, R., Vermetten, E., Loewenstein, R. J., & Spiegel, D. (2012). Where are we going? An update on assessment, treatment, and neurobiological research in dissociative disorders as we move toward the DSM-5. *Journal of Trauma & Dissociation, 13*(1), 9–31.

Brereton, A. V., Tonge, B. J., & Einfeld, S. L. (2006). Psychopathology in children and adolescents with autism compared to young people with intellectual disability. *Journal of Autism and Developmental Disorders, 36*, 862–870.

Brown, J. R., & Rogers, S. J. (2003). Cultural issues in autism. In R. L. Hendren, S. Ozonoff, & S. Rogers (Eds.), *Autism spectrum disorders* (pp. 209–226). Washington, DC: American Psychiatric Press.

Brugha, T. S., McManus, S., Bankart, J., Scott, F., Purdon, S., Smith, J., et al. (2011). Epidemiology of autism spectrum disorders in adults in the community in England. *Archives of General Psychiatry, 68*(5), 459–466.

Bryson, S. A., Corrigan, S. K., McDonald, T. P., & Holmes, C. (2008). Characteristics of children with autism spectrum disorders who received services through community mental health centers. *Autism, 12*, 65–82.

Burgess, A. F., & Gutstein, S. E. (2007). Quality of life for people with autism: Raising the standard for evaluating successful outcomes. *Child and Adolescent Mental Health, 12*, 80–86.

Camarena, P. M., & Sarigiani, P. A. (2009). Postsecondary educational aspirations of high-functioning adolescents with autism spectrum disorders and their parents. *Focus on Autism and Other Developmental Disabilities, 24*(2), 115–128.

Cederlund, M., Hagberg, B., Billstedt, E., Gillberg, I. C., & Gillberg, C. (2008). Asperger syndrome and autism: A comparative longitudinal follow-up study more than 5 years after original diagnosis. *Journal of Autism and Developmental Disorders, 38*, 72–85.

Cederlund, M., Hagberg, B., & Gillberg, C. (2010). Asperger syndrome in adolescent and young adult males. Interview, self – And parent assessment of social, emotional, and cognitive problems. *Research in Developmental Disabilities, 31*, 287–298.

Centers for Disease Control and Prevention (CDC). (2014). Prevalence of Autism Spectrum disorder among children aged 8 years — Autism and Developmental disabilities monitoring network, 11 sites, United States, 2010. *Morbidity and Mortality Weekly Report, 63*(SS02), 1–21.

Chang, H. L., Juang, Y. Y., Wang, W. T., Huang, C. I., Chen, C. Y., & Hwang, Y. S. (2003). Screening for autism spectrum disorder in adult psychiatric outpatients in a clinic in Taiwan. *General Hospital Psychiatry, 25*, 284–288.

Chawarska, K., Klin, A., & Volkmar, F. R. (2008). Autism spectrum disorders in infants and toddlers: diagnosis, assessment, and treatment. *Autism spectrum disorders in infants and toddlers: Diagnosis, assessment, and treatment* (pp. 327–336, 348). New York: Guilford Press.

Chiang, H.-M., Cheung, Y. K., Hickson, L., Xiang, R., & Tsai, L. Y. (2012). Predictive factors of participation in postsecondary education for high school leavers with autism. *Journal of Autism and Developmental Disorders, 42*, 685–696. doi:10.1007/s10803-011-1297-7.

Chiri, G., & Warfield, M. E. (2012). Unmet needs and problems accessing core health care services for children with autism spectrum disorders. *Journal of Child and Maternal Health, 16*, 1081–1091.

Cimera, R. E., & Cowan, R. J. (2009). The costs of services and employment outcomes achieved by adults with autism in the US. *Autism, 13*(3), 285–302.

Constantino, J. N., Zhang, Y., Frazier, T., Abbacchi, A. M., & Law, P. (2010). Sibling recurrence and the genetic epidemiology of autism. *The American Journal of Psychiatry, 167*(11), 1349–1356.

Creak, M. (1961). Schizophrenic syndrome in childhood. *Developmental Medicine and Child Neurology, 3*, 501–504.

Daniels, A. M., Rosenberg, R. E., Law, J. K., Lord, C., Kaufmann, W. E., & Law, P. A. (2011). Stability of initial disorder diagnoses in community settings. *Journal of Autism and Developmental Disorders, 41*(1), 110–121.

Dawson, G., & Bernier, R. (2013). A quarter century of progress on early detection and treatment of autism spectrum disorder. *Development and Psychopathology, 25*, 1455–1472.

Dawson, G., Jones, E. J., Merkle, K., Venema, K., Lowy, R., Faja, S., et al. (2012). Early behavioral intervention is associated with normalized brain activity in young children with autism. *Journal of the American Academy of Child & Adolescent Psychiatry, 51*, 1150–1159.

DeMyer, M. K., Barton, S., DeMyer, W. E., Norton, J. S., Allen, J., & Steele, R. (1973). Prognosis in autism: A follow-up study. *Journal of Autism and Childhood Schizophrenia, 3*, 199–246.

Devlin, B., & Scherer, S. W. (2012). Genetic architecture in autism spectrum disorder. *Current Opinion in Genetics and Development, 22*, 229–237.

Devlin, B., Melhem, N., & Roeder, K. (2011). Do common variants play a role in risk for autism? Evidence and theoretical musings. *Brain Research, 1380*, 78–84.

Drmic, I., Aljunied, M., & Reaven, J. (2017). Facing your fears in schools: Implementing CBT for teens with ASD and anxiety in Singapore. *Journal of Autism and Developmental Disabilities*. doi:10.1007/s10803-016-3007-y.

Drmic, I., & Szatmari, P. (2014). Emotional dysregulation and comorbidity in Autism Spectrum Disorder. *Invited review for Cutting Edge Psychiatry in Practice – Autism Issue, 1*, 119–131.

Eaves, L. C., & Ho, H. H. (2008). Young adult outcomes of autism spectrum disorders. *Journal of Autism and Developmental Disorders, 38*, 739–747.

Eisenberg, L. (1956). The autistic child in adolescence. *The American Journal of Psychiatry, 112*, 607–612.

Elsabbagh, M., Divan, G., Koh, Y.-J., Kim, Y. S., Kauchali, S., Marcin, C., et al. (2012). Global prevalence of autism and other pervasive developmental disorders. *Autism Research, 5*(3), 160–179. doi: http://dx.doi.org/10.1002/aur.239.

Engstrom, I., Ekstrom, L., & Emilsson, B. (2003). Psychosocial functioning in a group of Swedish adults with Asperger syndrome or high-functioning autism. *Autism, 7*(1), 99–110.

Faja, S., Webb, S. J., Jones, E., Merkle, K., Kamara, D., Bavaro, J., et al. (2012). The effects of face expertise training on the behavioral performance and brain activity of adults with high functioning autism spectrum disorders. *Journal of Autism and Developmental Disorders, 42*, 278–293.

Farley, M. A., McMahon, W. M., Fombonne, E., Jenson, W. R., Miller, J., Gardner, M., et al. (2009). Twenty-year outcome for individuals with autism and average or near-average cognitive abilities. *Autism Research, 2*, 109–118.

Fombonne, E. (2005a). Epidemiology of autistic disorder and other pervasive developmental disorders. *Journal of Clinical Psychiatry, 66*(Suppl 10), 3–8.

Fombonne, E. (2005b). The changing epidemiology of autism. *Journal of Applied Research in Intellectual Disabilities, 18*(4), 281–294. doi: http://dx.doi.org/10.1111/j.1468-3148.2005.00266.x.

Frank, A. R., & Siltington, P. L. (2000). Young adults with mental disbailities – Does transition planning make a difference? *Education and Training in Mental Retardation and Developmental Disabilities, 35*, 119–134.

Fussell, E., & Furstenberg, F. F. (2005). The transition to adulthood during the twentieth century. In R. A. Settersten, F. F. Furstenberg, & R. G. Rumbaut (Eds.), *On the frontier of adulthood: Theory, research and public policy* (pp. 29–75). Chicago: University of Chicago Press.

García-Villamisar, D. A., & Dattilo, J. (2010). Effects of a leisure pro-gramme on quality of life and stress of individuals with ASD. *Journal of Intellectual Disability Research, 54*, 611–619.

Garcia-Villamisar, D., Ross, D., & Wehman, P. (2000). Clinical differential analysis of persons with autism in a work setting: A follow-up study. *Journal of Vocational Rehabilitation, 14*, 183–185.

García-Villamisar, D., Wehman, P., & Navarro, M. D. (2002). Changes in the quality of autistic people's life that work in supported and sheltered employment: A 5-year follow-up study. *Journal of Vocational Rehabilitation, 17*, 309–312.

Gardener, H., Spiegelman, D., & Buka, S. L. (2009). Prenatal risk factors for autism: Comprehensive meta-analysis. *British Journal of Psychiatry, 195*(1), 7–14.

Gerber, F., Bessero, S., Robbiani, B., et al. (2011). Comparing residential programmes for adults with autism spectrum disorders and intellectual disability: Outcomes of challenging behaviour and quality of life. *Journal of Intellectual Disability Research, 55*, 918–932.

Geschwind, D.H., & State, M.W. (2015). Gene hunting in autism spectrum disorder: on the path to precision medicine. *Lancet Neurology*, Published online http://dx.doi.org/10.1016/S1474-4422(15)00044-7.

Ghaziuddin, M., & Zafar, S. (2008). Psychiatric comorbidity in adults with autism spectrum disorders. *Clincial Neuropsychiatry, 5*, 9–12.

Ghaziuddin, M., Weidmer-Mikhail, E., & Ghaziuddin, N. (1998). Comorbidity of Asperger syndrome: A preliminary report. *Journal of Intellectual Disability Research, 42*, 278–283.

Gillberg, C. (1991). Outcome in autism and autistic-like conditions. *Journal of the American Academy of Child and Adolescent Psychiatry, 30*, 375–382.

Gillberg, C., & Steffenburg, S. (1987). Outcomes and prognostic factors in infantile autism and similar conditions: A population-based study of 46 cases followed through puberty. *Journal of Autism and Developmental Disorders, 17*, 272–288.

Gillespie-Lynch, K., Sepeta, L., Wang, Y., Marshall, S., Gomez, L., Sigman, M., & Hutman, T. (2012). Early childhood predictors of the social competence of adults with autism. *Journal of Autism and Developmental disorder, 42*, 161–174.

Gilotty, L., Kenworthy, L., Sirian, L., Black, D. O., & Wagner, A. E. (2012). Adaptive skills and executive function in autism spectrum disorders. *Child Neuropsychology, 8*(4), 241–248.

Gjevik, E., Eldevik, S., Fjaeran-Granum, T., & Sponheim, E. (2011). Kiddie-SADS reveals high rates of DSM-IV disorders in children and adolescents with autism spectrum disorders. *Journal of Autism and Developmental Disorders, 41*, 761–769.

Glennon, T. J. (2001). The stress of the university experience for students with Asperger syndrome. *Work: Journal of Prevention, Assessment & Rehabilitation, 17*(3), 183–190.

Gulsrud, A. C., Hellemann, G. S., Freeman, F. N., & Kasari, C. (2014). Two to ten years: Developmental trajectories of joint attention with ASD who received targeted social communication interventions. *Autism Research, 7*, 207–215.

Hagner, D., & Cooney, B. F. (2005). "I do that for everybody": Supervising employees with autism. *Focus on Autism and Developmental Disabilities, 20*(2), 91–97.

Halfon, N., & Forrest, C. B. (2017). The emerging theoretical framework of life course health development. In N. Halfon, C. B. Forrest, R. M. Lerner, & E. Faustman (Eds.), *Handbook of life course health-development science*. Cham: Springer.

Halfon, N., Larson, K., Lu, M., Tullis, E., & Russ, S. (2014). Lifecourse health development: Past, present and future. *Journal of Maternal Child Health, 18*, 344–365.

Hallmayer, J., Cleveland, S., Torres, A., Phillips, J., Cohen, B., Torigoe, T., et al. (2011). Genetic heritability and shared environmental factors among twin pairs with autism. *Archives of General Psychiatry, 68*(11), 1095–1102. doi:10.1001/archgenpsychiatry.2011.76.

Harris, L. J., & Handelman, J. S. (Eds.). (2000). *Preschool education programs for children with autism* (2nd ed.). Austin: PRO-ED.

Henninger, N. A., & Taylor, J. L. (2012). Outcomes in adults with autism spectrum disorders: A historical perspective. *Autism, 0*(0), 1–14. doi:10.1177/1362361312441266.

Hermelin, B. (2001). *Bright Splinters of the mind: A personal story of research with Autistic savants*. London: Jessica Kingsley.

Hofvander, B., Delorme, R., Chaste, P., Nyden, A., Wentz, E., Stahlberg, O., et al. (2009). Psychiatric and psychosocial problems in adults with normal-intelligence autism spectrum disorders. *BMC Psychiatry, 9*, 35. doi:10.1186/1471-244X-9-35.

Holden, B., & Gitlesen, J. P. (2006). A total population study of challenging behavior in the country of Hedmark, Norway: Prevalence, and risk markers. *Research in Developmental Disabilities, 27*(4), 456–465.

Howlin, P. (1998). *Children with autism and Asperger syndrome. A guide for practitioners and carers*. Chichester: John Wiley & Sons.

Howlin, P. (2000). Outcome in adult life for more able individuals with Autism or Asperger Syndrome. *Autism, 4*(1), 63–83.

Howlin, P. (2003). Outcome in high-functioning adults with autism with and without early language delays: Implications for the differentiation between autism and Asperger syndrome. *Journal of Autism and Developmental Disorders, 33*, 3–13.

Howlin, P. (2005). Outcomes in autism spectrum disorders. In P. Howlin (Ed.), *Handbook od autism and pervasive developmental disorder, volume 1: Diagnosis, development, neurobiology, and behavior* (3rd ed.). Hoboken: John Wiley & Sons.

Howlin, P. (2013). Outcomes in adults with autism spectrum disorders. In F. Volkmar, S. Rogers, R. Paul, & K. Pelphrey (Eds.), *Handbook of autism* (4th ed.). Hoboken: Wiley.

Howlin, P., & Goode, S. (1998). Outcomes in adult life for individuals with autism. In F. Volkmar (Ed.), *Autism and developmental disorders*. New York: Cambridge University Press.

Howlin, P., & Moss, P. (2012). Adults with autism spectrum disorders. *Canadian Journal of Psychiatry, 57*(5), 275–283.

Howlin, P., Alcock, J., & Burkin, C. (2005). An 8 year follow-up of a specialist supported employment service for high-ability adults with autism or Asperger syndrome. *Autism, 9*(5), 533–549.

Howlin, P., Goode, J., Hutton, J., & Rutter, M. (2004). Adult outcomes for children with autism. *Journal of Child Psychology and Psychiatry, 45*, 212–229.

Huerta, M., Bishop, S. L., Duncan, A., Hus, V., & Lord, C. (2012). Application of the DSM-5 criteria for autism spectrum disorder to three samples of children with DSM-IV diagnoses of pervasive developmental disorders. *American Journal of Psychiatry, 169*(10), 1056–1064.

Jobe, L., & White, S. W. (2007). Loneliness, social relationships, and a broader autism phenotype in college students. *Personality and Individual Differences, 42*, 1479–1489.

Joshi, G., Petty, C., Wozniak, J., Henin, A., Fried, R., Galdo, M., et al. (2010). The heavy burden of psychiatric comorbidity in youth with autism spectrum disorders: A large comparative study of psychiatrically referred population. *Journal of Autism and Developmental Disorders, 40*, 1361–1370.

Kamio, Y., Inada, N., & Koyama, T. (2012). A nationwide survey on quality of life and associated factors of adults with high-functioning autism spectrum disorders. *Autism, 17*, 15–26.

Kamp-Becker, I., Schröder, J., Muehlan Remschmidt, H., et al. (2011). Health-related quality of life in children and adolescents with autism spectrum disorder. *Zeitschrift für Kinder - und Jugendpsychiatrie und Psychotherapie, 39*(2), 123–131.

Kanner, L. (1943). Autistic disturbances of affective contact. *Nervous Child, 2*, 217–250.

Kanner, L. (1971). Follow-up study of eleven autistic children originally reported in. *Journal of Autism & Childhood Schizophrenia, 1*(2), 119–145.

Kasari, C., Gulsrud, A. C., Wong, C., Kwon, S., & Locke, J. (2010). Randomized controlled caregiver mediated joint engagement intervention for toddlers with autism. *Journal of Autism Developmental Disorders, 40*(9), 1045–1056.

Keel, J. H., Mesibov, G. B., & Woods, A. V. (1997). TEACCH-supported employment program. *Journal of Autism and Developmental Disabilities, 27*(1), 3–9.

Keogh, B. K., Bernheimer, L. P., & Guthrie, D. (2004). Children with developmental delays twenty years later: Where are they? How are they? *American Journal on Mental Retardation, 109*(3), 219–230.

Kim, S.H., Macari, S., Koller, J., & Chawarska, K. (2015). Examining the phenotypic heterogeneity of early autism spectrum disorder: Subtypes and short-term outcomes. *Journal of Child Psychology and Psychiatry*. doi:10.1111/jcpp.12448.

King, M., & Bearman, P. (2009). Diagnostic change and the increased prevalence of autism. *International Journal of Epidemiology, 38*(5), 1224–1234. Epub 2009 Sep 7. PubMed PMID: 19737791.

Kleinman, J., Ventola, P., Pandey, J., Verbalis, A., Barton, M., Hodgson, S., et al. (2008). Diagnostic stability in very young children with autism spectrum disorder. *Journal of Autism and Developmental Disorders, 38*(4), 606–615. doi:10.1007/s10803-007-0427-8.

Klin, A., Volkmar, F. R., Sparrow, S. S., Cicchetti, D. V., & et al. (1996). Validity and neuropsychological characterization of Asperger syndrome: Convergence with nonverbal learning disabilities syndrome. *Annual Progress in Child Psychiatry & Child Development*, 241–259.

Kobayashi, R., Murata, T., & Yoshinaga, K. (1992). A follow-up study of 201 children with autism in Kyushu and Yamaguchi areas, Japan. *Journal of Autism and Developmental Disorders, 22*, 395–411.

Kraemer, B. R., & Blacher, J. (2001). Transition for young adults with severe mental retardation: School preparation, parent expectations, and family involvement. *Mental Retardation, 39*, 432–455.

Kraemer, B. R., McIntyre, L. L., & Blacher, J. (2003). Quality of life for young adults with mental retardation during transition. *Mental Retardation, 41*, 250–262.

Kim, J., Szatmari, P., Bryson, S. E., & Wilson, F. J. (2000). Prevalence of anxiety and mood problems among children with autism and Asperger syndrome. *Autism, 4*, 117–132.

LaFramboise, T., Winckler, W., & Thomas, R. K. (2009). A flexible rank-based framework for detecting copy number aberrations from array data. *Bioinformatics, 25*(6), 722–728.

La Malfa, G., Lassi, S., Salvini, R., Giganti, C., Bertelli, M., & Albertini, G. (2007). The relationship between autism and psychiatric disorders in intellectually disabled adults. *Research in Autism Spectrum Disorders, 1*, 218–228.

Landa, R. J., & Kalb, L. G. (2012). Long-term outcomes of toddlers with autism spectrum disorders exposed o short-term intervention. *Pediatrics, 130*(2), S186–S190. doi:10.1542/peds.2012-0900Q.

Landa, R. J., Holman, K. C., & Garrett-Mayer, E. (2007). Social and communication development in toddlers with early and later diagnosis of autism spectrum disorders. *Archives of General Psychiatry, 64*(7), 853–864.

Landa, R. J., Holman, K. C., O'Neill, A. H., & Stuart, E. A. (2011). Intervention targeting development of socially synchronous engagement in toddlers with autism spectrum disorder: A randomized controlled trial. *Journal of Child Psychology and Psychiatry, 52*(1), 13–21.

Larsen, F. W., & Mouridsen, S. E. (1997). The outcome in children with childhood autism and Asperger syndrome originally diagnosed as psychotic. A 30-year follow-up study of subjects hospitalized as children. *European Child and Adolescent Psychiatry, 6*(4), 181–190.

Lee, G. K., & Carter, E. W. (2012). Preparing transition-age students with high-functioning autism spectrum disorders for meaningful work. *Psychology in the Schools, 49*(10), 988–1000. doi:10.1002/pits.21651.

Leekam, S. R., Nieto, C., Libby, S. J., Wing, L., & Gould, J. (2006). Describing the sensory abnormalities of children and adults with autism. *Journal of Autism and Developmental Disorders, 37*, 894–910. doi:10.1007/s10803-006-0218-7.

Levy, A., & Perry, A. (2011). Outcome in adolescents and adults with autism: A review of the literature. *Research in Autism Spectrum Disorders, 5*, 1271–1282.

Levy, S. E., Mandell, D. S., & Schultz, R. T. (2009). Autism. *Lancet, 374*, 1627–1638.

Leyfer, O. T., Folstein, S. E., Bacalman, S., Davis, N. O., Dinh, E., Morgan, J., et al. (2006). Comorbid psychiatric disorders in children with autism: Interview development and rates of disorders. *Journal of Autism and Developmental Disorders, 36*, 849–861.

Li, X., Zou, H., & Brown, W. T. (2012). Genes associated with autism spectrum disorder. *Brain Research Bulletin, 88*(6), 543–552.

Liptak, G. S., Benzoni, L. B., Mruzek, D. W., Nolan, K. W., Thingvoll, M. A., Wade, C. M., & Fryer, G. E. (2008). Disparities in diagnosis and access to health services for children with autism: Data from the national survey of children's health. *Journal of Developmental & Behavioral Pediatrics, 29*(3), 152–160.

Lockyer, L., & Rutter, M. (1969). A five- to fifteen-year follow-up study of infantile psychosis: III. *Psychological aspects. The British Journal of Psychiatry, 115*, 865–882.

Lockyer, L., & Rutter, M. (1970). A five- to fifteen-year follow-up study of infantile psychosis: IV. Patterns of cognitive ability. *British Journal of Social and Clinical Psychology, 9*(2), 152–163.

Loke, Y. J., Hannan, A. J., & Craig, J. M. (2015). The role of epigenetic change in autism spectrum disorders. *Frontiers in Neurology, 6*, 107. doi:10.3389/fneur.2015.00107.

Lord, C., & Bailey, A. (2002). Autism spectrum disorders. In M. Rutter & E. Taylor (Eds.), *Child and adolescent psychiatry* (4th ed., pp. 664–681). Oxford, MA: Blackwell Scientific.

Lord, C., & Schopler, E. (1989). The role of age at assessment, developmental level, and test in the stability of intelligence scores in young autistic children. *Journal of Autism and Developmental Disorders, 19*(4), 483–499.

Lotter, V. (1974). Social adjustment and placement of autistic children in Middlesex: A follow-up study. *Journal of Autism and Childhood Schizophrenia, 4*, 11–32.

Lotter, V. (1978). Follow-up studies. In M. Rutter & E. Schopler (Eds.), *Autism: A reappraisal of concepts and treatment* (pp. 475–495). New York: Plenum Press.

Lounds Taylor, J., Dove, D., Veenstra-VanderWeele, J., Sathe, N.A., McPheeters, M.L., Jerome, R.N., Warren, Z.. (2012). *Interventions for adolescents and young Adults with Autism Spectrum disorders*. Comparative effectiveness review no. 65. (Prepared by the Vanderbilt evidence-based practice Center under contract no. 290–2007-10065-I.) AHRQ publication no. 12-EHC063-EF. Rockville, MD: Agency for Healthcare Research and Quality. www.effectivehealthcare.ahrq.gov/reports/final.cfm

Lovaas, I. (1987). Behavioral treatment and normal educational and intellectual functioning in young autistic children. *Journal of Consulting and Clinical Psychology, 55*(1), 3–9.

LoVullo, S. V., & Matson, J. L. (2009). Comorbid psychopathology in adults with autism spectrum disorders and intellectual disabilities. *Research in Developmental Disabilities, 30*, 1288–1296. doi:10.1016/j.ridd.2009.05.004.

Lugnegard, T., Hallerback, M. U., & Gillberg, C. (2011). Psychiatric comorbidity in young adults with a clinical diagnosis of Asperger syndrome. *Research in Developmental Disabilities, 32*, 1910–1917.

Lunsky, Y., Gracey, C., & Bradley, E. (2009). Adults with autism spectrum disorders using psychiatric hospitals in Ontario: Clinical profile and service needs. *Research in Autism Spectrum Disorders, 3*, 1006–1013.

Luxford, S., Hadwin, J. A., & Kovshoff, H. (2016). Evaluating the effectiveness of a school-based cognitive behavioural therapy intervention for anxiety in adolescents diagnosed with autism spectrum disorder. *Journal of Autism and Developmental Disorders*, doi:http://dx.doi.org/10.1007/s10803-016-2857-7

Magiati, I., Moss, J., Charman, T., & Howlin, P. (2011). Patterns of change in children with autism spectrum disorders who received community based comprehensive interventions in their pre-school years: A seven year follow-up study. *Research in Autism Spectrum Disorders, 5*(3), 1016–1027.

Malhotra, D., & Sebat, J. (2012). Copy number variants: Harbingers of a rare variant revolution in psychiatric genetics. *Cell, 148*(6), 1223–1241.

Mattila, M.-L., Hurtig, T., Haapsamo, H., Jussila, K., Kuusikko-Gauffin, S., Kielinen, M., et al. (2010). Comorbid psychiatric disorders associated with Asperger syndrome/high functioning autism: A community and clinic-based study. *Journal of Autism and Developmental Disorders, 40*, 1080–1093.

Mattilla, M.-L., Kielinen, M., Linna, S.-L., Jussilla, K., Ebeling, H., Bloigu, R., et al. (2011). Autism Spectrum disorders According to DSM-IV-TR and comparison with DSM-5 draft criteria an epidemiological study. *Journal of the American Academy of Child & Adolescent Psychiatry, 50*(6), 583–592.

MacNeil, B. M., Lopes, V. A., & Minnes, P. M. (2009). Anxiety in children and adolescents with autism spectrum disorders. *Research in Autism Spectrum Disorders, 3*, 1–21. doi:10.1016/j.rasd.2008.06.001.

Mandell, D. (2008). Psychiatric hospitalization among children with autism spectrum disorders. *Journal of Autism and Developmental Disorders, 38*, 1059–1065.

Marshall, C. R., Noor, A., Vincent, J. B., Lionel, A. C., Feuk, L., Skaug, J., et al. (2008). Structural variation of chromosomes in autism spectrum disorder. *American Journal of Human Genetics, 82*(2), 477–488.

Matson, J. L., Wilkins, J., & Ancona, M. (2008). Autism in adults with severe intellectual disability: An empirical study of symptom presentation. *Journal of Intellectual & Developmental Disability, 33*, 36–42. doi:10.1080/13668250701829837.

Mawhood, L., & Howlin, P. (1999). The outcome of a supported employment scheme for high functioning adults with autism or Asperger syndrome. *Autism, 3*, 229–254.

Mawhood, L., Howlin, P., & Rutter, M. (2000). Autism and developmental receptive language disorder-a comparative follow-up in early adult life I: Cognitive and language outcomes. *Journal of Child Psychology and Psychiatry, 41*, 547–559.

Mazefsky, C. A., Folstein, S. E., & Lainhart, J. E. (2008). Overrepresentation of mood and anxiety disorders in adults with autism and their first degree relatives: What does it mean? *Autism Research, 1*, 193–197.

McGrew, S. G., Peters, B. R., Crittendon, J. A., & Veenstra-VaderWeele, J. (2012). Diagnostic yield of chromosomal microarray analysis in autism primary care practice: Which guidelines to implement? *Journal of Autism and Developmental Disorders, 42*(8), 1582–1591.

McDougle, C. J., Erickson, C. A., Stigler, K. A., & Posey, D. J. (2005). Neurochemistry in the pathophysiology of autism. *Journal of Clinical Psychiatry, 66*(Suppl 10), 9–18.

Meyer, J. A., & Minshew, N. J. (2002). An update on neurocognitive profiles in Asperger syndrome and high-functioning autism. *Focus on Autism and Other Developmental Disabilities, 17*(3), 152–160. http://dx.doi.org/10.1177/10883576020170030501.

Moseley, D. S., Tonge, B. J., Brereton, A. V., & Einfeld, S. L. (2011). Psychiatric comorbidity in adolescents and young adults with autism. *Journal of Mental Health Research in Intellectual Disabilities, 4*, 229–243.

Mouridsen, S. E., Rich, B., Isager, T., & Nedergaard, N. J. (2008). Psychiatric disorders in individuals diagnosed with infantile autism as children: A case control study. *Journal of Psychiatric Practice, 14*, 5–12.

Muller, N., Myint, A., & Schwarz, M. J. (2015). *Immunology and psychiatry: From basic research to therapeutic interventions*. Cham: Springer International Publishing.

Mundy, P., & Jarrold, W. (2010). Infant joint attention, neural networks and social cognition. *Neural Networks, 23*, 985–997. doi:10.1016/j.neunet.2010.08.009.

Mundy, P., Sullivan, L., & Mastergeorge, A. M. (2009). A parallel and distributed processing model of joint attention, social cognition, and autism. *Autism Research, 2*, 2–21.

Muris, P., Steerneman, P., Merckelbach, H., Holdrinet, I., & Meesters, C. (1998). Comorbid anxiety symptoms in children with pervasive developmental disorders. *Journal of Anxiety Disorders, 12*, 387–393.

Narendorf, S. C., Shattuck, P. T., & Sterzing, P. R. (2011). Mental health services among adolescents with an autism spectrum disorder. *Psychiatric Services, 62*, 975–978.

National Autism Center. (2015). *Findings and conclusions: National standards project, phase 2*. Randolph, MA: Author.

National Autism Center. (2009). *National Standards Report – Addressing the need for evidence-based practice guidelines for Autism Spectrum Disorders*. Massachusetts: National Autism Center.

National Research Council. (2001). *Educating young children with autism*. Washington, DC: National Academy Press.

Newman, L., Wagner, M., Knokey, A. M., Marder, C., Nagle, K., Shaver, D., & Wei, X. (2011). *The posy-high school outcomes of young adults with disabilities up to 8 years after high school*. Menlo Park: SRI International.

Nordin, V., & Gillberg, C. (1998). The long-term course of autistic disorders: Update on follow-up studies. *Acta Psychiatrica Scandinavica, 97*, 99–108.

Noterdaeme, M., Wriedt, E., & Höhne, C. (2010). Asperger's syndrome and high-functioning autism: Language, motor and cognitive profiles. *European Child & Adolescent Psychiatry, 19*(6), 475–481.

Palac, S., & Meador, K. J. (2011). Antiepileptic drugs and neurodevelopment: An update. *Current Neurology and Neuroscience Reports, 11*(4), 423–427.

Palucka, A. M., Bradley, E., & Lunsky, Y. (2008). A case of unrecognized intellectual disability and autism misdiagnosed as schizophrenia: Are there lessons to be learned? *Mental Health Aspects of Developmental Disabilities, 11*(2), 55–60.

Parr, J. R., Le Couteur, A., Baird, G., Rutter, M., Pickles, A., Fombonne, E., Bailey, A. J., & International Molecular Genetic Study of Autism Consortium. (2011). Early developmental regression in autism spectrum disorder: Evidence from an international multiplex sample. *Journal of Autism & Developmental Disorders, 41*(3), 332–340.

Paul, R. (2008). Communication development and assessment. In K. Chawarska, A. Klin, & F. Volkmar (Eds.), *Autism Spectrum disorders in infants and toddlers: Diagnosis, Assessment, and treatment* (pp. 76–103). New York: Guilford Press.

Pinto, D., Pagnamenta, A. T., Klei, L., Anney, R., Merico, D., Regan, R., et al. (2010). Functional impact of global rare copy number variation in autism spectrum disorders. *Nature, 466*(7304), 368–372.

Piven, J., & Rabins, P. (2011). Autism spectrum disorders in older adults: Toward defining a research agenda. *Journal of the American Geriatrics Society, 59*(11), 2151–2155.

Perkins, E. A., & Berkman, K. A. (2012). Into the unknown: Aging with autism spectrum disorders. *American Journal on Intellectual and Developmental Disabilities, 117*(6), 478–496.

Perlman, L. (2000). Adults with Asperger disorder misdiagnosed as schizophrenic. *Professional Psychology: research & Practice, 31*(2), 221–225. False.

Peters-Scheffer, N., Didden, R., Hubert, K., & Sturmey, P. (2011). A meta-analytic study on the effectiveness of comprehensive ABA-based early intervention programs for children with Autism Spectrum disorders. *Research in Autism Spectrum Disorders, 5*(1), 60–69.

Polloway, E. A., Patton, J. R., & Serna, L. (2001). *Strategies for teaching learners with special needs*. Upper Saddle River: Merrill Prentice Hall.

Potvin, M. C., Snider, L., Prelock, P. A., Wood-Dauphinee, S., & Kehayia, E. (2015). Health-related quality of life in children with high-functioning autism. *Autism, 19*(1), 14–19.

Power, R. A., Kyaga, S., Uher, R., Maccabe, J. H., Långström, N., Landen, M., et al. (2012). Fecundity of patients with schizophrenia, Autism, bipolar disorder, depression, anorexia nervosa, or substance abuse vs their unaffected siblings. *Archives of General Psychiatry, 12*, 1–8.

Raphael, D., Brown, I., Renwick, R., & Rootman, I. (1996). Assessing the quality of life of persons with developmental disabilities: Description of a new model, measuring instruments, and initial findings. *International Journal of Diability, 43*(1), 25–42.

Reichow, B. (2012). Overview of meta-analyses on early intensive behavioral intervention for young children with autism spectrum disorders. *Journal of Autism and Developmental Disorders, 42*, 512–520.

Reichow, B., & Wolery, M. (2009). Comprehensive synthesis of early intensive behavioral interventions for young children with autism based on the UCLA young Autism Project model. *Journal of Autism and Developmental Disorders, 39*(1), 23–41.

Renty, J., & Roeyers, H. (2006). Quality of life in high-functioning adults with autism spectrum disorder: The predictive value of disability and support characteristics. *Autism, 10*, 511–524.

Ritvo, E. R., Jorde, L. B., Mason-Brothers, A., Freeman, B. J., Pingree, C., Jones, M. B., et al. (1989). The UCLA-University of Utah epidemiologic survey of autism: Recurrence risk estimates and genetic counseling. *American Journal of Psychiatry, 146*(8), 1032–1036.

Robinson, S., Goddard, L., Dritschel, B., Wisley, M., & Howlin, P. (2009). Executive functions in children with autism spectrum disorders. *Brain and Cognition, 71*(3), 362–368. http://dx.doi.org/10.1016/j.bandc.2009.06.007

Rogers, S. J. (2009). What are infant siblings teaching us about autism in infancy? *Autism research : Official Journal of the International Society for Autism Research, 2*(3), 125–137.

Rondeau, E., Klein, L. S., Masse, A., Bodeau, N., Cohen, D., & Guile, J.-M. (2011). Is pervasive developmental disorder not otherwise specified less stable than autistic disorder? A meta-analysis. *Journal of Autism and Developmental Disorders, 41*, 1267–1276.

Ruble, L. A., & Dalrymple, N. J. (1996). An alternative view of outcome in autism. *Focus on Autism and Other Developmental Disabilities, 11*(1), 3–14.

Rumsey, J. M., Rapoport, J. L., & Sceert, W. R. (1985). Autistic children as adults: Psychiatric, social, and behavioral outcomes. *Journal of the American Academy of Child Psychiatry, 24*(4), 465–473.

Russ, S. A., Larson, K., Tullis, E., & Halfon, N. (2014). A lifecourse approach to health development: Implications for the maternal and child health research agenda. *Maternal and Child Health Journal, 18*(2), 497–510.

Russell, E., & Sofronoff, K. (2005). Anxiety and social worries in children with Asperger syndrome. *Australian and New Zealand Journal of Psychiatry, 39*, 633–638.

Rutter, M. (1967). The autistic child. *Royal Institute of Public Health & Hygiene Journal, 30*(4), 130–132.

Rutter, M. (1973). Why are London children so disturbed? *Proceedings of the Royal Society of Medicine, 66*(12), 1221–1225.

Rutter, M. (1978). Diagnosis and definition of childhood autism. *Journal of Autism & Childhood Schizophrenia, 8*(2), 139–161.

Rutter, M. (1982). Prevention of children's psychosocial disorders: Myth and substance. *Pediatrics, 70*(6), 883–894.

Rutter, M. (2005). Environmentally mediated risks for psychopathology: Research strategies and findings. *Journal of the American Academy of Child & Adolescent Psychiatry, 44*(1), 3–18.

Rutter, M., & Lockyer, L. (1967). A five to fifteen year follow-up study of infantile psychosis I. Description of sample. *British Journal of Psychiatry, 113*(504), 1169–1182.

Rutter, M., Greenfield, D., & Lockyer, L. (1967). A five to fifteen year follow-up of infantile psychosis II social and behavioral outcome. *The British Journal of Psychiatry, 113*, 1183–1199.

Schreibman, L., Dawson, G., Stahmer, A. C., Landa, R., Rogers, S., et al. (2015). Naturalistic developmental behavioral interventions: Empirically validated treatments for autism spectrum disorder. *Journal of Autism and Developmental Disorders, 45*(8), 2411–2428.

Saxena, S., & Orley, J. (1997). Quality of life assessment: The world health organization perspective. *European Psychiatry, 12*, 263s–266s.

Schumann, C. M., Bloss, C. S., Barnes, C. C., Wideman, G. M., Carper, R. A., Akshoomoff, N., et al. (2010). Longitudinal magnetic resonance imaging study of cortical development through early childhood in autism. *Journal of Neuroscience, 30*, 4419–4427.

Seltzer, M. M., Krauss, M. W., Shattuck, P. T., Orsmond, G., Swe, A., & Lord, C. (2003). The stmptoms of autism spectrum disorders in adolescents and adulthood. *Journal of Autism and Developmental Disorders, 33*, 565–581.

Seltzer, M. M., Shattuck, P., Abbeduto, L., & Greenberg, J. S. (2004). Trajectory of development in adolescents and adults with autism. *Mental Retardation and Developmental Disabilities, 10*, 234–247.

Shattuck, P. T., Durkin, M., Maenner, M., Newschaffer, C., Mandell, D. S., Wiggins, L., et al. (2009). Timing of identification among children with an autism spectrum disorder: Findings from a population-based surveillance study. *Journal of the American Academy of Child & Adolescent Psychiatry, 48*(5), 474–483.

Shattuck, P. T., Roux, A. M., Hudson, L. E., Taylor, J. L., Maenner, M. J., & Trani, J.-F. (2012). Services for adults with autism spectrum disorder. *Canadian Journal of Psychiatry, 57*(5), 284–291.

Shattuck, P. T., Seltzer, M. M., Greenberg, J. S., Orsmond, G. I., Bolt, D., Kring, S., et al. (2007). Change in autism symptoms and maladaptive behaviors in adolescents with an autism spectrum disorder. *Journal of Autism and Developmental Disorders, 37*, 1735–1747.

Shelton, J. F., Tancredi, D. J., & Hertz-Picciotto, I. (2010). Independent and dependent contributions of advanced maternal and paternal ages to autism risk. *Autism Research, 3*(1), 30–39.

Sigman, M., & Kasari, C. (1995). *Joint attention across contexts in normal and autistic children.* (pp. 189–203). Hillsdale: Lawrence Erlbaum Associates, Inc. Retrieved from http://search.proquest.com/docview/618769168?accountid=14771

Sigman, M., & McGovern, C. W. (2005). Improvement in cognitive and language skills from preschool to adolescence in autism. *Journal of Autism and Developmental Disorders, 35*(1), 15–23.

Sigman, M., & Ruskin, E. (1999). Continuity and change in the social competence of children with autism, down syndrome, and developmental delays. *Monographs of the Society for Research in Child Development, 64*(1), 1–139.

Simonoff, E., Pickles, A., Charman, T., Chandler, S., Loucas, T., & Baird, G. (2008). Psychiatric disorders in children with autism spectrum disorders: Prevalence, comorbidity, and associated factors in a population-derived sample. *Journal of the American Academy of Child and Adolescent Psychiatry, 47*, 921–929.

Skokauskas, N., & Gallagher, L. (2010). Psychosis, affective disorders, and anxiety in autistic spectrum disorder: Prevalence and nosological considerations. *Psychopathology, 43*, 8–16.

Smith, M., & Paulippen, L. (1999). Community integration and supported employment. In D. Zager (Ed.), *Autism: Identification, education, treatment* (pp. 301–319). Mahwah: Erlbaum.

State, M. W. (2010). The genetics of child psychiatric disorders: Focus on autism and Tourette syndrome. *Neuron, 68*(2), 254–269.

Sterling, L., Dawson, G., Estes, A., & Greenson, J. (2008). Characteristics associated with presence of depressive symptoms in adults with autism spectrum disorder. *Journal of Autism and Developmental Disorders, 38*, 1011–1018.

Stoner, J. B., Angell, M. E., House, J. J., & Bock, S. J. (2007). Transitions: Perspectives from parents of young children with autism spectrum disorders (ASD). *Journal of Developmental Disabilities, 19*, 23–39.

Strauss, K., Mancini, F., & Fava, L. (2013). Parent inclusion in early intensive behavior interventions for young children with ASD: A synthesis of meta-analyses from 220 to 2011. *Reseach in Developmental Disabilities, 34*(9), 2967–2985.

Sullivan, P. F., Daly, M. J., & O'Donovan, M. (2012). Genetic architectures of psychiatric disorders: The emerging picture and its implications. *Nature Reviews Genetics, 13*(8), 537–551.

Sun F, Oristaglio J, Levy SE, Hakonarson H, Sullivan N, Fontanarosa J, Schoelles KM. 2015. Genetic testing for developmental disabilities, intellectual disability, and Autism Spectrum disorder. Technical brief no. 23. (prepared by the ECRI institute–Penn medicine evidence-based practice Center under contract no. 290–2012-00011-I.) AHRQ publication no.15-EHC024-EF. Rockville, MD: Agency for Healthcare Research and Quality. www.effectivehealthcare.ahrq.gov/reports/final.cfm.

Szatmari, P. (2011). New recommendations on autism spectrum disorder shifting the focus from subtypes to dimensions carriers potential costs and benefits. *BMJ, 342*. doi:10.1136/bmj.d2456.

Szatmari, P., & McConnell, B. (2011). Anxiety and mood disorders in individuals with autism spectrum disorder. In D. G. Amaral, G. Dawson, & D. H. Geschwind

(Eds.), *Autism spectrum disorders* (pp. 330–338). New York: Oxford University Press, Inc.

Szatmari, P., Bartolucci, G., Brenner, R., Bond, S., & Rich, S. (1989). A follow-up study of high-functioning autistic children. *Journal of Autism and Developmental Disorders, 19*, 213–225.

Szatmari, P., Bryson, S. E., Boyle, M. H., Streiner, D. L., & Duku, E. (2003). Predictors of outcome among high functioning children with autism and Asperger syndrome. *Journal of Child Psychology and Psychiatry, 44*(4), 529–528.

Szatmari, P., Georgiades, S., Duku, E., Bennett, T. A., Bryson, S., et al. (2015). Developmental trajectories of symptom severity and adaptive functioning in an inception cohort of preschool children with autism spectrum disorder. *JAMA Psychiatry, 72*(3), 276–283.

Szatmari, P., Jones, M. B., Zwaigenbaum, L., & MacLean, J. E. (1998). Genetics of autism: Overview and new directions. *Journal of Autism and Developmental Disorders, 28*(5), 351–368.

Szatmari, P., Paterson, A. D., Zwaigenbaum, L., Roberts, W., Brian, J., Autism Genome Project Consortium, et al. (2007). Mapping autism risk loci using genetic linkage and chromosomal rearrangements. *Nature Genetics, 39*(3), 319–328.

Taylor, J. L. (2009). The transition out of high school and into adulthood for individuals with autism and for their families. *International Review of Research in Mental Retardation, 38*, 1–32. doi:10.1016/S0074-7750(08)38001-X.

Taylor, J. L., & Seltzer, M. M. (2010). Changes in the autism behavioral phenotype during the transition to adulthood. *Journal of Autism and Developmental Disorders, 40*, 1431–1446.

Taylor, J. L., & Seltzer, M. M. (2011a). Changes in the mother-child relationship during the transition to adulthood for youth with autism spectrum disorders. *Journal of Autism and Developmental Disorders, 41*, 1397–1410. doi:10.1007/s10803-010-1166-9.

Taylor, J. L., & Seltzer, M. M. (2011b). Employment and post-secondary educational activities for young adults with autism spectrum disorders during the transition to adulthood. *Journal of Autism and Developmental Disorders, 41*, 566–574.

Taylor, J. L., McPheeters, M. L., Sathe, N. A., Dove, D., Veenstra-VanderWeele, J., & Warren, Z. (2012). A systematic review of vocational interventions for young adults with autism spectrum disorders. *Pediatrics, 130*(3), 531–538. doi:10.1542/peds.2012-0682.

Thomas, K. C., Ellis, A. R., McLaurin, C., Daniels, J., & Morrissey, J. P. (2007). Access to care for autism-related services. *Journal of Autism and Developmental Disorders, 37*, 1902–1912.

Totsika, V., Flece, D., Kerr, M., & Hastings, R. P. (2010). Behavior problems, psychiatric symptoms, and quality of life for older adults with intellectual disability with and without autism. *Journal of Autism and Developmental Disorders, 40*, 1171–1178.

Tomasello, M. (1995). Joint attention as social cognition. In C. Moore, & P. J. Dunham (Eds.), *Joint attention: Its origins and role in development; joint attention: Its origins and role in development* (pp. 103-130, Chapter vii, 286 Pages). Hillsdale: Lawrence Erlbaum Associates, Inc.

Towbin, K. E. (2005). Pervasive developmental disorder not otherwise specified. In F. R. Volkmar, A. Klin, R. Paul, & D. J. Cohen (Eds.), *Handbook of autism and pervasive developmental disorders* (Vol. 1, 3rd ed., pp. 165–200). Hoboken: Wiley.

Tsakanikos, E., Costello, H., Holt, G., Bouras, N., Sturmey, P., & Newton, T. (2006). Psychopathology in adults with autism and intellectual disability. *Journal of Autism and Developmental Disorders, 36*, 1123–1129.

Tsakanikos, E., Costello, H., Holt, G., Sturmey, P., & Bouras, N. (2007a). Behavior management problems as predictors of psychotropic medication and use of psychiatric services in adults with autism. *Journal of Autism and Developmental Disorders, 37*, 1080–1085.

Tsakanikos, E., Sturmey, P., Costello, H., Holt, G., & Bouras, N. (2007b). Referral trends in mental health services for adults with intellectual disability and autism spectrum disorders. *Autism, 11*, 9–17.

Turner, L. M., & Stone, W. L. (2007). Variability in outcome for children with an ASD diagnosis at age 2. *The Journal of Child Psychology and Psychiatry, 48*(8), 793–802.

Van Acker, R., Loncola, J. A., & Van Acker, E. Y. (2005). Rett syndrome: A pervasive developmental disorder. In F. R. Volkmar, R. Paul, A. Klin & D. Cohen (Eds.), Handbook of autism and pervasive developmental disorders: Diagnosis, development, neurobiology, and behavior (vol. 1) (3rd ed) (pp. 126–164, Chapter xxv, 703 Pages). Hoboken: John Wiley & Sons Inc.

VanBergeik, E., Klin, A., & Volkmar, F. (2008). Supporting more able students on the autism spectrum: College and beyond. *Journal of Autism and Developmental Disorders, 38*, 1359–1370. doi:10.1007/s10803-007-0524-8.

van Heijst, B. F. C., & Geurts, H. M. (2015). Quality of life in autism across the lifespan: A meta-analysis. *Autism, 19*(2), 158–167. doi:10.1177/1362361313517053.

Vaughan Van Hecke, A., Mundy, P., Acra, C. F., Block, J. J., Delgado, C. E. F., Parlade, M. V., et al. (2007). Infant joint attention, temperament, and social competence in preschool children. *Child Development, 78*(1), 53–69.

Veltman, J. A., & Brunner, H. G. (2012). De novo mutations in human genetic disease. *Nature Reviews Genetics, 13*(8), 565–575.

Venter, A., Lord, C., & Schopler, E. (1992). A follow-up study of high-functioning autistic children. *Journal of Child Psychology and Psychiatry, 33*(3), 489–507.

Volkmar, F. R. (2004). Adolescence and sexuality. In F. R. Volkmar & L. A. Wiesner (Eds.), *Healthcare for children on the autism spectrum* (pp. 245–260). New York: Harbour House.

Volkmar, F. R., & McPartland, J. (2014). From Kanner to DSM-5: Autism as an evolving diagnostic concept. *Annual Review of Clinical Psychology, 10*, 193–212.

Volkmar, F. R., & Cohen, D. J. (1991). Comorbid association of autism and schizophrenia. *The American Journal of Psychiatry, 148*(12), 1705–1707.

Volkmar, F. R., Koenig, K., & State, M. (2005). Childhood disintegrative disorder. In F. R. Volkmar, A. Klin, R. Paul, & D. J. Cohen (Eds.), *Handbook of autism and pervasive developmental disorders* (Vol. 1, 3rd ed., pp. 70–78). Hoboken: Wiley.

Volkmar, F. R., Klin, A., & McPartland, J. (2014). Asperger's syndrome: An overview. In J. McPartland, A. Klin, & F. Volkmar (Eds.), *Asperger syndrome: Assessing and treating high-functioning autism spectrum disorders* (pp. 1–42). New York: Guilford Press.

Watts, G. (2012). More psychiatrists attack plans for DSM-5. *BMJ, 344*, e3357. http://dx.doi.org/10.1136/bmj.e3357

Weitlauf, A.S., McPheeters, M.L., Peters, B., Sathe, N., Travis, R., Aiello, R., Williamson, E., Veenstra-VanderWeele, J., Krishnaswami, S., Jerome, R., Warren, Z. (2014). Therapies for Children With Autism Spectrum Disorder: Behavioral Interventions Update. Comparative Effectiveness Review No. 137. (Prepared by the Vanderbilt Evidence-based Practice Center under Contract No. 290–2012-00009-I.) AHRQ Publication No. 14-EHC036-EF. Rockville, MD: Agency for Healthcare Research and Quality. www.effectivehealthcare.ahrq.gov/reports/final.cfm

Wing, L. (1980). Childhood autism and social class: a question of selection? *British Journal of Psychiatry, 137*, 410–417.

White, S., Oswald, D., Ollendick, T., & Scahill, L. (2009). Anxiety in children and adolescents with ASD. *Clinical Psychology Review, 29*, 216–229.

Wolff, J. J., Gu, H., Elison, J. T., Styner, M., Gouttard, S., et al. (2012). Differences in white matter fiber tract development present from 6 to 24 months in infants with autism. *The American Journal of Psychiatry, 169*, 589–600.

Woodbury-Smith, M. R., & Volkmar, F. R. (2009). Asperger syndrome. *European Child & Adolescent Psychiatry, 18*(1), 2–11.

Woolfenden, S., Sarkozy, V., Ridley, G., & Williams, K. (2012). A systematic review of the diagnostic stability of autism spectrum disorder. *Research in Autism Spectrum Disorders, 6*, 345–354. doi:10.1016/j.rasd.2011.06.008.

Zachor, D. A., & Itzchak, E. B. (2010). Treatment approach, autism severity and intervention outcomes in young children. *Research in Autism Spectrum Dosorders, 4*(3), 425–432.

Zwaigenbaum, L., Bryson, S. E., Szatmari, P., Brian, J., Smith, I. M., Roberts, W., et al. (2012). Sex differences in children with autism spectrum disorder identified within a high-risk infant cohort. *Journal of Autism and Developmental Disorders, 42*(12), 2585–2596.

Self-Regulation

Megan McClelland, John Geldhof, Fred Morrison, Steinunn Gestsdóttir, Claire Cameron, Ed Bowers, Angela Duckworth, Todd Little, and Jennie Grammer

1 Self-Regulation

Self-regulation has received enormous attention in recent years as a key predictor of a variety of outcomes, including obesity (Evans et al. 2012), school readiness (Blair and Razza 2007; McClelland et al. 2007; Morrison et al. 2010), academic achievement in adolescence (Duckworth et al. 2010b), and long-term health and educational outcomes (McClelland et al. 2013; Moffitt et al. 2011). Although researchers have focused on self-regulation from a diverse set of perspectives (Geldhof et al. 2010; McClelland et al. 2010), there is consensus that self-regulation has important implications for individual trajectories of health and well-being across the life course. Indeed, over a decade ago, it was suggested that "understanding self-regulation is the single most crucial goal for advancing the understanding of development" (Posner and Rothbart, 2000, p. 427).

Self-regulation is fundamental to successful accomplishment of adaptive developmental tasks at all stages of life. In the field of maternal and child health, a recent emphasis utilizing a life course health development (LCHD) perspective has shed new light on how these trajectories are shaped by dynamic mechanisms such as self-regulation. This perspective is captured by the seven LCHD principles—as described by Halfon and Forrest (2017)—which are also consistent with the relational developmental

M. McClelland (✉)
Human Development and Family Sciences, 245 Hallie E. Ford Center for Healthy Children and Families, Oregon State University, Corvallis, OR 97331, USA
e-mail: megan.mcclelland@oregonstate.edu

J. Geldhof
Oregon State University, Human Development and Family Sciences, Corvallis, OR, USA

F. Morrison
University of Michigan, Department of Psychology, Ann Arbor, MI, USA

S. Gestsdóttir
University of Iceland, Department of Psychology, Reykjavik, Iceland

C. Cameron
University at Buffalo, SUNY, Learning and Instruction, Buffalo, NY, USA

E. Bowers
Clemson University, Youth Development Leadership, Clemson, SC, USA

A. Duckworth
University of Pennsylvania, Department of Psychology, Philadelphia, PA, USA

T. Little
Texas Tech University, Department of Educational Psychology and Leadership, Lubbock, TX, USA

J. Grammer
University of California, Los Angeles, Graduate School of Education and Information Studies, Los Angeles, CA, USA

N. Halfon et al. (eds.), *Handbook of Life Course Health Development*,
DOI 10.1007/978-3-319-47143-3_12

systems (RDS) perspective in the field of human development.

The development of self-regulation is a prime example of many of the LCHD principles in action. For example, the notion that health develops continuously over the life span would imply that individual pathways in self-regulation skills are formed partly through life course transitions and turning points or the points in a person's life which can influence developmental pathways in either positive (protective) or negative (maladaptive) ways, and in fact this is the case. Similarly, the notion that the timing and structure of environmental exposures are important for health development applies very well to self-regulation, the development of which is significantly and adversely affected by persistent and chronic stress, especially prenatally and in the first few years of life. (Conversely, protective factors such as sensitive and engaged caregiving can be a buffer for a child's development of these skills during this time.) Additionally, the LCHD notion that the rhythm of human development is a result of synchronized timing of molecular, physiological, behavioral, and evolutionary processes and that the synchronization of these processes contributes to the enormous individual variability in health development over time is also relevant to self-regulation.

Another illustration of the degree to which the development of self-regulation serves as a powerful example of the LCHD framework and its underlying principles in action is the fact that, at a time in history when the importance of children's self-regulation is perhaps greater than in previous decades due to an increasing academic focus in school settings, children and youth are using media to a much greater extent than ever before, a trend which could be detrimental to the development of these essential skills. This mismatch between the demands of the environment and the capacities of the developing individual is well described by the LCHD principles, which emphasize how evolution enables and constrains health development pathways and plasticity, how different aspects of development are intertwined over time (e.g., biobehavioral development is connected to sociocultural development), and how efforts to promote more optimal health development can promote survival and enhance thriving by countering the negative impact of these kinds of mismatches.

Finally, the LCHD principles capture the dynamic and complex nature of health development and emphasize that development emerges as a result of person interactions at multiple levels. This speaks to the importance of integrating interventions both vertically—meaning along primary, secondary, and tertiary care continua—and horizontally, that is, across domains of function (i.e., biological, behavioral, social), as well as longitudinally (e.g., across life stages and/or generations). This is especially relevant here because the capacity for self-regulation has been shown to be highly malleable and because interventions to promote such skills have been shown to be more effective when they are integrated across different levels and contexts (Diamond and Lee 2011; Raver et al. 2011).

Together, the LCHD principles will guide our discussion of self-regulation, which are also consistent with an RDS perspective. After providing a theoretical framework based on RDST, we will view the seven principles of LCHD to better understand the determinants and pathways of self-regulation, methods for studying self-regulation, and translational issues. We conclude by providing recommendations for better integrating the principles of LCHD with the study of self-regulation.

1.1 Relational Developmental Systems Theory as a Framework for Self-Regulation

While many processes currently subsumed under the "self-regulation" moniker have been studied from the earliest days of psychology (e.g., James 1890), the modern study of self-regulation truly emerged as psychologists moved away from the mechanistic neopositivism that dominated their field during the middle part of the twentieth century. Work by Bandura (1969) and Mischel (1968), for instance, rejected the notion of the "black box" and instead emphasized the self (and vicariously behavioral regulation by the self) as the object of valid scientific inquiry. This renewed focus on the self has made way for many of the core concepts that frame modern developmental science (e.g., that individuals are proactive agents capable of influencing their own development; Lerner 1982). Much of the recent work on self-regulation can be subsumed under the meta-theoretical stance that Overton (e.g., 2010, 2013) has termed relational developmental systems ((RDS) theory.

Similar to the principles of LCHD, RDS represents an approach to human development that rejects the dualistic separation of individual and context (Overton 2013). Instead, like the principles of LCHD, RDST specifies that the individual is completely embedded as a locally self-organized component of his or her larger context. Development of the individual therefore necessarily influences and is influenced by his or her surrounding environment. These mutual influences can be thought of co-regulation (i.e., action and development of the individual partially "regulate" and are partially "regulated" by the surrounding context), resulting in what Brandstädter (e.g., 2006) has called developmental regulations. Similarly, Lerner (e.g., 1985; Lerner et al. 2011) has heuristically decomposed this person-context system and has described developmental regulations as mutually influential, bidirectional person-context interactions—similar to LCHD Principle 3. Accordingly, across the life span, individuals are active agents in the mutually influential interactions among the variables from the integrated biological, social, cultural, and historical (or temporal) levels of the dynamic developmental system (as in LCHD Principles 1, 2, 7).

The co-regulative nature of the person-context system described in RDST directly informs the contemporary study of self-regulation. While person and context are truly inseparable from the RDST perspective, Gestsdottir and Lerner (e.g., 2008) note that we can heuristically separate developmental regulations into those that primarily arise from the individual (i.e., the self) and those that primarily arise from the context. Using this logic, they proceed to define self-regulation as comprised of "the attributes involved in and the means through which the individual contributes to developmental regulations…" (p. 203). As a broadly defined construct, self-regulation therefore entails cognitions, emotions, and actions that arise within the individual and do not differentiate between conscious and subconscious (or even automatic) action.

Differentiating between consciousness and sub- or (non)conscious behavior has been a recurring issue in the study of self-regulation, and it is now widely acknowledged that all self-regulated action falls along a continuum ranging from fully intentional to fully automatic. For instance, work done by Bargh and colleagues (e.g., Bargh et al. 2001) clearly shows that subconscious goals can influence (i.e., regulate) behavior outside of the actor's explicit awareness. Similarly, Gestsdottir and Lerner (2008) differentiate between organismic and intentional self-regulation. Here, organismic self-regulation occurs below the threshold of consciousness and includes diverse actions ranging from the cardiovascular regulation of blood oxygen levels to the regulation of outwardly directed behavior through automatized goal structures. In contrast, intentional self-regulation includes behavior that the individual is consciously aware of, representing an agent's intentional influence over the person-context system. The remainder of this chapter focuses specifically on intentional self-regulation. In total, self-regulation may be defined as "the ability to flexibly activate, monitor, inhibit, persevere and/or adapt one's behavior, attention, emotions and cognitive strategies in response to directions from internal cues, environmental stimuli and feedback from others, in an attempt to attain personally-relevant goals" (Moilanen 2007, p. 835).

2 Definitions of Self-Regulation

The study of self-regulation lacks integration across the life span. Theories that approach self-regulation within a given period of the life span are often not integrated with each other nor are they usually integrated with theories that focus on subsequent or preceding life periods. In this section, we briefly review several of the major conceptualizations of self-regulation in an attempt to highlight the complexity of self-regulated processes in children and youth. Inherent in these conceptualizations and definitions are the seven principles of LCHD, which have important implications for the concepts of turning points and transitions, how mismatches can occur in development, and the need to integrate interventions across multiple levels of influence.

2.1 Executive Functioning

As an instantiation of self-regulation, the study of executive function (EF) emphasizes the fluid, cognitive processes that underlie self-regulated action. While the precise definition of which skills and processes constitute EF may vary across studies, researchers studying self-regulation have emphasized a few key skills. In particular, researchers have studied the importance and development of agentic control over one's attention, inhibitory control, and working memory (McClelland et al. 2010). Research addressing the development of attentional control describes the transition from simple arousal to fully endogenous attention across the first few years of life (e.g., Colombo 2001) and the subsequent development of attentional capacities from childhood to late life (e.g., Posner and Rothbart 1998). Attentional processes play a major role in self-regulated action (e.g., Norman and Shallice's (1986) Supervisory Attentional System) and may especially relate to emotion regulation in infants and children (Sheese et al. 2008). Children begin to display inhibitory control by approximately 3 years of age (Posner and Rothbart 1998), a time that corresponds to the onset of endogenous attention and also corresponds to the transition out of Piaget's preoperational stage (see Geldhof et al. 2010 for a brief discussion). Inhibitory control continues to develop throughout childhood (e.g., Backen Jones et al. 2003) and continues to increase throughout adolescence and into early adulthood (e.g., Hooper et al. 2004). Finally, working memory is an aspect of executive functioning that includes the ability to actively work on and process information. In young children, it is demonstrated by children's ability to remember and follow instructions (Gathercole et al. 2004; Kail 2003).

The early years are a sensitive period of brain development, which closely parallel the development of EF. Understanding how EF develops during this developmental window has important implications for biological, cognitive, and social development.

2.2 Self-Regulation Versus Self-Control

The literature does not consistently distinguish between the concepts of self-regulation and self-control, with many authors using the terms interchangeably. Other authors consider self-regulation and self-control as distinct processes, which follow a sensitive period of development in infancy. For instance, Kopp (1982) describes self-control as developing at around 24 months of age and as including the ability to behave according to a caregiver's requests and to adhere to social expectations in the absence of external monitors. She distinguishes this from self-regulation, which instead develops when a child is approximately 36 months old and represents an internalization of self-control that allows for a degree of flexibility, allowing children to meet the changing demands of a dynamic context. According to Kopp, the distinction between self-control and self-regulation is therefore "a difference in degree, not in kind" (Kopp 1982, p. 207). In other words, self-regulation is an outgrowth of self-control that allows for flexible adaptation to real-world demands but which develops rapidly over the infant and toddler years. As such, this progression reflects the principles of LCHD especially for our understanding of how transitions and sensitive periods influence self-regulation development.

2.3 Effortful Control

In addition to the terms executive functions, self-regulation, and self-control, effortful control is a related construct that stems from the temperament literature. Rothbart and colleagues have defined the effortful control dimension of childhood temperament as “the ability to inhibit a dominant response to perform a subdominant response” (Rothbart and Bates 1998, p.137). Measures of effortful control for preschool children encompass several facets, including attention focusing and inhibitory control over inappropriate impulses (Rothbart et al. 2001). Rothbart distinguishes effortful control from two temperament factors that encompass more reactive (i.e., less voluntary) tendencies: surgency/extraversion and negative affect. Moreover, effortful control seems highly related, both conceptually and empirically, to self-control and conscientiousness in adolescents and adults (Eisenberg et al. (2012), under review). While this definition closely reflects cognitive inhibition, effortful control is instead considered an aspect of children’s temperament that develops in tandem with the development of endogenous attention. Research on infant temperament has not found a complete analogue to effortful control, for instance, with factor analyses instead uncovering a factor called orienting/regulation (e.g., Garstein and Rothbart 2003). Orienting/regulation contains many “regulatory” components similar to effortful control (e.g., orienting, soothability) but lacks a truly effortful component.

Effortful control incorporates the influence of temperament that infants are born with, along with the influence of the environment, including quality of caregiving. This dynamic coaction can be seen in the temperamental concept of “goodness of fit.” Goodness of fit refers to the match (or mismatch) between children’s temperamental states and the quality of caregiving and temperament of their parents/caregivers. When there is a positive fit or match between children and caregivers, children’s development of self-regulation is optimized. In contrast, when a mismatch occurs, there is greater potential for difficulty with self-regulation and related outcomes. Thus, effortful control is especially relevant to understanding self-regulation through an LCHD framework.

2.4 Delay of Gratification

Delay of gratification is another approach to self-regulation with close ties to both inhibition and attention. Mischel and colleagues (e.g., Mischel and Ebbesen 1970) originally studied delay of gratification using the now-famous delay of gratification task with children. In this task, a researcher shows a child two rewards (e.g., a single marshmallow versus several marshmallows) and asks the child which reward he or she would prefer. Subsequent research has adapted this task for adults by varying the value of the rewards—sometimes making them hypothetical—and by extending the delay time to a month or longer (e.g., Fortsmeier et al. 2011; Duckworth and Seligman 2005).

Regardless of the delivery, inherent in the construct is the integration of emotion with cognition in their understanding of self-regulation. Mischel’s research especially links the ability to delay gratification to endogenous attention through what he and his colleagues have called the cognitive-affective processing system (e.g., Mischel and Ayduk 2004). This work has shown that when the rewards are visible to children during the delay period, children who distract their attention away from the reward delay longer than children that do not (Mischel et al. 1972). Similarly, children who attend only to the cool, non-motivating, features of the reward (e.g., by treating the actual reward as if it is instead a picture of the reward) delay longer than children who do not (Moore et al. 1976). Delay of gratification thus complements the principles of LCHD by assuming that self-regulated behavior includes the transactional processes of emotion and cognition.

2.5 Emotion Regulation

Although the study of emotion regulation is a complete area of the literature unto itself, there is some important overlap with the study of self-regulation more generally defined. Infants' early regulatory tasks involve regulating their reactions to stimuli, including affective, temperament-based reactions that fall under the emotion regulation umbrella (Eisenberg et al. 2004). Emotion regulation means that children can modulate their strong emotional reactions with an appropriate strategy or combination of strategies (Bridges et al. 2004). Stansbury and Zimmerman (1999) describe four types of emotion regulatory strategies: instrumental or trying to change the situation (e.g., bidding for caregiver attention), comforting or soothing oneself without changing the situation (e.g., thumb-sucking), distraction or redirecting attention elsewhere (e.g., looking away), or cognitive, which is thought to be the most sophisticated and includes reframing the situation in a positive light, bargaining, or compromising. Importantly, children use different strategies depending on their individual characteristics as well as the situational context (Zimmermann and Stansbury 2003). This line of work demonstrates that the regulation of attention and emotion is closely interrelated and also reflects the principles of LCHD.

Together, the different definitions of self-regulation share many common conceptual underpinnings and are relevant to how these skills develop in individuals across the life span. They also apply to the key principles of LCHD. In the next section, we apply these principles to the developmental processes of self-regulation.

3 Developmental Processes of Self-Regulation

As noted above, the principles of LCHD can help to inform our understanding of the development of self-regulation. We orient our discussion around these principles by employing three lenses through which to view the development of self-regulation: (1) the lens of transitions and turning points, (2) the lens of mismatches, and (3) the lens of intervention integration. We include important individual, contextual, and sociocultural factors that influence the development of these skills over time since such information is critical for developing effective ways to help promote strong self-regulation in individuals.

3.1 Transitions and Turning Points in the Development of Self-Regulation

Because of the malleability in self-regulation evident throughout the life course, there are many transitions and turning points for the development of these skills. The early childhood years represent one important time in the life course because they constitute a sensitive period for the development of self-regulation and underlying executive function skills. This makes it especially important for children's early biological, cognitive, and social-emotional development (Diamond 2002; Carlson et al. 2013). As noted above, children's self-regulation undergoes rapid change during early childhood, which parallels brain development, especially of the prefrontal cortex (e.g., Diamond 2002). The translation of this development can be seen in turning points in development, one of which is the transition to formal schooling for young children.

3.1.1 The Transition to Schooling as a Turning Point for Self-Regulation

Several lines of research point to relations between schooling and self-regulation as a developmental turning point for children. Evidence points to bidirectional relations between the biological and cognitive factors predicting development of self-regulation as well as the influence of context such as the schooling environment (e.g., Diamond 2002; Carlson et al. 2013; Morrison et al. 2010). Although much research focuses on how individual factors influence self-regulation (e.g., temperament, neurodevelopment of the prefrontal cortex), research has also examined how contextual factors such as schooling may influence self-regulation. For example, researchers have suggested that differences in self-regulation across cultures may be due to early instructional environments (Morrison et al. 2010) as well as other factors such as temperamental variables (Hsu et al. 1981) or the prevalence of particular genes (Chang et al. 1996) that might contribute to observed advantages in self-regulation (Sabbagh et al. 2006).

Research looking at the transition to formal schooling has also used a natural experiment (designated "school cutoff") design, which examines children whose birth dates cluster closely on either side of the cutoff date for entering formal schooling (e.g., kindergarten in the United States). This method effectively equates the two groups of children on age (Morrison et al. 2010). Using this methodology, results from recent quasi-experimental and experimental investigations have provided further evidence for the importance of schooling in the development of self-regulation. For example, Burrage et al. (2008) examined the influence of experience in preschool on growth of word decoding, working memory, and inhibitory control. This quasi-experimental work suggests that schooling, and more specifically the years of prekindergarten and kindergarten, improves working memory for children who attend school compared with same-age peers who, because of arbitrary school cutoff dates, do not attend at the same time (Burrage et al. 2008). Together this research suggests that the early childhood years provide a sensitive period for the development of self-regulation, which is influenced by both individual and contextual factors.

3.1.2 Adolescence as a Turning Point for Self-Regulation

In adolescence, children experience another sensitive period of development, especially for self-regulation. Adolescence, the second decade of life, is a period of ontogeny characterized by extraordinary biological, social, and ecological changes (Lerner and Steinberg 2009). Cognitive and social development means that the capacities necessary for advanced, adult-like self-regulation may for the most part emerge in adolescence. This is in large part due to the gradual maturation of the prefrontal context. In particular, as the frontal lobe develops, so does higher-order, regulation-relevant cognition, such as metacognition and internalized control. In turn, these skills enable adolescents to make better interpretations, choices, and decisions about how to interact with their environment, especially in accordance with long-term goals (Brandstädter 2006; Larson 2011; Steinberg 2010). In addition, the formulation of an adaptive identity, which is a major developmental task of adolescence, allows for the construction of a personal future that informs long-term decision-making and goal pursuit (Brandtstädter 2006; McClelland et al. 2010). After all, it is impossible to formulate a plan to reach a long-term goal that has not yet been determined. Finally, during adolescence, young people may, for the first time, face decreased probabilities of achieving major life goals (e.g., graduating from high school) that have long-term consequences. This fact makes self-regulation particularly pertinent during the adolescent period (McClelland et al. 2010).

A growing body of research has confirmed the relation between adolescents' self-regulation skills and positive and problematic behaviors. In the last decade, a body of research has advanced our understanding of how adolescents regulate their own learning (Zimmerman 2002; Zimmerman and Schunk 2001). Self-regulated learning involves many goal-related skills, such as the ability to set proximal learning goals, use appropriate strategies for attaining the goal, self-evaluate the method one has chosen to achieve a goal, and monitor one's performance toward that goal. The use of self-regulated learning skills has repeatedly been related to school achievement (Miller and Byrnes 2001; Zimmerman and Schunk 2001). Similarly, the use of self-regulatory behaviors of youth is positively related to other positive outcomes, such as measures of social competence and mental well-being, and negatively related to indicators of problematic development, such as sexual risk behaviors, substance abuse, depression, and anxiety (e.g., Gestsdottir et al. 2009; Massey et al. 2008; Quinn and Fromme 2010). In addition, self-regulatory skills may have particular significance for youth living in high-risk environments. For instance, Buckner et al. (2009) found that youth from very low-income families fared better on a wide range of developmental outcomes, ranging from academic achievement to anxiety, if they had adaptive self-regulation skills. The authors emphasize that such skills help youth to cope with stressful life events, making them less likely to be overwhelmed by the difficulties that they are faced with, and as such, high levels of self-regulation are considered a key factor in supporting youth's resiliency (Buckner et al. 2009; Quinn and Fromme 2010). In spite of the growing evidence that self-regulation has important implications for healthy functioning in adolescence, as it does in childhood, there has been limited developmental research on how such important, adult-like processes develop in adolescence.

In sum, although the understanding about the nature and development of self-regulatory processes is not complete, recent research confirms the contribution of adaptive self-regulation to the healthy development of children and youth. Furthermore, some recent findings point to an emerging theme and match both the principles of LCHD and the RDS framework: complex, adult-like, self-regulatory processes appear to develop in middle adolescence and continue to grow through adolescence and early adulthood. In addition, the function of self-regulation in adolescence may differ in function from that of childhood and adulthood. As such, the structure and function of self-regulation may be specific to this age period and constitute a sensitive period in development.

3.2 Mismatches (and Matches) in the Development of Self-Regulation

In addition to research pointing to the importance of examining the transaction of how self-regulation develops across multiple levels of analysis, the match (or mismatch) between different aspects of development is also important. This can be seen in the notion of goodness of fit, taken from the child temperament literature, where an individual's characteristics and skills may not fit with those of the environment, such as the characteristics of caregivers. In the development of self-regulation, a child's individual characteristics and skills may be adversely influenced by the aspects of their environment, such as adverse childhood experiences, stress, poor parenting, maternal depression, and the influence of the media and technology use.

3.2.1 Adverse Childhood Experiences and Cumulative Risk

Recent research on adverse childhood experiences (ACEs) and toxic stress suggests that multiple and chronic environmental stressors can have significant and adverse effects on the development of a host of outcomes throughout the life span (Blair and Raver 2012; Shonkoff et al. 2012). For example, the early and chronic stress experienced by children living in poverty can have a profound influence on areas of the brain most involved in the development of self-regulation (the prefrontal cortex [PFC]; e.g., Blair 2010; Blair and Raver 2012). One study found that low-income children exhibited lower prefrontal functioning compared to higher-income children. Specifically, the PFC functioning of low-income children in the study was similar to the level of functioning of individuals with damage to the PFC (Kishiyama et al. 2009).

In addition to effects on the developing brain, ACEs are related to poorer executive function and self-regulation, increased substance use, obesity, and risk-taking behaviors in adolescents and adults (see Table 1). For example, one study found that children with cumulative risk exposure (e.g., poverty, family turmoil, substandard housing) gain more weight during the transition to adolescence than their more advantaged peers, an effect mediated by lower levels of self-regulation (Evans et al. 2012). Such pernicious effects were predicted by Walter Mischel and colleagues, whose hot/cool model of self-control specified that stressful life events would potentiate impulsive ("hot") system activity and attenuate slower, more reflective and voluntary ("cool") system activity (Metcalfe and Mischel 1999).

Research has also indicated that children from low-income families are more likely to experience family and housing instability, a lack of resources,

Table 1 Examples of direct and/or indirect relations between self-regulation and health-related outcomes

Predictor	Health-related outcomes
Self-regulation	Obesity
	Weight gain and loss
	Addiction and substance use
	Risk-taking behaviors
	Cardiovascular disease
	Asthma
	Autoimmune diseases
	Depression
	Liver cancer
	Academic achievement
	School readiness
	Educational attainment
	Economic well-being (savings behavior, financial security, occupational prestige)
	Lack of criminal convictions
	Health behaviors
	Physical activity
	Nutritious eating
	ADHD

and lower-quality learning environments in the home (e.g., Gershoff et al. 2007; Mistry et al. 2010; Obradovic 2010; Sektnan et al. 2010), all of which have been linked to lower levels of self-regulation. For example, children facing cumulative risk factors may experience significant difficulty with self-regulation in early childhood (Wanless et al. 2011).

Partly because of this, children with chronic environmental stressors are more likely to experience school failure, unemployment, poverty, violent crime, and incarceration as adults. Moreover, and perhaps most important for the long-term implications of ACEs, these children are less likely as adults to provide supportive environments for their own children, who in turn are at significant risk of demonstrating some of these same issues. In addition to behavioral and economic effects, chronic and toxic stresses have been linked to biological changes including premature aging and death, alterations in immune functioning, and significant increases in inflammatory markers. Related to this, ACEs have been associated with a host of physical health outcomes, including cardiovascular disease, liver cancer, asthma, autoimmune diseases, and depression (Committee on Psychosocial Aspects of Child and Family Health et al. 2012; Shonkoff et al. 2012).

Together, this research suggests that ACEs, toxic stress, and cumulative risk can significantly impair the development of self-regulation in children. This is also an example of a potential mismatch between children's own development and the context in which they live. For example, it is possible that children facing cumulative risk have parents who provide fewer opportunities to practice self-regulation (Fuller et al. 2010; Wachs et al. 2004). These children may also have higher levels of stress, which interfere with the development of prefrontal cortex, experience more family and housing instability, and have fewer learning and economic resources (Blair 2010; Blair and Raver 2012). Thus, there may be few opportunities for children to experience a positive match between their own developing skills and those of the environment in which they live.

3.2.2 Parenting and Caregiving

As the research above indicates, poor parenting can have significant and detrimental effects on their children's own self-regulation. For example, extensive research documents the negative effects that maternal depression can have on a range of child outcomes, including self-regulation (Center on the Developing Child 2011).

In contrast to the conflicted and non-supportive parent-child relationships that undermine children's ability to self-regulate, organized and predictable home environments and emotionally positive parent-child relationships provide a context that allows for the development of self-regulatory competencies (e.g., Bowers et al. 2011; Brody and Ge 2001; Grolnick et al. 2000; Lewin-Bizan et al. 2010; Moilanen et al. 2010). For example, parenting that includes a focus on supporting autonomy and setting limits has significantly predicted stronger self-regulation in children compared to parenting that is more controlling and focused on compliance (Bernier et al. 2010; Lengua et al. 2007). A similar line of work in early childhood classrooms has established the importance of orienting and organizing teacher behaviors for children's self-regulation, engagement, and academic outcomes (Cameron and Morrison, 2011; Cameron Ponitz et al. 2009). Taken together, this work indicates the importance of structured and predictable environments for helping children's emerging self-regulatory capacities. It also demonstrates the importance of matches between children's characteristics and parenting characteristics and behaviors, which complement the principles of the LCHD perspective.

3.2.3 Media and Technology Use

Another example of a possible mismatch is the increasing structure in school settings paired with the high prevalence of media and television use by children and adults. Children's media and technology use is rapidly increasing, but there remains little evidence on the positive effects of such media on children's development, especially for very young children (Radesky et al. 2014). Many studies have found persistent negative effects of extended television and media viewing on children's short- and long-term development (Robertson et al. 2013), including inattention and attention deficit hyperactivity disorder (ADHD)-related behaviors (Christakis et al. 2004; Nikkelen et al. 2014). These findings indicate that media use is related to poorer self-regulation and that households with heavy media use may be a poor context for supporting children's self-regulatory development. Thus, children's increased media use may run counter to the increased demands for self-regulated behavior in schools and society.

In addition to the issue of child media use is the high prevalence of media use by adults and parents. For example, parents who are distracted by texting and being on mobile devices may not be able to adequately respond to and parent their children. Although limited research exists, one study found that caregivers who used mobile devices at a restaurant while with their children were most often highly absorbed in the content and were less attentive to the children they were with. Those caregivers who were highly absorbed in their mobile devices were also more likely to respond harshly to child misbehavior (Radesky et al. 2014). Thus, an increased inattention and distraction on the part of parents and caregivers may provide children with fewer opportunities to learn how to self-regulate themselves. Moreover, it is possible that although children's self-regulation is needed to successfully navigate increasing structured school settings, children and parents are using media to a much greater extent than ever before, which could be detrimental to the development of these skills. This potential mismatch may have significant long-term implications and is an area ripe for additional research.

3.3 Integrating Levels of Influence in Self-Regulation Interventions

Another LCHD lens through which to view self-regulation processes is the importance of integration across multiple levels of influence, especially in the context of interventions. This integration includes lateral integration or integration across subject domains, vertical integration or integration across levels of analysis, and developmental integration or integration across time. Because of the evidence pointing to the malleability of self-regulation, there has been an explosion in recent years in interventions aiming to foster the development of these skills.

Accumulating evidence suggests that interventions targeting children's self-regulation at various levels can be effective at improving self-regulation and other outcomes. For example, at the sociocultural level, preschool curricula, such as Tools of the Mind, focus on social, emotional, and executive function skills in addition to literacy and math. Research suggests that program participation is related to significant improvement in children's self-regulation (Blair and Raver 2014; Diamond et al. 2007), social behavior (Barnett et al. 2008), academic outcomes (Blair and Raver 2014), and neuroendocrine function (e.g., levels of salivary cortisol and alpha amylase; Blair and Raver 2014).

Some work, however, has not found significant intervention effects (Farran et al. 2013), suggesting that more work is needed to fully understand the key components of intervention effectiveness.

Other interventions that include multiple levels of integration (e.g., at the parent, teacher, and child level) are the Promoting Alternative Thinking Strategies (PATHS) and the Head Start REDI (Research-based, Developmentally Informed) programs (Bierman et al. 2008a), which focus on social-emotional skills and self-regulation. Children receiving these interventions have demonstrated more socially competent behavior (Domitrovich et al. 2007) and significant improvements in self-regulation (Bierman et al. 2008b) compared to children in a control group. Another recent study examining a broad intervention targeting social-emotional learning and literacy development found that children in intervention schools demonstrated improvements in a variety of social behaviors and self-regulation skills (e.g., attention). Improvements were also found in children's early math and reading achievement for those initially most at risk for behavior problems (Jones et al. 2011).

Further evidence from a school-based intervention that included multiple levels of integration with teachers, mental health consultants, and children (Raver et al. 2011) reveals that preschool children participating in the Chicago School Readiness Project exhibited significantly higher performance on self-regulation tasks than did their peers in a control group. Moreover, there was a mediating role of children's EF on pre-academic literacy and math skills. These findings complement those of Connor and colleagues (2010) who also found that an instructional intervention—which emphasized teacher planning, organization, classroom management, and opportunities for students to work independently—was most beneficial for children who started first grade with weaker self-regulation. Similarly, a recent intervention focusing on aspects of self-regulation (attentional flexibility, working memory, and inhibitory control) integrated into classroom games found that participation in the intervention was significantly related to gains in self-regulation skills and academic achievement compared to children in the control group (Tominey and McClelland 2011; Schmitt et al. 2015).

For children with ADHD, research has also documented that interventions that focus on strengthening aspects of self-regulation and underlying executive function skills can be beneficial (Reid et al. 2005). Such interventions have been found to help children improve on task behavior, decrease inappropriate behavior, and increase academic achievement, although results have been somewhat weaker for lasting improvement in academic skills (DuPaul et al. 2011).

Overall, results from a growing number of randomized control trials suggest that interventions designed to strengthen self-regulation can improve children's self-regulation, social behavior, and academic achievement. It is not known, however, if these effects persist over time. More research is needed on the long-term effects of such interventions and how interventions may work for different subgroups of children (e.g., those most at risk). Moreover, following the principles of LCHD, interventions tend to be most effective when they include multiple levels of influence and are integrated across domains of functioning and over time (Jones and Bouffard 2012).

4 Self-Regulation and Health-Related Outcomes

Although self-regulation has been conceptualized differently in a variety of fields and at different developmental periods, accumulating evidence demonstrates the importance of self-regulation for a variety of outcomes. Moreover, our view of self-regulation reflects both the principles of LCHD and the RDS perspective. Below we review research on predictive relations between self-regulation and important outcomes such as academic achievement and educational attainment and health and well-being (see also Table 1).

4.1 Academic Achievement, Educational Attainment, and Economic Well-Being

Over a century ago, in a series of lectures for schoolteachers near his home institution of Harvard University, William James (1899) declared that much of schoolwork was necessarily "dull and unexciting" in comparison with other things children might be doing (pp. 104–105). Consequently, James reasoned that students who could voluntary control their attention enjoyed a distinct advantage over students who regularly succumbed to the "temptation to serve aside to other subjects" (p.112). Alfred Binet, Charles Spearman, and David Wechsler all made similar observations. That three of the most important figures in the history of intelligence testing would individually highlight the importance of "will" as a necessary complement to talent is somewhat ironic, given that intellectual aptitude, rather than self-regulation, was until very recently given disproportionate emphasis in the educational psychology literature.

Prospective longitudinal studies have confirmed James's earlier intuitions. For young children, a large body of evidence now demonstrates that self-regulation sets the stage for learning in children even prior to formal schooling. For example, self-regulation in preschool and during the transition to kindergarten has uniquely predicted gains in academic achievement after controlling for child IQ and initial achievement levels (von Suchodoletz et al. 2013; Blair and Razza 2007; McClelland et al. 2007). In elementary school, strong kindergarten learning-related skills (including self-regulation and social competence) significantly predicted higher reading and mathematics achievement between kindergarten and sixth grade and growth in literacy and mathematics from kindergarten to second grade after controlling for prior achievement levels, child IQ, and a host of background variables (McClelland et al. 2006; see also Duncan et al. 2007; McClelland et al. 2006; McClelland et al. 2007; McClelland et al. 2000). Studies have also documented the long-term contributions of self-regulation to practically significant outcomes such as high school graduation and college completion (McClelland et al. 2013; Moffitt et al. 2011). In one recent study, a 4-year-old child with one standard deviation higher ratings of attention (one aspect of self-regulation) than average had 49% greater odds of completing college by age 25 (McClelland et al. 2013).

In terms of economic well-being, the best evidence for the importance of self-regulation comes from a longitudinal study by Moffitt et al. (2011). Self-regulation was assessed using parent, teacher, observer, and self-report ratings at multiple time points in the first decade of life in a nationally representative sample of New Zealanders who were followed into adulthood. Childhood self-regulation predicted income, savings behavior, financial security, occupational prestige, lack of substance use, and lack of criminal convictions. These benefits were partially mediated by better decisions in adolescence, including staying in high school, not becoming a teenage parent, and not smoking. For a review of the relevance of self-regulation to academic achievement, including school readiness and lifetime educational attainment, see Duckworth and Allred (2012).

4.2 Health and Well-Being

Self-regulation has been shown to be related to a variety of health behaviors, including recovery from physical illness or disabilities (e.g., exercise during and after cardiac rehabilitation (Blanchard et al. 2002), functional activity of patients undergoing surgical replacement of the hip or knee (Orbell and Sheeran 2000), physical activity for individuals in orthopedic rehabilitation (e.g., Ziegelmann et al. 2006, 2007), disease prevention (e.g., attendance for cervical cancer screenings, Sheeran and Orbell 2000; performance of breast self-examinations, Orbell et al. 1997), and general health (e.g., regulation of body weight via dieting and exercising/sport activities, Bagozzi and Edwards 1998; and increased consumption of nutritious foods and other dietary behaviors [Anderson et al. 2001; Calfas et al. 2002; Jackson et al. 2005]). Many of these studies are framed by Gollwitzer's model of action phases (Gollwitzer 1990, 1996).

As an action theory, Gollwitzer's model of action phases focuses on the factors that determine how effective one is during the process of setting a goal to actual goal attainment. A key construct distinction within this model—and ultimately in predicting one's success in behavior change or goal attainment—is between goal intentions and implementation intentions. A goal intention indicates a desired behavior or outcome and is a declaration of one's commitment to a goal. Implementation intentions, on the other hand, specify the "when, where, and how of responses leading to goal attainment…and thus link anticipated opportunities with goal-directed responses" (Gollwitzer 1999, p. 494). As a goal intention states an individual's commitment to a specific goal, the implementation intention states the individual's commitment to certain actions in an effort to attain that particular goal. Gollwitzer's model also highlights the contention that self-regulated actions fall along an intentional-automatic continuum; forming implementation intentions allows people to "strategically switch from conscious and effortful control of their goal-directed behaviors to being automatically controlled by selected situational cues" (Gollwitzer 1999, p. 495). In turn, implementation intentions promote goal attainment by helping to initiate action, above and beyond the effects of goal intentions alone.

Studies applying Gollwitzer's model to health behavior have indicated that it is not only important for participants to have goal intentions, but it is also imperative for them to form implementation intentions and make subsequent planning strategies to work toward their goals. These strategies allow individuals to pinpoint when, where, and how they will enact specific goal-related behaviors. For example, Luszczynska (2006) examined how well patients who suffered a myocardial infarction utilized physical activity planning strategy and performed moderate physical activity after engaging in an implementation intention intervention program. The results indicated that as compared to controls, patients who participated in the implementation intention intervention more frequently used their planning strategies and maintained the same levels of physical activity at 8 months after their infarction as they did at 2 weeks after rehabilitation. Furthermore, implementation intentions (as compared to goal intentions) may be more predictive of health behaviors at later time points (Orbell and Sheeran 2000; Ziegelmann et al. 2007). When participants were asked to perform breast self-examinations, those who made such planning strategies were more likely to perform the behavior in the manner in which they originally specified (i.e., time and place) and were less likely to report forgetting to perform the behavior (e.g., Orbell et al. 1997). Likewise, the formation of such plans for breast self-examinations or to attend cervical cancer screenings can lead to earlier enactment of goal intentions even among a sample of highly motivated individuals (Orbell and Sheeran 2000; Sheeran and Orbell 2000) and influence motivation and adherence (Levack et al. 2006).

Another work examining the role of intentional self-regulation in health-related behaviors also focuses on specific self-regulatory cognitions and behaviors. Many studies have highlighted the importance of developing action and coping plans for successful adoption and maintenance of healthy behaviors such as physical activity and nutritious eating (e.g., Calfas et al. 2002; Sniehotta et al. 2005; Zeigelmann and Lippke 2007). Behavioral interventions aimed at initiating or increasing certain health behaviors—or aiding participants in reaching certain health goals—were often more effective when they included the creation of "action plans" (e.g., Calfas et al. 2002). The development of these plans often included having the participant explicitly identify the goals to pursue and sources for social support or resources to be utilized for achieving those goals. In some cases, the action plans also included identifying possible obstacles or barriers that might interfere with the implementation of their plans and solutions to overcome them (e.g., Calfas et al. 2002), but separate "coping plans" were also used for that purpose. For example, in a sample of 352 cardiac patients undergoing rehabilitation, Sniehotta et al. (2005)

provided evidence that action planning and coping planning can be identified as distinct strategies; in addition, the combination of forming both action plans and coping plans was more effective in increasing health behaviors over time than forming action plans alone. The additive benefit of action and coping plans was replicated in experimental designs (Sniehotta et al. 2006; Sniehotta et al. 2005; Scholz et al. 2007).

A large body of research also points to the importance of self-regulation for weight gain and loss (e.g., Evans et al. 2012; Francis and Susman 2009; Hofmann et al. 2014), addiction (Baumeister and Vonasch 2014), and other health-related outcomes (Moffitt et al. 2011). Several recent studies have demonstrated that poor self-regulation predicts unhealthy weight gain, particularly in adolescence, a period marked by pubertal changes that influence adiposity and greater latitude to make diet and exercise choices independent of parental control (Duckworth et al. 2010a; Tsukayama et al. 2010). In one study, children exposed to a number of risk factors were significantly more likely to gain weight during adolescence, which was mediated by having significantly lower levels of self-regulation (Evans et al. 2012). Adiposity, in turn, is a robust predictor of physical vitality later in life, suggesting one causal pathway linking childhood self-regulation to adult physical health and, ultimately, mortality.

Issues with self-regulation have also been implicated in ADHD, with ADHD often characterized as a disorder of self-regulation and underlying executive function components (Barkley 1997, 2011). For example, many individuals with ADHD exhibit significant difficulties with the core executive function components of self-regulation, including attentional or cognitive flexibility, working memory, and inhibitory control. This can be seen in individuals who are inattentive, who lack behavioral inhibition, and who have difficulty with planning, organizing, and being goal-oriented. These issues can also lead to difficulty with emotion regulation. Thus, individuals with ADHD are more likely to have problems with impulse control, be more reactive, and have diminished social perspective taking abilities (Barkley 2011; Berwid et al. 2005). This means that children with ADHD may have a harder time stopping and thinking about a situation before reacting and illustrates why these children are more at risk for peer rejection and other behavior problems (Molina et al. 2009). Children with ADHD also demonstrate significant problems with academic achievement, which can also be linked back to difficulties with behavioral and emotional aspects of self-regulation (DuPaul and Kern 2011).

5 Methods for Studying Self-Regulation

As demonstrated by how self-regulation relates to the principles of LCHD and RDS, self-regulation shows important transitions and sensitive periods, multiple levels of influence, and person-context fit in the form of matches or mismatches that can affect health development. Our understanding of these issues, however, hinges on how self-regulation is measured and analyzed in health-related research. In this section, we examine recent research on ways to measure and analyze self-regulation.

5.1 Measuring Self-Regulation

Self-regulation is generally treated as a slowly developing phenomenon, meaning studies that target the development of self-regulation can easily take advantage of the large sample, small time point analyses that dominate research in health-related fields. Self-regulation research can accordingly draw on the strengths of modern statistical methods such as latent variable structural equation modeling, multilevel modeling, and mixture modeling. In this vein, researchers readily acknowledge that one size rarely fits all people. Advances in mixture modeling have allowed us to appropriately model theories that stem from the person-centered movement and systems theories. Large sample research can be facilitated by utilizing advances in modern missing data procedures to incorporate planned missing data collection designs. Such designs allow researchers to collect all the data needed to utilize modern analytic methods without burdening parents, teachers, or individuals with excessively long surveys.

It is also important to note, however, that challenges exist with some of these methods because self-regulation measures change over the developmental years and are often not strongly related with each other. Thus, developing self-regulation measures that are reliable and valid over a broad age range and at important points of transition is of particular importance. Some progress, however, has been made on this front. For example, the National Institutes of Health (NIH) Toolbox has developed brief assessments for a variety of skills, including aspects of self-regulation, which are appropriate to use with individuals throughout the life span (Zelazo et al. 2013).

In addition to measures that span a large age range, other measures capture a broad set of children's developmental skills, especially at school entry. Some research has focused on population-based measures that are based on teacher or caregiver ratings. One example is the Early Developmental Instrument (EDI; Janus and Offord 2007), which measures five developmental domains: social, emotional, physical, cognitive, and communicative. Although not specifically focused on measuring self-regulation, the measure includes items tapping aspects of self-regulation mostly in the social and emotional domains. The measure has been shown to be reliable and valid and significantly related to broad measures of school readiness, although less strongly related to direct assessments of children's skills (Hymel et al. 2011). A strength of this type of measure is the potential to capture a range of children's skills. A weakness, however, is that there may be considerable construct overlap and variability in how teachers rate children.

An example of a more targeted measure is the Head-Toes-Knees-Shoulders (HTKS) task (McClelland et al. 2014), which specifically measures behavioral aspects of self-regulation. The HTKS taps children's ability to pay attention, use working memory, and demonstrate inhibitory control by doing the opposite of what was asked. The task is most appropriate for young children during the transition to formal schooling, which is important because this time is a crucial period for the development of self-regulation. A number of studies have shown that the HTKS is reliable and valid and significantly predicts academic achievement in diverse groups of children in the US, Asian, and European countries (McClelland et al. 2007, 2014; von Suchodoletz et al. 2013; Wanless et al. 2011).

In youth and adults, self-regulation is often measured either using self-report, parent-report, or teacher-report questionnaires, delay of gratification tasks, or, ideally, a multi-method battery of measures. Such measures predict report card grades and changes in report card grades over time (Duckworth and Seligman 2005), but the predictive validity of self-regulation for standardized achievement test scores, in contrast, is less dramatic (Duckworth et al. 2012). One reason that report card grades are differentially sensitive to self-regulation may be their relatively greater emphasis on effort on the part of the student, to complete homework assignments on time and with care, to come to class prepared and pay attention when present, and to study for quizzes and tests from provided materials. Notably, report card grades predict persistence through college better than standardized test scores, a testament to the continued importance of self-regulation as students move through the formal education system (Bowen et al. 2009).

5.1.1 Construct Diversity

The major limitation to measure self-regulation stems from the fact that self-regulation is not a single globally measurable construct. Instead, self-regulation represents an individual's agentic attempts to reach distal outcomes by influencing what Lerner (e.g., Gestsdottir and Lerner 2008) has called person-context relations. The extant diversity of theories and measures of self-regulation suggest that the apparently unitary domain of self-regulation actually consists of many oblique fragments that differentially influence behavior as a function of context. We therefore need refinements in the measures of and theories about context-specific self-regulation. Here, better measurement of the parts will better inform the whole.

5.1.2 Complementing Nomothetic Analyses with Idiographic Analyses

In addition, if we truly see self-regulation as part of an ongoing process that is unique to each individual, we must begin to complement our existing analyses with more idiographic examinations of self-regulation over a variety of time spans (e.g., moments, days). Idiographic analyses such as dynamic factor analysis and p-technique have a place in research, and it is important that self-regulation researchers begin to acknowledge this role. We currently have a poor understanding of self-regulation as an idiographic phenomenon. A better understanding of intraindividual differences will allow greater insight into interindividual phenomena related to self-regulation as well as its intraindividual development.

6 Issues for Future Research

The previous sections demonstrate that, across a broad spectrum of disciplines, interest has steadily mounted in self-regulation and related constructs—executive function (EF), self-control, and effortful control. A growing body of research has shown the importance of self-regulation for children's success in school, as well as for subsequent health, wealth, and criminality (e.g., Moffitt et al. 2011). In addition, the study of self-regulation can be informed by a closer appreciation of the principles of LCHD and RDS, including how turning points and transitions, mismatches, and intervention integration influence self-regulation trajectories. Despite advances in many areas, our understanding of aspects of self-regulation, including the neurological underpinnings of these skills, and efforts to intervene in the development of self-regulation for children at risk remains limited. In this section, we suggest key issues and next steps for self-regulation research.

6.1 Integration in Conceptualizing and Measuring Self-Regulation

When studied from multiple perspectives and fields, differences in how self-regulation is defined and conceptualized arise in part because its study stems from diverse research traditions that use distinct methods to examine phenomena across the life course. For example, research has burgeoned in basic investigations of self-regulation, including understanding the underlying neurological and behavioral mechanisms driving these skills in children, adolescents, and adults (Blair and Raver 2012). It is also the case that the particular domain of inquiry informs where and how phenomena and individuals are studied. Scholars sometimes refer to different levels of analysis (e.g., neurological activation, physiological responses, observed behavior, or self-report) to clarify some of these differences. More could be done, however, to provide better integration across different disciplines and contexts to study the development and measurement of these skills. For example, although the knowledge base of research on different aspects of self-regulation is deep, it lacks breadth, and most of the work in this area has been conducted in convenience samples of middle-SES North Americans. More research is needed on how self-regulation develops within different groups and populations especially as it relates to the principles of LCHD.

Another critical issue is the need to move away from deficit models of self-regulation (e.g., attribution of undesirable outcomes to having "poor" self-regulation) and instead take a strength-based perspective. Each individual carries a unique set of self-regulatory strengths. By understanding how to maximize these strengths and the fit between these strengths and an individual's contextual resources, the continued study of self-regulation will help researchers promote thriving and positive outcomes across the life course.

6.2 Examining Developmental Changes in Self-Regulation Over Time

In addition to issues with conceptualization, it is also not clear if constructs, as operationalized across disciplines, are all measuring the same underlying skills. In addition, longitudinal measurement of the developmental course (both behavioral and neurological) of the underlying components of self-regulation over different transitions and turning points is lacking at present. Although a number of recent investigations provide insight into the structure of self-regulation in young children (i.e., unitary vs. componential), very little of this work has involved repeated assessments over time. As a result, we know a great deal about the performance of children before and early in preschool (e.g., Carlson 2005) but much less about self-regulation as children move through formal schooling. It is also important to examine whether and how these changing abilities relate to behavior in real-world contexts. Indeed, it could be the case that children who come into school with stronger self-regulation skills—as assessed from using tasks derived from cognitive neuroscience—also exhibit stronger self-regulation on classroom-based measures (Rimm-Kaufman et al. 2009). It is also possible that the relations between these sets of skills are more limited than anticipated and that these different types of tasks tap into different abilities altogether. Finally, the malleability of self-regulation—and its components, such as working memory, inhibitory control, and attention control, and particularly the impact of different intervention efforts on these abilities—has not been extensively charted. We turn to this next.

6.3 Improving Intervention Efforts

As the research reviewed suggests, there has been a sharp increase in the number of applied investigations targeting self-regulation, including a plethora of new programs for young children (Bierman et al. 2008a; Diamond and Lee 2011; Jones et al. 2011; Raver et al. 2011; Schmitt et al. 2015; Tominey and McClelland 2011). Along with these changes, there has been an increase in interdisciplinary collaborations. These collaborations have led to new developments in measurements, analyses, and interventions related to understanding and promoting self-regulation skills early in the life course as a way to optimize development and prevent future difficulties. Moreover, researchers have started to examine the complex and dynamic relations among self-regulation and important variables that together influence individual health and well-being across the life course (McClelland et al. 2010).

Although research has documented the stability of self-regulation trajectories over time, the malleability of these skills is also evident. Thus, although more research is needed to examine the key components of effective interventions to promote self-regulation and the long-term effects of such interventions, a few recommendations can be made. First, in accordance with the principles of LCHD, self-regulation interventions are likely most effective when administered to individuals at turning points or sensitive periods of development, such as the early childhood years (Blair and Raver 2012). In addition, interventions are most effective when they integrate multiple levels of influence across different contexts (e.g., Jones and Bouffard 2012) and involve repeated practice of skills that are relevant to behavior in everyday settings and which increase in complexity over time (e.g., Diamond and Lee 2011). There is also support for interventions to be most effective for groups of children who are at the most risk, such as those living in poverty and/or experiencing toxic stress and ACEs (Blair and Raver 2014; Schmitt et al. 2015). Finally, recent work has examined the impact of additional intervention components, such as mindfulness practices and yoga, on children's self-regulation, with some encouraging results (Diamond and Lee 2011; Zelazo and Lyons 2012).

It is also clear that more needs to be done to translate research and interventions into practice. From a public health perspective, clinicians and pediatricians need better tools for assessing children's self-regulation especially in the early childhood years. Based on the importance of developing strong self-regulation, it seems plausible that well-child visits include screening of self-regulation starting when children are 3 years of age. There are some measures available that assess aspects of self-regulation such as the EDI (Janus and Offord 2007), but more work is needed in this area. In the research realm, some progress has been made in developing ecologically valid and sensitive measures of self-regulation and in recognizing the roles of context in the development of these skills (e.g., McClelland and Cameron 2012). As noted above, however, it is unclear if self-regulation measured in one context relates to self-regulation in another context and how these relations change over time.

Finally, it is critical that the results of basic and applied research get translated into policy. Some efforts are ongoing to bridge the science of self-regulation and child development with policy and between a diverse number of fields (see, e.g., Halfon 2012; Halfon and Inkelas 2003; Shonkoff 2011; Shonkoff and Bales 2011; Shonkoff et al. 2012). Thus, there is great momentum in this arena. Although more work remains, there is an increasing energy around translating the importance of self-regulation for important health and developmental outcomes into policy and practice. Framing our understanding of self-regulation within the principles of LCHD and the RDS perspective is a promising way to improve research and translational efforts and promote healthy development across the life span.

References

Anderson, E. S., Winett, R. A., Wojcik, J. R., Winett, S. G., & Bowden, T. (2001). A computerized social cognitive intervention for nutrition behavior: Direct and mediated effects on fat, fiber, fruits, and vegetables, self-efficacy, and outcome expectations among food shoppers. *Annals of Behavioral Medicine, 23*(2), 88–100.

Backen Jones, L., Rothbart, M. K., & Posner, M. I. (2003). Development of executive attention in preschool children. *Developmental Science, 6*(5), 498–504.

Bagozzi, R. P., & Edwards, E. A. (1998). Goal setting and goal pursuit in the regulation of body weight. *Psychology and Health, 13*(4), 593–621.

Baker, C. E., Cameron, C. E., Rimm-Kaufman, S. E., & Grissmer, D. W. (2012). Family and sociodemographic predictors of school readiness among African American boys in kindergarten. *Early Education and Development, 23*, 833–854.

Bandura, A. (1969). *Principles of behavior modification*. New York, NY: Holt, Rinehart & Winston.

Bargh, J. A., Gollwitzer, P. M., Lee-Chai, A., Barndollar, K., & Trötschel, R. (2001). The automated will: Nonconscious activation and pursuit of behavioral goals. *Journal of Personality and Social Psychology, 81*(6), 1014–1027.

Barkley, R. A. (1997). Behavioral inhibition, sustained attention, and executive functions: Constructing a unifying theory of ADHD. *Psychological Bulletin, 121*, 65–94.

Barkley, R. A. (2011). Attention-deficit/hyperactivity disorder, self-regulation, and executive functioning. In K. D. V. R. F. Baumeister (Ed.), *Handbook of self-regulation: Research, theory, and applications* (2nd ed., pp. 551–563). New York, NY: Guilford Press.

Barnett, W. S., Jung, K., Yarosz, D. J., Thomas, J., Hornbeck, A., Stechuk, R., & Burns, S. (2008). Educational effects of the tools of the mind curriculum: A randomized trial. *Early Childhood Research Quarterly, 23*(3), 299–313. doi:10.1016/j.ecresq.2008.03.001.

Baumeister, R. F., & Vonasch, A. J. (2014). Uses of self-regulation to facilitate and restrain addictive behavior. *Addictive Behaviors, 44*, 3–8. doi:10.1016/j.addbeh.2014.09.011.

Bernier, A., Carlson, S. M., & Whipple, N. (2010). From external regulation to self-regulation: Early parenting precursors of young children's executive functioning. *Child Development, 81*(1), 326–339. doi:10.1111/j.1467-8624.2009.01397.x.

Berwid, O. G., Curko Kera, E. A., Marks, D. J., Santra, A., Bender, H. A., & Halperin, J. M. (2005). Sustained attention and response inhibition in young children at risk for attention deficit/hyperactivity disorder. *Journal of Child Psychology & Psychiatry, 46*(11), 1219–1229.

Bierman, K. L., Domitrovich, C. E., Nix, R. L., Gest, S. D., Welsh, J. A., Greenberg, M. T., Blair, C., Nelson, K. E., & Gill, S. (2008a). Promoting academic and social-emotional school readiness: The Head Start REDI program. *Child Development, 79*(6), 1802–1817.

Bierman, K. L., Nix, R. L., Greenberg, M. T., Blair, C., & Domitrovich, C. E. (2008b). Executive functions and school readiness intervention: Impact, moderation, and mediation in the Head Start REDI program. *Development and Psychopathology, 20*(03), 821–843. doi:10.1017/S0954579408000394.

Blair, C. (2010). Stress and the development of self-regulation in context. *Child Development Perspectives, 4*(3), 181–188. doi:10.1111/j.1750-8606.2010.00145.x.

Blair, C., & Raver, C. C. (2012). Child development in the context of adversity: Experiential canalization of brain and behavior. *American Psychologist, 67*(4), 309–318. doi:10.1037/a0027493.

Blair, C., & Raver, C. C. (2014). Closing the achievement gap through modification of neurocognitive and neuroendocrine function: Results from a cluster randomized controlled trial of an innovative approach to the education of children in kindergarten. *PLoS One, 9*(11), e112393. doi:10.1371/journal.pone.0112393.

Blair, C., & Razza, R. P. (2007). Relating effortful control, executive function, and false belief understanding to emerging math and literacy ability in kindergarten. *Child Development, 78*(2), 647–663. doi:10.1111/j.1467-8624.2007.01019.x.

Blanchard, C. M., Courneya, K. S., Rodgers, W. M., Daub, B., & Knapik, G. (2002). Determinants of exercise intention and behavior during and after phase 2 cardiac rehabilitation: An application of the theory of planned behavior. *Rehabilitation Psychology, 47*(3), 308–323.

Bowen, W. G., Chingos, M. M., & McPherson, M. S. (2009). *Test scores and high school grades as predictors. Crossing the finish line: Completing college at America's public universities* (pp. 112–133). Princeton, NJ: Princeton University Press.

Bowers, E. P., Gestsdottir, S., Geldhof, G., Nikitin, J., von Eye, A., & Lerner, R. M. (2011). Developmental trajectories of intentional self-regulation in adolescence: The role of parenting and implications for positive and problematic outcomes among diverse youth. *Journal of Adolescence, 34*(6), 1193–1206.

Brandstädter, J. (2006). Action perspectives on human development. In W. Damon (Series Ed.), & R. Lerner (Vol. Ed.), *Handbook of child psychology* (Theoretical models of human development). (Vol. 1, pp. 516–568). Hoboken, NJ: Wiley.

Bridges, L. J., Denham, S. A., & Ganiban, J. M. (2004). Definitional issues in emotion regulation research. *Child Development, 75*(2), 340–345.

Brody, G. H., & Ge, X. (2001). Linking parenting processes and self-regulation to psychological functioning and alcohol use during early adolescence. *Journal of Family Psychology, 15*(1), 82–94. doi:10.1037/0893-3200.15.1.82.

Buckner, J. C., Mezzacappa, E., & Beardslee, W. R. (2009). Self-regulation and its relations to adaptive functioning in low income youths. *American Journal of Orthopsychiatry, 79*(1), 19–30. doi:10.1037/a0014796.

Burrage, M. J., Ponitz, C. C., McCready, E. A., Shah, P., Sims, B. C., Jewkes, A. M., & Morrison, F. J. (2008). Age- and schooling-related effects on executive functions in young children: A natural experiment. *Child Neuropsychology, 14*(6), 510–524. doi:10.1080/09297040701756917.

Calfas, K. J., Sallis, J. F., Zabinski, M. F., Wilfley, D. E., Rupp, J., Prochaska, J. J., et al. (2002). Preliminary evaluation of a multicomponent program for nutrition and physical activity change in primary care: PACE for adults. *Preventive Medicine, 34*, 153–161.

Cameron, C. E., & Morrison, F. J. (2011). Teacher activity orienting predicts preschoolers' academic and self-regulatory skills. *Early Education & Development, 22*(4), 620–648.

Cameron Ponitz, C. E., Rimm-Kaufman, S. E., Grimm, K. J., & Curby, T. W. (2009). Kindergarten classroom quality, behavioral engagement, and reading achievement. *School Psychology Review, 38*(1), 102–120.

Carlson, S. M. (2005). Developmentally sensitive measures of executive function in preschool children. *Developmental Neuropsychology, 28*(2), 595–616. doi:10.1207/s15326942dn2802_3.

Carlson, S. M., Zelazo, P. D., & Faja, S. (2013). Executive function. In P. D. Zelazo (Ed.), *The Oxford handbook of developmental psychology, Body and mind* (Vol. 1, pp. 706–743). New York, NY: Oxford University Press.

Center on the Developing Child. (2011). Building the brain's "Air Traffic Control" system: How early experiences shape the development of executive function. (Working Paper No. 11). Retrieved from http://www.developingchild.harvard.edu.

Chang, F., Kidd, J. R., Livak, K. J., Pakstis, A. J., & Kidd, K. K. (1996). The world-wide distribution of allele frequencies at the human dopamine D4 receptor locus. *Human Genetics, 98*(1), 91–101. doi:10.1007/s004390050166.

Christakis, D. A., Zimmerman, F. J., DiGiuseppe, D. L., & McCarty, C. A. (2004). Early television exposure and subsequent attentional problems in children. *Pediatrics, 113*(4), 708–713.

Colombo, J. (2001). The development of visual attention in infancy. *Annual Review of Psychology, 52*, 337–367.

Committee on Psychosocial Aspects of Child and Family Health, Committee on Early Childhood, Adoption, Dependent Care, Section on Developmental Behavioral Pediatrics, Garner, A. S., Shonkoff, J. P., Siegel, B. S., et al. (2012). Early childhood adversity, toxic stress, and the role of the pediatrician: Translating developmental science into lifelong health. *Pediatrics, 129*(1), e224–e231. doi:10.1542/peds.2011-2662.

Connor, C., Ponitz, C., Phillips, B. M., Travis, Q., Glasney, S., & Morrison, F. J. (2010). First graders' literacy and self-regulation gains: The effect of individualizing student instruction. *Journal of School Psychology, 48*(5), 433–455.

Diamond, A. (2002). Normal development of prefrontal cortex from birth to young adulthood: Cognitive functions, anatomy, and biochemistry. In D. T. Stuss & R. T. Knight (Eds.), *Principles of frontal lobe function* (pp. 466–503). London, England: Oxford University Press.

Diamond, A., Barnett, W. S., Thomas, J., & Munro, S. (2007). Preschool program improves cognitive control. *Science, 318*, 1387–1388. doi:10.1126/science.1151148.

Diamond, A., & Lee, K. (2011). Interventions shown to aid executive function development in children 4 to 12 years old. *Science, 333*, 959–964. doi:10.1126/science.1204529.

Domitrovich, C. E., Cortes, R. C., & Greenberg, M. T. (2007). Improving young children's social and emotional competence: A randomized trial of the preschool 'PATHS' curriculum. *Journal of Primary Prevention, 28*(2), 67–91.

Duckworth, A. L., & Allred, K. M. (2012). Temperament in the classroom. In R. L. Shiner & M. Zentner (Eds.), *Handbook of temperament* (pp. 627–644). New York, NY: Guilford Press.

Duckworth, A. L., & Seligman, M. E. P. (2005). Self-discipline outdoes IQ in predicting academic performance of adolescents. *Psychological Science, 16*(12), 939–944.

Duckworth, A. L., Tsukayama, E., & Geier, A. B. (2010a). Self-controlled children stay leaner in the transition to adolescence. *Appetite, 54*(2), 304–308.

Duckworth, A. L., Tsukayama, E., & May, H. (2010b). Establishing causality using longitudinal hierarchical linear modeling: An illustration predicting achievement from self-control. *Social Psychology and Personality Science, 1*(4), 311–317. doi:10.1177/1948550609359707.

Duckworth, A. L., Quinn, P. D., & Tsukayama, E. (2012). What no child left behind leaves behind: A comparison of standardized achievement test score and report card grades. *Journal of Educational Psychology, 104*(2), 439–451. doi:10.1037/a0026280.

Duncan, G. J., Dowsett, C. J., Claessens, A., Magnuson, K., Huston, A. C., Klebanov, P., et al. (2007). School readiness and later achievement. *Developmental. Psychology, 43*(6), 1428–1446. doi:10.1037/0012-1649.43.6.1428.

DuPaul, G. J., & Kern, L. (2011). *Promotion of academic skills Young children with ADHD: Early identification and intervention (pp. 107–125)*. Washington, DC: American Psychological Association.

DuPaul, G. J., Kern, L., Gormley, M. J., & Volpe, R. J. (2011). Early intervention for young children with ADHD: Academic outcomes for responders to behavioral treatment. *School Mental Health, 3*(3), 117–126. doi:10.1007/s12310-011-9053-x.

Eisenberg, N., Smith, C. L., Sadovsky, A., & Spinrad, T. L. (2004). Effortful control: Relations with emotion regulation, adjustment, and socialization in childhood. In R. F. Baumeister & K. D. Vohs (Eds.), *Handbook of self-regulation: Research, theory, and applications* (pp. 259–282). New York, NY: Guilford.

Eisenberg, N., Duckworth, A. L., Spinrad, T. L., & Valiente, C. (2014). Conscientiousness: Origins in childhood? *Developmental Psychology, 50*(5), 1331–1349. http://dx.doi.org/10.1037/a0030977.

Evans, G. W., Fuller-Rowell, T. E., & Doan, S. N. (2012). Childhood cumulative risk and obesity: The mediating role of self-regulatory ability. *Pediatrics, 129*(1), e68–e73. doi:10.1542/peds.2010-3647.

Farran, D., Wilson, S. J., & Lipsey, M. (2013). *Effects of a curricular attempt to improve self- regulation and achievement in prekindergarten children.* Paper presented at the biennial meeting for the Society for Research in Child Development in Seattle, WA.

Fortsmeier, S., Drobetz, R., & Maercker, A. (2011). The delay of gratification test for adults: Validating a behavioral measure of self-motivation in a sample of older people. *Motivation and Emotion, 35*(2), 118–134.

Francis, L. A., & Susman, E. J. (2009). Self-regulation and rapid weight gain in children from age 3 to 12 years. *Archives of Pediatrics & Adolescent Medicine, 163*(4), 297–302. doi:10.1001/archpediatrics.2008.579.

Fuller, B., Bein, E., Bridges, M., Halfon, N., Jung, S., Rabe-Hesketh, S., et al. (2010). Maternal practices that influence Hispanic infants' health and cognitive growth. *Pediatrics, 125*(2), e324–e332. doi:10.1542/peds.2009-0496.

Garstein, M. R., & Rothbart, M. K. (2003). Studying infant temperament via the revised infant behavior questionnaire. *Infant Behavior and Development, 26*(1), 64–86.

Gathercole, S. E., Pickering, S. J., Ambridge, B., & Wearing, H. (2004). The structure of working memory from 4 to 15 years of age. *Developmental Psychology, 40*(2), 177–190. doi:10.1037/0012-1649.40.2.177.

Geldhof, G. J., Little, T. D., & Colombo, J. (2010). Self-regulation across the life span. In *The handbook of life-span development, Social and emotional development* (Vol. 2, pp. 116–157). Hoboken, NJ: Wiley.

Gershoff, E. T., Aber, J. L., Raver, C. C., & Lennon, M. C. (2007). Income is not enough: Incorporating maternal hardship into models of income associations with parenting and child development. *Child Development, 78*(1), 70–95.

Gestsdottir, S., & Lerner, R. M. (2008). Positive development in adolescence: The development and role of intentional self-regulation. *Human Development, 51*, 202–224.

Gestsdottir, S., Lewin-Bizan, S., von Eye, A., Lerner, J. V., & Lerner, R. M. (2009). The structure and function of selection, optimization, and compensation in adolescence: Theoretical and applied implications. *Journal of Applied Developmental Psychology, 30*(5), 585–600.

Gollwitzer, P. M. (1990). Action phases and mind-sets. In E. T. Higgins & R. M. Sorrentino (Eds.), *Handbook of motivation and cognition: Foundations of social behavior* (Vol. 2, pp. 53–92). New York, NY: Guilford Press.

Gollwitzer, P. M. (1996). The volitional benefits of planning. In P. M. Gollwitzer & J. A. Bargh (Eds.), *The psychology of action* (pp. 287–312). New York, NY: Guilford.

Gollwitzer, P. M. (1999). Implementation intentions: Strong effects of simple plans. *American Psychologist, 54*(7), 493–503.

Grolnick, W. S., Kurowski, C. O., Dunlap, K. G., & Hevey, C. (2000). Parental resources and the transition to junior high. *Journal of Research on Adolescence, 10*(4), 465–488. doi:10.1207/SJRA1004_05.

Halfon, N. (2012). Addressing health inequalities in the US: A life course health development approach. *Social Science & Medicine, 74*(5), 671–673. doi:10.1016/j.socscimed.2011.12.016.

Halfon, N., & Forrest, C. B. (2017). The emerging theoretical framework of life course health development. In N. Halfon, C. B. Forrest, R. M. Lerner, & E. Faustman (Eds.), *Handbook of life course health-development science*. Cham: Springer.

Halfon, N., & Inkelas, M. (2003). Optimizing the health and development of children. *JAMA: The Journal of the American Medical Association, 290*(23), 3136–3138. doi:10.1001/jama.290.23.3136.

Hofmann, W., Adriaanse, M., Vohs, K. D., & Baumeister, R. F. (2014). Dieting and the self-control of eating in everyday environments: An experience sampling study. *British Journal of Health Psychology, 19*(3), 523–539. doi:10.1111/bjhp.12053.

Hooper, C. J., Luciana, M., Conklin, H. M., & Yarger, R. S. (2004). Adolescents' performance on the Iowa gambling task: Implications for the development of decision making and ventromedial prefrontal cortex. *Developmental Psychology, 40*(6), 1148–1158.

Hsu, C., Soong, W., Stigler, J. W., Hong, C., & Liange, C. (1981). The temperamental characteristics of Chinese babies. *Child Development, 52*(4), 1337–1340. doi:10.2307/1129528.

Hymel, S., LeMare, L., & McKee, W. (2011). The early development Instrument: An examination of convergent and discriminant validity. *Social Indicators Research, 103*(2), 267–282. doi:10.1007/s11205-011-9845-2.

Jackson, C., Lawton, R., Knapp, P., Raynor, D. K., Conner, M., Lowe, C., & Closs, S. J. (2005). Beyond intention: Do specific plans increase health behaviours in patients in primary care? A study of fruit and vegetable consumption. *Social Science & Medicine, 60*(10), 2383–2391.

James, W. (1890). *The principles of psychology*. New York, NY: Henry Holt and Company.

James, W. (1899). *Talks to teachers on psychology and to students on some of life's ideals*. New York, NY: Holt and Company.

Janus, M., & Offord, D. R. (2007). Development and psychometric properties of the early development Instrument (EDI): A measure of children's school readiness. *Canadian Journal of Behavioural Science/Revue canadienne des sciences du comportement, 39*(1), 1–22. doi:10.1037/cjbs2007001.

Jones, S. M., & Bouffard, S. M. (2012). Social and emotional learning in schools: From programs to strategies. *Society for Research in Child Development Social Policy Report, 26*, 1–33. http://files.eric.ed.gov/fulltext/ED540203.pdf.

Jones, S. M., Brown, J. L., & Aber, J. L. (2011). Two-year impacts of a universal school-based social- emotional and literacy intervention: An experiment in translational developmental research. *Child. Development, 82*(2), 533–554. doi:10.1111/j.1467-8624.2010.01560.x.

Kail, R. V. (2003). Information processing and memory. In M. H. Bornstein, L. Davidson, C. L. M. Keyes, & K. A. Moore (Eds.), *Crosscurrents in contemporary psychology* (pp. 269–279). Mahwah, NJ: Lawrence Erlbaum.

Kishiyama, M. M., Boyce, W. T., Jimenez, A. M., Perry, L. M., & Knight, R. T. (2009). Socioeconomic disparities affect prefrontal function in children. *Journal of Cognitive Neuroscience, 21*(6), 1106–1115.

Kopp, C. (1982). Antecedents of self-regulation: A developmental perspective. *Developmental Psychology, 18*(2), 199–214.

Larson, R. W. (2011). Adolescents' conscious processes of developing regulation: Learning to appraise challenges. *New Directions for Child and Adolescent Development, 2011*(133), 87–97.

Lengua, L. J., Honorado, E., & Bush, N. R. (2007). Contextual risk and parenting as predictors of effortful control and social competence in preschool children. *Journal of Applied Developmental Psychology, 28*(1), 40–55.

Lerner, R. M. (1982). Children and adolescents as producers of their own development. *Developmental Review, 2*(4), 342–370.

Lerner, R. M. (1985). Adolescent maturational changes and psychosocial development: A dynamic interactional perspective. *Journal of Youth and Adolescence, 14*(4), 355–372.

Lerner, R. M., & Steinberg, L. D. (2009). The scientific study of adolescent development: Historical and contemporary perspectives. In R. M. Lernerog & L. D. Steinberg (Eds.), *Handbook of adolescent psychology* (pp. 3–15). Hoboken, N.J: Wiley.

Lerner, R. M., Lerner, J. V., von Eye, A., Bowers, E. P., & Lewin-Bizan, S. (2011). Individual and contextual bases of thriving in adolescence: A view of the issues. *Journal of Adolescence, 34*(6), 1107–1114.

Levack, W. M. M., Taylor, K., Siegert, R. J., Dean, S. G., McPherson, K. M., & Weatherall, M. (2006). Is goal planning in rehabilitation effective? A systematic review. *Clinical Rehabilitation, 20*(9), 739–755.

Lewin-Bizan, S., Bowers, E. P., & Lerner, R. M. (2010). One good thing leads to another: Cascades of positive youth development among American adolescents. *Development and Psychopathology, 22*(4), 759–770. doi:10.1017/S0954579410000441.

Luszczynska, A. (2006). An implementation intentions intervention, the use of a planning strategy, and physical activity after myocardial infarction. *Social Science & Medicine, 62*(4), 900–908.

Massey, E. K., Gebhardt, W. A., & Garnefski, N. (2008). Adolescent goal content and pursuit: A review of the literature from the past 16 years. *Developmental Review, 28*(4), 421–460.

McClelland, M. M., Acock, A. C., & Morrison, F. J. (2006). The impact of kindergarten learning-related skills on academic trajectories at the end of elementary school. *Early Child Research Quarterly, 21*(4), 471–490.

McClelland, M. M., & Cameron, C. E. (2012). Self-regulation in early childhood: Improving conceptual clarity and developing ecologically-valid measures. *Child Development Perspectives, 6*(2), 136–142. doi:10.1111/j.1750–8606.2011.00191.x.

McClelland, M. M., Cameron, C. E., Connor, C. M., Farris, C. L., Jewkes, A. M., & Morrison, F. J. (2007). Links between behavioral regulation and preschoolers' literacy, vocabulary and math skills. *Developmental Psychology, 43*(4), 947–959. doi:10.1037/0012-1649.43.4.947.

McClelland, M. M., Cameron Ponitz, C. C., Messersmith, E., & Tominey, S. (2010). Self-regulation: The integration of cognition and emotion. In R. Lerner (Series Ed.) & W. Overton (Vol. Ed.), *Handbook of life-span development* (Cognition, biology and methods) (Vol. 1, pp. 509–553). Hoboken, NJ: Wiley.

McClelland, M. M., Acock, A. C., Piccinin, A., Rhea, S. A., & Stallings, M. C. (2013). Relations between preschool attention span-persistence and age 25 educational outcomes. *Early Childhood Research Quarterly, 28*, 314–324. doi:10.1016/j.ecresq.2012.07.008.

McClelland, M. M., Cameron, C. E., Duncan, R., Bowles, R. P., Acock, A. C., Miao, A., & Pratt, M. E. (2014). Predictors of early growth in academic achievement: The Head-toes-knees-shoulders task. *Frontiers in Psychology, 5*, 1–14. doi:10.3389/fpsyg.2014.00599.

Metcalfe, J., & Mischel, W. (1999). A hot/cool-system analysis of delay of gratification: Dynamics of willpower. *Psychological Review, 106*(1), 3–19.

Miller, D. C., & Byrnes, J. P. (2001). Adolescents' decision making in social situations. A self-regulation perspective. *Journal of Applied Developmental Psychology, 22*(3), 237–256.

Mischel, W. (1968). *Personality and assessment*. Hoboken, NJ: Wiley.

Mischel, W., & Ayduk, O. (2004). Willpower in a cognitive-affective processing system: The dynamics of delay of gratification. In R. F. Baumeister & K. D. Vohs (Eds.), *Handbook of self-regulation: Research, theory, and applications* (pp. 99–129). New York, NY: Guilford.

Mischel, W., & Ebbesen, E. B. (1970). Attention in delay of gratification. *Journal of Personality and Social Psychology, 16*(2), 329–337.

Mischel, W., Ebbesen, E. B., & Zeiss, A. R. (1972). Cognitive and attentional mechanisms in delay of gratification. *Journal of Personality and Social Psychology, 21*(2), 204–218.

Mistry, R. S., Benner, A. D., Biesanz, J. C., Clark, S. L., & Howes, C. (2010). Family and social risk, and parental investments during the early childhood years as predictors of low-income children's school readiness outcomes. *Early Childhood Research Quarterly, 25*(4), 432–449. doi:10.1016/j.ecresq.2010.01.002.

Moffitt, T. E., Arseneault, L., Belsky, D., Dickson, N., Hancox, R. J., Harrington, H., et al. (2011). A gradient of childhood self-control predicts health, wealth, and public safety. *Proceedings of the National Academy of Sciences, 108*(7), 2693–2698. doi:10.1073/pnas.1010076108.

Moilanen, K. L. (2007). The adolescent self-regulatory inventory: The development and validation of a questionnaire of short-term and long-term self-regulation. *Journal of Youth and Adolescence, 36*(6), 835–848.

Moilanen, K. L., Shaw, D. S., & Fitzpatrick, A. (2010). Self-regulation in early adolescence: Relations with mother-son relationship quality and maternal regulatory support and antagonism. *Journal of Youth and Adolescence, 39*(11), 1357–1367. doi:10.1007/s10964-009-9485-x.

Molina, B. S. G., Hinshaw, S. P., Swanson, J. M., Arnold, L. E., Vitiello, B., Jensen, P. S., Epstein, J. N., Hoza, B., Hechtman, L., Abikoff, H. B., Elliott, G. R., Greenhill, L. L., Newcorn, J. H., Wells, K.C., Wigal, T., Gibbons, R. D., Hur, K., Houck, P. R., Houck, P. R. (2009). The MTA at 8 years: Prospective follow-up of children treated for combined-type ADHD in a multisite study. Journal of the American Academy of Child & Adolescent Psychiatry, 48(5), 484–500. doi:10.1097/CHI.0b013e31819c23d0.

Moore, B., Mischel, W., & Zeiss, A. (1976). Comparative effects of the reward stimulus and its cognitive representation in voluntary delay. *Journal of Personality and Social Psychology, 34*(3), 419–424.

Morrison, F. J., Ponitz, C. C., & McClelland, M. M. (2010). Self-regulation and academic achievement in the transition to school. In S. D. Calkins & M. Bell (Eds.), *Child development at the intersection of emotion and cognition* (pp. 203–224). Washington, DC: American Psychological Association.

Nikkelen, S. W. C., Valkenburg, P. M., Huizinga, M., & Bushman, B. J. (2014). Media use and ADHD-related behaviors in children and adolescents: A meta-analysis. *Developmental Psychology, 50*(9), 2228–2241. doi:10.1037/a0037318.

Norman, D. A., & Shallice, T. (1986). Attention to action: Willed and automatic control of behavior. In R. J. Davidson, G. E. Schwartz, & D. Shapiro (Eds.), *Consciousness and self-regulation: Advances in research and theory* (Vol. 4, pp. 1–18). New York, NY: Plenum Press.

Obradovic, J. (2010). Effortful control and adaptive functioning of homeless children: Variable-focused and person-focused analyses. *Journal of Applied Developmental Psychology, 31*(2), 109–117. doi:10.1016/j.appdev.2009.09.004.

Orbell, S., & Sheeran, P. (2000). Motivational and volitional processes in action initiation: A field study of the role of implementation intentions. *Journal of Applied Social Psychology, 30*(4), 780–797.

Orbell, S., Hodgkins, S., & Sheeran, P. (1997). Implementation intentions and the theory of planned behavior. *Personality and Social Psychology Bulletin, 23*(9), 945–954.

Overton, W. F. (2010). Life-span development: Concepts and issues. In W. F. Overton (Ed). Cognition, biology, and methods across the lifespan. In R. M. Lerner (Ed.), *Handbook of life-span development* (pp. 1–29). Hoboken, NJ: Wiley.

Overton, W. F. (2013). Relationism and relational developmental systems: A paradigm for developmental science in the post-Cartesian era. In R. M. Lerner & J. B. Benson (Eds.), *Advances in child development and behavior, Embodiment and epigenesis: Theoretical and methodological issues in understanding the role of biology within the relational developmental system* (Vol. 44, pp. 21–64). San Diego, CA: Academic Press.

Posner, M. I., & Rothbart, M. K. (1998). Attention, self-regulation, and consciousness. *Philosophical*

Transactions of the Royal Society of London B, 353(1377), 1915–1927.

Posner, M. I., & Rothbart, M. K. (2000). Developing mechanisms of self-regulation. *Development and Psychopathology, 12*(3), 427–441.

Quinn, P. D., & Fromme, K. (2010). Self-regulation as a protective factor against risky drinking and sexual behavior. *Psychology of Addictive Behaviors, 24*(3), 376–385. doi:10.1037/A0018547.

Radesky, J. S., Kistin, C. J., Zuckerman, B., Nitzberg, K., Gross, J., Kaplan-Sanoff, M., et al. (2014). Patterns of mobile device use by caregivers and children during meals in fast food restaurants. *Pediatrics, 133*(4), e843–e849. doi:10.1542/peds.2013-3703.

Raver, C. C., Jones, S. M., Li-Grinning, C., Zhai, F., Bub, K., & Pressler, E. (2011). CSRP's impact on low- income preschoolers' preacademic skills: Self-regulation as a mediating mechanism. *Child Development, 82*(1), 362–378. doi:10.1111/j.1467-8624.2010.01561.x.

Reid, R., Trout, A. L., & Schartz, M. (2005). Self-regulation interventions for children with attention deficit/hyperactivity disorder. *Exceptional Children, 71*, 361–377.

Rimm-Kaufman, S. E., Curby, T. W., Grimm, K. J., Nathanson, L., & Brock, L. L. (2009). The contribution of children's self-regulation and classroom quality to children's adaptive behaviors in the kindergarten classroom. *Developmental Psychology, 45*(4), 958–972.

Robertson, L. A., McAnally, H. M., & Hancox, R. J. (2013). Childhood and adolescent television viewing and antisocial behavior in early adulthood. *Pediatrics, 131*(3), 439–446. doi:10.1542/peds.2012-1582.

Rothbart, M. K., & Bates, J. E. (1998). Temperament. In W. Damon (Series Ed.) & N. Eisenberg (Ed.), *Handbook of child psychology* (Social, emotional, and personality development) (Vol. 3). Hoboken, NJ: Wiley.

Rothbart, M. K., Ahadi, S. A., Hersey, K. L., & Fisher, P. (2001). Investigations of temperament at three to seven years: The Children's behavior questionnaire. *Child Development, 72*(5), 1394–1408.

Sabbagh, M. A., Xu, F., Carlson, S. M., Moses, L. J., & Lee, K. (2006). The development of executive functioning and theory of mind: A comparison of Chinese and U.S. preschoolers. *Psychological Science, 17*(1), 74–81.

Schmitt, S. A., McClelland, M. M., Tominey, S. L., & Acock, A. C. (2015). Strengthening school readiness for head start children: evaluation of a self-regulation intervention. *Early Childhood Research Quarterly 30*(A), 20–31.doi: http://dx.doi.org/10.1016/j.ecresq.2014.08.001.

Scholz, U., Sniehotta, F. F., Burkert, S., & Schwarzer, R. (2007). Increasing physical exercise levels: Age-specific benefits of planning. *Journal of Aging and Health, 19*(5), 851–866.

Sektnan, M., McClelland, M. M., Acock, A. C., & Morrison, F. J. (2010). Relations between early family risk, children's behavioral regulation, and academic achievement. *Early Childhood Research Quarterly, 25*(4), 464–479. doi:10.1016/j.ecresq.2010.02.005.

Sheeran, P., & Orbell, S. (2000). Using implementation intentions to increase attendance for cervical cancer screening. *Health Psychology, 19*(3), 283–289.

Sheese, B. E., Rothbart, M. K., Posner, M. I., White, L. K., & Fraundorf, S. H. (2008). Executive attention and self-regulation in infancy. *Infant Behavior & Development, 31*(1), 501–510.

Shonkoff, J. P. (2011). Protecting brains, not simply stimulating minds. *Science, 333*(6045), 982–983. doi:10.1126/science.1206014.

Shonkoff, J. P., & Bales, S. N. (2011). Science does not speak for itself: Translating child development research for the public and its policymakers. *Child Development, 82*(1), 17–32. doi:10.1111/j.1467-8624.2010.01538.x.

Shonkoff, J. P., Garner, A. S., The Committee on Psychosocial Aspects of Child Family Health, Committee on Early Childhood, Adoption, Dependent Care, Section on Developmental Behavioral Pediatrics, Siegel, B. S., et al. (2012). The lifelong effects of early childhood adversity and toxic stress. *Pediatrics, 129*(1), e232–e246. doi:10.1542/peds.2011-2663.

Sniehotta, F. F., Schwarzer, R., Scholz, U., & Schüz, B. (2005). Action planning and coping planning for long-term lifestyle change: Theory and assessment. *European Journal of Social Psychology, 35*(4), 565–576.

Sniehotta, F. F., Scholz, U., & Schwarzer, R. (2006). Action plans and coping plans for physical exercise: A longitudinal intervention study in cardiac-rehabilitation. *British Journal of Health Psychology, 11*(1), 23–37.

Stansbury, K., & Zimmermann, L. K. (1999). Relations among child language skills, maternal socializations of emotion regulation, and child behavior problems. *Child Psychiatry & Human Development, 30*(2), 121–142.

Steinberg, L. (2010). A behavioral scientist looks at the science of adolescent brain development. *Brain and Cognition, 72*(1), 160–164. doi:10.1016/j.bandc.2009.11.003.

von Suchodoletz, A., Gestsdottir, S., Wanless, S. B., McClelland, M. M., Birgisdottir, F., Gunzenhauser, C., et al. (2013). Behavioral self-regulation and relations to emergent academic skills among children in Germany and Iceland. *Early Childhood Research Quarterly, 28*(1), 62–73. doi:10.1016/j.ecresq.2012.05.003.

Tominey, S. L., & McClelland, M. M. (2011). Red light, purple light: Findings from a randomized trial using circle time games to improve behavioral self-regulation in preschool. *Early Education & Development, 22*(3), 489–519. doi:10.1080/10409289.2011.574258.

Tsukayama, E., Toomey, S. L., Faith, M., & Duckworth, A. L. (2010). Self-control as a protective factor against overweight status in the transition to adolescence. *Archives of Pediatrics and Adolescent Medicine, 164*(7), 631–635.

Wachs, T. D., Gurkas, P., & Kontos, S. (2004). Predictors of preschool children's compliance behavior in early childhood classroom settings. *Journal of Applied Developmental Psychology, 25*(4), 439–457.

Wanless, S. B., McClelland, M. M., Tominey, S. L., & Acock, A. C. (2011). The influence of demographic risk factors on children's behavioral regulation in prekindergarten and kindergarten. *Early Education & Development, 22*(3), 461–488.

Zelazo, P. D., & Lyons, K. E. (2012). The potential benefits of mindfulness training in early childhood: A developmental social cognitive neuroscience perspective. *Child Development Perspectives, 6*(2), 154–160. doi:10.1111/j.1750–8606.2012.00241.x.

Zelazo, P. D., Anderson, J. E., Richler, J., Wallner-Allen, K., Beaumont, J. L., & Weintraub, S. (2013). II. NIH toolbox cognition battery (CB): Measuring executive function and attention. *Monographs of the Society for Research in Child Development, 78*(4), 16–33. doi:10.1111/mono.12032.

Ziegelmann, J. P., Lippke, S., & Schwarzer, R. (2006). Adoption and maintenance of physical activity: Planning interventions in young, middle-aged, and older adults. *Psychology and Health, 21*(2), 145–163.

Ziegelmann, J. P., Luszczynska, A., Lippke, S., & Schwarzer, R. (2007). Are goal intentions or implementation intentions better predictors of health behavior? A longitudinal study in orthopedic rehabilitation. *Rehabilitation Psychology, 52*(1), 97–102.

Ziegelmann, J. P., & Lippke, S. (2007). Planning and strategy use in health behavior change: A life span view. *International Journal of Behavioral Medicine, 14*(1), 30–39. doi:10.1007/BF02999225.

Zimmerman, B. J. (2002). Becoming a self-regulated learner: An overview. *Theory Into Practice, 41*(2), 64–70.

Zimmerman, B. J., & Schunk, D. H. (2001). *Self-regulated learning and academic achievement: Theoretical perspectives* (2nd ed.). Mahwah, NJ: Erlbaum.

Zimmermann, L. K., & Stansbury, K. (2003). The influence of temperamental reactivity and situational context on the emotion-regulatory abilities of 3-year-old children. *Journal of Genetic Psychology, 164*(4), 389–409.

A Life Course Health Development Perspective on Oral Health

James J. Crall and Christopher B. Forrest

1 Introduction

1.1 Life Course Health Development Concepts and Principles

Life Course Health Development(LCHD) is a conceptual framework that helps to explain how health develops over an individual's lifetime and emphasizes the need to treat health development as a long-term investment, beginning early and continuing throughout life (Halfon and Hochstein 2002). LCHD provides a powerful approach to understanding diseases and conditions and how risk factors, protective factors, critical life experiences, and environments affect long-term health and disease outcomes. LCHD also can help examine and explain how health and disease patterns, particularly health disparities, develop across populations and over time (Halfon and Hochstein 2002; Ben-Shlomo and Kuh 2002; Keating and Hertzman 1999).

J.J. Crall (✉)
Division of Public Health and Community Dentistry, University of California Los Angeles (UCLA) School of Dentistry, Los Angeles, CA, USA
e-mail: jcrall@dentistry.ucla.edu

C.B. Forrest
Applied Clinical Research Center, Children's Hospital of Pennsylvania, Philadelphia, PA, USA

Efforts to relate the life course perspective or life course theory to the field of maternal and child health (Fine and Kotelchuck, 2010) have emphasized the following key concepts:

Pathways or Trajectories Health pathways or trajectories are constructed and modified throughout the life span. While individual trajectories vary, general patterns can be predicted for populations and communities based on social, economic, and environmental exposures and experiences. A life course does not reflect a series of discrete steps or stages, but rather an integrated, dynamic, and continuous set of exposures and experiences. The set of possible trajectories that a person can experience is constrained by evolutionary forces and is highly determined by exposure to various environmental contexts.

Importance of Early Life Exposures Early experiences can markedly influence an individual's future health development. Of particular salience are exposures that occur prenatally (i.e., exposures in utero) and intergenerationally (i.e., factors related to the health of the mother prior to conception). While adverse events and exposures can have an impact at any point in a person's life course, the impact may be greatest at specific critical or sensitive periods when developing biological systems are most readily modified (e.g., during fetal development, in early childhood, during adolescence).

N. Halfon et al. (eds.), *Handbook of Life Course Health Development*,
DOI 10.1007/978-3-319-47143-3_13

Cumulative Impact Cumulative experiences also can influence an individual's future health and development, even though any individual experience may not impact health development. For example, individuals may adapt with minimal impact to each episode of stress; however, the cumulative impact of multiple stresses over time (also referred to as "weathering" or "allostatic load") may have a profound direct impact on health development by altering biological function and human behavior.

Risk and Protective Factors Throughout the life span, protective factors improve health and contribute to health development, while risk factors diminish health and make it more difficult to reach full health potential. Moreover, pathways are changeable, and risk and protective factors are not limited to individual behavioral patterns or receipt of health-care and social services, but also include factors related to family, neighborhood, community, and social policy.

The LCHD theoretical framework (presented more thoroughly in Chap. 2) incorporates and expands these concepts into a robust explanatory synthesis of how health in individuals and populations is produced and modified. In this chapter, we use the LCHD principles to guide our review of oral health development. The Table 1 illustrates each LCHD principle's relevance to oral health.

1.2 Previous Efforts to Apply Life Course Concepts to Oral Health

The multifactorial etiology of oral conditions, their chronic nature and occurrence over the life span, and inherent features of their expression make oral health well suited to studies which seek to apply life course concepts. For example, Nicolau and colleagues (Nicolau et al. 2007) have highlighted several features that make oral conditions amenable to life course epidemiological studies, the first of which is their observability—i.e., once these conditions develop, they are readily detectable during assessments as opposed to conditions that resolve or go unnoted if study participants fail to report them. A second feature relates to their being cumulative conditions, which allows for comparisons of the degree of disease development among individuals so that, rather than all who develop the disease being enumerated together, distinctions can be made among them with respect to the extent or severity of their disease. Third, oral conditions can be reliably measured and validly diagnosed without sophisticated or costly technology. Fourth, these conditions are moderately prevalent; thus, the required sample size for cohort studies is manageable. And, finally, oral health conditions have a public health importance that makes their study justifiable on both ethical and economic grounds.

Despite growing interest in using life course concepts as the basis for various oral health-related scientific studies, robust applications have been rather limited. A PubMed search conducted as part of the literature review for this chapter using the terms "life course and oral health" yielded over 500 citations. However, a substantial portion of the publications examined in this and other literature searches were found to have one or more of the following limitations: studies focused on a single condition, used cross-sectional data, or analyzed a relatively narrow portion of the life span, studies were based on relatively small sample sizes, and studies were predicated on retrospective analyses that frequently relied on recall of rather distant events.

Furthermore, efforts to examine oral health from the perspective of LCHD concepts and principles have not been pursued. Therefore, the goals of this chapter are to (a) examine the concept of oral health and major oral diseases and conditions from a LCHD perspective using the key concepts and principles noted in the table, (b) assess what is (and what is not) known about the development of oral health and its impact on general health and well-being across the life course, and (c) offer recommendations for future research. In light of the evidence-based literature shortcomings noted in the preceding paragraph, assessments of what is known about applications of life course research approaches to studies of oral health are limited to research publications consistent with the life course epidemiology

Table 1 Life Course Health Development principles

	Principle	Brief description	Oral health illustrations
1	Health Development	Health development integrates the concepts of health and developmental processes into a unified whole. Health enables adaptation to the environment, task execution, participation in desired activities, and attainment of thriving. Development refers to the mechanisms by which health changes over time. Health development, then, comprises trajectories of health assets and integrated sets of health resources that emerge as a result of a person's continuous and relational interactions with their environments.	Oral health is not merely the absence of oral diseases. Instead, oral health refers to the capacity to adapt to ubiquitous environmental and microbial challenges, maintaining the robustness of teeth and other structures in the mouth, and oral health development refers to the pathways and trajectories of change of these assets over the life course.
2	Unfolding	Health development unfolds continuously over the lifespan, from conception to death, and is shaped by prior experiences and environmental interactions. For human health development, there are four major functional phases: (1) *generativity*, preconception and prenatal period; (2) *acquisition of capacity*, the early years; (3) *maintenance of capacity*, the middle years; and (4) *managing decline*, the later years. Each is conceptually distinct but can be overlapping.	Prenatal conditions can predispose developing teeth to elevated risk of early childhood caries, which is in turn a risk factor for caries later in life, which can lead to tooth loss and associated negative impacts on oral and overall health.
3	Complexity	Health development results from adaptive, multilevel, and reciprocal interactions between individuals and their physical, natural, and social environments. There is a dynamic interplay between individual and multiple physical, biochemical, psychological, social, and cultural networks which enable adaptation and individual robustness. Each level is both a part and a whole, nested and hierarchically aligned to optimize health development.	Oral health is strongly influenced by nutritional intake and changes in the microbiome. These effects in turn impact health development of individuals as well as their energy levels, healing, behavior, and cognitive development.

(continued)

Table 1 (continued)

	Principle	Brief description	Oral health illustrations
4	Timing	Health development is sensitive to the timing and social structuring of environmental exposures and experiences. Time-specific health development pathways refer to biological embedding that occurs during sensitive or critical periods, when developing systems are most alterable, and exogenous and endogenous influences can result in different adaptive responses. Socially structured pathways link experiences and exposures in ways that create recursive and mutually reinforcing patterns of risk, protection, and promotion.	Oral cancers result from the dynamic interaction of genetic, physical, biochemical, psychological, behavioral, social, and cultural factors. Risk for these conditions is highest for individuals who use alcohol, use tobacco, are exposed to human papilloma virus or Epstein-Barr virus, or are exposed to x-radiation before the age of 50 years
5	Plasticity	Health development phenotypes are systematically malleable and enabled and constrained by evolution to enhance adaptability to diverse environments. Heredity transmits evolutionary signals through genetic, epigenetic, behavioral, and symbolic dimensions, which establish health phenotypes that depending on environmental circumstances may or may not be selected and optimized to produce desirable outcomes. At the microlevel, a range of strategies introduce variable types and levels of plasticity to optimize adaptability from the molecular to the behavioral level. At a macrolevel, strategies organize health development phases and life stages into functional entities.	The human jaw developed over millennia among our human ancestors who spent hours each day chewing their food. The interaction between chewing of tough food and bone development may have been responsible for the lack of malocclusion observed in the hominid fossil record. Today a softer diet has contributed to smaller jaws and smaller teeth in modern humans, leading to the large numbers of individuals with malocclusion and need for orthodontic treatment.
6	Thriving	Optimal health development promotes survival, enhances well-being, and protects against disease. Health development can also be perturbed to create suboptimal states that are precursors to fully formed disease—so-called endophenotypes that represent intermediate phase transitions toward a fully manifest phenotypic expression of a disease or disorder.	Diabetes perturbs oral health development by increasing risk for periodontal disease, which when present causes pain, chewing difficulties, and tooth loss. Dry mouth, often a symptom of undetected diabetes, can cause sores, ulcers, infections and tooth decay. Smoking makes these problems worse. Conversely, reducing diabetes risk and reducing or eliminating smoking can promote oral health.
7	Harmony	Health development results from the balanced interactions of molecular, physiological, behavioral, cultural, and evolutionary processes. Genetic modulations that occur in molecular time frames measured in nanoseconds are linked to biochemical modulation measured in milliseconds, homeostatic mechanisms measured in seconds to days, social norms that evolve over years and decades, cultural processes that change from years to centuries, and ecological processes that until recently took millennia. Harmonization of these processes produces rhythms and variability that characterize health. Loss of coordination of these processes results in less robustness of the human system with negative consequences.	Analysis of the DNA from ancient humans has demonstrated shifts in oral bacterial species ecology following dietary pattern changes and reductions in the diversity of the oral ecosystem, a possible factor in the rise of dental caries and periodontal disease in modern humans whose oral health may be better matched to circumstances in our evolutionary history than to modern environments.

standard and LCHD framework. Furthermore, because of the diverse nature of the major oral health-related conditions noted above, assessments are largely limited to "dental conditions" (i.e., dental caries, periodontal diseases, and tooth loss), with limited additional examples pertaining to craniofacial abnormalities, oral cancers, or temporomandibular joint dysfunction.

2 Conceptualizing Oral Health and Overview of Major Conditions

2.1 Conceptualizing Oral Health

Concepts and definitions of oral health have varied over time, often paralleling broader conceptualizations of health. Concepts of how oral health changes over time also often parallel more general paradigms. For example, many recent concepts of oral health have been based on the biopsychosocial model, which focuses on how the integration of various aspects of biological, psychological, and social domains influence individuals' health in different contexts and over time (Borrell-Carrio et al. 2004).

The US Surgeon General's Report on Oral Health (SGROH), issued in 2000, and ensuing initiatives have emphasized two major themes regarding the concept of oral health—i.e., oral health means much more than healthy teeth, and oral health is integral to general health (US Department of Health and Human Services 2000). Interestingly, the SGROH embraced the World Health Organization (WHO) definition of oral health as "a state of being free from mouth and facial pain, oral and throat cancer, oral infection and sores, periodontal (gum) disease, tooth decay, tooth loss, and other diseases and disorders that limit an individual's capacity in biting, chewing, smiling, speaking, and psychosocial wellbeing." This definition espoused by both the WHO and SGROH is deficient in that it does not positively define what oral health is, but rather presents the concept as the absence of detrimental conditions or disorders. Conflating oral health and oral disorders is contrary to the WHO definition of overall health which states that health is more than just the absence of disease and represents a state of complete physical, mental, and social well-being. Researchers working to develop measures related to oral health and its impact on quality of life also have concluded that health and disease are different domains of human experience, which vary both over time and among individuals, and are dependent on context (Locker and Slade 1994; Gregory et al. 2005).

A recent development in the conceptualization and definition of oral health has emerged from the FDI World Dental Federation in late 2016. According to the new FDI definition, "Oral health is multifaceted and includes the ability to speak, smile, smell, taste, touch, chew, swallow, and convey a range of emotions through facial expressions with confidence and without pain, discomfort, and disease of the craniofacial complex. The core elements of oral health in the FDI framework are as follows: *disease and condition status* refers to a threshold of severity or a level of progression of disease, which also includes pain and discomfort; *physiological function* refers to the capacity to perform a set of actions that include, but are not limited to, the ability to speak, smile, chew, and swallow; and *psychosocial function* refers to the relationship between oral health and mental state that includes, but is not limited to, the capacity to speak, smile, and interact in social and work situations without feeling uncomfortable or embarrassed." (Glick et al. 2016).

LCHD theoretical principles conceptualize health as an emergent set of integrated assets that enable adaptation and pursuit of meaning and happiness, reflect broader notions of the impact of various health determinants over time, and consider health in a more positive context (see Table 1). Applying LCHD concepts, individuals with disease (e.g., diabetics or persons living with AIDS) can also be considered healthy if they have developed assets which enable adaptation to their environment, task execution, participation in desired activities, and an ability to thrive; health and disease are distinct, albeit interrelated concepts.

LCHD builds and expands upon the basic tenets of the biopsychosocial and other ecological models and establishes a conceptual foundation for a future era of health care that moves beyond systems focused on management of acute and chronic diseases and conditions to systems whose focus is on optimizing lifelong health for individuals and populations (Halfon et al. 2014). Using LCHD concepts and principles to conceptualize and define oral health has the potential to move practitioners, researchers, policy makers, and the public beyond their historical limited focus on the physical form and function of structures in and surrounding the oral cavity and the clinical consequences of oral/dental diseases to a new paradigm—one which fully embraces LCHD tenets and the development of more robust LCHD-based policies and systems for optimizing the oral health of individuals and populations.

2.2 Major Oral Health-Related Diseases and Conditions

Clinical conditions that have major significance with respect to oral health in terms of prevalence, impact on health, development and well-being, and economic considerations include *dental diseases and their consequences* (dental caries, periodontal diseases, tooth loss), *craniofacial developmental disorders* (e.g., cleft lip, cleft palate, malocclusion), *oral cancers* (including pharyngeal and salivary gland cancers), and *facial pain* (distinct from dental pain) generally associated with temporomandibular joint and muscular disorders. Brief overviews of these conditions are provided below.

Dental Conditions Despite significant progress during the latter portion of the twentieth century, *dental caries (tooth decay)* remains the most common chronic disease of childhood and a major cause of tooth loss in children and adults. In the United States, approximately 25% of 2–5-year-olds and over 50% of 6–8-year-old children experience dental caries in their primary teeth, and over 50% of 12–15-year-olds and 67% of 16–19-year-olds experience caries in their permanent teeth (Dye et al. 2011a). Although substantial declines in the average number of teeth and tooth surfaces affected by caries have been documented in recent decades, particularly in developed countries, according to the WHO, the prevalence of tooth decay in school-age children globally ranges from 60% to 90% (WHO, The World Oral Health Report 2008).

Significant disparities in childhood caries experience also persist. On average, US children from lower-income households and children of color are three to five times more likely than their white more affluent counterparts to experience caries and exhibit more severe forms of tooth decay (Dye et al. 2011a; Vargas et al. 1998). Of interest from a LCHD perspective, many children from high-risk population groups do not exhibit severe forms of dental caries, presumably because the balance between individual's risk and protective factors (e.g., diet, toothbrushing habits, fluoride exposure, oral microflora or other unidentified characteristics) is conducive to maintaining a healthy dentition (Feathersone 2000).

Caries affects dentate individuals across the life span (Fig. 1), with over 90% of US adults with natural teeth experiencing dental caries in their permanent teeth (Dye et al. 2011a, b). According to the WHO (WHO, The World Oral Health Report, 2008) nearly 100% of dentate adults globally are affected by dental caries, making it the most prevalent chronic condition of people worldwide. From a life course perspective, early childhood caries can have a profound deleterious lifelong effect on an individual's dentition status, as ECC often is a precursor of caries and its consequences in adults.

Periodontal disease mainly results from infections and inflammation of the gingiva (gums) and bone that surround and support the teeth. In its early stage, called gingivitis, the gums can become swollen and red and may bleed. In its more serious form, called periodontitis, the gums can pull away from the teeth, bone can be lost, and teeth may loosen or even fall out. Thirty percent of US adults 30+ years of age have moderate periodontal disease, and 8.5% have severe periodontitis (Thornton-Evans 2013). Males, older adults, Black and Hispanic adults, current smokers, and those with lower incomes and less education are more likely to have moderate or severe

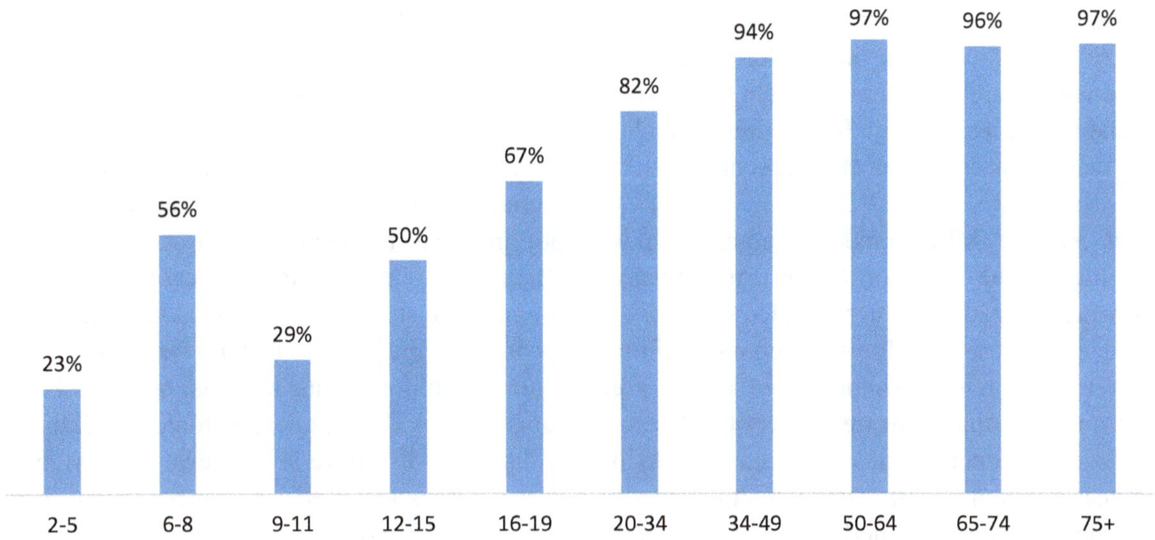

Fig. 1 Proportion of the US population with caries experience (percentages for 2–5- and 6–8-year-olds reflect the percentage of individuals with caries experience in primary teeth; for ages 9 and above, percentages reflect the percentage with caries experience in permanent teeth) by age (years) (Data Source: National Health and Nutrition Examination Survey, 2011–2012. National Center for Health Statistics, CDC)

periodontal disease (Thornton-Evans 2013). Globally, severe periodontal disease is found in 15–20% of adults aged 35–44 years and increases in prevalence with advancing age (WHO, The World Oral Health Report 2008).

Dental caries and periodontal disease are the primary reasons for *tooth loss* (Dye et al. 2011b; Thornton-Evans 2013) which in its more severe forms (loss of multiple teeth) can have negative psychological, social, nutritional, and physical effects. A person's quality of life is diminished as a result of tooth loss due to reductions in their ability to chew and speak and reduced social interactions and self-esteem (US Department of Health and Human Services 2000; Hollister & Weintraub 1993; Brennan et al. 2008). National survey data indicate that approximately 50% of US adults have lost at least one tooth. Approximately 5% of US adults overall and 25% of adults aged 65+ are completely edentulous (have no natural teeth) (Dye et al. 2011b). Worldwide, about 30% of people aged 65–74 have no natural teeth, with considerable disparities across countries (WHO, The World Oral Health Report 2008).

Total US spending for dental services has been relatively flat at approximately $111 billion since 2010 (Wall 2013). The bulk of dental care spending is related to diagnosis, prevention and treatment of dental caries and periodontal disease, and treatment related to removal and replacement of lost teeth.

Craniofacial Conditions Craniofacial defects such as *cleft lip and cleft palate (CLP)* are among the most common of all birth defects. The US incidence of cleft palate is 6 per 10,000 live births, and the incidence for cleft lip with or without cleft palate is 11 per 10,000 live births (Center for Disease Control and Prevention (CDC) 2014). CLP can occur as an isolated condition or may be a component of an inherited disease or syndrome. Cleft lip and cleft palate are thought to be caused by a combination of genes and other factors, such as things the mother comes in contact with in her environment, what the mother eats or drinks, or certain medications she uses during pregnancy. Maternal smoking, alcohol use, steroid use, and anticonvulsants are associated with increased risk for cleft lip and palate (Kohli and Kohli 2012). The incidence of CLP also varies by race, with Asians and Native Americans having higher rates and African-Americans having lower rates. According to the Centers for Disease Control and Prevention

(CDC), in the United States, cleft lip and palate is the third most common birth defect, and health expenditures are approximately eight times higher in the first 10 years of life for children with clefting than for those without (Boulet et al. 2009).

Malocclusion Misalignment or abnormal positioning of the teeth or an incorrect relation between the teeth in the upper and lower jaws—is neither a disease nor a life-threatening condition. Nevertheless, growing numbers of people seek and undergo orthodontic treatment, often because of esthetic concerns and other quality of life issues (Liu et al. 2009). Although children make up the majority of orthodontic patients, adults increasingly are seeking treatment for malocclusion and now comprise one-fifth of all orthodontic patients in the US. Orthodontic services account for approximately one-eighth of US dental care expenditures (Agency for Healthcare Research and Quality 2015).

Oral Cancers Approximately 45,000 Americans and over 450,000 people worldwide are diagnosed each year with cancers that affect the mouth and/or pharynx. Oral cancers comprise 85% of all head and neck cancers and have relatively high mortality rates (5-year survival = 63%) (The Oral Cancer Foundation 2015; American Cancer Society 2015). Oral cancer occurrence rates are significantly higher for males than for females (except in American Indians/Alaska Natives) and higher for black males than for white males up to age 70. Oral cancer rates increase with age, increase more rapidly after age 50, and peak between ages 70 and 80 (Fig. 2) (Ram et al. 2011). Extensive case-control and longitudinal studies have implicated tobacco and alcohol as major risk factors for oral cancer. Human papillomavirus, syphilis, oro-dental factors, dietary deficiencies, chronic candidiasis, and viruses also have been shown to be significantly associated with oral cancer (Ram et al. 2011). Findings of a recent study (Jacobson et al. 2012) suggest that oral cancers may be among the most costly forms of cancer to treat in the United States.

Facial Pain Associated with Temporomandibular Joint Disorders The most common cause of facial pain is a group of conditions called temporomandibular joint and muscle disorders (TMJD). These disorders cause recurrent or chronic pain and dysfunction in the jaw joint and its associated muscles and supporting tissues. TMJD are the second most commonly occurring musculoskeletal condition resulting in pain and disability (after chronic low back pain), affecting

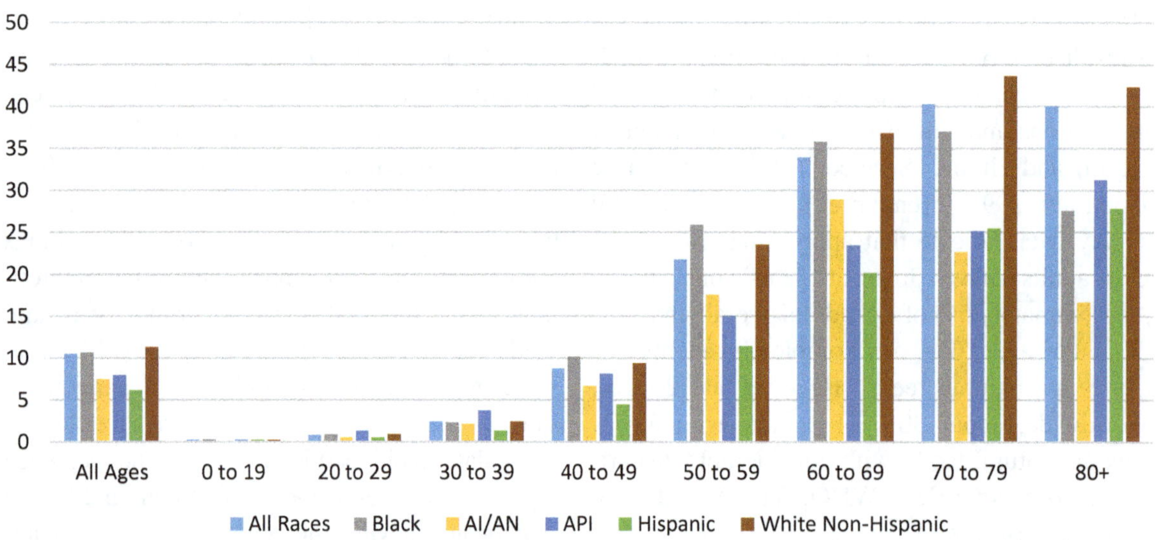

Fig. 2 Incidence of oral cancer cases per 100,000 among different age and racial groups (Data Source: Oral Cancer Incidence by Age, Race and Gender, 2009. National Institute of Dental and Craniofacial Research)

approximately 5–12% of the population, with an annual cost estimated at $4 billion. About half to two-thirds of those with TMJD seek treatment; among those seeking treatment, approximately 15% develop chronic TMJD (NIDCR 2003).

3 Evolution of Oral Health Paradigms

The evolution of concepts regarding oral health and associated analytical models designed to measure oral health in the aggregate and its various components have paralleled the evolution of general health concepts, albeit frequently with a variable time lag. Ancient theories and hypotheses have given way to more scientifically grounded concepts reflecting changing scientific paradigms, initially based on biomedical models of disease causation, followed by biopsychosocial models that attempted to incorporate a wider range of factors influencing health and, more recently, Life Course Health Development. The following section provides a broad overview of that progression, focusing primarily on concepts regarding dental conditions.

3.1 Changing Concepts of Dental Disease: From Worms to Germs to Chronic Disease Terms

Tooth Worm Theory The concept of a tooth worm which according to prevailing popular beliefs caused caries and periodontitis existed in diverse cultures across the ages and, despite being labeled by medical doctors as superstition during the time of the Enlightenment, persisted in some cultures into the twentieth century. Numerous popular "therapies" were applied to eradicate the tooth worm, including fumigations with henbane seeds, magical formulas, and oaths (Gerabek 1999).

Chemo-Parasitic and Focal Infection Theories In 1890, W.D. Miller (an American dentist and the first oral microbiologist), building on Pasteur's discovery that bacteria can ferment sugars into lactic acid, formulated the chemo-parasitic theory of caries. This theory held that tooth decay is caused by acids, produced by oral bacteria following fermentation of ingested sugars, which lead to loss of mineral from teeth (demineralization) (Miller 1890). Miller's second major contribution was the focal infection theory, which hypothesized that oral microorganisms or their products have a role in the development of a variety of diseases in sites removed from the oral cavity, including brain abscesses, pulmonary diseases, and gastric problems (Miller 1891). Later work by Keyes in the 1960s led to explanations of the mechanisms by which dental caries develops based on the interaction of cariogenic bacteria in biofilm/dental plaque and dietary substrates that lead to acid production, which in turn leads to demineralization of tooth structure (illustrated in the Venn diagram in Fig. 5).

Concept of Caries as a Specific and Transmissible Infection The concept of dental caries being infectious and transmissible is based on the biomedical model of disease causation, and grew out of well-designed rodent studies performed by Keyes (Keyes 1960) showing that caries only developed in rodents when they were caged with or ate the fecal pellets of groups of caries-active rodents. Further proof emerged when certain streptococci isolated from caries lesions in hamsters, unlike other types of streptococci, caused rampant decay in previously caries-inactive animals (Fitzgerald and Keyes 1961). The bacteria, later identified as *Streptococcus mutans* (SM), gave rise to the concept of caries being due to a specific infection with mutans streptococci (MS), a concept that has gained wide support within the field of caries microbiology (Fejerskov 2004). Subsequent studies conducted from the mid-1970s through the 1990s demonstrated that infants acquire MS from their mothers and that MS can colonize the mouths of infants even before teeth erupt (Berkowitz 2006).

Conceptualizing Caries as a Complex, Chronic Disease More recently, Featherstone (Feathersone 2000) used a modification of the chronic disease model, referred to as the "caries balance," to describe caries as a dynamic process that depends on the balance between constellations of risk factors (e.g., high levels of cariogenic bacteria, reduced salivary function, cariogenic dietary practices, tooth structure anomalies) and protective factors (e.g., salivary components and flow, exposure to fluorides, anti-cariogenic dietary components). Although the caries balance concept highlights the importance of risk factors and protective factors and the potential for dynamic changes over time, published examples generally depict factors related to biomedical models rather than broader biopsychosocial models.

The shift from conceptualizing dental caries based on biomedical models to models based on biopsychosocial theory represents a relatively recent paradigm change. These newer models recognize that caries expression not only depends on the complex interplay between saliva, dietary habits, and many biological determinants related to biofilm composition and metabolism; it also depends on those factors acting in concert with innumerable other biological, behavioral, and social factors acting at the level of individuals and populations. In summarizing the implications of this paradigm shift, Fejerskov (Fejerskov 2004) highlighted the following:

> By appreciating that dental caries belongs to the group of common diseases considered as 'complex' or 'mulifactorial' such as cancer, heart diseases, diabetes, and certain psychiatric illnesses, we have to realize that there is no simple causation pathway. It is not a simplistic problem such as 'elimination of one type of microorganism', or a matter of improving 'tooth resistance'. Complex diseases cannot be ascribed to mutations in a single gene or to a single environmental factor. Rather they arise from the concerted action of many genes, environmental factors, and risk-conferring behaviors. … [This concept also] explains why dental caries has to be controlled lifelong if a functional dentition is to be maintained.
>
> These new concepts explain why . . . several of the 'old' recommended preventive programs are no longer effective. It is of course not because the agents we used in prevention are no longer efficacious. They just become ineffective because the caries incidence rate has changed as the environment has changed.

This brief overview highlights changes in popular and scientific concepts regarding the etiology of common dental diseases and methods for preventing or minimizing their consequences over time. Nevertheless, the persistence of relatively high levels of dental disease in sizeable segments of the population and substantial disparities within and across populations serve to highlight the limitations of traditional concepts and approaches.

3.2 Common Risk Factors, Social Determinants, and Ecological Models

Common Risk Factors As noted above, there is growing recognition that major oral health-related conditions are complex (multifactorial), chronic conditions whose occurrence and severity across the lifespan depend on interactions of a broad array of biological, behavioral, social, and environmental factors, which also are implicated in other chronic diseases and conditions as indicated in Fig. 3 (Fejerskov 2004; Sheiham and

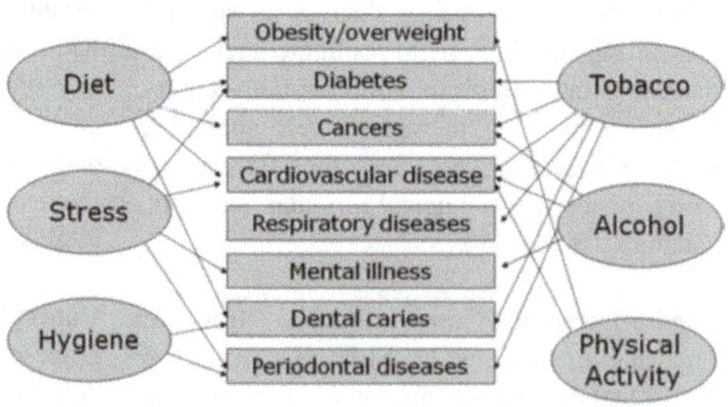

Fig. 3 Common risk factor model of oral disease and other chronic diseases (Source: Tomar 2012)

Watt 2000; Larson et al. 2008; Tomar 2012). We now realize that different types of organisms are involved in the etiology of dental caries and periodontal diseases and that the ecology of the oral microbiome is influenced by an array of common biological and biopsychosocial factors. We recognize that craniofacial disorders are caused by developmental disturbances that occur in utero and are influenced by genetic and environmental factors. We know that oral cancers result from mutations in genes that control cell behavior and are influenced by exposure to carcinogens (most notably tobacco) and biological factors, including viruses and fungi. Evidence also indicates that risk factors implicated in TMJD include poor alignment of teeth, stress, parafunctional habits, arthritis, trauma, and structural developmental abnormalities.

Cumulative Impact of Multiple Social Determinants Larson et al. (Larson et al. 2008) highlighted the cumulative impact of multiple social risk factors (limited parental education, low family income, single-parent household, race, being uninsured, family conflict, poor maternal mental health, living in an unsafe neighborhood) on various aspects of children's health, including their oral health. As shown in Fig. 4, the percentage of parents who reported that their children had suboptimal oral health and other indicators of poor health rises with increases in the number of prevailing social risk factors, with the relationship between social risk factors and poor oral health demonstrating the steepest linear gradient. The proportion reporting less than very good teeth ranged from 14% for children with no social risk factors to 64% for children with ≥6 social risk factors. Analyses that controlled for child age, gender, and number of children in the household showed an almost 11-fold increase in the odds for less than very good teeth in children with ≥6 versus no social risks, underscoring the importance of social structure to healthy development.

Ecological Models of Caries and Periodontal Disease Figure 5 depicts a multidimensional

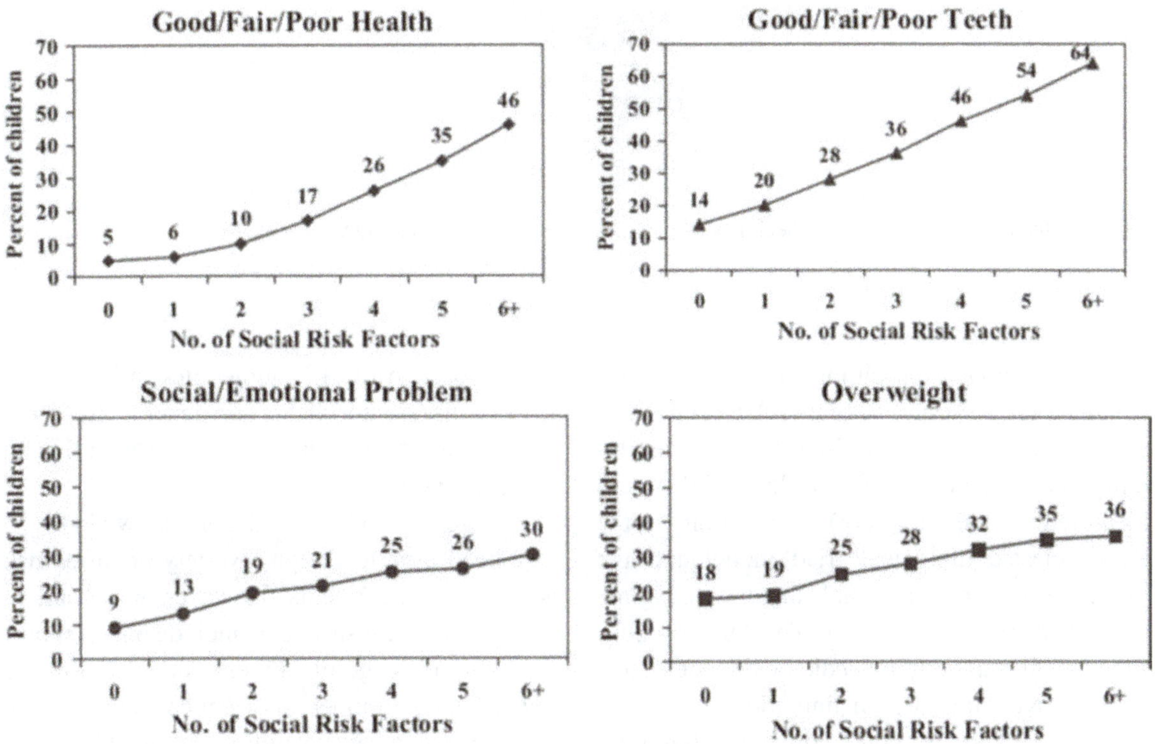

Fig. 4 Percentage of children in worse health by number of social risk factors (Source: Larson et al. 2008)

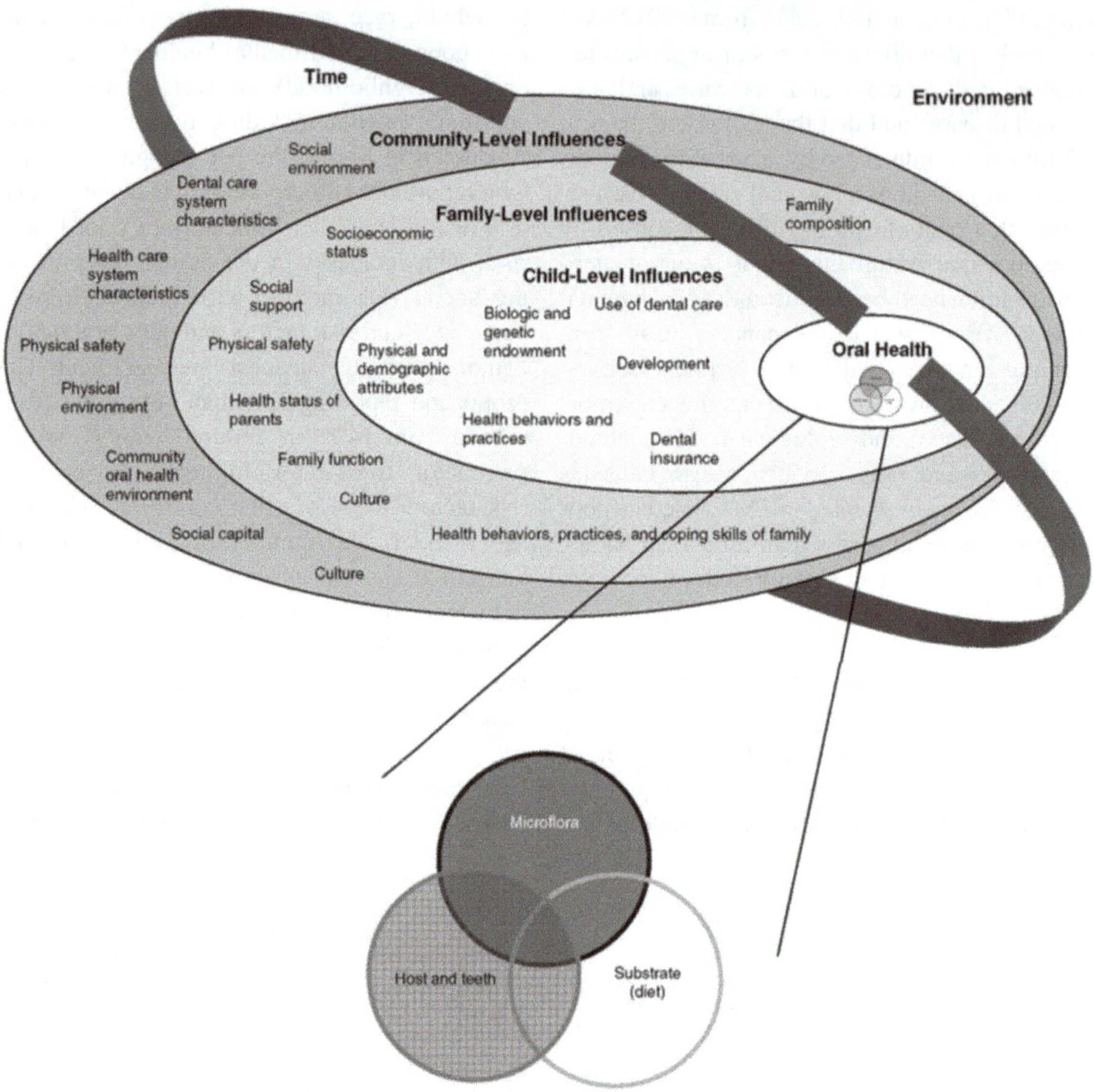

Fig. 5 Influences on children's oral health: a conceptual model (Source: Fisher-Owens et al. 2007)

ecological model for childhood dental caries, enumerating an array of biopsychosocial influences (including six child-level, eight family-level, and eight community-level influences identified in the literature) in addition to the Keyes classic biological triad model and the influence of environmental factors and time (Fisher-Owens et al. 2007). The bulk of published studies underlying ecological models such as this have study design limitations similar to those identified in conducting the literature review for this chapter. Accordingly, their utility with respect to LCHD studies lies in helping to identify disease correlates and generate hypotheses, not in establishing oral disease or health development pathways.

Ecological models like the one shown in Fig. 5 have been used to design a variety of caries-risk assessment instruments. However, most caries-risk assessment instruments include only a subset of the broad range of influences depicted in the Fisher-Owens model and generally have not undergone extensive validity testing (Quinonez and Crall 2009).

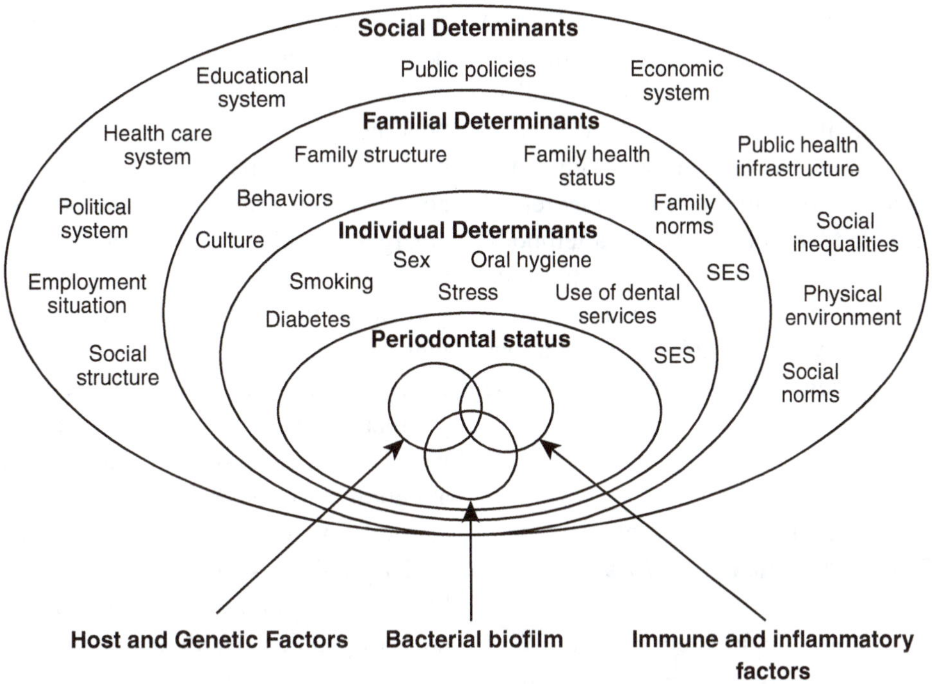

Fig. 6 Social determinants of oral health and disease in US men (Source: Tomar 2012)

Figure 6 depicts an ecological conceptual model for periodontal disease using a framework similar to the Fisher-Owens et al. model for childhood caries (Tomar 2012). In this case, the biological model emphasizes the interactions among host and genetic factors, bacteria associated with periodontal disease (different and distinct from cariogenic bacteria), and immune and inflammatory factors—reflecting a different pathogenic mechanism for periodontal disease than for dental caries. Constellations of individual, familial, and social influences are identified within categories of social, behavioral, and contextual factors in this model.

Ecological models like those shown in Figs. 5 and 6 are useful for depicting the complex array of etiological factors that potentially influence disease development, but are of limited value for explaining disease mechanisms or pathways as they do not explicitly incorporate developmental mechanisms or time into the frameworks. LCHD principles address these gaps by building on ecological models, adding time dimensions and developmental pathways to the models.

4 Research Applications of Life Course Concepts to Oral Health

4.1 Life Course Epidemiology

Life course epidemiology adds the time dimension to disease causation models, moving beyond the limitations of models such as those shown in the preceding section which depict an unspecified, essentially cross-sectional interplay among nested layers of environmental and individual factors. According to Kuh and Ben-Shlomo (Ben-Shlomo and Kuh 2002), "Life course epidemiology is defined as 'the study of long-term effects on chronic disease risk of physical and social exposures during gestation, childhood, adolescence, young adulthood and later adult life. It seeks to understand causal links between exposures and outcomes, taking into consideration the importance of time (duration) and timing in the disease development." In a recent paper on concepts and theoretical models of life course epidemiology and its relevance to chronic oral conditions, Nicolau et al. (Nicolau et al. 2007) noted that "The life course approach to studying chronic disease etiology is not merely a collection of longitudinal data or the use of a particular study design or analytical method. Rather, the unique feature of this approach is a theoretical framework which assumes and tests a temporal ordering of exposure variables and their interrelationship with a specific outcome." The following section provides several examples of applications of life course epidemiology to studies of chronic oral diseases and conditions.

4.2 Oral Health Trajectories: Dunedin Cohort Studies

A number of studies published since the turn of the twenty-first century have begun to more fully embrace life course research methodologies and examine a broader array of life course influences. Foremost among them from the standpoint of assessing changes in oral health status over time and the influence of socioeconomic influences beginning in early childhood is the Dunedin Multidisciplinary Health and Development Study—a longitudinal investigation of health and behavior in a complete birth cohort of study members born in Dunedin, New Zealand, between April, 1972 and March, 1973. Findings of several Dunedin studies are summarized below.

Poulton et al. (Poulton et al. 2002) assessed a number of health outcomes, including dental caries, dental plaque scores, gingival bleeding, and periodontal disease status in a cohort of 1000 26-year-old Dunedin Study subjects whose socioeconomic status (SES) had been documented at birth and at ages, 3, 5, 7, 9, 11, 13, and 15 years. All dental health measures at age 26 years showed a graded relation with childhood SES. As SES increased, the amount of plaque and gingival bleeding and the proportion of individuals with periodontal disease and decayed surfaces decreased. The adverse influence of low childhood socioeconomic status was seen after controlling for infant health and contemporaneous adult SES. Additionally, the results showed that low adult SES had a significant effect on poor adult dental health after controlling for low childhood SES. The authors concluded that their "findings document that the social gradient in health—which has been amply documented among middle-aged and older adults—actually emerges in childhood. Whereas clinical and research interest in the social gradient has been generated mostly by studies of adults, the findings from this study suggest that the social gradient can be scrutinised in paediatric and adolescent populations as well. Further, whereas most studies of the social gradient have narrowed their attention to specific diseases, such as cardiovascular diseases, we document that the social gradient is far more ubiquitous and troubling. Low social class adversely affects many areas of people's health, including their physical, dental and mental health" (Poulton et al. 2002). This finding concerning children's dental health is highly noteworthy because there are few pediatric conditions that show a substantial SES gradient, which raises the possibility that body systems that develop rapidly and dramatically during childhood, such as the structures and physiological systems of the oral cavity, are more vulnerable to, and perhaps dependent on, environmental exposures.

Thomson et al. (2004) analyzed data on 789 Dunedin Study subjects at ages 5 and 26 years to investigate whether adult oral health status is influenced by (a) childhood socioeconomic advantage or disadvantage (controlling for childhood oral health) or (b) oral health in childhood (controlling for childhood socioeconomic advantage or disadvantage) and whether oral health in adulthood is affected by changes in SES. With respect to the question of whether poor adult oral health is predicted by socioeconomic disadvantage in childhood, after controlling for childhood oral health, analyses revealed that oral health inequalities present at age 5 years were also apparent at age 26 years when the early childhood SES categories were used, suggesting that early socioeconomic inequalities in a number of important oral health indicators do persist well into the third decade of life. Concerning the question of whether poor adult oral health is predicted by poor oral health in childhood, after controlling for childhood socioeconomic status, the evidence was unequivocal regarding dental caries: having high caries disease experience early in life predicted having greater disease experience in adulthood, other factors being equal. The pattern was not as clear with respect to periodontal disease, however. Finally, in examining the impact of individuals' SES at ages 5 and 26, Thomson and colleagues (Thomson et al. 2004) found that, for nearly all oral health indicators, a clear gradient for disease severity and prevalence was observed across socioeconomic trajectory groups in the following ascending order: "high (at age 5)–high (at age 26)," "low–high" (upwardly mobile), "high–low" (downwardly mobile), and "low–low." These findings led the authors to conclude that adult oral health is predicted by not only childhood socioeconomic advantage or disadvantage but also by oral health in childhood. Changes in socioeconomic advantage or disadvantage between ages 5 and 26 were associated with differing levels of oral health in adulthood. Also of interest from the standpoint of LCHD is the possibility that oral health may represent a sentinel system, with early manifestations of disease serving as a harbinger for elevated risk of other chronic diseases (e.g., obesity, diabetes).

Broadbent et al. (2008) investigated longitudinal patterns of caries experience in a birth cohort of 955 Dunedin Study subjects in order to identify and describe developmental trajectories of caries experience in the permanent dentition using data collected from dental examinations at ages 5, 9, 15, 18, 26, and 32 years. Three caries experience trajectory classes were identified: "high" (15% of subjects), "medium" (43%), and "low" (42%) with respect to decayed, missing, and filled (tooth) surfaces (DMFS). All trajectories were relatively linear, although the higher trajectories were more "S-shaped" (Fig. 7). This effect disappeared following adjustment for the number of unaffected surfaces remaining at each age, suggesting that, among individuals following a similar caries trajectory, the caries rate is relatively constant across time. This finding is

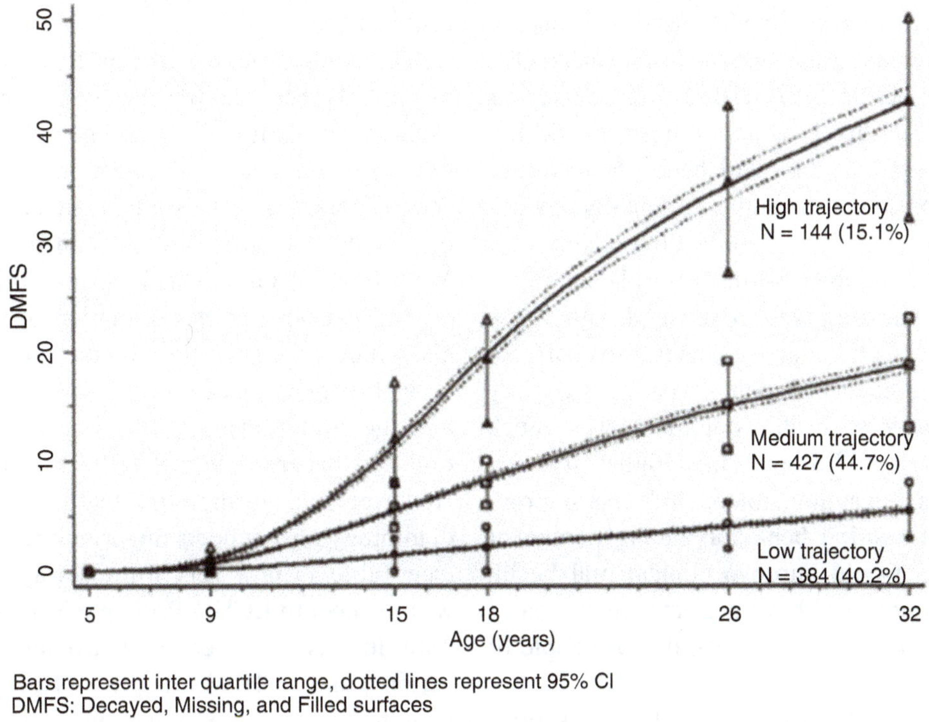

Fig. 7 Trajectory patterns of dental caries experience in the permanent dentition to the fourth decade of life (Source: Broadbent et al. 2008)

consistent with observations by Fejerskov (2004) that the caries incidence rate in a group of individuals appears fairly constant throughout life if no special efforts to control lesion progression are made. Broadbent et al. (2008) concluded that these results did not support the commonly held belief among dentists that childhood and adolescence are periods of special risk for dental caries or that caries "immunity" may be acquired during late adolescence or early adulthood. In fact, other studies have reported that ECC is one of the most reliable predictors of elevated risk of caries experience later in life.

Crocombe et al. (2011) also analyzed data from 833 participants in the Dunedin Study to assess the impact of dental visiting trajectory patterns on clinical oral health and oral health-related quality of life measures. Information on the use of dental services was collected at ages 15, 18, 26, and 32. Dental visiting trajectories were significantly associated with both measures of self-reported oral health and three of the four dental clinical indicators. The regular dental attendance group had less than half the mean number of missing teeth, a lower mean DMFS score, and a lower mean decayed surfaces (DS) than those defined as "opportunists" and "decliners." The regular group had the lowest mean Oral Health Impact Profile (OHIP-14) score and was nearly twice as likely as opportunists and decliners to report that they had better-than-average oral health. Low SES and being dentally anxious were associated with worse health outcomes for all outcome variables, while "poor plaque trajectory" and smoking were associated with worse outcomes for all variables except filled surfaces (FS). The influence of dental visiting trajectory on clinical oral health outcomes was much higher at lower SES levels than higher SES levels, leading the authors to conclude that improving dental visiting behavior among people of lower SES would improve clinical oral health outcomes more and have a greater reduction of oral health impacts than it would for people of higher SES.

A number of additional studies of shorter duration and/or employing retrospective methods of data collection (which may be subject to some degree of recall bias) have been conducted in other countries, most notably Brazil, Norway, the United Kingdom, and Hong Kong (Lu et al. 2011; Holst; Peres et al. 2011; Mason et al. 2006). Collectively, these studies generally affirm the findings from analyses conducted as part of the Dunedin Study, with some variation that likely reflects varying levels of SES (particularly poverty) and differences in the types of oral health-care systems and programs available across countries. Many of these studies are limited to adolescents (starting at age 15) or adults. An exception is the work of (Holst and Schuller 2011) which examined different birth cohorts in Norway and found that the health environment in childhood was important for adults' oral health during most of the twentieth century. Attention from parents and the local environment lead to better oral health outcomes in adulthood. Social status measured by length of education also was associated with choices leading to better oral health. Regular dental visits were important especially for the eldest birth cohort. Good oral health behaviors early and during adulthood were important for oral health.

The studies summarized in this section represent advances in our understanding of the impacts of various influences on oral health over the life course. Interest in using a life course perspective to study various aspects of oral health has grown steadily in recent times. Main lines of pursuit include investigations of critical periods and accumulation of risk models, which have shed light on the importance of early life experiences, oral health trajectories, and the importance of social determinants to oral and general health (Heilman et al. 2015). However, it is worth noting that life course epidemiology only reflects the principles of LCHD (see Table 1) in a very limited way, primarily with respect to LCHD Principle 3 (Complexity: multidimensional person-environmental interactions) and LCHD Principle 5 (Timing: health is highly sensitive to timing and social structuring of environmental exposures).

4.3 Relating Oral Health, General Health, and Quality of Life

Summarizing what is known about the influences of oral health and oral health problems on life course outcomes, general health and overall quality of life is a daunting challenge that goes beyond the scope of this chapter. In lieu of attempting such a synopsis, the reader is referred initially to the US Surgeon General's Report on Oral Health (US Department of Health and Human Services 2000) for a broad introduction to the literature. Chapters 5 and 6 of that extensively researched and widely vetted document are summarized below.

Chapter 5 of the SGROH examines multiple linkages between oral and general health, noting that the mouth and the face reflect signs and symptoms of health and disease that can serve as an adjunct for diagnosis for some conditions. Diagnostic tests using oral cells and fluids—especially saliva—are available to detect drug abuse, hormonal changes, and specific diseases, and more are being developed. The mouth also is a portal of entry for pathogens and toxins, which can affect the mouth and, if not cleared by the many defense mechanisms that have evolved to protect the oral cavity, may spread to the rest of the body. Recent epidemiologic and experimental animal research provides evidence of possible associations between oral infections—particularly periodontal disease—and diabetes, cardiovascular disease, and adverse pregnancy outcomes. The review in Chapter 5 of the SGROH also highlights the need for an aggressive research agenda to better delineate the specific nature of these associations and the underlying mechanisms of action.

Chapter 6 of the SGROH looks at the impact of oral health problems on quality of life and includes examples of the kinds of questionnaires used to measure oral-health-related quality of life. Oral health generally is highly valued by society and individuals, and the chapter begins with a brief description of the reflections of those values in myth and folklore concerning facial appearance and the meaning of teeth. It then explores dimensions beyond the biological and the physical to examine how oral diseases and disorders can interfere with the functions of daily living, including participation in work or school, and what is known about their psychosocial impacts and economic costs. The deleterious effects of facial disfigurement and tooth loss may be magnified in modern societies that celebrate youth and beauty. Self-reported impacts of oral conditions on social functions include limitations in communication, social interactions, and intimacy. Additional research on oral-health-related quality of life is recommended to permit further exploration of the dimensions of oral health and well-being.

Sheiham (2005) also has provided a commentary on the relationships among oral health, general health, and quality of life. Many of the points highlighted in this commentary relate to LCHD Principle 1 (Health Development) that health is an emergent property and that oral health is a component of and contributes to overall health. Sheiham's summary ultimately reiterates the SGROH's call for cessation of "the compartmentalization involved in viewing the mouth separately from the rest of the body, noting that oral health affects general health by causing considerable pain and suffering and by altering what people eat, their speech, and their quality of life and well-being."

Additional excerpts from Sheiham's commentary include the following. "Oral health also has an effect on other chronic diseases, and failure to tackle social and material determinants and incorporate oral health into general health promotion means that millions suffer intractable toothache and poor quality of life, and end up with few teeth.

Oral diseases are the most common of the chronic diseases and are important public health problems because of their prevalence, their impact on individuals and society, and the expense of their treatment. The general determinants of oral diseases are known and include risk factors common to a number of chronic diseases: diet, inadequate hygiene practices, smoking, alcohol, risky behaviors causing injuries, and stress. Moreover, effective methods are available to prevent or reduce the impact of major oral diseases.

Oral health affects people physically and psychologically and influences how they grow, enjoy life, look, speak, chew, taste food and socialize, as well as their feelings of social well-being. Severe caries detracts from children's quality of life: they experience pain, discomfort, disfigurement, acute and chronic infections, and eating and sleep disruption as well as higher risk of hospitalization, high treatment costs and loss of school days with the consequently diminished ability to learn. Caries affects nutrition, growth and weight gain. Children of three years of age with nursing caries weigh about 1 kg less than control children because toothache and infection alter eating and sleeping habits, dietary intake and metabolic processes. Disturbed sleep affects glucocorticoid production. In addition, there is suppression of hemoglobin from depressed erythrocyte production.

Chronic diseases such as obesity, diabetes and caries are increasing in developed and developing countries, with the implication that quality of life related to oral health, as well as general quality of life, may deteriorate. Because oral and other chronic diseases have determinants in common, more emphasis should be on the common risk factor approach. The key concept underlying future oral health strategies is integration with this approach, a major benefit being the focus on improving health conditions in general for the whole population and for groups at high risk, thereby reducing social inequities."

5 Relating Oral Health and LCHD Concepts

5.1 Relating Oral Health Research Findings to Key LCHD Concepts

Pathways and Trajectories Analyses based on the Dunedin prospective, longitudinal birth cohort studies have distinguished three oral health trajectory groupings (high, medium, low) that emerge as early as age 5, remain relatively constant over time, and exhibit increasing divergence through the third decade of life. Authors of the Dunedin Study acknowledge that aggregating their findings into three trajectory 'groups' is an analytical convenience that may mask the heterogeneity of individuals within each group. To that point, LCHD suggests that a focus on intraindividual trajectories rather than on "group" means may prove more insightful because it allows for careful ascertainment of temporal exposure-outcome relationships and allows the analysis to take advantage of the diversity and complexity of these interactions rather than masking variability by aggregation into a few classes. Classes assume homogeneity of persons within a group, an assumption that is generally not supported. Little if any investigations of intraindividual change with detailed ascertainment of exposure and outcome over time have been reported in the dental/oral health literature.

Additional Dunedin cohort studies have examined the effect of SES in childhood and adulthood on adult oral health, and the effect of early childhood oral health on adult oral health, and found that the highest oral health trajectories are exhibited by those who have higher SES and better oral health in childhood; the lowest trajectories are found in those who have low SES and poor oral health in childhood; and those whose SES changed (either upwardly or downwardly) between childhood and adulthood fall between the other two trajectories. Oral health-care utilization and other personal, family, and community factors (e.g., oral hygiene, diet, dental anxiety, emphasis placed on oral health within one's family or community) also appear to exert influences on oral health trajectories throughout the life course.

Early Programming Evidence concerning the impact of early programming on oral health over the lifespan is less well defined, in part because many studies focus on adolescents or adults. Developmental disturbances that result in structural anomalies of tooth structure represent one documented example of early programming influences that can increase risk for dental disease (Targino et al. 2011). Findings from studies conducted by Holst and Schuller (2011) and Alm (Alm et al. 2008) suggest that good oral hygiene habits, including the use of fluoride toothpaste, established in early childhood provide a foundation for a low risk of proximal caries in adolescents. Evidence for the influence of less direct influences such as low birth weight is more equivocal, but represents an area of growing research interest (Nicolau et al. 2007). Evidence of intergenerational programming has been documented, particularly with respect to maternal-child oral health relationships (Shearer and Thomson, 2010; Shearer et al. 2011).

Critical or Sensitive Periods Some evidence, including studies cited above, supports the critical or sensitive period hypothesis with respect to the impact of various influences during fetal, early childhood, and later stages on life course oral health development and the determinants of oral health disparities. The importance and etiological mechanisms of disturbances arising during the prenatal period on craniofacial developmental problems such as cleft lip and/or cleft palate have been extensively documented. However, much remains to be elucidated with respect to the effects of different influences, at different times, on other oral health-related conditions (dental caries, periodontal disease, cancer, TMJD) (Hallqvist et al. 2004).

Cumulative Impact Substantial evidence also exists to support the hypothesis that the impact of major oral health-related conditions is a function of cumulative experiences or episodes of disease over time. Clearly, it is well established that dental caries is a chronic, cumulative disease and that the caries status of an individual develops and is subject to biological, behavioral, social, and environmental influences over time. Caries occurs at any stage in life, provided that an individual has susceptible teeth (and surfaces) remaining (Broadbent et al. 2008). The same case can be made for periodontal disease and tooth loss resulting from caries and periodontal diseases (Shearer et al. 2011; Watt 2007).

Risk and Protective Factors Considerable evidence has been compiled with respect to the biological and, to a lesser extent, behavioral risk and protective factors for major dental conditions (see Figs. 5 and 6). The influence of genetic, epigenetic, family, community, social, and environmental risk factors, in individual populations or across populations, is less well documented and understood.

5.2 Gaps in Knowledge Concerning Oral Health from a LCHD Perspective

Researchers involved in studying life course influences on oral health have identified a number of gaps in the current knowledge base. Using the lens of the LCHD principles, we have compiled research needs for future studies on oral health:

- Evaluate the contribution of social isolation, social relationships, and social support to oral health.
- Obtain more information on the economic, political, social, and environmental causes of individual behaviors related to oral health.
- Increase the number of longitudinal studies assessing the long-term effects of early childhood caries (ECC) and treatment on the health and quality of life of preschool children.
- Longitudinal studies are needed in order to obtain more knowledge about causative factors and the possible relationships between dental caries and overweight/obesity in children.
- Conceptual work that articulates a definition of oral health motivated by the LCHD principles is needed.
- Theoretical explanations for health inequalities are limited and biased due to the types of data collected in modern epidemiological studies, which are geared toward identifying and quantifying risk factors for disease and intended as a basis for description (of disease), not explanation (of causal pathways). This raises questions about the validity of current explanations. Current epidemiological approaches are widely criticized for neglecting broad social factors and failing to dig below the surface into issues such as how differ-

ent social class groups live their lives and what factors influence their lifestyle decisions. Current explanations are based largely on what epidemiological researchers can see and measure; factors that are harder to assess (such as culture), but which may be critically important to advancing our understanding of social inequalities in health, are frequently neglected.

- Epidemiologists have largely persisted in the use of disease-based measures to assess inequalities in health and oral health. The most significant advance to our understanding of social inequalities in health may come from the creation of a data set that measures oral health as defined by the FDI or oral-health-related quality of life.
- To date there is no research exploring how members of the population understand and account for inequalities in oral health, which remains a significant omission as it could offer promising new insights.
- Further research is needed to clarify the apparently differing oral health beliefs, attitudes, and practices of lower and higher SES groups.
- Much work remains to be done to establish which biological, social, and environmental factors are determinants of oral health or disease and which are merely markers, "proxies," or confounders.
- The process by which social stratification translates to poor oral health beginning in earliest childhood, especially for groups at higher risk for disease, is not well understood.
- There is a need for future research to move beyond traditional risk factors and more closely examine the impact of the social environment on oral health beliefs, behavior, and outcomes.
- A number of oral health problems have been shown to be associated with other health conditions (e.g., low birth weight, cardiovascular disease, respiratory disease); however, the demonstration of actual causal connections or pathways, such as the bidirectional relationship between diabetes and periodontal disease, has been modest.

5.3 Recommendations for Research and Policy Priorities

The knowledge gaps noted above give rise to a number of recommendations for research priorities to better understand oral health life course influences and policy changes to help reduce the impact of oral health problems and reduce oral health inequalities, which can be summarized as follows:

- Greater support for longer-term longitudinal oral health life course studies with detailed and frequent data collection to allow for the construction of intraindividual trajectories
- Replication of true oral health life course studies in different populations to assess whether findings apply across diverse settings
- Greater emphasis on research delineating relationships among oral health determinants to identify causal pathways
- Greater emphasis on identifying and addressing broader influences on oral health (i.e., family, community, social, and environmental influences)

6 Summary

This chapter has outlined major concepts embodied in the Life Course Health Development framework, examined evidence relating various aspects of major oral health-related conditions to this framework, and produced recommendations for advancing research and policy concerning oral health. LCHD provides a highly useful approach for understanding oral health determinants, disparities, and influences on general health and well-being and for advancing knowledge, policies, and programs to optimize health across individuals and populations.

References

Agency for Healthcare Research and Quality. 2015. Dental Services Mean and Median Expenses per Person With Expense and Distribution of Expenses by Source of Payment: United States, 2012. Medical Expenditure

Panel Survey Household Component Data. Generated interactively. (3 Mar 2015).

Alm, A., et al. (2008). Oral hygiene and parent-related factors during early childhood in relation to approximal caries at 15 years of age. *Caries Research, 42*(1), 28–36.

American Cancer Society. (2015). Cancer Facts & Figures 2015. Atlanta: American Cancer Society.

Ben-Shlomo, Y., & Kuh, D. (2002). A life course approach to chronic disease epidemiology: Conceptual models, empirical challenges and interdisciplinary perspectives. *International Journal of Epidemiology, 31*, 285–293.

Berkowitz, R. J. (2006). Mutans steptococci: Acquistion and transmission. *Pediatric Dentistry, 28*, 106–109.

Borrell-Carrio, F., Suchman, A. L., & Epstein, R. M. (2004). The biopsychosocial model 25 years later: Principles, practice, and scientific inquiry. *Annals of Family Medicine, 2*, 576–582.

Boulet, S. L., Grosse, S. D., Honein, M. A., & Correa-Villasenor, A. (2009). Children with orofacial clefts: Health care use and costs among a privately insured population. *Publ Health Reports, 124*, 447–453.

Brennan, D. S., Spencer, A. J., & Roberts-Thomson, K. F. (2008). Tooth loss, chewing ability and quality of life. *Quality of Life Research, 17*, 227–235.

Broadbent, J. M., Thomson, W. M., & Poulton, R. (2008). Trajectory patterns of dental caries experience in the permanent dentition to the fourth decade of life. *Journal of Dental Research, 87*, 69–72.

Center for Disease Control and Prevention (CDC). (2014). Prevalence (number of cases) of cleft lip and cleft palate. Available at: http://www.nidcr.nih.gov/DataStatistics/FindDataByTopic/CraniofacialBirthDefects/PrevalenceCleft%20LipCleftPalate.htm.

Crocombe, L. A., et al. (2011). Dental visiting trajectory patterns and their antecedents. *Journal of Public Health Dentistry, 71*(1), 23–31.

Dye, B. A., Thornton-Evans, G., Li, X., & Iafolla, T. J. (2015a). *Dental caries and sealant prevalence in children and adolescents in the United States, 2011a–2012. NCHS data brief, no 191*. Hyattsville: National Center for Health Statistics.

Dye, B. A., Thornton-Evans, G., Li, X., & Iafolla, T. J. (2015b). *Dental caries and tooth loss in adults in the United States, 2011b–2012. NCHS data brief, no 197.* Hyattsville: National Center for Health Statistics.

Feathersone, J. B. D. (2000). The science and practice of caries prevention. *Journal of the American Dental Association (Chicago, IL), 131*, 887–899.

Fejerskov, O. (2004). Changing paradigms in concepts on dental caries: Consequences for oral health care. *Caries Research, 38*, 182–191.

Fine, A., & Kotelchuck, M. (2010). *Rethinking MCH: The life course model as an organizing framework.* Washington, DC: US Department of Health and Human Services, Health Resources and Services Administration, Maternal and Child Health Bureau.

Fisher-Owens, S. A., Gansky, S. A., Platt, L. J., et al. (2007). Influences on children's oral health: A conceptual model. *Pediatrics, 120*, e510–e520.

Fitzgerald, R. J., & Keyes, P. H. (1961). Demonstration of the etiologic role of streptococci in experimental caries in the hamster. *Journal of the American Dental Association (Chicago, IL), 61*, 9–19.

Gerabek, W. E. (1999). The tooth-worm: Historical aspects of a popular medical belief. *Clin Oral Invest, 3*, 1–6.

Glick, M., et al. (2016). A new definition for oral health developed by the FDI World dental federation opens the door to a universal definition of oral health. *Journal of the American Dental Association (Chicago, IL), 147*, 915–917.

Gregory, J., Gibson, B., & Robinson, P. G. (2005). Variation and change in the meaning of oral health related quality of life: A 'grounded' systems approach. *Social Science & Medicine, 60*, 1859–1868.

Halfon, N., & Hochstein, M. (2002). Life course health development: An integrated framework for developing health, policy, and research. *The Milbank Quarterly, 80*, 433–479.

Halfon, N., Larson, K., Lu, M., Tullis, E., & Russ, S. (2014). Lifecourse health development: Past, present and future. *Maternal and Child Health Journal, 18*, 344–365.

Hallqvist, J., et al. (2004). Can we disentangle life course processes of accumulation, critical period and social mobility? An analysis of disadvantaged socio-economic positions and myocardial infarction in the Stockholm heart epidemiology program. *Social Science & Medicine, 58*(8), 1555–1562.

Heilman, A., et al. (2015). Oral health over the life course. In C. Burton-Jeangros, S. Cullati, & A. Sacker (Eds.), *A life course perspective on health trajectories and transitions [Internet]*. Cham (CH): Springer. doi:10.1007/9783319204840_3.

Hollister, M. C., & Weintraub, J. A. (1993). The association of oral status with systemic health, quality of life, and economic productivity. *Journal of Dental Education, 57*(12), 901–912.

Holst, D., & Schuller, A. A. (2011). Equality in adults' oral health in Norway. Cohort and cross-sectional results over 33 years. *Community Dent Oral Epidemiol, 39*(6), 488–497. doi:10.1111/j.1600-0528.2011.00624.x.

Jacobson, J. J., et al. (2012). The cost burden of oral, oral pharyngeal, and salivary gland cancers in three groups: Commercial insurance, Medicare, and Medicaid. *Head & Neck Oncology, 4*, 15.

Keating, D. P., & Hertzman, C. (1999). *Developmental health and the wealth of nations : Social, biological, and educational dynamics.* New York, NY: Guilford Press.

Keyes, P. H. (1960). The infectious and transmissible nature of experimental dental caries. *Archives of Oral Biology, 1*, 304–320.

Kohli, S. S., & Kohli, V. S. (2012). A comprehensive review of the genetic basis of cleft lip and palate. *J Oral Maxillofac Pathol., 16*, 64–72. doi:10.4103/0973-029X.92976.

Larson, K., Russ, S. A., Crall, J. J., & Halfon, N. (2008). Influence of multiple social risks on children's health. *Pediatrics, 121*, 337–344.

Liu, Z., et al. (2009). The impact of malocclusion/orthodontic treatment need on the quality of life: A systematic review. *The Angle Orthodontist, 79*, 585–591.

Locker, D., & Slade, G. (1994). Association between clinical and subjective indicators of oral health status in an older adult population. *Gerodontology, 11*, 108–114.

Lu, H. X., et al. (2011). Trends in oral health from childhood to early adulthood: A life course approach. *Community Dentistry and Oral Epidemiology, 39*(4), 352–360.

Mason, J., et al. (2006). How do factors at different stages of the lifecourse contribute to oral-health-related quality of life in middle age for men and women? *Journal of Dental Research, 85*(3), 257–261.

Miller, W. D. (1890). *The micro-organisms of the human mouth*. Philadelphia: S.S. White Publishing Co..

Miller, W. D. (1891). The human mouth as a focus of infection. *Dental Cosmos, 33*, 689–706.

Nicolau, B., et al. (2007). Life-course epidemiology: Concepts and theoretical models and its relevance to chronic oral conditions. *Community Dentistry and Oral Epidemiology, 35*(4), 241–249.

NIDCR. (2003). Prevalence of TMJD and its signs and symptoms; Available from: http://www.nidcr.nih.gov/DataStatistics/FindDataByTopic/FacialPain/PrevalenceTMJD.htm.

Peres, M. A., et al. (2011). The influence of family income trajectories from birth to adulthood on adult oral health: Findings from the 1982 Pelotas birth cohort. *American Journal of Public Health, 101*(4), 730–736.

Poulton, R., et al. (2002). Association between children's experience of socioeconomic disadvantage and adult health: A life-course study. *Lancet, 360*(9346), 1640–1645.

Quinonez, R., & Crall, J. J. (2009). Caries-risk assessment in early childhood. In J. H. Berg & R. Slayton (Eds.), *Early childhood oral health*. Hoboken: Wiley-Blackwell.

Ram, H., Kumar, H., Konwar, R., Bhatt, M. L. B., & Mohammad, S. (2011). Oral cancer: Risk factors and molecular pathogenesis. *J Maxillofac Oral Surg, 10*, 132–137.

Shearer, D. M., & Thomson, W. M. (2010). Intergenerational continuity in oral health: A review. *Community Dentistry and Oral Epidemiology, 38*(6), 479–486.

Shearer, D. M., et al. (2011). Maternal oral health predicts their children's caries experience in adulthood. *Journal of Dental Research, 90*(5), 672–677.

Sheiham, A. (2005). Oral health, general health and quality of life. *Bulletin of the World Health Organization, 83*(9), 644–644.

Sheiham, A., & Watt, R. G. (2000). The common risk factor approach: A rational basis for promoting oral health. *Community Dentistry and Oral Epidemiology, 28*, 399–406.

Targino, A. G. R., et al. (2011). The relationship of enamel defects and caries: A cohort study. *Oral Diseases, 17*(4), 420–426.

The Oral Cancer Foundation. (2015). Oral cancer facts. Available at: http://www.oralcancer.org/facts/.

Thomson, W. M., et al. (2004). Socioeconomic inequalities in oral health in childhood and adulthood in a birth cohort. *Community Dentistry and Oral Epidemiology, 32*, 345–353.

Thornton-Evans, et al. (2013). Periodontitis among adults aged > United States, 2009–2010. *MMWR, 62*(3), 129–135.

Tomar, S. L. (2012). Social determinants of oral health and disease in US men. *Journal of Mens Health, 9*, 113–119.

U.S. Department of Health and Human Services. (2000). Oral Health in America: A Report of the Surgeon General. Rockville: U.S. Department of Health and Human Services, National Institute of Dental and Craniofacial Research, National Institutes of Health.

Vargas, C. M., Crall, J. J., & Schneider, D. A. (1998). Sociodemographic distribution of pediatric dental caries: NHANES III, 1988-1994. *Journal of the American Dental Association (1939), 129*(9), 1229–1238.

Wall, T., & Vujicic M. (2014). No growth in U.S. dental spending in 2013. Health policy Institute research brief. American Dental Association. December 2014. Available from: http://www.ada.org/~/media/ADA/Science%20and%20Research/HPI/Files/HPIBrief_1214_4.ashx.

Watt, R. G. (2007). From victim blaming to upstream action: Tackling the social determinants of oral health inequalities. *Community Dentistry and Oral Epidemiology, 35*(1), 1–11.

WHO, The World Oral Health Report 2003. (2008). Continuous improvement of oral health in the 21st century–the approach of the WHO global oral health Programme. *Community Dent Oral Epidemiol, 31*(s1), 3–24.

Life Course Health Development Outcomes After Prematurity: Developing a Community, Clinical, and Translational Research Agenda to Optimize Health, Behavior, and Functioning

Michael E. Msall, Sarah A. Sobotka, Amelia Dmowska, Dennis Hogan, and Mary Sullivan

Definitions Late preterm infants (LPIs) $34^{0/7}$–$36^{6/7}$ week infants; moderate preterm infants (MPI) $32^{0/7}$–$33^{6/7}$ week infants; very preterm infants (VPI) $28^{0/7}$–$31^{6/7}$ weeks; extreme preterm infants (EPI) $<28^{0/7}$ weeks; cerebral palsy (CP); normal birth weight (NBW) $\geq$2500 g; low birth weight (LBW) 1500–2499 g; very low birth weight (VLBW) 1000–1499 g; extremely low birth weight (ELBW) <1000 g; *IQ* = intelligence quotient; *ID* = intellectual disability

1 Introduction

National vital statistics from 2013 estimate that the rate of preterm birth (<37 weeks of gestation) involves approximately 1 in 10 infants in the United States each year (Hamilton et al. 2015). An estimated 68 per 1000 US live births, over 270,000 annually, are born at late preterm gestation (34–36 weeks). Currently, 28 per 1000 US live births, more than 100,000 infants annually,

M.E. Msall, MD (✉)
Developmental and Behavioral Pediatrics University of Chicago, Comer and LaRabida Children's Hospitals, Chicago, IL, USA

JP Kennedy Research Center on Intellectual and Developmental Disabilities, University of Chicago Comer Children's Hospital, Section of Developmental and Behavioral Pediatrics, 950 East 61St Street, SSC Room 207, Chicago, IL 60637, USA
e-mail: mmsall@peds.bsd.uchicago.edu

S.A. Sobotka, MD, MS • A. Dmowska, BA
Section of Developmental and Behavioral Pediatrics, University of Chicago Comer Children's Hospitals, Chicago, IL, USA

D. Hogan, PhD
Sociology and Demography, Population Research and Training Center, Brown University, Providence, RI, USA

M. Sullivan, PhD, RN
University of Rhode Island, College of Nursing, Women and Infants Hospital, Providence, RI, USA

N. Halfon et al. (eds.), *Handbook of Life Course Health Development*,
DOI 10.1007/978-3-319-47143-3_14

are born <34 weeks of gestation, and 56,000 are born at very low birth weight status (<1500 g). These infants have high risks for long-term neurodevelopmental disabilities such as intellectual disability (ID), blindness, sensorineural hearing loss, and cerebral palsy (CP). There are several biomedical causes for these high rates of preterm birth, such as the role of assisted reproductive technologies increasing the rate of multiple births (twins, triplets, or quadruplets) and maternal age. Teenage pregnancy, also a risk factor for prematurity, has instead been decreasing over the past decade (Hamilton et al. 2015; The March of Dimes Data Book for Policy Makers 2012). However, it is very critical to remember that both very preterm infants (VPI) and extreme preterm infants (EPI) are heterogeneous, and our understanding of causal pathways that lead to successful interventions is at an early scientific stage (Rubens et al. 2014). For example, the same factors that create the biological risk in the mothers for prematurity may be the same factors that influence the inflammatory, hormonal, and neurochemical regulators that influence the mothers' caregiving capacity once their premature infant is born. Therefore, ascribing causality to biomedical, behavioral, or neuro-regulatory factors is difficult and does not allow for the complex systems understanding required to advance life course-oriented prevention and intervention strategies. In addition, despite increased access to prenatal care, there still remain limitations on our ability to prevent all moderate and late preterm birth (Requejo et al. 2013).

Estimates of the economic impact of prematurity typically factor in acute care medical costs, early childhood intervention expenditures, long-term special education, special health care, and disability costs. A report released by the Institute of Medicine in 2007 estimated that the economic burden associated with preterm birth was at least $26.2 billion in 2005, equivalent to $51,600 per infant born preterm. These estimates included $16.9 billion in medical care costs, $1.9 billion in maternal delivery costs, $611 million for early intervention services, $1.1 billion for special education services, and $5.7 billion in lost household and labor market productivity (Preterm Birth: Causes, Consequences, and Prevention 2007). Importantly, each premature/LBW baby costs employers an average of $54,149 in payments for newborn medical care during the first year of life, about twelve times that of an uncomplicated newborn (Preterm Birth: Causes, Consequences, and Prevention 2007). In addition to medical care, children born preterm are more likely to experience learning and behavior disabilities later in life, often resulting in poor test scores, grade repetition, and increased utilization of special education services. The Institute of Medicine estimates the costs of special education at $2200 per year per child (Preterm Birth: Causes, Consequences, and Prevention 2007), though for children with major neurodevelopmental disabilities, the special cost per child can exceed $50,000 per academic year.

High-quality early childhood intervention programs, however, may minimize the later need for special education and drastically reduce these additional costs (Aron and Loprest 2012). Model programs like the Infant Health Development Program (IHDP) are successful in improving educational, behavioral, and life course outcomes for preterm infants experiencing poverty, thereby decreasing children's need for special education (Aron and Loprest 2012). Economic modeling estimates the impact of comprehensive early intervention services on long-term special education costs as having a direct savings of $2.60 for every dollar invested in early intervention, early childcare services, and Early Head Start (Dmowska et al. 2016). When considering costs incurred from school dropouts, reentry to school, and additional weight on mental health-care services and the criminal justice system, the savings would likely double (Dmowska et al. 2016). Increased access to comprehensive family-centered early intervention services, therefore, may substantially reduce special education costs for children born preterm as well as long-term behavioral and social health costs.

There have been dramatic improvements in long-term survival for infants born premature and low birth weight, but developmental outcomes are far from optimized. Survival has increased dramatically with the regionalization of neonatal intensive care and the application of obstetrical and neonatal biomedical interventions for optimizing growth, lung maturity, cardiopulmonary functioning, and infection control. Overall, these efforts resulted in decreased rates of major neurodevelopmental disabilities in survivors in the 1980s and 1990s from 25–40% to 15–25%. For those born with extreme prematurity (<28 weeks of gestation) and extremely low birth weight status (<1000 g), survival has increased dramatically from <50% to >80%. However, there remain high rates of cognitive impairment and intellectual disability (ID), with over 50% of survivors requiring special education services.

Growing inequality in the United States hits families with young children very hard. Close to 50% of children younger than 5 are growing up in households living below 200% of the poverty level. Research shows that families with this level of income do not have the economic, social, educational, and community assets they need to support optimal health development (Crouter and Booth 2014). So many of the 8% premature babies, who start off life with higher levels of inherent vulnerabilities, are increasingly facing a family, social, and community landscape that cannot support their optimal development.

In addition, there is increased recognition that both moderate and late preterm births (32–36 weeks of gestation), which account for over 8% of live births or approximately 325,000 children yearly, have increased risk for long-term health, developmental, and behavioral challenges (Table 1). In spite of these biomedical advances, environmental and social conditions that can deleteriously affect the health and well-being of these already vulnerable children have not only improved in the United States; there are some indications that they have in fact worsened. Additionally, there are major gaps in accessing comprehensive family supports and quality health, early childhood, and educational and community experiences for recent cohorts of children at the highest biomedical and social risks.

The purpose of this paper is to apply a life course health development perspective in order to identify factors that promote more optimal health and developmental trajectories and the mechanisms that underlie resilience for children with prematurity from a life course health development perspective. We will describe some research findings about the role of social and environmental factors among VPI and EPI survivors in aggravating or moderating neonatal risks for suboptimal developmental and behavioral outcomes. We will also discuss available evidence from longitudinal studies of preterm children at psychosocial disadvantage and what lessons can be learned from the bidirectional impacts of prematurity and poverty. Longitudinal studies will be evaluated for health, disability, and community outcome trajectories for children with prematurity across preschool, middle childhood, adolescent, and young adult epochs. Our review will highlight important opportunities on a community level for systematically optimizing population-based prevention strategies for individuals with the double jeopardy of prematurity and social adversity and the long-term impact of failing to optimize these outcomes.

1.1 Approach

Two frameworks will inform our analysis. The first framework will be the International Classification of Functioning, Disability, and Health (ICF) model (World Health Organization

Table 1 Life course impact of prematurity

Weeks gestation	Children special health-care needs	Major neurodevelopmental disability	Educational supports	Behavioral disorders
<28	50%	20%	50%	20%
28–31	40%	15%	40%	15%
32–36	30%	10%	25%	10%
37+	20%	5%	15%	5%

Morse et al. (2009), Allen et al. (2011), Stephens and Vohr (2009), B. Vohr (2013), Saigal and Doyle (2008)

2007), which we will use to comprehensively describe the diverse outcomes occurring in preterm survivors. This framework goes beyond dichotomous classification of impairments (e.g., cerebral palsy, yes or no; intellectual disability, yes or no) and instead describes a spectrum of functioning at body structure and body function levels. For example, activities in whole-person tasks include running, reading, and dancing and participation in children's roles with peers including being on a team; participating in church, temple, or mosque; or meeting friends for a movie.

The second framework will be the *life course health development (LCHD) model,* which holds that the trajectories of children are influenced by the dynamic interaction of multiple risk, protective, and promoting factors, especially during sensitive periods of health development. From the standpoint of fetal development, due to critical human brain development in the second and third trimesters, a focus on premature infants must consider complex maternal, placental, and fetal dynamic interactions. Likewise, infant, toddler, and childhood periods of development are indelibly influenced by multilevel, multidirectional, transactional, and long-lasting interactions and critically emphasize the importance of timing. Using a LCHD framework to analyze the origins and impact of prematurity and the opportunities to optimize health development outcomes suggest the following considerations:

- Children who are born prematurely are assumed to be more developmentally vulnerable and are potentially more sensitive to a wide range and nested array of dynamic interacting influences.
- Because the alterations in evolutionarily influenced and developmentally determined adaptive mechanisms are well documented, lags in developmental processes, as well as catch-up and feed-forward processes that are specific to premature infants, may influence the nature and dynamic of their health and developmental trajectories.
- Understanding how the caregiving environment of premature infants interacts with emerging developmental capacities and how different types of exposures, levels of support, and adversity influence these emergent developmental trajectories is important if specific and targeted interventions are to be designed to modify developmental pathways based on specific risk profiles to shift the health and developmental curves for the entire population of premature infants.
- In order to implement a broader approach to improve the health and developmental outcomes of diverse preterm populations, it is important to determine what is known about the special development vulnerabilities of premature infants, how that vulnerability manifests (timing, context, specific risks), and whether the mechanisms involved are phase or period specific, modifiable, or one of cumulative risk.

2 Framing Our Inquiry and Agenda

On a population level, it is important to acknowledge the diversity of both the underlying causes and life course effects of prematurity and the gaps in proactive and comprehensive medical, developmental, and behavioral supports. This is occurring within the context of recognizing that current community systems are under-resourced to systematically audit barriers and facilitators to home visiting, medical homes, early interventions, parenting supports, and coordinated services for children with special health-care needs (CSHCN). In particular, we must go from a crisis-oriented response system for the few with the severest impairments to an optimization system for all at risk for less than optimal health development.

To address these systemic needs, the following themes will be highlighted that require increased research and policy efforts:

- We must better understand the role of and need to engage mothers and other caregivers in developmentally optimizing interactions from the neonatal period through school entry. This includes how they gain and utilize their knowledge about their child's health and development, as well as how to optimally serve as their child's first teacher and advocate. This requires understanding ways that early parent involvement and developmental activities can be part of everyday childcare tasks.

- We must explore how social environments are best tailored to maximally support positive growth, child regulatory behaviors, and developmental competencies. This includes how all children can access comprehensive preschool services and how health, developmental, and behavioral competencies are measured, monitored, and accounted for from birth to kindergarten entry. In keeping with a two-generation model of optimizing health development, close attention to caregiver physical and behavioral health and supports that help vulnerable children access quality childcare and early child education have the potential to ensure that children's social-emotional, communicative, and cognitive competencies are supported so that children enter kindergarten healthy and ready to learn.
- We must clarify the roles that preconception maternal, physical, and behavioral health play on maternal and child vulnerabilities and on epigenetic programming. This includes a better understanding of how maternal mental health stressors (depression, anxiety, isolation, and violence) increase vulnerability of children when they do not receive quality early childhood social, learning, and behavioral supports.
- We must determine the optimum and appropriate role and function of community outreach strategies that promote parental physical and behavioral health, child development, and social competencies.
- We should pursue evidence-based strategies to promote resiliency and positive adult health trajectories which include independent living, employment, and family formation while minimizing physical risk factors that increase early-onset adult chronic diseases (e.g., cardiac, pulmonary, mental illness, substance abuse) (Figs. 1 and 2).

Our cases illustrate how the interaction of positive home, preschool, and educational supports can increase thriving and reduce adverse long-term adult health conditions.

3 Risk Factors for Poor Birth Outcomes

3.1 Social Risks

An important determinant of preterm birth is social risk. Social risk factors include suboptimal home and community environments. Poverty, domestic violence, drug addiction, crime, hunger, and poor-quality housing are some of the features of social risks (Holzmann and Jørgensen 2001). Mothers who live in adverse environments often experience multiple stressors and are prone to nutritional deficiency, suboptimal prenatal care, single parenthood, and frequent tobacco and alcohol use compared to mothers from non-poor backgrounds (Jiang 2015). Several studies have also shown that rates of marijuana, cocaine, tobacco, and alcohol use are higher for women who are unmarried, unemployed, and have less than a college education, indicating that substance abuse and poverty are closely related (Huston 1991). It has been suggested that the prevalence of substance abuse, illicit drug use, and smoking among women from impoverished or low SES background is largely due to the sense of helplessness, low self-esteem, difficulties coping with stress, and pressure from coping with difficult financial situations in everyday living (Huston 1991; Weitzman et al. 2002).

When mothers receive late prenatal care (or not at all), the opportunity to identify and intervene on maternal reproductive complications or health problems that jeopardize fetal growth is limited. Also, late or no prenatal care decreases the chances of maternal access to educational and support services (such as counseling, community health, and education services) (The March of Dimes Data Book for Policy Makers 2012).

3.2 Race and Social Disadvantage

Race in the United States is closely related to SES; thus, it is not surprising to see racial discrepancies in preterm births (Table 2). African-American infants are more than 1.5 times likely than whites to be born preterm and 2.5 times likely to be very premature than their white peers

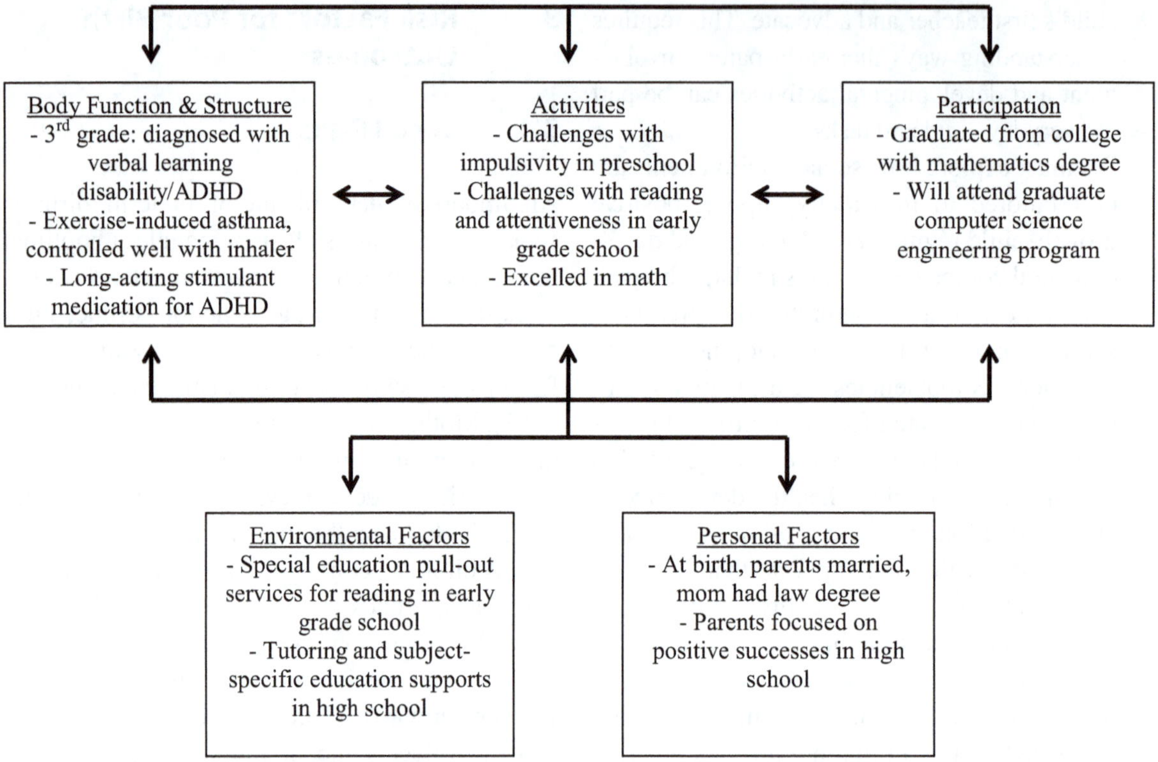

Fig. 1 Case 1. James was born late preterm at 34 weeks of gestation due to preeclampsia. His parents were married and mother completed law school. She had some challenges with impulsivity in preschool, and reported significant job-related stressors during pregnancy. The immediate newborn period was complicated by immature lungs leading to respiratory distress syndrome; however, ultimately James was discharged at 38 weeks of gestational age without a need for oxygen in the home. He was enrolled in full-day daycare and preschool since the age of 2 years. James was found to have some challenges with impulsivity in preschool, which his parents addressed with occupational and behavioral therapies. He entered kindergarten without an Individualized Education Program and in early grade school was found to struggle with reading and inattentiveness. He received a formal diagnosis of verbal learning disability and ADHD in third grade. James received special education pull-out services for reading and language arts and was starting on a long-acting stimulant medication for ADHD with the guidance of a Developmental and Behavioral Pediatrician. James received tutoring and subject-specific special education supports throughout high school. His parents focused on his positive successes, such as his strong performance in math. James went to college and pursued a math and engineering program. His adult health is complicated by exercise-induced asthma, well-controlled on an inhaler

(The March of Dimes Data Book for Policy Makers 2012). These data on preterm birth rates correlate with disparities in wealth distribution, with African-American families experiencing the lowest 3-year average median income (2003–2005) among US racial groups (Income, Poverty, and Health Insurance Coverage in the United States: 2005–2006). These data on higher rates of prematurity in women experiencing social disadvantage from poverty and minority status also hold across both developing and developed countries. The role of maternal health, educational, behavioral, and social competencies during her own childhood and how they impact on her child's health and development require systematically measuring both maternal and child allostatic load. These data can help understand what factors promote positive adaptations.

4 Prematurity and Developmental Outcomes

Prematurely born infants have long-term vulnerabilities on multiple outcomes, including physical and developmental health, behavioral and adaptive well-being, as well as social functioning. Over the past decade, much has been learned

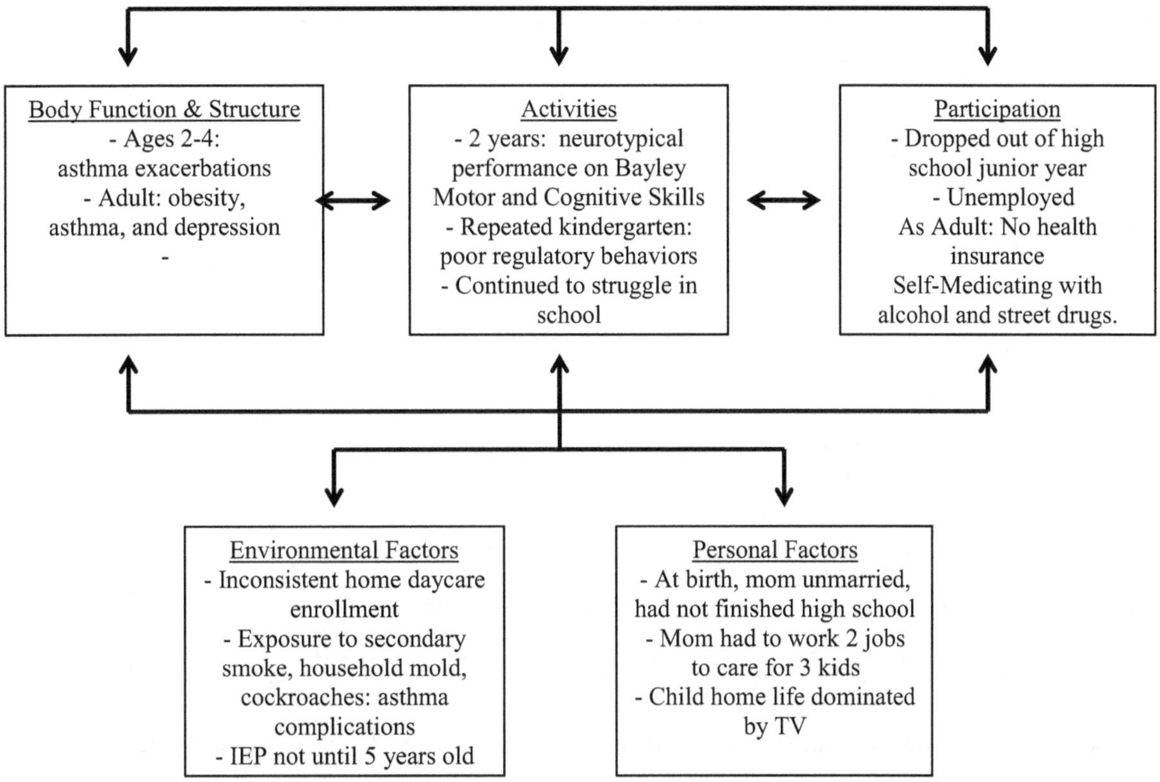

Fig. 2 Case 2. Michael was born at 28 weeks due to pre-eclampsia and preterm labor. His mother was unmarried and did not finish high school. His NICU course was complicated by intubation for the first 4 weeks of life, but he did not experience additional medical complications and was able to be slowly transitioned to room air and oral feedings. At 2 years of age, he tested within age appropriate range on the Bayley Scales of Toddler Development. Between ages 2 and 4, he experienced asthma exacerbations complicated by environmental exposures to secondary tobacco smoke, household mold, and cockroach infestation and was hospitalized about 2–3 times a year. Until the age of 5 years, Michael was enrolled in inconsistent home daycare programs and did not receive early intervention services because he was considered less than 30% delayed and thereby was deemed not eligible for services. He enrolled in kindergarten at age 5 years. However, he had to repeat kindergarten due to poor regulatory behaviors, which interfered with learning. Throughout his early childhood education, he continued to struggle in school. His home life was largely dominated by television watching while his mom worked two jobs to help care for him and his two siblings. In school he was supported by an Individual Education Plan, but did not access pharmacotherapies for ADHD. He dropped out of high school in his junior year. His adult health is complicated by obesity, asthma, and depression. Because of unemployment, he does not have health insurance. His state has not expanded Medicaid access

in the management of preterm infants and the interventions required to stabilize their immature organ system functioning.

Table 2 Rate (%) of preterm birth by maternal race and trimester of first prenatal visit

Trimester of first prenatal visit	Non-Hispanic black	Non-Hispanic white	Hispanic
First	14.7	8.3	9.7
Second	17.6	10.2	10.0
Third	16.0	10.0	10.0
None	33.4	21.7	19.8

Lang and Iams (2009)

4.1 Cerebral Palsy and Neurosensory Impairment

Table 3 highlights rates of CP and neurodevelopmental disabilities in early childhood among extremely preterm cohorts born into the medical era, which had both prenatal maternal corticosteroid and surfactant replacement interventions available. These studies demonstrate that, despite common misconceptions, the overwhelming majority of children who survive extreme prematurity do not experience CP. These data

Table 3 Major neurodevelopmental disabilities at age 2 years among survivors of ELBW in the 1990s

Study	Sample	% CP	% DD	% HI	% VI
Schmidt et al. (1996–1998)	*N* = 944 500–999 g	12	27	2	2
Mikkola et al. (1996–1998)	*N* = 206 <1000 g	14	9	4	2.6
Vohr et al. (1993–1998)	*N* = 2291 22–26 weeks	19	30	2	2
	N = 1494 27–32 weeks GA	11.6	26	1	0.7
Wood et al. (1995)	*N* = 283 22–25 weeks GA	16	30	2	2
Doyle et al. (1997)	*N* = 170 500–999 g	11	22	1.8	2.4
Mestan et al. (1998–2001)	*N* = 138 27.4 weeks GA	9.5	27.3	0.8	1.5
Shankaren et al. (1993–1999)	*N* = 246; ≤750 g ≤24 weeks; API ≤3	30	46	5	5
Wilson-Costello et al. (1990–1998)	*N* = 417 500–999 g	14	26	7	1
Fily et al. (1997)	*N* = 545 <33 weeks GA	9	4.7	0.8	0.2

DD developmental disability as defined as mental developmental index < 70, *HI* hearing impairment, *VI* visual impairment
AP1 Apgar 1 min
GA gestational age

complement population registries, which dramatically highlight the increased rate of CP among preterm survivors with decreasing gestational age. In Sweden, EPI have rates of CP at 71 per 1000, VPI 40 per 1000, and LPI (32–36 weeks) 6.4 per 1000, compared to term births at 1.1 per 1000 (Himmelmann and Uvebrant 2014).

Although there are many types of CP with varying degrees of difficulty with motor control and higher cortical function, the two most common types among preterm survivors are spastic diplegia and spastic hemiplegia. These CP syndromes affect the motor control of lower extremities (diplegia) or one side of the body (hemiplegia) and increase risks for communicative, perceptual, learning, and attention disorders (Allen et al. 2011). However, an examination of these broader outcomes for recent VPI and EPI cohorts at ages 5–8 years has not occurred in large United States regional or multicenter cohorts. Furthermore, functional measures of gross motor, manual ability, and communication activities offer more detailed descriptions of performance in everyday activities than topographical classifications of CP.

Over the past decade, there has been an increased appreciation of a wider range of motor challenges that have been characterized as developmental coordination disorders. A developmental coordination disorder is defined by acquisition and execution of coordinated motor skills below what would be expected at a given chronologic age. Difficulties are manifested as clumsiness, slowness, and inaccuracy of performance of motor skills. These motor skill deficits persistently interfere with activities of daily living appropriate to the chronologic age (*Diagnostic and Statistical Manual of Mental Disorders: DSM-5* 2013). A systematic analysis of 14 studies of children <33 weeks of gestation and <1501 g demonstrated 41% had mild developmental coordination disorder (characterized by motor standard scores 1–2 standard deviations below the mean) and 19% had moderate developmental coordination disorder (≥2 standard deviations below the mean) (Williams et al. 2010).

The second column in Table 3 reviews rates of developmental disability. These studies demonstrated rates of cognitive disability ranging between 9 and 46% among those EPI and 5% when VPI and EPI were combined. It must be emphasized that their early cognitive disabilities do not fully capture long-term educational impact.

Among ELBW survivors, there are high rates of neurosensory impairments. Severe hearing impairment ranges from 1% to 7%. This is also substantially higher than the 1 per 1000 rate in term infants. Another neurodevelopmental disability after prematurity is visual loss or blindness caused by retinopathy of prematurity (ROP). This disorder primarily affects premature infants weighing 1250 g or less and those born before 31 weeks of gestation. ROP in the current era of neonatology reaches its severest stages in those who are most immature and medically fragile. Severe visual impairment occurs in 1–2% of <27-week preemies, 20–40 times higher than in term infants. In a multicenter study on cryosurgery for ROP, increased severity of ROP was linked to motor, self-care, and communicative disability at kindergarten entry (Msall et al. 2000). Children with severe ROP, but with favorable visual acuity, had a motor disability rate of 5% compared to 43% of children with severe ROP and unfavorable visual acuity (eyesight worse than 6.4 cycles per degree on Teller Cards includes legal and total blindness). In this cohort, neonatal risk factors for severe disability involving multiple motor, self-care, and communicative domains included severe ROP, gestational age <27 weeks, birth weight <750 g, and poverty as reflected by the absence of private health insurance. A protective factor associated with a significant risk reduction for severe disability was African-American race. In middle childhood, children with severe ROP had substantial differences in cognitive and educational outcomes (Msall et al. 2004). Children with severe ROP and unfavorable visual status had a 3 in 5 chance of ID (57%) and a 3 in 5 chance of needing special education services. Children with severe ROP and favorable visual skills had a 1 in 5 chance of ID (22%) and a 1 in 4 chance of needing special education. More than 4 in 5 children with unfavorable vision (84%) but less than half of children with favorable vision (48%) were below grade level in school performance. Lower socioeconomic status (SES) and minority status were associated with lower-grade performance and utilization of special education services across both visual outcome groups. Table 3 also highlights that over 95% of extremely preterm survivors do not experience blindness.

4.2 Cognitive Outcomes

The assessment of cognitive outcomes can focus on three related domains: intelligence testing, achievement testing, and neuropsychological testing. The latter includes evaluation of specific higher cortical processes such as executive function, working memory, and information processing. Assessment of toddlers and young children combines precursors of verbal and nonverbal intelligence and cognitive processes (e.g., object permanency, symbolic play), whereas school-age assessment and beyond require more complex testing to assess problem-solving, literacy, and numeracy. There is increased recognition that Bayley II and III scores <70 predict complex cognitive and learning challenges among school-age children. However, among children with 2-year Bayley scores of 71–84 (1–2 standard deviations below the mean), they may be uniquely vulnerable to the lack of quality early childhood education and preschool experiences, especially in socially disadvantaged families (Patrianakos-Hoobler et al. 2009). Therefore, one needs to be cautious in using developmental assessments in the first 2 years of life to fully assess the spectrum of cognitive and learning disorders in all children, not only those preterm and growing up in vulnerable circumstances. The limitations in Bayley assessments are due to the dynamic processes of higher cortical functioning in childhood. Additionally, the assessment of developmental delay is intertwined with perceptual and sensory skills as well as early learning experiences and neuroplasticity. Learning, communication, and social challenges may not be apparent until there is increased complexity of tasks for academic skills and behavioral/attention regulatory capacity required by school environments.

In order to address higher-level skills at school entry, one strategy is to examine children's status at kindergarten entry. EPI cohorts born in the 1980s from Hamilton, Ontario, Melbourne, Australia, Buffalo, New York, and Chicago, Illinois, have demonstrated that 44–56% require special education resources and 21–29% have major neurodevelopmental impairments (Baek et al. 2002; Vohr and Msall 1997). These studies indicate that, in addition to planning for major developmental disabilities, resources are required to ensure success with peers in the classroom.

Gross and colleagues followed infants born very preterm and found that 41% of preterm infants were performing at grade level versus 70% of term children. These preterm children were more likely to receive special education services and three times as likely to be diagnosed with learning disabilities. In this cohort, parental marital status and educational attainment were significantly related to educational outcomes (Gross et al. 2001). Nearly three times as many preterm children achieved grade-level performance if parents were married as compared to children from single-parent homes. Thus, preterm survivors with limited family resources are further disadvantaged and vulnerable.

In Cleveland, Litt and colleagues prospectively followed 219 surviving ELBW children born between 1992 and 1995 through middle childhood and adolescence. Surviving children had a mean birth weight of 815 g, a mean GA of 26.4 weeks; and almost 1 in 5 was from multiple birth gestations. Neonatal morbidities included bronchopulmonary dysplasia in 41%, sepsis in 29%, and sonographic parenchymal brain injury in 24% (IVH3–IVH4/PVL by cranial ultrasound). Importantly, 115 term controls from the extremely preterm survivor's community classroom were assessed at 14 years. Both the extremely preterm survivors and a prospectively recruited term control group underwent a comprehensive neuropsychological battery that included reading and mathematics and neuropsychological skills of processing speed, attention, visual memory, working memory, and planning. In addition, social capital as determined by maternal education and median household income as well as gender and minority status was used as covariates when analyzing predictors of high school functioning (Litt et al. 2012).

Though major neurosensory disabilities occurred in approximately 1 in 6 of ELBW survivors (CP 15%, blindness in 0.5%, and hearing loss requiring amplification in 1.7%), a far greater number of children experienced ID and cognitive impairments. More than 1 in 6 (18%) had ID (IQ <70), a 4.5-fold greater risk than for term peers. More than 1 in 3 (37%) were cognitively impaired (IQ 71–84), a 2.3-fold greater risk than for term peers. Most importantly, almost 1 in 2 (49%) of ELBW survivors required an individualized educational plan, a fivefold higher rate than term peers. The educational resources required for managing these highly prevalent disorders would require an additional $50,000 per child during their high school years for tutoring, smaller class size, and specific curriculum modifications (Msall 2012).

Of concern were the achievement challenges of extremely preterm survivors who experienced socioeconomic adversity. These children not only demonstrated a 6.6-point lower IQ but had standard scores that were 10 points lower in reading and 8 points lower in mathematics. Importantly, both executive function and visual memory challenges were associated with academic struggles in reading and mathematics (Johnson et al. 2009, 2011; Simms et al. 2015; Wolke et al. 2015).

4.2.1 What Does This Mean?

The first lesson brings optimism: the large majority of ELBW survivors (83%) are free of neurosensory disability. Thus, unprecedented survival without major neurosensory disability can be expected. However, despite antenatal corticosteroids, surfactant replacement, improved nutrition, and infection control, the rates of CP are over 100-fold greater than for term infants. Thus, ongoing efforts in neuroprotection remain a scientific, clinical, and political priority.

The second lesson is sobering: the majority of ELBW survivors experience ongoing and serious challenges in learning, coordination, and executive function. These children benefit from quality and comprehensive interventions and special educational accommodations with continued review of how these services promote literacy, numeracy, and life skills. Litt and colleagues' outcomes suggest that evidence-based psychoeducational management strategies for executive function and specific learning disorders may be key areas for maintaining children on positive developmental trajectories (Litt et al. 2012). An important challenge in the upcoming decade is to comprehensively implement, at a population level, appropriately targeted developmental and educational optimization strategies for all preterm survivors. With more developmentally appropriate individual- and population-level supports, their neurodevelopmental risks that currently result in costly and adverse long-term physical, behavioral, educational, and social health outcomes could be dramatically reduced.

4.2.2 Behavioral/Emotional Disorders

Behavioral and emotional disorders are more prevalent among children born premature compared to their term birth peers. Meta-analysis of behavioral outcomes by Bhutta and colleagues revealed that children born preterm have a 2.6-fold risk for developing attention-deficit hyperactivity disorder (ADHD) during school age (Bhutta et al. 2002). These children are also at high risk for externalization problems such as aggression, oppositionality, and disruptive behaviors, which also are major obstacles in establishing friendships or other social relationships (e.g., lack of patience in waiting for their turn in group play) (Farooqi et al. 2007; Saigal et al. 2003). In these studies, birth weight, family function, gender, and SES predicted the behavioral adjustment of adolescents who survived ELBW status in the 1980s or the middle childhood behavioral and childhood behavioral and social adjustment of children who survived 23–25 weeks of gestation in the 1990s.

An important discovery occurred over the past decade whereby it was noted that very and extremely preterm infants were at high risk for delays in social-emotional behavioral regulation that manifested as hyperactivity, impulsivity, and difficulty with social competencies in the preschool years (Jones et al. 2013). Importantly, those children receiving appropriate quality preschool education experiences were more ready for kindergarten both cognitively and behaviorally than those who did not access these services (Arpi and Ferrari 2013; Treyvaud et al. 2013). There has also been increased recognition that late preterm survivors are at risk for regulatory and social challenges. Recent comparative investigations of toddler outcomes for LPI versus other premature infants demonstrate more externalizing, oppositional, and aggressive behaviors, suggesting a unique vulnerability for LPIs (Shah et al. 2013). Infants more prone to distress who also experienced more critical parenting styles in infancy were more likely to demonstrate externalizing behaviors at age 3, suggesting that characteristics of both infants and parents influence preterm vulnerability (Poehlmann et al. 2012).

There has also been an increased awareness of the vulnerability of adolescent and adult survivors of very and extremely preterm birth to increased rates of behavior and mental health disorders (Gardner et al. 2004). This is highlighted in Table 4. An important review by Johnson and Marlow emphasized a life course health development framework and highlighted the increased risk of attention, socio-communicative (including autism spectrum disorder), and emotional difficulties among extremely preterm survivors (Johnson et al. 2011). Importantly they highlighted rates of autism spectrum disorder (ASD) as high as 1 in 12 EPI survivors as they enter adolescence (Johnson et al. 2011). A New Jersey cohort found a rate of 1 in 20 for ASD in moderate LBW at school exit (Pinto-Martin et al. 2011). Most recently, in a large US cohort of 889 EPI survivors born in 2002–2004, Joseph and colleagues found a rate of ASD in males at age 10 of 9% and in females of 5%. Rates of ASD were 15% at 23–24 weeks of gestation, 6.5% at 25–26 weeks of gestation, and 3.4% at 27 weeks of gestation (Joseph et al. 2016).

Table 4 Adolescent and adult behavioral health outcomes

Authors	Cohort	Age at assessment	Developmental outcome
Botting et al. (1997)	1980–1983 Liverpool, England 138 VLBW and 108 matched controls	12 years	1. Any psychiatric disorder: 28% VLBW vs. 9% controls had any psychiatric disorder 2. ADHD: 23% VLBW vs. 6% controls
Dahl et al. (2006)	1978–1989 Norway 99 VLBW	13–18 years	1. VLBW adolescents report less externalizing behaviors than NBW adolescents 2. Parents of VLBW adolescents report more externalizing behaviors and emotional problems than NBW adolescents.
Grunau et al. (2004)	1981–1986 British Columbia 79 <800 g vs. 31 term	17 years	1. No differences for focus and attention 2. Significantly more parental reported internalizing, externalizing, and problem behaviors
Jong et al. (2012)	Meta-analysis of moderate and late preterm (32–36 weeks) 28 papers reviewed	Not reported (meta-analysis)	30% higher psychiatric disorders
Kunugi et al. (2001)	Meta-analysis of LBW and schizophrenia prevalence; 750 with schizophrenia and 29,000 control subjects	Not reported (meta-analysis)	LBW prevalence: 9.5% of schizophrenics and 3.9% of controls
Levy-Shiff et al. (1994)	Israel 90 VLBW and 90 NBW	13–14 years	Significantly increased hyperactive behavior among VLBW. However paternal involvement was as predictive as birth weight for hyperactivity in childhood
Saigal et al. (2006)	1977–1982 Ontario, Canada 166 ELBW and 145 NBW	22–25 years	1.3% of ELBW had autism vs. 0% controls
Saigal et al. (2007)	Ontario, Canada 149 ELBW and 133 NBW	23 years	14.1% ELBW vs. 6% on antidepressants

4.2.3 What Does This Mean?

The current understanding of the vulnerabilities of the preterm infant brain to challenges in coordination, learning, attention, and social skills offers opportunities for understanding cumulative risk and protective strategies linked to biomarkers and neurometrics. The goal of understanding what supports are needed to protect the vulnerable preterm infant brain for learning regulatory, attention, executive function, and social competencies will require increased attention to how active health and developmental experiences shape these developmental processes and what proactive informed interventions support success academically, behaviorally, and socially. Revolutionary strategies in developmental neuroscience will help inform an evidence-based approach to early identification and intervention so that children stay on track in development. In many ways, children with prematurity can help inform a shift from categorizing children's delays as leading to low learning expectations. We can examine how attention, regulatory, and social skills can be modified and lead to pathways of resilience in academic achievement and social-emotional behavioral competencies.

5 Chronic and Acute Stress

Recent studies have produced a large body of evidence that stress is significantly correlated with the occurrence of adverse birth outcomes, including prematurity and low birth weight (Graignic-Philippe et al. 2014). Prenatal stressors can include physical and psychological stress, infections, nutritional deficiencies, and drug exposures (Bock et al. 2015). In a prospective study, Killingworth-Rein et al. combined three variables into a single stress indicator comprised of state anxiety, perceived chronic stress, and life event distress. Higher scores on this aggregated factor predicted a shortened gestation and lower birth weight (Rini et al. 1999). Torche and Kleinhaus (2012) found that females who were exposed to earthquakes in early pregnancy had higher rates of preterm delivery (Torche and Kleinhaus 2012). In a study in the southern Israeli town of Sderot (4 km away from the Gaza Strip), Wainstock et al. hypothesized that the frequent exposure to rocket attacks in this community would be associated with adverse birth outcomes when compared to Kiryat Gat, a similar town without constant rocket attack exposure. Researchers found that women living in Sderot gave birth to more babies born preterm and at low birth weight, confirming the hypothesis that stress in pregnancy increases adverse birth outcomes (Wainstock et al. 2014).

A number of other studies have demonstrated an association between prenatal stress and adverse pregnancy and birth outcomes, including effects on birth weight, gestational age, and preterm birth (Bock et al. 2015). Chronic stress and acute stress may exert different effects on fetal development and perinatal outcomes. Several authors have reported lower birth weight and shortened gestation in children born to mothers exposed to chronic stress compared to acute stress (Chrousos and Gold 1992; Rini et al. 1999; Sable and Wilkinson 2000; Wadhwa et al. 1996).

Likewise, there is increasing evidence that exposure to forms of toxic stress in early life alters stress responses in adulthood. A case-controlled longitudinal study of preterm and term infants with and without medical complications demonstrated dysregulation of the hypothalamic-pituitary-adrenal axis in adult survivors of prematurity, particularly survivors also exposed to socioeconomic disadvantage (Winchester et al. 2016).

There is also a strong association between specific early pregnancy events, such as complications in the first trimester, and increased risk of preterm delivery and very preterm delivery (van Oppenraaij et al. 2009). An increased risk of low birth weight and very low birth weight was associated with first-trimester bleeding in a large prospective study (M. A. Williams et al. 1991). These adverse infant outcomes were associated with threatened miscarriage in the first trimester in another large retrospective study (Wijesiriwardana et al. 2006).

6 Epigenetic Mechanisms

Although the mechanisms of prenatal stress are not precisely known, it has been proposed that the hypothalamic-pituitary-adrenal (HPA) axis and sympathetic nervous system stress responses could lead to complications in pregnant women during pregnancy and delivery (Graignic-Philippe et al. 2014). In particular, McLean et al. (1995) suggest that high levels of neurohormones in the HPA axis as well as placental neurohormones could induce prematurity. A growing body of evidence suggests that epigenetic mechanisms induce transient and permanent alterations in gene function, resulting in altered developmental processes in the brain that result in long-term changes in emotional and cognitive behaviors (Bock et al. 2015).

The main function of the epigenome is to regulate gene transcription and compaction of DNA into the cell nucleus through mechanisms such as DNA methylation and hydroxymethylation, histone modifications, ATP-dependent chromatin remodeling, and noncoding RNAs (Provencal and Binder 2015). Prenatal stress has been shown to reduce the expression and activity of the enzyme 11-β-hydroxysteroid dehydrogenase type 2, an enzyme that converts glucocorticoids into inactive metabolites (Bock et al. 2015). An alteration in placental permeability may lead to excess exposure to maternal stress hormones, thereby promoting developmental dysregulation. Maternal intake of steroid hormones (Marciniak et al. 2011), maternal depression (O'Connor et al. 2014), and maternal anxiety (Kane et al. 2014) have been shown to alter maternal glucocorticoid levels, with a high correlation between maternal and fetal plasma glucocorticoids (Provencal and Binder 2015). In addition to affecting birth outcomes, stressful experiences in utero or during early life may also increase the risk of neurodevelopmental and behavioral disorders later in life due to alterations in epigenetic regulation (Babenko et al. 2015).

Pregnant mothers who have anxiety disorders, post-traumatic stress disorder (PTSD), depressive disorders, or major psychoses are at higher risk of adverse birth outcomes including preterm birth, low birth weight, and small-for-gestational-age infants. Mothers with bipolar disorder are at twice the risk for these adverse outcomes (MacCabe et al. 2007). Importantly, pregnant mothers with both PTSD and major depressive episode have four times the risk of having a preterm birth (Yonkers et al. 2014).

These risks occur because the brain and placenta are closely linked by a number of peptides and proteins, including oxytocin, somatostatin, neurotensin, encephalin, cortisol, insulin-like growth factor 1, vascular endothelial growth factor, and cyclic AMP response element binding factor. Individuals with mental illness often have a tendency toward coagulation and low activity of tissue plasminogen activator, potentially contributing to placental insufficiency that may lead to increased exposure of the fetus to maternal hormones. Hyperemesis gravidarum, a condition more common in women with eating disorders and anxiety than in controls, is another risk factor for pregnancy complications which may increase the risk of miscarriage, low birth weight infants, and preterm infants (Hoirisch-Clapauch et al. 2015).

7 Prenatal Stress Reduction Strategies

Intervention programs aimed at reducing stress should be considered to potentially lower the rates of unfavorable pregnancy outcomes (Wainstock et al. 2014). Feinberg et al. examined the effects of family foundation (FF), a transition to parenthood program, through a randomized control study of 148 expectant mothers. Researchers showed that the intervention significantly reduced the negative impact of maternal cortisol on birth weight, gestational age, and days in hospital in infants, thereby decreasing the risk for adverse birth outcomes (Feinberg et al. 2015). Follow-up at age 5–7 years demonstrated improved outcomes in behavior regulation and children's school adjustment (Feinberg et al. 2014). It is important to recognize the extent to which a child is affected by a mother's stress, and mental health heavily depends on moderating factors that include quality of parenting, social support, and the length and severity of the parental disorder (Howard et al. 2014). In this respect, early identification and interventions are essential (Stein et al. 2014). A recent report estimated that the long-term economic costs of perinatal mental disorders for each annual cohort exceed 8 billion euros in the UK alone (Bauer et al. 2014). Early interventions for perinatal mental disorders could produce great economic benefits and improve maternal and child physical and mental health (Howard et al. 2014) via impacting on child's regulatory behaviors and learning opportunities.

8 The Impact of Fetal Environment and Prematurity on Adult Health Outcomes

Exposure to an unfavorable environment in early life is closely associated with an increased tendency to develop adult disease. In 1992, David Barker hypothesized that the period of pregnancy and the intrauterine environment have a profound impact on risk of developing diseases like hypertension; diabetes; cardiac, pulmonary, and renal diseases; and mental illness (Capra et al. 2013). Intrauterine environment and early postnatal life are now generally accepted as important factors that may lead to increased risk for disease in adulthood (Hofman et al. 2004). In particular, low birth weight, a marker of poor fetal growth, is linked to vascular disease, hypertension, obesity, and insulin resistance (Calkins and Devaskar 2011).

Although several studies have reported an association between low birth weight and poor adult health outcomes, it remains unclear whether this association exists for children with poor fetal growth born small for gestational age as well as premature babies whose weight is appropriate for gestational age. In a retrospective study, Kaijser et al. identified subjects born preterm or with a low birth weight at four major delivery units in Sweden from 1925 to 1945. Researchers found that future risk for ischemic heart disease was most closely mediated by fetal growth restriction instead of preterm birth without growth restriction. Of note, these results came from a 1925 to 1949 birth cohort, a period when infants did not benefit from modern neonatal care. During more recent decades, infant survival has improved substantially for children born very preterm. It may not be appropriate, therefore, to generalize these results to preterm and growth-restricted infants being born today (Kaijser et al. 2008).

Babies born prematurely, whether or not they have intrauterine growth restriction (IUGR), are also at risk as adults for poor cardiovascular health outcomes (Irving et al. 2000). In a study of mothers of 72 LBW and 54 NBW infants born in Edinburgh between November 1973 and February 1975, LBW premature babies had higher adult blood pressure and fasting plasma glucose than NBW controls born at term. Babies born prematurely also had trends for an adverse metabolic profile and were at risk for hypertension and hyperglycemia as adults. Infants with IUGR were not measurably more disadvantaged than preterm infants with birth weight appropriate for gestational age (Irving et al. 2000).

A prospective follow-up study of 458 adults at age 30 in New Zealand also aimed to distinguish the relative contributions of gestation length and fetal growth to cardiovascular risk factors in adulthood. Preterm birth, rather than poor fetal growth, was shown to be the major determinant of the association between early environment and adult health outcomes; adults born preterm had increased systolic blood pressure and insulin resistance at age 30. Birth weight, independent of gestational age, was not associated with increased adult systolic blood pressure and insulin resistance, suggesting that length of gestation may be the major contribution to cardiovascular risk in adulthood (Dalziel et al. 2007).

Adult-onset insulin resistance, an early marker for type 2 diabetes, is also associated with premature birth (Hofman et al. 2004). Exposure to an adverse environment may be responsible for this reduction to insulin sensitivity, whether during intrauterine life in infants small for gestational age or a primarily adverse postnatal environment in premature infants (Hofman et al. 2004).

For the most part, mechanisms to explain the associations between intrauterine and postnatal environments and adult health outcomes are unknown. It is hypothesized that alterations to the HPA axis may explain the link between low birth weight and later increased blood pressure (Dalziel et al. 2007). Furthermore, it is theorized that earlier maturation of organ system exposure to nutritional, metabolic, hormonal, sensory, and respiratory environments at earlier time points in premature babies may also lead to abnormal development of organ systems involved in cardiovascular health (Curhan et al. 1996). Preterm infants and small-for-gestational-age infants often experience a period of "catchup growth" in the postnatal period, which may influence changes in their metabolism that are related to increased risk for these diseases (Smith and Ryckman 2015).

Increasing preterm infant survival has critical implications on the burden of adult diseases such as diabetes and cardiovascular disease. In fact, the historic trends in preterm survival and birth may be playing a critical, yet underappreciated, role in the population trend toward increasing prevalence of diabetes and cardiovascular disease (Dalziel et al. 2007).

9 Postnatal and Social Risk

Despite knowledge that supports that intervention in early childhood can positively impact disability trajectories, large gaps in services exist and disproportionally impact disadvantaged families. A 1997–2000 study looked at access to early intervention services among a population of infants aged birth to 3 years. Even in the highest risk neonates, access to community and early intervention supports was problematic and fragmented at best (>40% not enrolled in early intervention). Those toddlers with higher rates of disability were more likely to receive more services, yet a significant unmet need for services was documented among milder cases (Hintz et al. 2008).

Second, a Chicago-based cohort was followed after NICU discharge and demonstrated that less than 60% of VLBW infants living in extreme poverty (<50% federal poverty level) were receiving early intervention (EI) services despite having access to a medical home and legal advocacy. Of the 415 infants deemed not automatically eligible by EI, 95% had child and family impairments (e.g., gastrostomy, feeding delays, income <$10 K per year, parental mental or developmental disorder) that met EI inclusion criteria. This data confirms that a substantial number of infants with multiple medical and social risks do not receive ongoing developmental surveillance or early intervention services (Weiss et al. 2007).

Third, in a recent analysis of the Early Childhood Longitudinal Survey-Birth Cohort, it was found that eligibility for Part C varied widely between states (2–78%), yet the proportion of children receiving services remained consistently low (1.5–7%). There is significant state-by-state variability between eligibility criteria, yet there is also a clear national trend of insufficient enrollment for children with qualifying delays (Rosenberg et al. 2008). Given that in elementary school years 10–20% of children nationally have Individual Educational Plans, early intervention rates less than 5% reflect significant missed opportunities for secondary and tertiary prevention.

Among both VLBW and ELBW survivors, disproportionate numbers live in communities with high rates of school dropouts and poorly performing schools. This will result in barriers to accessing quality early and middle childhood educational experiences. The combination of developmental vulnerability due to LBW and preterm birth with social and family distress has shown to have cumulative impacts (Hille et al. 1994). In an 8–10-year follow-up study of infants who were the sickest and tiniest and had the most medical complications in the newborn period, Msall and colleagues found that not only were favorable vision and functional motor status at kindergarten entry associated with significantly lower rates of special education and below-grade-level educational achievement, but higher SES was also associated with positive academic and developmental outcomes. Factors strongly associated with increased risk for special education services included minority status, poverty, lack of access to a car, and Supplemental Social Security Income because of disability and poverty (Msall et al. 2004).

9.1 Adolescent and Adult Outcomes

Clinical research to date on the outcomes for preterm infants during adolescence and adulthood reveals a spectrum of strengths and challenges in physical and behavioral health, educational achievement and supports, and community participation. However, the social, educational/vocational, and independent adaptive life skills required for adulthood are inherently more quantitatively and qualitatively complex than basic developmental milestones in an infant or school achievement in middle childhood. A few crude measures of adult success have been used to examine adolescent and adult outcomes, but much work remains to unveil more meaningful multidimensional measures of adult physical and behavioral health, daily functioning, social participation, family formation, and economic well-being.

Educational attainment is a frequently examined adult outcome in the literature. The studies highlighted in Table 5 demonstrate lower rates of academic achievement, high school completion, and postsecondary education among preterm survivors. Premature survivors show high rates of

Table 5 Cognitive, executive function and academic achievement in adolescence and adulthood

Authors	Cohort	Assessment age	Developmental outcome
Botting et al. (1998)	1980–1983 Liverpool, England 138 VLBW 108 matched controls	12 years	1. VLBW lower IQ 2. Lower math and reading comprehension
Saigal et al. (2000)	1977–1982 Ontario, Canada 141 ELBW 124 matched controls	12–16 years	1. 28% reported neurosensory impairments 2. 25% of ELBW vs. 6% repeated a grade 3. 49% of ELBW vs. 10% required special education services 4. 22% ELBW required full-time educational assistance (vs. 0%) 5. Lower mean WISC-R DQ 6. Lower mean WRAT-R
Rushe et al. (2001)	1979–1980 London, England <33 weeks; 75 premature and 53 FT	14–15 years	1. No differences for tests of executive function, verbal memory, attention 2. Preterm group had impaired verbal fluency
Lefebvre et al. (2005)	1976–1981 Montreal, Canada 57 ELBW and 44 NBW	18 years	1. 56.1% ELBW vs. 84.6% controls completed HS 2. 33% vs. 9% required special education 3. Significant differences in low IQ (<85)
Hack et al. (2002)	1977–1979 Cleveland, Ohio 242 VLBW and 233 controls	20 years	1. 74% VLBW graduated HS vs. 83% NBW 2. 30% pursued secondary education vs. 53% NBW 3. 40% repeated grade vs. 27% NBW 4. Scored 1/3 SD lower on WAIS-R
Lindstrom et al. (2009)	1973–1979 Sweden 24–28 weeks vs. FT	1987–2002 national registry	71% vs. 78.6% completed 12 or more years of school
Moster et al. (2008)	1976–1983 Norway 325 preterm (23–27 weeks) vs. 828,227 FT	20–36 years	1. 67.7 preterm vs. 75.4% completed HS 2. 4.4% preterm vs. 0.1% fullterm with ID
Nomura et al. (2009) Johns Hopkins Collaborative Perinatal Study	1960–1965 Baltimore 226 near-term and 1393 FT	27–33 years	1. Near-term birth associated with lower adult educational attainment only for those living below poverty line 2. SGA had no association with educational attainment
Saigal et al. (2006)	1977–1982 Ontario, Canada 166 ELBW and 145 controls	22–25 years	No significant difference in: 1. % graduation from high school 2. Pursuit of postsecondary education

HS high school, *SD* standard deviation, *WAIS-R* Wechsler Adult Intelligence Scale-Revised, *WISC-R* Wechsler Intelligence Scale for Children-Revised, *DQ* deviation quotient, *WRAT-R* Wide Range Achievement Test-Revised, *FT* full term

need for special education supports, both in general special education services and with individual assistants, and have higher rates of grade repetition than their normal birth weight peers (Saigal et al. 2003). Furthermore, preterm survivors are less likely to graduate high school and pursue secondary education (Hack et al. 2002; Moster et al. 2008).

However, this outcome is also influenced by contextual factors. When high school graduation rates are adjusted for parental SES, there is evidence of mitigation of the difference in educational attainment. In a study by Nomura et al., it was found that in near-term survivors, only those living at incomes close to poverty line differed from full-term peers on educational attainment. The relationship between cognitive testing in adulthood and gestational age has also been significantly mitigated by socioeconomic factors (Ekeus et al. 2010). There is compelling evidence that the same risk factors disproportionately distributing premature birth to poorer, less educated mothers are also at play with the long-term outcomes of low birth weight progeny, compounding the disadvantage of the disadvantaged.

IQ outcomes have been repeatedly tested and show consistently lower scores for ELBW adults compared to matched peers. However, many studies are unable to match for socioeconomic status or parental IQ which arc highly influential mediating factors. Maternal education and income have been shown consistently to predict IQ within these cohorts, indeed often with stronger correlation coefficients than LBW status (Drillien 1961; Drillien et al. 1980). There is evidence that IQ in middle childhood is strongly predictive of IQ at adolescence, suggesting that, on this measure, there is neither increasing gap nor improved catch-up to normal birth weight peers. Alternatively, one study highlighted a widening IQ gap in later childhood (Botting et al. 1998), which may be due to the complexity of the involved intellectual task in testing at older ages or the additional components of social/emotional intelligence, which are not entirely captured by younger measures of IQ. Furthermore, studies that evaluate both educational and professional attainment do not consistently demonstrate strong correlation; 50% of preterm adults in the 1983 Dutch cohort who reported poor educational attainment during the school years held full-time employment as young adults (Hille et al. 2007). How this translates to US cohorts in the ongoing economic crisis for those without college degrees is yet unknown. Other educational outcomes, such as reading and math achievement, have shown significant gaps in core educational outcomes between VLBW and age-matched peers. However given that many term children in low-income urban or rural communities in the United States also are struggling with reading, mathematics, science, and social studies performance, it is difficult to make international comparisons.

Additional evidence demonstrates the power of socioeconomic status in modifying the effect of prematurity; Lefebvre et al. assessed the cognitive and academic achievement outcomes in early adulthood of a cohort of 82 ELBW subjects in Montreal (Lefebvre et al. 2005). There were significant differences between ELBW and NBW groups in full-scale IQ (94 versus 108), verbal IQ (93 versus 106), and performance IQ (97 versus 109). However, father's low socioeconomic status contributed significantly to the prevalence of IQ <85 (19% versus 2%, $p = 0.012$), schooling in mainstream education with a regular curriculum for age (36% versus 68%), requirement for special classes or schools (33% versus 9%), and high school graduation for those 18 years or older (56% versus 85%).

Adolescent/adult self-perceptions of health, quality of life, and overall functioning are important outcomes, which may guide our clinical understanding and facilitate improved anticipatory guidance to families of premature neonates. A socioeconomically diverse cohort of adolescents born in 1983–1984 at <801 g (Brown et al. 2003) reported themselves and was reported by their parents as having lower functional status than normal birth weight peers; however, overall these health concerns did not significantly interfere with tasks of daily living. On rating scales of externalizing and internalizing problems, however, (The Behavioral Assessment System for Children- BASC), there were no differences between preterm and comparison groups. Additionally, using a self-perception profile, which included domains of scholastic competence, social acceptance, athletic competence, and global self-worth, responses did not significantly differ. In a similar cohort of adults (born at weight <1250 g in Zurich), preterm and term controls did not differ on overall physical health

Table 6 Adult outcomes after very preterm birth

Authors	Cohort	Age at assessment	Developmental outcome
Baumgardt et al. (2012)	1983–1985 Zurich, Switzerland 52 preterm (<1250 g) 75 controls	23 years	No difference in overall self-reported quality of life
Hack et al. (2007)	1977–1979 Cleveland, Ohio 241 VLBW 232 NBW	20 years	1. No difference on self-reported health satisfaction 2. No difference on self-reported comfort (physical or emotional) 3. Decreased self-reported resiliency 4. Increased self-reported risk avoidance
Hille et al. (2008)	1983 Netherlands 959 adult survivors of prematurity (<32 weeks or VLBW)	19 years	1. 11.4% had moderate/severe problem with profession 2. ½ of individuals with moderate/severe problems in education had full-time employment
Moster et al. (2008)	1976–1983; Norway 325- 23–27 weeks 1608- 28–30 weeks 6363- 31–33 weeks 31,169- 34–36 weeks 828,227- full term	20–36 years	1. 10.6% vs. 1.7% receiving disability pension 2. Lower gestation less likely to have found life partner 3. Lower gestation less likely to have children
Saigal et al. (2006)	1977–1982 Ontario, Canada 166 ELBW and 145 controls	22–25 years	No significant difference in rates of: 1. Employment 2. Independent living 3. Married/cohabitation 4. Parenthood

VLBW very low birth weight (<1500 g), *ELBW* extremely low birth weight (<1000 g), *NBW* normal birth weight (>2500 g), *CPT* Conners' continuous performance task

or mental health scores on the Short Form 36 Health Survey (Baumgardt et al. 2012) (Table 6).

Adult males who survived prematurity rated themselves significantly lower than male term adults on the "physical functioning domain," but females did not differ from matched controls in any subset. Patterns of high risk and protective health habits varied: the use of marijuana was significantly lower among adults who survived prematurity, yet significantly more control adults practiced sports and more males exercised. The overall trend appears that adolescents and adult survivors of prematurity, by and large, consider themselves similar to normal term survivors on self-ratings of physiologic and psychological functioning. Some studies suggest that females may be more similar to full-term peers than males, suggesting that males may be somewhat more vulnerable to the long-term effects of prematurity and LBW. It deserves mentioning that the discrepancy between self-reported health and external measures of health has been reported in other health conditions; overall persons with a health condition rate the impact of that condition more positively than health professionals may surmise (Groot 2000).

Research on long-term consequences of low birth weight has focused on adolescent and early adult life – especially the negative impact of low birth weight on academic achievement, high school graduation and years of school completion, and college attendance. Low birth weight has been linked to these outcomes through the effects of low birth weight on kindergarten preparedness and weak performance in the first few years of schooling. Poor educational performance in subsequent years is negatively linked to both poor school readiness and accomplishment on subsequent school performance and the lingering health effects of low birth weight. The latter often includes not only growth and respiratory sequelae but increased vulnerability to a spectrum of neurobehavioral disorders that impact attention and mood. Importantly, buffers for these disorders include attention to caregiver mental health and child behavior health in the context of increasing school and community successes. While longer-term effects of low birth weight, mediated by poor educational performance and continued weak health, are hypothesized, little research has examined the midlife consequences of low birth weight and what factors contribute to thriving.

An additional complexity of measuring adolescent and adult outcomes is the shift of health status reporting from the parent of a premature survivor to the adolescent or adult himself/herself. In an adolescent follow-up of 99 very low birth weight babies born in Norway, there was found to be a significant discrepancy between adolescent and parental reporters, with the overall trend being parents reporting significantly more emotional and behavior problems than the adolescents reported in themselves (Dahl et al. 2006). In these later stages of follow-up, investigators must consider the inherent bias in asking parents vs. adolescents to report on health and behavior.

This research limitation can be remedied through analysis of data from two population datasets that include information on weight at birth and current health and well-being – the Wisconsin Longitudinal Study (WLS) and the Midlife in the United States: A National Study of Health and Well-Being (MIDUS). Additionally, utilizing these cohorts from the United States may help remedy the current data gap between well-tracked international cohorts and the dearth of longitudinal US data. International cohorts, which have lower rates of single parenthood and more homogenous racial ethnic and socioeconomic composition as compared to the United States, dominate the current knowledge base of long-term outcomes for premature babies. Extrapolating from their long-term outcomes likely vastly underestimates the need for social support throughout the life course in the United States. Additionally, international countries with single-payer systems tend to diagnose and provide more consistent social support for persons with disabilities when compared to the fragmented nature of health care in the United States.

The Wisconsin Longitudinal Study (WLS) is a long-term study of a random sample of 10,317 men and women who graduated from Wisconsin high school in 1957. The WLS provides an opportunity to study the life course, intergenerational transfers and relationships, family functioning, physical and mental health and well-being, and morbidity and mortality from late adolescence (in 1957) through early geriatric (in 2008). WLS data also cover social background, youthful aspirations, schooling, military service, labor market experiences, family characteristics and events, social participation, psychological characteristics, and retirement. Survey data were collected from the original respondents or their parents in 1957, 1964, 1975, 1992, and 2004 (when they were approximately at age 64 or 65). The WLS includes end-of-life data for members of the cohort who have died. Sibling and twin data for the original respondents, as well as gene-environment interactions from late adolescent to the retirement years, will permit models that separate the effects of family origins from the impact of low birth weight at retirement age.

The first national representative survey of Midlife Development in the United States (MIDUS) was conducted in 1995–1996. MIDUS is a 1994 national sample survey of 7189 randomly chosen adults ages 25–74 years, as well as 1914 respondents to a separate nationally representative sample of twin pairs. The wide age range of the sample was intended to permit comparisons on persons in their early adult life to those in midlife and old age. The survey permits the assessment of many psychological factors such as personality traits, sense of control, and goal commitments and their linkages to marital status, family structure, socioeconomic standing, social participation, social support, employment status, health status, and health-care utilization. MIDUS respondent follow-ups were conducted from 2002 to 2006, and there were a third round of interviews from 2006 to 2011. This dataset, including sibling data, will permit models that separate the effects of family origins and early life experiences from the impact of low birth weight at retirement age and beyond.

10 Conclusion

The interdependent challenges of prematurity and socioeconomic risk create numerous hurdles for achieving optimal physical, developmental, and emotional health. With over 50,000 surviving extremely preterm and very preterm infants per year in the United States, we have the equivalent of an ongoing annual polio crisis in the pre-vaccination era. Not only are many of these children growing up in families that are strapped for material resources, services and time, but our current early intervention and preschool systems are not delivering child health, developmental, and behavioral supports on a population basis. Therefore, there is decreased likelihood that the 325,000 late preterm survivors who annually enter kindergarten will be healthy and ready to learn. Nor will they stay on track during the first three grades, achieving adequate levels of literacy, numeracy, information handling, and social participation; they will need to succeed in school and life. As their development lags and their academic performance falters, there is too often a response of educational systems, especially during the middle school years, to divert children by using grade repetition, expulsions, and nonevidence-based remediation that only increase the likelihood that the child will leave school or be classified with behavioral problems. Importantly, unlike their middle-class and affluent counterparts, low-income children with a spectrum of neurodevelopmental dysfunction will have less access to high-quality medical care, appropriately targeted and responsive parent-child interactions, quality educational accommodations and explicit strategies for promoting basic competencies, and extracurricular activities.

Although potentially detrimental to a child's future, his/her gestational age and birth weight are rarely the major determining factors when long-term educational, social, and behavioral outcomes are considered. In this chapter we have examined several research studies that emphasized the importance of family, social, and economic environmental factors, which can either aggravate or moderate neonatal risks caused by premature birth. Much is to be gained by attention to how adversity impacts allostatic load, and through epigenetic mechanisms and complex protective buffers of parenting, health promotion, and social supports, leads to long-term outcomes of thriving across physical, behavioral, and social health outcomes. With so much to lose while living under suboptimal conditions, it is of critical importance that both health and educational professionals create systems for enhancing access to early childhood learning experiences, parenting supports, quality preschool education services, and biopsychosocial strategies in middle childhood to help children achieve basic educational, behavioral, and social competencies and adolescent supports of mentoring, preparation for independent living, and proactive behavioral health strategies for stress, time management, mood disorders, and self-efficacy. We need more research about how to spread and scale successful biopsychosocial health development strategies at a community level to insure that VLBW and ELBW survivors do not miss out on the critical experiences, which have potential to compensate for birth disadvantage, and are critical for long-term adult success. A summary of the gaps and recommendations for increasing research in life course health development after prematurity follows.

Research in life course health development for children who survive prematurity has made the following advances:

1. *Medical advances in pregnancy*: Over the past decades, there has been improved management of high-risk pregnancy disorders such as hypertension, diabetes, multiple gestation, intrauterine growth restriction, prenatal infections, and fetal malformations. There has been growing awareness that women's health involving the use of tobacco, alcohol, illicit drugs, anticonvulsants, and antidepressants has subtle neurobehavioral consequences on child development. Additionally, society has

had greater recognition that poverty, social adversity involving basic resources as well as lack of partner/family supports, previous preterm birth, minority status, limited education, and low health literacy increase the risk of low birth weight, prematurity, and early childhood health and developmental impairments.

2. *Medical advances in the neonatal period*: Over the last decades, there has been remarkable improvement in the management of premature labor and delivery. In particular, the widespread screening for and treatment of Group B *Streptococcus* colonization and the use of maternal corticosteroids when preterm labor presents have had marked improvements in premature survival and sequelae of neonatal infections. We have had improved resuscitation and neonatal transport to tertiary care centers. Throughout the vulnerable neonatal course, improved respiratory support (the use of positive pressure and noninvasive ventilator techniques after surfactant), evidence-based nutritional interventions, and infection control management have improved neonatal survival.

Although there is increased recognition that very and extremely preterm survivors experience a variety of health (e.g., growth, pulmonary), neurological (e.g., sensory impairments, seizures), neurodevelopmental (e.g., CP, ID, ASD), and learning and behavior impairment, the population-level risks have not been systematically measured. In order to improve life course health development, we propose seven theme research agenda.

11 Recommendations for an After Prematurity Life Course Health Disparities Research Agenda

1. Establish national registries.

   It is imperative to create national registries for children from birth to 5 years old who are at highest risk of CP and neurodevelopmental disabilities such as intellectual disability, neurosensory disability, and autism spectrum disorders. These registries would not only include preterm infants but also include term infants with history of critical illness from cardiac, pulmonary, infectious, neurological, or genetic disorders. Such registries would allow for the investigation of diverse interventions and link health, early intervention, special education, and rehabilitation services to long-term outcomes across the life course. Most importantly attention must be paid to maternal health, adversity, and mental health. Registries ought to include placental samples as well as cord blood and newborn screening blood spots, in order to allow for the evaluation of early biomarkers of toxic stress during early childhood.

2. Build population-based datasets.

   To understand health across the life course, it is imperative to create population-based datasets which originate at delivery and during newborn primary care visits. We must be able to link information on birth certificates with early childhood health, developmental, and educational outcomes through collaborative arrangements between public health, regional neonatal follow-up, early intervention, and district-wide educational testing. We should use these population databases to engage in ongoing health and developmental surveillance of all children with all degrees of prematurity requiring neonatal intensive care, especially those with seizures, neonatal encephalopathy, congenital heart disease, malformation requiring surgery, and abnormalities in newborn genetic and hearing screening. We should model our US efforts on the Longitudinal Study of Australian Children to understand diverse trajectories of health, development, and behavior for those with and without special health-care needs.

   Preterm infants need the establishment of longitudinal data collection registries that can collect information that is similar to the National Survey of Children's Health and NHIS disability follow-up studies. We must determine the risk factors for trajectories of positive and negative outcomes across cohorts of middle childhood, adolescence, and adulthood for sequential preterm survivors who were <28 weeks of gestation, 29–31 weeks of gestation, 32–36 weeks of gestation, and term gestation. Only with informed, collaborative, and comprehensive life course health development registries will we determine ways to support resiliency among preterm offspring of high-risk mothers with respect to health, developmental, educational, and social outcomes over the life course.

3. Expansion and evaluation of comprehensive health and developmental surveillance interventions on a population level.

   We need to improve population surveillance for children exposed to high-risk maternal conditions such as hypertension, diabetes, obesity, asthma, seizure disorders, depression, ADHD, anxiety, and maternal use of tobacco, alcohol, and illegal substances. In the setting of these risk factors, we must evaluate what factors promote maternal and child resiliency and promote positive newborn and developmental outcomes. We must understand which factors mitigate the negative effect of these exposures on growth, obesity, developmental delays, and regulatory disorders. We should seek to determine the impact of positive parenting, quality early child education (early intervention, head start preschool programming), and pediatric medical homes especially using neonatal and epigenetic biomarkers.

   Surveillance should extend beyond the neonatal period into preschool (ages 2–4 years) to identify young children who lack the basic numeracy, literacy, and social and emotional maturity needed to enter kindergarten ready to learn. Kindergarten is also a key transition for measuring health and developmental status, yet there are no systematic screening modalities in place at kindergarten entry across diverse biomedical and social risks.

4. Integration of twenty-first-century technologies to improve care coordination and integrated health and engage families in time-efficient interventions.

   Diagnostic tools such as fidgety movements are shown to have high reliability in detection of future motor delays; texting has been shown to improve parental engagement with early childhood development; and telemedicine has enabled the delivery of highly specialized care to remote or mobility-challenged populations. These growing technologies, increasingly available across socioeconomic populations, must be fully embraced and leveraged for population surveillance and therapeutic interventions.

5. Shift research methodology from antiquated methods studying individuals and parent-child dyads to novel techniques examining clusters of families and communities.

   Increasingly we need to better understand the power of parent-child interactions on determining developmental trajectories in conjunction with genetic and epigenetic biomarkers. Furthermore, siblings certainly impact health and development of one another, yet most research fails to consider the contribution of sibling factors. We must seek to develop and improve our research modalities, which look beyond a single child as the unit of measure and examine interrelatedness among family and community factors.

6. Research on impacting parent-child interventions.

   A critical need is to formally evaluate the caregiving environment of premature infants and determine how cumulative parent-child interactions impact the child's developmental capacities and parental health and well-being. Examine developmental activities as a part of everyday childcare tasks to promote early parent involvement and positive health and regulatory trajectories.

7. Determine what types of interventions effectively impact maternal mental health in the setting of adversities.

It is incompletely known how maternal mental health stressors (depression, anxiety, isolation, and violence) increase vulnerability of children when they do not receive quality early childhood social learning and behavioral supports. Strategies for integrating maternal and child physical and behavioral health have the potential to increase resilience for high-risk populations.

By combining themes from this research agenda to populations involving life course health development and the ICF model for promoting health, functioning, and participation, we have the opportunities to improve thriving after prematurity and measure our impact on long-term health, education, and community costs.

Acknowledgments This work was supported in part by NIH NINR03095 (Sullivan, Msall). Dr. Msall was also supported in part by NIH/NICHD Grant P30 HD0544275 JP Kennedy Intellectual and Developmental Disabilities Research Center and HRSA-DHHS T73 MC 11047 Leadership Education in Neurodevelopmental and Related Disorders Training Program (LEND).

References

Allen, M. C., Cristofalo, E. A., & Kim, C. (2011). Outcomes of preterm infants: Morbidity replaces mortality. *Clinics in Perinatology, 38*(3), 441–454. doi:10.1016/j.clp.2011.06.011.

Aron, L., & Loprest, P. (2012). Disability and the education system. *The Future of Children, 22*(1), 97–122.

Arpi, E., & Ferrari, F. (2013). Preterm birth and behaviour problems in infants and preschool-age children: A review of the recent literature. *Developmental Medicine and Child Neurology, 55*(9), 788–796. doi:10.1111/dmcn.12142.

Babenko, O., Kovalchuk, I., & Metz, G. A. (2015). Stress-induced perinatal and transgenerational epigenetic programming of brain development and mental health. *Neuroscience and Biobehavioral Reviews, 48*, 70–91. doi:10.1016/j.neubiorev.2014.11.013.

Baek, Y., Vohr, B. R., Alksninis, B., Cashore, W. J., Hogan, D. P., & Msall, M. E. (2002). Kindergarten readiness in very low birth weight (VLBW) children. *Pediatric Research, 51*(4), 293A.

Bauer, A., Parsonage, M., Knapp, M., Iemmi, V., & Adelaja, B. (2014). *The costs of perinatal mental health problems*. London: Cemtre for Mental Health and London School of Economics.

Baumgardt, M., Bucher, H. U., Mieth, R. A., & Fauchere, J. C. (2012). Health-related quality of life of former very preterm infants in adulthood. *Acta Paediatrica, 101*(2), e59–e63. doi:10.1111/j.1651-2227.2011.02422.x.

Bhutta, A. T., Cleves, M. A., Casey, P. H., Cradock, M. M., & Anand, K. J. (2002). Cognitive and behavioral outcomes of school-aged children who were born preterm: A meta-analysis. *JAMA, 288*(6), 728–737.

Bock, J., Wainstock, T., Braun, K., & Segal, M. (2015). Stress in utero: Prenatal programming of brain plasticity and cognition. *Biological Psychiatry*. doi:10.1016/j.biopsych.2015.02.036.

Botting, N., Powls, A., Cooke, R. W., & Marlow, N. (1998). Cognitive and educational outcome of very-low-birthweight children in early adolescence. *Developmental Medicine and Child Neurology, 40*(10), 652–660.

Brown, K. J., Kilbride, H. W., Turnbull, W., & Lemanek, K. (2003). Functional outcome at adolescence for infants less than 801 g birth weight: Perceptions of children and parents. *Journal of Perinatology, 23*(1), 41–47. doi:10.1038/sj.jp.7210850.

Calkins, K., & Devaskar, S. U. (2011). Fetal origins of adult disease. *Current Problems in Pediatric and Adolescent Health Care, 41*(6), 158–176. doi:10.1016/j.cppeds.2011.01.001.

Capra, L., Tezza, G., Mazzei, F., & Boner, A. L. (2013). The origins of health and disease: The influence of maternal diseases and lifestyle during gestation. *Italian Journal of Pediatrics, 39*, 7. doi:10.1186/1824-7288-39-7.

Chrousos, G. P., & Gold, P. W. (1992). The concepts of stress and stress system disorders. Overview of physical and behavioral homeostasis. *JAMA, 267*(9), 1244–1252.

Crouter, A. C., & Booth, A. (Eds). (2014). *Work-family challenges for low-income parents and their children*. Routledge. Abingdon, UK.

Curhan, G. C., Willett, W. C., Rimm, E. B., Spiegelman, D., Ascherio, A. L., & Stampfer, M. J. (1996). Birth weight and adult hypertension, diabetes mellitus, and obesity in US men. *Circulation, 94*(12), 3246–3250.

Dahl, L. B., Kaaresen, P. I., Tunby, J., Handegard, B. H., Kvernmo, S., & Ronning, J. A. (2006). Emotional, behavioral, social, and academic outcomes in adolescents born with very low birth weight. *Pediatrics, 118*(2), e449–e459. doi:10.1542/peds.2005-3024.

Dalziel, S. R., Parag, V., Rodgers, A., & Harding, J. E. (2007). Cardiovascular risk factors at age 30 following pre-term birth. *International Journal of Epidemiology, 36*(4), 907–915. doi:10.1093/ije/dym067.

Diagnostic and Statistical Manual of Mental Disorders: DSM-5. (2013). (5th ed.). Washington, DC: American Psychiatric Association.

Dmowska, A., Andrews, B., Schreiber, M., & Msall, M. E. (2016). Preterm survivors: Community support to lessen health disparities. In J. Merrick & L. Rubin (Eds.), *Environmental health disparities: Costs and benefits of breaking the cycle*. Hauppauge, NY: Nova Publishers.

Drillien, C. M. (1961). A longitudinal study of the growth and development of prematurely and maturely born children. VIII. Morbidity in the age period 2-5 years. *Archives of Disease in Childhood, 36*, 515–525.

Drillien, C. M., Thomson, A. J., & Burgoyne, K. (1980). Low-birthweight children at early school-age: A longitudinal study. *Developmental Medicine and Child Neurology, 22*(1), 26–47.

Ekeus, C., Lindstrom, K., Lindblad, F., Rasmussen, F., & Hjern, A. (2010). Preterm birth, social disadvantage, and cognitive competence in Swedish 18- to 19-year-old men. *Pediatrics, 125*(1), e67–e73. doi:10.1542/peds.2008-3329.

Farooqi, A., Hagglof, B., Sedin, G., Gothefors, L., & Serenius, F. (2007). Mental health and social competencies of 10- to 12-year-old children born at 23 to 25 weeks of gestation in the 1990s: A Swedish national prospective follow-up study. *Pediatrics, 120*(1), 118–133. doi:10.1542/peds.2006-2988.

Feinberg, M. E., Jones, D. E., Roettger, M. E., Solmeyer, A., & Hostetler, M. L. (2014). Long-term follow-up of a randomized trial of family foundations: Effects on children's emotional, behavioral, and school adjustment. *Journal of Family Psychology, 28*(6), 821–831. doi:10.1037/fam0000037.

Feinberg, M. E., Roettger, M. E., Jones, D. E., Paul, I. M., & Kan, M. L. (2015). Effects of a psychosocial couple-based prevention program on adverse birth outcomes. *Maternal and Child Health Journal, 19*(1), 102–111. doi:10.1007/s10995-014-1500-5.

Gardner, F., Johnson, A., Yudkin, P., Bowler, U., Hockley, C., Mutch, L., et al. (2004). Behavioral and emotional adjustment of teenagers in mainstream school who were born before 29 weeks' gestation. *Pediatrics, 114*(3), 676–682. doi:10.1542/peds.2003-0763-L.

Graignic-Philippe, R., Dayan, J., Chokron, S., Jacquet, A. Y., & Tordjman, S. (2014). Effects of prenatal stress on fetal and child development: A critical literature review. *Neuroscience and Biobehavioral Reviews, 43*, 137–162. doi:10.1016/j.neubiorev.2014.03.022.

Groot, W. (2000). Adaptation and scale of reference bias in self-assessments of quality of life. *Journal of Health Economics, 19*(3), 403–420.

Gross, S. J., Mettelman, B. B., Dye, T. D., & Slagle, T. A. (2001). Impact of family structure and stability on academic outcome in preterm children at 10 years of age. *The Journal of Pediatrics, 138*(2), 169–175. doi:10.1067/mpd.2001.111945.

Hack, M., Flannery, D. J., Schluchter, M., Cartar, L., Borawski, E., & Klein, N. (2002). Outcomes in young adulthood for very-low-birth-weight infants. *The New England Journal of Medicine, 346*(3), 149–157. doi:10.1056/NEJMoa010856.

Hamilton, B. E., Martin, J. A., Osterman, M. J., Curtin, S. C., & Matthews, T. J. (2015). Births: Final data for 2014. *National Vital Statistics Reports, 64*(12), 1–64. Retrieved from http://www.ncbi.nlm.nih.gov/pubmed/26727629.

Hille, E. T., den Ouden, A. L., Bauer, L., van den Oudenrijn, C., Brand, R., & Verloove-Vanhorick, S. P. (1994). School performance at nine years of age in very premature and very low birth weight infants: Perinatal risk factors and predictors at five years of age. Collaborative project on preterm and small for gestational age (POPS) infants in The Netherlands. *The Journal of Pediatrics, 125*(3), 426–434.

Hille, E. T., Weisglas-Kuperus, N., van Goudoever, J. B., Jacobusse, G. W., Ens-Dokkum, M. H., de Groot, L., et al. (2007). Functional outcomes and participation in young adulthood for very preterm and very low birth weight infants: The Dutch project on preterm and small for gestational age infants at 19 years of age. *Pediatrics, 120*(3), e587–e595. doi:10.1542/peds.2006-2407.

Himmelmann, K., & Uvebrant, P. (2014). The panorama of cerebral palsy in Sweden. XI. Changing patterns in the birth-year period 2003-2006. *Acta Paediatrica, 103*(6), 618–624. doi:10.1111/apa.12614.

Hintz, S. R., Kendrick, D. E., Vohr, B. R., Poole, W. K., & Higgins, R. D. (2008). Community supports after surviving extremely low-birth-weight, extremely preterm birth: Special outpatient services in early childhood. *Archives of Pediatrics & Adolescent Medicine, 162*(8), 748–755. doi:10.1001/archpedi.162.8.748.

Hofman, P. L., Regan, F., Jackson, W. E., Jefferies, C., Knight, D. B., Robinson, E. M., et al. (2004). Premature birth and later insulin resistance. *The New England Journal of Medicine, 351*(21), 2179–2186. doi:10.1056/NEJMoa042275.

Hoirisch-Clapauch, S., Brenner, B., & Nardi, A. E. (2015). Adverse obstetric and neonatal outcomes in women with mental disorders. *Thrombosis Research, 135*(Suppl 1), S60–S63. doi:10.1016/s0049-3848(15)50446-5.

Holzmann, R., & Jørgensen, S. (2001). Social risk management: A new conceptual framework for social protection, and beyond. *International Tax and Public Finance, 8*(4), 529–556. doi:10.1023/A:1011247814590.

Howard, L. M., Piot, P., & Stein, A. (2014). No health without perinatal mental health. *The Lancet, 384*(9956), 1723–1724. doi:10.1016/S0140-6736(14)62040-7.

Huston, A. C. (1991). *Children in poverty : Child development and public policy*. Cambridge, NY: Cambridge University Press.

Income, Poverty, and Health Insurance Coverage in the United States: 2005 (2006). In U. S. C. Bureau (Ed.).

Irving, R. J., Belton, N. R., Elton, R. A., & Walker, B. R. (2000). Adult cardiovascular risk factors in premature babies. *Lancet, 355*(9221), 2135–2136. doi:10.1016/s0140-6736(00)02384-9.

Jiang Y. E. M., & Skinner C. (2015). Basic facts about low-income children: Children under 3 Years, 2013 (trans: D. o. H. P. Management). Columbia University: National Center for Children in Poverty.

Johnson, S., Hennessy, E., Smith, R., Trikic, R., Wolke, D., & Marlow, N. (2009). Academic attainment and special educational needs in extremely preterm children at 11 years of age: The EPICure study. *Archives of Disease in Childhood. Fetal and Neonatal Edition, 94*(4), F283–F289. doi:10.1136/adc.2008.152793.

Johnson, S., Wolke, D., Hennessy, E., & Marlow, N. (2011). Educational outcomes in extremely preterm children: Neuropsychological correlates and predictors of attainment. *Developmental Neuropsychology, 36*(1), 74–95. doi:10.1080/87565641.2011.540541.

Jones, K. M., Champion, P. R., & Woodward, L. J. (2013). Social competence of preschool children born very preterm. *Early Human Development, 89*(10), 795–802. doi:10.1016/j.earlhumdev.2013.06.008.

Joseph, R. M., O'Shea, T. M., Allred, E. N., Heeren, T., Hirtz, D., Paneth, N., Leviton, A., & Kuban, K. C. (2016). Prevalence and associated features of autism spectrum disorder in extremely low gestational age newborns at age 10 years. *Autism Research, 10*(2), 224–232. doi:10.1002/aur.1644.

Kaijser, M., Bonamy, A. K., Akre, O., Cnattingius, S., Granath, F., Norman, M., et al. (2008). Perinatal risk factors for ischemic heart disease: Disentangling the roles of birth weight and preterm birth. *Circulation, 117*(3), 405–410. doi:10.1161/circulationaha.107.710715.

Kane, H. S., Dunkel Schetter, C., Glynn, L. M., Hobel, C. J., & Sandman, C. A. (2014). Pregnancy anxiety and prenatal cortisol trajectories. *Biological Psychology, 100*, 13–19. doi:10.1016/j.biopsycho.2014.04.003.

Lang, C. T., & Iams, J. D. (2009). Goals and strategies for prevention of preterm birth: An obstetric perspective. *Pediatric Clinics of North America, 56*(3), 537–563.

Lefebvre, F., Mazurier, E., & Tessier, R. (2005). Cognitive and educational outcomes in early adulthood for infants weighing 1000 grams or less at birth. *Acta Paediatrica, 94*(6), 733–740. doi:10.1080/08035250510025987.

Litt, J. S., Gerry Taylor, H., Margevicius, S., Schluchter, M., Andreias, L., & Hack, M. (2012). Academic achievement of adolescents born with extremely low birth weight. *Acta Paediatrica, 101*(12), 1240–1245. doi:10.1111/j.1651-2227.2012.02790.x.

MacCabe, J. H., Martinsson, L., Lichtenstein, P., Nilsson, E., Cnattingius, S., Murray, R. M., et al. (2007). Adverse pregnancy outcomes in mothers with affective psychosis. *Bipolar Disorders, 9*(3), 305–309. doi:10.1111/j.1399-5618.2007.00382.x.

Marciniak, B., Patro-Malysza, J., Poniedzialek-Czajkowska, E., Kimber-Trojnar, Z., Leszczynska-Gorzelak, B., & Oleszczuk, J. (2011). Glucocorticoids in pregnancy. *Current Pharmaceutical Biotechnology, 12*(5), 750–757.

McLean, M., Bisits, A., Davies, J., Woods, R., Lowry, P., & Smith, R. (1995). A placental clock controlling the length of human pregnancy. *Nature Medicine, 1*(5), 460–463.

Morse, S. B., Zheng, H., Tang, Y., & Roth, J. (2009). Early school-age outcomes of late preterm infants. *Pediatrics, 123*(4), e622–e629. doi:10.1542/peds.2008-1405.

Moster, D., Lie, R. T., & Markestad, T. (2008). Long-term medical and social consequences of preterm birth. *The New England Journal of Medicine, 359*(3), 262–273. doi:10.1056/NEJMoa0706475.

Msall, M. E. (2012). Academic achievement after extreme prematurity: Optimizing outcomes for vulnerable children in times of uncertainty. *Acta Paediatrica, 101*(12), 1196–1197. doi:10.1111/apa.12038.

Msall, M. E., Phelps, D. L., DiGaudio, K. M., Dobson, V., Tung, B., McClead, R. E., et al. (2000). Severity of neonatal retinopathy of prematurity is predictive of neurodevelopmental functional outcome at age 5.5 years. Behalf of the Cryotherapy for retinopathy of prematurity cooperative group. *Pediatrics, 106*(5), 998–1005.

Msall, M. E., Phelps, D. L., Hardy, R. J., Dobson, V., Quinn, G. E., Summers, C. G., et al. (2004). Educational and social competencies at 8 years in children with threshold retinopathy of prematurity in the CRYO-ROP multicenter study. *Pediatrics, 113*(4), 790–799.

O'Connor, T. G., Monk, C., & Fitelson, E. M. (2014). Practitioner review: Maternal mood in pregnancy and child development--implications for child psychology and psychiatry. *Journal of Child Psychology and Psychiatry, 55*(2), 99–111. doi:10.1111/jcpp.12153.

van Oppenraaij, R. H., Jauniaux, E., Christiansen, O. B., Horcajadas, J. A., Farquharson, R. G., & Exalto, N. (2009). Predicting adverse obstetric outcome after early pregnancy events and complications: A review. *Human Reproduction Update, 15*(4), 409–421. doi:10.1093/humupd/dmp009.

Patrianakos-Hoobler, A. I., Msall, M. E., Marks, J. D., Huo, D., & Schreiber, M. D. (2009). Risk factors affecting school readiness in premature infants with respiratory distress syndrome. *Pediatrics, 124*(1), 258–267. doi:10.1542/peds.2008-1771.

Pinto-Martin, J. A., Levy, S. E., Feldman, J. F., Lorenz, J. M., Paneth, N., & Whitaker, A. H. (2011). Prevalence of autism spectrum disorder in adolescents born weighing <2000 grams. *Pediatrics, 128*(5), 883–891. doi:10.1542/peds.2010-2846.

Poehlmann, J., Hane, A., Burnson, C., Maleck, S., Hamburger, E., & Shah, P. E. (2012). Preterm infants who are prone to distress: Differential effects of parenting on 36-month behavioral and cognitive outcomes. *Journal of Child Psychology and Psychiatry, 53*(10), 1018–1025. doi:10.1111/j.1469-7610.2012.02564.x.

Preterm Birth: Causes, Consequences, and Prevention (2007). In R. E. Behrman, & A. S. Butler (Eds.). Washington, DC: Committee on Understanding Premature Birth and Assuring Healthy Outcomes, Institute of Medicine of the Academies.

Provencal, N., & Binder, E. B. (2015). The effects of early life stress on the epigenome: From the womb to adulthood and even before. *Experimental Neurology, 268*, 10–20. doi:10.1016/j.expneurol.2014.09.001.

Requejo, J., Merialdi, M., Althabe, F., Keller, M., Katz, J., & Menon, R. (2013). Born too soon: Care during pregnancy and childbirth to reduce preterm deliveries and improve health outcomes of the preterm baby. *Reproductive Health, 10*(Suppl 1), S4. doi:10.1186/1742-4755-10-s1-s4.

Rini, C. K., Dunkel-Schetter, C., Wadhwa, P. D., & Sandman, C. A. (1999). Psychological adaptation and birth outcomes: The role of personal resources, stress, and sociocultural context in pregnancy. *Health Psychology, 18*(4), 333–345.

Rosenberg, S. A., Zhang, D., & Robinson, C. C. (2008). Prevalence of developmental delays and participation in early intervention services for young children. *Pediatrics, 121*(6), e1503–e1509. doi:10.1542/peds.2007-1680.

Rubens, C. E., Sadovsky, Y., Muglia, L., Gravett, M. G., Lackritz, E., & Gravett, C. (2014). Prevention of preterm birth: Harnessing science to address the global epidemic. *Science Translational Medicine, 6*(262), 262sr265. doi:10.1126/scitranslmed.3009871.

Sable, M. R., & Wilkinson, D. S. (2000). Impact of perceived stress, major life events and pregnancy attitudes on low birth weight. *Family Planning Perspectives, 32*(6), 288–294.

Saigal, S., & Doyle, L. W. (2008). An overview of mortality and sequelae of preterm birth from infancy to adulthood. *Lancet, 371*(9608), 261–269. doi:10.1016/s0140-6736(08)60136-1.

Saigal, S., Pinelli, J., Hoult, L., Kim, M. M., & Boyle, M. (2003). Psychopathology and social competencies of adolescents who were extremely low birth weight. *Pediatrics, 111*(5 Pt 1), 969–975.

Shah, P. E., Robbins, N., Coelho, R. B., & Poehlmann, J. (2013). The paradox of prematurity: The behavioral vulnerability of late preterm infants and the cognitive susceptibility of very preterm infants at 36 months post-term. *Infant Behavior & Development, 36*(1), 50–62. doi:10.1016/j.infbeh.2012.11.003.

Simms, V., Gilmore, C., Cragg, L., Clayton, S., Marlow, N., & Johnson, S. (2015). Nature and origins of mathematics difficulties in very preterm children: A different etiology than developmental dyscalculia. *Pediatric Research, 77*(2), 389–395. doi:10.1038/pr.2014.184.

Smith, C. J., & Ryckman, K. K. (2015). Epigenetic and developmental influences on the risk of obesity, diabetes, and metabolic syndrome. *Diabetes Metab Syndr Obes, 8*, 295–302. doi:10.2147/dmso.s61296.

Stein, A., Pearson, R. M., Goodman, S. H., Rapa, E., Rahman, A., McCallum, M., et al. (2014). Effects of perinatal mental disorders on the fetus and child. *Lancet, 384*(9956), 1800–1819. doi:10.1016/s0140-6736(14)61277-0.

Stephens, B. E., & Vohr, B. R. (2009). Neurodevelopmental outcome of the premature infant. *Pediatric Clinics of North America, 56*(3), 631–646., Table of Contents. doi:10.1016/j.pcl.2009.03.005.

The March of Dimes data book for policy makers: Maternal, infant, and child health in the United States (2012). Washington, DC: March of Dimes.

Torche, F., & Kleinhaus, K. (2012). Prenatal stress, gestational age and secondary sex ratio: The sex-specific effects of exposure to a natural disaster in early pregnancy. *Human Reproduction, 27*(2), 558–567. doi:10.1093/humrep/der390.

Treyvaud, K., Ure, A., Doyle, L. W., Lee, K. J., Rogers, C. E., Kidokoro, H., et al. (2013). Psychiatric outcomes at age seven for very preterm children: Rates and predictors. *Journal of Child Psychology and Psychiatry, 54*(7), 772–779. doi:10.1111/jcpp.12040.

Vohr, B. (2013). Long-term outcomes of moderately preterm, late preterm, and early term infants. *Clinics in Perinatology, 40*(4), 739–751. doi:10.1016/j.clp.2013.07.006.

Vohr, B. R., & Msall, M. E. (1997). Neuropsychological and functional outcomes of very low birth weight infants. *Seminars in Perinatology, 21*(3), 202–220.

Wadhwa, P. D., Dunkel-Schetter, C., Chicz-DeMet, A., Porto, M., & Sandman, C. A. (1996). Prenatal psychosocial factors and the neuroendocrine axis in human pregnancy. *Psychosomatic Medicine, 58*(5), 432–446.

Wainstock, T., Anteby, E. Y., Glasser, S., Lerner-Geva, L., & Shoham-Vardi, I. (2014). Exposure to life-threatening stressful situations and the risk of preterm birth and low birth weight. *International Journal of Gynaecology and Obstetrics, 125*(1), 28–32. doi:10.1016/j.ijgo.2013.09.035.

Weiss, E. L., Msall, M.E., & Muhammad, C. (2007). Barriers to receipt of early intervention. *Passages*. doi:E-PAS2007:616311.10.

Weitzman, M., Byrd, R. S., Aligne, C. A., & Moss, M. (2002). The effects of tobacco exposure on children's behavioral and cognitive functioning: Implications for clinical and public health policy and future research. *Neurotoxicology and Teratology, 24*(3), 397–406.

Wijesiriwardana, A., Bhattacharya, S., Shetty, A., Smith, N., & Bhattacharya, S. (2006). Obstetric outcome in women with threatened miscarriage in the first trimester. *Obstetrics and Gynecology, 107*(3), 557–562. doi:10.1097/01.AOG.0000199952.82151.de.

Williams, M. A., Mittendorf, R., Lieberman, E., & Monson, R. R. (1991). Adverse infant outcomes associated with first-trimester vaginal bleeding. *Obstetrics and Gynecology, 78*(1), 14–18.

Williams, J., Lee, K. J., & Anderson, P. J. (2010). Prevalence of motor-skill impairment in preterm children who do not develop cerebral palsy: A systematic review. *Developmental Medicine and Child Neurology, 52*(3), 232–237. doi:10.1111/j.1469-8749.2009.03544.x.

Winchester, S. B., Sullivan, M. C., Roberts, M. B., & Granger, D. A. (2016). Prematurity, birth weight, and socioeconomic status are linked to atypical diurnal hypothalamic-pituitary-adrenal Axis activity in young adults. *Research in Nursing & Health, 39*(1), 15–29.

Wolke, D., Strauss, V. Y., Johnson, S., Gilmore, C., Marlow, N., & Jaekel, J. (2015). Universal gestational age effects on cognitive and basic mathematic processing: 2 cohorts in 2 countries. *J Pediatr, 166*(6), 1410–1416. doi:10.1016/j.jpeds.2015.02.065.

World Health Organization. (2007). *ICF-CY, international classification of functioning, disability, and health: Children & Youth version*. Geneva: World Health Organization.

Yonkers, K. A., Smith, M. V., Forray, A., Epperson, C. N., Costello, D., Lin, H., et al. (2014). Pregnant women with posttraumatic stress disorder and risk of preterm birth. *JAMA Psychiatry, 71*(8), 897–904. doi:10.1001/jamapsychiatry.2014.558.

A Life Course Approach to Hearing Health

Shirley A. Russ, Kelly Tremblay, Neal Halfon, and Adrian Davis

1 Introduction

Challenges to hearing health are a significant public health problem.

At least ten million Americans have a hearing loss that interferes with the understanding of normal speech (Mitchell 2005). If lesser degrees of loss are included, the number rises to 28 million (US DHHS 2010). Sensorineural hearing loss (SNHL) is the commonest sensory deficit in more developed societies (Davis 1989). The term "deaf" is usually reserved for individuals with severe (>60–90 dBHL) or profound (>90 dBHL) losses, representing half a million Americans, while those with mild (<40 dBHL) or moderate (40–60 dBHL) losses are referred to as "hard of hearing" (Smith et al. 2005; Blanchfield et al. 2001). Congenital losses sufficient to adversely affect speech and language development are seen in at least one per thousand newborns (Fortnum et al. 2001; Russ et al. 2003; Van Naarden et al. 1999), and if lesser degrees of loss and unilateral losses are included, this number rises to up to five per thousand. Only 4% cases of hearing loss nationwide are accounted for by children under the age of 18 years, while 50% cases occur in persons 65 years of age or older (Russ 2001). The cumulative prevalence of hearing loss within the US population rises with age, as has been demonstrated in other countries (Russ 2001; Parving and Christensen 1996), with the sharpest rise in prevalence occurring in old age, when 50–80% are ultimately affected (see Table 1). The relative contributions of delayed diagnosis of congenital losses, progression of existing losses, and acquisition of new losses to the rising prevalence of hearing loss with age are uncertain. Improvements to the prevention, diagnosis, and management of hearing loss across all age groups are public health priorities (Reavis et al. 2016; Davis et al. 2016).

S.A. Russ, MD, MPH (✉)
UCLA Center for Healthier Children, Families and Communities, Department of Pediatrics, David Geffen School of Medicine, UCLA, Los Angeles, CA, USA
e-mail: shirlyruss@cox.net

K. Tremblay
Speech & Hearing Sciences College of Arts & Sciences, University of Washington, Seattle, WA, USA

N. Halfon
Department of Pediatrics, David Geffen School of Medicine, UCLA, Los Angeles, CA, USA

Department of Health Policy and Management, Fielding School of Public Health, UCLA, Los Angeles, CA, USA

Department of Public Policy, Luskin School of Public Affairs, UCLA, Los Angeles, CA, USA

Center for Healthier Children, Families, and Communities, UCLA, Los Angeles, CA, USA

A. Davis
University College London, NHS Newborn Hearing Screening Program, London, UK

N. Halfon et al. (eds.), *Handbook of Life Course Health Development*,
DOI 10.1007/978-3-319-47143-3_15

Table 1 Prevalence of hearing loss in the USA across the life span

Age	Estimated prevalence of hearing loss % (95% CI)	Case definition	Author and year of study	Place of study and sample size	Data source
Newborn	0.14%	Bilateral loss >35 dBHL requiring amplification	Mason, Herrman 1992–1997	Honolulu, HI, 10,372	Kaiser Permanente Honolulu, HI, NHSP
Newborn	0.19%	Loss ≥35 dBHL in one or both ears	Mehl, Thompson 1992–1999	Colorado 63,590	Colorado NHSP
Newborn	0.31%	Unilateral and bilateral sensorineural and conductive losses	Finitzo, Albright, O'Neal 1994–1997	Texas 54,228	Texas Newborn Hearing Screening Data
Newborn	0.33%	Unilateral and bilateral sensorineural hearing loss	Barsky-Firsker, Sun 1993–1995	Livingston, New Jersey, 15,749	St. Barnabas Medical Center Newborn Hearing Screening Data
3 years	0.067% (0.053–0.085)	Bilateral PTA loss at 0.5, 1, and 2 KHz ≥40dBHL in better unaided ear	Van Naarden, Decoufle, Caldwell 1991–1993	Metropolitan Atlanta 255,742	Metropolitan Atlanta Developmental Disabilities Surveillance Program (MADDSP)
10 years	0.14% (0.12–0.16)				
8 years	0.14% 0.12%	Bilateral PTA loss at 0.5, 1, and 2 KHz ≥40 dBHL in better unaided ear	Karapurkar Bhasin, Brocksen, Avchen, Van Naarden Braun 1996 and 2000	Metropolitan Atlanta 36,749 (1996) 43,593 (2000)	MADDSP
6–19 years	0.4%	Bilateral loss at low (0.5, 1, and 2 kHZ) frequencies PTA ≥26 dBHL	Niskar, Kieszak, Holmes, et al. 1988–1994	USA 5249	NHANES III
	0.7%	Bilateral loss at high (3, 4, and 6 kHZ) frequencies PTA ≥26 dBHL			
	14.9%	Unilateral or bilateral loss PTA >16 dBHL at low or high frequencies			
18–34 years	3.4%	Self-reported hearing trouble	National Center for Health Statistics (1990 and 1991)	USA 239,663	National Health Interview Survey (NHIS)
35–44 years	6.3%	Self-reported hearing trouble	National Center for Health Statistics (1990 and 1991)	USA 239,663	National Health Interview Survey (NHIS)
45–54 years	10.3%	Self-reported hearing trouble	National Center for Health Statistics (1990 and 1991)	USA 239,663	National Health Interview Survey (NHIS)
48–59 years	21%	PTA 0.5, 1, 2, and 4 KHz >25 dBHL in the worst ear	Cruickshanks, Wiley, Tweed, et al.	Beaver Dam, WI, (EHLS) 4541	Epidemiology of Hearing Loss Study (EHLS)
70–79 years	66%				
80 years	90%				

(continued)

Table 1 (continued)

Age	Estimated prevalence of hearing loss % (95% CI)	Case definition	Author and year of study	Place of study and sample size	Data source
60–90 years	29%	PTA 0.5, 1, and 2 KHz >26 dBHL in the better ear	Gates, Cooper, Kannel, et al. 1983–1985	Framingham 1662	Framingham Heart Study
73–84 years	59.9%	Hearing loss: two averages of thresholds 0.5, 1, and 2 KHz >25 dBHL	Helzner, Cauley, Pratt, et al. 1997–1998	Pittsburgh, Pennsylvania, and Memphis, Tennessee, 2052	Health, Aging, and Body Composition (ABC) Study
	76.9%	High-frequency hearing loss >40 dBHL 2, 4, and 8 KHz			

Although there have been considerable advances in understanding the etiology of hearing loss, with genetic causes now thought to account for up to 50% of congenital losses (Mitchell 2005), in many individual cases, the cause of hearing loss remains unknown. Even where genetic causes have been identified, discovery of the abnormal gene does not necessarily lead to an understanding of the mechanism whereby the gene's product exerts its effect. Similarly, genetic and environmental causes of hearing losses that have their onset later in life have not been well defined. This lack of knowledge of the basic pathophysiology of hearing difficulties hampers prevention and treatment efforts.

Hearing health has important implications for general health and well-being. Both children and adults with hearing loss face significant educational and social challenges. For children who are profoundly deaf, language and academic levels at high school graduation have been reported historically to correspond to those of fourth grade students with normal hearing (Holt 1993). Adults with hearing loss are reported to have higher levels of unemployment (Parving and Christensen 1993) and lower quality of life than their hearing peers (Appollonio et al. 1996). For older individuals, hearing disability is associated with accelerated cognitive decline, depression, increased risk of dementia, poorer balance, falls, hospitalizations, and early mortality (for a review, see Davis et al. 2016). In addition to these medical consequences, there are also social functioning implications including social isolation due to reduced communication, loss of autonomy, and financial decline. Traditionally, hearing losses in childhood and in adult life have been considered as separate issues.

Growing interest in life course theory has led to suggestions that it could prove useful to apply a life course lens to the study of hearing loss, and of hearing health, throughout the life span. The early years of life, especially the period from conception through to 3 years of age, are now understood to impact lifelong health. Childhood conditions and early experiences can become "embedded" into emerging biological systems, altering health trajectories. The Life Course Health Development (LCHD) model posits that health is an emergent capacity of human beings that dynamically develops over time in response to multiple-nested, ever-changing genetic, biological, behavioral, social, and economic contexts. Multiple risk and protective factors influence development of key biological systems, including the anatomic and biochemical determinants of hearing ability, during critical and sensitive periods of development (see Table 2). Health, at individual and population levels, is also influenced by the timing and sequence of biological,

Table 2 Risk and protective factors for hearing loss across the life span

Life stage	Risk factor	Protective factor
Prenatal	1. Syndrome association with HL 2. Family history of permanent childhood SNHL 3. Craniofacial anomalies 4. In utero TORCH	1. Maternal rubella immunization
Perinatal	1. NICU >48 h 2. Jaundice-exchange Tx 3. Ototoxic medications 4. Meningitis	1. Prompt treatment for neonatal jaundice. 2. Avoid/monitor ototoxic medications. 3. Prompt antibiotic treatment for meningitis
Early childhood	Pre- and Perinatal risk factors, plus: 1. Parent/caregiver concern 2. Persistent pulmonary hypertension with ventilation. 3. Conditions requiring ECMO 4. Syndromes associated with progressive hearing loss (e.g., neurofibromatosis, osteopetrosis, Usher's) 5. Neurodegenerative disorder (e.g., Hunter's, sensorimotor neuropathies, Friedreich's ataxia, Charcot-Marie-Tooth) 6. Head trauma 7. Recurrent/persistent OME for ≥ 3 months	1. Immunization 2. Avoid/monitor ototoxic medications. 3. Prompt antibiotic treatment for meningitis 4.Head injury prevention 5.Noise avoidance/protection
Middle childhood, adolescence, and adulthood	Early childhood risk factors plus: Noise Drug/chemical exposure Head trauma Otosclerosis	1. Noise avoidance/protection 2. Avoid/monitor ototoxic drugs 3. Head injury prevention 4. Immunizations 5. Higher family income 6. Education

cultural, and historic events and experiences. Application of the LCHD model to hearing health challenges predominantly biomedical models and suggests that there are multiple potential avenues for improving hearing health. As hearing losses in childhood and in adult life have been considered as separate issues, investigations into adult hearing loss largely ignore early-life exposures. However, the LCHD model highlights the importance of studying these links.

In this paper we consider the implications of the LCHD model for understanding the mechanisms, pathways, and determinants of hearing ability. We consider the implications of early hearing loss for health development over the life course and the factors through the life course that contribute to hearing ability in adult life. We consider the concept not just of hearing loss but of "hearing health" and how to achieve it, the research priorities that are suggested by this review, and the implications for policy and practice.

2 The Life Course Health Development Model and the Mechanisms, Pathways, and Determinants of Hearing Ability

According to Halfon and Forrest (2017), the LCHD model is grounded in the following seven principles:

1. *Health development*: Health development integrates the concepts of health and developmental processes into a unified whole.

2. *Unfolding*: Health development unfolds continuously over the life span, from conception to death, and is shaped by prior experiences and environmental interactions.
3. *Complexity*: Health development results from adaptive, multilevel, and reciprocal interactions between individuals and their physical, natural, and social environments.
4. *Timing*: Health development is sensitive to the timing and social structuring of environmental exposures and experiences.
5. *Plasticity*: Health development phenotypes are malleable and enabled and constrained by evolution to enhance adaptability to diverse environments.
6. *Thriving*: Optimal health development promotes survival, enhances well-being, and protects against disease.
7. *Harmony*: Health development results from the balanced interactions of molecular, physiological, behavioral, cultural, and evolutionary processes.

Taken together, these seven principles suggest that in order to understand the mechanisms underlying hearing loss and hearing health from a life course standpoint, it is essential to explore the role of multiple risk and protective factors operating at multiple levels to influence hearing-related outcomes. In addition, scientists must study the emergence and development of hearing health trajectories over extended time frames, including the pivotal role of social relationships in the development of functional hearing capacity. Researchers must consider the critical importance of timing in relation to sensitive periods and turning points in the development of hearing abilities. All of these principles point to the importance of adopting a developmental perspective on hearing health. The following section takes each of these issues in turn, providing a review of the evidence pertaining to each.

2.1 Multiple Risk and Protective Factors

Traditional approaches to investigation of the etiology of hearing loss have focused on finding a single or principal cause for clinically observed losses; however, etiology of hearing loss remains unknown in 35–55% most reported case series (Das 1996).

2.1.1 Genetics

Over the past two decades, there has been an explosion in understanding of the genetic basis of deafness. Over half of newborns with SNHL are now believed to have a genetic cause for their loss. Over 120 independent genes for deafness have been identified (Nance 2003). More than 40 are associated with nonsyndromic dominant deafness and more than 30 with autosomal recessive nonsyndromic deafness (Bitner-Glindzicz 2002). Most newborns with inherited forms of hearing loss are born to hearing parents and have recessive, nonsyndromic losses (Russ et al. 2003). Mutations in a single gene—GJB2, coding for the connexin 26 protein which contributes to gap junctions in inner ear cells—are now believed to account for almost half of cases of hereditary nonsyndromic SNHL in America (Davis et al. 1990; Kelley et al. 2000; Cohn and Kelley 1999), with autosomal dominant, X-linked and mitochondrial mutations accounting for the remainder (Russ et al. 2003). Frequently, hearing loss occurs alongside associated conditions. The commonest form of syndromic SNHL is Pendred syndrome, where hearing loss is associated with thyroid abnormalities. Other syndromic losses include Usher's syndrome, Waardenburg syndrome, Alport syndrome, and branchio-oto-renal syndrome. Not all genetic losses are expressed at birth. For example, although the mutation in the pendrin gene is present at birth, Pendred syndrome may be missed in the neonatal period as initial loss may be mild and progress over time, while the thyroid abnormality may not present at birth (Russ et al. 2003). In Usher's syndrome, hearing loss may precede accompanying vision loss by several years.

2.1.2 Gene-Environment Interactions and Epigenetics

It is becoming increasingly clear that even well-described single-gene mutations known to result in hearing loss have a variety of expressed phenotypes. Clinical phenotypes may vary depending on either the effects of modifier genes or on gene-environment interactions. Functional modifications to the genome, referred to as "epigenetics," may result from DNA methylation, histone protein modification, and other mechanisms, and may occur only under certain environmental conditions. For some individuals, a genetic predisposition to hearing loss may only result in phenotypic expression under certain environmental circumstances, and in others, hearing loss may only be manifest in late childhood, adolescence, or adult life.

One of the best-described gene-environment mechanisms leading to expression of hearing loss is that involving the mitochondrial mutation, A1555G, where hearing loss in some individuals occurs only after exposure to aminoglycosides (Gurtler et al. 2005; Fischel-Ghodsian 2003). Epigenetic modifications may result in either temporary or permanent upregulation or downregulation of transcription of certain genes. The timing and duration of key environmental triggers may greatly influence the clinical phenotype. It is not yet known whether there are times in the life span beyond the prenatal period and the first years of life, such as puberty and menopause which are particularly sensitive to environmental effects.

2.1.3 Environmental Causes of Hearing Loss

Environmental causes of congenital hearing loss include congenital TORCH infections (toxoplasmosis, rubella, cytomegalovirus and herpes), prematurity, birth asphyxia, jaundice, and ototoxic drugs. Although prematurity and low birthweight are known to be associated with congenital hearing loss, the causal pathway has not been clearly delineated. One study in Atlanta showed elevated relative risks of bilateral sensorineural hearing impairment among children with lower birthweights: prevalence was 0.4/1000 in children weighing ≥4000 g, compared with 1.27/1000 for 1500–1499 g and 5.1/1000 for those <1500 g (Van Naarden and Decoufle 1999). Admission to a Neonatal Intensive Care Unit (NICU) is a known risk factor for hearing loss, with prolonged mechanical ventilation, birth asphyxia, jaundice, extracorporeal membrane oxygenation (ECMO), and ototoxic medications all contributing risk. While a principal cause for hearing loss might be identifiable in individual cases, infants at this sensitive stage of aural development might be particularly susceptible to the *cumulative effects of multiple risks* on the infant's hearing ability and to *interactions* between risk factors (Fligor et al. 2005, Marlow et al. 2000). For infants who have undergone ECMO, hearing loss may not be detected immediately but appears later in infancy or childhood, implying that the effects of the environmental agent in some way continue even after the period of exposure. Similarly, the influence of these early risk factors for hearing loss may not operate solely during childhood, but may *continue throughout the life course*. One recent study has shown a higher risk of SNHL in males aged 18 who were born small for gestational age (Barrenas et al. 2005b) and in males of short stature (Barrenas et al. 2005a). This interesting finding has led to the hypothesis that fetal programming arising from intrauterine growth retardation might result in delayed cell cycles during development of the cochlea which eventually leads to development of SNHL in adulthood (Niskar et al. 2001). If this is the case, then some newborns who have normal hearing thresholds at birth may have underlying auditory system compromise which only becomes clinically apparent in later life.

Hearing ability in the newborn period, then, may be best conceptualized as a spectrum, with the subsequent hearing trajectory followed by each child depending both on baseline hearing capacity together with the effects of multiple hearing risk and protective factors operating through the life course (see Fig. 1).

Prolonged otitis media in childhood is known to be associated with transient conductive hearing loss; however, its role in the pathogenesis of permanent hearing loss is uncertain. In one series, self-reported hearing loss was recorded in 30% of young patients who had had secretory otitis media for more than 6 years (Ryding et al. 2005), while in another study only boys who had been treated with tympanostomy tubes were at increased risk of loss >20 dBHL for at least one

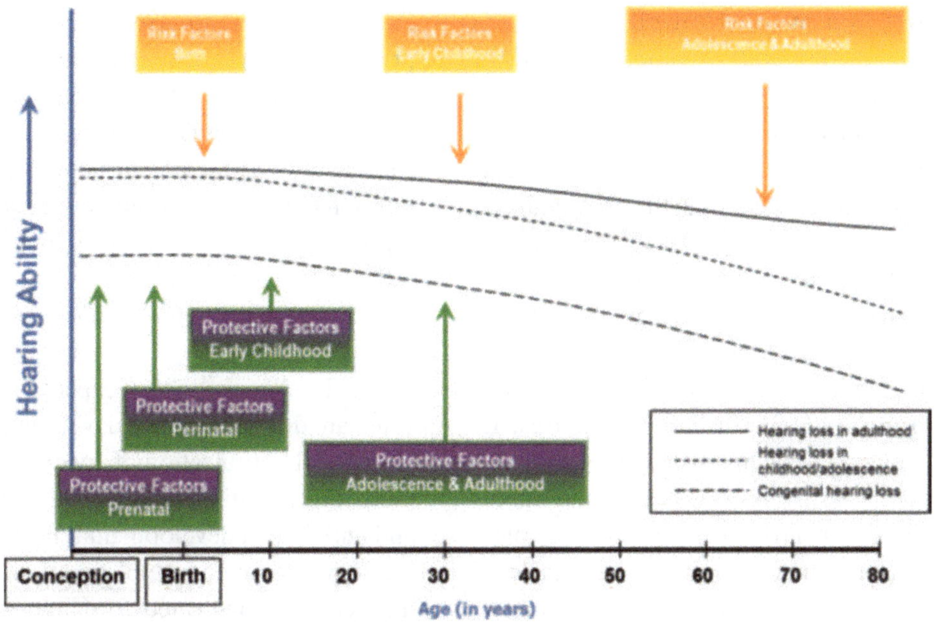

Fig. 1 Hearing loss trajectories

frequency at the age of 18 years (Augustsson and Engstrand 2005).

The environmental risk factor most closely studied for hearing loss in adulthood is noise exposure. Over 11 million Americans have regular exposure to sound levels which have the potential to damage hearing (National Institute in Deafness and Other Communication Disorders 2002), and many of these exposures are related to occupations, e.g., mining, farm work, entertainment industry, or recreational activities, e.g., rock concerts or motorcycles. While noise-induced hearing loss is typically gradual and insidious, starting with a notched loss in the high frequencies, sudden hearing loss has also been reported in response to acoustic trauma, e.g., gunshot or explosion (Danielson 2005). With that said, noise exposure can manifest itself even without the presence of an observed audiometric impact, making the prevalence much greater than originally thought. For example, Tremblay et al. (2015) reported a history of noise exposure, to be a primary risk factor among adults' self-reporting hearing difficulties, even when there was no audiometric evidence of hearing loss.

Interactions between noise exposure and other risk factors for hearing loss, such as those present from infancy and childhood, have not been well studied, though smoking has been shown to increase risk of high-frequency loss and to exert an additive risk effect with noise exposure (Uchida et al. 2005). Evidence is emerging that exposure to leisure-time noise in young adults results in detectable changes to hearing capacity, indicated by decreased transient evoked otoacoustic emission (TEOAE) levels and reproducibility even when hearing thresholds remain normal (>20 dBHL) (Rosanowski et al. 2006). Noise-induced threshold shifts have been observed in up to 12.5% children ages 6–19 years (Niskar et al. 2001). Of young people who responded to a recent web-based survey, 61% reported experiencing tinnitus or hearing loss following attendance at loud music concerts (Chung et al. 2005). Compliance with recommendations regarding use of ear protection for those at risk of occupational exposure or for leisure-related exposures is generally low.

Despite the high prevalence of presbycusis, or age-related hearing loss, in the USA, the mechanism of pathogenesis has not been fully elucidated and appears to be multifactorial (Gates and Mills 2005), involving genetic and environmental influences. A Danish study of twins aged

75 and older estimated a heritability factor of 40% for self-reported reduced hearing (Christensen et al. 2001) and suggested that even older adults with hearing loss should be asked about familial risk factors. Interestingly, in a genome-wide linkage analysis in the Framingham Heart Study, several of the chromosome locations linked to presbycusis overlapped with loci known to cause congenital hearing loss, raising the possibility that the same genes might cause presbycusis and congenital hearing loss (DeStefano et al. 2003). In individual cases, it can be challenging to distinguish age-related and noise-induced hearing loss, and in some cases both factors may contribute to the clinical picture. Adults, too, remain at risk of hearing loss secondary to bacterial meningitis, head injuries, and exposure to ototoxic medications.

While multiple risk and protective factors contribute to defined hearing deficits and elevated hearing thresholds, additional factors operating at multiple levels influence functional outcomes for individuals with hearing loss. It is well recognized that two individuals with the same hearing loss etiologies may have identical audiometric thresholds, yet one is apparently asymptomatic while the other reports significant difficulties with hearing. Contributing factors may include different hearing environments—one individual may work or attend school in a less optimal acoustic environment than the other—or subtle differences in hearing pathology affecting, e.g., speech discrimination. Differences in speech understanding, among individuals with similar audiograms, also appear along the aging trajectory. Individuals with similar chronological ages show differences in the ability to conduct sound along central auditory pathways (Clinard and Tremblay 2013). For children with congenital hearing loss, functional communication outcomes are sensitive to age at diagnosis of hearing loss, age at onset of intervention, socioeconomic status, and degree of family engagement.

2.2 Hearing Health Trajectories

Baltes, Lindenberger, and Staudinger (2007) describe four distinct phases of health development:

- Phase 1—Generativity: Preconception and prenatal period is dedicated to the formation of the organism, within the context in which the developing fetus will emerge. This phase can include the nutritional inputs and neural-hormonal contexts that influence the mother's reproductive health trajectory, including early influences on the eggs that are developing in her ovaries years before she is reproductively able.
- Phase 2—Acquisition of capacity: The early years are dedicated to the development, acquisition, and optimization of specific capacities, including investing in future health potential and anticipated developmental reserves.
- Phase 3 – Maintenance of function: The middle years are dedicated to maintaining function of these capacities in the face of accumulating risks and ongoing weathering.
- Phase 4 – Managing decline: The later years are dedicated to managing, adjusting, and adapting to functional decline of various body and regulatory systems.

These Phases are readily applicable to the study of the development of hearing health.

2.2.1 Generativity

Outside of genetic factors, there have been few studies addressing women's preconception health and future risk of hearing loss in any children she might conceive. There has been little research into maternal preconception nutritional factors or neurohormonal variants that might pose a risk for future fetal auditory system development and function. The prenatal period has been more intensively studied, and multiple genetic and environmental factors contributing to disruption of hearing ability have been described. However, too often, underlying pathophysiologic mechanisms have not been fully delineated. Formation of the auditory system in the fetus is a complex process, apparently sensitive to the effects of multiple gene products and environmental variants. In addition, hearing loss frequently occurs alongside other developmental effects either as part of a defined syndrome or for reasons that are obscure. Abnormalities can arise in the absence of a gene product, the formation of an abnormal gene product, and/or in the regulation of a gene's expression. Pathology can occur at the molecular, subcellular, cellular, or organ formation stages. Environmental effects may operate via disruption to the normal process of genetic transcription and translation or through mechanisms that are independent of the genome, e.g., direct disruption of developing tissues. Environmental factors may act through more than one mechanism, and clinical effects may vary significantly based on timing of exposure in relation to gestation. Effects on different organs of a single genetic or environmental factor may be similar or quite different. Consequently, elucidation of the pathophysiology of hearing loss requires a cooperative effort across multiple disciplines and approaches.

2.2.2 Acquisition of Capacity

Study of hearing ability during the early years has largely been limited to measurement of auditory thresholds, yet children with identical thresholds may have very different hearing reserves, hearing potential, and hearing function. There is moderately good evidence that auditory input in the first 6 months of life is important for the development of functional hearing ability, suggesting that in some way the stimulation of auditory neurons in early postnatal life is necessary for the acquisition of full hearing capacity (Levine et al. 2016). Among children with congenital hearing loss, adaptations such as the early use of hearing aids or acquisition of lip-reading skills may affect either physiologic hearing ability or functional hearing through stimulation of higher auditory pathways. Similarly, early acquisition of sign language may circumvent auditory difficulties by providing an alternate route to functional communication. Life course models suggest that many factors contribute to an individual's functional hearing capacity, in ways that are currently poorly understood.

2.2.3 Maintenance of Function

In the middle years, adults attempt to maintain hearing function in the face of new risk factors such as occupational noise exposure, alcohol, smoking, etc. Many adults make conscious or subconscious adaptations to maintain function in the face of clinical or subclinical hearing threshold drops (e.g., avoiding noisy environments, sitting at the front of lecture halls, turning up the TV volume). The impact of early-life factors on hearing ability in the middle years has not been well studied, and the potential biochemical or cellular mechanisms whereby some individuals may be able to "buffer" a failing auditory pathway while others cannot are unclear.

2.2.4 Managing Decline

In old age the emphasis is on functional adaptation to decline in hearing ability. In addition to cogent biochemical and cellular mechanisms underlying the response to falling auditory capacity, social and cultural factors play a large role in acceptance of and accommodations for reduced hearing ability.

To date, there have been no studies documenting hearing ability from birth through to death either at individual or population level, so hearing trajectories can only be estimated using data from separate studies over different phases of the life course (see Fig. 1). We know surprisingly little about how slowly or rapidly hearing ability deteriorates both at individual and population level at different age ranges. We do not know to what degree recognized risk factors for hearing loss in the prenatal and early childhood periods continue to act as risk factors for hearing loss in later childhood, adolescence, and throughout adult life. What is more, there is evidence from animal studies to suggest that an early history of noise exposure can impact auditory function later in life (Fernandez et al. 2015). However, there is little longitudinal data to help determine whether hearing loss in middle and old age is preceded by threshold shifts earlier in life nor whether deteriorations in hearing ability in this middle phase of life occur continuously, or in a stepwise fashion.

Studies that approach hearing loss from a life course perspective are starting to emerge. Wisconsin teenagers actively involved in farm work have been demonstrated to have a higher prevalence of hearing loss compared with their peers who were not engaged in farm work, suggesting that the hearing loss observed in adult farmers may, in fact, begin in childhood and adolescence (Broste et al. 1989). A recent study of over 2000 adults from Tennessee and Pennsylvania aged 73–84 years revealed a prevalence of hearing loss (>25 dBHL) of 59% at low frequencies and 76.9% at high frequencies. In a multivariate model, older age, white race, diabetes mellitus, cerebrovascular disease, smoking, poorer cognitive status, occupational noise exposure, and ear surgery were all associated with hearing loss. Possible protective factors included salicylate use (black men) and moderate alcohol intake (black women). National Health Interview Survey analyses have indicated that lower educational levels (less than high school) and lower family income are also associated with higher prevalences of hearing loss (Gates and Mills 2005). Recent animal study data suggest that pathological changes caused by early noise exposure in young mice might actually render inner ears more vulnerable to aging (Kujawa and Liberman 2006), while a retrospective clinical study suggested that noise-induced hearing loss before old age may reduce the effects of aging at noise-associated frequencies but accelerate deterioration at adjacent frequencies (Gates et al. 2000).

Analysis of short-term longitudinal data from the UK and Denmark reveals that in adult life, hearing ability gradually and continuously deteriorates, at an average rate of 3 dB per decade for those under 55 and 9 dB/decade for those over 55 (Davis et al. 1990). A recent short-term US longitudinal study found a similar hearing threshold increase of 1 dB per year for adults age 60 years and over (Lee et al. 2005). Most US studies report a higher prevalence of hearing loss for men than women across all age ranges; however, more recent studies suggest gender differences might be starting to diminish because of changes in lifestyle (Homans et al. 2016). More boys than girls are born each year with congenital hearing loss, and this increased vulnerability of males to hearing loss continues through the life course. Increased genetic susceptibility and higher rates of exposure to noise, especially occupational exposures, have been proposed as potential causes for the observed gender differences, while estrogen has been hypothesized as exerting potential protective effects against hearing loss for premenopausal women (Hultcrantz et al. 2006). For females in the rural Midwest study, there was a rapid increase in prevalence of hearing loss sufficient to interfere with the understanding of speech in the sixth decade, whereas for males it was earlier—in the fourth decade (Flamme et al. 2005), possibly reflecting different environmental exposures, genetic susceptibilities, or both. The Baltimore Longitudinal Study of Aging also showed that hearing sensitivity declines twice as fast in men as in women at most ages and frequencies, with age of onset of decline being later in women. Although women have more sensitive hearing than men at frequencies above 1000 Hz, men have more sensitive hearing than women at lower frequencies (Pearson et al. 1995), an interesting finding which has been replicated in other studies.

Although some studies appear to show a rising prevalence of hearing loss in the USA over time, even after adjusting for age (Wallhagen et al. 1997, Benson and Marano 1994), this has not been confirmed in others (Lee et al. 2004). There is general agreement, however, that with the aging of the "baby boomers," the absolute numbers of individuals who are deaf or hard of hearing in the USA are set to rise. While prevention of hearing loss in old age remains an important goal, life course models emphasize that there are multiple routes to managing such hearing losses, although they require adaptations both at individual population levels. Evidence suggests that powerful social and cultural factors may be limiting these adaptations. For example, less than 15% for those who would benefit from aids series and only 55% for those with more severe losses (Popelka et al. 1988) accepted aiding despite good evidence from randomized trials that hearing aids improve outcomes (Yueh et al. 2003). High rates of nondisclosure of hearing loss by students to institutions of higher education (Richardson et al. 2004) and in the workplace have also been reported, suggesting that there may be a stigma attached to disclosure of hearing loss.

2.3 Social Relationships

Hearing ability is closely related to ability to communicate via the spoken word and as such has the capacity to impact multiple social relationships. Most children with hearing loss are born to hearing parents who have no experience of living with and adapting to hearing difficulties. Parents face early decisions regarding whether or not to pursue use of hearing aids and choice of language modality. Historically, intervention programs were divided into signing or oral/aural approaches. Parents faced the difficult decision of choosing one or other route. In more recent years, programs have emerged that address multiple communication modalities, and it is not unusual for children and families to trial several approaches before deciding on a principal course of action. Nonetheless, parents face the sometimes daunting task of acquiring a new language, sign language, in midlife to aid communication with their child. Not surprisingly, studies of language development among children that are deaf or hard of hearing have identified family engagement and maternal sensitivity as important factors influencing outcomes from interventions and maternal sensitivity (Pressman et al. 1999). These findings are very much in tune with life course models that emphasize the importance of social relationships at every stage of health development. Early decisions have a potential for lifelong impact. For example, there may be less-immediate imperative for fathers to become fluent in sign language if mother is the primary caregiver, but in the long-term this is essential for the development of one of the child's pivotal social relationships if sign language is a chosen mode of communication. Parents' abilities to access resources to support communication and relationship building with their child are dependent on factors at multiple levels including financial resources, services offered in their geographic location, parents' ability to take necessary leave from work or limit work hours, support of the wider family including grandparents, aunts, and uncles, and willingness of the local community to make adaptations (e.g., close-captioned TV and interpreter services).

2.4 Sensitive Periods and Turning Points

The LCHD model posits that individuals are most susceptible to the effects of multiple risk and protective factors during critical and sensitive time periods in development. Many of these sensitive periods occur before birth and in the first years of life, when physiological systems are being initialized and programmed. Health, or lack of health, results from both genetic makeup and both the timing and sequence of biological, psychological, cultural, and historic events.

For example, cytomegalovirus (CMV) infection in the first or second trimester may result in widespread organ damage affecting cognitive and neurological function in addition to hearing loss, while infection later in pregnancy may result only in a progressive hearing loss which develops later in childhood (Rivers et al. 2002), when CMV may not be identified as causative (Pass 2005). Prelingual deafness, occurring prior to the development of language, has far more profound impact than postlingual deafness.

There is considerable debate, however, about the nature of critical and sensitive time periods for early language development. The balance of evidence currently supports early identification of and intervention for hearing loss prior to the sixth month of life as being advantageous for future language development. Consequently, identification of hearing loss no later than age 3 months and commencement of intervention no later than 6 months are important goals of the National Newborn Hearing Screening program; however, some experts suggest that optimal diagnosis and intervention should begin even earlier.

Parents of children with profound losses face another decision with long-term implications when they determine whether they wish their child to receive cochlear implantation. There is some evidence to suggest that early implantation, before the second year of life, results in an advantage of language acquisition over later implantation and that bilateral implantation is advantageous to unilateral. Balanced against this is the desire by some providers and parents to leave one ear free for potential future technologically advanced adaptations and the difficulties inherent in making a decision for the child before they are old enough to express their own view. These difficulties are compounded when the evidence base on which families make these decisions is uncertain at best. Life course models emphasize the importance of professional working in partnership with families, providing unbiased information and ensuring they are fully informed about the state of evidence.

Critical timing decisions are not confined to the early years. Young adults with hearing loss often find their need for aiding and hearing supports increase as they progress through the educational system and on to higher education. Older adults entering more acoustically challenging work environments may also need additional supports for the first time. Failure to identify and address these needs could result in unnecessary withdrawal from education or employment.

2.5 A Developmental Perspective on Hearing Health

The LCHD model regards health as a "capacity for life," envisaging a continuous dynamic process during which each individual interacts with her environment in ways that either support or inhibit the development of health. Accordingly, a diagnosis of profound hearing loss does not necessarily commit that person to a state of "poor health." Rather, with appropriate adaptations, high levels of communication and interpersonal relationships can be achieved. In fact, many members of the deaf community feel strongly that their condition is not a deficit, do not choose to use assistive technology, and view their choices as quite simply an alternate way of living.

Hearing loss poses particular challenges early in life, especially if it goes undetected. Deprived of auditory input and lacking alternatives such as sign language, infants are challenged to develop a structure or "scaffolding" for language. Evidence suggests that this can affect many other aspects of development including social pragmatics. The impact of hearing loss is closely related to the developmental stage in which it occurs, being strongest when onset is in the prelingual years. Even moderate losses with onset at adolescence can impact social development and academic attainment. Life course models stress the importance of viewing hearing loss in developmental context and ensuring that interventions are developmentally appropriate. In recent years early intervention has shifted from models in which interventionists worked primarily 1:1 with children to one in which the therapist works with the family to support their interactions and interventions with their own child, mirroring the primacy of parent-child interactions at this developmental stage.

A health development perspective emphasizes the importance of considering the individual's developmental stage when tailoring interventions and promoting hearing health. For example, in infancy the emphasis must be on facilitating early communication and primary relationship development; in the preschool and early school years, it will be on communication for wider relationship development and hearing for early learning; in adolescence issues of identity and peer acceptance come to the fore; in adulthood adaptation to the workplace, projection of a competent professional image, romantic relationships, and finding a life partner are prime concerns, followed by becoming a good parent. In old age the focus is on avoidance of being a burden to family and society and maintaining close relationships and quality of life. Each stage requires a related yet focused response from public and individual health services.

3 Implications of Early Hearing Loss for Health Development over the Life Course

We have already described how early hearing loss sufficient to interfere with speech and language development can negatively impact communication and social skills and education and occupational attainment. However, even mild degrees of loss have been associated with educational challenges including greater likelihood of grade repetition and attention difficulties in school (Bess 1998), while slight bilateral hearing loss, frequently unrecognized by parents, has been associated with lower reading scores (Byrd 2002). Recent studies suggest that many factors impact the expressive vocabularies of children with congenital hearing loss in the first 2 years of life, but that diagnosis and commencement of early intervention prior to the age of 3 months has a sustained beneficial effect (Vohr et al. 2011). Children diagnosed early, without significant comorbidities and who receive a cochlear implant up to 45%, are reported to have normal to slightly delayed language development (Verhaert et al. 2008). While cochlear implantation is not the only route to language development, and many factors in addition to age at intervention contribute to language abilities, this finding underscores the importance of the child's experience very early in the life course for future language development.

The quality of studies that investigate developmental effects of early hearing loss varies considerably. Some are confined to those children that have hearing loss as their only condition and have an IQ within the normal range, while others do not exclude children with either additional or related conditions. Consequently, caution must be exercised in ascribing developmental effects solely to the impact of hearing loss. In addition, there are special difficulties inherent in estimating the IQ of children that are deaf or hard of hearing (Vernon 2005), including capacity for testing in the child's language (e.g., sign language). Nonetheless, there is good evidence that children who are hard of hearing find it much more difficult than children with normal hearing to learn vocabulary, grammar, word order, idiomatic expressions, and other aspects of verbal communication (Mohr et al. 2000).

Communication difficulties that persist into adolescence and adult life affect later education, employment, and well-being, and pose significant challenge for day-to-day life (NIDCD Plain Language Strategic Plan 2003). High levels of intelligence do not necessarily protect against significant life challenges. In one study of 57 intellectually gifted deaf and hard of hearing subjects followed longitudinally, almost half graduated from a four-year college, but 39% experienced mental illness of sufficient severity to warrant inpatient hospitalization or outpatient therapy, and a surprising 30% were unemployed (Vernon and LaFalce-Launders 1993). Similar (31%) unemployment rates were found in a group of young Danish adults, aged 20–35 years, with congenital hearing loss versus 12% in the age-matched hearing population (Parving and Christensen 1993). Disappointingly, a recent Australian study using historic data on the employment of deaf school leavers demonstrated that deaf adults continue to have poor employment outcomes despite access to higher education and legislation prohibiting discrimination. The authors suggested that programs addressing community attitudes to deafness might be needed to bring about change (Winn 2007). This conclusion is consistent with a life course approach to understanding outcomes, as it emphasizes the importance of considering multiple levels of contributory factors, including community attitudes, when investigating well-being at all stages of life. In contrast, a more recent study from the USA of 46 young adults that attended a nonpublic agency school for the deaf reported high levels of college completion and employment (Appelman et al. 2012).

There is mixed evidence regarding the effects of hearing loss on mental health at different stages of the life course. Australian children have been demonstrated to have lower parent-reported psychological well-being than their hearing peers, while those with mild losses actually had poorer health-related quality of life (HRQoL), possibly reflecting added stress resulting from unrealistic expectations of hearing ability (Wake et al. 2004). Dutch youth with auditory disabilities had two to three times higher prevalence of mental health problems than the normative sample in one series (Van Eldik 2005), while elderly prelingually deaf people in Sweden who used sign language showed a greater frequency of depressive symptoms and insomnia than hearing peers, though there was no significant difference in perceived well-being. Interestingly, age-associated acquired hearing loss has been reported to lead to more emotional issues and social isolation than lifelong hearing loss (Gething 2000), possibly reflecting adjustment and coping issues. In a recent qualitative study, deaf and hard of hearing US adults reported difficulties with access to adequate mental health services, largely due to communication barriers, along with feelings of isolation and stigma (Cabral et al. 2013). In a Lancet review of the mental health of deaf people, the authors concluded that early access to effective communication with family members and peers was a protective factor for mental health and that provision of specialist services by professional trained to communicate with deaf people and with sign language interpreters could improve access to both mental health and more general health services. Such access is particularly important for the 25% of deaf individuals reported to have additional disabilities and a high probability of complex mental health needs (Fellinger et al. 2012). Discussing mental health issues through interpreters is not easy—studies also suggest that careful training is needed to reduce possible role conflicts and ensure conceptual equivalence in real-time translating (Sheppard 2011). Professional services must be culturally competent. Deaf adults report feeling that interpreters were not welcome during mental health encounters and were generally not asked about depressive symptoms even when manifesting signs of depression (Sheppard and Badger 2010).

Deaf and hard of hearing people also report difficulties with access to general health services, and are frequently excluded from health research. Recent community-based participatory research has identified some glaring health inequalities in the deaf community, notably obesity, partner violence, and suicide (Barnett et al. 2012), while other studies have demonstrated inconsistent knowledge of common health issues such as cardiovascular health related to difficulties with communication during health education (McKee et al. 2011). Fewer than one in ten deaf women report fully understanding what the doctor tells them when visiting the doctor's office alone (Ubido 2002).

The relationship between congenital hearing loss and mortality is uncertain. One study showed no excess of mortality among prelingually deaf people compared with hearing controls, although a small excess in mortality was observed for postlingually deafened individuals (Barnett and Franks 1999), again possibly reflecting adjustment and coping difficulties. In the USA, Schubert et al. (2017) studied the associations between hearing, visual, and olfactory impairments with mortality and somewhat surprisingly found that olfactory impairment, but not hearing or visual impairment, was associated with an increased risk of mortality. In Iceland, older men with hearing impairment or dual sensory impairment (vision + hearing loss) had a greater risk of dying from any cause and particularly cardiovascular causes within a median 5-year follow-up. Women with hearing impairment, however, had a nonsignificantly elevated risk (Fisher et al. 2014).

4 Achieving Hearing Health

Health is increasingly conceptualized not just as the absence of disease but as a positive capacity for life. Achieving "hearing health," then, means more than just avoiding "poor" outcomes. At each stage of life, hearing capacity needs to be sufficient for the functional needs of the individual and for successful interaction with the broader environment. Interventions are no longer aimed at simply remediating deficits but must be tailored to ensure that each individual can meet her needs, develop her full potential, and, regardless of adaptations adopted or chosen method of communication, interact successfully socially with the broader population (Lin et al. 2016). In early childhood, during the period of language acquisition, children with severe and profound hearing loss face significant communication challenges. Early diagnosis, prompt intervention, and ready access to the family's choice of communication modality appear to offer the best hope for successful outcomes. Throughout childhood, optimum hearing capacity needs to be maintained through continuous use of high-quality assistive listening devices such as hearing aids and use of frequency modulation (FM) classroom systems. Access to teachers of the deaf and to sign language and sign language interpreters needs to be provided if children are to meet increasing school curricular demands.

As children who are deaf or hard of hearing transition into higher education or the workforce, they need to have the same range of occupational choices as their hearing peers. The acoustic demands of the workplace may be more challenging than structured classroom settings, presenting difficulties even for those with mild or minimal hearing loss. For older adults with age-related or noise-induced hearing loss, the ability to maintain social and occupational functioning is an important goal of habilitation, as even mild degrees of hearing loss may result in difficulties with conversational speech under adverse listening conditions such as the presence of background noise or reverberation (Gordon-Salant 2005). Understanding of accented speech is particularly challenging for the elderly, so the changing demographics of the USA with increasing diversity of accents may pose added challenges in future years. Adoption of a positive functional framework for hearing health implies that assessments of hearing ability at all ages should not be limited to documentation of hearing thresholds under testing conditions but need to measure the individual's functional hearing capacity in their everyday life—an area where even mild limitations may have negative consequences before significant threshold shifts are observed. Similarly, amplification to a specified threshold level may not be sufficient in and of itself to ensure an individual's ability to maintain a prior job function, or to manage social situations in a way that achieves true hearing health.

Hearing health may be achieved in different ways by different individuals—a person with a profound hearing loss who is fluent in sign language and able to communicate successfully with both deaf and hearing peers through the use of readily available translators has found one route to hearing health. For others, it may come with the use of hearing aids. Conversely, the middle-aged construction worker who develops a noticeable hearing loss, is unable to afford a hearing aid, and reluctantly avoids social situations due to his communication difficulties is not achieving hearing health. Optimization of hearing health—both at individual and population levels—could yield significant benefits in quality of communication and social interactions.

Current evidence suggests that many Americans, across all stages of life, are not achieving full hearing health. Until recently, late diagnosis of congenital hearing loss was the norm, with a reported mean age at diagnosis of 24–30 months in 1989 (Gustason 1989; Moore et al. 1990). Consequently, many children (who are now in adulthood) missed the opportunity for very early intervention during a critical and sensitive time period for language acquisition.

Although Universal Newborn Hearing Screening programs have made great strides in reducing ages at diagnosis and intervention, some children still "fall through the cracks," or fail to return for follow-up appointments, and are diagnosed late. The Centers for Disease Control (CDC) Early Hearing Detection and Intervention (EHDI) program aims to promote communication from birth for all children and to ensure that children with hearing loss achieve communication and social skills commensurate with their cognitive ability (National EHDI Goals). Screening of all newborns by 1 month of age, diagnostic evaluations for all screen "refers" by 3 months of age, and commencement of early intervention by 6 months of age are core EHDI goals. However, a 2004 (UPDATE) survey of screening program administrators revealed that only 55% of infants needing diagnostic audiologic evaluations are receiving them by 3 months of age, and only 48% of infants confirmed with hearing loss commence early intervention services by age 6 months (Van Naarden and Decoufle 1999). Similar experience has been reported in the UK in a follow-up to the Wessex study, where fitting of aids and commencement of early intervention did not occur in approximately half of cases until the child was over 18 months old (Kennedy et al. 2005). Factors cited by EHDI administrators as contributing to follow-up challenges include shortages of pediatric audiologists, delays in obtaining necessary insurance authorizations, and lack of knowledge of the EHDI system by primary care physicians. Parents too may be reluctant to accept the results of a computerized test of hearing in a baby who appears normal, while cultural biases and negative perceptions of deaf people might contribute to lack of acceptance of diagnosis and lack of compliance with the use of hearing aids (Mutton and Peacock 2005).

While the vast majority of children with moderate or greater degrees of hearing loss will be detected by current newborn screening protocols, many cases of milder loss, both bilateral and unilateral, will be missed. When screen protocols reliant only on otoacoustic emissions (OAEs) are used, cases of auditory neuropathy will also be missed. The question of how much benefit results from early detection of mild and unilateral losses remains unanswered, but there is evidence that even mild losses may be associated with academic difficulties, while in one series unilateral losses were demonstrated to be associated with scholastic or behavioral problems in school in up to 30% affected children (Brookhouser et al. 1991). These findings raise the question of whether earlier intervention for these types of loss might also improve long-term outcomes. Ongoing audiological surveillance throughout childhood is needed if children with late-onset, progressive, or acquired hearing loss are to be identified at the earliest possible time (National EHDI Goals). Although hearing assessment is recommended at each preventive health visit in childhood, the method of the assessment, pass/fail criteria, and follow-up protocols have not been clearly delineated. Joint Committee on Infant Hearing recommends that any infant with risk indicators for progressive or delayed-onset hearing loss receive audiological monitoring every 6 months until age 3 years, yet risks will probably persist beyond this age. Of children ages 3–19 years, 10% are reported to "refer" on audiometric screening at pediatrician visits, of whom less than half report receiving any follow-up services (Halloran et al. 2005), limiting the effectiveness of these screening efforts. Although school-entry hearing screening and intermittent screening throughout the school years are performed through most school districts, there are few published data on the outcomes of these screening programs. For adults, screening is recommended every decade after age 18 years with more frequent monitoring after age 50 or if there are risk factors such as occupational noise exposure. In practice, however, compliance with screening recommendations is low. Acceptance rates of hearing aids in adults are also low—less than 15% for those who would benefit in one series and only 55% for those with more severe losses (Popelka et al. 1998)—despite good evidence from high rates of nondisclosure of hearing loss by students to institutions of higher education (Richardson et al. 2004) and in the workplace have also been reported, suggesting that there may be a stigma attached to disclosure of hearing loss.

These findings all suggest that powerful social and cultural factors may act throughout the life course as strong disincentives for the identification and treatment of hearing loss. Indeed, data suggest that the identification of hearing losses later in life is far less complete than in the early years at population level. Hearing aids do not appear to be as well accepted by the population as, for example, glasses—this may reflect issues of cost, availability, and ease of use, but may also reflect negative cultural attitudes. Many health plans, for example, do not cover the provision of hearing aids despite the fact that hearing loss is the third most prevalent chronic condition in older adults (Yueh et al. 2003). In the USA, where hearing aids can cost approximately $5000 US dollars, efforts are being made to make hearing technology more affordable and more accessible. In their report, the National Academies of Sciences, Engineering, and Medicine and their task force recommended key institutional, technological, and regulatory changes that would enable consumers to find and fully use appropriate, affordable, and high-quality services and technologies (National Academies 2016). One such recommendation is to implement a new Food and Drug Administration (FDA) device category for over-the-counter wearable hearing devices. Another is to improve affordability of hearing health care by actions across federal, state, and private sectors.

5 Research Priorities

The Life Course Health Development (LCHD) model provides a comprehensive conceptual framework for understanding both how hearing loss develops and how hearing health can be achieved throughout the life span. This framework can be used to guide formation of a research agenda incorporating study of early developmental influences and genetic, environmental, social, societal, and cultural contributors to hearing health. Here we consider priorities for this agenda arising from this application of the model to hearing health. These include the need for a comprehensive knowledge synthesis, adoption of longitudinal interdisciplinary study designs, place of hearing loss registries, better measures of positive hearing health, further development of investigation of pathophysiology of hearing loss, involvement of the deaf and hard of hearing communities in the design and conduct of the research agenda, and more translational research in how best to move evidence into practice.

5.1 Knowledge Synthesis

Existing knowledge of auditory pathology resides in multiple disciplinary silos, with few attempts to draw all of the knowledge together into one area. Epidemiologists do not generally read cell biology journals, while psychologists and teachers of the deaf seldom read publications on epigenetics. Yet, each may have knowledge that could prove useful if not invaluable to the other. The LCHD model indicates how diverse factors, being studied by quite separate groups of individuals, contribute to a cohesive whole, with the relationships between factors too often ignored in research studies. The challenge is to gather relevant materials together in such a way that it is comprehensible and readily accessible across disciplines. This paper represents one attempt to move across multiple disciplinary lines and consider, using the life course framework, the myriad of potential factors operating at multiple levels to contribute to hearing ability at individual and population levels.

5.2 Study Design

The preceding discussion of a life course view of hearing health makes a strong argument for a need to shift from cross-sectional to longitudinal study designs, and from a uni- or limited disciplinary approach to one in which multiple disciplines contribute to the same study. An "ideal" study would involve following a large cohort prospectively, preferably starting prior to conception and continuing throughout the life span. The study would incorporate detailed measures of hearing health at multiple points during the life course, together with a wide range of additional genetic, epigenetic, biological, general health, environmental, psychological, social, and educational measures. No existing studies fulfill all aspects of the ideal, but a few longitudinal studies do exist that embody some of these features. For example, the National Child Development Study (NCDS; UK) (1958), the British Birth Cohort Study (1970), and the Avon Longitudinal Study of Parents and Children (ALSPAC) each includes some measures of hearing ability. However, even large cohort studies will include only 100–200 children with congenital hearing loss, and the amount of additional data of most interest to hearing researchers will be limited by the length of the study protocol that subjects can reasonably be expected to complete. Large de novo longitudinal studies that are focused on addressing hearing-related hypotheses will likely be costly and take, potentially, decades to deliver results. The challenge is to develop new approaches that will allow for the study of hearing from a life course perspective in a less costly fashion. Approaches could include addition of follow-forward or follow-back components to existing cross-sectional studies such as National Health and Nutrition Examination Survey (NHANES), which already includes detailed measures of subjects hearing ability; addition of hearing-related data to existing longitudinal studies such as NCDS (UK), Biorepository and Bioanalysis Centre (BBC), ALSPAC, National Longitudinal Survey of Children and Youth (NLSCY), and the National Children's Study (NCS); addition of hearing-related biological data from selected subjects in cross-sectional studies such as NSCH; and voluntary collection of historical and biological data using approaches such as a hearing loss registry (see below). Any of these approaches would require dedicated funding streams, as they would fall outside of the traditional scope of R01s.

5.3 Hearing Loss Registries

Researchers have traditionally been reluctant to develop disease-specific registries owing to legitimate concerns about confidentiality and a reluctance to ask potential subjects to participate, especially at sensitive times such as shortly after diagnosis. Recently, however, highly successful registries for conditions such as autism have been developed on a voluntary basis, incorporating both detailed patient/family reported data and biological specimens for genetic and biochemical analysis. In addition to subjects with hearing loss, hearing subjects could contribute vital control data. While a voluntary approach undoubtedly introduces bias, the reality is that any existing approach to population study involves some forms of bias both known and unknown. Provided that biases can be documented, there is now potential to address them statistically. Similarly, missing data can be inferred using techniques such as multiple imputations. Experience with other registries suggests that a community-based participatory research approach involving members of the deaf and hard of hearing community working alongside professionals to develop and implement the registry and determine the ways in which data can be accessed is most likely to be successful. Subjects could determine whether they wished to contribute data alone, biological specimens alone, or both, and whether they wished to interface with the registry at a single time point or would be willing to return at intervals. Much of the data collection could be performed online at times convenient for the registry participants. Participants would be free to withdraw at any time. Depending on content, parts of the registry could potentially be made publicly available for analysis provided individual subjects could not be recognized from released data. Most likely, some parts of the dataset would be made available only to researchers who agreed to comply with confidentiality restrictions. Funding for such a registry could be from private or public sources or both. A US-based registry could either interface with similar registries in other countries that were independently run, or an international initiative could be launched aimed at uniformity of approach and data collection in multiple countries, greatly increasing the number of available subjects and potentially accelerating research.

This type of data collection effort also falls outside of traditional research-funding mechanisms and shifts the focus from hypothesis-driven research to one of "big data" collection, where the emphasis is on examining large amounts of data looking for new types of patterns and relationships. While there are legitimate concerns that this type of "data trawling" could lead to "false positives" with recognition of associations occurring by chance, many researchers now argue that this concern could be at least partially overcome by employing more stringent criteria for significance testing, e.g., employing p values of <0.005 rather than 0.05. While some researchers fear a move away from hypothesis-testing, many others now view it as the way forward. In fact there are fears that continuing with strict hypothesis-driven approaches will delay useful research potentially by decades and involve vast amounts of unnecessary expense. Resolving these tensions will be key to establishing a functioning registry.

5.4 Measures of Positive Hearing Health

The LCHD model emphasizes that the goal of health development should be to optimize hearing health, not just avoid disease. Life course models view hearing health as a capacity for life, so optimal health incorporates hearing ability that is sufficient for each hearing function that person requires in their daily life, not just reaching a defined threshold on a single hearing test. This might include hearing well even in a noisy work environment, or being able to converse with friends without missing some words in the conversation. Existing audiometrics appear insufficiently sensitive to identify early functional hearing challenges. Researchers need operational measures of positive hearing health, both for better measurement of treatment outcomes and of functional hearing ability. These measures should be developed and trailed by multidisciplinary teams with representation from deaf, hard of hearing, and hearing consumers across a range of ages. In addition, more sensitive measures of environmental noise exposure are needed.

5.5 Investigating the Pathophysiology of Hearing Loss

Further elucidation of the pathophysiology of hearing loss will require a combination of bench and clinical research across multiple disciplines including genetics, biochemistry, cell biology, physiology, and audiology. Greater synthesis of existing knowledge could link information on known genetic variants associated with hearing loss, with suspected polymorphisms that could be related to hearing loss, and with what is known about abnormalities at metabolic, biochemical, subcellular, and cellular processes in individuals with different types of hearing loss. Epidemiologic data on identified clinical associations with hearing loss should be linked with genetic and biochemical data repositories in ways that facilitate the identification of potentially important relationships. More work is needed on elucidating the mechanisms that underlie observed associations, e.g., low socioeconomic status in childhood and later hearing loss, smoking and adult hearing loss, and noise exposure and hearing loss at all ages.

5.6 Involvement of Deaf and Hard of Hearing Communities in Research

Widespread understanding of the importance of involving members of the deaf and hard of hearing communities and their families in research on the etiology, diagnosis, and management of hearing loss is driving new efforts to find effective ways to ensure productive partnerships between consumers and researchers. Funding bodies are beginning to invite members of the deaf and hard of hearing community to contribute to boards that set funding agendas and to invite them to review grant applications and new program proposals. Community-based participatory research (CBPR) models envisage the deaf and hard of hearing as integral members of research teams, often suggesting research questions that they, as a community, would like to see answered and suggesting ways to engage deaf and hard of hearing (DHH) subjects in the research. These efforts must be inclusive. Where distinct groups of DHH communities exist, each must be invited to participate fully, even if there will be more than one view on priorities and conduct of research. Input from each of these groups is more likely to lead to a study protocol that will be embraced by a majority of DHH subjects, reducing inherent biases. This work is not easy and would benefit from use of professional facilitators. Metrics must be developed to monitor progress toward true, rather than token, involvement, e.g., reporting of number of DHH individuals on research boards, invited to key meetings, contributing to possible research questions. Life course theory acknowledges the multiple contributors to health at social and community levels, suggesting that there may be much to learn from DHH individuals who have successfully overcome communication, educational, and occupational challenges.

5.7 Translational Research

The translation of evidence into practice does not occur automatically and itself requires study. As evidence accrues for the mechanisms underlying hearing health trajectories, investigators will need to test their potential mutability and consider implications for clinical practice. Promising interventions, whether they be pharmacological, surgical, or social, then need to undergo clinical trials (T1) and trials in community-based programs (T2) and then be trialed as new systems of care (T3). Finally, researchers need to test ways to scale and spread successful interventions (T4) before incorporating them into state and national MCH programs and policies. While funding for T1 research can be obtained through traditional National Institute on Deafness and Other Communication Disorders (NIDCD) R01 mechanisms, funding of other types of translational research falls at the intersection of NIDCD and other agencies such as Agency for Healthcare Research and Quality (AHRQ). The reality is that funding for this type of research is very limited. In addition, life course models indicate that successful interventions will likely have both "medical" and "social" components, potentially making them less likely to be funded through traditional health mechanisms. Public-private partnerships may provide innovative ways to fund this type of research, which may cut across traditional barriers between health and education, or health and occupational development.

6 Implications for Policy and Practice

6.1 Impact Studies

Life course models acknowledge that policies affecting women of childbearing age and young children can have profound direct and indirect effects on the health of the next generation. Infrastructure and funding must be developed for studying the impact of existing and proposed policy changes on hearing health. For example, fiscal challenges have resulted in a number of states offering early intervention services to children with moderate or greater bilateral hearing loss, while children with mild and unilateral losses are deemed ineligible, despite the existence of at least moderately good evidence that these children also face additional challenges with school performance. This type of policy may prove to be a "false economy" if children that missed out on early intervention ultimately, as adults, lack skills that they would have acquired had intervention been available to them. Balancing the evidence may require additional studies, or use of computer simulation models, to make a best estimate of cost-benefits.

6.2 Integrated Services

Services for children and adults that are DHH are separated into "medical" interventions including auditory surgery and cochlear implantation, "developmental" interventions such as early intervention, "social" interventions such as family support services, and "mental health" interventions such as counseling. Life course models suggest that in order to achieve optimal hearing health trajectories, these services must be integrated into a cohesive whole, preferably with a single point of entry, rather than operated and run independently with minimal communications between providers. While electronic medical records may help with information flow, the provision of community-based services poised to address all the needs of DHH individuals will require a transformation of the present system of care and a blurring of the boundaries between health, educational, and social services.

6.3 Public Information Campaign

The LCHD model acknowledges that cultural and social pressures can have a major impact on health. Many deaf people report feeling marginalized in society, while reluctance to wear hearing aids among some individuals that are hard of hearing stems from a desire to keep their condition hidden. These cultural issues are powerful barriers to the achievement of full hearing health for many. A national and international campaign is needed to inform the general public about the nature of deafness and the importance of respecting deaf culture and communication choices. For people who are hard of hearing and who choose to wear hearing aids, use of hearing aids must be destigmatized. Use of accommodations such as closed captioning and telephone interpreter services should be strongly encouraged even for those that can function, albeit imperfectly, without them. Involvement of the DHH community in the planning and execution of this campaign is essential. The internet and social media including Facebook and Twitter offer ideal venues to distribute information and challenge cultural assumptions.

6.4 Costs and Cost-Effectiveness

Hearing loss has profound economic implications for individuals, families, and society as a whole. Comprehensive economic studies are needed to address the true costs of hearing loss at all levels. New policies must incorporate strong consideration of cost-effectiveness in preventive and treatment measures across all stages of the life span. The provision of amplification aids to a much wider proportion of the population in a cost-effective manner is a research and policy priority (National Academies 2016).

7 Conclusions

The Life Course Health Development model offers a conceptual framework for understanding the many genetic, biological, social, psychological, and cultural factors that contribute to hearing health over a lifetime. Early life events and experiences can have profound effects on hearing trajectories with lifelong consequences. Shifting trajectories involves altering the balance between risk and protective factors, especially during critical and sensitive periods of development including fetal life and the prelingual period in the first 6 months of postnatal life. Early diagnosis and intervention, early exposure to language whether signed or oral, warm reciprocal parent-infant relationships regardless of communication modality, broad family support, responsive school and work environments, and policies that enable lifelong supports can combine to lead to good outcomes. The goal of management is optimal hearing health, not just avoidance of poor auditory function. New measures of positive hearing health are needed to drive research on optimal hearing function.

Universal Newborn Hearing Screening has achieved early diagnosis and intervention for many, but loss to follow-up threatens the success of the program and can have long-reaching consequences in individual cases. People who are deaf and/or hard of hearing face continuing challenges with educational achievement and workplace function. Addressing hearing loss later in life will require multiple approaches including a greater focus on early prevention, reduction to noise exposure throughout the life span, reductions in smoking and excessive alcohol consumption, and avoidance of excessive weight gain. The focus of research must shift from uni- and bi-disciplinary cross-sectional designs to interdisciplinary longitudinal cohort studies that incorporate both historical and biological data. Voluntary hearing loss registries, both national and international, could provide "big data" for new research approaches to studying the etiology and management of hearing loss. Transdisciplinary knowledge synthesis, potentially adopting a wiki-type framework, could provide a resource for use across disciplines by providers, researchers, and consumers. Research into the pathophysiology of hearing loss must cut across traditional boundaries, embracing genetic, epigenetic, biological, and cellular mechanisms incorporating a health development perspective.

There is considerable wisdom in the deaf and hard of hearing communities that should be utilized both in assisting newly diagnosed DHH individuals in achieving optimal functioning and in driving the research and service improvement agenda. Focused studies must address the impact of existing and proposed policies on hearing health, while management of established hearing loss requires a more integrated approach across health education and social services. Achieving optimal hearing health for all will require cultural and societal shifts in which deafness is destigmatized and an inclusive agenda actively pursued for the deaf and hard of hearing across all stages of the life span. Optimal hearing health in childhood must be prioritized as the foundation for lifelong hearing health in the US population.

References

Appelman, K. I., Callahan, J. O., Mayer, M. H., Luetke, B. S., & Stryker, D. S. (2012). Education, employment and independent living of young adults who are deaf and hard of hearing. *Am Ann Deaf, 157*(3), 264–275.

Appollonio, I., Carabellese, C., Frattola, L., & Trabucchi, M. (1996). Effects of sensory aids on the quality of life and mortality of elderly people: A multivariate analysis. *Age and Ageing, 25*(2), 89–96.

Augustsson, I., & Engstrand. (2005). Hearing loss as a sequel of secretory and acute otitis media as reflected by audiometric screening of Swedish conscripts. *International Journal of Pediatric Otorhinolaryngology, 70*(4), 703–710.

Baltes, P. B., Lindenberger, U., & Staudinger, U. M. (2007). Life span theory in developmental psychology. In *Handbook of child psychology* (Vol. 1, p. 11). Hoboken: John Wiley and Sons. Accessed onlinelibrary.wiley.com.

Barnett, S., & Franks, P. (1999). Deafness and mortality: Analysis of linked data from the National Health Interview Survey and National Death Index. *Public Health Rep, 114*(4), 330–336.

Barrenas, M. L., Brathall, A., & Dahlgren, J. (2005a). The association between short stature and sensorineural hearing loss. *Hearing Research, 205*(1–2), 123–130.

Barrenas, M. L., Jonsson, B., Tuvemo, T., Hellstrom, P. A., & Lundgren, M. (2005b). High risk of sensorineural hearing loss in men born small for gestational age with and without obesity or height catch up growth: A prospective longitudinal register study on birth size in 245,000 Swedish conscripts. *The Journal of Clinical Endocrinology and Metabolism, 90*(8), 4452–4456.

Benson, V., & Marano, M. A. (1994). Current estimates from the National Health Interview Survey, 1993, vital health stat **3.** Tackling inequality: Get them while they're young. *British Medical Journal, 340*, c346–c348. 190: DHHS Publication PHS 95-1518.

Bhasin, T. K., Brocksen, S., Avchen, R. N., & Van Naarden Braun, K. (2006). Prevalence of four developmental disabilities among children aged 8 years – Metropolitan Atlanta developmental disabilities surveillance program, 1996 and 2000. *MMWR Surveillance Summaries, 55*(1), 1–9. Erratum in MMWR Morb Mortal Wkly Rep. (2006) Feb 3, 55(4):105–6.

Bess, F. H., Dodd-Murphy, J., & Parker, R. A. (1998). Children with minimal sensorineural hearing loss: Prevalence, educational performance, and functional status. *Ear Hear, 19*(5), 339–354.

Bitner-Glindzicz, M. (2002). Hereditary deafness and phenotyping in humans. *British Medical Bulletin, 63*, 73–94.

Blanchfield, B. B., Feldman, J. J., Dunbar, J. L., & Gardner, E. N. (2001). The severely to profoundly hearing-impaired population in the United States: Prevalence estimates and demographics. *Journal of the American Academy of Audiology, 12*(4), 183–189.

Brookhouser, P. E., Worthington, D. W., & Kelly, W. J. (1991). Unilateral hearing loss in children. *Laryngoscope, 101*(12Pt 1), 1264–1272.

Broste, S. K., Hansen, D. A., Strand, R. L., & Stueland, D. T. (1989). Hearing loss among high school farm students. *American Journal of Public Health, 79*(5), 619–622.

Cabral, L., Muhr, K., & Savageau, J. (2013). Perspectives of people who are deaf and hard of hearing on mental health, recovery, and peer support. *Community Ment Health J, 49*(6), 649–657. Epub 2012 Nov 13.

Christensen, K., Fredericksen, H., & Hoffman, H. J. (2001). Genetic and environmental influences on self-reported reduced hearing in the old and oldest old. *Journal of the American Geriatrics Society, 49*(11), 1512–1517.

Chung, J. H., DesRoches, C. M., Meunier, J., & Eavey, R. D. (2005). Evaluation of noise-induced hearing loss in young people using a web-based survey technique. *Pediatrics, 115*, 861–867.

Clinard, C. G., & Tremblay, K. L. (2013). Aging degrades the neural encoding of simple and complex sounds in the human brainstem. *Journal of the American Academy of Audiology, 24*(7), 590–599. quiz 643-4.

Cohn, E. S., & Kelley, P. M. (1999). Clinical phenotype and mutations in connexin 26 (DFNB1/GJB2), the most common cause of childhood hearing loss. *American Journal of Medical Genetics, 89*(3), 130–136.

Cruickshanks, K. J., Wiley, T. L., Tweed, T. S., et al. (1998). Prevalence of hearing loss in older adults in Beaver dam, Wisconsin: The Epidemiology of hearing loss study. *American Journal of Epidemiology, 148*(9), 879–886.

Danielson, R W. (2005). Hearing loss prevention-prevention of hearing loss from noise exposure. Better hearing Institute http://www.betterhearing.org/hearing_loss_prevention. Accessed 12/29/05.

Das, V. K. (1996). Aetiology of bilateral sensorineural hearing impairment in children: A 10 year study. *Archives of Disease in Childhood, 74*(1), 8–12.

Davis, A., McMahon, C. M., Pichora-Fuller, K. M., Russ, S., Lin, F., Olusanya, B. O., Chadha, S., & Tremblay, K. L. (2016). Aging and hearing health: The life-course approach. *The Gerontologist, 56*(Suppl 2), S256–S267.

Davis, A. C. (1989). The prevalence of hearing impairment and reported hearing disability among adults in Great Britain. *International Journal of Epidemiology, 18*, 911–917. Cited in Smith, R J., Bale, J F., White, K R. (2005) Sensorineural hearing loss in children. *Lancet, 365*, 879–90.

Davis, A. C., Ostri, B., & Parving, A. (1990). Longitudinal study of hearing. *Acta Oto-Laryngologica. Supplementum, 476*, 12–22.

DeStefano, A. L., Gates, G. A., Heard-Costa, N., & Myers, R. H. (2003). Baldwin CT. *Archives of Otolaryngology – Head & Neck Surgery, 129*(3), 285–289.

Fernandez, K. A., Jeffers, P. W., Lall, K., Liberman, M. C., & Kujawa, S. G. (2015). Aging after noise exposure: Acceleration of cochlear synaptopathy in "recovered" ears. *The Journal of Neuroscience, 35*(19), 7509–7520.

Finitzo, T., Albright, K., & O'Neal, J. (1998). The newborn with hearing loss: Detection in the nursery. *Pediatrics, 102*(6), 1452–1460.

Fischel-Ghodsian, N. (2003). Mitochondrial deafness. *Ear and Hearing, 24*(4), 303–313.

Fisher, D., Li, C. M., Chiu, M. S., Themann, C. L., Petersen, H., Jónasson, F., Jónsson, P. V., Sverrisdottir, J. E., Garcia, M., Harris, T. B., Launer, L. J., Eiriksdottir, G., Gudnason, V., Hoffman, H. J., & Cotch, M. F. (2014). Impairments in hearing and vision impact on mortality in older people: The AGES-Reykjavik study. *Age and Ageing, 43*(1), 69–76.

Flamme, G. A., Mudipalli, V. R., Reynolds, S. J., Kelly, K. M., Stromquist, A. M., Zwerling, C., Burmeister, L. F., Peng, S. C., & Merchant, J. A. (2005). Prevalence of hearing impairment in a rural midwestern cohort :

Estimates from the Keokuk county rural health study, 1994 to 1998. *Ear and Hearing, 26*(3), 350–360.

Fligor, B. J., Neault, M. W., Mullen, C. H., Feldman, H. A., & Jones, D. T. (2005). Factors associated with sensorineural hearing loss among survivors of extracorporeal membrane oxygenation therapy. *Pediatrics, 115*(6), 1519–1528.

Fellinger, J., Holtzinger, D., & Pollard, R. (2012). Mental health of deaf people. *Lancet, 379*(9820), 1037–1044.

Fortnum, H. M., Summerfield, A. Q., Marshall, D. H., Davis, A. C., & Bamford, J. M. (2001). Prevalence of permanent childhood hearing impairment in the United Kingdom and implications for universal neonatal hearing screening: Questionnaire based ascertainment study. *British Medical Journal, 323*(7312), 536–540.

Gates, G. A., & Mills, J. H. (2005). Presbycusis. *Lancet, 366*(9491), 1111–1120.

Gates, G. A., Cooper, J. C. J. R., Kannel, W. B., et al. (1990). Hearing in the elderly: The Framingham cohort, 1983-1985. Part 1. Basic audiometric test results. *Ear and Hearing, 11*(4), 247–256.

Gates, G. A., Schmid, P., Kujawa, S. G., Nam, B., & D'Agostino, R. (2000). Longitudinal threshold changes in older men with audiometric notches. *Hearing Research, 141*(1–2), 220–228.

Gething, L. (2000). Ageing with long-standing hearing impairment and deafness. *International Journal of Rehabilitation Research, 23*(3), 209–215.

Gordon-Salant. (2005). Hearing loss and aging: New research findings and clinical implications. *Journal of Rehabilitation Research and Development, 42*(4), 9–24.

Gurtler, N., Schmuziger, N., Kim, Y., Mhatre, A. N., Jungi, M., & Lalwani, A. K. (2005). Audiologic testing and molecular analysis of 12S rRNA in patients receiving aminoglycosides. *The Laryngoscope, 115*(4), 640–644.

Gustason, G. (1989). Early identification of hearing impairment in infants: A review of Israeli and American progress. *Volta Review, 91*, 291–295.

Halfon, N., & Forrest, C. B. (2017). The emerging theoretical framework of life course health development. In N. Halfon, C. B. Forrest, R. M. Lerner, & E. Faustman (Eds.), *Handbook of life course health-development science*. Cham: Springer.

Helzner, E. P., Cauley, J. A., Pratt, S. R., Wisniewski, S. R., Zmuda, J. M., Talbott, E. O., de Rekeneire, N., Harris, T. B., Rubin, S. M., Simonsick, E. M., Tylavsky, F. A., & Newman, A. B. (2005). Race and sex differences in age-related hearing loss: The health, aging and body composition study. *Journal of the American Geriatrics Society, 53*(12), 2119–2127.

Hertzman, C., Siddiqi, A., Hertzman, E., Irwin, L., Vaghri, Z., Houweling, T. A., Bell, R., Tinajero, A., & Marmo, M. (2010). Tackling inequality: Get them while they're young. *British Medical Journal, 340*, c346–c348.

Halloran, D. R., Wall, T. C., Evans, H. H., Hardin, J. M., & Woolley, A. L. (2005). Hearing screening at well-child visits. *Arch Pediatr Adolesc Med, 159*(10), 949–955.

Holt, JA. (1993) Stanford Achievement Test. 8th Ed: Reading Comprehension Subgroup Results. Am Ann Deaf. 138, 172–5 cited in Durieux-Smith A. Chapter VII in Early Hearing and Communication Development accessed at http://www.phac-aspc.gc.ca/publicat/eh-dp/chap7_e.html 11/10/–05.

Homans, N. C., Metselaar, R. M., Dingemanse, J. G., van der Schroeff, M. P., Brocaar, M. P., Wieringa, M. H., Baatenburg de Jong, R. J., Hofman, A., & Goedegebure, A. (2016). Prevalence of age-related hearing loss, including sex differences, in older adults in a large cohort study. *Laryngoscope, 127*(3), 725–730.

Hultcrantz, M., Simonoska, R., & Stenberg, A. E. (2006). Estrogen and hearing: A summary of recent investigations. *Acta Oto-Laryngologica, 126*(1), 10–14.

Kelley, P. M., Cohn, E., & Kimberling, W. J. (2000). Connexin 26: Required for normal auditory function. *Brain Research. Brain Research Reviews, 32*(1), 184–188.

Kennedy, C., McCann, D., Campbell, M., Kimm, L., & Thornton, R. (2005). Universal newborn screening for permanent childhood hearing impairment: An 8 year follow-up of a controlled trial. *Lancet, 366*, 660–662.

Kujawa, S. G., & Liberman, M. C. (2006). Acceleration of age-related hearing loss by early noise exposure: Evidence of a misspent youth. *The Journal of Neuroscience, 26*(7), 2115–2123.

Kuzawa, C. W., & Thayer, Z. M. (2011). Timescales of human adaptation: The role of epigenetic processes. *Epigenomics, 3*(2), 221–234.

Lee, D. J., Gomez-Martin, O., Lam, B. L., & Zheng, D. D. (2004). Trends in hearing impairment in United States adults: The national health interview survey, 1986-1995. *Journal of Gerentol. A. Biological Medical Science, 59*(11), 1186–1190.

Lee, F. S., Matthews, L. J., Dubno, J. R., & Mills, J. H. (2005). Longitudinal study of pure tone thresholds in older persons. *Ear and Hearing, 26*(1), 1–11.

Levine, D., Strother-Garcia, K., Golinkoff, R. M., & Hirsh-Pasek, K. (2016). Language development in the first year of life: What deaf children might be missing before Cochlear implantation. *Otology & Neurotology, 37*(2), e56–e62.

Lin, F. R., Hazzard, W. R., & Blazer, D. G. (2016). Priorities for improving hearing health Care for Adults: A report from the National Academies of Sciences, Engineering, and Medicine. *Journal of the American Medical Association, 316*(8), 819–820.

Low, F. M., Gluckman, P. D., & Hanson, M. A. (2011). Developmental plasticity and epigenetic mechanisms underpinning metabolic and cardiovascular diseases. *Epigenomics, 3*(3), 279–294.

Mason, J. A., & Herrmann, K. R. (1998). Universal infant hearing screening by automated auditory brainstem response measurement. *Pediatrics, 101*(2), 221–228.

Marlow, E. S., Hunt, L. P., & Marlow, N. (2000). Sensorineural hearing loss and prematurity. *Archives of Disease in Childhood. Fetal and Neonatal Edition, 82*, F141–F144.

Mehl, A. L., & Thomson, V. (2002). The Colorado newborn hearing screening project, 1992–1999: On the threshold of effective population-based universal newborn hearing screening. *Pediatrics, 109*(1), E7.

McKee, M., Schlehofer, D., Cuculick, J., Starr, M., Smith, S., & Chin, N. P. (2011). Perceptions of cardiovascular health in an underserved community of deaf adults using American Sign Language. *Disabil Health J, 4*(3), 192–197.

Mitchell, R. E. (2005). How many deaf people are there in the United States: Estimates from the survey of income and program participation. *Journal of Deaf Studies and Deaf Education, 11*(1), 112–119. [Epub].

Mohr, P. E., Feldman, J. J., Dunbar, J. L., McConkey-Robbins, A., Niparko, J. K., Rittenhouse, R. K., & Skinner, M. W. (2000). The societal costs of severe to profound hearing loss in the United States. *Int J Technol Assess Health Care, 16*(4), 1120–1135.

Moore, W. G., Josephson, J. A., & Mauk, G. W. (1990). Identification of children with hearing impairments: A baseline survey. *The Volta Review, 93*, 187–196.

Mutton, P., & Peacock, K. (2005). Neonatal hearing screens: Wessex re-visited. *Lancet, 366*, 612–613.

Nance, W. E. (2003). The genetics of deafness. *Mental Retardation and Developmental Disabilities Research Reviews, 9*(2), 109–119.

National Academies of Sciences, Engineering and Medicine (2016). Hearing Health Care for Adults: Priorities for Improving Access and Affordability. http://nationalacademies.org/hmd/reports/2016/Hearing-Health-Care-for-Adults.aspx.

National Center for Health Statistics, Data from the National Health Interview Survey 1994, Series 10, Number 188. National EHDI Goals http://www.cdc.gov/ncbdd/ehdi/nationalgoals.htm.

National Institute in Deafness and Other Communication Disorders. Noise-induced hearing loss (2002). NIH Pub. NO. 97–4233 Bethesda MD cited in The prevalence and Incidence of hearing Loss in Children http://www.asha.org/public/hearing/disorders/children.htm.

National Institute on Deafness and other Communication Disorders (NIDCD) Strategic Plan: Plain Language Version FY 2003-2005 2017. Accessed July 6th 2017 at https://www.nidcd.nih.gov/about/strategic-plan/2003-2005/strategic-plan-plain-language-version-fy-2003-2005

Niskar, A. S., Kieszak, S. M., Holmes, A. E., Esteban, E., Rubin, C., & Brody, D. J. (2001). Estimated prevalence of noiseinduced hearing threshold shifts among children 6 to 19 years of age: The third National Health and Nutrition Examination Survey, 1998–1994, United States. *Pediatrics, 108*(1), 40–43.

Park, J., Lombardino, L. J., & Ritter, M. (2013). Phonology matters: A comprehensive investigation of reading and spelling skills of school-age children with mild to moderate sensorineural hearing loss. *Am Ann Deaf, 158*(1), 20–40.

Parving, A., & Christensen, B. (1993). Training and employment in hearing-impaired subjects at 20-35 years of age. *Scandinavian Audiology, 22*(2), 133–139.

Parving, A., & Christensen, B. (1996). Epidemiology of permanent hearing impairment in children in relation to costs of a hearing health surveillance program. *International Journal of Pediatric Otorhinolaryngology, 34*, 9–23.

Pass, R. F. (2005). Congenital cytomegalovirus infection and hearing loss. *Herpes, 12*(2), 50–55.

Pearson, J. D., Morrell, C. H., Gordon-Salant, S., Brant, L. J., Metter, E. J., Klein, L. L., & Fozard, J. L. (1995). Gender differences in a longitudinal study of age-associated hearing loss. *Journal of the Acoustical Society of America, 97*(2), 1196–1205.

Popelka, M. M., Cruickshanks, K. J., Wiley, T. L., Tweed, T. S., Klein, B. E., & Klein, R. (1998). Low prevalence of hearing aid use among older adults with hearing loss: The Epidemiology of hearing loss study. *Journal of the American Geriatrics Society, 46*(9), 1168–1169.

Pressman, L., Pipp-Siegel, S., Yoshinaga-Itano, C., & Deas, A. (1999). Maternal sensitivity predicts language gain in preschool children who are deaf and hard of hearing. *Journal of Deaf Studies and Deaf Education, 4*($), 294–304.

Reavis, K. M., Tremblay, K. L., & Saunders, G. (2016). How can public health approaches and perspectives advance hearing health care? *Ear and Hearing, 37*(4), 376–380.

Richardson, J. T., Long, G. L., & Woodley, A. (2004). Students with an undisclosed hearing loss: A challenge for academic access, progress, and success? *Journal of Deaf Studies and Deaf Education, 9*(4), 427–441.

Rivers, B., Boppana, S. B., Fowler, K. B., Britt, W. J., Stagno, S., & Pass, R. F. (2002). Predictors of hearing loss in children with symptomatic congenital cytomegalovirus infection. *Pediatrics, 110*, 762–767.

Rosanowski, F., Eysholdt, U., & Hoppe, U. (2006). Influence of leisure-time noise on outer hair cell activity in medical students. *Int Arch Occup Environ health, 80*(1), 25–31.

Russ, S. (2001). Measuring the prevalence of permanent childhood hearing impairment. *British Medical Journal, 323*(7312), 725–726.

Russ, S. A., Poulakis, Z., Barker, M., Wake, M., Rickards, F., & Saunders, K. (2003). Oberklaid F Epidemiology of congenital hearing loss in Victoria. *Australia International Journal Audiology, 42*, 385–390.

Ryding, M., White, P., & Kalm, O. (2005). Course and long-term outcome of "refractory" secretory otitis media. *The Journal of Laryngology and Otology, 119*(2), 113–118.

Schubert, C. R., Fischer, M. E., Pinto, A. A., Klein, B. E. K., Klein, R., Tweed, T. S., & Cruickshanks, K. J. (2017). Sensory impairments and risk of mortality in older adults. *The Journals of Gerontology Series A: Biological Sciences and Medical Sciences, 72*(5), 710–715.

Sheppard, K., & Badger, T. (2010). The lived experience of depression among culturally Deaf adults. *J Psychiatr Ment Health Nurs, 17*(9), 783–789.

Sheppard, K. (2011). Using American sign language interpreters to facilitate research among deaf adults: Lessons learned. *J Transcult Nurs, 22*(2), 129–134.

Smith, R. J., Bale, J. F., & White, K. R. (2005). Sensorineural hearing loss in children. *Lancet, 365*, 879–890.

Tremblay, K. L., Pinto, A., Fischer, M. E., Klein, B. E., Klein, R., Levy, S., Tweed, T. S., & Cruickshanks, K. J. (2015). Selfreported hearing difficulties among adults with normal audiograms: The beaver dam offspring study. *Ear Hear, 36*(6), e290–e299.

Ubido, J., Huntington, J., & Warburton, D. (2002). Inequalities in access to healthcare faced by women who are deaf. *Health Soc Care Community, 10*(4), 247–253.

Uchida, Y., Nakshimat, T., Ando, F., Niino, N., & Shimokata, H. (2005). Is there a relevant effect of noise and smoking on hearing? A population-based aging study. *International Journal of Audiology, 44*(2), 86–91.

US Department of Health and Human Services Healthy Hearing 2010 Progress Report. (2010). www.healthypeople.gov/data/2010prog/focus28 Accessed 2/21/06.

Van Eldik, T. (2005). Mental health problems of Dutch youth with hearing loss as shown on the youth self report. *American Annals of the Deaf, 150*(1), 11–16.

Van Naarden, K., & Decoufle, P. (1999). Relative and attributable risks for moderate to profound bilateral sensorineural hearing impairment associated with lower birth weight in children 3 to 10 years old. *Pediatrics, 104*(4 Pt 1), 905–910.

Van Naarden, K., Decoufle, P., & Caldwell, K. (1999). Prevalence and characteristics of children with serious hearing impairment in metropolitan Atlanta, 1991-1993. *Pediatrics, 103*, 570–575.

Verheart, N., Willems, M., Van Kerschaver, E., & Desloovere, C. (2008). Impact of early hearing screening and treatment on language development and education level: Evaluation of 6 years of universal newborn hearing screening (ALGO) in Flanders, Belgium. *Int J Pediatr Otorhinolaryngol, 72*(5), 599–608.

Vernon, M., & LaFalce-Landers, E. (1993). A longitudinal study of intellectually gifted deaf and hard of hearing people. Educational, psychological and career outcomes. *Am Ann Deaf, 138*(5), 427–434.

Vernon, M. (2005). Fifty years of research on the intelligence of deaf and hard-of-hearing children: A review of literature and discussion of implications. *J Deaf Stud Deaf Educ Summer, 10*(3), 225–231.

Vohr, B., Jodoin-Krauzyk, J., Tucker, R., Topol, D., Johnson, M. J., Ahlgren, M., & Pierre, L. S. (2011). Expressive vocabulary of older children with hearing loss in the first 2 years of life; Impact of early intervention. *J Perinatol, 31*(4), 274–280.

Wake, M., Hughes, E. K., Collins, C. M., & Poulakis, Z. (2004). Parent-reported health-related quality of life in children with congenital hearing loss: A population study. *Ambulatory Pediatrics, 4*(5), 411–417.

Wallhagen, M. I., Strawbridge, W. J., Cohen, R., & Kaplan, G. A. (1997). An increasing prevalence of hearing impairment and associated risk factors over three decades of the Alameda County study. *American Journal Public Heaith, 87*(3), 440–442.

Winn, S. (2007). Employment outcomes for people in Australia who are congenitally deaf: Has anything changed? *Am Ann Deaf, 152*(4), 382–390.

Yueh, B., Shapiro, N., MacLean, C. H., & Shekelle, P. G. (2003). Screening and management of adult hearing loss in primary care: Scientific review. *JAMA, 289*(15), 1976–1985.

Chronic Kidney Disease: A Life Course Health Development Perspective

Patrick D. Brophy, Jennifer R. Charlton,
J. Bryan Carmody, Kimberly J. Reidy,
Lyndsay Harshman, Jeffrey Segar, David Askenazi,
David Shoham, and Susan P. Bagby

1 Introduction

Chronic kidney disease (CKD) impacts approximately 650,000 Americans, and health-related costs exceed 28 billion dollars per year (USRDS 2003; Wyld et al. 2015; Feldman et al. 2003; Furth et al. 2006). Given that many patients receive kidney transplants between 20 and 71, it is likely that some of these individuals (particularly the young adults) developed the initial stages of CKD early in life (USRDS 2003; Wyld et al. 2015; Feldman et al. 2003; Furth et al. 2006). Infants and children who develop CKD are at significant risk for associated health problems beyond those directly attributable to kidney disease because of the manifold effects of CKD on health development (Furth et al. 2006).

The risk factors and natural history for CKD progression in infants and children are not well understood (Furth et al. 2006). Currently, North American and European investigators are monitoring childhood cohorts of patients with CKD in order to better understand the natural progression and treatment of CKD and to identify significant risk factors for developing progressive CKD (Furth et al. 2006; Wong et al. 2012; Querfeld et al. 2010; ESCAPE Trial Group et al. 2009). In the same manner, the Chronic Renal Insufficiency Cohort Study (Lash et al. 2011) is identifying characteristics of patients associated with CKD among patients 21–74 years old. These population-based studies are providing data that will enable research to elucidate variables associated with progression of CKD, thereby permitting development of early intervention strategies.

P.D. Brophy, MD, MHCDS (✉)
University of Iowa Stead Family Children's Hospital, Pediatric Nephrology, Iowa City, IA, USA
e-mail: patrick-brophy@uiowa.edu

J.R. Charlton, MD, MSc • J. Bryan Carmody, MD
University of Virginia, Department of Pediatrics, Division of Nephrology, Charlottesville, VA, USA

K.J. Reidy, MD
Albert Einstein College of Medicine, Montefiore Medical Center, Pediatric Nephrology, Bronx, NY, USA

L. Harshman, MD
University of Iowa Children's Hospital, Pediatrics, Iowa City, IA, USA

J. Segar, MD
University of Iowa Children's Hospital, Neonatology, Iowa City, IA, USA

D. Askenazi, MD
University of Alabama Children's Hospital, Pediatric Nephrology, Birmingham, AL, USA

D. Shoham, PhD, MSPH
Department of Public Health Sciences, Loyola University Chicago, Maywood, IL, USA

S.P. Bagby, MD
Division of Nephrology & Hypertension, Department of Medicine, Moore Institute for Nutrition and Wellness, Oregon Health & Science University, Portland, OR, USA

N. Halfon et al. (eds.), *Handbook of Life Course Health Development*,
DOI 10.1007/978-3-319-47143-3_16

Given that the risk of mortality from cardiovascular diseases increases with a declining renal function status in individuals, any insights on reducing the risks or rates of CKD may have also influence cardiac morbidity and mortality in this population (Thompson et al. 2015).

Longitudinal studies of CKD progression and consequences are critical. Renal functional plasticity is substantial in infants, children, and even adults, although it peaks during fetal development. This means that it is possible to alter the negative effects of environmental and other inimical factors that threaten kidney development and function. In adult patients, early identification of modifiable risk factors (including diet) for CKD progression may have profound effects on their outcomes.

The life course health development principles (see Halfon and Forrest 2017) when applied to CKD suggest a set of mechanisms of disease progression and health development, which we will explore more fully throughout this chapter. These include:

1. The need to develop measures of kidney health and developmental plasticity to provide outcome measures that can be evaluated with respect to prevention efforts (Principle 1)
2. The importance of evaluating how kidney health and chronic kidney disease change over the life span (Principle 2)
3. The relationships between gene regulation, environmental exposures, and change in CKD risk over time, as they dynamically interact with one another (Principle 3)
4. Studying how social factors, particularly those related to risk for premature delivery and low birth rate, influence kidney health and chronic kidney disease risk (Principle 4)
5. Understanding the constraints that evolution places on the range of developmental pathways for kidney development and plasticity (Principle 5)
6. The effects of optimal kidney health development on long-term well-being and quality of life for individuals and populations (Principle 6)
7. Elucidating how the synchronization of biological "clocks" with cultural and environmental exposures influences the health development of kidney function (Principle 7)

Life course health development points to the need to study the dynamic interactions between individuals and their physical and social environmental exposures from gestation through to adult life. The principles also suggest that studies on cross-generational as well as individual biological, behavioral, psychosocial, and environmental determinants are important in understanding the development of kidney health and kidney disease (Ben-Shlomo and Kuh 2002).

The CKD framework as defined by the Kidney Disease Outcomes Quality Initiative (KDOQI) provides evidence-based guidelines for management of CKD (National Kidney Foundation; KDOQI (Kidney Disease Outcomes Quality Initiative) 2012). Given the already significant healthcare and societal costs of CKD, there is a need to reframe how we investigate the life course health development determinants of this chronic disease and the ways in which we deliver care in terms of prevention as well as management of extant disease. A clear understanding of these determinants can inform prevention and disease management programs which will have beneficial effects on patient health outcomes and costs of care.

Although diabetes is the single most important cause of CKD and end-stage renal disease in the adult population in the USA, congenital abnormalities of the kidney and urinary tract and reduced nephron endowment secondary to prematurity, intrauterine growth retardation, or early renal injury are the biggest risk factors for CKD that emerges during childhood (NAPRTCS 2011). The following sections of this chapter employ a life course health development framework to guide future research and public policy regarding CKD. The ability to use health services and outcomes research approaches to test public policy effects on health determinants along with the traditional basic, clinical, and translational science methods including the "omics" approach (Chen et al. 2012) provides a path forward within the innovative framework of the life course health development approach (Fig. 1).

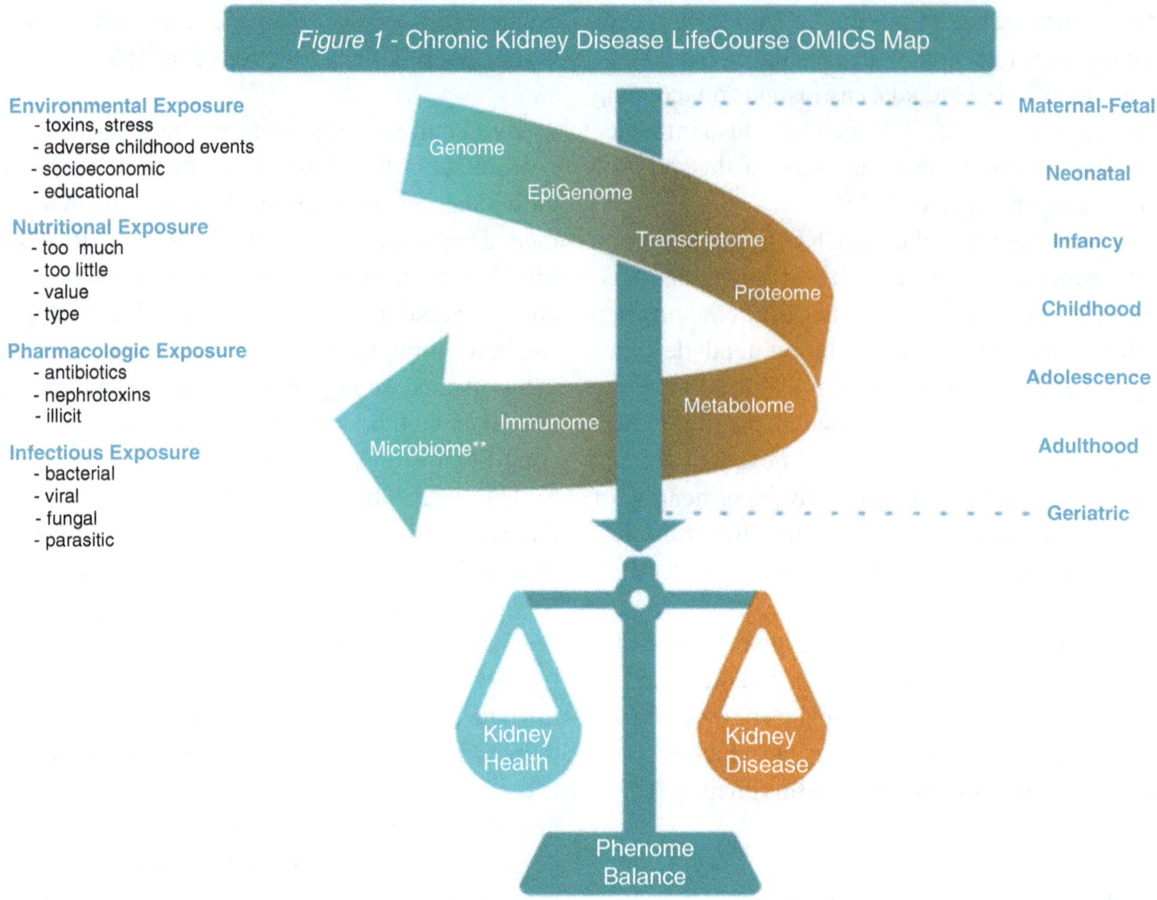

Fig. 1 Chronic kidney disease life course omics map

2 Preconceptional and Gestational Determinants of CKD

2.1 Preconception

The influence of the intrauterine environment in supporting optimal fetal development, including the developing kidney and metabolic regulatory processes, has lifelong implications for hypertension risk and renal health in later life (Bagby 2015). The impact of nutritional state appears to be multigenerational. In fact, the nutritional state of a woman from the time of her own conception (hence her mother's nutritional status) can influence how well she can nourish a fetus. Animal studies demonstrate that poor preconceptual nutrition and certain medication exposures both can alter allocation of kidney cell mass and yield reduced nephron number in offspring (Bagby 2015). Key considerations for prevention include developing ways to motivate young girls and women to adopt nutritional supplementation in the preconception period when there are clear benefits for doing so. There is increasing evidence (human and animal studies) that even modest levels of vitamin A deficiency can reduce nephron number in developing fetuses (Puddu et al. 2009). These simple and easily treated risks should not be overlooked. In fact, a recently published hospital-based, case-control study found an association among plasma lycopene, analgesic use, and CKD. This study showed that the higher the plasma lycopene was, the lower the CKD risk, whereas elevated retinol levels were associated with a higher risk of CKD in the context of analgesic use. Thus, while there may be clear benefits in preconception and early fetal life of adequate vitamin A levels, these same micronutrient levels may have differential effects in adult patients at risk for CKD development or progression. Further research on micronutrients and how and when they are delivered (either enterally or parenterally) is an important and cost-effective method of understanding the development of CKD (Chiang et al. 2010).

In a recent landmark study, a group of investigators hypothesized that the risk of CKD may be influenced prenatally. These investigators conducted a population-based, case-control study with 1994 patients with childhood CKD (<21 years of age at diagnosis) and 20,032 controls in order to examine the association of childhood CKD with prenatal risk factors, including fetal growth, maternal diabetes mellitus, and maternal overweight/obesity. Maternal and infant hospital discharge records were linked from 1987 to 2008. Results showed that CKD prevalence in this cohort was 127 cases per 100,000 births. The adjusted odds ratios for CKD associated with prenatal factors were 2.9 (95% CI, 2.3–3.6) for low birth weight, 1.5 (95% CI, 1.1–2.1) for maternal gestational diabetes mellitus, 1.2 (95% CI, 1.1–1.5) for maternal overweight/obesity, and 1.3 (95%CI, 1.05–1.52) for maternal obesity. CKD subtype analysis revealed low birth weight and maternal pregestational diabetes mellitus were associated with increased risk of renal dysplasia/aplasia, whereas poor fetal growth, maternal gestational diabetes mellitus, and maternal overweight/obesity were associated with obstructive uropathy. These findings suggest that targeted modification of these risk factors may reduce the risk of childhood CKD. Such interventions should be a focus of future investigations (Hsu et al. 2014).

Theoretical, experimental, and observational data suggest that there is an increased risk of CKD for infants born prematurely without specific renal birth defects. Indeed, a recent study evaluated 426 participants of the Chronic Kidney Disease in Children study cohort to determine whether low birth weight (<2500 grams), prematurity (gestational age < 36 weeks), small for gestational age (birth weight < 10th percentile for gestational age), or requirement for intensive care unit (ICU) care at birth were risk factors for poor growth outcomes in children identified with subsequent CKD – defined as a median baseline glomerular filtration rate (GFR) of 42.9 ml/min per 1.73 m2. The study found higher than expected prevalences of these risk factors: small for gestational age (14%), low birth weight (17%), prematurity (12%), and neonatal intensive care unit stays (40%) in patients from this CKD cohort. These results led investigators to conclude that small for gestational age and low birth weight are novel risk factors for CKD (Greenbaum et al. 2011).

2.2 Evidence from Animal Models

In rodents, in which nephrogenesis normally continues for 5–7 days postnatally, premature birth has a profound effect on kidney development. Mice born 1–2 days prematurely develop a CKD phenotype by the time they are 5 weeks old, exhibiting hypertension, albuminuria, and reduced nephron number (Stelloh et al. 2012). In other mouse studies, prenatal exposure to low protein and low vitamin A supply, perinatal exposure to gentamicin, and antenatal exposure to steroids all reduce nephron number in offspring (Gilbert et al. 1990; Lelievre-Pegorier et al. 1998; Sutherland et al. 2012a; Ortiz et al. 2001). Rats with 5/6 nephrectomy have been used as a model system to study the mechanisms by which low nephron number results in glomerular hyperfiltration, hypertension, albuminuria, and glomerulosclerosis (Brenner and Anderson 1987). Glomerular hyperfiltration and mechanical stress may contribute to podocyte loss and apoptosis (Reidy and Kaskel 2007; Fogo 2007). Activation of the renin-angiotensin system and TGF-beta has been implicated in podocyte loss and progressive glomerulosclerosis (Reidy and Kaskel 2007; Lopez-Hernandez and Lopez-Novoa 2012).

Other intriguing evidence comes from the baboon model of prematurity in which animals are delivered prematurely and maintained under conditions that very closely approximate the neonatal intensive care unit – including mechanical ventilation and treatment with nephrotoxins such as gentamicin for infections (Gubhaju et al. 2009) and ibuprofen for patent ductus arteriosus (PDA) closure (Sutherland et al. 2012b). Analogous to human studies, the nephrons of the premature baboons continue to develop postnatally, but with a high percentage of histological abnormalities (Gubhaju et al. 2009).

2.3 Prematurity: An Under-recognized Risk Factor for CKD

To date, there have been no prospective, longitudinal population-based prospective cohort studies to confirm the association between prematurity and CKD. However, evidence from well-designed retrospective, longitudinal studies has become increasingly abundant. A systematic review of 31 retrospective cohort or case-control studies found a 70% increase in the risk of CKD by adulthood for infants with a birth weight of <2.5 kg (White et al. 2009).

Clinical signs of oligonephropathy (i.e., low nephron number and mass) among patients born prematurely can often be detected in childhood. Two case series (each including 50 infants born at less than 30–32 weeks gestation) found that children born prematurely had smaller kidneys and higher blood pressure compared with full-term controls, even though their GFR remained normal (Bacchetta et al. 2009; Keijzer-Veen et al. 2010). Microalbuminuria – an early and sensitive indicator of kidney disease and a marker for future cardiovascular morbidity (Rademacher and Sinaiko 2009) – is also common among children 8–11 years old who were born prematurely or with low birth weight (Salgado et al. 2009) (Centers for Disease Control and Prevention (CDC) 2007).

A single case series of six patients with a history of prematurity who developed secondary focal glomerulosclerosis at an average age of 32 years old has been published (Hodgin et al. 2009a), providing an example of prematurity's association with CKD later in life. These individuals were all noted to be born prematurely (gestational ages of 22–30 weeks) and at the time of their presentation had nephrotic-range proteinuria, hypoalbuminemia, and lack of edema without any other risk factors for secondary focal glomerulosclerosis, suggesting that the premature infants are at higher risk for developing focal glomerulosclerosis later in life and raising the possibility of closer renal follow-up for such patients.

In infancy/childhood, the most overt cause of CKD and end-stage renal disease is birth defects or congenital anomalies of the kidney and urinary tract that result in inadequate renal mass to provide internal physiologic homeostasis for the provision of growth and development (NAPRTCS 2011; Chen et al. 2012; Bagby 2015; Puddu et al. 2009; Chiang et al. 2010; Hsu et al. 2014; Greenbaum et al. 2011; Horbar et al. 2012; Hack et al. 2002; Stelloh et al. 2012; Gilbert et al. 1990; Lelievre-Pegorier et al. 1998; Sutherland et al. 2012a; Ortiz et al. 2001; Brenner and Anderson 1987; Reidy and Kaskel 2007; Fogo 2007; Lopez-Hernandez and Lopez-Novoa 2012; Gubhaju et al. 2009; Sutherland et al. 2012b; White et al. 2009; Bacchetta et al. 2009; Keijzer-Veen et al. 2010; Rademacher and Sinaiko 2009; Salgado et al. 2009; Centers for Disease Control and Prevention (CDC) 2007; Hodgin et al. 2009a; Harambat et al. 2012; Warady and Chadha 2007; Tabel et al. 2010; Sanna-Cherchi et al. 2009). The long-term consequences of prematurity on renal mass are more subtle but, as mentioned above, are becoming increasingly clear. The advances in neonatal intensive care in the past 50 years have been nothing less than remarkable: according to the most recent data from the Vermont Oxford Network, nearly 90% of infants born weighing 501–1500 grams survive to neonatal intensive care unit (NICU) discharge, and nearly 60% of these very low birth weight survivors leave the NICU without any major neonatal morbidity (Horbar et al. 2012). It is clear that today, premature infants who in another era would have died within a matter of hours are now surviving to adulthood. While there has been a great deal of research into the neurodevelopmental outcomes of premature infants (Hack et al. 2002), the impact of premature birth on other organ systems is less well understood. There is emerging evidence from basic science and clinical research to suggest that both prematurity and medical treatment for its consequences may have serious long-term effects on kidney health development (Greenbaum et al. 2011). The implications of these studies are that the development of CKD and subsequent growth are influenced by maternal preconceptual nutritional status, premature birth, low birth weight, and small for gestational age. These early risk factors merit much more animal and human subject research to understand the specific mechanisms by which they influence the health development of the kidney. Indeed, the conceptualization of gestational renal mass development and its impact on later renal function and sequelae of CKD development continues to be an area of some controversy as well as active investigation.

2.4 Renal Development and Genetic Abnormalities

The congenital anomalies of the kidney and urinary tract spectrum represent relatively common birth defects, present in up to 1 in 500 live births, and are the leading causes of chronic kidney and end-stage renal disease in childhood. Hypoplastic or dysplastic kidneys, obstructive uropathy, and vesicoureteral reflux (VUR) account for 30% of children on dialysis in the USA (NAPRTCS 2011; Chen et al. 2012; Bagby 2015; Puddu et al. 2009; Chiang et al. 2010; Hsu et al. 2014; Greenbaum et al. 2011; Horbar et al. 2012; Hack et al. 2002; Stelloh et al. 2012; Gilbert et al. 1990; Lelievre-Pegorier et al. 1998; Sutherland et al. 2012a; Ortiz et al. 2001; Brenner and Anderson 1987; Reidy and Kaskel 2007; Fogo2007; Lopez-Hernandez and Lopez-Novoa 2012; Gubhaju et al. 2009; Sutherland et al. 2012b; White et al. 2009; Bacchetta et al. 2009; Keijzer-Veen et al. 2010; Rademacher and Sinaiko 2009; Salgado et al. 2009; Centers for Disease Control and Prevention (CDC) 2007; Hodgin et al. 2009a; Harambat et al. 2012; Warady and Chadha 2007; Tabel et al. 2010; Sanna-Cherchi et al. 2009). The development of end-stage renal disease in infancy/childhood results in poor growth and altered health development. Mortality rates among children with end-stage renal disease are 30–150 times higher than age-matched children in the general population (Warady and Chadha 2007). Moreover, kidney and urinary tract malformations that do not result in end-stage renal disease during childhood are risk factors for CKD during adulthood and contribute to significant healthcare and societal costs (Sanna-Cherchi et al. 2009; Westland et al. 2011; Spencer et al. 2011). Genetic studies of children with congenital anomalies of the kidney and urinary tract and animal studies have enabled investigators to identify multiple molecular signaling pathways that are required for normal kidney and urinary tract development. These include Wnts, bone morphogenetic proteins (BMPs), fibroblast growth factor (FGF), sonic hedgehog, RET/glial cell-derived neurotrophic factor, and Notch pathways (Horbar et al. 2012; Hack et al. 2002; Stelloh et al. 2012; Gilbert et al. 1990; Lelievre-Pegorier et al. 1998; Sutherland et al. 2012a; Ortiz et al. 2001; Brenner and Anderson 1987; Reidy and Kaskel 2007; Fogo 2007; Lopez-Hernandez and Lopez-Novoa 2012; Gubhaju et al. 2009; Sutherland et al. 2012b; White et al. 2009; Bacchetta et al. 2009; Keijzer-Veen et al. 2010; Rademacher and Sinaiko 2009; Salgado et al. 2009; Centers for Disease Control and Prevention (CDC) 2007; Hodgin et al. 2009a; Harambat et al. 2012; Warady and Chadha 2007; Tabel et al. 2010; Sanna-Cherchi et al. 2009; Westland et al. 2011; Spencer et al. 2011; Bertoli-Avella et al. 2008; Nishimura et al. 1999; Song and Yosypiv 2011; Paces-Fessy et al. 2012; Reidy and Rosenblum 2009). These signaling pathways regulate the outgrowth of the ureteric bud (from the Wolffian duct), the subsequent ureteric bud branching, and the reciprocal interactions between the tips of the ureteric bud and metanephric mesenchyme that lead to nephron and hence kidney formation. Abnormalities in these pathways lead to the spectrum of congenital anomalies of the kidney and urinary tract (Reidy and Rosenblum 2009). While the majority of over 70 genes identified are associated with syndromes involving multiple congenital anomalies, human genetic studies have confirmed a role for defects in several genes in non-syndromic congenital anomalies of the kidney and urinary tract, including HNF1, PAX2, ROBO2, GDNF, RET, SPRY1, FREM, FRET, and the angiotensin receptor 2 gene (Horbar et al. 2012;

Hack et al. 2002; Stelloh et al. 2012; Gilbert et al. 1990; Lelievre-Pegorier et al. 1998; Sutherland et al. 2012a; Ortiz et al. 2001; Brenner and Anderson 1987; Reidy and Kaskel 2007; Fogo 2007; Lopez-Hernandez and Lopez-Novoa 2012; Gubhaju et al. 2009; Sutherland et al. 2012b; White et al. 2009; Bacchetta et al. 2009; Keijzer-Veen et al. 2010; Rademacher and Sinaiko 2009; Salgado et al. 2009; Centers for Disease Control and Prevention (CDC) 2007; Hodgin et al. 2009a; Harambat et al. 2012; Warady and Chadha 2007; Tabel et al. 2010; Sanna-Cherchi et al. 2009; Westland et al. 2011; Spencer et al. 2011; Bertoli-Avella et al. 2008; Nishimura et al. 1999; Song and Yosypiv 2011; Paces-Fessy et al. 2012; Chatterjee et al. 2012; Nakayama et al. 2010; Saisawat et al. 2012; Weber et al. 2006). In addition to genetic mutations, prenatal environmental influences such as exposures to renin-angiotensin inhibition or antiepileptic medications may lead to congenital anomalies of the kidney and urinary tract (Carta et al. 2007; Serreau et al. 2005). Mouse models have revealed that the interactions between different signaling pathways are complex and the effects of loss of gene function are time and cell-lineage specific (Paces-Fessy et al. 2012; Reidy and Rosenblum 2009; Sims-Lucas et al. 2012; Schedl and Hastie 2000).

Polycystic kidney disease is the most common and best-studied genetic disease associated with CKD. Autosomal recessive polycystic kidney disease, a relatively rare genetic disorder, occurs in approximately 1 in 20,000 individuals, affecting males and females equally; it commonly presents in the perinatal period; and, it has a high morbidity and mortality rate in the first month of life (Cramer and Guay-Woodford 2015). Autosomal-dominant polycystic kidney disease is the most prevalent inherited renal disease and one of the most common life-threatening genetic diseases.

Autosomal-dominant polycystic kidney disease affects approximately 1 in 500 individuals and does not skip generations. It is often characterized by multiple renal cysts that can eventually lead to kidney failure and may present from birth all the way through to old age. This presentation may be impacted by underlying genetic, epigenetic, and environmental modifying factors. Given the variable phenotypic presentation, autosomal-dominant polycystic kidney disease provides a visual framework for the life course health development approach to care including targets for research and associations with cardiovascular disease and hypertension (see Fig. 2 (Takamitsu and Darwin Bell 2015)).

The second leading cause of CKD in childhood is focal glomerulosclerosis, comprising 14% of children with end-stage renal disease in the USA (NAPRTCS 2011). Populations such as Aboriginal Australians that have low nephron numbers at birth have increased susceptibility to glomerular diseases, especially focal glomerulosclerosis, and there are reports of focal glomerulosclerosis in isolated patients with decreased nephron mass due to oligonephronia or traumatic injury (Hoy et al. 1999, 2010; 2012; Mallick 2003; Hodgin et al. 2009b), suggesting that low nephron number may increase the risk for glomerular disease and CKD (Lackland et al. 2000; Furth et al. 2011; Hallan et al. 2008; Zandi-Nejad et al. 2006).

2.5 Fetal Origins of Adult Disease

David Barker is credited with the observation that many "adult" diseases in fact have their origins in fetal life (Barker and Sir Richard Doll Lecture 2012). To survive in a stressful or resource-poor environment, a fetus must make "choices" about how to utilize scarce resources in a way that maximizes the likelihood of survival in early life in order to reproduce, even at the expense of increased susceptibility to chronic illnesses in later life. This kind of developmental programming among low birth weight infants has been suggested to be an important risk factor for adulthood hypertension (Barker et al. 2007), insulin resistance (Barker 2005), and coronary artery disease (Barker 1995). The so-called Barker hypothesis implicates a reduction in nephron mass from either congenital abnormalities or environmental stressors resulting in CKD. Nephrologist Barry Brenner first substantiated Barker's theory in the development of CKD. Building on the observation that human

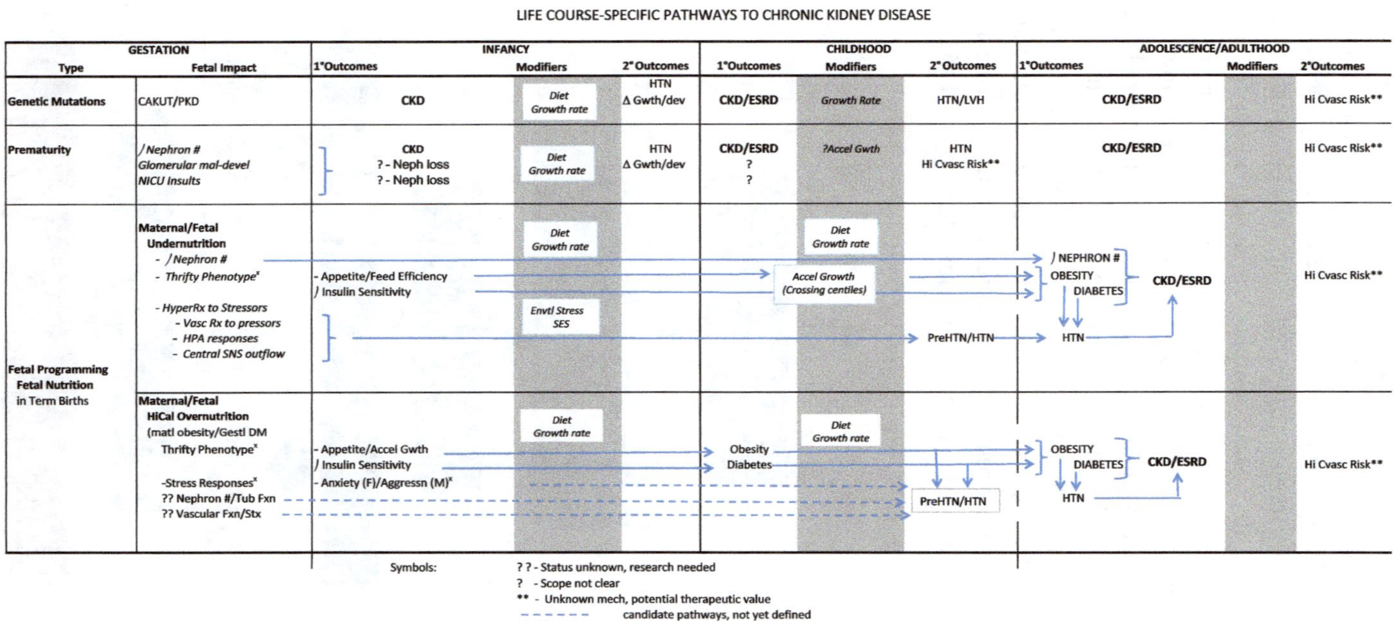

Fig. 2 Life course specific pathways to chronic kidney disease

nephron number is widely variable (with current best estimates showing a range of glomeruli from 210,000 to 1.8 million per kidney (Hoy et al. 2003)), Brenner proposed that either a congenital or developmentally programmed reduction in nephron number might explain why some individuals are more susceptible to hypertension and CKD (Brenner et al. 1988). Brenner suggested that, among persons with a decreased complement of nephrons, a normal GFR can be maintained initially as individual nephrons enlarge to increase the total surface area available for renal work (Luyckx and Brenner 2005). This leads to a further decrease in nephron number and requires even more hyperfiltration, leading to more rapid nephron dropout and perpetuating renal injury in a vicious cycle (Brenner et al. 1982) (see Fig. 3 (Carmody and Charlton 2013; Brenner et al. 1996; Brenner and Chertow 1994).

Indeed, low nephron number may result from defects in some of the same signaling pathways involved in congenital anomalies of the kidney and urinary tract, as nephron number is ultimately determined by the degree of ureteric bud branching, as nephrons are induced by the tips of the ureteric bud (Reidy and Rosenblum 2009).

The mechanisms by which intrauterine growth retardation and low birth weight result in low nephron number have been studied in rats exposed to resource-poor intrauterine environments. Adverse intrauterine environments can be induced experimentally by caloric or protein restriction or uterine artery ligation and placental insufficiency (Schröder 2003). Offspring develop

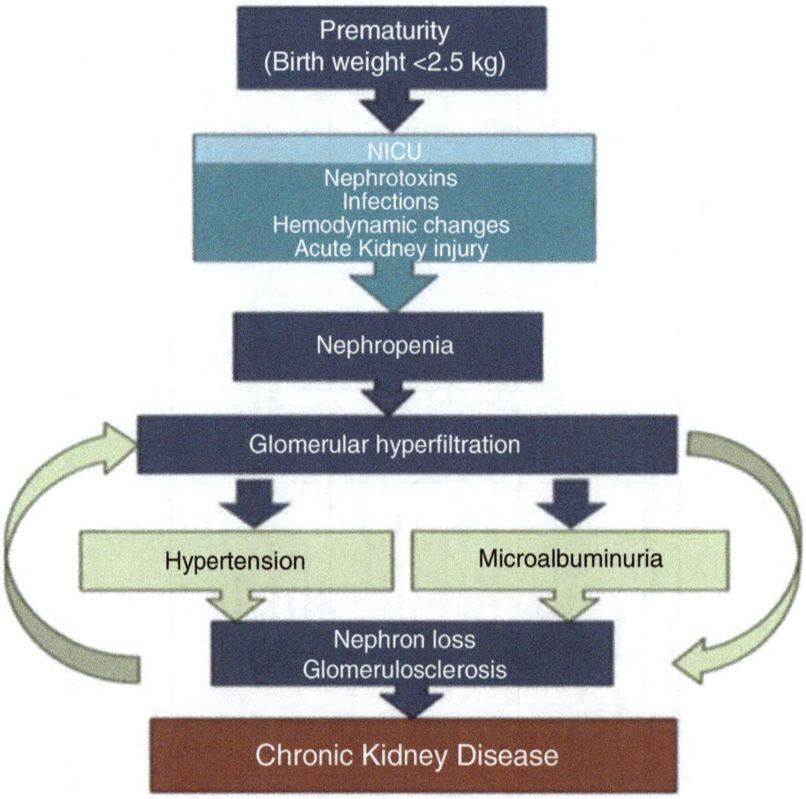

Fig. 3 This figure demonstrates the impact of cumulative insults on final nephron number in a premature infant. A combination of preterm birth (failure to develop a full functional set of nephrons) in addition to treatment and hemodynamic changes often seen in the treatment of premature infants can lead to increasing workload on the remaining functional nephrons and over the course of years these nephrons begin to scar which leads to subsequent high blood pressure, microalbuminuria, progressive nephron loss and ultimately progressive chronic kidney disease.

low nephron number with adult-onset hypertension, proteinuria, and glomerulosclerosis, especially in the setting of additional postnatal stressors such as high-protein diet or additional glomerular injury (Schreuder and Nauta 2007; Baserga et al. 2009, 2010; Merlet-Benichou et al. 1994; Schreuder et al. 2005; Shen et al. 2011; Plank et al. 2010). Alterations in expression of ureteric bud branching factors including downregulation of Pax2, GDNF, FGF7, BMP4, WNT4, and WNT11 mRNAs have been identified and may contribute to the decrease in nephron number (Abdel-Hakeem et al. 2008; Buffat et al. 2007). In addition, increased glomerular apoptosis has been observed (Pham et al. 2003). Studies of the mechanism by which intrauterine growth retardation may induce hypertension have suggested a role for the renin-angiotensin system, renal sympathetic activation, maternal glucocorticoid and fetal kidney 11beta-hydroxysteroid dehydrogenase type 2 activation, and increased sodium retention (Baserga et al. 2010; Ojeda et al. 2007; Grigore et al. 2007; Langley-Evans 1997; Sanders et al. 2005; Franco et al. 2012). Several studies have indicated that altered gene expression may be the result of epigenetic regulation (Baserga et al. 2010; Pham et al. 2003; Woroniecki et al. 2011).

2.6 Late Gestation Is Critical for Nephrogenesis

Although nephrogenesis in humans begins around 9 weeks gestation (Chevalier 1996; Engle 1986), the majority of nephrons (60%) are formed during the third trimester (Hinchliffe et al. 1991). The nephron complement of a human kidney is determined and fixed by 36 weeks gestation (Osathanondh and Potter 1963). Nephrons do not have the ability to regenerate; even in healthy persons, the number of functional nephrons gradually declines over time (leading to the natural age-dependent decline in GFR seen in older and elderly adults (Winearls and Glassock, 2011)).

For infants born prematurely, nephrons continue to form postnatally, but data from an autopsy study of 56 premature infants (birth weight < 1000 g) suggests that postnatal glomerulogenesis ceases after 40 days (Rodriguez et al. 2004). In an ex utero environment, these "potential" and youngest nephrons seem to be particularly vulnerable to maldevelopment and dysfunction: another study showed that up to 13% of postnatal glomeruli are morphologically abnormal (Sutherland et al. 2011).

3 Acute Kidney Injury as a Risk Factor for CKD

Acute kidney injury in the neonatal intensive care unit is common and often poorly recognized. While its overall incidence is difficult to determine given the lack of multicenter studies and variable definitions of acute kidney injury, one recent study from a single center that used the Acute Kidney Injury Network criteria (Mehta et al. 2007) found that nearly one of every five infants with birth weight < 1500 g who survived to discharge experienced acute kidney injury (Koralkar et al. 2011). Because the majority of infants that develop acute kidney injury are discharged home with a normal creatinine for their gestational age and size, the significance of their renal injury is underappreciated.

Until recently, it was believed that acute kidney injury was completely reversible (Kiley et al. 1960). Although this may be true for prerenal acute kidney injury caused by volume depletion, it is now clear that other forms of acute kidney injury cause irreversible damage and that the more severe the injury, the more likely the progression to CKD. Animal models of acute kidney injury induced by ischemia (Basile et al. 2001), aminoglycoside toxicity (Mingeot-Leclercq and Tulkens 1999), and sepsis (Holly et al. 2006) all exhibit permanent histologic changes even if the serum creatinine returns to normal. Such models of renal injury may be particularly applicable to the premature population, in which hemodynamic instability, antibiotic exposure, and systemic infections are common. As serum creatinine is a poor marker of acute kidney injury risk and represents a better marker for the resulting damage

(Askenazi et al. 2012), the emergence of new biomarkers for acute kidney injury has promising potential for predicting risk, damage, progression, and recovery.

Clinical evidence in neonatal and childhood cohorts linking acute kidney injury to the development of CKD is strengthening and well established in adults, leading some authors to even suggest that the rising incidence of acute kidney injury may be partly responsible for the nationwide increase in CKD and end-stage renal disease (Hsu 2007). A recent meta-analysis of adult trials found a substantial and exposure-dependent risk for developing CKD following acute kidney injury, with patients who experienced more severe acute kidney injury developing CKD and end-stage renal disease more frequently (Coca et al. 2012). While there are inherent risks in extrapolating the results of adult studies to pediatric patients, it is worth considering that nephron loss in a newborn infant may have far greater impact on future quality of life than it might for an older adult. Moreover, the limited number of pediatric observational studies undertaken has found similar results. In a single-center pediatric intensive care unit study, approximately 10% of patients with acute kidney injury subsequently developed significant CKD within the next 1–3 years (Mammen et al. 2012a). Alarmingly, nearly 50% of this cohort were deemed "at risk" for CKD based on the presence of hypertension, a reduced GFR (60–90 ml/min/1.73 m^2), or hyperfiltration (GFR >150 ml/min/1.73 m^2) during the follow-up period (Mammen et al. 2012a).

It could be argued that patients who are predisposed to the development of CKD may also be predisposed to the development of acute kidney injury (Rifkin et al. 2012). However, for pediatricians caring for premature infants who have suffered acute kidney injury, this distinction is likely an academic one. Whether acute kidney injury identifies a subgroup of infants most at risk of CKD or in fact leads independently to CKD, the implications for the child are the same, and the long-term implications of acute kidney injury ought not be ignored. Infants born prematurely (or with congenital anomalies of the kidney and urinary tract) begin life in the neonatal intensive care unit with an incomplete complement of nephrons. They are then exposed to a variety of external stressors that can hinder kidney development or cause additional nephron loss (see Fig. 4, (Brophy et al. 2015)). But unlike respiratory or infectious diseases, kidney disease is seldom a proximate cause of life-threatening illness for premature infants while they are in the NICU.

Although general pediatricians are attuned to the short-term risks associated with prematurity such as chronic lung disease, they often miss the implications of acute kidney injury on the long-term renal health of their patients. Indeed, recent analyses have identified the risk factors and repercussions of the use of nonsteroidal anti-inflammatory agents in pediatric patients (Misurac et al. 2013) along with other known nephrotoxins in an inpatient noncritical care environment (Kirkendall et al. 2014; Menon et al. 2014). There is a clear impact of over-the-counter medications alone and in combination with prescription medications on the development of acute kidney injury or worsening of CKD. (Onuigbo and Agbasi 2014) In particular, the geriatric population may be at very high risk for this effect (Mizokami and Mizuno 2015). Across the life span, medications can have a significant impact on the development of acute kidney injury. This in particular may be a very easy target for quality improvement initiatives that target reducing unnecessary use of medications (Goldstein et al. 2013).

4 CKD and Sequelae Beyond the First Year of Life

The interval between the newborn period and the first year of life among individuals with CKD or end-stage renal disease has conventionally been the highest risk period. Recent data has demonstrated improvement in outcomes in this age group in terms of survival (Carey et al. 2007). This appears due to better clinical management and understanding of the underlying renal pathology. The significant impact on families and early

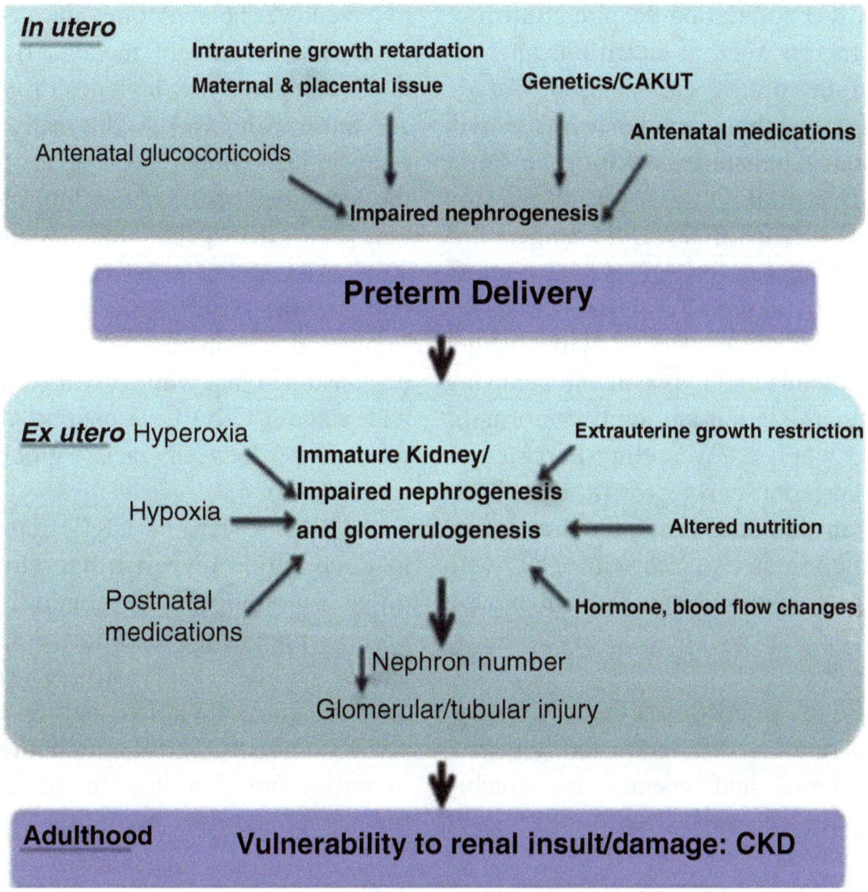

Fig. 4 This figure demonstrates some of the possible risks and insults that can occur in utero and ex utero to the renal system in infants, particularly those at higher risk, i.e. premature infants. The in-utero or maternal factors are often major contributors to antenatal renal function and yet may be overlooked during gestation. The impact of ex-utero damage is still not well vetted, but either alone or in combination with in utero insults, may lead to an increased vulnerability to subsequent renal damage as the patient ages and lead to progressive chronic kidney disease

child development cannot be underestimated. This is an intense and high-risk period for infants with CKD (Wedekin et al. 2008).

The development of CKD in children ages 1 through 17 years is strongly linked to the presence of congenital anomalies of the kidney and urinary tract diagnosed in infancy, infections, prematurity, glomerular disorders (most often diagnosed in preadolescence), and hereditary causes of renal dysfunction (National Kidney Foundation; KDOQI (Kidney Disease Outcomes Quality Initiative) 2012; Mong Hiep et al. 2010). New emphasis has also been placed on the long-term complications of acute kidney injury in the pediatric intensive care unit population as data suggests as many as 10% of children with kidney injury in this setting will progress to CKD within 1–3 years after injury (Mammen et al. 2012b).

Much of the recent data on the significance of CKD on life course health development outcomes in children springs from the Chronic Kidney Disease in Children (CKiD) prospective cohort study (Feldman et al. 2003). This study has enrolled children ages 1–16 years in a multicenter study aimed at determining the factors associated with progression through the CKD stages and onto end-stage renal disease and to investigate the impact of CKD on growth, cardiovascular complications, and neurodevelopmental outcomes in children.

Growth less than the third percentile has been noted in approximately 35% of children at the point of entry into the North American Pediatric Renal Trials and Collaborative Studies database of children with CKD (Seikaly et al. 2003), with poor growth pervasive in the CKD population despite control of modifiable factors such as nutrition, anemia, and hypoparathyroidism (Mahan and Warady 2006). Initial metabolic evidence of growth failure includes phosphate wasting in early CKD (Ben-Dov et al. 2007) with progression to decreasing calcitriol levels in stages 2–3 CKD resulting later in low 1,25(OH)2 vitamin D levels and hyperparathyroidism in stages 3–4 (Heidbreder et al. 1997), with further hyperphosphatemia and hypocalcemia causing defective mineralization and bony abnormalities as CKD worsens (Wesseling-Perry et al. 2012). Furthermore, early growth and development is an important marker for future growth prediction as children with CKD who are small for gestational age at birth have a higher risk for poor weight gain in childhood (Greenbaum et al. 2011).

With regard to cardiovascular outcomes, diagnoses of hypertension, left ventricular hypertrophy, dyslipidemia, and anemia are notably increased in children with CKD. A majority of children in CKiD are noted to have hypertension with a systolic blood pressure > 95th percentile on at least one occasion with a large number of children with blood pressure >90th percentile not receiving pharmacotherapy (Flynn et al. 2008). A minority of children with CKD have left ventricular hypertrophy as diagnosed by echocardiography. In this study, independent predictors for development of LVH include hypertension, female gender, and lower hemoglobin (Mitsnefes et al. 2010). Dyslipidemia is strongly associated with poor cardiovascular health, and dyslipidemia becomes more notable in those children with a comparatively lower GFR (<30 ml/min per 1.73 m2) and in the presence of nephrotic-range proteinuria (Saland et al. 2010). Even in moderate-stage CKD, anemia is a prevalent finding. Anemia worsens in patients with a GFR less than 43 mL/min per 1.73 m2 and glomerular causes of CKD (Fadrowski et al. 2008; Atkinson et al. 2010a).

Specific effort has been directed toward understanding differences in hemoglobin levels between Caucasian and African-American children. African-American children have been noted to have lower hemoglobin values at diagnosis of CKD, independent of the underlying cause of CKD, compared with both healthy white children and those with CKD. Additionally, racial differences in hemoglobin levels appear to increase at the lower end of the hemoglobin level distribution in a CKD population (Robins and Blum 2007; Atkinson et al. 2010b). Further research utilizing the North American Pediatric Renal Trials and Collaborative Studies CKD registry demonstrated that while the majority of children with stage 3 CKD have anemia, there were no differences between racial groups (Atkinson et al. 2010b).

A 2011 review of CKiD data specific to neurocognition revealed that while neurocognitive functioning was generally within the average range for the cohort, a large percentage of children demonstrated scores at least one standard deviation below the mean in areas such as IQ, academic achievement, and executive functioning with specific predictors for worse outcomes including decline in GFR and proteinuria (Hooper et al. 2011). Additionally, research from outside of the CKiD study has found that young age of disease onset and increasing length of disease and disease severity predict poorer neurocognitive performance (Slickers et al. 2007). Although much has been discovered to date regarding the etiology and pathogenesis of CKD in childhood and adolescence, there remain several areas to expand knowledge in the field. Great strides have been made to improve nutrition and slow worsening of mineral-bone disease in children with CKD. Despite this, there still remains debate regarding therapeutic targets, such as optimal parathyroid levels, as well as differing diagnostic approaches and use of pharmacologic agents in the treatment of mineral-bone disease; thus, much can be gained from research further validating more uniform treatment approaches to optimize patient outcomes.

Much evidence regarding treatment of hypertension utilizing management of volume status via intensive dialysis in CKD progressing to end-stage renal disease is derived from the adult nephrology literature. More research is needed in this domain to further solidify potential benefits on the cardiovascular system in this population using intensified dialysis in the time leading to transplant. Little is known about mechanisms aside from deficient erythropoietin synthesis in the progression of anemia, and further investigation into this topic may yield new clinical interventions to augment the use of erythropoietin-stimulating agents in CKD (Robins and Blum 2007; Atkinson et al. 2010b; Hooper et al. 2011; Slickers et al. 2007; Marciano et al. 2010). Lastly, the field of neurocognition in CKD holds many opportunities for future research – particularly, as survival continues to improve in this population leading to more patients successfully completing college and entering the workforce. In particular, much remains to be gained in understanding the health development course of executive function on both a functional and neuroanatomical basis and the possibility for reversal of dysfunction and neural remodeling following transplantation.

5 Life Course Health Development Origins of Adolescent and Adult CKD

Although the tenets of early-life onset CKD are vitally important to understanding the context of life course impact on this disease process, other pathways likely impact the development of late adolescent and adult CKD. The association of diabetes on the development of CKD is clear. The impact of obesity itself is an area of active investigation (Hall et al. 2015). Other risk factors like hypertension also provide early intervention targets for reducing the incidence and slowing the progression of CKD.

Numerous large clinical databases have been developed over the years that have allowed investigators to better understand the sociodemographic diversity associated with CKD development in adulthood. The Chronic Renal Insufficiency Cohort Study has published multiple articles (Ricardo et al. 2015; Sandsmark et al. 2015), and there are multiple excellent reviews available to better appreciate the relationships among risk factors for adult-onset CKD. Notably, the relationship between CKD and cardiovascular disease is complex and reciprocal. The origins of cardiovascular diseases (including hypertension and obesity) are rooted in the genetic makeup of the individual and, like CKD, are impacted by preconception maternal status, intrauterine environment, and manifold other person ⇔ environmental interactions. Although there are many determinants of CKD progression in late adolescence and adults, an example of one of the emerging prototypical diseases that clearly reflects the early environmental impact on longer-term CKD is metabolic syndrome. The metabolic syndrome is known to be associated with cardiovascular risk, mortality, type 2 diabetes mellitus, and stroke, but its relationship to CKD is an emerging area of research. Patients with metabolic syndrome have a 2.5-fold higher risk of developing CKD, compared to individuals without the syndrome. Renal dysfunction, manifesting as such signs as early microalbuminuria, becomes apparent long before the appearance of hypertension or diabetes. Compared with healthy controls, individuals with metabolic syndrome have increased microvascular disease-tubular atrophy, interstitial fibrosis, arterial sclerosis, and global and segmental sclerosis. The etiology of the renal fibrosis associated with individuals with metabolic syndrome might be caused through a combination of inflammation, insulin resistance, hypertension, and dyslipidemia (Thomas et al. 2011a). The resulting overexpression of inflammatory cytokines, adipocytokines, and hormones such as angiotensin moves the balance from intrarenal homeostasis toward fibrosis pathways. The impact of early dietary intervention and regular exercise are unclear. What is clear is that the requirement for earlier evaluation of these patients by pediatricians speaks to the "epidemic" this has become.

6 Life Course Health Development Origins of Geriatric CKD

Given the aging of developed nations and the ever-increasing expenditures on renal care, estimated to be in the billions worldwide, understanding the opportunities for early recognition and prevention of renal disease development among the aging adult population is imperative (Nitta et al. 2013). Although it is clear that diabetes and hypertension are risk factors for development of CKD, in general CKD is a "silent" disease often going unrecognized until patients are well beyond possible modifiable stages of disease using dietary of medical intervention (Zhang and Rothenbacher 2008).

7 Socioeconomic Status and Race

A variety of socioeconomic determinants of CKD have been identified, including parental social class, living in a resource constrained neighborhoods, and membership in a marginalized or minority group (Shoham et al. 2005). These findings have been replicated in several populations in the USA (Shoham et al. 2005), Canada (Zacharias et al. 2012), and Australia (Cass et al. 2004), although socioeconomically disadvantaged groups in the USA may be at greatest risk (White et al. 2008). Although numerous studies have examined the association between adult socioeconomic status and CKD (Crews et al. 2012; McClellan et al. 2010; Volkova et al. 2008; Cass et al. 2002; Fored et al. 2003; Martins et al. 2006; Merkin et al. 2005; Merkin et al. 2007; Patzer and McClellan 2012; Perneger et al. 1995), few have examined the contribution of early-life socioeconomic determinants of CKD (Shoham et al. 2007; Shoham et al. 2008).

Premature birth often occurs in the context of poverty and social marginalization (Messer et al. 2008a). In the USA, preterm delivery is more common among racial minorities (Messer et al. 2008b). Although racial segregation explains some of the disparity, neighborhoods with a greater proportion of African-Americans show increased premature delivery among both black and white residents (Mason et al. 2009), suggesting that socioeconomic factors may be causative. The understanding of these dynamics is poor, given the complexity of the variables at play. The opportunity for research into better understanding these variables is rich, and the potential return on investment is high, yet targeted funding for research into these socioeconomic factors has not been a major national priority to date. One particular area they may have almost immediate dividends may be a better understanding of the role of maternal drug abuse in offspring risk for renal and hypertensive diseases. This line of investigation does not appear to have been widely addressed but has potential for significant impact via immediate returns on improved understanding of fetal development and longer-term population studies and their effects in the adult population.

Recently, Vart and colleagues performed a meta-regression analysis to identify study-level characteristics related to the strength of the socioeconomic status (SES) associations with CKD. They found that low SES was associated with low estimated glomerular filtration rate (eGFR) (odds ratio (OR) = 1.4, 95% CI = 1.2–1.6), high albuminuria (OR = 1.5, 95% CI = 1.2–1.8), low eGFR/high albuminuria (OR = 1.4, 95% CI = 1.0–1.7), and renal failure (OR = 1.6, 95% CI = 1.4, 1.7) and that variations in the strength of the associations were related to the covariate adjustment, particularly for low eGFR and high albuminuria. Overall, they noted that SES disparities in CKD were robust, irrespective of how SES was measured (Vart et al. 2015).

8 Quality-of-Life Effects of CKD

The social implications, medical regimen adherence, and impact on quality of life for children and families of children with CKD are enormous. The general improvement in survival of children with CKD has also been accompanied by an increased awareness of the effects of this disease on the quality of life of children and their families (Marciano et al. 2010; Soliday et al. 2000). Dietary and fluid management, complex hospital treatments and investigations, and disruption of normative school attendance place the children at risk for significant behavioral and psychiatric disorders, risk that is present into adulthood (Marciano et al. 2010). Childhood CKD also significantly affects family functioning (Mong Hiep et al. 2010). The development of a variety of quality-of-life assessment instruments has improved our understanding of some of the issues facing children with CKD, their parents, and siblings. Despite the availability of these types of assessment tools, there remains a paucity of data across the life course, and this area is rich in research opportunity (Marciano et al. 2010).

9 Implications for Practice

Worldwide, almost 13 million infants are born prematurely each year (Beck et al. 2010). It is unlikely that this entire population is at significant risk for developing CKD due to congenital or acquired nephropenia, but there is currently no test or biomarker for identifying the infants most at risk. No specific clinical management guidelines exist on how to follow low birth weight and intrauterine growth-retarded infants in order to identify those at risk for CKD. One in eight infants is born prematurely in the USA, and there is evidence that ex utero renal growth may be insufficient. Yet, it is not well understood how modifiable factors in postnatal care, such as nutrition and activation of retinoic acid signaling pathways, could optimize renal growth (Thomas and Kaskel 2009). The clinician must therefore rely on historical factors and subtle clinical signs of a low nephron endowment when evaluating infants with a history of prematurity.

A careful review of the neonatal history is the most important procedure to identify infants who deserve the closest follow-up. Note should be made of the infant's birth weight and gestational age as well as any history of acute kidney injury. Given the long-term implications of the latter, it is important that appropriate follow-up is in place (the specific timing requirements for this are also unclear).

Current American Academy of Pediatrics recommendations call for measuring blood pressure at health maintenance examinations beginning at 3 years among healthy children (National High Blood Pressure Education Program Working Group on High Blood Pressure in Children and Adolescents 2004). All premature infants should be considered a high-risk group in which blood pressure screening should be performed routinely at earlier visits. Hypertension may be the earliest clinical indicator of nephropenia, as the overworked nephrons require more forceful filtration to maintain an effective GFR. Careful assessment of linear growth at every well child check is also important, as children with CKD have poor linear growth, even when the GFR is only mildly impaired (Kleinknecht et al. 1983).

It is essential that these assessments continue into adolescence, a time when many children see their pediatrician less frequently. Rapid growth in puberty often unmasks renal dysfunction, as vulnerable kidneys are less able to clear an increasing burden of waste products. It is also critical that adolescent patients – particularly those nearing transition to adult practitioners – be made aware of their history of prematurity, the increased long-term risk for CKD, and modifiable risk factors for CKD progression (such as smoking, hypertension, or obesity).

Although an abnormal creatinine at NICU discharge or in childhood carries an ominous prognosis, the serum creatinine is not a sensitive indicator of long-term CKD risk. Clinicians must therefore not be falsely reassured by normal values. The functional redundancy of the kidneys and the ability of individual nephrons to hyperfilter mean that significant disease can be hidden beneath a normal or near-normal creatinine. Routine measurement of serum creatinine should be considered especially if other signs of kidney disease are present.

Microalbuminuria (urine albumin/creatinine of 30–300 mg/g) is also an early indicator of CKD and represents a therapeutic target for CKD progression (Taal and Brenner 2008). Standard urine dipsticks detect only overt albuminuria, but targeted screening of infants and children could result in earlier detection of CKD. Such screening is already standard of care in certain other high-risk groups, such as children with insulin-dependent diabetes mellitus and sickle cell disease.

Any recommendation for increased population-based screening must be tempered with the acknowledgment that presently there is no specific therapy to slow or arrest the progression of CKD. However, risk-based screening appears justified. There are modifiable therapeutic targets for CKD progression (such as hypertension (ESCAPE Trial Group et al. 2009), microalbuminuria (Taal and Brenner 2008), and dyslipidemia (Taal and Brenner 2008)). Additionally, because patients with stage 1 and stage 2 CKD are asymptomatic, there is an opportunity to intervene before complications of CKD have developed. At the very least, identification of patients with early CKD could facilitate education for the child and parents about the treatments for CKD and allow the opportunity to provide counseling on avoiding risk factors that may accelerate its progression (dehydration, nephrotoxic medications, recurrent urinary tract infections, coexisting urologic issues).

10 Implications for Research

Our scientific understanding of the significance of nephron number is advancing rapidly, but there remain significant gaps in our knowledge. We need a better understanding, on the molecular level, of the mechanism of nephrogenesis and its disruptors. Are there strategies that can be used in the NICU to optimize postnatal nephrogenesis for infants born prematurely? Would the clinical use of more sensitive proteomic/metabolomic biomarkers of renal injury result in earlier identification of infants with acute kidney injury and improve their care? Indeed, among low birth weight infants, we lack biomarkers to quantify risk of CKD. Furthermore, once those at risk are identified, we lack knowledge of effective interventions to combat the fetal environment: adult environment imbalance with the goal of preventing CKD. Could a targeted screening program for CKD among NICU graduates improve outcomes or be cost-effective?

Currently, the only direct means of assessing nephron number in humans is through autopsy. Perhaps the most useful research development would be a mechanism to measure the number of nephrons in a living patient. Recently, Bennett et al. have successfully used cationic ferritin to label the glomerular basement membrane, allowing an accurate count of glomeruli in rodents using magnetic resonance imaging (MRI) (Beeman et al. 2011). Though not ready for in vivo use in humans, such techniques would allow the real-time measurement of glomerular counts in the clinical arena in the future and serve as a gold standard for research studies.

Children with CKD secondary to congenital anomalies of the kidney and urinary tract are at risk for hypertension, including masked hypertension. The ESCAPE trial has shown that strict blood pressure control in conjunction with ACE inhibition is reno-protective for these children (ESCAPE Trial Group et al. 2009; Mitsnefes et al. 2010). Beyond this, there is limited data on interventions to delay progression of disease.

Screens for known kidney and urinary gene mutations in populations with non-syndromic and nonfamilial congenital anomalies of the kidney and urinary tract were able to identify mutations in only 10–20% of the sample population. This indicates that the majority of patients with isolated congenital anomalies of the kidney and urinary tract either have mutations in genes not yet identified or have other causes such as epigenetic changes (Weber et al. 2006; Thomas et al. 2011b; Weber et al. 2011). It is also unclear to what extent congenital anomalies of the kidney and urinary tract is oligogenic or the result of interactions between multiple genetic abnormalities (Weber et al. 2006). Studies in mice and humans suggest that gene mutations can result in diverse renal/urologic phenotypes, suggesting there are modifier genes or gene-environment interactions that contribute to congenital anomalies of the kidney and urinary tract but remain incompletely understood (Weber 2012). The genetics of the formation of the lower urinary tract and the potential contribution of epigenetic or genetic abnormalities to the development of posterior urethral valves, one of the leading causes of childhood end-stage renal disease, remains unknown. The study of genetics of congenital anomalies of the kidney and urinary tract may be complicated in that it can result from difficult-to-detect microdeletions and genome-wide association studies may not be able to detect defects if the mutations involved are rare or are of a low effect size (Weber et al. 2011; Hoshi et al. 2012; van Eerde et al. 2012). Exome sequencing may be helpful to identify novel genes. One of the major challenges to understanding the mechanisms of congenital anomalies of the kidney and urinary tract is the interaction between gene networks and a need to better understand time and cell specificity of gene mutations. The GenitoUrinary Development Molecular Anatomy Project (GUDMAP) has developed a molecular atlas of gene expression in the genitourinary tract (Yu et al. 2012) and is now developing tools to delete genes from specific compartments of the developing kidney and urinary tract using Cre-recombinase technology. This will allow investigators to dissect out functions of genes in these distinct cell compartments. In addition, system-based analysis may be necessary to understand the interactions between gene networks (Gallegos et al. 2012).

Epigenetic modifications are likely mechanisms by which the prenatal environment and genetic factors may interact to engender the increased risk of CKD. Limited data is available on the role of epigenetics in the development of CKD.

While glomerular hypertrophy is thought to be maladaptive, there are conflicting data on the benefit of interventions designed to block renal hypertrophy, such as with mTOR inhibition (Vogelbacher et al. 2007; Kurdian et al. 2012; Fukuda et al. 2012). While the ESCAPE trial (which included children with congenital anomalies of the kidney and urinary tract) showed strict blood pressure control in conjunction with ACE inhibition was beneficial, retrospective analyses were unable to identify a benefit from ACE inhibition in children with congenital anomalies of the kidney and urinary tract (Ardissino et al. 2007; Neild 2009). Interestingly, recent studies have suggested that an imbalance between podocyte and nephron growth can induce glomerulosclerosis (Fukuda et al. 2012). Further studies are needed to better understand the developmental determinants of nephron and podocyte growth and whether imbalance of podocyte and glomerular growth contributes to glomerulosclerosis in genetic forms of focal glomerulosclerosis.

A key question for cases of both congenital anomalies of the kidney and urinary tract and low nephron number is whether the advent of stem cell technologies and gene delivery techniques can result in interventions that can alter or rescue abnormal renal development. Reports of improvement in renal function in rat remnant kidney by injections of the mesenchyme make pursuit of stem cell technologies promising (Cavaglieri et al. 2009; Semedo et al. 2009). However, better understanding of the epigenetic and genetic factors regulating cell types may be necessary to program and tailor stem cells to renal compartments (Hendry and Little 2012).

One of the challenges of congenital anomalies of the kidney and urinary tract is how to use increasing knowledge of genotypes to optimize care of patients. One issue is a need to correlate genotypes with phenotypes and to identify modifiers. In particular, this may be relevant for potential prenatal diagnosis or screening of siblings/relatives. Despite our increased understanding of the genetics of congenital anomalies of the kidney and urinary tract, a major concern is whether there is a potential for intervention. Identification of genetic and epigenetic causes of congenital anomalies of the kidney and urinary tract may improve patient care by improving screening for extrarenal manifestations.

The identification and consistent monitoring of individuals at risk for CKD should not stop after the childhood period. Indeed, it is precisely the aging process and the lifestyle and SES effects on aging populations and particularly females of childbearing age that necessitate the educational, population health and nutritional efforts of our society if we are to impact significantly the incidence and prevalence of CKD.

10.1 Specific Research Recommendations

Clinical Research

1. Nutritional-based studies to better understand the impact and optimization of maternal nutrition and the possible impact on fetal/neonatal renal health.
2. Evaluation of the impact of public education and maternal intervention for nutrition, medication, and lifestyle impact on fetal/neonatal renal health.
3. Examine maternal/environmental exposures that may contribute to congenital anomalies of the kidney and urinary tract and low nephron number.
4. Research on factors that will optimize renal growth in premature infants.
5. Develop research networks of patients with congenital anomalies of the kidney and urinary tract and CKD using global registries to facilitate both cohort studies and interventional studies and to develop bio-repositories.
6. In the USA, facilitate broad-based collaboration between pediatric nephrology centers to enable implementation of clinical and translational studies on congenital anomalies of the kidney and urinary tract, low nephron number, and CKD. Utilize and expand upon existing resources, such as the networks of North American Pediatric Renal Trials and Collaborative Studies (NAPRTCS), Pediatric Clinical and Translation Science Award (CTSA) sites, and the PCORI-funded clinical data research networks, such as PEDSnet.
7. Collate the data from major adult and geriatric CKD and cardiovascular trials, and drive to identify improved biomarkers for progression and associations with CKD.
8. Interventional trials to test optimal timing and efficacy of angiotensin-converting enzyme inhibition in the setting of CKD secondary to congenital anomalies of the kidney and urinary tract and in the adult and geriatric population.
9. Develop national research strategies on the utilization of social media and eHealth to improve adherence and social acceptance of children with CKD.

Translational Research

1. Examine genetic and epigenetic factors that may contribute to nephropenia/congenital anomalies of the kidney and urinary tract using exome sequencing, DNA copy number variant analyses, and histone methylation/acetylation patterns.
2. Examine epigenetic and genetic factors necessary to program kidney stem cells.
3. Develop technologies to deliver stem cells to kidneys and possible gene therapy.
4. Use existing pediatric CKD cohorts, such as those in the CKiD and focal glomerulosclerosis studies, to develop genotype/phenotype correlations and to examine modifiers of renal outcomes.
5. Develop metabolomic and proteomic biomarkers to identify who is at higher risk among those born with intrauterine growth retardation or prematurely.
6. Research on determining nephron number using noninvasive technology.
7. Define best healthcare delivery practices in pediatric and transitional settings.
8. Define acute kidney injury in neonates, and develop strategies to identify high-risk patients whereby premature intervention may prevent development of CKD.

Basic Science Research

1. Time and cell compartment-specific effects of developmental renal gene mutations.
2. Develop system-based ("omics") approaches to integrate data on multiple gene interactions, incorporating time and cell compartment specificity – identify pathways that contribute to CKD progression, and examine potential drug repurposing.

3. Examine epigenetic mechanisms by which renal developmental programming may lead to risk of CKD.
4. Assess factors that contribute to glomerular and podocyte development and growth.
5. Assemble the necessary tools to begin to build and/or regenerate a kidney.

Translational Priorities: Recommendations for Translating Existing Research into Practice and Policy

1. Develop recommendations for renal follow-up of premature/IUGR infants, and consider recommendations to monitor renal growth and for screening urinalyses in addition to blood pressure assessments.
2. Develop recommendations for use of ambulatory blood pressure monitoring in diagnosis of masked hypertension and optimization of blood pressure control in children with congenital anomalies of the kidney and urinary tract and CKD.
3. Develop innovative healthcare delivery models that improve patient health while reducing health system costs.
4. Focus on improved surveillance systems and access to healthcare providers across regional boundaries.
5. Employ telemedicine for Medicaid and Medicare patients for improved healthcare accessibility.

References

Abdel-Hakeem, A. K., Henry, T. Q., Magee, T. R., Desai, M., Ross, M. G., Mansano, R. Z., et al. (2008). Mechanisms of impaired nephrogenesis with fetal growth restriction: Altered rena transcription and growth factor expression. *American Journal of Obstetrics and Gynecology, 199*(3), 252 e1–252 e7.

Ardissino, G., Vigano, S., Testa, S., Dacco, V., Paglialonga, F., Leoni, A., et al. (2007). No clear evidence of ACEi efficacy on the progression of chronic kidney disease in children with hypodysplastic nephropathy--report from the ItalKid project database. *Nephrology, Dialysis, Transplantation : Official Publication of the European Dialysis and Transplant Association - European Renal Association., 22*(9), 2525–2530.

Askenazi, D. J., Koralkar, R., Hundley, H. E., Montesanti, A., Parwar, P., Sonjara, S., & Ambalavanan, N. (2012). Urine biomarkers predict acute kidney injury in newborns. *The Journal of Pediatrics, 161*(2), 270–275.

Atkinson, M. A., Pierce, C. B., Zack, R. M., et al. (2010a). Hemoglobin differences by race in children with CKD. *American Journal of Kidney Diseases, 55*(6), 1009–1017.

Atkinson, M. A., Martz, K., Warady, B. A., & Neu, A. M. (2010b). Risk for anemia in pediatric chronic kidney disease patients: A report of NAPRTCS. *Pediatric Nephrology, 25*(9), 1699–1706.

Bacchetta, J., Harambat, J., Guy, B., Putet, G., Cochat, P., & Dubourg, L. (2009). Long term renal outcome of children born preterm: A regular follow-up is needed. *Archives of Pediatrics, 16*(Suppl 1), S42–S48.

Bagby, S. P. (2015). Prenatal origins of chronic kidney disease. In P. Kimmel & M. Rosenberg (Eds.), *Chronic renal disease* (pp. 783–801). New York: Elsevier.

Barker, D. J. (1995). Fetal origins of coronary heart disease. *BMJ, 311*, 171–174.

Barker, D. J. (2005). The developmental origins of insulin resistance. *Hormone Research, 64*(Suppl 3), 2–7.

Barker, D. J., & Sir Richard Doll Lecture. (2012). Developmental origins of chronic disease. *Public Health, 126*, 185–189.

Barker, D. J., Osmond, C., Forsen, T. J., Kajantie, E., & Eriksson, J. G. (2007). Maternal and social origins of hypertension. *Hypertension, 50*, 565–571.

Baserga, M., Bares, A. L., Hale, M. A., Callaway, C. W., McKnight, R. A., Lane, P. H., et al. (2009). Uteroplacental insufficiency affects kidney VEGF expression in a model of IUGR with compensatory glomerular hypertrophy and hypertension. *Early Human Development, 85*(6), 361–367.

Baserga, M., Kaur, R., Hale, M. A., Bares, A., Yu, X., Callaway, C. W., et al. (2010). Fetal growth restriction alters transcription factor binding and epigenetic mechanisms of renal 11beta-hydroxysteroid dehydrogenase type 2 in a sex-specific manner. *American Journal of Physiology. Regulatory, Integrative and Comparative Physiology, 299*(1), R334–R342.

Basile, D. P., Donohoe, D., Roethe, K., & Osborn, J. L. (2001). Renal ischemic injury results in permanent damage to peritubular capillaries and influences long-term function. *American Journal of Physiology. Renal Physiology, 281*, F887–F899.

Beck, S., Wojdyla, D., Say, L., Betran, A. P., Merialdi, M., Requejo, J. H., et al. (2010). The worldwide incidence of preterm birth: A systematic review of maternal mortality and morbidity. *Bulletin of the World Health Organization, 88*, 31–38.

Beeman, S. C., Zhang, M., Gubhaju, L., Wu, T., Bertram, J. F., Frakes, D. H., et al. (2011). Measuring glomerular number and size in perfused kidneys using MRI. *American Journal of Physiology. Renal Physiology, 300*, F1454–F1457.

Ben-Dov, I. Z., Galitzer, H., Lavi-Moshayoff, V., et al. (2007). The parathyroid is a target organ for FGF23 in rats. *The Journal of Clinical Investigation, 117*(12), 4003–4008.

Ben-Shlomo, Y., & Kuh, D. (2002). A life course approach to chronic disease epidemiology: Conceptual models, empirical challenges and interdisciplinary perspectives. *International Journal of Epidemiology, 31*, 285–293.

Bertoli-Avella, A. M., Conte, M. L., Punzo, F., de Graaf, B. M., Lama, G., La Manna, A., et al. (2008). ROBO2 gene variants are associated with familial vesicoureteral reflux. *Journal of the American Society of Nephrology, 19*(4), 825–831.

Brenner, B. M., & Anderson, S. (1987). The Gordon Wilson lecture. Why kidneys fail: An unifying hypothesis. *Transactions of the American Clinical and Climatological Association, 98*, 59–70.

Brenner, B. M., & Chertow, G. M. (1994). Congenital oligonephropathy and the etiology of adult hypertension and progressive renal injury. *American Journal of Kidney Diseases, 23*, 171–175.

Brenner, B. M., Meyer, T. W., & Hostetter, T. H. (1982). Dietary protein intake and the progressive nature of kidney disease: The role of hemodynamically mediated glomerular injury in the pathogenesis of progressive glomerular sclerosis in aging, renal ablation, and intrinsic renal disease. *The New England Journal of Medicine, 307*, 652–659.

Brenner, B. M., Garcia, D. L., & Anderson, S. (1988). Glomeruli and blood pressure. Less of one, more the other? *American Journal of Hypertension, 1*, 335–347.

Brenner, B. M., Lawler, E. V., & Mackenzie, H. S. (1996). The hyperfiltration theory: A paradigm shift in nephrology. *Kidney International, 49*, 1774–1777.

Brophy, P. D., Shoham, D. A., CKD Life Course Group, Charlton, J. R., Carmody, J., Reidy, K. J., Harshman, L., Segar, J., & Askenazi, D. (2015). Early-life course socioeconomic factors and chronic kidney disease. *Advances in Chronic Kidney Disease, 22*(1), 16–23.

Buffat, C., Boubred, F., Mondon, F., Chelbi, S. T., Feuerstein, J. M., Lelievre-Pegorier, M., et al. (2007). Kidney gene expression analysis in a rat model of intrauterine growth restriction reveals massive alterations of coagulation genes. *Endocrinology, 148*(11), 5549–5557.

Carey, W. A., Talley, L. I., Sehring, S. A., Jaskula, J. M., & Mathias, R. S. (2007). Outcomes of dialysis initiated during the neonatal period for treatment of end-stage renal disease: A North American pediatric renal trials and collaborative studies special analysis. *Pediatrics, 119*(2), e468.

Carmody, J. B., & Charlton, J. R. (2013). Short-term gestation, long-term risk: Prematurity and chronic kidney disease. *Pediatrics, 131*(6), 1168–1179.

Carta, M., Cimador, M., Giuffre, M., Sergio, M., Di Pace, M. R., De Grazia, E., et al. (2007). Unilateral multicystic dysplastic kidney in infants exposed to antiepileptic drugs during pregnancy. *Pediatric Nephrology, 22*(7), 1054–1057.

Cass, A., Cunningham, J., & Hoy, W. (2002). The relationship between the incidence of end-stage renal disease and markers of socioeconomic disadvantage. *New South Wales Public Health Bulletin, 13*(7), 147–151.

Cass, A., et al. (2004). Exploring the pathways leading from disadvantage to end-stage renal disease for indigenous Australians. *Social Science & Medicine, 58*(4), 767–785.

Cavaglieri, R. C., Martini, D., Sogayar, M. C., & Noronha, I. L. (2009). Mesenchymal stem cells delivered at the subcapsule of the kidney ameliorate renal disease in the rat remnant kidney model. *Transplantation Proceedings, 41*(3), 947–951.

Centers for Disease Control and Prevention (CDC). (2007). Prevalence of chronic kidney disease and associated risk factors—United States, 1999–2004. *MMWR. Morbidity and Mortality Weekly Report, 56*, 161–165.

Chatterjee, R., Ramos, E., Hoffman, M., Vanwinkle, J., Martin, D. R., Davis, T. K., et al. (2012). Traditional and targeted exome sequencing reveals common, rare and novel functional deleterious variants in RET-signaling complex in a cohort of living US patients with urinary tract malformations. *Human Genetics, 131*(11), 1725–1738.

Chen, R., Mias, G. I., Li-Pook-Than, J., Jiang, L., Lam, H. Y., Chen, R., Miriami, E., et al. (2012). Personal omics profiling reveals dynamic molecular and medical phenotypes. *Cell, 148*(6), 1293–1307.

Chevalier, R. L. (1996). Developmental renal physiology of the low birth weight pre-term newborn. *The Journal of Urology, 156*, 714–719.

Chiang, S. S., Tai, C. W., Chung, C. J., Shiue, H. S., Chen, J. B., Su, C. T., & Hsueh, Y. M. (2010). Micronutrients and lifestyles in Taiwanese patients with stage 3 to 5 chronic kidney disease. *Nutrition, 26*(3), 276–282.

Coca, S. G., Singanamala, S., & Parikh, C. R. (2012). Chronic kidney disease after acute kidney injury: A systematic review and meta-analysis. *Kidney International, 81*, 442–448.

Cramer, M. T., & Guay-Woodford, L. M. (2015). Cystic kidney disease: A primer. *Advances in Chronic Kidney Disease, 22*(4), 297–305.

Crews, D. C., McClellan, W. M., Shoham, D. A., Gao, L., Warnock, D. G., Judd, S., Muntner, P., Miller, E. R., & Powe, N. R. (2012). Low income and albuminuria among REGARDS (reasons for geographic and racial differences in stroke) study participants. *American Journal of Kidney Diseases, 60*(5), 779–786.

van Eerde, A. M., Duran, K., van Riel, E., de Kovel, C. G., Koeleman, B. P., Knoers, N. V., et al. (2012). Genes in the ureteric budding pathway: Association study on vesico-ureteral reflux patients. *PloS One, 7*(4), e31327.

Engle, W. D. (1986). Development of fetal and neonatal renal function. *Seminars in Perinatology, 10*, 113–124.

ESCAPE Trial Group, Wuhl, E., Trivelli, A., Picca, S., Litwin, M., Peco-Antic, A., et al. (2009). Strict blood-pressure control and progression of renal failure in children. *The New England Journal of Medicine, 361*, 1639–1650.

Fadrowski, J. J., Pierce, C. B., Cole, S. R., Moxey-Mims, M., Warady, B. A., & Furth, S. L. (2008). Hemoglobin decline in children with chronic kidney disease: Baseline results from the chronic kidney disease in children prospective cohort study. *Clinical Journal of the American Society of Nephrology : CJASN., 3*(2), 457–462.

Feldman, H. I., Appel, L. J., Chertow, G. M., Cifelli, D., Cizman, B., Daugirdas, J., Fink, J. C., Franklin-Becker, E. D., Go, A. S., Hamm, L. L., He, J., Hostetter, T., Hsu, C. Y., Jamerson, K., Joffe, M., Kusek, J. W., Landis, J. R., Lash, J. P., Miller, E. R., Mohler, E. R., III, Muntner, P., Ojo, A. O., Rahman, M., Townsend, R. R., & Wright, J. T. (2003). The chronic renal insufficiency cohort (CRIC) study: Design and methods. *Journal of the American Society of Nephrology, 14*(Suppl), S148–S153.

Flynn, J. T., Mitsnefes, M., Pierce, C., et al. (2008). Blood pressure in children with chronic kidney disease: A report from the chronic kidney disease in children study. *Hypertension, 52*(4), 631–637.

Fogo, A. B. (2007). Mechanisms of progression of chronic kidney disease. *Pediatric Nephrology, 22*(12), 2011–2022.

Fored, C. M., et al. (2003). Socio-economic status and chronic renal failure: A population-based case-control study in Sweden. *Nephrology, Dialysis, Transplantation, 18*(1), 82–88.

Franco, M. C., Oliveira, V., Ponzio, B., Rangel, M., Palomino, Z., & Gil, F. Z. (2012). Influence of birth weight on the renal development and kidney diseases in adulthood: Experimental and clinical evidence. *International Journal of Nephrology, 2012*, 608025.

Fukuda, A., Chowdhury, M. A., Venkatareddy, M. P., Wang, S. Q., Nishizono, R., Suzuki, T., et al. (2012). Growth-dependent podocyte failure causes glomerulosclerosis. *Journal of the American Society of Nephrology : JASN., 23*(8), 1351–1363.

Furth, S. L., Cole, S. R., Moxey-Mims, M., Kaskel, F., Mak, R., Schwartz, G., Wong, C., Munoz, A., & Warady, B. A. (2006). Design and methods of the chronic kidney disease in children (CKiD) prospective cohort study. *Clinical Journal of the American Society of Nephrology : CJASN., 1*(5), 1006–1015.

Furth, S. L., Abraham, A. G., Jerry-Fluker, J., Schwartz, G. J., Benfield, M., Kaskel, F., et al. (2011). Metabolic abnormalities, cardiovascular disease risk factors, and GFR decline in children with chronic kidney disease. *Clinical Journal of the American Society of Nephrology : CJASN., 6*(9), 2132–2140.

Gallegos, T. F., Kouznetsova, V., Kudlicka, K., Sweeney, D. E., Bush, K. T., Willert, K., et al. (2012). A protein kinase a and Wnt-dependent network regulating an intermediate stage in epithelial tubulogenesis during kidney development. *Developmental Biology, 364*(1), 11–21.

Gilbert, T., Lelievre-Pegorier, M., & Merlet-Benichou, C. (1990). Immediate and long-term renal effects of fetal exposure to gentamicin. *Pediatric Nephrology, 4*, 445–450.

Goldstein, S. L., Kirkendall, E., Nguyen, H., Schaffzin, J. K., Bucuvalas, J., Bracke, T., Seid, M., Ashby, M., Foertmeyer, N., Brunner, L., Lesko, A., Barclay, C., Lannon, C., & Muething, S. (2013). Electronic health record identification of nephrotoxin exposure and associated acute kidney injury. *Pediatrics, 132*(3), e756–e767.

Greenbaum, L. A., Muñoz, A., Schneider, M. F., Kaskel, F. J., Askenazi, D. J., Jenkins, R., Hotchkiss, H., Moxey-Mims, M., Furth, S. L., & Warady, B. A. (2011). The association between abnormal birth history and growth in children with CKD. *Clinical Journal of the American Society of Nephrology, 6*, 14–21.

Grigore, D., Ojeda, N. B., Robertson, E. B., Dawson, A. S., Huffman, C. A., Bourassa, E. A., et al. (2007). Placental insufficiency results in temporal alterations in the renin angiotensin system in male hypertensive growth restricted offspring. *American Journal of Physiology. Regulatory, Integrative and Comparative Physiology, 293*(2), R804–R811.

Gubhaju, L., Sutherland, M. R., Yoder, B. A., Zulli, A., Bertram, J. F., & Black, M. J. (2009). Is nephrogenesis affected by preterm birth? Studies in a non-human primate model. *American Journal of Physiology. Renal Physiology, 297*, F1668–F1677.

Hack, M., Flannery, D. J., Schluchter, M., Cartar, L., Borawski, E., & Klein, N. (2002). Outcomes in young adulthood for very-low-birth-weight infants. *The New England Journal of Medicine, 346*, 149–157.

Halfon, N., & Forrest, C. B. (2017). The emerging theoretical framework of life course health development. In N. Halfon, C. B. Forrest, R. M. Lerner, & E. Faustman (Eds.), *Handbook of life course health-development science*. Cham: Springer.

Hall, J. E., do Carmo, J. M., da Silva, A. A., Wang, Z., & Hall, M. E. (2015). Obesity-induced hypertension: Interaction of neurohumoral and renal mechanisms. *Circulation Research, 116*(6), 991–1006.

Hallan, S., Euser, A. M., Irgens, L. M., Finken, M. J., Holmen, J., & Dekker, F. W. (2008). Effect of intrauterine growth restriction on kidney function at young adult age: The Nord Trondelag health (HUNT 2) study. *American Journal of Kidney Diseases: The Official Journal of the National Kidney Foundation, 51*(1), 10–20.

Harambat, J., van Stralen, K. J., Kim, J. J., & Tizard, E. J. (2012). Epidemiology of chronic kidney disease in children. *Pediatric Nephrology, 27*(3), 363–373.

Heidbreder, E., Naujoks, H., Brosa, U., & Schramm, L. (1997). The calcium-parathyroid hormone regulation in chronic renal failure investigation of its dynamic secretion pattern. *Hormone and Metabolic Research, 29*(2), 70–75.

Hendry, C. E., & Little, M. H. (2012). Reprogramming the kidney: A novel approach for regeneration. *Kidney International, 82*(2), 138–146.

Hinchliffe, S. A., Sargent, P. H., Howard, C. V., Chan, Y. F., & van Velzen, D. (1991). Human intrauterine renal growth expressed in absolute number of glomeruli assessed by the disector method and Cavalieri principle. *Laboratory Investigation, 64*, 777–784.

Hodgin, J. B., Rasoulpour, M., Markowitz, G. S., & D'Agati, V. D. (2009a). Very low birth weight is a risk factor for secondary focal segmental glomerulosclerosis. *Clinical Journal of the American Society of Nephrology, 4*, 71–76.

Holly, M. K., Dear, J. W., Hu, X., Schechter, A. N., Gladwin, M. T., Hewitt, S. M., et al. (2006). Biomarker and drug-target discovery using proteomics in a new rat model of sepsis-induced acute renal failure. *Kidney International, 70*, 496–506.

Hooper, S. R., Gerson, A. C., Butler, R. W., et al. (2011). Neurocognitive functioning of children and adolescents with mild-to-moderate chronic kidney disease. *Clinical Journal of the American Society of Nephrology : CJASN., 6*(8), 1824–1830.

Horbar, J. D., Carpenter, J. H., Badger, G. J., Kenny, M. J., Soll, R. F., Morrow, K. A., et al. (2012). Mortality and neonatal morbidity among infants 501 to 1500 grams from 2000 to 2009. *Pediatrics, 129*, 1019–1026.

Hoshi, M., Batourina, E., Mendelsohn, C., & Jain, S. (2012). Novel mechanisms of early upper and lower urinary tract patterning regulated by RetY1015 docking tyrosine in mice. *Development, 139*(13), 2405–2415.

Hoy, W. E., Rees, M., Kile, E., Mathews, J. D., & Wang, Z. (1999). A new dimension to the Barker hypothesis: Low birthweight and susceptibility to renal disease. *Kidney International, 56*(3), 1072–1077.

Hoy, W. E., Douglas-Denton, R. N., Hughson, M. D., Cass, A., Johnson, K., & Bertram, J. F. (2003). A stereological study of glomerular number and volume: Preliminary findings in a multiracial study of kidneys at autopsy. *Kidney International. Supplement, 83*, S31–S37.

Hoy, W. E., Kincaid-Smith, P., Hughson, M. D., Fogo, A. B., Sinniah, R., Dowling, J., et al. (2010). CKD in aboriginal Australians. *American Journal of Kidney Diseases the Official Journal of the National Kidney Foundation, 56*(5), 983–993.

Hoy, W. E., Samuel, T., Mott, S. A., Kincaid-Smith, P. S., Fogo, A. B., Dowling, J. P., et al. (2012). Renal biopsy findings among indigenous Australians: A nationwide review. *Kidney International, 82*(12), 1321–1331.

Hsu, C. Y. (2007). Linking the population epidemiology of acute renal failure, chronic kidney disease and end-stage renal disease. *Current Opinion in Nephrology and Hypertension, 16*, 221–226.

Hsu, C. W., Yamamoto, K. T., Henry, R. K., De Roos, A. J., & Flynn, J. T. (2014). Prenatal risk factors for childhood CKD. *American Society of Nephrology, 25*, 2105–2111.

Keijzer-Veen, M. G., Dulger, A., Dekker, F. W., Nauta, J., & van der Heijden, B. J. (2010). Very preterm birth is a risk factor for increased systolic blood pressure at a young adult age. *Pediatric Nephrology, 25*, 509–516.

Kiley, J. E., Powers, S. R., Jr., & Beebe, R. T. (1960). Acute renal failure: Eighty cases of renal tubular necrosis. *The New England Journal of Medicine, 262*, 481–486.

Kirkendall, E. S., Spires, W. L., Mottes, T. A., Schaffzin, J. K., Barclay, C., & Goldstein, S. L. (2014). Development and performance of electronic acute kidney injury triggers to identify pediatric patients at risk for nephrotoxic medication-associated harm. *Applied Clinical Informatics, 5*(2), 313–333.

Kleinknecht, C., Broyer, M., Huot, D., Marti-Henneberg, C., & Dartois, A. M. (1983). Growth and development of nondialyzed children with chronic renal failure. *Kidney International. Supplement, 15*, S40–S47.

Koralkar, R., Ambalavanan, N., Levitan, E. B., McGwin, G., Goldstein, S., & Askenazi, D. (2011). Acute kidney injury reduces survival in very low birth weight infants. *Pediatric Research, 69*, 354–358.

Kurdian, M., Herrero-Fresneda, I., Lloberas, N., Gimenez-Bonafe, P., Coria, V., Grande, M. T., et al. (2012). Delayed mTOR inhibition with low dose of everolimus reduces TGFbeta expression, attenuates proteinuria and renal damage in the renal mass reduction model. *PloS One, 7*(3), e32516.

Lackland, D. T., Bendall, H. E., Osmond, C., Egan, B. M., & Barker, D. J. (2000). Low birth weights contribute to high rates of early-onset chronic renal failure in the southeastern United States. *Archives of Internal Medicine, 160*(10), 1472–1476.

Langley-Evans, S. C. (1997). Hypertension induced by foetal exposure to a maternal low-protein diet, in the rat, is prevented by pharmacological blockade of maternal glucocorticoid synthesis. *Journal of Hypertension, 15*(5), 537–544.

Lash, J. P., Go, A. S., Appel, L. J., He, J., Ojo, A., Rahman, M., Townsend, R. R., Xie, D., Cifelli, D., Cohan, J., Fink, J. C., Fischer, M. J., Gadegbeku, C., Hamm, L. L., Kusek, J. W., Landis, J. R., Narva, A., Robinson, N., Teal, V., Feldman, H. I., & Chronic Renal Insufficiency Cohort (CRIC) Study Group. (2009). Chronic renal insufficiency cohort (CRIC) study: Baseline characteristics and associations with kidney function. *Clinical Journal of the American Society of Nephrology, 4*(8), 1302–1311. 2011;6(10):2548-53.

Lelievre-Pegorier, M., Vilar, J., Ferrier, M. L., Moreau, E., Freund, N., Gilbert, T., et al. (1998). Mild vitamin a deficiency leads to inborn nephron deficit in the rat. *Kidney International, 54*, 1455–1462.

Lopez-Hernandez, F. J., & Lopez-Novoa, J. M. (2012). Role of TGF-beta in chronic kidney disease: An integration of tubular, glomerular and vascular effects. *Cell and Tissue Research, 347*(1), 141–154.

Luyckx, V. A., & Brenner, B. M. (2005). Low birth weight, nephron number, and kidney disease. *Kidney International. Supplement, 97*, S68–S77.

Mahan, J. D., & Warady, B. A. (2006). Assessment and treatment of short stature in pediatric patients with chronic kidney disease: A consensus statement. *Pediatric Nephrology, 21*(7), 917–930.

Mallick, N. (2003). Secondary focal glomerulosclerosis not due to HIV. *Nephrology, Dialysis, Transplantation, 18*(90006), 64vi–64v7.

Mammen, C., Al Abbas, A., Skippen, P., Nadel, H., Levine, D., Collet, J. P., et al. (2012a). Long-term risk of CKD in children surviving episodes of acute kidney injury in the intensive care unit: A prospective cohort study. *American Journal of Kidney Diseases, 59*, 523–530.

Marciano, R. C., Bouissou Soares, C. M., Santos Diniz, J. S., Lima, E. M., Penido Silva, J. M., Ribeiro Canhestro, M., Gazzinelli Oliveira, A., Duarte Melo, C., Santos Dias, C., Correa, H., & Araujo de Oliveira, E. (2010). Mental disorders and quality of life in pediatric patients with chronic kidney disease. *Jornal Brasileiro de Nefrologia, 32*(3), 309–315.

Martins, D., et al. (2006). The association of poverty with the prevalence of albuminuria: Data from the third National Health and nutrition examination survey (NHANES III). *American Journal of Kidney Diseases, 47*(6), 965–971.

Mason, S. M., et al. (2009). Segregation and preterm birth: The effects of neighborhood racial composition in North Carolina. *Health & Place, 15*(1), 1–9.

McClellan, W. M., Newsome, B. B., McClure, L. A., Howard, G., Volkova, N., Audhya, P., & Warnock, D. G. (2010). Poverty and racial disparities in kidney disease: The REGARDS study. *American Journal of Nephrology, 32*(1), 38–46.

Mehta, R. L., Kellum, J. A., Shah, S. V., Molitoris, B. A., Ronco, C., Warnock, D. G., et al. (2007). Acute kidney injury network: Report of an initiative to improve outcomes in acute kidney injury. *Critical Care, 11*, R31.

Menon, S., Kirkendall, E. S., Nguyen, H., & Goldstein, S. L. (2014). Acute kidney injury associated with high nephrotoxic medication exposure leads to chronic kidney disease after 6 months. *The Journal of Pediatrics, 165*(3), 522–527.

Merkin, S. S., et al. (2005). Area socioeconomic status and progressive CKD: The atherosclerosis risk in communities (ARIC) study. *American Journal of Kidney Diseases, 46*(2), 203.

Merkin, S. S., et al. (2007). Individual and neighborhood socioeconomic status and progressive chronic kidney disease in an elderly population: The cardiovascular health study. *Social Science & Medicine, 65*(4), 809–821.

Merlet-Benichou, C., Gilbert, T., Muffat-Joly, M., Lelievre-Pegorier, M., & Leroy, B. (1994). Intrauterine growth retardation leads to a permanent nephron deficit in the rat. *Pediatric Nephrology, 8*(2), 175–180.

Messer, L. C., et al. (2008a). Socioeconomic domains and associations with preterm birth. *Social Science & Medicine, 67*(8), 1247–1257.

Messer, L. C., et al. (2008b). Black-white preterm birth disparity: A marker of inequality. *Annals of Epidemiology, 18*(11), 851–858.

Mingeot-Leclercq, M. P., & Tulkens, P. M. (1999). Aminoglycosides: Nephrotoxicity. *Antimicrobial Agents and Chemotherapy, 43*, 1003–1012.

Misurac, J. M., Knoderer, C. A., Leiser, J. D., Nailescu, C., Wilson, A. C., & Andreoli, S. P. (2013). Nonsteroidal anti-inflammatory drugs are an important cause of acute kidney injury in children. *The Journal of Pediatrics, 162*(6), 1153–1159.

Mitsnefes, M., Flynn, J., Cohn, S., et al. (2010). Masked hypertension associates with left ventricular hypertrophy in children with CKD. *Journal of American Society of Nephrology, 21*(1), 137–144.

Mizokami, F., & Mizuno, T. (2015). Acute kidney injury induced by antimicrobial agents in the elderly: Awareness and mitigation strategies. *Drugs & Aging, 32*(1), 1–12.

Mong Hiep, T. T., Ismaili, K., Collart, F., et al. (2010). Clinical characteristics and outcomes of children with stage 3-5 chronic kidney disease. *Pediatric Nephrology, 25*(5), 935–940.

Nakayama, M., Nozu, K., Goto, Y., Kamei, K., Ito, S., Sato, H., et al. (2010). HNF1B alterations associated with congenital anomalies of the kidney and urinary tract. *Pediatric Nephrology, 25*(6), 1073–1079.

NAPRTCS. Annual Report. 2011. http://www.kidney.org/professionals/kdoqi/guidelines_ckd/toc.htm

National High Blood Pressure Education Program Working Group on High Blood Pressure in Children and Adolescents. (2004). The fourth report on the diagnosis, evaluation, and treatment of high blood pressure in children and adolescents. *Pediatrics, 114*, 555–576.

National Kidney Foundation; KDOQI (Kidney Disease Outcomes Quality Initiative) (2012). Clinical Practice Guidelines for Chronic Kidney Disease: Evaluation, Classification and Stratification. Part 4. definition and classification of stages of chronic kidney disease. https://www.kidney.org/professionals/guidelines

Neild, G. H. (2009). What do we know about chronic renal failure in young adults? I. Primary renal disease. *Pediatric Nephrology, 24*(10), 1913–1919.

Nishimura, H., Yerkes, E., Hohenfellner, K., Miyazaki, Y., Ma, J., Hunley, T. E., et al. (1999). Role of the angiotensin type 2 receptor gene in congenital anomalies of the kidney and urinary tract, CAKUT, of mice and men. *Molecular Cell, 3*(1), 1–10.

Nitta K, Okada K, Yanai M,· Takahashi S. (2013). Aging and chronic kidney disease. Kidney & Blood Pressure Research 38:109-120.

Ojeda, N. B., Johnson, W. R., Dwyer, T. M., & Alexander, B. T. (2007). Early renal denervation prevents development of hypertension in growth-restricted offspring. *Clinical and Experimental Pharmacology & Physiology, 34*(11), 1212–1216.

Onuigbo, M. A., & Agbasi, N. (2014). "Quadruple whammy"- a preventable newly described syndrome of post-operative AKI in CKD II and CKD III patients on combination "triple whammy" medications: A Mayo Clinic health system, Eau Claire, Wisconsin experience. *Nigerian Journal of Clinical Practice, 17*(5), 649–654.

Ortiz, L. A., Quan, A., Weinberg, A., & Baum, M. (2001). Effect of prenatal dexamethasone on rat renal development. *Kidney International, 59*, 1663–1669.

Osathanondh, V., & Potter, E. (1963). Development of human kidney as shown by microdissection. III. Formation and interrelationship of collecting tubules and nephrons. *Archives of Pathology, 76*, 290–302.

Paces-Fessy, M., Fabre, M., Lesaulnier, C., & Cereghini, S. (2012). Hnf1b and Pax2 cooperate to control different pathways in kidney and ureter morphogenesis. *Human Molecular Genetics, 21*(14), 3143–3155.

Patzer, R. E., & McClellan, W. M. (2012). Influence of race, ethnicity and socioeconomic status on kidney disease. *Nature Reviews. Nephrology, 8*(9), 533–541.

Perneger, T. V., Whelton, P. K., & Klag, M. J. (1995). Race and end-stage renal disease. Socioeconomic status and access to health care as mediating factors. *Archives of Internal Medicine, 155*(11), 1201–1208.

Pham, T. D., MacLennan, N. K., Chiu, C. T., Laksana, G. S., Hsu, J. L., & Lane, R. H. (2003). Uteroplacental insufficiency increases apoptosis and alters p53 gene methylation in the full-term IUGR rat kidney. *American Journal of Physiology. Regulatory, Integrative and Comparative Physiology, 285*(5), R962–R970.

Plank, C., Nusken, K. D., Menendez-Castro, C., Hartner, A., Ostreicher, I., Amann, K., et al. (2010). Intrauterine growth restriction following ligation of the uterine arteries leads to more severe glomerulosclerosis after mesangioproliferative glomerulonephritis in the offspring. *American Journal of Nephrology, 32*(4), 287–295.

Puddu, M., Fanos, V., Podda, F., & Zaffanello, M. (2009). The kidney from prenatal to adult life: Perinatal programming and reduction of number of nephrons during development. *American Journal of Nephrology, 30*(2), 162–170.

Querfeld, U., Anarat, A., Bayazit, A. K., Bakkaloglu, A. S., Bilginer, Y., Caliskan, S., Civilibal, M., Doyon, A., Duzova, A., Kracht, D., Litwin, M., Melk, A., Mir, S., Sözeri, B., Shroff, R., Zeller, R., Wühl, E., Schaefer, F., & 4C Study Group. (2010). The cardiovascular comorbidity in children with chronic kidney disease (4C) study: Objectives, design, and methodology. *Clinical Journal of the American Society of Nephrology, 5*(9), 1642–1648.

Rademacher, E. R., & Sinaiko, A. R. (2009). Albuminuria in children. *Current Opinion in Nephrology and Hypertension, 18*, 246–251.

Reidy, K., & Kaskel, F. J. (2007). Pathophysiology of focal segmental glomerulosclerosis. *Pediatric Nephrology, 22*(3), 350–354.

Reidy, K. J., & Rosenblum, N. D. (2009). Cell and molecular biology of kidney development. *Seminars in Nephrology, 29*(4), 321–337.

Rengo, F., Parisi, V., Rengo, G., Femminella, G. D., Rengo, C., Zincarelli, C., Pagano, G., Festa, G., De Lucia, C., & Leosco, D. (2012). Instruments for geriatric assessment: New multidimensional assessment approaches. *Journal of Nephrology, 25* Suppl 19, S73–8.

Ricardo, A. C., Roy, J. A., Tao, K., Alper, A., Chen, J., Drawz, P. E., Fink, J. C., Hsu, C. Y., Kusek, J. W., Ojo, A., Schreiber, M., Fischer, M. J., & CRIC Study Investigators. (2015). Influence of nephrologist care on management and outcomes in adults with chronic kidney disease. *Journal of General Internal Medicine, 31*, 22. [Epub ahead of print].

Rifkin, D. E., Coca, S. G., & Kalantar-Zadeh, K. (2012). Does AKI truly lead to CKD? *Journal of The American Society of Nephrology, 23*, 979–984.

Robins, E. B., & Blum, S. (2007). Hematologic reference values for African American children and adolescents. *American Journal of Hematology, 82*(7), 611–614.

Rodriguez, M. M., Gomez, A. H., Abitbol, C. L., Chandar, J. J., Duara, S., & Zilleruelo, G. E. (2004). Histomorphometric analysis of postnatal glomerulogenesis in extremely preterm infants. *Pediatric and Developmental Pathology, 7*, 17–25.

Saisawat, P., Tasic, V., Vega-Warner, V., Kehinde, E. O., Gunther, B., Airik, R., et al. (2012). Identification of two novel CAKUT-causing genes by massively parallel exon resequencing of candidate genes in patients with unilateral renal agenesis. *Kidney International, 81*(2), 196–200.

Saland, J. M., Pierce, C. B., Mitsnefes, M. M., et al. (2010). Dyslipidemia in children with chronic kidney disease. *Kidney International, 78*(11), 1154–1163.

Salgado, C. M., Jardim, P. C., Teles, F. B., & Nunes, M. C. (2009). Influence of low birth weight on microalbuminuria and blood pressure of school children. *Clinical Nephrology, 71*, 367–374.

Sanders, M. W., Fazzi, G. E., Janssen, G. M., Blanco, C. E., & De Mey, J. G. (2005). High sodium intake increases blood pressure and alters renal function in intrauterine growth-retarded rats. *Hypertension, 46*(1), 71–75.

Sandsmark, D. K., Messé, S. R., Zhang, X., Roy, J., Nessel, L., Lee Hamm, L., He, J., Horwitz, E. J., Jaar, B. G., Kallem, R. R., Kusek, J. W., Mohler, E. R., 3rd, Porter, A., Seliger, S. L., Sozio, S. M., Townsend, R. R., Feldman, H. I., & Kasner, S. E. (2015). Proteinuria, but not eGFR, predicts stroke risk in chronic kidney disease: Chronic renal insufficiency cohort study. *Stroke, 46*, 2075. [Epub ahead of print].

Sanna-Cherchi, S., Ravani, P., Corbani, V., Parodi, S., Haupt, R., Piaggio, G., et al. (2009). Renal outcome in patients with congenital anomalies of the kidney and urinary tract. *Kidney International, 76*(5), 528–533.

Schedl, A., & Hastie, N. D. (2000). Cross-talk in kidney development. *Current Opinion in Genetics and Development, 10*(5), 543–549.

Schreuder, M. F., & Nauta, J. (2007). Prenatal programming of nephron number and blood pressure. *Kidney International, 72*(3), 265–268.

Schreuder, M. F., Nyengaard, J. R., Fodor, M., van Wijk, J. A., & Delemarre-van de Waal, H. A. (2005). Glomerular number and function are influenced by spontaneous and induced low birth weight in rats. *Journal of the American Society of Nephrology: JASN., 16*(10), 2913–2919.

Schröder, H. J. (2003). Models of fetal growth restriction. *European Journal of Obstetrics, Gynecology, and Reproductive Biology, 110*, S29–S39.

Seikaly, M. G., Ho, P. L., Emmett, L., Fine, R. N., & Tejani, A. (2003). Chronic renal insufficiency in children: The 2001 Annual report of the NAPRTCS. *Pediatric Nephrology, 18*(8), 796–804.

Semedo, P., Correa-Costa, M., Antonio Cenedeze, M., Maria Avancini Costa Malheiros, D., Antonia dos Reis, M., Shimizu, M. H., et al. (2009). Mesenchymal stem cells attenuate renal fibrosis through immune modulation and remodeling properties in a rat remnant kidney model. *Stem Cells, 27*(12), 3063–3073.

Serreau, R., Luton, D., Macher, M. A., Delezoide, A. L., Garel, C., & Jacqz-Aigrain, E. (2005). Developmental toxicity of the angiotensin II type 1 receptor antagonists during human pregnancy: A report of 10 cases. *BJOG : An International Journal of Obstetrics and Gynaecology, 112*(6), 710–712.

Shen, Q., Xu, H., Wei, L. M., Chen, J., & Liu, H. M. (2011). Intrauterine growth restriction and postnatal high-protein diet affect the kidneys in adult rats. *Nutrition, 27*(3), 364–371.

Shoham, D. A., Vupputuri, S., & Kshirsagar, A. V. (2005). Chronic kidney disease and life course socioeconomic status: A review. *Advances in Chronic Kidney Disease, 12*(1), 56–63.

Shoham, D. A., et al. (2007). Kidney disease in life-course socioeconomic context: The atherosclerosis risk in communities (ARIC) study. *American Journal of Kidney Diseases, 49*(2), 217–226.

Shoham, D. A., et al. (2008). Kidney disease and the cumulative burden of life course socioeconomic conditions: The atherosclerosis risk in communities (ARIC) study. *Social Science & Medicine, 67*(8), 1311–1320.

Sims-Lucas, S., Di Giovanni, V., Schaefer, C., Cusack, B., Eswarakumar, V. P., & Bates, C. M. (2012). Ureteric morphogenesis requires Fgfr1 and Fgfr2/Frs2alpha signaling in the metanephric mesenchyme. *Journal of the American Society of Nephrology, 23*(4), 607–617.

Slickers, J., Duquette, P., Hooper, S., & Gipson, D. (2007). Clinical predictors of neurocognitive deficits in children with chronic kidney disease. *Pediatric Nephrology, 22*(4), 565–572.

Soliday, E., Kool, E., & Lande, M. B. (2000). Psychosocial adjustment in children with kidney disease. *Journal of Pediatric Psychology, 25*(2), 93–103.

Song, R., & Yosypiv, I. V. (2011). Genetics of congenital anomalies of the kidney and urinary tract. *Pediatric Nephrology, 26*(3), 353–364.

Spencer, J. D., Schwaderer, A., McHugh, K., Vanderbrink, B., Becknell, B., & Hains, D. S. (2011). The demographics and costs of inpatient vesicoureteral reflux management in the USA. *Pediatric Nephrology, 26*(11), 1995–2001.

Stelloh, C., Allen, K. P., Mattson, D. L., Lerch-Gaggl, A., Reddy, S., & El-Meanawy, A. (2012). Prematurity in mice leads to reduction in nephron number, hypertension, and proteinuria. *Translational Research, 159*, 80–89.

Sutherland, M. R., Gubhaju, L., Moore, L., Kent, A. L., Dahlstrom, J. E., Horne, R. S., et al. (2011). Accelerated maturation and abnormal morphology in the preterm neonatal kidney. *Journal of American Society of Nephrology, 22*, 1365–1374.

Sutherland, M. R., Yoder, B. A., McCurnin, D., Seidner, S., Gubhaju, L., Clyman, R. I., et al. (2012a). Effects of ibuprofen treatment on the developing preterm baboon kidney. *American Journal of Physiology. Renal Physiology, 302*(10), F1286–F1292.

Taal, M. W., & Brenner, B. M. (2008). Renal risk scores: Progress and prospects. *Kidney International, 73*, 1216–1219.

Tabel, Y., Haskologlu, Z. S., Karakas, H. M., & Yakinci, C. (2010). Ultrasonographic screening of newborns for congenital anomalies of the kidney and the urinary tracts. *Urology Journal, 7*(3), 161–167.

Takamitsu, S., & Darwin Bell, P. (2015). Molecular pathways and therapies in autosomal-dominant polycystic kidney disease. *Physiology, 30*(3), 195–207.

Thomas, R., & Kaskel, F. J. (2009). It's not over till the last glomerulus forms. *Kidney International, 76*(4), 361–363.

Thomas, G., Sehgal, A. R., Kashyap, S. R., Srinivas, T. R., Kirwan, J. P., & Navaneethan, S. D. (2011a). Metabolic syndrome and kidney disease: A systematic review and meta-analysis. *Clinical Journal of the American Society of Nephrology, 6*(10), 2364–2373.

Thomas, R., Sanna-Cherchi, S., Warady, B. A., Furth, S. L., Kaskel, F. J., & Gharavi, A. G. (2011b). HNF1B and PAX2 mutations are a common cause of renal hypodysplasia in the CKiD cohort. *Pediatric Nephrology, 26*(6), 897–903.

Thompson, S., James, M., Wiebe, N., Hemmelgarn, B., Manns, B., Klarenbach, S., Tonelli, M., & for the Alberta Kidney Disease Network. (2015). Cause of death in patients with reduced kidney function. *Journal of the American Society of Nephrology, 26*, 2504.

USRDS. (2003). *2003 Annual data report: Atlas of end stage renal disease in the United States*. Bethesda: National Institutes of Health, National Institute of Diabetes and Digestive and Kidney Diseases.

Vart, P., Gansevoort, R. T., Joosten, M. M., Bültmann, U., & Reijneveld, S. A. (2015). Socioeconomic disparities in chronic kidney disease: A systematic review and meta-analysis. *American Journal of Preventive Medicine, 48*(5), 580–592.

Vogelbacher, R., Wittmann, S., Braun, A., Daniel, C., & Hugo, C. (2007). The mTOR inhibitor everolimus induces proteinuria and renal deterioration in the remnant kidney model in the rat. *Transplantation, 84*(11), 1492–1499.

Volkova, N., et al. (2008). Neighborhood poverty and racial differences in ESRD incidence. *Journal of the American Society of Nephrology, 19*(2), 356–364.

Warady, B. A., & Chadha, V. (2007). Chronic kidney disease in children: The global perspective. *Pediatric Nephrology, 22*(12), 1999–2009.

Weber, S. (2012). Novel genetic aspects of congenital anomalies of kidney and urinary tract. *Current Opinion in Pediatrics, 24*(2), 212–218.

Weber, S., Moriniere, V., Knuppel, T., Charbit, M., Dusek, J., Ghiggeri, G. M., et al. (2006). Prevalence of mutations in renal developmental genes in children with renal hypodysplasia: Results of the ESCAPE study. *Journal of the American Society of Nephrology, 17*(10), 2864–2870.

Weber, S., Landwehr, C., Renkert, M., Hoischen, A., Wuhl, E., Denecke, J., et al. (2011). Mapping candidate regions and genes for congenital anomalies of the kidneys and urinary tract (CAKUT) by array-based comparative genomic hybridization. *Nephrology, Dialysis, Transplantation : Official Publication of the European Dialysis and Transplant Association - European Renal Association., 26*(1), 136–143.

Wedekin, M., Ehrich, J. H. H., Offner, G., & Pope, L. (2008). Aetiology and outcome of acute and chronic renal failure in infants. *Nephrology, Dialysis, Transplantation, 23*, 1575–1580.

Wesseling-Perry, K., Pereira, R. C., Tseng, C. H., et al. (2012). Early skeletal and biochemical alterations in pediatric chronic kidney disease. *Clinical Journal of the American Society of Nephrology : CJASN., 7*(1), 146–152.

Westland, R., Schreuder, M. F., Bokenkamp, A., Spreeuwenberg, M. D., & van Wijk, J. A. (2011). Renal injury in children with a solitary functioning kidney--the KIMONO study. *Nephrology, Dialysis, Transplantation: Official Publication of the European Dialysis and Transplant Association - European Renal Association, 26*(5), 1533–1541.

White, S. L., et al. (2008). Socioeconomic disadvantage and kidney disease in the United States, Australia, and Thailand. *American Journal of Public Health, 98*(7), 1306–1313.

White, S. L., Perkovic, V., Cass, A., Chang, C. L., Poulter, N. R., Spector, T., et al. (2009). Is low birth weight an antecedent of CKD in later life?. A systematic review of observational studies. *American Journal of Kidney Diseases, 54*, 248–261.

Winearls, C. G., & Glassock, R. J. (2011). Classification of chronic kidney disease in the elderly: Pitfalls and errors. *Nephron. Clinical Practice, 119*(Suppl 1), c2–c4.

Wong, C. J., Moxey-Mims, M., Jerry-Fluker, J., Warady, B. A., & Furth, S. L. (2012). CKiD (CKD in children) prospective cohort study: A review of current findings. *American Journal of Kidney Diseases, 60*(6), 1002–1011.

Woroniecki, R., Gaikwad, A. B., & Susztak, K. (2011). Fetal environment, epigenetics, and pediatric renal disease. *Pediatric Nephrology, 26*(5), 705–711.

Wyld, M. L., Lee, C. M., Zhuo, X., White, S., Shaw, J. E., Morton, R. L., Colagiuri, S., & Chadban, S. J. (2015). Cost to government and society of chronic kidney disease stage 1-5: A national cohort study. *Internal Medicine Journal, 45*(7), 741–747.

Yu, J., Valerius, M. T., Duah, M., Staser, K., Hansard JK, Guo, J. J., et al. (2012). Identification of molecular compartments and genetic circuitry in the developing mammalian kidney. *Development, 139*(10), 1863–1873.

Zacharias, J. M., et al. (2012). Prevalence, risk factors and awareness of albuminuria on a Canadian first nation: A community-based screening study. *BMC Public Health, 12*, 290.

Zandi-Nejad, K., Luyckx, V. A., & Brenner, B. M. (2006). Adult hypertension and kidney disease: The role of fetal programming. *Hypertension, 47*(3), 502–508.

Zhang, Q.-L., & Rothenbacher, D. (2008). Prevalence of chronic kidney disease in population-based studies: Systematic review. *BMC Public Health, 8*, 117.

Part IV

Crosscutting Topics in Life Course Health Development

Growth and Life Course Health Development

Amanda Mummert, Meriah Schoen,
and Michelle Lampl

1 Introduction

Physical growth is an indicator and predictor of both present and future health. Auxology, the science of physical growth, has historical roots in studies noting that poor social conditions harm children's health and well-being as reflected by their size (Tanner 1981). Subsequent epidemiologic studies linking infant size to health risks emerging later in life identify that growth is a translational embodiment of health (Barker 2012). The full spectrum of biological processes by which size accrual translates life course health development remains to be clarified. Present challenges standing in the way of better understanding the nexus between growth and health include distinctions between public health information derived from population-level epidemiologic assessments and research evidence based on the study of growth biology of individuals; the current focus on attained size rather than the process of growth, or change in size, with a reliance on weight in lieu of length/height and body composition; and a tendency to interpret patterns derived from growth charts rather than understanding growth trajectories as they occur during individual biological processes.

Research approaches to human physical growth have largely been driven by public health efforts. Auxologically based epidemiology documented smaller size among individuals subjected to the rigors of child labor in Britain, contributing to the nineteenth-century Factory Acts aimed at regulating children's working conditions. By the twentieth century, it was recognized that such measurements were useful for population- and community-level growth surveillance. The prevalence of stunting and wasting, using age-adjusted measures of low height and weight, respectively, is currently a key component of international criteria for assessing health and well-being on a global scale (UNICEF 2014). Similarly, growth screening at an individual level became commonplace, and plotting size for age across infancy and childhood is now part of nationally and internationally endorsed guidelines for pediatric clinical medicine. Children are compared with peers of similar age and background for perspective on how they are faring relative to one another on "growth charts" produced, for example, by the US

A. Mummert, PhD (✉) • M. Lampl, MD, PhD
Department of Anthropology, Emory University, Atlanta, GA, USA

Center for the Study of Human Health, Emory University, Atlanta, GA, USA
e-mail: amanda.mummert@alumni.emory.edu

M. Schoen
Center for the Study of Human Health, Emory University, Atlanta, GA, USA

Department of Nutrition, Georgia State University, Atlanta, GA, USA

N. Halfon et al. (eds.), *Handbook of Life Course Health Development*,
DOI 10.1007/978-3-319-47143-3_17

Centers for Disease Control and Prevention (CDC) (Kuczmarski et al. 2000) and assessed for how they should be growing under optimal circumstances, as proposed by the World Health Organization (WHO) (WHO MGRS 2006). It is important to note that these assessments actually compare size, an indication of how much growth has occurred previously, but do not provide information on growth itself as represented by the pathway taken to achieve current size (Lampl and Thompson 2007) and are often mistakenly assumed to provide details of growth biology (Lampl 2012a). Growth is an emergent process at the individual level; trajectories of growth in height, weight, and body composition offer a phenotypic reflection of the complex interactions between macro- and microlevel processes that influence life course health development.

This chapter reviews environmental and biological factors that influence physical growth, concentrating primarily on gestation through early childhood which temporally sets the stage for disease risk in later life (Barker et al. 2013). First, we describe how growth is fundamentally an emergent process reflecting the embodiment of a complex network of social, biological, and environmental interactions. Here we assess how the diversity of body size and shape reflects developmental plasticity that is evolutionarily and historically influenced. Second, we describe the importance of timing for growth biology and briefly discuss theoretical frameworks that leverage auxological research. Third, we describe macro- and micropathways affecting growth in a global perspective. Fourth, we reflect upon data and methodological challenges for understanding how attained size and/or growth rate predicts life course health development, including issues of validity and actionable clinical recommendations. Finally, we consider approaches for future research and policies to advance the science of growth biology as it may contribute to improvements in human health across the life course.

2 Growth Is an Emergent Process

As a record of individual health experiences, the process of growth reflects many of the life course health development principles presented by Halfon and Forrest (2017). The process of human growth unfolds as a complex adaptive system (Holland 1992). Increases in size across time occur as nodally mediated interactions among multiple pathways, reiteratively changing in response to novel environmental inputs (Lampl 2009). This sensitivity to changing conditions enables a wide bandwidth of pathways by which individuals actually grow. Variability in growth patterns is an evolutionarily robust strategy for the fundamental goal of transforming one cell to a fully functional and reproductively capable organism, necessary for preservation of the species. The human body emerges through growth (increases in size) and maturation (acquisition of adult features) as an expression of molecular and physiological processes with developmental time specificity for organ construction and functional pathway regulation.

This is well illustrated by the growth of the skeleton. Skeletal growth expresses a chronobiological program whereby length/height accrual occurs through discontinuous, aperiodic saltatory spurts at long bone growth plates, intermittently punctuating durations of no growth (Lampl et al. 1992; Noonan et al. 2004) within a species-specific maturational time frame until final height is achieved (e.g., several decades for humans). The mechanism(s) driving episodic growth saltations, permitting skeletal growth to emerge from a stasis period, remains to be discovered. This pulsatile system of growth increments, proceeding with variability in amplitude and frequency, is the underlying complex adaptive system (Lampl and Johnson 1998). This is the mechanism by which individual growth trajectories vary in response to reiterative readings of the environment as "novel surroundings," interpreted as macro- and micropathways following the life course health development terminology proposed by Halfon and Hochstein (2002). Similar complex cellular interactions and environmental exposures govern the expansion and distribution of adipose tissue depots (Ibrahim 2010), which influence weight and fat mass accrual across the life course. Growth has a cadence, with facultative processes providing for plasticity within the bounds of critical or sensitive periods, leading to a final adult form that summarizes biological events across developmental time.

Advances in skeletal biology research have expanded an appreciation of the complex system that regulates the timing and progression of skeletal growth. Initial studies described long bone length accrual as a system controlled by simple "condition/action" commands directed by growth hormone (GH) effects on the cartilaginous growth plate (Isaksson et al. 1982). Research in the following decades demonstrated that bone growth represents the outcome of multiple nodes of cellular communication orchestrated by GH and insulin-like growth factor 1 (IGF-1) interacting with factors such as thyroid hormones, sex steroids, and inflammatory cytokines (Sederquist et al. 2014; Wit and Camacho-Hubner 2011). These are not simply additive processes but rather work as feedback loops among pathways by which the skeleton integrates environmental information. In this way, genetic predispositions underlying bone growth are influenced by environmental signals that culminate in adult stature. For example, inputs from both brain- and gut-derived serotonin act directly on the bone building and remodeling cells, osteoblasts, and osteoclasts, respectively, providing several paths by which skeletal growth reflects the interaction between nutrition and the social environment (Karsenty and Yadav 2011).

The outcome of this multiple input system is a wide bandwidth of growth patterns and considerable phenotypic variation in human height, from the very tall Dutch to the relatively short Mbuti peoples (Eveleth and Tanner 1990). Intergenerational changes, with taller offspring by comparison with their parents, are not uncommon accompaniments to public health improvements in many different environments and ecologies (Malina 2004). For example, among four cohorts born between 1883 and 1999 in Sweden, adult stature increased on average by 16 cm (6.3 inches) for males and 8 cm (3.2 inches) for females (Stinson 2012). Recent secular increases have occurred predominantly in developing regions as compared to developed regions (Cole 2003), reflecting contemporary changes in determinants of growth such as improved nutrition, reduced disease burden, and social conditions. Examples include the increased height among children and adolescents from Oaxaca, Mexico, between the 1970s and late 2000s that are attributed to improvements in local infrastructure in the form of healthcare services, dietary variety, and potable water (Malina et al. 2011). Nonetheless, these individuals remain significantly shorter than individuals born and raised in the United States, with a high proportion of stunting in relation to WHO growth standards. This may reflect intergenerational and/or genetic effects, including maternal size, as well as sustained challenges from the local environment on final height. Indeed, a trend toward taller individuals is not a universal historic trend, and stature attenuation, stagnation, or even decline has been observed among women in the poorest countries (Subramanian et al. 2011). As childhood height predicts longevity (Barker et al. 2011), these growth-based differences have important implications for life course health development.

Secular changes are not reserved for height; high-income countries saw increases in body mass index [BMI – height (m)/weight (km)^2] beginning in the 1970s. These trends came to characterize middle- and low-income countries globally (Swinburn et al. 2011) with approximately 1.46 billion adults overweight (BMI $\geq$ 25) as of 2008 (Finucane et al. 2011). Increasing overweight and obesity prevalence extends to children and adolescents, with only some plateaus emerging (Olds et al. 2011). These types of morphological fluctuations are not new and have been described as signaling epidemiologic or nutritional transitions, whereby historical changes in ecological and sociocultural factors alter major risks facing human health (Harper and Armelagos 2010; Omran 1971; Popkin et al. 2012) that are expressed through alterations in growth and body size. Overall, interpopulation variability in height and weight is a sensitive reflection of diversity in local conditions (Paciorek et al. 2013).

3 The Importance of Timing for Health and Well-Being

Humans have a relatively lengthy period of physiologic immaturity among mammals, presenting a window of environmental sensitivity with the potential for considerable phenotypic plasticity (Johnston 1998). While experiences in the juvenile and adolescent phases affect developmental trajectories (Cameron and Demerath 2002), by all present accounts, the earliest growth periods are most formative for growth and life course health development. Indeed, the effects of malnutrition and chronic infectious diseases occurring during infancy and early childhood can have greater predictive power for height than genetics (Delgado et al. 1982; Martorell et al. 1977). This reflects the cadence of development in which attained height results from bone growth during critical periods in early life. By contrast, weight and body composition are responsive to short-term effects from nutrition and physical activity across the life course.

The body grows through cumulative cell division, expansion, and reorganization. While gene regulatory networks lay down the basic human body form and function (Peter and Davidson 2011), functional pathways and organs are modified by intrinsic biological mechanisms influenced by maternal conditions. The term *programming mechanisms* has been utilized to describe factors that lead to permanent changes in physiology during critical or sensitive periods and have long-term implications for life course health development (Ben-Shlomo and Kuh 2002). Programming opportunities start prior to conception. Obese women, for example, accumulate metabolites such as insulin, lactate, and triglycerides within their ovarian follicles, increasing the likelihood that their offspring will develop certain diseases, such as diabetes, cardiovascular disease, or cancer later in life (Robker et al. 2009). Subsequently, trophoblast cell invasion of the uterine wall and remodeling of the uterine spiral arteries are among the earliest critical moments of development as the pathway for fetal blood supply is established (Gude et al. 2004). Thereafter, the expansion of the functional placenta takes on a mediating role. Once regarded as merely a filter protecting the fetus from environmental insults (Susser and Stein 1994), the placenta is now recognized as a fundamental source of significant life course health programming (Barker and Thornburg 2013).

Numerous studies document the importance of early life for health, with intrauterine growth predicting outcomes spanning multiple domains. One of the most clarifying human data sets comes from a group of individuals exposed to famine conditions at different periods of pregnancy in Amsterdam during World War II. Biomarkers of chronic disease progression document more prominent atherogenic lipid profiles among the offspring of mothers with early exposure (Roseboom et al. 2000), while the odds of microalbuminuria, a prognostic marker for kidney disease, are greater among those with mid-gestational exposure (Painter et al. 2005b), and glucose intolerance has been associated with late exposure (Ravelli et al. 1998). These effects were not only confined to the generation who were fetuses during the war but also extended to the children of those individuals. Among women exposed to malnutrition as fetuses late in gestation, their own pregnancies were characterized by increased twinning (Painter et al. 2008b) as well as excess perinatal mortality (Lumey and Stein 1997). While birth weight in the second generation was not associated with maternal gestational exposure to famine, length at birth was decreased, and ponderal index was increased, even when adjusting for other maternal characteristics (Painter et al. 2008a), suggesting persistent effects. Several sex-specific morbidity and mortality trends have also emerged. For men, early gestational exposure was associated with obesity at age 19 (Ravelli et al. 1976), although this risk attenuated by age 50 (Ravelli et al. 1999). Meanwhile, among women, early exposure was associated with higher BMI at age 50 (Ravelli et al. 1999), and the relative severity of famine exposure increased the hazard ratio for type 2 diabetes by 51% (van Abeelen et al. 2012a). The age at sequelae emergence also reflects sex-specific interactions. While earlier studies documented no association between mortality risk and famine exposure (Painter et al. 2005a; Roseboom et al. 2001), a reexamination of the aging cohort 7 years later found sex-specific mortality trends (van Abeelen et al. 2012b; Ekamper et al. 2015).

The evidence from the Dutch Hunger Winter cohort draws attention to the importance of timing for life course health development in two key ways. First, the timing of famine exposure had discrete effects during specific developmental windows for organ development. For example, kidney nephron number increases slowly from gestational weeks 10 to 18, after which proliferation increases rapidly until formation permanently terminates at about the 32nd week (Gasser et al. 1993; Hinchliffe et al. 1991). Individuals with famine exposure within this discrete window display biomarkers of glomerular impairment, and in utero exposure to the famine increased the odds of hypertension at age 59 by 1.44 (Stein et al. 2006). This was not the case among individuals exposed only during midgestation (Roseboom et al. 1999). Thus, time-specific famine exposure may have inhibited glomerular expansion leading to long-term kidney function inefficiencies and subsequent increased blood pressure, a contributor to multiple chronic conditions documented among this cohort (Roseboom et al. 2011). With the recognition of previously unidentified disease sequelae later in life (van Abeelen et al. 2012b; Ekamper et al. 2015), these data also demonstrate the importance of long-term longitudinal research for investigating life course health development. Risk profiles reflecting aberrant growth during earliest development may not emerge for decades and may continue to be expressed in future generations.

The data from the Dutch Hunger Winter cohort identify an array of health outcomes sourced to a common exposure and validate the robust literature, encompassing both historical and contemporary prospective cohorts, that relates birth weight and/or the tempo of postnatal weight and length accrual as mechanistically linked to adult health and well-being. These findings have been reviewed elsewhere (Barker 2012; Gluckman et al. 2008) and include altered risk for a wide range of chronic morbidities such as type 2 diabetes and metabolic syndrome (Eriksson et al. 2006), cardiovascular disease (Kelishadi and Poursafa 2014), hypertension and kidney disease (Barker et al. 2006), chronic obstructive lung disease (Duijts et al. 2014), and osteoporosis (Cooper et al. 2006), in addition to heightened risks for multimorbidity (Hack 2006) and early mortality (Barker et al. 2011). Surveys of the literature have also identified long-term associations between poor early life conditions and social capital indicators, ranging from cognitive ability (Shenkin et al. 2004) and behavioral traits suggestive of poor mental health (Schlotz and Phillips 2009) to differential employment and wages (Barker et al. 2005).

Most of the research included in these reviews, however, was not privy to information about specific exposures and/or exposure timing comparable to the temporally defined events endured by the Dutch Hunger Winter cohort. This has led to a series of methodological critiques, including remarks noting the limited incorporation of considerations stemming from cumulative life course adversity (Elford et al. 1991), the use of an inductive approach without attempts at refutation (Paneth and Susser 1995), and concerns that the results of some studies reflect an explanatory framework-guided statistical modeling influence on outcomes, in alignment with "Simpson's paradox" (Weinberg 2005; Tu et al. 2005).

The life course health data have also fueled controversy stemming from evolutionary perspectives on modern disease trends, with Ellison and Jasienska (2007) arguing for the necessity to develop and test alternative hypotheses in order to investigate if the reported outcomes actually represent inherent biological constraints, pathologies, or adaptations. Similarly, Hanson and Gluckman (2014) encourage distinction between outcomes of what they term *developmental conditioning*, namely, that some effects are potentially adaptive in the sense of conferring a fitness advantage (e.g., epigenetic influences on fetal growth rates and placental perfusion), whereas others are pathophysiological or nonadaptive and arise through exposure to environmental attributes that are novel in comparison to human evolutionary time (e.g., human-produced endocrine disruptors that alter neural and behavioral development). These critiques reflect the depth and breadth to which the research community has embraced the importance of early life experiences for health and have led to several distinct, yet interrelated, explanatory frameworks, including the life course health development framework.

4 Explanatory Frameworks for Understanding Early Growth and Later-Life Health Outcomes

The impact of maternal conditions and the greater environment on offspring health has been long recognized. For example, scientific description of "critical" and "sensitive" periods can be traced to at least the 1920s and 1930s in studies documenting temporal specificity between exposures and physiological and behavioral attributes (Lorenz 1935; Stockard 1921). Epidemiological interest in factors driving adult mortality, including an appreciation for how changes to child welfare would have long-term benefits emerging in adulthood, was similarly present by at least the 1930s (Kermack et al. 1934). Later, the severe birth defects resulting from thalidomide exposure, a drug prescribed to pregnant women to reduce morning sickness in the late 1950s and 1960s (McBride 1961), provided an unfortunate example of fetal sensitivity that demonstrated the phenotypic effects of environmental insults. From this earlier work, multiple disciplines and frameworks have emerged to describe and theorize why and how developmental outcomes in the pre- and perinatal period affect later health outcomes.

Epidemiologists, for example, have utilized and developed the *life course health development* framework which identifies health as a function of environmental, social, psychological, and biological factors that interact across the life span, which can more generally be described as macro- and micropathways (Halfon and Hochstein 2002). This framework draws attention to the correlation between macropathways fundamental to growth biology. For example, poverty and food insecurity have shared outcomes, including growth faltering (Cook and Frank 2008). In other epidemiologic literature, macropathways have been described as *social determinants of health* (Wilkinson and Marmot 2003), although here poverty was specifically excluded because increased gross national product and income equality are not consistently tied to reduced neonatal and infant mortality or increased life expectancy (Regidor et al. 2012). *Biological embedding*, meanwhile, emphasizes how systematic differences in social environments alter developmental processes and physiological attributes that influence health, well-being, learning, and behavior across the life course (Hertzman 2012). In this framework, gradients of exposure within three domains of child development (physical, social-emotional, and language-cognitive) reflect the timing and persistence of early social experiences and correspond to how the signature unfolds as latent, pathway, and cumulative effects.

Multiple disciplines, ranging from neuroendocrinology to anthropology, have embraced the concept of *allostatic load* to explain how one's cumulative life experience, including perceived and actual challenges to physiology, contributes to health outcomes. Allostasis is the process of achieving homeostasis by modulating physiological systems or behaviors and is considered an adaptive short-term response to acute stressors (McEwen and Wingfield 2003). Allostatic overload occurs when an individual's adaptive range is exceeded after chronic stress exposure. This is expressed as a differential risk for poor physical and mental health outcomes resulting from, for example, chronic activation of the hypothalamic-pituitary-adrenal (HPA) axis (Worthman 2009; Krieger and Smith 2004). Using this framework, Worthman and Panter-Brick (2008) constructed a measure of allostatic load to assess how psychosocial stress and markers of developmental adversity, including physical growth, are mediated by individual-level factors among Nepali children. They observed that village residence posed a greater risk for low height-for-age *Z*-scores compared to both homeless and squatter boys, who reported lower psychosocial stress, typically considered protective of health. Further, their measure of allostatic load consistently distinguished between the three living conditions, suggesting that mixed methods approaches combining biomarkers, field epidemiology, and ethnography are important for contextualizing developmental research.

The notion of a *mismatch* between the environment in which the human body evolved and that in which we live today has been invoked to explain the recent rise in chronic disease prevalence (Gluckman and Hanson 2006), a concept that was earlier an underlying feature of several developmental biology frameworks. The idea of diseases emerging across time as legacies from once useful genes, later interacting with novel environments, was originally tagged as the *thrifty gene hypothesis* (Neel 1962). A similar concept appeared decades later as the *thrifty phenotype hypothesis* (Hales and Barker 2001) to describe the emergence of modern disease patterns as reflections of discontinuities between what the human body expects from the environment and what the environment delivers (Nesse 2005). A more recent proposal defined *predictive adaptive responses* (*PARs*) as anticipatory adaptive phenotypic traits that offer a fitness advantage between the postnatal period and onset of reproductive competence, such as increased insulin sensitivity that promotes accelerated growth and adipose tissue deposition to potentially improve survivorship in early life (Gluckman et al. 2005; Hanson and Gluckman 2014). While a PAR may increase reproductive fitness in the short term, it could have longer-term consequences for the health of individuals if the phenotype is not aligned with the later-life environment. The association between maternal vitamin D deficiency and poor perinatal outcomes is a compelling example of how modern health trends might be explained within these "mismatch" frameworks. Vitamin D deficiency among ethnic minority women with darker complexions living in northern latitudes is highly prevalent (Prentice 2008) and has been interpreted as reflecting the intersection of biological adaptations to limit ultraviolet radiation exposure and sociocultural veiling practices (Jablonski and Chaplin 2000), which in combination have been posited to underlie heightened risks for maternal/infant health including low birth weight (LBW), gestational diabetes, and preeclampsia (Aghajafari et al. 2013). As vitamin D is essential for skeletal growth and bone strength (DeLuca 2004) and influences chronic disease risk (Souberbiellea et al. 2010), low maternal vitamin D may alter offspring initial bone set points and increase the risk of osteoporosis and skeletal fractures across the life span.

Understanding that early growth is a fundamental source of life course health is the result of considerable work describing the *developmental origins of health and disease* (DOHaD), launched by the geographic and social epidemiologic work of David Barker (2012), and building on previous insights of the importance of maternal and environmental conditions for body size and growth (e.g., McKeown and Record 1954; Ounsted 1965) and their relationship to later disease risk (e.g., Forsdahl 1977; Gennser et al. 1988). Recognizing that intrauterine growth and growth rates in infancy and childhood serve as cumulative markers of early life experience, several longitudinal cohorts have provided data across multiple generations from both Europe (e.g., Boyd et al. 2013; Wijnstok et al. 2013) and developing regions globally (e.g., Adair et al. 2011; Richter et al. 2007) documenting that birth weight and growth trajectories predict a number of later-life health outcomes, including type 2 diabetes, stroke, and osteoporosis (Barker 2012). This framework has been a primary driver in stimulating the discovery of mechanisms that permanently alter metabolism, physiology, or the structure of growing organs and, thus, result in a predisposition to adult health risks (Barker and

Thornburg 2013). Research supporting the macro- and micropathways involved in these relationships are emerging.

5 Macropathways Affecting Growth Outcomes Across the Life Course

While family studies document heritability as a determinant of height and BMI (Silventoinen et al. 2010), phenotypic variability among individuals as they grow is more influenced by the local context into which one is born and subsequently develops than by one's genome (Frongillo et al. 1997). Whether environmental influences are additive or synergistic is difficult to ascertain (Bart van der Worp et al. 2010), but growth and its outcome, size, are clearly biosensors of population health (Tanner 1981; Cameron 2007). Historical studies concentrated on environmental challenges associated with insufficiency (e.g., malnutrition) and resultant size reduction, while present populations face overabundance, mirroring increasing ill-health associated with overweight globally. External factors influencing physical growth reflect national-, state-, community-, and individual-level resource availability (Eveleth and Tanner 1976; 1990). Here we focus on a selection of macropathways that influence growth with implications for subsequent life course health.

5.1 Nutrition and Feeding Practices

Among the best-documented pathways affecting growth outcomes and life course health development are maternal nutrition during preconception, gestation, and postnatal infant feeding practices (Ramakrishnan et al. 2012; Wiedmeier et al. 2011). Maternal nutritional well-being, either in terms of her actual intake or as summarized by her own size and body composition, influences her offspring's health through effects on fetal growth and birth size (Barker et al. 2013). Fetal nutritional adequacy is often assessed by proxy, based on maternal weight and weight gain during pregnancy, which positively predict fetal limb, head, and abdominal growth (Thame et al. 2012; Neufeld et al. 2004) as well as subcutaneous fat at birth (Yajnik et al. 2003): within the normal range, larger mothers have larger babies. Maternal diet during pregnancy likewise affects neonatal outcomes, such that lower average birth weights have been reported following pregnancies among British women who consumed high carbohydrate intake in early pregnancy and those who consumed less dairy and meat protein in late pregnancy (Godfrey et al. 1996). Similarly, proportionate birth weight increases were found in relation to maternal protein consumption across gestation in South Australia (Moore et al. 2004). A meta-analysis of 29 randomized controlled trials – conducted in both low- and high-income countries – found that maternal nutritional supplementation reduced the incidence of LBW and interventions that increased macronutrient intake increased average birth weight and length (Gresham et al. 2014). Maternal overnutrition as assessed by obesity, in contrast, is associated with both small and large size at birth with consequences for life course metabolic health (Schmatz et al. 2010; Dabelea et al. 2000).

Infant and postnatal feeding clearly alter the tempo of growth with size outcomes: low weight is generally indicative of short-term nutritional insufficiency, while shorter length/stature reflects cumulative exposures to undernutrition. Specific effects of breastfeeding on growth and size are mixed, with greater life course gains in weight and length/height associated with longer exclusive breastfeeding durations in developing countries, particularly among boys (Juez et al. 1983; Ricco et al. 2001), while smaller size is found among exclusively or predominantly breastfed as opposed to formula-fed infants in some environments (Saleemi et al. 2001; Victora et al. 1998). This may reflect differences in breast milk composition (Gidrewizc and Fenton 2014), secondary to maternal physiology and/or local ecology. A pooled analysis of outcomes in developed countries from nearly 300,000 infants represented in 28 studies found that breastfeeding in early infancy reduces the risk of obesity among older children and adults (Owen et al. 2005). Similar results have been obtained from studies in developing countries where, for example, breastfeeding was inversely associated with BMI among young adolescents in Iran (Kelishadi et al. 2007). These outcomes may reflect the benefit of breastfeeding for self-regulation beyond the content of the milk itself (Li et al. 2010). After the weaning transition, during which growth often falters (McDade and Worthman 1998), feeding patterns and dietary choices continue to affect growth. For example, sweetened beverage intake (Fiorito et al. 2009) and energy-dense diets low in fiber and high in fat (Johnson et al. 2009) in childhood predict later adiposity and obesity.

5.2 Psychosocial Stress

Animal models document that psychosocial stress influences on physical growth begin at the earliest ages. The human experience of psychosocial stress is more difficult to quantify due to the complexity of isolating factors empirically. One pathway is mediated by effects on birth size: both acute and chronic maternal psychosocial stress increase the risk for intrauterine growth restriction (IUGR) and LBW (Beydoun and Saftlas 2008), including a dose/response decrease in infant birth weight associated with serial prenatal stress events (Wadhwa et al. 1993). Chronic stress has been found to explain a high proportion of birth weight disparities among Latinas, African Americans, and Caucasians (Strutz et al. 2014). Specific sources of stress associated with infant size include parental job displacement (Lindo 2011), while maternal distress and depression have been linked to increased risk of LBW, as reported among both urban Brazilian (Rondo et al. 2003) and rural Pakistani (Rahman et al. 2007) mothers, respectively. Conversely, social support during pregnancy is protective; birth weight buffering occurs as social network size increases among white and Latina women from Utah (Dyer et al. 2011) and with higher perceived social support among pregnant displaced women in Thailand (Sanguanklin et al. 2014).

Various data sources document that psychosocial stress experienced during infancy and childhood has lasting effects on health. Family conflict doubled the odds of short stature at age 7 among a British cohort (Mongomery et al. 1997), and physical growth deficits escalate with increasing time in institutional care and age at adoption (Dobrova-Krol et al. 2008). These outcomes tend to persist regardless of socioeconomic status (SES) (Peck and Lundberg 1995). Stress from geopolitical circumstances is also significant, as shown by the reduced growth across infancy and childhood accompanying segregation and the concomitant living conditions among black South Africans (Cameron 2003). Similarly, shorter adult height has been associated with the total number of lifetime displacement experiences among Laotian adult refugees (Clarkin 2012).

5.3 Acute and Chronic Disease

Life course health development also reflects direct effects from the local ecology on growth. Disease burden can exacerbate poor nutrition-expressed growth outcomes (Dewey and Mayers 2011), as demonstrated by the association between both chronic intestinal and respiratory infections and reduced stature. Chronic diarrheal disease often accompanies a failure to gain and maintain weight (Bhutta et al. 2004), with a dose/response relationship between diarrheal days and the likelihood of stunting reported among a pooled cohort of 2-year-old children from nine prospective studies representing five developing countries (Checkley et al. 2008). Similarly, an increased risk of stunting at age two was independently predicted by both febrile respiratory infection and diarrhea history (Adair and Guilkey 1997). These are effects comparable to those documented among South African maternally HIV-infected children, who exhibit reduced length-for-age and weight-for-age *Z*-scores across the first year of life (Bobat et al. 2011).

5.4 Altitude

Ecological effects on birth size and subsequent growth include oxygen tension and other environmental challenges associated with living at varied altitudes. Compared to their low-altitude (300 m) counterparts, Bolivian infants born at high altitude (3600 m) weigh approximately 300 g less with a concomitant higher occurrence of IUGR (Keyes et al. 2003). Comparable differences between low- and high-altitude dwelling populations have been documented in the Himalayas (Wiley 1994) and the Rocky Mountains in the United States (Unger et al. 1988). These patterns persist across childhood and adulthood. For example, even when controlling for confounding factors like SES, the odds of stunting and underweight are significantly increased among Tibetan children living at higher altitudes (>3500 m) (Dang et al. 2008). Stunting continues to be a defining feature of children in the Peruvian highlands despite relative improvements in political and economic stability, which may impact future secular trends in the region (Pawson and Huicho 2010).

5.5 Environmental Contaminants

Industrialization has introduced a number of environmental contaminants, including but not limited to air pollution, lead, and polychlorinated biphenyls (PCBs) that have observable effects on skeletal growth and body composition outcomes, particularly through gestational exposure (Schell et al. 2006). Ambient air pollution is related to birth weight and IUGR (Sram et al. 2005), as seen among Californian (Salam et al. 2005) and rural Guatemalan cohorts (Thompson et al. 2011). Lead exposure has effects on multiple dimensions of body size. Among a New York cohort, infants of mothers with mid-gestational lead levels $\geq 3\ \mu g/dL$ had reduced head circumference at 6 and 12 months, and weight-for-length and upper arm circumference-for-age *Z*-scores declined as maternal lead concentrations increased (Schell et al. 2009). Additionally, maternal consumption of PCB-contaminated fish or cooking oil has been linked to reduced birth weight near Lake Michigan (Fein et al. 1984) and shortened stature and reduced lean mass in older children from Taiwan (Guo et al. 1994).

5.6 Income, Social Status, and Educational Attainment

Social inequalities have long been tied to differential health outcomes, including growth trajectories, in studies using various indicators of SES, including parental education or income (Wilkinson and Pickett 2006). A systematic review found a consistent relationship between socioeconomic disadvantage and an increased risk for adverse birth outcomes, particularly among racial/ethnic minorities (Blumenshine et al. 2010). Among British infants, a mean height deficit of approximately 1.5 cm was observed among those whose mothers had low education levels, with comparable results obtained in relation to occupation and father's education (Howe et al. 2012). Social standing and body composition show similar associations, irrespective of ethnicity. For example, among both white and black South African children, being in the lowest SES tertile at birth was associated with decreased lean mass index [LMI – lean mass (kg)/height $(m)^2$] at 9 and 10 years of age, while higher current SES was associated with increased BMI (Griffiths et al. 2008). A multinational investigation conducted among 4- to 6-year-old children found location-specific associations between maternal educational attainment and offspring height and obesity. While among children in the United States, Sweden, and China higher maternal education was associated with taller child height, it was only protective against obesity in American and Swedish children (Lakshman et al. 2013). In addition to formal maternal education, instruction on topics such as feeding strategies has been associated with increased length gain in a cluster randomized controlled trial conducted among rural Indian families (Vazir et al. 2013), suggesting that education is a tangible target for improving global well-being (Simkhada et al. 2008).

5.7 Healthcare Resources and Urban/Rural Status

Healthcare resources are unequally distributed globally, with additional significant differences in access to care in urban versus rural locations that contribute to growth outcomes. Lavy et al. (1996) found that increased access to healthcare services had positive benefits on both height-for-age and weight-for-height in rural Ghana. They estimated that if rural children had access to health services equal to those received by urban children (11.5 h per week), their life span would increase by 9.3%, and health disparities would become nearly absent. Likewise, Frankenberg et al. (2005) reported that children born into a village with a midwife in Indonesia were on average 1.5 cm taller than their peers at age 4; the effect was greatest among children with mothers who had less education relative to her community which suggests that the midwife was increasing access to perinatal care. Similar differences are observed in developed countries. In the United States, 21.6% of rural children in eastern Kentucky were low in height-for-age, and 13% met the criteria for stunting (Crooks 1999), while Lutfiyya et al. (2007) found that rural residency in the United States increased the odds of overweight or obesity by 25% among children over 5. In contrast, Martorell et al. (2000) found rural residence protective of overweight and obesity among children 12–60 months of age in a survey of developing nations. These differences reflect the underlying complexity of these indicators, particularly in relation to global nutrition transitions (Popkin et al. 2012).

6 Micropathways from the Cell to the Organism

The preceding section described relationships between socio-structural conditions and body size with examples intended to demonstrate that similar outcomes in terms of size stem from disparate sources, whether assessed by income, the burden of stress or disease, or environmental contaminants. Mechanisms or micropathways that enable these factors to become embodied are beginning to be elucidated. Unlike the observational studies conducted among global human populations, much of the mechanistic work is based on findings from animal models and cell-level research.

6.1 Cell-Level Controls

The tempo of fetal and postnatal growth fundamentally reflects coordinated cellular events, influenced by nutrition and overall energetic balance (Yanagida et al. 2011). Among humans, cell-level underpinnings of morphologic features may underlie the link between decreased birth weight and growth velocity among Kenyan infants with maternal diets low in animal protein, zinc, and iron (Neumann and Harrison 1994), for example. Here, protein restriction may be operating to downregulate cell cycling and, together with iron deficiency, upregulating apoptotic genes (Swali et al. 2011), resulting in reduced size. One of the more enigmatic human health challenges is a relationship between poor gestational nutrition and obesity risk (Ong and Dunger 2002). Animal models suggest cell differentiation pathways as contributory. Reduced size observed through the first 12 weeks of life among rats with gestational, but not postnatal, protein restriction can reflect delayed mesenchymal stem cell differentiation, as well as modulation of osteoblast proliferation and differentiation by IGF-1 and GH (Oreffo et al. 2003). Subsequently, by 16 weeks of age, the gestationally protein-restricted rats' growth rates were significantly increased by comparison with control animals, suggesting a "catch-up" response during the postnatal period. Similarly, maternal protein restriction was associated with both increased preadipocyte proliferation in 28-day rat pups (Bol et al. 2008) and obesity in adult rats (Bol et al. 2009). Hence, maternal diet may translate to offspring size by multiple pathways from cell cycle control to gene transcription with long-term consequences on cell size and differentiation potential (Fowden et al. 2006).

6.2 Hormonal, Inflammatory, Metabolic, and Immune Signaling

A broad range of hormones, immune cells, and inflammatory compounds influence growth outcomes through signaling cascades of fetal and maternal origin. Maternal stress illustrates one circuit. Chronic maternal HPA axis activation, and subsequent cortisol production, moderates IGF-1 and GH exposure (Cooper 2004), central pathways in skeletal biology (Hall 2005). Fetoplacental 11β-hydroxysteroid dehydrogenase type 2 (11β-HSD2), which catalyzes the metabolism of active cortisol and corticosterone to more inert forms, turns up and down the volume on potential fetal glucocorticoid exposure. This permits fetal levels to be lower than maternal levels (Mastorakos and Ilias 2003), a potentially protective effect. The efficiency of 11β-HSD2 is variable, however, and reduced 11β-HSD2 activity is associated with IUGR and LBW (Kajantie et al. 2003; Mericq et al. 2009).

Maternal diet modulates metabolic hormones, with effects on fetal skeletal growth and body composition. In a rat model, maternal dietary protein restriction was associated with decreased concentrations of maternal IGF-1, insulin, and leptin, accompanied by downregulated placental amino acid transporters, decreasing nutrient delivery to the fetus with subsequent LBW (Jansson et al. 2006). Conversely, obese human mothers with high BMI and elevated leptin levels showed upregulation of placental amino acid transporters associated with increased birth weight (Jansson et al. 2008).

Maternal influences on postnatal growth continue via the immunostimulatory effects of breastfeeding. Breast milk contains growth signaling compounds, ranging from leptin to inflammatory cytokines such as TNF-α and IL-6, with effects on skeletal, fat, and lean mass accrual. Increasing breast milk leptin levels have been associated with lower infant weight gain through the sixth postnatal month (Schuster et al. 2011) and increasing IL-6 levels with lower infant weight-for-length Z-score and fat mass at 1 month of age (Fields and Demerath 2012), effects that attenuate at later ages (Brunner et al. 2015). The leptin and IL-6 effects on weight gain and fat mass accrual may reflect influences on appetite and/or digestive processes via gastrointestinal epithelial cell receptors (Savino et al. 2009), or changing patterns of adipocyte cell size and/or differentiation potential (Morrison and Farmer 2000).

Likewise, a wide range of common environmental exposures influences growth hormones and sex steroids. A common contaminant, lead exposure, disrupts the pituitary gland, directly attenuating the release of GH (Berry et al. 2002) and thereby diminishing skeletal growth, with indirect effects of appetite suppression (Hammond et al. 1989) reducing weight gain in rat pups. Further, pre- and postnatal lead exposure is associated with subsequent delayed menarche and alterations in body morphology across the pre- and postpubertal period (Denham et al. 2005).

6.3 Microbiome

Microbial communities are a significant source of metabolic influences on growth. Comparisons between germ-free and normal mice reveal that the microbiome is largely responsible for circulating metabolites (Wikoff et al. 2009), offering a mechanism by which environmental exposures have differential effects among individuals. Distinct microbiome compositions are found in the gastrointestinal tracts of monozygotic twins (Turnbaugh et al. 2010), and phylum-level differences in microbiota and bacterial diversity distinguish between obese and lean individuals within twin pairs (Turnbaugh et al. 2009). Infant microbiome colonization reflects maternal vaginal and fecal microbiota, with maternal factors including weight and pregnancy-associated weight gain altering bacterial content (Funkhouser and Bordenstein 2013). While it remains to be described, it is plausible that even the earliest of maternal-to-fetal bacterial exposure via the placental microbiome (Aagaard et al. 2014) is a source of both direct and indirect life course health development influences.

The microbiome is not static; in fact, microbial composition has been shown to be sensitive to dietary change (David et al. 2014) and antibiotic exposure (Theriot et al. 2014). In the postnatal period, microbiome content changes with the transition from breast milk to complementary food and is influenced by caretaking practices and other social environmental factors (Guarner and Malagelada 2003; Thompson et al. 2015). Bacteria that are highly efficient at processing milk oligosaccharides are abundant during early infancy, with the profile shifting to a more adult-like composition as weaning occurs (Koenig et al. 2011). Temporal fluctuations of the microbial diversity during infancy are highly individualized (Palmer et al. 2007) and, in comparison to adult microbiomes, exhibit more interpersonal variation in functional genes (Kurokawa et al. 2007). As these factors may influence aspects of metabolism and in turn energy availability, this variation may offer personalized pathways by which various exposures encountered across development are incorporated and reflected phenotypically in terms of body size. For example, evidence of reduced levels of *Bacteroides* and increased levels of *Firmicutes* among obese individuals in samples of both humans (Turnbaugh and Gordon 2009) and mice (Ley et al. 2005) suggests microbial contributions to weight regulation.

6.4 Epigenetics

The mechanisms by which environmental factors influence phenotypic outcomes during development include genetic polymorphisms involved in growth and metabolism, such as those reported for *Igf1* or *PPARγ* (Dos Santos et al. 2004; Arends et al. 2002), with risks that may change across the life course via epigenetic modifications (Waterland et al. 2006). While these modifications are concentrated during gametogenesis and early embryogenesis (Vickaryous and Whitelaw 2005), the epigenome continues to be altered across the life span with known effects from nutrition and endocrine factors (Ozanne and Constancia 2007), among others. The direct effects of maternal dietary modulation on phenotype are well illustrated by the agouti mouse model in terms of both body size (Dolinoy et al. 2006) and coat color (Dolinoy 2008). Among humans, epigenotypes are influenced by health states as illustrated by the association between impaired maternal glucose tolerance and decreased placental leptin gene expression induced by hypermethylation (Bouchard et al. 2010). Likewise, epigenetic effects secondary to maternal dietary intake are a mechanistic source for variation in fetal and postnatal adiposity and growth (Lee et al. 2014).

6.5 Structural Changes in Organs

The separate and overlapping periods of organ development provide windows of susceptibility with long-term consequences for life course health. Gestational protein restriction may differentially influence not only development of the kidney, as noted previously, but also the pancreas. Associated with a predisposition to type 2 diabetes, gestational protein restriction may underlie decreased β-cell proliferation, increased β-cell apoptosis, and thereby smaller functional islets in the pancreas (Petrik et al. 1999). Similarly, lifelong cardiac health has prenatal origins with several intrauterine factors leading to postnatal endothelial dysfunction that increase heart disease and stroke risk (Thornburg 2004). In comparison to rats fed a normal protein diet, those with low-protein exposure during gestation exhibited LBW and low heart weight, as well as significantly reduced numbers of cardiomyocytes (Corstius et al. 2005). The heart may be most sensitive to stressors in late gestation when cardiomyocytes become binucleated and permanently leave the cell cycle. A similar outcome is observed in relation to reduced placental gas exchange and hypoxemia, where the combination of increased cortisol and decreased IGF-1 also reduces cardiomyocyte binucleation (Thornburg et al. 2011). When combined later in life with hypertension, the reduction in cardiomyocytes may explain increased risks of heart failure. Organ structural integrity established early in development likely puts individuals at risk for adult disease susceptibility with age (e.g., Rinaudo and Wang 2012).

7 Data and Methodological Challenges: Growth as a Predictor of Life Course Health Development

Progress in understanding causality underlying the empirical associations between growth and life course health development depends on clarifying mechanistic links embedded in the growth process. A fundamental challenge is the wide range of data that are glossed to represent "growth" in these studies. First, a number of studies rely on assessments of size, not growth itself. Second, studies in this area rely on many different assessments of size, which do not assess the same biological processes. Third, many studies rely on proxies for growth or growth rate, such as patterns that emerge from size as plotted on growth charts.

7.1 The Fallacy of Size as Growth

While size is a cumulative outcome of previous growth, size alone does not reveal the path taken by an individual to achieve a particular size, and it is the path itself that embodies predictive forerunners (Eriksson et al. 2006). Growth is change in size over time within an individual; this is not captured by summary statistics of sample data. Hence, study design is critical: causality between growth and health outcomes requires within-individual repeated measures studies. These are more challenging to undertake in terms of sampling, subject compliance, and funding needs and demand unique analytic approaches (Lampl 2012b).

7.2 Measurement Considerations

Body size measurements are not interchangeable. A commonly measured parameter is weight, a relatively simple assessment to take. Weight is a nonspecific summary of mass, however, and does not differentiate lean mass and fat mass. Changes in weight are not a sensitive marker of growth in the developmental sense but can simply reflect the accumulation of tissue as energy intake exceeds utilization. A lack of appreciation for the not subtle differences between weight and length, or fat and lean mass, in their predictive power for later health outcomes is common. Taken together with different assessment periods, these differences may underlie discrepancies between studies (Baird et al. 2005; Monteiro and Victora 2005).

More specific issues for size assessment include the methodological need for attention to sources of error, including the precision (Cameron 2012) and reliability of measurement (Lampl et al. 2001) of the human body. This is essential when the object of study is growth, or the significant difference between sequential measurements unencumbered by measurement unreliability. Precision scales and specially constructed length/height tools, including recumbent measuring boards for infants, are gold standard research tools required for longitudinal studies of individuals. By contrast, clinical and community-based screening measurements are less rigorous in their approaches for efficiency. Not infrequently, a lack of standardization between facilities reflects an absence of evidence-based clinical practice guidelines (Foote et al. 2011) with no small margins of error. A specific example includes methods for assessing adiposity, of particular importance in view of present health challenges. The primary technique for body fat estimation employs subcutaneous skinfold measures, while whole-body approaches, based on bioelectrical impedance analysis (BIA) and dual-energy X-ray absorptiometry (DXA), among others (Zemel 2012), are more common in research contexts. These methods are not, however, interchangeable, and variations in approach may explain reported inconsistencies in health outcomes based on size in early life. For example, fat mass as measured by DXA is highly correlated with BMI as a categorical variable (using ≥ 30 kg/m^2 as an indicator of obesity) (Flegal et al. 2009), while results comparing BMI and BIA outcomes show high specificity but not sensitivity (Romero-Corral et al. 2008).

Furthermore, phenomena such as secular changes in size make size-based assessments particularly problematic, with markers of the "normal" shifting through time as evidenced by demographic trends of increasing obesity. It is increasingly unclear whether one BMI criterion for obesity, for example, is appropriate globally (Deurenberg et al. 1998), further complicating interpretations of studies employing categorical outcomes.

7.3 Proxies of Growth and Definitions of Normal Growth Trajectories

A number of studies use patterns of "growth trajectories" that emerge when repeated measures data are plotted on growth curves over time as a study predictor or outcome. While a common diagnostic approach in the clinical setting, this is problematic. Growth charts are merely summary statistics of size for age and are not designed to represent growth paths followed by individuals (Lampl and Thompson 2007); any "pattern" only reflects how an individual's size compares to peers of similar age, who themselves are not staying the same relative to one another. The WHO child growth standards, widely implemented in clinical practice for identifying pathological growth (Grummer-Strawn et al. 2010), were developed from data collected by international sampling among "healthy" breastfed infants, with the goal of representing optimal growth trajectories (WHO MGRS 2006). These standards are not without criticism in achieving their prescriptive mission. Concerns include the validity of pathological interpretations applied to observed differences in weight gain trajectories between breastfed and non-breastfed infants (Griffiths et al. 2009), particularly in light of the actual rates of breastfeeding globally (Cai et al. 2012; Allen et al. 2013). It remains unclear what "optimal" growth patterns mean or if, indeed, such universals are appropriate goals.

Clinicians commonly diagnose pathological growth as a change in size for age of more than two major growth chart-based percentile lines between clinical assessments. While upward crossing of two or more major growth chart percentiles (often tagged "rapid growth") has been reported as increasing the odds of obesity in childhood and adolescence (Taveras et al. 2011; Ekelund et al. 2006), it is not always clear in studies whether "rapid growth" reflects exposure resulting from prior growth restriction, that is, "catch-up growth," or whether it is an outcome, as a shift in the tempo of growth prompted by another factor. "Percentile crossing" in weight-for-length is common during early development and may reflect more about normal variability in individual growth rates than pathology (Mei et al. 2004). Indeed, strategies for intervention that derive from proxies of growth rates may not serve individuals well. In general, the use of growth charts depends on the education of healthcare workers and their effectiveness when communicating with parents (Frongillo and Habicht 1997).

8 Research Recommendations

8.1 Major Themes and Findings

Three major themes emerge to guide future research efforts:

- Early growth trajectories are associated with life course health. The mechanistic understanding of these relationships is limited among humans; further research is required to discern micropathways that translate macropathways.
- Growth measurements need to be linked to their local context. As growth is an emergent process, the notion of optimal growth deserves reconsideration. Optimality of the system is a property reflecting flexibility under a variety of challenges, not a particular size or pattern of change under theoretical conditions.
- Prenatal healthcare services and the health of young girls and women must be a global public health priority (Barker et al. 2013). The true benefits of interventions in these realms may only be evident when measured at generational or intergenerational timescales, which may require new methods for evaluation and funding.

8.2 Key Research Priorities

8.2.1 Basic/Mechanism Research

- Refine our understanding of tissue differentiation timing and influences to delineate the specific effects of exposures during development and their influence on life course health.
- Integrate new technologies to assist in identifying how exogenous exposures affect endogenous processes in the short and long term [e.g., metabolomics (Jones et al. 2012), exposomics (Miller 2014)].
- Clarify how sex differences shape growth and body composition trajectories.

8.2.2 Clinical Research

- Explore alternate models of health promotion across female development, in particular

methods that foster healthy nutrition and change family conditions, such as moving them out of adverse and impoverished environments.
- Incorporate new and creative technologies to document lifestyle effects on growth, in particular fostering the widespread availability of devices that can transmit data in real time via Internet-based telecommunication.

8.2.3 Population/Epidemiologic Research

- Prioritize funding to continue well-developed studies that already have long-term observations. This is of particular importance given the need to understand how intervention benefits unfold at generational and intergenerational timescales.
- Apply complex statistical modeling techniques to existing epidemiological data to examine individual variability in outcomes. Biological variation is a signature characteristic of mankind that must be embraced, rather than ignored, if we are to find meaningful ways to improve life course health.

8.2.4 Translational Research

- Ensure that appropriate animal models are utilized (e.g., Kilborn et al. 2002) and that experimental protocols are transparent to improve replication and accelerate their movement from bench to bedside.
- Share research findings with the communities in which observations are made, and develop educational materials that can benefit society at large. This will promote both the importance of science as a whole and mobilization of ingenuity and resourcefulness at local and national levels.

8.3 Data and Method Development Priorities

- Refine study design and methods to enhance collaborations between basic scientists, clinicians, and social scientists to deliver coherent, evidence-based research plans.

8.3.1 Translational Priorities

- Continue policy efforts aimed at ameliorating poor growth with attention to desired outcomes; increased weight attainment has different ends by comparison with length promotion (Adair et al. 2013). Given the current global obesity crisis and our already robust understanding of how excess weight and fat mass impact intergenerational well-being, such an effort can offer significant gains for current and future public health wellness.
- Improve public health messaging regarding what growth standards represent to help individual families implement health-promoting activities. Such an effort could include both family- and practitioner-based education programs to understand growth charts, as well as more robust efforts surrounding nutrition and exercise recommendations.

8.3.2 Barriers to an Understanding of Growth and Life Course Health Development

- Declining research budgets necessitate interdisciplinary projects that maximize yield. By encouraging collaboration to meet common goals, we can prioritize research programs that target several domains encompassed by the life course health development framework, ranging from the basic mechanistic level to how well-being crosses generational and intergenerational timespans.
- Increased participation is needed among family-focused studies, as it is clear that maternal and paternal factors influence health, as do the environments in which children are raised. Incentivizing participation by emphasizing health benefits will enable researchers to capture data at an intergenerational scale.
- Today's ecosystem is novel when conceptualized across evolutionary timescales, and our manmade environment poses new biological challenges. The major structural issues that affect health – poverty, deprivation, and inequality – require state- and nation-level attention, and the improvements in these areas can only be observed if we pay attention to outcomes over larger timespans.

References

Aagaard, K., Ma, J., Antony, K. M., Ganu, R., Petrosino, J., & Versalovic, J. (2014). The placenta harbors a unique microbiome. *Science Translational Medicine, 6*(237), 237ra65.

Adair, L. S., & Guilkey, D. K. (1997). Age-specific determinants of stunting in Filipino children. *Journal of Nutrition, 127*(27), 314–320.

Adair, L. S., Popkin, B. M., Akin, J. S., Guilkey, D. K., Guliano, S., Borja, J., et al. (2011). Cohort profile: The Cebu longitudinal health and nutrition survey. *International Journal of Epidemiology, 40*(3), 619–625.

Adair, L. S., Fall, C. H., Osmond, C., Stein, A. D., Martorell, R., Ramirez-Zea, M., et al. (2013). Associations of linear growth and relative weight gain during early life with adult health and human capital in countries of low and middle income: Findings from five birth cohort studies. *The Lancet, 362*(9891), 525–534.

Aghajafari, F., Nagulesapillai, T., Ronksley, P. E., Tough, S. C., O'Beirne, M., & Rabi, D. M. (2013). Association between maternal serum 25-hydroxyvitamin D level and pregnancy and neonatal outcomes: Systematic review and meta-analysis of observational studies. *British Medical Journal, 346*, f1169.

Allen, J. A., Li, R., Scanlon, K. S., Perrine, C. G., & Chen, J. (2013). Progress in increasing breastfeeding and reducing racial/ethnic differences – United States, 2000–2008 births. *Morbidity and Mortality Weekly Report, 62*(5), 77–80.

Arends, N., Johnston, L., Hokken-Koelega, A., van Duijn, C., de Ridder, M., Savage, M., et al. (2002). Polymorphism in the IGF-1 gene: Clinical relevance for short children born small for gestational age. *Journal of Clinical Endocrinology and Metabolism, 87*(6), 2720–2724.

Baird, J., Fisher, D., Lucas, P., Kleignen, J., Roberts, H., & Law, C. (2005). Being big or growing fast: Systematic review of size and growth in infancy and later obesity. *British Medical Journal, 331*(7522), 929.

Barker, D. J. P. (2012). Sir Richard Doll Lecture: Developmental origins of chronic disease. *Public Health, 126*(3), 185–189.

Barker, D. J. P., & Thornburg, K. (2013). The obstetric origins of health for a lifetime. *Clinical Obstetrics and Gynecology, 56*(3), 511–519.

Barker, D. J. P., Eriksson, J. G., Forsen, T., & Osmond, C. (2005). Infant growth and income 50 years later. *Archives of Disease in Childhood, 90*, 272–273.

Barker, D. J. P., Bagby, S. P., & Hanson, M. A. (2006). Mechanisms of disease: In utero programming in the pathogenesis of hypertension. *Nature Clinical Practice Nephrology, 2*(12), 700–707.

Barker, D. J. P., Kajantie, E., Osmond, C., Thornburg, K., & Ericksson, J. G. (2011). How boys grow determines how long they live. *American Journal of Human Biology, 23*(3), 412–416.

Barker, D. J. P., Barker, M., Fleming, T., & Lampl, M. (2013). Developmental biology: Support mothers to secure future public health. *Nature, 504*(7479), 209–211.

Bart van der Worp, H., Howells, D. W., Sena, E. S., Porritt, M. J., Rewell, S., O'Collins, V., et al. (2010). Can animal models of disease reliably inform human studies? *PLoS Medicine, 7*(3), e1000245.

Ben-Shlomo, Y., & Kuh, D. (2002). A life course approach to chronic disease epidemiology: Conceptual models, empirical challenges and interdisciplinary perspectives. *International Journal of Epidemiology, 31*(2), 285–293.

Berry, W. D. J., Moriarty, C. M., & Lau, Y.-S. (2002). Lead attenuation of episodic growth hormone secretion in male rats. *International Journal of Toxicology, 21*(2), 93–98.

Beydoun, H., & Saftlas, A. F. (2008). Physical and mental health outcomes of prenatal maternal stress in human and animal studies: A review of recent evidence. *Paediatric and Perinatal Epidemiology, 22*(5), 438–466.

Bhutta, Z. A., Ghishan, F., Lindley, K., Memon, I. A., Mittal, S., & Rhoads, J. M. (2004). Persistent and chronic diarrhea and malabsorption. *Journal of Pediatric Gastroenterology and Nutrition, 39*(Suppl 2), S711–S716.

Blumenshine, P., Egerter, S., Barclay, C. J., Cubbin, C., & Braveman, P. A. (2010). Socioeconomic disparities in adverse birth outcomes: A systematic review. *American Journal of Preventive Medicine, 39*(3), 263–272.

Bobat, R., Coovadia, H., Moodley, D., Coutsoudis, A., & Gouws, E. (2011). Growth in early childhood in a cohort of children born to HIV-1-infected women from Durban, South Africa. *Annals of Tropical Paediatrics, 21*(3), 203–210.

Bol, V. V., Reusens, B. M., & Remacle, C. A. (2008). Postnatal catch-up growth after fetal protein restriction programs proliferation of rat preadipocytes. *Obesity, 16*(12), 2760–2763.

Bol, V., Delattre, A., Reusens, B., Raes, M., & Remacle, C. (2009). Forced catch-up growth after fetal protein restriction alters the adipose tissue gene expression program leading to obesity in adult mice. *American Journal of Physiology. Regulatory, Integrative and Comparative Physiology, 297*, R291–R299.

Bouchard, L., Thibault, S., Guay, S.-P., Santure, M., Monpetit, A., St. Pierre, J., et al. (2010). Leptin gene epigenetic adaptation to impaired glucose metabolism during pregnancy. *Diabetes Care, 33*(11), 2436–2441.

Boyd, A., Golding, J., Macleod, J., Lawlor, D. A., Fraser, A., Henderson, J., et al. (2013). Cohort profile: The 'Children of the 90s' – the index offspring of the Avon Longitudinal Study of Parents and Children. *International Journal of Epidemiology, 42*(1), 111–127.

Brunner, S., Schmid, D., Zang, K., Much, D., Knoeferi, B., Kratzsch, J., et al. (2015). Breast milk leptin and adiponectin in relation to infant body composition up to 2 years. *Pediatric Obesity, 10*(1), 67–73.

Cai, X., Wardlaw, T., & Brown, D. W. (2012). Global trends in exclusive breastfeeding. *International Breastfeeding Journal, 7*(1), 12.

Cameron, N. (2003). Physical growth in a transitional economy: The aftermath of South African apartheid. *Economics and Human Biology, 1*(1), 29–42.

Cameron, N. (2007). Growth patterns in adverse environments. *American Journal of Human Biology, 19*(5), 615–621.

Cameron, N. (2012). The measurement of human growth. In N. Cameron & B. Bogin (Eds.), *Human growth and development* (2nd ed., pp. 487–513). New York: Academic Press.

Cameron, N., & Demerath, E. W. (2002). Critical periods in human growth and their relationship to diseases of aging. *Yearbook of Physical Anthropology, 45*, 159–184.

Checkley, W., Buckley, G., Gilman, R. H., Assis, A. M. O., Guerrant, R. L., Morris, S. S., et al. (2008). Multi-country analysis of the effects of diarrhoea on childhood stunting. *International Journal of Epidemiology, 37*(4), 816–830.

Clarkin, P. F. (2012). War, forced displacement and growth in Laotian adults. *Annals of Human Biology, 39*(1), 36–45.

Cole, T. J. (2003). The secular trend in human physical growth: A biological view. *Economics and Human Biology, 1*(2), 161–168.

Cook, J. T., & Frank, D. A. (2008). Food security, poverty, and human development in the United States. *Annals of the New York Academy of Sciences, 1136*, 193–209.

Cooper, C., Westlake, S., Harvey, N., Javaid, K., Dennison, E., & Hanson, M. (2006). Review: Developmental origins of osteoporotic fracture. *Osteoporosis International, 17*(3), 337–347.

Cooper, M. S. (2004). Sensitivity of bone to glucocorticoids. *Clinical Science, 107*(2), 111–123.

Corstius, H. B., Zimanyi, M. A., Maka, N., Herath, T., Thomas, W., van der Laarse, A., et al. (2005). Effect of intrauterine growth restriction on the number of cardiomyocytes in rat hearts. *Pediatric Research, 57*(6), 796–800.

Crooks, D. L. (1999). Child growth and nutritional status in a high-poverty community in eastern Kentucky. *American Journal of Physical Anthropology, 109*(1), 129–142.

Dabelea, D., Hanson, R. L., Lindsay, R. S., Pettitt, D. J., Imperatore, G., Gabir, M. M., et al. (2000). Intrauterine exposure to diabetes conveys risks for type 2 diabetes and obesity: A study of discordant sibships. *Diabetes, 49*(12), 2208–2211.

Dang, S., Yan, H., & Yamamoto, S. (2008). High altitude and early childhood growth retardation: New evidence from Tibet. *European Journal of Clinical Nutrition, 62*(3), 342–348.

David, L. A., Maurice, C. F., Carmody, R. N., Gootenberg, D. B., Button, J. E., Wolfe, B. E., et al. (2014). Diet rapidly and reproducibly alters the human gut microbiome. *Nature, 505*(7484), 559–563.

Delgado, H., Valverde, V., Martorell, R., & Klein, R. (1982). Relationship of maternal and infant nutrition to infant growth. *Early Human Development, 6*(3), 273–286.

DeLuca, H. F. (2004). Overview of general physiologic features and functions of vitamin D. *American Journal of Clinical Nutrition, 80*(6), 1689S–1696S.

Denham, M., Schell, L. M., Deane, G., Gallo, M. V., Ravenscroft, J., & DeCaprio, A. P. (2005). Relationship of lead, mercury, mirex, dichlorodiphenyldichloroethylene, hexachlorobenzene, and polychlorinated biphenyls to timing of menarche among Akwesanse Mohawk girls. *Pediatrics, 115*(2), e127–e134.

Deurenberg, P., Yap, M., & van Staveren, W. (1998). Body mass index and percent body fat: A meta-analysis among different ethnic groups. *International Journal of Obesity and Related Metabolic Disorders, 22*(12), 1164–1171.

Dewey, K. G., & Mayers, D. R. (2011). Early child growth: How do nutrition and infection interact? *Maternal & Child Nutrition, 7*(S3), 129–142.

Dobrova-Krol, N. A., van IJzendoorn, M. H., Bakersmans-Kranenburg, M. J., Cyr, C., & Juffer, F. (2008). Physical growth delays and stress dysregulation in stunted and nonstunted Ukrainian institution-reared children. *Infant Behavior & Development, 31*(3), 539–553.

Dolinoy, D. C. (2008). The agouti mouse model: An epigenetic biosensor for nutritional and environmental alterations on the fetal epigenome. *Nutrition Reviews, 66*(Suppl 1), S7–S11.

Dolinoy, D. C., Weidman, J. R., Waterland, R. A., & Jirtle, R. L. (2006). Maternal genistein alters coat color and protects Avy mouse offspring from obesity by modifying the fetal epigenome. *Environmental Health Perspectives, 114*(4), 567–572.

Dos Santos, C., Essioux, L., Teinturier, C., Tauber, M., Goffin, V., & Bougneres, P. (2004). A common polymorphism of the growth hormone receptor is associated with increased responsiveness to growth hormone. *Nature Genetics, 36*(7), 720–724.

Duijts, L., Reiss, I. K., Brusselle, G., & de Jongste, J. C. (2014). Early origins of chronic obstructive lung diseases across the life course. *European Journal of Epidemiology, 29*(12), 871–885.

Dyer, J. M., Hunter, R., & Murphy, P. A. (2011). Relationship of social network size to infant birth weight in Hispanic and Non-Hispanic women. *Journal of Immigrant and Minority Health, 13*(3), 487–493.

Ekamper, P., van Poppel, F., Stein, A. D., Bijwaard, G. E., & Lumey, L. H. (2015). Prenatal famine exposure and adult mortality from cancer, cardiovascular disease, and other causes through age 63 years. *American Journal of Epidemiology*. doi:10.1093/aje/kwu288.

Ekelund, U., Ong, K., Linne, Y., Neovius, M., Brage, S., Dunger, D. B., et al. (2006). Upward weight percentile crossing in infancy and early childhood independently predicts fat mass in young adults: The Stockholm Weight Development Study (SWEDES). *American Journal of Clinical Nutrition, 83*(2), 324–330.

Elford, J., Whincup, P., & Shaper, A. G. (1991). Early life experience and adult cardiovascular disease: Longitudinal and case-control studies. *International Journal of Epidemiololy, 20*(4), 833–844.

Ellison, P. T., & Jasienska, G. (2007). Constraint, pathology, and adaptation: How can we tell them apart? *American Journal of Human Biology, 19*(5), 622–630.

Eriksson, J. G., Osmond, C., Kajantie, E., Forsen, T. J., & Barker, D. J. P. (2006). Patterns of growth among children who later develop type 2 diabetes or its risk factors. *Diabetologia, 49*(12), 2853–2858.

Eveleth, P., & Tanner, J. M. (1976). *Worldwide variation in human growth* (1st ed.). Cambridge: Cambridge University Press.

Eveleth, P., & Tanner, J. M. (1990). *Worldwide variation in human growth* (2nd ed.). Cambridge: Cambridge University Press.

Fein, G. G., Jacobson, J. L., Jacobson, S. W., Schwartz, P. M., & Dowler, J. K. (1984). Prenatal exposure to polychlorinated biphenyls: Effects on birth size and gestational age. *Journal of Pediatrics, 105*(2), 315–332.

Fields, D. A., & Demerath, E. W. (2012). Relationship of insulin, glucose, leptin, IL-6 and TNF-α in human breast milk with infant growth and body composition. *Pediatric Obesity, 7*(4), 304–312.

Finucane, M. M., Stevens, G. A., Cowan, M. J., Danaei, G., Lin, J. K., Paciorek, C. J., et al. (2011). National, regional, and global trends in body-mass index since 1980: Systematic analysis of health examination surveys and epidemiological studies with 960 country-years and 9.1 million participants. *The Lancet, 377*(9765), 557–567.

Fiorito, L. M., Marini, M., Francis, L. A., Smiciklas-Wright, H., & Birch, L. L. (2009). Beverage intake of girls at age 5 y predicts adiposity and weight status in childhood and adolescence. *American Journal of Clinical Nutrition, 90*(4), 935–942.

Flegal, K. M., Shepherd, J. A., Looker, A. C., Graubard, B. I., Borrud, L. G., Ogden, C. L., et al. (2009). Comparisons of percentage body fat, body mass index, waist circumference, and waist-stature ratio in adults. *American Journal of Clinical Nutrition, 89*(2), 500–508.

Foote, J. M., Brady, L. H., Burke, A. L., Cook, J. S., Dutcher, M. E., Gradoville, K. M., et al. (2011). Development of an evidence-based clinical practice guideline on linear growth measurement of children. *Journal of Pediatric Nursing, 26*(4), 312–324.

Forsdahl, A. (1977). Are poor living conditions in childhood and adolescence an important risk factor for arteriosclerotic heart disease? *British Journal of Preventive & Social Medicine, 31*(2), 91–95.

Fowden, A. L., Giussani, D. A., & Forhead, A. J. (2006). Intrauterine programming of physiological systems: Causes and consequences. *Physiology, 21*(1), 29–37.

Frankenberg, E., Suriastini, W., & Thomas, D. (2005). Can expanding access to basic healthcare improve children's health status? Lessons from Indonesia's 'midwife in the village' programme. *Population Studies, 59*(1), 5–19.

Frongillo, E. A., & Habicht, J. P. (1997). Investigating the weanling's dilemma: Lessons from Honduras. *Nutrition Reviews, 55*(11), 390–395.

Frongillo, E. A., de Onis, M., & Hanson, K. M. P. (1997). Socioeconomic and demographic factors are associated with worldwide patterns of stunting and wasting of children. *Journal of Nutrition, 127*(12), 2302–2309.

Funkhouser, L. J., & Bordenstein, S. R. (2013). Mom knows best: The universality of maternal microbial transmission. *PLoS Biology, 11*(8), e1001631.

Gasser, B., Mauss, Y., Ghnassia, J. P., Favre, R., Kohler, M., Yu, O., et al. (1993). A quantitative study of normal nephrogenesis in the human fetus: Its implication in the natural history of kidney changes due to low obstructive uropathies. *Fetal Diagnosis and Therapy, 8*(6), 371–384.

Gennser, G., Rymark, P., & Isbert, P. (1988). Low birth weight and risk of high blood pressure in adulthood. *British Medical Journal, 296*, 1498–1500.

Gidrewizc, D. A., & Fenton, T. R. (2014). A systematic review and meta-analysis of the nutrient content of preterm and term breast milk. *BMC Pediatrics, 14*, 216.

Gluckman, P. D., & Hanson, M. A. (2006). *Mismatch: The lifestyle diseases timebomb*. Oxford: Oxford University Press.

Gluckman, P. D., Hanson, M. A., & Spencer, H. G. (2005). Predictive adaptive responses and human evolution. *TRENDS in Ecology and Evolution, 20*(10), 527–533.

Gluckman, P. D., Hanson, M. A., Cooper, C., & Thornburg, K. (2008). Effect of in utero and early-life conditions on adult health and disease. *New England Journal of Medicine, 359*(1), 61–73.

Godfrey, K., Robinson, S., Barker, D. J., Osmond, C., & Cox, V. (1996). Maternal nutrition in early and late pregnancy in relation to placental and fetal growth. *British Medical Journal, 312*(7028), 410–414.

Gresham, E., Byles, J. E., Bisquera, A., & Hure, A. J. (2014). Effects of dietary interventions on neonatal and infant outcomes: A systematic review and meta-analysis. *American Journal of Clinical Nutrition, 100*(5), 1298–1321.

Griffiths, P. L., Rousham, E. K., Norris, S. A., Pettifor, J. M., & Cameron, N. (2008). Socio-economic status and body composition outcomes in urban South African children. *Archives of Disease in Childhood, 93*(10), 862–867.

Griffiths, L. J., Smeeth, L., Sherburne Hawkins, S., Cole, T. J., & Dezateux, C. (2009). Effects of infant feeding practice on weight gain from birth to 3 years. *Archives of Disease in Childhood, 94*(8), 577–582.

Grummer-Strawn, L. M., Reinold, C., & Krebs, N. F. (2010). Use of World Health Organization and CDC growth charts for children aged 0–59 months in the United States. *Morbidity and Mortality Weekly Report, 59*(RR09), 1–15.

Guarner, F., & Malagelada, J. R. (2003). Gut flora in health and disease. *The Lancet, 361*(9356), 512–519.

Gude, N. M., Roberts, C. T., Kalionis, B., & King, R. G. (2004). Growth and function of the normal human placenta. *Thrombosis Research, 114*(5–6), 397–407.

Guo, Y. L., Lin, C. J., Yao, W. J., Ryan, J. J., & Hsu, C. C. (1994). Musculoskeletal changes in children prenatally exposed to polychlorinated biphenyls and related compounds (Yu-Cheng children). *Journal of Toxicology and Environmental Health, 41*(1), 83–93.

Hack, M. (2006). Young adult outcomes of very-low-birth-weight children. *Seminars in Fetal and Neonatal Medicine, 11*(2), 127–137.

Hales, C. N., & Barker, D. J. (2001). The thrifty phenotype hypothesis. *British Medical Bulletin, 60*, 5–20.

Halfon, N., & Forrest, C. B. (2017). The emerging theoretical framework of life course health development. In N. Halfon, C. B. Forrest, R. M. Lerner, & E. Faustman (Eds.), *Handbook of life course health-development science*. Cham: Springer.

Halfon, N., & Hochstein, M. (2002). Life course health development: An integrated framework for developing health, policy, and research. *Milbank Quarterly, 80*(3), 433–479.

Hall, B. K. (2005). *Bones and cartilage: Developmental and evolutionary skeletal biology*. New York: Elsevier Academic Press.

Hammond, P. B., Chernausek, S. D., Succop, P. A., Shukla, R., & Bornschein, R. L. (1989). Mechanisms by which lead depresses linear and ponderal growth in weanling rats. *Toxicology and Applied Pharmacology, 99*(3), 474–486.

Hanson, M. A., & Gluckman, P. D. (2014). Early developmental conditioning of later health and disease: Physiology or pathophysiology? *Physiology Reviews, 94*, 1027–1094.

Harper, K., & Armelagos, G. J. (2010). The changing disease-scape in the third epidemiological transition. *International Journal of Environmental Research and Public Health, 7*(2), 675–697.

Hertzman, C. (2012). Putting the concept of biological embedding in historical perspective. *Proceedings of the National Academy of Sciences, 109*(Suppl 2), 17160–17167.

Hinchliffe, S. A., Sargent, P. H., Howard, C. V., Chan, Y. F., & van Velzen, D. (1991). Human intrauterine renal growth expressed in absolute number of glomeruli assessed by the dissector method and Cavalieri principle. *Laboratory Investigation, 64*(6), 777–784.

Holland, J. H. (1992). Complex adaptive systems. *Daedalus, 121*(1), 17–30.

Howe, L. D., Tilling, K., Galobardes, B., Davey Smith, G., Gunnell, D., & Lawlor, D. A. (2012). Socioeconomic differences in childhood growth trajectories: At what age do height inequalities emerge? *Journal of Epidemiology and Community Health, 66*(2), 143–148.

Ibrahim, M. M. (2010). Subcutaneous and visceral adipose tissue: Structural and functional differences. *Obesity Reviews, 11*(1), 11–18.

Isaksson, O. G. P., Jansson, J.-O., & Gause, I. A. M. (1982). Growth hormone stimulates longitudinal bone growth directly. *Science, 216*(4551), 1237–1239.

Jablonski, N. G., & Chaplin, G. (2000). The evolution of human skin coloration. *Journal of Human Evolution, 39*(1), 57–106.

Jansson, N., Pettersson, J., Haafiz, A., Ericsson, A., Palmberg, I., Tranberg, M., et al. (2006). Downregulation of placental transport of amino acids precedes the development of intrauterine growth restriction in rats fed a low protein diet. *Journal of Physiology, 576*(Pt 3), 935–946.

Jansson, N., Nilsfelt, A., Gellerstedt, M., Wennergren, M., Rossander-Hulthen, L., Powell, T. L., et al. (2008). Maternal hormones linking maternal body mass index and dietary intake to birth weight. *American Journal of Clinical Nutrition, 87*(6), 1743–1749.

Johnson, L., Mander, A. P., Jones, L. R., Emmett, P. M., & Jebb, S. A. (2009). Energy-dense, low-fiber, high-fat dietary pattern is associated with increased fatness in childhood. *American Journal of Clinical Nutrition, 87*(4), 846–854.

Johnston, F. E. (1998). The ecology of postnatal growth. In S. J. Ulijaszek, F. E. Johnston, & M. A. Preece (Eds.), *Cambridge Encyclopedia of human growth and development* (pp. 315–319). Cambridge: Cambridge University Press.

Jones, R. L., Cederberg, H. M., Wheeler, S. J., Poston, L., Hutchison, C. J., Seed, P. T., et al. (2010). Relationship between maternal growth, infant birthweight and nutrient partitioning in teenage pregnancies. *British Journal of Obstetrics & Gynecology, 117*, 200–211.

Jones, D. P., Park, Y., & Ziegler, T. R. (2012). Nutritional metabolomics: Progress in addressing complexity in diet and health. *Annual Review of Nutrition, 32*, 183–202.

Juez, G., Diaz, S., Casado, M., Duran, E., Salvatierra, A., Peralta, O., et al. (1983). Growth pattern of selected urban Chilean infants during exclusive breast-feeding. *American Journal of Clinical Nutrition, 38*(3), 462–468.

Kajantie, E., Dunkel, L., Turpeinen, U., Stenman, U.-H., Wood, P. J., Nuutila, M., et al. (2003). Placental 11β-hydroxysteroid dehydrogenase-2 and fetal cortisol/cortisone shuttle in small preterm infants. *Journal of Clinical Endocrinology and Metabolism, 88*(1), 493–500.

Karsenty, G., & Yadav, V. (2011). Regulation of bone mass by serotonin: Molecular biology and therapeutic implications. *Annual Review of Medicine, 62*, 323–331.

Kelishadi, R., & Poursafa, P. (2014). A review on the genetic, environmental, and lifestyle aspects of the early-life origin of cardiovascular disease. *Current Problems in Pediatric and Adolescent Health Care, 44*(3), 54–72.

Kelishadi, R., Ardalan, G., Gheiratmand, R., Gouya, M. M., Razahi, E. M., Delavari, A., et al. (2007). Association of physical activity and dietary behaviours in relation to the body mass index in a national sample of Iranian children and adolescents: CASPIAN Study. *Bulletin of the World Health Organization, 85*(1), 19–26.

Kermack, W. O., McKendrick, A. G., & McKinlay, P. L. (1934). Death-rates in Great Britain and Sweden. Some general regularities and their significance. *The Lancet, 223*(5770), 698–703.

Keyes, L. E., Armaza, J. F., Niermeyer, S., Vargas, E., Young, D. A., & Moore, L. G. (2003). Intrauterine growth restriction, preeclampsia, and intrauterine mortality at high altitude in Bolivia. *Pediatric Research, 54*(1), 20–25.

Kilborn, S. H., Trudel, G., & Uhthoff, H. (2002). Review of growth plate closure compared with age at sexual maturity and lifespan in laboratory animals. *Contemporary Topics in Laboratory Animal Science, 41*(5), 21–26.

Koenig, J. E., Spor, A., Scalfone, N., Fricker, A. D., Stombaugh, J., Knight, R., et al. (2011). Succession of microbial consortia in the developing infant gut microbiome. *Proceedings of the National Academy of Sciences, 108*(Suppl 1), 4578–4585.

Krieger, N. S., & Smith, G. (2004). "Bodies count," and body counts: Social epidemiology and embodying inequality. *Epidemiology Reviews, 26*, 92–103.

Kuczmarski, R. J., Ogden, C. L., Grummer-Strawn, L. M., Flegal, K. M., Guo, S. S., Wei, R., et al. (2000). *CDC growth charts: United States* (Vol. Vol. 314). Hyattsville: National Center for Health Statistics.

Kurokawa, K., Itoh, T., Kuwahara, T., Oshima, K., Toh, H., Toyoda, A., et al. (2007). Comparative metagenomics revealed commonly enriched gene sets in human gut microbiomes. *DNA Research, 14*(4), 169–181.

Lakshman, R., Zhang, J., Zhang, J., Koch, F. S., Marcus, C., Ludvigsson, J., et al. (2013). Higher maternal education is associated with favourable growth of young children in different countries. *Journal of Epidemiology and Community Health, 67*(7), 595–602.

Lampl, M. (2009). Human growth from the cell to the organism: Saltations and integrative physiology. *Annals of Human Biology, 36*(5), 478–495.

Lampl, M. (2012a). Limitation of growth chart curves in terms of individual growth biology. In V. R. Preedy (Ed.), *Handbook of growth and growth monitoring in health and disease* (pp. 3013–3029). New York: Springer.

Lampl, M. (2012b). Perspectives on modelling human growth: Mathematical models and growth biology. *Annals of Human Biology, 39*(5), 342–351.

Lampl, M., & Johnson, M. L. (1998). Normal human growth as saltatory: Adaptation through irregularity. In K. Newell & P. Molenaar (Eds.), *Dynamical systems in development* (pp. 15–38). Hillsdale: Lawrence Erlbaum, Inc..

Lampl, M., & Thompson, A. L. (2007). Growth chart curves do not describe individual growth biology. *American Journal of Human Biology, 19*(5), 643–653.

Lampl, M., Veldhuis, J. D., & Johnson, M. L. (1992). Saltation and stasis: A model of human growth. *Science, 258*(5083), 801–803.

Lampl, M., Birch, L., Picciano, M. F., Johnson, M. L., & Frongillo, E. A., Jr. (2001). Child factor in measurement dependability. *American Journal of Human Biology, 13*(4), 548–557.

Lavy, V., Strauss, J., Thomas, D., & de Vreyer, P. (1996). Quality of health care, survival, and health outcomes in Ghana. *Journal of Health Economics, 15*(3), 333–357.

Lee, H.-S., Barraza-Villarreal, A., Biessy, C., Duarte-Salles, T., Sly, P. D., Ramakrishnan, U., et al. (2014). Dietary supplementation with polyunsaturated fatty acid during pregnancy modulates DNA methylation at *IGF2/H19* imprinted genes and growth of infants. *Physiological Genomics, 46*(23), 851–857.

Ley, R. E., Backhed, F., Turnbaugh, P., Lozupone, C. A., Knight, R. D., & Gordon, J. I. (2005). Obesity alters gut microbial ecology. *Proceedings of the National Academy of Sciences, 102*(31), 11070–11075.

Li, R., Fein, S. B., & Grummer-Strawn, L. M. (2010). Do infants fed from bottles lack self-regulation of milk intake compared with directly breastfed infants? *Pediatrics, 125*(6), e1386–e1393.

Lindo, J. M. (2011). Parental job loss and infant health. *Journal of Health Economics, 30*(5), 869–879.

Lorenz, K. (1935). The companion in the bird's world: The fellow-member of the species as releasing factor of social behavior. *Journal fur Ornithologie Beiblatt (Leipzig), 83*, 137–213.

Lumey, L. H., & Stein, A. D. (1997). In utero exposure to famine and subsequent fertility: The Dutch Famine Birth Cohort Study. *American Journal of Public Health, 87*(12), 1962–1966.

Lutfiyya, M. N., Lipsky, M. S., Wisdom-Behounek, J., & Inpanbutr-Martinkus, M. (2007). Is rural residency a risk factor for overweight and obesity for U.S. children? *Obesity, 15*(9), 2348–2356.

Malina, R. M. (2004). Secular trends in growth, maturation and physical performance: A review. *Anthropology Reviews, 67*, 3–31.

Malina, R. M., Pena Reyes, M. E., Bali Chavez, G., & Little, B. B. (2011). Secular change in height and weight of indigenous school children in Oaxaca, Mexico, between the 1970s and 2007. *Annals of Human Biology, 38*(6), 691–701.

Martorell, R., Yarbrough, C., Lechtig, A., Delgado, H., & Klein, R. E. (1977). Genetic-environmental interactions in physical growth. *Acta Pædiatrica Scandinavia, 66*(5), 579–584.

Martorell, R., Kettel Khan, L., & Grummer-Strawn, L. M. (2000). Overweight and obesity in preschool children from developing countries. *International Journal of Obesity and Related Metabolic Disorders, 24*(8), 959–967.

Mastorakos, G., & Ilias, I. (2003). Maternal and fetal hypothalamic-pituitary-adrenal axes during pregnancy and postpartum. *Annals of the New York Academy of Sciences, 997*, 136–149.

McBride, W. G. (1961). Thalidomide and congenital abnormalities. *The Lancet, 278*(7216), 1358.

McDade, T., & Worthman, C. M. (1998). The weanling's dilemma reconsidered: A biocultural analysis of breastfeeding ecology. *Developmental and Behavioral Pediatrics, 19*(4), 286–299.

McEwen, B. S., & Wingfield, J. C. (2003). The concept of allostasis in biology and biomedicine. *Hormones and Behavior, 43*(1), 2–15.

McKeown, T., & Record, R. (1954). Influence of pre-natal environment on correlation between birth weight and parental height. *American Journal of Human Genetics, 6*(4), 456–463.

Mei, Z., Grummer-Strawn, L. M., Thompson, D., & Dietz, W. H. (2004). Shifts in percentiles of growth during early childhood: Analysis of longitudinal data from the California Child Health and Development Study. *Pediatrics, 113*(6), e617–e627.

Mericq, V., Medina, P., Kakarieka, E., Marquez, L., Johnson, M. C., & Iniguez, G. (2009). Differences in expression and activity of 11β-hydroxysteroid dehydrogenase type 1 and 2 in human placentas of term pregnancies according to birth weight and gender. *European Journal of Endocrinology, 161*(3), 419–425.

Miller, G. W. (2014). *The exposome: A primer*. Waltham: Academic Press.

Mongomery, S. M., Bartley, M. J., & Wilkinson, R. G. (1997). Family conflict and slow growth. *Archives of Disease in Childhood, 77*(4), 326–330.

Monteiro, P. O. A., & Victora, C. G. (2005). Rapid growth in infancy and childhood and obesity in later life – A systematic review. *Obesity Reviews, 6*(2), 143–154.

Moore, V. M., Davies, M. J., Willson, K. J., Worsley, A., & Robinson, J. S. (2004). Dietary composition of pregnancy women is related to size of the baby at birth. *Journal of Nutrition, 134*(7), 1820–1826.

Morrison, R. F., & Farmer, S. R. (2000). Hormonal signaling and transcriptional control of adipocyte differentiation. *Journal of Nutrition, 130*(12), 3116S–3121S.

Neel, J. V. (1962). Diabetes Mellitus: A "thrifty" genotype rendered detrimental by "progress"? *American Journal of Human Genetics, 14*(4), 353–362.

Nesse, R. M. (2005). Maladaptation and natural selection. *The Quarterly Review of Biology, 80*(1), 62–70.

Neufeld, L. M., Haas, J. D., Grajeda, R., & Martorell, R. (2004). Changes in maternal weight from the first to second trimester of pregnancy are associated with fetal growth and infant length at birth. *American Journal of Clinical Nutrition, 79*(4), 646–652.

Neumann, C., & Harrison, G. (1994). Onset and evolution of stunting in infants and children. Examples from the Human Nutrition Collaborative Research Support Program. Kenya and Egypt studies. *European Journal of Clinical Nutrition, 48*(Suppl1), S90–S102.

Noonan, K. J., Farnum, C. E., Leiferman, E. M., Lampl, M., Markel, M. D., & Wilsman, N. J. (2004). Growing pains: Are they due to increased growth during recumbency as documented in a lamb model? *Journal of Pediatric Orthopedics, 24*(6), 726–731.

Olds, T., Maher, C., Zumin, S., Peneau, S., Lioret, S., Castebon, K., et al. (2011). Evidence that the prevalence of childhood overweight is plateauing: Data from nine countries. *International Journal of Pediatric Obesity, 6*(5–6), 342–360.

Omran, A. R. (1971). The epidemiologic transition. A theory of the epidemiology of population change. *The Milbank Memorial Fund Quarterly, 49*(4), 509–538.

Ong, K. K., & Dunger, D. B. (2002). Perinatal growth failure: The road to obesity, insulin resistance and cardiovascular disease in adults. *Best Practice & Research. Clinical Endocrinology & Metabolism, 16*(2), 191–207.

Oreffo, R. O., Lashbrooke, B., Roach, H. I., Clarke, N. M., & Cooper, C. (2003). Maternal protein deficiency affects mesenchymal stem cell activity in the developing offspring. *Bone, 33*(1), 100–107.

Ounsted, M. (1965). Maternal constraint of foetal growth in man. *Developmental Medicine and Child Neurology, 7*(5), 479–491.

Owen, C. G., Martin, R. M., Whincup, P. H., Davey Smith, G., & Cook, D. G. (2005). Effect of infant feeding on the risk of obesity across the life course: A quantitative review of published evidence. *Pediatrics, 115*(5), 1367–1377.

Ozanne, S. E., & Constancia, M. (2007). Mechanisms of disease: The developmental origins of disease and the role of the epigenotype. *Nature Clinical Practice Endocrinology & Metabolism, 3*(7), 539–546.

Paciorek, C. J., Stevens, G. A., Finucane, M. M., Ezzati, M., & Nutrition Impact Model Study Group. (2013). Children's height and weight in rural and urban populations in low-income and middle-income countries: A systematic analysis of population-representative data. *The Lancet Global Health, 1*(5), e300–e309.

Painter, R. C., Roseboom, T. J., Bossuyt, P. M., Osmond, C., Barker, D. J. P., & Bleker, O. P. (2005a). Adult mortality at age 57 after prenatal exposure to the Dutch famine. *European Journal of Epidemiology, 20*(8), 673–676.

Painter, R. C., Roseboom, T. J., van Montfrans, G. A., Bossuyt, P. M. M., Krediet, R. T., Osmond, C., et al. (2005b). Microalbuminuria in adults after prenatal exposure to the Dutch Famine. *Journal of the American Society of Nephrology, 16*(1), 189–194.

Painter, R. C., Osmond, C., Gluckman, P. D., Hanson, M. A., Phillips, D. I. W., & Roseboom, T. J. (2008a). Transgenerational effects of prenatal exposure to the Dutch famine on neonatal adiposity and health in later life. *BJOG, 115*(10), 1243–1249.

Painter, R. C., Westendorp, R. G. J., de Rooij, S. R., Osmond, C., Barker, D. J. P., & Roseboom, T. J. (2008b). Increased reproductive success of women after prenatal undernutrition. *Human Reproduction, 23*(11), 2591–2595.

Palmer, C., Bik, E. M., DiGiulio, D. B., Relman, D. A., & Brown, P. O. (2007). Development of the human infat intestinal microbiota. *PLoS Biology, 5*, e177.

Paneth, N., & Susser, M. (1995). Early origin of coronary heart disease (the "Barker hypothesis"). *British Medical Journal, 310*(6977), 411–412.

Pawson, I. G., & Huicho, L. (2010). Persistence of growth stunting in a Peruvian high altitude community, 1964–1999. *American Journal of Human Biology, 22*(3), 367–374.

Peck, M. N., & Lundberg, O. (1995). Short stature as an effect of economic and social conditions in childhood. *Social Science & Medicine, 41*(5), 733–738.

Peter, I. S., & Davidson, E. H. (2011). Evolution of gene regulatory networks controlling body plan development. *Cell, 144*(6), 970–985.

Petrik, J., Reusens, B., Arany, E., Remacle, C., Coelho, C., Hoet, J. J., et al. (1999). A low protein diet alters the balance of islet cell replication and apoptosis in the fetal and neonatal rat and is associated with a reduced pancreatic expression of insulin-like growth factor-II. *Endocrinology, 140*(10), 4861–4873.

Popkin, B. M., Adair, L. S., & Wen Ng, S. (2012). Global nutrition transition and the pandemic of obesity in developing countries. *Nutrition Reviews, 70*(1), 3–21.

Prentice, A. (2008). Vitamin D deficiency: A global perspective. *Nutrition Reviews, 66*(S2), S153–S164.

Rahman, A., Bunn, J., Lovel, H., & Creed, F. (2007). Association between antenatal depression and low birthweight in a developing country. *Acta Psychiatrica Scandinavica, 115*(6), 481–486.

Ramakrishnan, U., Grant, F., Goldenberg, T., Zongrone, A., & Martorell, R. (2012). Effect of women's nutrition before and during early pregnancy on maternal and infant outcomes: A systematic review. *Paediatric and Perinatal Epidemiology, 26*(Suppl 1), 285–301.

Ravelli, A. C., van der Meulen, J. H., Osmond, C., Barker, D. J. P., & Bleker, O. P. (1999). Obesity at the age of 50 y in men and women exposed to famine prenatally. *American Journal of Clinical Nutrition, 70*(5), 811–816.

Ravelli, A. C. J., van der Meulen, J. H. P., Michels, R. P. J., Osmond, C., Barker, D. J. P., Hales, C. N., et al. (1998). Glucose tolerance in adults after prenatal exposure to famine. *The Lancet, 351*(9097), 173–177.

Ravelli, G. P., Stein, Z. A., & Susser, M. W. (1976). Obesity in young men after famine exposure in utero and early infancy. *New England Journal of Medicine, 295*(7), 349–353.

Regidor, E., Martinez, D., Santos, J. M., Calle, M. E., Ortega, P., & Astasio, P. (2012). New findings do not support the neomaterialist theory of the relation between income inequality and infant mortality. *Social Science & Medicine, 75*(4), 752–753.

Ricco, R., Nogueira-de-Almeida, C., Del Ciamp, L., Daneluzzi, J., Ferlin, M., & Muccillo, G. (2001). Growth of exclusively breast-fed infants from a poor urban population. *Archivos Latinoamericanos de Nutrición, 51*, 122–126.

Richter, L., Norris, S., Pettifor, J., Yach, D., & Cameron, N. (2007). Cohort profile: Mandela's children: The 1990 birth to twenty study in South Africa. *International Journal of Epidemiology, 36*(3), 504–511.

Rinaudo, P., & Wang, E. (2012). Fetal programming and metabolic syndrome. *Annual Review of Physiology, 74*, 107–130.

Robker, R. L., Akison, L. K., Bennett, B. D., Thrupp, P. N., Chura, L. R., Russell, D. L., et al. (2009). Obese women exhibit differences in ovarian metabolites, hormones, and gene expression compared with moderate-weight women. *The Journal of Clinical Endocrinology and Metabolism, 94*(5), 1533–1540.

Romero-Corral, A., Somers, V. K., Sierra-Johnson, J., Thomas, R. J., Collazo-Clavell, M. L., Korinek, J., et al. (2008). Accuracy of body mass index in diagnosing obesity in the adult general population. *International Journal of Obesity, 32*(6), 959–966.

Rondo, P. H. C., Ferreira, R. F., Nogueira, F., Ribeiro, M. C. N., Lobert, H., & Artes, R. (2003). Maternal psychological stress and distress as predictors of low birth weight, prematurity and intrauterine growth retardation. *European Journal of Clinical Nutrition, 57*(2), 266–272.

Roseboom, T. J., van der Meulen, J. H., Ravelli, A. C. J., van Montfrans, G. A., Osmond, C., Barker, D. J. P., et al. (1999). Blood pressure in adults after prenatal exposure to famine. *Journal of Hypertension, 17*(3), 325–330.

Roseboom, T. J., van der Meulen, J. H., Osmond, C., Barker, D. J. P., Ravelli, A. C., & Bleker, O. P. (2000). Plasma lipid profiles in adults after prenatal exposure to the Dutch famine. *American Journal of Clinical Nutrition, 72*(5), 1101–1106.

Roseboom, T. J., van der Meulen, J. H., Osmond, C., Barker, D. J. P., Ravelli, A. C., & Bleker, O. P. (2001). Adult survival after prenatal exposure to the Dutch famine 1944–45. *Paediatric and Perinatal Epidemiology, 15*(3), 220–225.

Roseboom, T. J., Painter, R. C., van Abeelen, A. F. M., Veenendaal, M. V. E., & de Rooij, S. R. (2011). Hungry in the womb: What are the consequences? Lessons from the Dutch famine. *Maturitas, 70*(2), 141–145.

Salam, M. T., Millstein, J., Li, Y. F., Lurmann, F. W., Margolis, H. G., & Filliland, F. D. (2005). Birth outcomes and prenatal exposure to ozone, carbon monoxide, and particulate matter: Results from the Children's Health Study. *Environmental Health Perspectives, 113*(11), 1638–1644.

Saleemi, M., Ashraf, R., Mellander, L., & Zaman, S. (2001). Determinants of stunting at 6, 12, 24 and 60 months and postnatal linear growth in Pakistani children. *Acta Paediatrica, 90*(11), 1304–1308.

Sanguanklin, N., McFarlin, B. L., Park, C. G., Giurgescu, C., Finnegan, L., White-Traut, R., et al. (2014). Effects of the 2011 flood in Thailand on birth outcomes and perceived social support. *Journal of Obstetric, Gynecologic, and Neonatal Nursing, 43*(4), 435–444.

Savino, F., Liguori, S. A., Fissore, M. F., & Oggero, R. (2009). Breast milk hormones and their protective effect on obesity. *International Journal of Pediatric Endocrinology, 2009*, e327505.

Schell, L. M., Gallo, M. V., Denham, M., & Ravenscroft, J. (2006). Effects of pollution on human growth and development: An introduction. *Journal of Physiological Anthropology, 25*(1), 103–112.

Schell, L. M., Denham, M., Stark, A. D., Parsons, P. J., & Schulte, E. E. (2009). Growth of infants' length, weight, head and arm circumferences in relation to low levels of blood lead measured serially. *American Journal of Human Biology, 21*(2), 180–187.

Schlotz, W., & Phillips, D. I. W. (2009). Fetal origins of mental health: Evidence and mechanisms. *Brain, Behavior, and Immunity, 23*(7), 905–916.

Schmatz, M., Madan, J., Marino, T., & Davis, J. (2010). Maternal Obesity: The interplay between inflammation, mother, and fetus. *Journal of Perinatology, 30*(7), 441–446.

Schuster, S., Hechler, C., Gebauer, C., Kiess, W., & Kratzsch, J. (2011). Leptin in maternal serum and breast milk: Association with infants' body weight gain in a longitudinal study over 6 months of lactation. *Pediatric Research, 70*(6), 633–637.

Sederquist, B., Fernandez-Vojvodich, P., Zaman, F., & Savendahl, L. (2014). Impact of inflammatory cytokines on longitudinal bone growth. *Journal of Molecular Endocrinology, 53*(1), T35–T44.

Shenkin, S. D., Starr, J. M., & Deary, I. J. (2004). Birth weight and cognitive ability in childhood: A systematic review. *Psychological Bulletin, 130*(6), 989–1013.

Silventoinen, K., Rokholm, B., Kaprio, J., & Sorensen, T. I. A. (2010). The genetic and environmental influences on childhood obesity: A systematic review of twin and adoption studies. *International Journal of Obesity, 34*(1), 29–40.

Simkhada, B., van Tejilingen, E. R., Porter, M., & Simkhada, P. (2008). Factors affecting the utilization of antenatal care in developing countries: Systematic review of the literature. *Journal of Advanced Nursing, 61*(3), 244–260.

Souberbiellea, J.-C., Body, J.-J., Lappe, J. M., Plebani, M., Shoenfeld, Y., Wang, T. J., et al. (2010). Vitamin D and musculoskeletal health, cardiovascular disease, autoimmunity and cancer: Recommendations for clinical practice. *Autoimmunity Reviews, 9*(11), 709–715.

Sram, R. J., Binkova, B. B., Dejmek, J., & Bobak, M. (2005). Ambient air pollution and pregnancy outcomes: A review of the literature. *Environmental Health Perspectives, 113*(4), 375–382.

Stein, A. D., Zybert, P. A., van der Pal-de Bruin, K. M., & Lumey, L. H. (2006). Exposure to famine during gestation, size at birth, and blood pressure at age 59 y: Evidence from the dutch famine. *European Journal of Epidemiology, 21*(10), 759–765.

Stinson, S. (2012). Growth variation: Biological and cultural factors. In S. Stinson, B. Bogin, & D. O'Rourke (Eds.), *Human biology: An evolutionary and biocultural perspective* (2nd ed., pp. 587–636). New York: John Wiley & Sons, Inc..

Stockard, C. R. (1921). Developmental rate and structural expression: An experimental study of twins, "double monsters" and single deformities, and the interaction among embryonic organs during their origin and development. *The American Journal of Anatomy, 28*(2), 115–277.

Strutz, K. L., Hogan, V. K., Siega-Riz, A. M., Suchindran, C. M., Halpern, C. T., & Hussey, J. M. (2014). Preconception stress, birth weight, and birth weight disparities among US women. *American Journal of Public Health, 104*(8), e125–e132.

Subramanian, S. V., Ozaltin, E., & Finlay, J. E. (2011). Height of nations: A socioeconomic analysis of cohort differences and patterns among women in 54 low- to middle-income countries. *PLoS ONE, 6*(4), e18962.

Susser, M., & Stein, Z. (1994). Timing in prenatal nutrition: A reprise of the Dutch Famine Study. *Nutrition Reviews, 52*(3), 84–94.

Swali, A., McMullen, S., Hayes, H., Gambling, L., McArdle, H. J., & Langley-Evans, S. C. (2011). Cell cycle regulation and cytoskeletal remodeling are critical processes in the nutritional programming of embryonic development. *PLoS One, 6*, e23189.

Swinburn, B., Sacks, G., Hall, K. D., McPherson, K., Finegood, D. T., Moodie, M. L., et al. (2011). The global obesity pandemic: Shaped by global drivers and local environments. *The Lancet, 378*(9793), 804–814.

Tanner, J. M. (1981). *A history of the study of human growth*. New York: Cambridge University Press.

Taveras, E. M., Rifas-Shiman, S. L., Sherry, B., Oken, E., Haines, J. L., Kleinman, K., et al. (2011). Crossing growth percentiles in infancy and risk of obesity in childhood. *Archives of Pediatrics and Adolescent Medicine, 165*(11), 993–998.

Thame, M., Osmond, C., & Trotman, H. (2012). Fetal growth and birth size is associated with maternal anthropometry and body composition. *Maternal & Child Nutrition*. doi:10.1111/mcn.12027.

Theriot, C. M., Koenigsknecht, M. J., Carlson, P. E. J., Hatton, G. E., Nelson, A. M., Li, B., et al. (2014). Antibiotic-induced shifts in the mouse gut microbiome and metabolome increase susceptibility to Clostridium difficile infection. *Nature Communications, 5*, 3114.

Thompson, L. M., Bruce, N., Eskenazi, B., Diaz, A., Pope, D., & Smith, K. R. (2011). Impact of reduced maternal exposures to wood smoke from an introduced chimney stove on newborn birth weight in rural Guatemala. *Environmental Health Perspectives, 119*(10), 1489–1494.

Thompson, A. L., Monteagudo-Mera, A., Cadenas, M. B., Lampl, M. L., & Azcarate-Peril, M. A. (2015). Milk- and solid-feeding practices and daycare attendance are associated with differences in bacterial diversity, predominant communities, and metabolic and immune function of the infant gut microbiome. *Frontiers in Cellular and Infection Microbiology, 5*(3), 1–15.

Thornburg, K. (2004). Fetal origins of cardiovascular disease. *NeoReviews, 5*(12), e527–e533.

Thornburg, K., Jonker, S., O'Tierney, P., Chattergoon, N., Louey, S., Faber, J., et al. (2011). Regulation of the cardiomyocyte population in the developing heart. *Progress in Biophysics and Molecular Biology, 106*(1), 289–299.

Tu, Y. K., West, R., Ellison, G. T., & Gilthorpe, M. S. (2005). Why evidence for the fetal origins of adult disease might be a statistical artifact: The "reversal paradox" for the relation between birth weight and blood pressure in later life. *American Journal of Epidemiology, 161*(1), 27–32.

Turnbaugh, P. J., & Gordon, J. I. (2009). The core gut microbiome, energy balance and obesity. *Journal of Physiology, 587*(17), 4153–4158.

Turnbaugh, P. J., Hamady, M., Yatsunenko, T., Cantarel, B. L., Duncan, A., Ley, R. E., et al. (2009). A core gut microbiome in obese and lean twins. *Nature, 457*(7228), 480–484.

Turnbaugh, P. J., Quince, C., Faith, J. J., McHardy, A. C., Yatsunenko, T., Niazi, F., et al. (2010). Organismal, genetic, and transcriptional variation in the deeply sequenced gut microbiomes of identical twins. *Proceedings of the National Academy of Sciences, 107*(16), 7503–7508.

Unger, C., Weiser, J. K., McCullough, R. E., Keefer, S., & Grindlay Moore, L. (1988). Altitude, low birth weight, and infant mortality in Colorado. *Journal of the American Medical Association, 259*(23), 3427–3432.

UNICEF. (2014). *The state of the world's children 2015: Reimagine the future: Innovation for every child. Department of communication*. New York: United Nations Children's Fund.

van Abeelen, A. F. M., Elias, S. G., Bossuyt, P. M. M., Grobbee, D. E., van der Schouw, Y. T., Roseboom, T. J., et al. (2012a). Famine exposure in the young and the risk of type 2 diabetes in adulthood. *Diabetes, 61*(9), 2255–2260.

van Abeelen, A. F. M., Veenendaal, M. V. E., Painter, R. C., de Rooij, S. R., Dijkgraaf, M. G. W., Bossuyt, P. M. M., et al. (2012b). Survival effects of prenatal famine exposure. *American Journal of Clinical Nutrition, 95*(1), 179–183.

Vazir, S., Engle, P., Balakrishna, N., Griffiths, P. L., Johnson, S. L., Creed-Kanashiro, H., et al. (2013). Cluster-randomized trial on complementary and responsive feeding education to caregivers found improved dietary intake, growth and development among rural Indian toddlers. *Maternal & Child Nutrition, 9*(1), 99–117.

Vickaryous, N., & Whitelaw, E. (2005). The role of early embryonic environment on epigeotype and phenotype. *Reproduction, Fertility, and Development, 17*(3), 335–340.

Victora, C., Morris, S., Barros, F., Horta, B., Weiderpass, E., & Tomasi, E. (1998). Breastfeeding and growth in Brazilian infants. *American Journal of Clinical Nutrition, 67*(3), 452–458.

Wadhwa, P. D., Sandman, C. A., Porto, M., Dunkel-Schetter, C., & Garite, T. J. (1993). The association between prenatal stress and infant birth weight and gestational age at birth: A prospective study. *American Journal of Obstetrics and Gynecology, 169*(4), 858–865.

Waterland, R. A., Lin, J. R., Smith, C. A., & Jirtle, R. L. (2006). Post-weaning diet affects genomic imprinting at the insulin-like growth factor 2 (Igf2) locus. *Human Molecular Genetics, 15*(5), 705–716.

Weinberg, C. R. (2005). Invited commentary: Barker meets Simpson. *American Journal of Epidemiology, 161*(1), 33–35.

WHO MGRS. (2006). *WHO child growth standards: Length/height-for-age, weight-for-age, weight-for-length, weight-for-height and body mass index-for-age: Methods and development*. Geneva: World Health Organization.

Wiedmeier, J. E., Joss-Moore, L. A., Lane, R. H., & Neu, J. (2011). Early postnatal nutrition and programming of the preterm neonate. *Nutrition Reviews, 69*(2), 76–82.

Wijnstok, N. J., Hoekstra, T., van Mechelen, W., Kemper, H. C. G., & Twisk, J. W. R. (2013). Cohort profile: The Amsterdam Growth and Health Longitudinal Study. *International Journal of Epidemiology, 42*(2), 422–429.

Wikoff, W. R., Anfora, A. T., Liu, J., Schultz, P. G., Lesley, S. A., Peters, E. C., et al. (2009). Metabolomics analysis reveals large effects of gut microflora on mammalian blood metabolites. *Proceedings of the National Academy of Sciences, 106*(10), 3698–3703.

Wiley, A. S. (1994). Neonatal and maternal anthropometric characteristics in a high-altitude population of the western Himalaya. *American Journal of Human Biology, 6*(4), 499–510.

Wilkinson, R., & Marmot, M. (Eds.). (2003). *Social determinants of health: The solid facts* (2nd ed.). Copenhagen: World Health Organization.

Wilkinson, R. G., & Pickett, K. E. (2006). Income inequality and population health: A review and explanation of the evidence. *Social Science & Medicine, 62*(7), 1768–1784.

Wit, J. M., & Camacho-Hubner, C. (2011). Endocrine regulation of longitudinal bone growth. *Endocrine Development, 21*, 30–41.

Worthman, C. (2009). Habits of the heart: Life history and the developmental neuroendocrinology of emotion. *American Journal of Human Biology, 21*(6), 772–781.

Worthman, C. M., & Panter-Brick, C. (2008). Homeless street children in Nepal: Use of allostatic load to assess the burden of childhood adversity. *Development and Psychopathology, 20*(1), 233–255.

Yajnik, C. S., Fall, C. H. D., Coyaji, K. J., Hirve, S. S., Rao, S., Barker, D. J. P., et al. (2003). Neonatal anthropometry: The thin-fat Indian baby. The Pune Maternal Nutrition Study. *International Journal of Obesity, 27*(2), 173–180.

Yanagida, M., Ikai, N., Shimanuki, M., & Sajiki, K. (2011). Nutrient limitations alter cell division control and chromosome segregation through growth-related kinases and phosphatases. *Philosophical Transactions of the Royal Society of London B, Biological Sciences, 366*, 3508–3520.

Zemel, B. S. (2012). Body composition during growth and development. In N. Cameron & B. Bogin (Eds.), *Human growth and development* (2nd ed., pp. 461–486). New York: Academic Press.

From Epidemiology to Epigenetics: Evidence for the Importance of Nutrition to Optimal Health Development Across the Life Course

Marion Taylor-Baer and Dena Herman

Nutrition is a desperately neglected aspect of maternal, newborn and child health. The reasons for this neglect are understandable, but not justifiable. Richard Horton BSc MB FRCP FMedSci, Editor-in-Chief, the Lancet (Horton 2008)

1 Introduction and Background

Nutrition is a young science. For thousands of years, foods and herbs were a major component in the armamentarium of the physician and his predecessors. Although built upon much earlier work in the sciences, as understood in centuries past (Carpenter 2003), nutrition science came into its own only a century or so ago with the discovery of certain micronutrients with an essential nature (needing to be provided in the diet) that were called vitamins. These discoveries were largely made in the context of finding a cure for, or the prevention of, serious diseases such as scurvy, beriberi, pellagra, rickets, and others. Following the recognition that these diseases were the result of dietary deficiencies, there also came an understanding of the major physiological functions of these nutrients; their other epigenetic and microbiological roles are still being elucidated.

In the mid-twentieth century, as technology advanced and research methodology became more sophisticated, it was discovered that insufficient amounts of some of the "trace" minerals, so called because of the small amounts and relative ubiquity in the diet, could also cause human deficiency disease. Zinc is a good illustration, "discovered" only in 1963 and, paradoxically, in the Middle East where zinc was adequate in the diet if considered only in terms of chemical analysis. However, the diet was also high in phytates, due to the consumption of unleavened bread, a staple of the Middle Eastern diet. The phytates, by binding to zinc in the gut, decreased its bioavailability, creating over time a deficiency syndrome characterized by short stature and delayed puberty, among other signs. Thus also began the understanding that other compounds in food can affect nutrient absorption and/or metabolism. The discovery of the essentiality of other trace

M. Taylor-Baer (✉)
Department of Community Health Sciences, Fielding School of Public Health, University of California Los Angeles, Los Angeles, CA, USA
e-mail: mtbaer@ucla.edu

D. Herman
Department of Family and Consumer Sciences, California State University Northridge, Northridge, CA, USA

N. Halfon et al. (eds.), *Handbook of Life Course Health Development*,
DOI 10.1007/978-3-319-47143-3_18

minerals soon followed, copper, selenium, nickel, etc., and in fact, the roles of new essential trace nutrients continue to be elucidated as laboratory techniques become more and more sensitive. Another important development is the ongoing discovery of other bioactive compounds in food and the emerging field of the microbiome and its relationship to diet, nutrition, and behavior.

The twenty-first century, following the mapping of the human genome and the rapid development of the relatively new field of epigenetics, where many of the epigenetic markers are nutrients or products thereof, promises to elucidate "new" biochemical and physiological functions for many of the nutrients whose non-genomic role was long ago understood. Perhaps food, or even selective nutrients, will again be part of the medical armamentarium and targeted with specificity to promote optimal health on both an individual and population basis. These concepts are presented in Fig. 1.

Today, nutrition is defined as a biological science, with physiological, genomic, medical, social, and environmental aspects (Beauman et al. 2005). Investigators have accumulated rigorous evidence about the importance of dietary intake, from preconception through old age, in shaping health trajectories across the lifespan and even into subsequent generations (Herman et al. 2014) through a process that is an interactive one, involving genes, environments, and behaviors. Being a field that crosses domains, nutrition epitomizes the need for an interdisciplinary approach to research and, certainly, to any intervention. Thus, when looking at the life course, nutrition must be seen through an integrative lens.

The purpose of this chapter is to use life course health development principles (as elaborated by Halfon and Forrest 2017) to organize a review of the current knowledge base regarding the crucial role nutrition plays in health development over the lifespan. There are time-specific health development pathways that result from particular nutritional exposures that occur during sensitive or critical periods, when developing biological systems are most alterable. Nutrition is an important determinant of health potential, such as reaching an individual's genetically endowed height. The

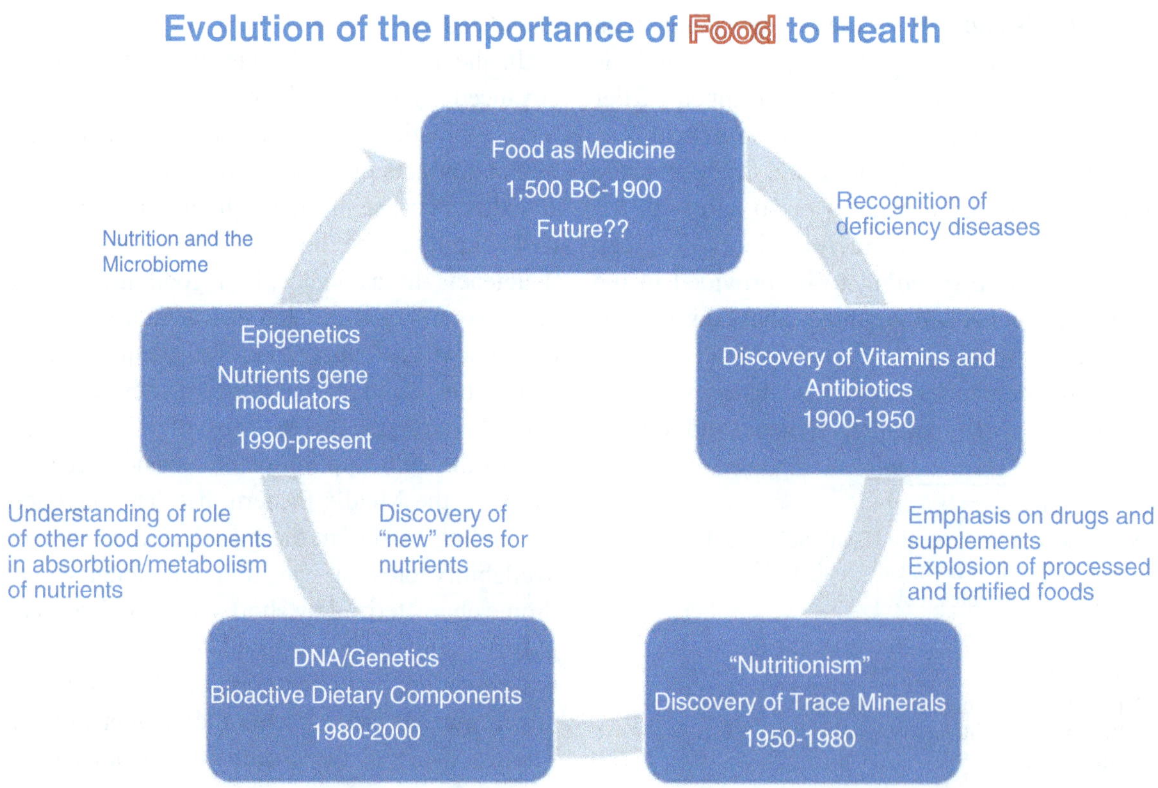

Fig. 1 Evolution of the Importance of Food to Health

effects of nutrition on human biology for individuals as children and then as adults are also constrained by evolutionarily determined adaptive responses to the perinatal nutritional milieu to which the developing fetus and infant are exposed. These generally stated links between nutrition and health development will be explored more specifically in each of the chapter's sections. We conclude with a discussion of the gaps in our knowledge that merit future research and attention from policy-makers.

1.1 Folate and Health Development

Our growing understanding of the importance of individual nutrients to optimal health development can be illustrated by the "story of folate," a trace nutrient that can be used to describe the role of certain nutrients that is increasingly being recognized as a basic mechanism for translating environmental cues into changes in gene expression that impact health development. Folate is the generic name for a group of related B vitamin, water-soluble compounds that have been known to be essential since being isolated in 1941. Folate acts as a cofactor in several reactions leading to the synthesis of deoxyribonucleic acid (DNA) and ribonucleic acid (RNA) and, along with vitamin B12, the amino acid methionine and other nutrients such as choline, to serve as a "methyl donor," providing one-carbon units for the methylation of a number of substances, including DNA, proteins, and neurotransmitters, thus influencing many functions at the cellular level. The exact mechanisms are still being worked out.

As early as the 1960s, epidemiological studies began focusing on geographic patterns that had been observed with regard to the incidence of neural tube defects, most commonly spina bifida, in newborns. Great Britain (specifically Wales, Northern England, Northern Ireland) was one of the sites of these studies. The initial approach to analyses of geographic clustering focused on a genetic cause. However, it soon became apparent that environmental factors and the timing of birth were important factors as well. The incidence of neural tube defects was lowest among babies conceived from April to June (Laurence et al. 1968). Social factors also emerged as potentially causal when it was observed that there was a social class gradient associated with the risk of developing a neural tube defect.

Since the neural tube develops very early in gestation, the suggestion was that women who conceived in late fall and winter, when there was very little access to fresh fruits and vegetables, might have been missing essential vitamins prior to, and during, the first month of their pregnancies, whereas those conceiving in late spring and summer would not have that dietary limitation. Women from higher social class groups may have had better access to fruits and vegetables during these months. The first intervention studies, in which women who had given birth to one child with a neural tube defect were given vitamin supplements (or not) prior to, or early in, their next pregnancies, provided further evidence that this was indeed likely to be the case; those who received the supplements had fewer subsequent children with a neural tube defect (Smithells et al. 1976).

Folate had been suspected early on (Laurence et al. 1968) as being the most likely vitamin because of the lack of green vegetables in winter and because it had been shown that there was a higher incidence of abnormal folate metabolism in mothers of babies with neural tube defects than in those with normal children (Hibbard et al. 1965). Several intervention studies followed, using periconceptional supplementation (Smithells et al. 1980, 1981). However, it took many years for the scientific community to declare the role of folate to be "fact" because the earlier studies had not been conclusive (Laurence et al. 1981) or were complicated by the inclusion of other vitamins in the supplement provided (Smithells et al. 1980, 1981). Finally, in the mid-1990s, after a large, well-designed clinical trial provided strong evidence in support of a protective role for folate (MRC 1991), the US government promulgated that in the interest of the public's health, white flour should be fortified with folic acid (the synthetic, more bioavailable form of folate). This was a controversial decision because of the population-wide aspects of the supplementation, targeting women of reproductive age in order to reduce risk to the developing fetus. Nonetheless, this program has proven to be successful (Williams et al. 2015).

Our current understanding of the next chapter in the "story" awaited the unraveling of the mystery of the human genome and the field of genomics. Nutritional genomics is the study of the interactions between our genes and the bioactive components—both nutrient and non-nutrient—of foods we consume and the resulting health outcomes. The ultimate goal is to understand the interactions well enough to be able to influence these outcomes by structuring diets to meet the genomic needs of certain populations, or even individuals, in order to prevent disease and promote optimal health.

1.2 Nutritional Genetics

Nutritional genetics, also known as nutrigenetics, is the study of changes in the *primary* sequencing of DNA that alter nutrient requirements or metabolism and the identification and description of human genetic variation that changes nutrient metabolism and food tolerances. The effects of certain mutations have been recognized for decades. The classic example is "inborn errors of metabolism," such as phenylketonuria (PKU), in which a mutation in a single gene alters the structure and function of an enzyme important in the metabolism of the essential amino acid phenylalanine, the toxic buildup of which results in severe intellectual disability. Now, infants are screened at birth, and those born with PKU, and many other metabolic disorders, can be treated by dietary means in order to promote normal development. Here is a clear example of a single gene-disease relationship that can be managed with a nutritional intervention which, if begun early enough, can have a dramatic, lifelong influence on the health of the individual.

As predicted by the life course health development principles, most disease causation is not as simple as one gene-one disease. The vast majority of diseases result from continuous interactions between individuals, inclusive of their genotype, with their environments over time. This multicausal and longitudinal paradigm requires new research tools for understanding etiological mechanisms.

1.3 Nutritional Epigenetics

More recently, geneticists recognized that the inheritance of traits was possible through mechanisms independent of genotype. Phenotypic changes where the sequence of DNA is *not* changed but *expression* of the gene is altered—turned on or off so to speak—are called epigenetic changes. The study of these phenomena is called *epigenomics*. Nutritional epigenetics is documenting how nutrition, one of the primary environmental factors that are in continuous interaction with individuals, may influence epigenetic changes with resultant consequences for health development (Jimenez-Chillaron et al. 2012).

Nutritional epigenetics examines the effects of nutrients on chromatin, a complex of DNA and histones; the latter is considered the superstructure or packaging (tertiary structure) of DNA which allows it to be contained in the nucleus of a cell by reducing its volume through chemical bonding. Regulation of the expression of proteins that function in metabolic or signaling pathways occurs through the opening and reforming of these bonds to allow transcription of DNA (through messenger RNA) and ultimately the formation of the protein coded in the DNA. Epigenetic regulation is mediated by means of methylation and demethylation that alters DNA, the histones that envelope DNA, and small RNA molecules. This type of epigenetic regulation depends on, or is influenced by, nutrients including, folate/choline, betaine, vitamin B12, vitamin B6, iron, selenium, methionine, and other bioactive components of food, such as resveratrol (red wine) and sulforaphane (broccoli) (Dolinoy et al. 2006). Polyunsaturated long-chain fatty acids (PUFA) have also been implicated in regulating gene expression in the brain as reviewed by Schuchardt et al. (2008). Thus, a growing body of evidence is pointing to an important link between food and gene regulation, with manifold effects on health.

Back to our folate story, it is currently believed that the epigenetic disruption caused by lack of, or insufficient, folate in the diets of pre-pregnant women and those in the first month of pregnancy can be overcome by sufficient, or additional, folate. Individual folate requirements vary, and it is further believed that women susceptible to neural tube defects have a greater than average need for folate—beyond two standard deviations of the population mean—or a metabolic impairment, perhaps due to epigenetic changes mitigated by the additional amount of folate. Maternal folic acid supplementation has been associated with higher rates of methylation of the IGF2 gene, increased intrauterine growth, but lower birth weights, demonstrating the potential to lower the risk of chronic disease as adults (Steegers-Theunissen et al. 2009).

In the space of half a century, we have progressed from the first epidemiological clues that the vitamin folate is linked to neural tube defects to an understanding, though not yet complete, of the probable mechanisms for that linkage, both as an essential cofactor for cell division and as a methyl donor involved in epigenetic regulation. Intriguingly, there are now suggestions that the paternal, as well as the maternal, folate status may influence pregnancy outcomes. A recent animal study found that the folate status of paternal rats plays an important role in regulating placental folate metabolism and transport (Kim et al. 2011). The contribution of fathers' nutritional status, prior to conception, to the life course health development of their offspring is another demonstration of the manifold ways in which environmental exposures can be transduced in ways that affect health development. Moreover, understanding these paternal effects is an area of research that merits much more attention.

Similar stories can be told and arguments made for the necessity of each of the known essential nutrients to the optimal development and functioning of an individual across the life course and beyond. However, we have chosen to highlight only a few to illustrate their crucial importance during sensitive periods of life course health development, or where improvement in the status of the nutrient would make a positive difference in life course health development beyond the early years, or where there is either current research activity or a need for such to advance our understanding of the contribution of nutrition to life course health development across the life trajectory and into future generations.

2 The Importance of Nutrition to Life Course Health Development: Selected Examples

2.1 Pre-conception and Pregnancy

The availability of an adequate supply of nutrients may be the most important environmental factor influencing pregnancy health outcomes. Although the woman's body adapts physiologically to meet the nutrient demands of both mother and fetus, these adaptations may not be sufficient if the mother is not well nourished. The placenta is recognized as a fundamental influence on life course health development (Barker and Thornburg 2013), and until rather recently, it was commonly thought that the placenta would provide for the nutrient needs of the fetus, even over those of the mother. Although some nutrients are actively transported across the placental barrier, others, including folate, pass by simple or mediated diffusion and are, therefore, much more dependent on the maternal diet and her available stores. Thus, the fetus should not be considered the "perfect parasite" (McNanley and Woods 2008).

Two groups at particular risk in this regard are adolescents within 2 years of menarche and women with inter-pregnancy intervals <18 months; both groups may have low nutrient reserves (King 2003). This underscores the importance of optimal nutritional status of women, from the preconception period and throughout pregnancy, detailed in a recent publication by the International Federation of Gynecologists and Obstetricians (FIGO), on optimal pregnancy outcomes and the prevention of low birth weight as well as defects such as neural tube defects (NTD) (Hanson et al. 2015). Current research interest is also turning to the role of the father's nutritional status/diet in influencing pregnancy outcomes, reflected in identified paternal epigenetic contributions in animal models (Siklenka et al. 2015; Donkin et al. 2016) as well as humans (Govic et al. 2016).

2.1.1 Birth Defects

In spite of the progress made in the prevention of neural tube defects worldwide, there are still approximately 300,000 infants born annually with neural tube defects (Christianson et al. 2006). Although the impact of folic acid fortification of the food supply has successfully lowered the incidence in the United States, there are still babies being born with neural tube defects. The latest Centers for Disease Control and Prevention data show the estimated prevalence has decreased from 10.7 per 10,000 live births in 1995–1996 (pre-fortification) to 6.5 per 10,000 in 2009–2011 (post-fortification) and that about 1326 fewer infants have been born over this 3-year period with a neural tube defect (Williams et al. 2015). However, Hispanic babies are affected disproportionately (4.17/10,000 live births) compared to either non-Hispanic Blacks (2.64/10,000) or Whites (3.22/10,000) (CDC, 2015; Parker et al. 2010), indicating that either this population is not being reached (e.g., only wheat flour, not corn, is fortified) or there are other factors in play such as genetic predispositions or other environmental exposures. In the case of Mexican-American women, there is some evidence that fumonisins, mycotoxins that contaminate corn, may be involved in the etiology (Missmer et al. 2006).

Incomplete uptake of folic acid, either from fortification or supplements (or folate from food), is suggested by recently published data (Tinker et al. 2015) from the 2007 to 2012 National Health and Nutrition Examination Survey (NHANES), which showed that 23% of women of childbearing age have red blood cell (RBC) folate concentrations below the recently established World Health Organization (WHO) recommended cutoff (i.e., 400 ng/mL or 906 nmol/L) for the prevention of neural tube defects (WHO 2015). On the other hand, another study has reported that one in ten women took folic acid supplements that exceeded the tolerable upper limits for that vitamin (Hoyo et al. 2011); more research into the possible effects of too much folate is also needed.

Even considering incomplete protection from dietary folate deficiencies in spite of the fortification program, not all cases of neural tube defects are preventable by folic acid alone (Heseker et al. 2009), indicating that there are other factors involved. Using the data (n = 954 with neural tube defects; n = 6268 controls) from the National Birth Defects Prevention Study (1997–2005), it was found that other micronutrients, related to methylation or oxidative pathways, in addition to folate and betaine, when present at higher levels in the maternal diet (thiamin, iron, and vitamin A), were associated with a decrease in anencephaly among some groups of women. In others, higher intakes of thiamin; riboflavin; vitamins B6, C, and E; niacin; and retinol were associated with decreased risk of spina bifida (Chandler et al. 2012). Vitamin A deficiency during pregnancy has also been associated with congenital diaphragmatic hernia (Beurskens et al. 2013).

Other birth defects, including cardiac anomalies, limb defects, cleft lip, and/or palate, have been prevented by provision of folate alone (Berry et al. 1999) or, in combination with other vitamins, urinary tract defects and congenital hydrocephalus, according to a meta-analysis (Goh et al. 2006).

Further evidence for the importance of other micronutrients has come from data collected by the Hungarian periconceptional service between 1984 and 1994 (Czeizel et al. 2004). In a randomized controlled trial (RCT) to test the efficacy of a multivitamin supplement containing folate (0.8 mg) in the prevention of neural tube defects, researchers were surprised to find that not only were neural tube defects reduced by about 90%, but there was a very significant reduction (21 per 1000 population versus 41 per 1000 population) in the incidence of other major anomalies as well, notably cardiovascular anomalies and urinary tract defects (Czeizel 2009). Even when the neural tube defect cases were removed, the results remained statistically significant. The Hungarian group has published several articles examining folate with and without multivitamin supplementation and, based on their results, has strongly recommended that folate be recognized as preventing cardiovascular malformations as well as neural tube defects (Czeisel 2011) and that multivitamins be included in periconceptional supplements (Czeizel and Bánhidy 2011).

The US Public Health Service currently recommends that women capable of becoming pregnant consume 400 μg of folic acid daily. Based on correlational data from Irish and Chinese studies (Cordero et al. 2015), the WHO recently recommended levels of maternal RBC folate >400 ng/ml in order to reduce the risk of neural tube defects. To determine optimal levels for supplementation to prevent birth defects, one approach would be to quantify the daily dietary amounts necessary to achieve a level in whatever biological sample is typically used to measure the status of the nutrient. For example, the next step in this case would be to examine the dietary intake necessary to produce those protective RBC folate levels.

In recognition of the importance of folate and zinc to the processes involved in cell division and DNA synthesis and that alcohol interferes with the metabolism of each of these nutrients, as well as providing calories devoid of any nutrients, it is not surprising that a recent publication (Young et al. 2014) has explored the nutritional etiology of fetal alcohol syndrome. Young and his colleagues provide a review of the current state of research on the effects of alcohol on folate and zinc metabolism, along with some of the other nutrients known to be essential to successful reproduction—vitamin A, docosahexaenoic acid (DHA), choline, vitamin E, and selenium—that have been studied in animal models in relation to fetal alcohol syndrome. The question these authors pose is an interesting one: What is the potential of preventing or at least mitigating the severity of the disorder, by providing nutrient supplementation for pregnant women who drink?

These findings provide support for the importance of optimal preconception nutritional status to long-term health development. According to the life course health development principles, we would predict that further research will implicate yet other nutrients and their interactions with the intrauterine environment in the development of a variety of birth defects. Even for conditions such as fetal alcohol syndrome, no single risk factor (such as alcohol) is likely to fully explain the development and severity of birth defects.

The complexity of intrauterine environmental interactions between nutrition and alcohol is further illustrated in a Danish National Birth Cohort study that found a lack of effect of mild to moderate alcohol intake (one to eight drinks/week; one drink = 12 gm pure alcohol) during early to mid-pregnancy on children's intelligence, executive function, or attention at age 5 (Kesmodel et al. 2012). It is possible that adequate nutritional status was a protective factor in these women. Although diet was considered in the study as a possible "confounding factor" (Olsen et al. 2001), the focus was on fish (omega 3s), iron, and breastfeeding. They did not evaluate how diet as a whole might have been a protective factor; the women sampled were largely middle class and so may be expected to have had adequate diets. Further research into diet as a protective factor among women who are moderate drinkers, as well as the implications of higher nutrient supplementation in an attempt to potentiate the damage to their fetuses in those whose alcohol intake is heavy is needed, particularly to confirm positive results, to determine optimal amounts of nutrients and types of nutrients that should be provided, and to investigate the collective effects of multiple-nutrient supplementation.

2.1.2 Low Birth Weight

Low birth weight has long been recognized as a risk factor for mortality and neurodevelopmental problems (Hack et al. 1995). When the infant is small for gestational age—that is, born either before or at term and weighing less than expected for his/her fetal "age"—it suggests that the fetus was malnourished in utero. Full-term low birth weight has an incidence of 5% of live births in the United States and is considered a proxy for intrauterine growth retardation (CDC 2011). Among women underweight preconceptionally, the prevalence of low weight gain during pregnancy is 23%, preterm birth 15%, and low birth weight 10%.

In 2009, the Institute of Medicine issued updated guidelines for weight gain during pregnancy based on World Health Organization body mass index categories (IOM 2009). (There were not enough data to recommend guidelines for adolescents, and this is an area needing to be examined.) A recommended action was to continue services, where needed, into the postpartum period to prepare women for the next pregnancy, assuring good nutrition and adequate weight gain. A recent meta-analysis has suggested that there are protective effects of maternal overweight or obesity on risk of delivering low birth weight infants, both in developed and developing countries, but especially the latter. However, there was also an increased risk of having an infant of very low birth weight (<1500 g) or extremely low birth weight (<1000 g); the heavier the woman, the higher the risk (McDonald et al. 2010). This seeming contradiction may be explained by a high risk for malnutrition due to a lack of micronutrients in obese women, as reported by Bodnar and Parrott (2012) and referenced earlier.

Two recent reviews of the potential effects of maternal multiple-micronutrient supplementation, as opposed to folate or iron alone, have clearly shown that there is a significant benefit on decreasing the incidence of low birth weight and babies born small for gestational age (Haider and Bhutta 2012; Zerfu and Avele 2013). Both reports recommend amassing more evidence through future, larger trials before moving to a universal policy change, as well as further studies to determine the optimal dosage and mix of the micronutrients to promote the best pregnancy outcomes.

The scope of this chapter does not extend to the examination of the literature concerning the many individual nutrients, or other environmental and social factors, that have been associated with the incidence of low birth weight. However, because of the current burgeoning interest in the effects of vitamin D beyond bone health (also related to undernutrition and deficiency in circulating concentrations of maternal vitamin D) (Javaid et al. 2005, 2006), it is worth mentioning that a recent study found an association between maternal vitamin D levels at 26 or fewer weeks of gestation and growth measures of newborns; serum vitamin D levels were positively related to birth weight and head circumference and negatively associated with the risk of an infant being born small for gestational age (Gernand et al. 2013).

2.1.3 Developmental Origins of Adult Disease

We now know that the embryo is particularly susceptible to "nutrient-induced adaptations in gene expression" (Waterland and Garza 1999). These adaptations, or developmental plasticity, have been defined as the ability of a single genotype to give rise to several different phenotypes which, teleologically speaking, allows organisms to adapt to their surrounding environmental conditions more rapidly than possible with evolutionary changes (Duncan et al. 2014). Some have suggested that the term "plasticity" was used to describe epigenetic phenomena before we had an understanding of epigenetics (Jablonski 2012). Whatever these phenomena are called, and some have suggested the term "evo-devo" (Jablonka 2012), there can be negative implications for life course health development when the prenatal and postnatal environmental conditions are dissimilar.

Beginning with the epidemiological observations of David Barker and his colleagues in England linking low birth weight to earlier adult mortality (Barker et al. 1989, 1993) and the subsequent fetal origins of adult disease hypothesis (Barker 1995), the consensus now is that undernutrition during the early stages of pregnancy results in epigenetic adaptations which prepare the fetus for survival in an extrauterine life where the environment is lacking in sufficient nutrients to support optimal development. If the infant, born with a low birth weight, is then exposed to an environment of plenty, there is a mismatch between the metabolic adaptations that took place prenatally and the demands of the extrauterine environment which can result in later chronic disease (Gluckman et al. 2008). For example, if the kidney develops with fewer nephrons in response to prenatal deprivation, the well-nourished adult may later be predisposed to hypertension (Stein et al. 2006). Christian and Stewart (2010) have published a conceptual framework (Fig. 2) that illustrates the pathways by which various organ systems may be affected by maternal micronutrient deficiency.

Barker's early hypothesis regarding the negative, lifelong consequences of poor nutrition during pregnancy, in spite of a presumably postnatal normal diet, has been supported by retrospective observations of life course health development of children prenatally exposed to starvation during the brief (6 months), but severe, Dutch famine during the winter of 1944–1945 when the Nazis laid siege to western Holland. Not only were these children more likely to experience coronary heart disease, decreased renal function, and decreased glucose tolerance in adulthood (Roseboom et al. 2006), but their offspring are shorter and heavier, which demonstrates the transgenerational effects of early nutritional insults on future health outcomes (Painter et al. 2008). This is possibly due to epigenetic changes occurring in fetuses exposed to the famine, which are then transmitted across generations (Tobi et al. 2009).

Similar findings of long-term health effects resulting from exposure to starvation during the developmental period have resulted from investigations following the Chinese famine of 1959–1961 during the "Great Leap Forward" (Huang et al. 2010). Over 35,000 young women (average age 32 years), exposed during this period, were studied. In the 1958 and 1959 cohorts, postnatal exposure (1.5–3 years of life) was associated with reduced height, increased body mass index, and a threefold increase in the odds of hypertension for the 1958 cohort. Body mass index increased for the same postnatal exposure for the 1957 cohort, but decreased for the 1960–1961 cohorts for those exposed during pregnancy and infancy. The authors note the young age of the subjects and hypothesize that later in life there might have been more significant effects. Interestingly, they also document negative effects on economic productivity as measured by labor and earning findings.

In a study of adults exposed as infants to undernutrition before, during, and after the Biafran famine of 1967, both women and men experienced a higher prevalence of overweight, hypertension, and impaired glucose tolerance at 40 years of age (Hult et al. 2010). This reinforces the above findings suggesting that fetal and infant undernutrition are closely associated with the development of chronic disease as adults and that nutritional challenges in early life can result in changes to epigenetic regulation of genes which are detectable up to 60 years later (Lillycrop 2011).

2.2 Growth and Obesity

2.2.1 Growth

Although adequate, if not optimal, nutrition is recognized universally as being important to growth and life course health development, nutritional evaluations are rarely considered in population-based studies because of the difficulties (i.e., time intensity, expense) in collecting the dietary and/or biochemical data that would reflect the inadequacies in dietary intake and/or decreases in nutrient stores that precede growth faltering, as the body adapts to the decreased nutrient intake. This continuum in nutritional status from optimal health to overt disease is depicted in Fig. 3, which also shows the typical measures used in assessing nutritional status, as well as their level of sensitivity. Dietary assessment is the most sensitive in predicting, and therefore preventing, nutritional problems, followed by biochemical assessment, a measure of nutrient stores. As these assessments are rarely included, many studies of children's health development use growth as a proxy for nutritional status. Although growth is a clinical/functional measure of nutritional status, it is not ideal, because it follows the usually chronic insufficient/poor nutrient intake which results in decreased nutrient stores. However, growth remains the most widely used and reported indicator of nutritional status and, if measurements are carefully taken, can be useful in monitoring growth rates in children or assessing nutritional health in populations.

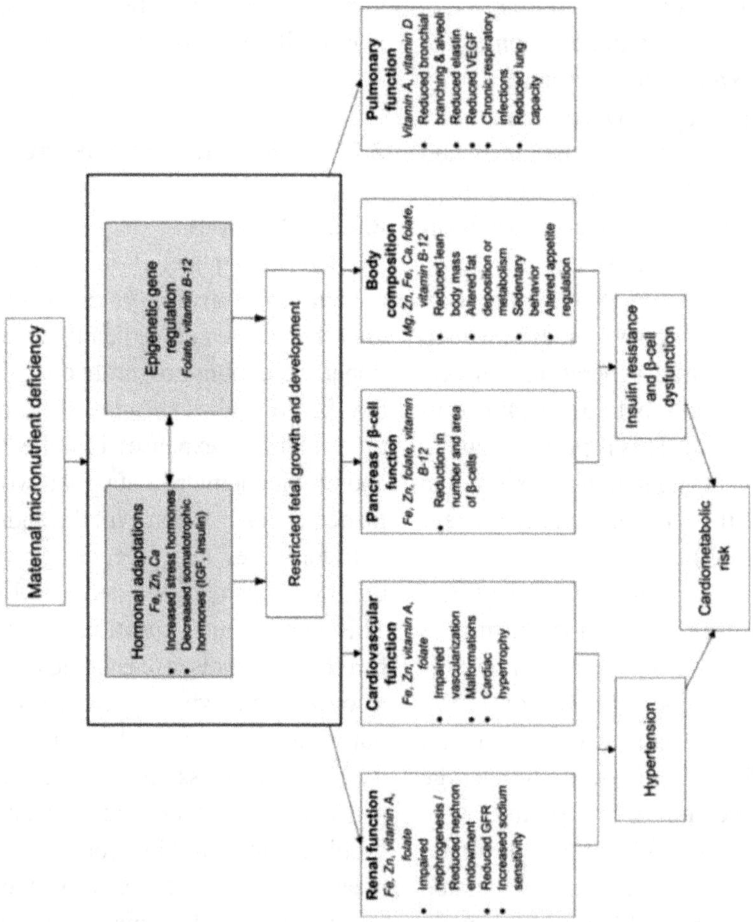

Fig. 2 Conceptual framework for the metabolic effects of maternal micronutrient deficiency (Christian and Stewart 2010)

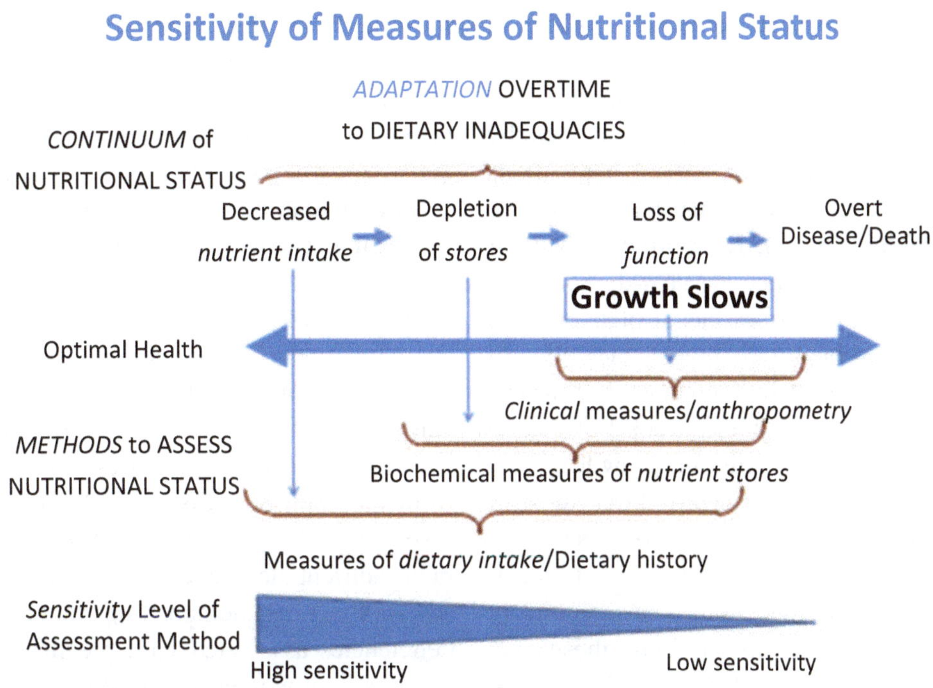

Fig. 3 Continuum of nutritional status and sensitivity of assessment methods to detect risk/signs of malnutrition

Reduced stature caused by a combination of poor diet and disease burden in childhood, called "net nutrition" by some (Steckel 1995; Silventoinen 2003), is modifiable. Data from the Organization for Economic Cooperation and Development (OECD) have shown an increase in stature, generally attributed to the improvement in net nutrition, for most of the 34 member countries (OECD 2009), although there do seem to be upper limits to growth potential, as evidenced by the apparent plateauing of the increases seen in the Dutch population (Schönbeck et al. 2012). Interestingly, the United States has not shown the same gains as the other countries (Komlos 2008), a finding not likely explained by the influx of immigrants of short stature (OECD 2009).

The Institute of Nutrition of Central America and Panama in Guatemala conducted a study from 1969 to 1977 in which women and children in entire villages were exposed to supplemental nutrition; findings showed significant improvements both in children's stature and in pregnancy outcomes in intervention, compared with control villages (Martorell 1992; Martorell et al. 1995). Follow-up studies (1988–2007) showed that the nutritional intervention for girls also increased the body size of their offspring, again demonstrating the intergenerational effects of nutritional status (Behrman et al. 2009).

The idea that there is a universal potential for growth, regardless of the environmentally sensitive phenotypic expression of that potential, led to a study (1997–2003), sponsored by WHO, of the growth of infants and children from six different continents who were healthy at birth and breastfed for at least 6 months (the Multicentre Growth Reference Study). The results strongly suggested that all human infants, regardless of racial or cultural background, have the genetic potential to achieve similar stature under optimal conditions (de Onis et al. 2004). These findings were considered robust enough for the WHO to adopt them as universal reference data for growth (WHO 2006); the international WHO Child Growth Standards, from 0 to 5 years of age, are now used in more than 140 countries worldwide (de Onis et al. 2015). In the United States, the Centers for Disease Control and Preventions have recommended their use for children 0–2 years, recognizing that the growth of breastfed infants should be the standard (Grummer-Strawn et al. 2010).

Data from the INTERGROWTH-21st Project (the International Fetal and Newborn Growth Consortium for the 21st Century), which assessed fetal growth and newborn size among healthy pregnant women in eight urban populations (Brazil, China, India, Italy, Kenya, Oman, the UK, and United States), have provided similar international convergence in growth potential. From 2009 to 2013, assessments of over 4600 women with problem-free pregnancies (out of 60,000) were done using ultrasound measurements at 5-week intervals from week 14 to delivery. Again, similar results in growth across ethnicities and countries suggested that most of the variation in the average size of babies born in different places around the world is due to nutritional and other socioeconomic and healthcare differences (Villar et al. 2014a). Thus, these data, representing optimal fetal growth, have been used to construct fetal growth charts to be used universally, in conjunction with the WHO charts, as a clinical tool to assess maternal, fetal, infant, and early childhood health and nutritional status on both the individual and population-based levels (Chatfield et al. 2013; Papageorghiou et al. 2014). For the newborn standards, meticulous measurements of weight, length, and head circumference for more than 20,000 babies born between 33 and 42 weeks' gestation during the same study were used to generate the charts, representing the first international standards for newborn growth under optimal conditions during pregnancy (Villar et al. 2014b).

2.2.2 Obesity

As the world goes through a "nutrition transition" from inadequate food to relative overabundance, adaptation to poor diets of a different sort in an age of "overnutrition" has no evolutionary precedent. Physiological constructs have been programmed from Paleolithic times, when we were hunters and gatherers, to conserve energy as fat in times of plenty to serve as energy stores for periods of relative food scarcity. At that time and up until the last century, most humans were very active physically and, because of their high-energy needs, consumed enough food to meet micronutrient needs as well. Today, a sedentary lifestyle means that we must be selective about our food choices to meet micronutrient needs with a lower energy intake. In fact, obese people may also be malnourished even while exceeding their energy needs if their diets are nutrient poor.

This double burden of malnutrition presents interesting challenges, with regard to which nutrients to supplement for optimal birth outcomes, when overweight or obese mothers coexist with underweight children in the same household. Until recently, the double burden was considered a phenomenon more common in low- and middle-income countries. However, data from the Danish National Birth Cohort studies reveal that obese women have a higher risk of micronutrient deficiencies (Bodnar and Parrott 2012). These data demonstrate that micronutrient deficiencies associated with pregnancy in overweight/obese women are becoming increasingly an issue in both affluent and lower- and middle-income countries and may further negatively impact birth outcomes, particularly the incidence of preeclampsia and low birth weight (Darnton-Hill and Mkparu 2015), and may explain the apparent contradiction mentioned earlier with regard to obesity being at the same time a potential protective factor for birth weight, but also a risk factor (McDonald et al. 2010).

There are many causes underlying the current worldwide "obesity epidemic," including many that are based in cultural, social, and political as well as biological factors. Genetics, epigenetics, and even causes related to the microbiome (discussed later in the chapter) are currently being studied intensely. However, the bottom line is that obesity is caused by increases in dietary energy (much of it nutrient-poor food) that is not compensated for by increased energy output.

Paradoxically, the increasing concern about obesity and its role in the predisposition to metabolic disease has resulted in the growing interest in the developmental origins of health and disease, discussed earlier.

The Newborn Epigenetics Study, a federally funded research project based at Duke University, is studying how pre- and postnatal environmental exposures, including nutrition, affect the epigenome, with a special interest in obesity. A paper, recently published by this group, examined the potential associations between DNA methylation patterns in newborns and parental preconception obesity and found that hypomethylation of the IGF2 gene in newborns is associated with paternal obesity (Soubry et al. 2013). The contribution of the father to pregnancy outcomes—mentioned earlier with regard to folate—is an area of research that has potentially important implications for the public health community with regard to the development of new and different population intervention strategies.

While an inverse relationship between total serum vitamin D and increased adiposity has been established in children, adolescents, and adults, the relationship between neonatal adiposity and vitamin D status has only recently been investigated. Researchers found that infants born to lean mothers had a third higher amount of vitamin D compared to infants born to obese mothers (Josefson et al. 2012). Obese women in this study transferred less vitamin D to offspring than normal weight women, despite similar serum levels, possibly due to sequestration of this fat-soluble vitamin in their adipose tissue. These findings underscore the evolving relationships between maternal obesity, vitamin D nutritional status, and adiposity in the neonatal period that may influence subsequent childhood and adulthood vitamin D-dependent processes (Josefson et al. 2012).

2.3 Neurological Development

The brain continues to grow rapidly after birth for the first 2–3 years of life, coinciding with a high iron requirement. Iron deficiency is the most prevalent nutritional problem worldwide, because after 6 months of age, even breastfed infants need an additional source of iron (WHO 2011). Multiple studies, dating back to the mid-twentieth century, have investigated the effects of iron deficiency and iron deficiency anemia on the development of infants and young children, which support the claim that there is a causal relationship between iron deficiency anemia and poor performance on measures of psychomotor and cognitive development, particularly when the anemia is severe (McCann and Ames 2007). In cases in which a child is iron deficient but not anemic, the findings are equivocal (Sachdev et al. 2005; Szajewska et al. 2010).

Other nutrient deficiencies in early childhood can also impact the ability to learn and affect school readiness, which in turn can alter lifelong achievement and increase inequalities in life course health development (WHO 2011). The importance of folate and iron to brain formation has already been mentioned. Another animal study has shown that offspring of pregnant rats fed a mildly zinc-deficient diet, compared to those of controls and supplemented rats, showed decreased learning and memory ability that was reflected in changes in the morphology of the hippocampus (Yu et al. 2013). Vitamin C has also been shown to be associated with fetal brain development. Unfortunately, the placental transport of vitamin C is not active, and it appears to be insufficient in the case of vitamin C deficiency (Norkus et al. 1979). In animal models, even marginal vitamin C deficiency in the mother stunts the development of the fetal hippocampus, the important memory center, permanently impeding optimal development of the brain even if guinea pig pups were given vitamin C after birth. (Tveden-Nyborg et al. 2012). This study has implications for the 10–20% of all adults in the developed world with vitamin C deficiency, including the most vulnerable populations who already suffer from health and socioeconomic disparities and who may also have poor dietary habits and perhaps smoke cigarettes, both of which increase the risk of vitamin C deficiency (Montez and Eschbach 2008).

Polyunsaturated fatty acids are essential nutrients for humans; omega-3 (synthesized from linolenic acid) and omega-6 (synthesized from linoleic acid) long-chain polyunsaturated fatty acids are involved in the development and maturation of neuronal structures, serve as structural and functional components of cell membranes, and are precursors of eicosanoids, which exert hormonal and immunological activity. The central role of the omega-3s DHA and eicosapentaenoic acid (EPA) in the development and functioning of the brain has met with growing research interest with regard to neurological development in children, including visual acuity (Schuchardt et al. 2008). In early studies, when it was recognized that infant formulas were lacking in DHA and EPA, it was shown that retinal development (Birch et al. 1992) and visual evoked potentials (Faldella et al. 1996) in very low birth weight infants were improved if they were supplemented with these omega-3 fatty acids. The effects of supplementation on visual acuity in term infants has also been shown (Birch et al. 2005), but not consistently. In addition, the effects of oral supplementation of omega-3 fatty acids during pregnancy on early childhood development, especially visual, were inconclusive (Gould et al. 2013). In a meta-analysis of 12 studies (1949 infants up to 12 months of age), omega-3 supplementation of infant formulas appeared to have possible effects on visual acuity as measured by evoked potential for infants 2 months of age and by behavioral methods at 12 months (Qawasmi et al. 2013). In another meta-analysis conducted by the same authors evaluating the effects of omega-3 supplementation of infant formula, no effects on general cognition were identified (Qawasmi et al. 2012).

Omega-6 fatty acids are also essential, but their metabolites are more inflammatory than those of omega-3, and some researchers believe that the ratio of omega-6 to omega-3 fatty acids that are consumed fall within a range of 1:1–1:4 (Lands 2005). Others believe that a ratio as high as 4:1, which is thought to approximate the ratio obtained in the diets, rich in animal meat and seafood, of our earliest ancestors, is still healthy (Simopoulos 2002). Currently, typical Western diets provide dramatically higher ratios of between 10:1 and 30:1, which may be of concern (Hibbeln et al. 2006; Schuchardt et al. 2010). The significance of these findings has been related to current dietary practices that result in an increased intake of omega-6 precursors (vegetable oils, processed and fast foods, meat) over those of omega-3 (fish, nuts, legumes).

A review of studies considering the significance of polyunsaturated fatty acids related to the development of behaviors in older children has found equivocal evidence in support of an association, although numerous observational studies have shown a link between omega-6 to omega-3 imbalances and some developmental disorders, including attention deficit hyperactivity disorder (ADHD) and autism (Schuchardt et al. 2010). In an RCT, conducted by Vaisman et al. (2008), among 60 children, aged 8–13, with impaired visual sustained attention, an improvement in performance test scores was seen in those supplemented with either EPA or EPA plus DHA compared to those receiving the placebo. Frensham and coworkers (2012) suggest that among children and adolescents, the greatest benefits of omega-3s in the diet are seen in trials with durations of at least 3 months and in subgroups of children with low socioeconomic status, learning disabilities, and ADHD or ADHD-type symptoms, which might explain the reported discrepancies.

2.4 Immune Function and Oxidative Stress

With respect to the development of the immune system, animal models show that exposure to omega-3s during gestation and lactation resulted in a more permeable gut, allowing new substances to pass through the lining and into the bloodstream more easily (De Quelen et al. 2011). The new substances then trigger the fetal immune response and the production of antibodies. This results in the potential for a more developed and mature immune system with better immune function, which could be important for the prevention of allergies as a child develops. Supporting this is a recent periconceptional multi-micronutrient supplementation intervention (vs. placebo) with malnourished Gambian women which led to differential methylation of genes, some of which were associated with the immune function, in their offspring at birth, and also at 9 months of age (Khulan et al. 2012).

Zinc has been shown to be required for the activation of at least 300 enzymes and for the gene expression of nearly 2000 transcription factors (Prasad 2012). It serves as an intracellular signaling molecule, playing an important role in cell-mediated immune function and oxidative stress (Prasad 2009). An estimated 17% of the global population is at risk for inadequate zinc intake, ranging from 8% in high-income regions to 30% in South Asia (Wessells and Brown 2012). Provision of zinc supplementation has been shown to decrease oxidative stress markers and inflammatory cytokines (Prasad 2008a, b). This is an interesting example of the dependence, as described by Hambidge (2000), of many metabolic processes important to life course health development, including the immune system, on the presence of a trace mineral. Certainly, the role of zinc, and other trace elements once thought to be insignificant, needs further investigation.

2.5 Healthy Aging

The aging process begins before birth with epigenetic changes that affect gene regulation. In addition to fundamental changes in organ structure, it has also been increasingly demonstrated that epigenetic mechanisms, which are susceptible to the presence or absence of certain nutrients during critical growth periods, establish long-lasting patterns of gene expression. Some of these have been discussed earlier in the chapter. The nutrient needs of individuals over 50 have only recently been explored; the oldest age category in the last edition of the Recommended Dietary Allowance (RDA), published in 1989, was 50 and over (Food and Nutrition Board 1989). This was largely because the studies carried out to determine nutrient needs used young subjects and were focused on deficiencies and extrapolating beyond the age of 50 was not deemed reasonable. With an aging population and an increased interest in the relationship between nutrition and chronic disease, there were calls to determine the RDAs for older adults (Russell 1997). In the newly defined series, the Dietary Reference Intakes, first published in 1997 and updated with regularity, the age categories were expanded to include 50–70 years and 70 and older (Food and Nutrition Board 1997), using data from the Jean Mayer USDA Human Nutrition Research Center on Aging at Tufts University. The following is a brief overview of some of the nutrients that the latest research has shown to be potentially important for healthy aging.

The traditional function of vitamin D is understood to involve the release of 1,25 vitamin D into the circulation, after which its effects are targeted on end organs involved in calcium and phosphorus homeostasis, such as the kidney, intestines, parathyroid, and bone (Jones 2007). However, we now know that there is a vast array of other biological functions in which vitamin D plays a role in and that these functions actually represent the bulk of daily metabolic utilization of vitamin D (Jones 2007; Heaney 2008). The recognition of these new pathways has led to newly ascribed paracrine functions of vitamin D that include multiple organ systems such as the cardiovascular (Heaney 2008; Verstuyf et al. 2010), renal, and immune systems. These systems are believed to activate vitamin D locally, via vitamin D receptors, to regulate cell and tissue growth and differentiation (Falkenstein et al. 2000), as well as to serve as precursors of enzyme cofactors, all integral to the intact functioning of numerous metabolic processes (Heaney 2008; Rostand and Warnock 2008). The widespread presence of vitamin D receptors supports the extensive range of physiological functions of 1,25 vitamin D (Dusso and Brown 1998). As such, vitamin D has a number of important effects on both developmental and lifelong health trajectories.

As an example of the role vitamin D plays in the development of long-term health outcomes, substantial evidence has linked low circulating vitamin D levels to increasing risk and incidence of cardiovascular disease (CVD) (Poole et al. 2006; Wang et al. 2008) and also suggests the possibility that vitamin D repletion may reverse or attenuate what remains the leading cause of mortality in the United States (Ford et al. 2011). In the cardiovascular system, the mechanisms responsible for vitamin D's effects appear to be mediated through the interaction of activated vitamin D with the intracellular vitamin D receptors within vascular smooth muscle, endothelium, and heart muscle cells. These mechanisms serve to modulate key processes involved with the pathogenesis of CVD including vascular inflammation (Rigby et al. 1987), platelet aggregation (Aihara et al. 2004) and vascular smooth cell proliferation, vascular calcification, and more (Artaza et al. 2009, 2010).

Age-related effects of vitamin D include its protective effects against Alzheimer's disease (Annweiler et al. 2012), improved cognitive health in older women (Annweiler et al. 2013), and improved mobility among older adults (Houston et al. 2013). Vitamin D plays an important role in the development and maintenance of muscle mass, particularly in institutionalized elderly, and is recommended for optimal musculoskeletal health (Mithal et al. 2012).

In addition to vitamin D, omega-3 fatty acid intake appears to influence the aging process. Adequate intake of omega-3 fatty acid supplements, to improve the balance of omega-3s to omega-6s, may slow a key biological process linked to aging. Among overweight middle-aged and older adults who took omega-3 supplements for 4 months, the ratio of their fatty acid consumption was altered in a way that helped preserve white blood cell telomeres, which normally shorten during the aging process (Kiecolt-Glaser et al. 2013). The improved omega ratio also resulted in reduced oxidative stress, caused by free radicals in the blood by about 15% compared to those in the placebo group. Other benefits of omega-3 intake for older adults include its putative role in the prevention of dementia and predementia. In the results from a meta-analysis of more than 2200 elderly subjects and matched controls with cognitive deficits, the latter had lower serum levels of EPA, DHA, and omega-3 fatty acids, while serum levels of EPA alone were significantly lower in those with pre-dementia. This indicates that EPA might not only be a disease state marker but may indicate increased risk for cognitive impairment as individuals age (Lin et al. 2012). All of these studies demonstrate that omega-3 fatty acid intake across all phases and stages of the life course is important and has the potential to alter health development outcomes, although there is some controversy regarding whether or not the omega 6/omega 3 ratio is important (Willett 2007).

There is also some evidence that vitamin E, with its antioxidant properties, may protect against memory loss in older adults. In a prospective study carried out in Finland, a sample of 140 over 65-year-olds with no memory impairment at the onset of the study was followed for 8 years, during which time it was found that higher total serum levels of vitamin E (alpha-tocopherol), as well as the other forms of the vitamin, seemed protective against memory disorders (Mangialasche et al. 2013). A recent study, using a zebra fish model, showed that a diet deficient in vitamin E—equivalent to a human lifelong deficiency—resulted in about 30% lower levels of DHA phosphatidylcholine (DHA-PC), which is a part of the cellular membrane in every brain cell or neuron, indicating that DHA-PC may be a good predictor of a higher risk for Alzheimer's disease (Choi et al. 2015). A recent meta-analysis found that patients with Alzheimer's disease, compared with cognitively intact elderly controls, had significantly lower plasma alpha-tocopherol concentrations (Lopes da Silva et al. 2013).

A recent large RCT involving over 500 patients with mild to moderate Alzheimer's disease at 14 Veterans Affairs medical centers found that 2000 IU/day of alpha-tocopherol compared to a placebo resulted in a slower cognitive functional decline (Dysken et al. 2014). Although supplements have been found to have benefit in slowing Alzheimer's disease progression, they do not seem to prevent Alzheimer's disease occurrence (Traber 2014). Because 96% of adult women and 90% of men in the United States do not receive adequate levels of vitamin E in their diet (Choi et al. 2015), it would seem that additional studies are needed to explore further risk reduction related to the development of cognitive impairment.

Further evidence of the preventive value of folate in reducing the risk of cardiovascular disease and stroke has been provided by recent studies. A meta-analysis of eight randomized trials which assessed the use of folic acid supplementation in the primary prevention of stroke showed beneficial effects, especially in trials that lasted longer than 3 years (Wang et al. 2007). The China Stroke Primary Prevention Trial, a large (n = 20,702) randomized, double-blind clinical trial that took place in 32 communities over 5 years, also examined folic acid's effects on cardiovascular disease (Huo et al. 2015). Participants were given either enalapril (a drug used to treat hypertension) alone or in combination with folic acid. The results showed that the combined use of enalapril and folic acid, compared with enalapril alone, significantly reduced the risk of first stroke. These examples (folate and vitamin E) both illustrate how the accumulation of a lifetime of inadequate intake of a nutrient may contribute to the development of a serious disease and also that improved nutrient intake can result in some degree of amelioration of chronic disease symptoms.

While adequate intake of specific nutrients has been shown to help preserve structure and function of the body with aging, a number of studies in model organisms have also demonstrated the benefits of caloric restriction. A 20–40% reduction in calorie intake reduces levels of insulin-like growth factor I and other growth factors, which has been consistently associated with increased lifespan, and prevents the development of age-associated cardiovascular functional and structural changes (Fontana et al. 2012; Wei et al. 2008). In animal models, caloric restriction is associated with reduced cancer risk (Longo and Fontana 2010), likely through similar mechanisms as described above, in addition to reduction in circulating levels of anabolic hormones, inflammatory cytokines, and oxidative stress markers (Hursting et al. 2003; Fontana and Klein 2007). Further, caloric restriction reduces glucose uptake and lactate concentration, which preserves vascular function. Therefore, the effects of caloric restriction appear to be neuroprotective (increased presence of ketone bodies, improved cerebral blood flow), which seems to play an important role in preserving brain physiology in aging (Lin et al. 2015).

3 The Importance of Food

3.1 Food Versus Nutritionism

We have highlighted the importance of individual nutrients to optimal health development. Nonetheless, we must emphasize that focusing on nutrients alone provides an incomplete picture. The tendency to isolate nutrients, to use them to fortify foods, and to manufacture supplements can lead to what Michael Pollan (2008) and others (Lang et al. 2009) have called "nutritionism," or the emphasis on individual nutrients rather than food. The science of nutrition has progressed to the point where we have amassed a great deal of information about nutrients, their metabolic roles, their influence on gene regulation, and ways that the physical and social environments interact with nutritional intake. The complexity of these interactions, which are dynamic, are continuous, and work on multiple levels, is typical of life course health development phenomena.

However, we cannot assume that we have no further discoveries to make regarding the thousands of bioactive compounds contained in food itself. Nutrition science is not yet able to "copy" nature; there remain elements, present in natural foods, that promote health development and which we are still just beginning to understand. An example of this is the ongoing attempt to emulate breast milk in infant formulas as newly recognized components of breast milk are uncovered. In the 1990s, it was shown experimentally that adding additional zinc than that found in breast milk to infant formula improved growth in male infants (Walravens and Hambidge 1976). Further investigation revealed that the zinc in breast milk is more biologically available than that in formula, due to the presence of previously unrecognized factors that enhance its absorption (Sandstrom et al. 1983; Blakeborough et al. 1986). DHA, one of the omega-3 acids, was not added to infant formula in this country until the mid-1990s, although we now know that this compound, present in breast milk, is critical to optimal infant health development. Thus, simply replicating the nutrient composition of breast milk, or of any other naturally occurring foods, cannot replicate all of the potentially bioactive compounds, as it is likely that there are as yet other unknown factors in all foods that positively affect health development.

There has been an evolution in the definition of dietary nutrient sufficiency in the past two decades. The Recommended Dietary Allowances were largely based on empirical criteria that established minimum nutrient requirements by assuming that individual requirements were normally distributed and recommending amounts that would meet the needs of 97.5% (two standard deviations above the mean) of the population. The newer Dietary Reference Intakes (DRI), besides being expanded to include older age categories as mentioned above, are based on the idea that optimal nutrient intakes should be the standard. As a part of establishing the DRI values, upper limits of intake are now also being recommended, along with the Estimated Average Requirement (EAR), recognizing that the new approach could lead to problems with exceeding safe intake level of some nutrients, particularly the fat-soluble vitamins, or nutrients like iron which are not readily excreted (see Fig. 4).

Going back to the "folate story" for another example, one of the objections to universal fortification in the United States was based on the fact that increased folate in the diet has the possibility of masking the pernicious anemia caused by a lack of vitamin B12. Deficiencies of vitamin B12 affect elders for whom its dietary absorption becomes less efficient and, if not recognized, can progress to severe neurological problems. Excess nutrient intake can also be an issue for young children because of the tendency of the food industry to "over-fortify" many of the foods intended for this age group. Most breakfast cereals, for example, have high levels of added nutrients, as do "snack foods," to make them more appealing to parents who often provide "vitamin pill" supplements to their children as well. The influence of excessive levels of certain nutrients on health development is an important area for research.

3.2 Food and Other Bioactive Compounds

As we delve more deeply into the biochemistry/metabolism of the individual nutrients, we are simultaneously realizing that our nutritional health depends not only on essential vitamins and minerals, as well as the optimal balance of the macronutrients that fuel our bodies, but also on the other bioactive compounds in our food, commonly referred to as phytochemicals or phytonutrients (Erdman et al. 2007; Beecher 1999). These include important subgroups such as carotenoids and phenolics, which are primarily derived from plant-based foods and are thought to convey

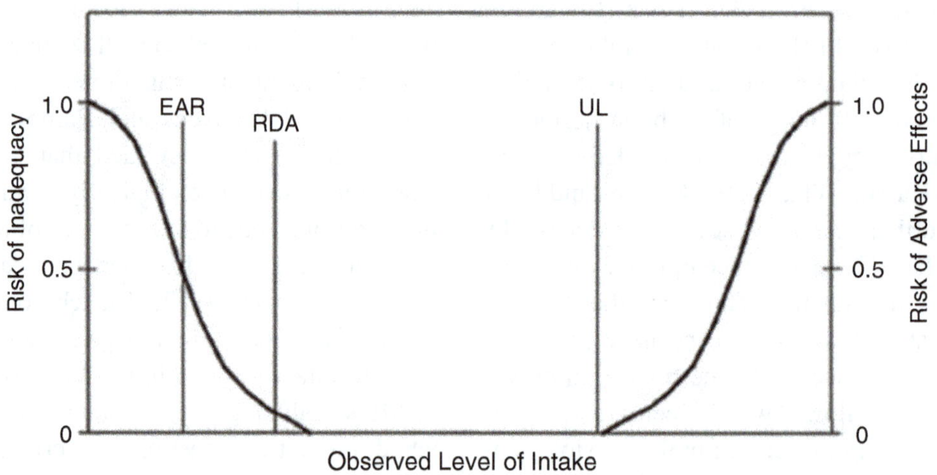

Fig. 4 Dietary Reference Intakes (Food and Nutrition Board 1997)

important health benefits. While there are more than 600 carotenoids identified in nature, nutrition research has focused primarily on just a handful, alpha-carotene, beta-carotene, beta-cryptoxanthin, lutein, zeaxanthin, and lycopene, because of their prevalence in both food and the body (Holden et al. 1999; Linus Pauling Institute 2015). Polyphenols are a diverse group of phytochemicals that include many of the molecules that give fruits and vegetables their colors. More than 8000 polyphenols have been distinctly identified to date (D'Archivio et al. 2007; Pandey and Rizvi 2009), and very little is known about the metabolic activity for the majority of them. Flavonoids, the most abundant of the polyphenols in the human diet, are comprised of many subclasses of compounds based on chemical structure (Scalbert and Williamson 2000; Mulvihill and Huff 2010). Flavonoids that have been well explored in the literature include anthocyanidins, found in red, blue, and purple fruits (Erdman et al. 2007) and vegetables, quercetin (Manach et al. 2004), and ellagic acid, primarily found in berries (Beecher 2009; Clifford and Scalbert 2000). Resveratrol, a polyphenol belonging to the group of stilbenoids, is found in the skin of wine grapes, both white and red. However, more frequent maceration in red winemaking allows the resveratrol to be released into red wine at a rate ten times higher than that of white wine.

Both carotenoids and polyphenols have potential health benefits. Carotenoids may reduce the risk for heart disease, particularly from intake of beta-carotene (Mente et al. 2009), while studies on lycopene show potential for the prevention of prostate cancer (Khan et al. 2010). Lutein and zeaxanthin may be instrumental in reducing the effects of oxidative injury that contribute to the development of age-related macular degeneration (Olson et al. 2011). Flavonoids have been studied for their anti-inflammatory characteristics (Garcia-Lafuente et al. 2009), while studies in animal models provide evidence that ellagic acid may reduce DNA damage (Aiyer et al. 2008). Stilbenoids such as resveratrol have been shown in animal models to prevent cancer, increase endurance, and lessen the consequences of obesity, including the loss of insulin sensitivity and increase in mortality rate (Jang et al. 1997; Baur et al. 2006; Lagouge et al. 2006). However, it should be noted that the amounts needed to produce such effects far exceed what could be obtained from usual dietary intake (Walle et al. 2004; Wenzel and Somoza 2005; Vitaglione et al. 2005).

In addition, recent analyses from national food consumption surveys in the United States (Murphy et al. 2012), Korea (Lee et al. 2013), and globally (Murphy et al. 2014) indicate that despite dietary recommendations that underscore the importance of increasing consumption of fruits and vegetables, intakes worldwide are lower than recommended. As a result, the diets of many individuals may be lacking in nutrients and phytonutrients typical of a diet rich in a variety of fruits and vegetables. Each of these studies demonstrates that individuals with the highest intakes of fruits and vegetables also have the highest intakes of phytonutrients, yet the sources of these phytonutrients in each of these studies are derived from just a few types of fruits and vegetables. This means that many of the essential nutrients already mentioned (e.g., vitamins A, C, and E and folate) that also play key roles in supporting optimal health are lacking in the diets of the majority of people. These data underscore one of the reasons why diets domestically and globally are suboptimal; without adequate access to fruits and vegetables, it is not possible to obtain essential nutrients let alone phytonutrients.

Optimizing the intake of specific foods and/or their bioactive components is a reasonable and cost-effective strategy for disease prevention. However, defining "the" ideal food pattern is challenging for a number of reasons including the difficulty in determining the required quantity of a particular food or nutrient to bring about the desired response as well as a host of nutrient-nutrient and nutrient-gene interactions that can occur (Milner 2008; Mariman 2008; Ferguson 2009; Ahmed et al. 2009; Simopoulos 2010). Even though there is not sufficient information to formulate the "ideal diet," there is sufficient knowledge to justify a call for future food-oriented health research (Milner 2008). In addition, it is becoming increasingly clear that individuals do not respond identically to the foods they consume. Therefore, as we begin to better understand the critical roles that multiple food components have in regulating cellular events and how these are influenced by genetic and epigenetic events, cultural and lifestyle differences, as well as our individual physical and social environments, the greater is our ability to develop a more individualized or personalized approach to our diets and to optimize our nutritional health (Kannan et al. 2008; da Costa et al. 2007; Kaput 2008). Since those compounds, which are growing in number, have yet to be fully understood, the importance of whole food itself, as opposed to simply the nutrients it provides, is becoming paramount again, as illustrated in Fig. 1.

3.3 Food and the Microbiome

An important area of emerging research focuses on the relationships between the microbiome and food and is helping to explain why individuals do not metabolize food in the same way. The human microbiome encompasses the collective genetic material of microbial communities found on several different sites on and inside the human body including the nasal passage, oral cavities, skin, urogenital tract, and the gastrointestinal (GI) tract and refers to the genetic information that these microorganisms carry (Ursell et al. 2012). In contrast, the human microbiota consists of 10–100 trillion symbiotic microbial cells, which are found primarily in the gut of every person (Turnbaugh et al. 2007). Evidence for a strong link between a person's microbiota, digestion, and metabolism is increasing. For example, in animal models, dietary changes have led to significant alterations in bacterial metabolism, especially small-chain fatty acids and amino acids, in as little as 1 week (Ley et al. 2008; Martin et al. 2010), and can lead to large changes after only 1 day (Turnbaugh et al. 2009). Perhaps most importantly, the genetic diversity found within our gut microbiota allows us to digest compounds via metabolic pathways not explicitly coded for in the mammalian genome, which greatly increases our ability to extract energy from our diverse diets. Therefore, these pathways are important linkages to understanding the individual differences in nutritional intake and how nutrients are utilized in our bodies to affect our health or risk for disease.

In addition to being an adjunct to the basic function of the human digestive system, the human microbiota have an important influence on the body's physiological, nutritional, and immunological processes and are able to modulate the expression of host genes that regulate diverse and fundamental physiological functions. Some of the ways in which the microbiome affects our health include its role in energy harvest from the gastrointestinal system, vitamin production, development and maintenance of the gut itself, metabolism of drugs and xenobiotics, deconjugation and metabolism of bile acids, and modulation of the immune system (Cerf-Bensussan and Gaboriau-Routhiau 2010; Young 2012; Maynard et al. 2012). However, despite the essential functions provided by the gut microbiome, the composition of each individual's microbiome is distinct (Costello et al. 2009). The individualized nature of the gut microbiome is related to a number of factors, including host genetics, age, diet, and health status and other processes like antibiotic use and birth delivery mode (Spor et al. 2011). To complicate things further, the amount of temporal stability in one's microbiome also appears to be personalized (Flores et al. 2014).

Nevertheless, a number of trends relating the composition of the microbiome to host health are beginning to emerge. In particular, changes in the dominant types of microorganisms living in the human gut have been associated with obesity in adults and model organisms (Backhed et al. 2004; Tremaroli and Backhed 2012; Ley et al. 2005, 2006; Turnbaugh et al. 2006). The relationship of the gut microbiome to obesity has become a focus of research. Although causality between the gut microbiome and obesity has yet to be established, findings from a number of studies suggest that the microbiome of obese individuals has an increased ability to extract energy from food. The gut microbiome has also been suggested to play a role in other inflammatory diseases (e.g., cardiovascular diseases, diabetes, and cancer) through the production of pro-inflammatory compounds that can cause chronic low-grade inflammation (Heilbronn and Campbell 2008; Tremaroli and Backhed 2012; van Olden et al. 2015; Hartstra et al. 2015).

Although several other factors play a role in the pathogenesis of obesity, the composition of the gut microbiome is now considered an important environmental factor and a potential therapeutic target for treatment of obesity (Tremaroli and Backhed 2012; Hartstra et al. 2015). Moreover, recent research suggests that not only are the metabolic products that result from carbohydrate digestion important in the etiology of obesity (e.g., short-chain fatty acids such as acetate, propionate, and butyrate) but that these factors may also have effects on appetite regulation through signaling of the hypothalamic region of the brain (Corfe et al. 2015).

The microbiome not only affects physical health but also our mental health across the life course. Patients with various mental health disorders appear to experience alterations in the stability, structure, and composition of fecal microbiota (Jiang et al. 2015; Mayer et al. 2014a), which in turn affect the severity of their disease. Scientists speculate that alterations in the gut microbiome may play a pathophysiological role in human brain diseases, including autism spectrum disorder, anxiety, depression, and chronic pain through bidirectional signaling between the brain and the gut microbiome involving multiple neurocrine and endocrine signaling mechanisms (Mayer et al. 2014b; Wang and Kasper 2014; Rosenfeld 2015). This research starts to bring together the effects that the microbiome has not only on physical health but also on mental and emotional health.

4 Conclusions and Future Directions

In this chapter, we have mainly considered population-based issues. However, if diet can be used to alter phenotypic expression of our genes, then nutritionists, food scientists, and physicians may also be able to work together to design personalized diets to prevent disease and optimize health development outcomes.

To affect maximum preventive benefit, dietary changes should begin early in life, ideally with breastfeeding, but, if not, with a formula more closely resembling breast milk than at present. Studies testing this hypothesis have already begun. The European Childhood Obesity Project, which has enrolled 1000 infants from five countries, tested an infant formula lower in protein, to more closely match that of breast milk, against the typically higher protein formula and a breastfed group, and found that the growth pattern of the infants more closely resembled that of the breastfed infants as well as the trajectory on the WHO growth charts referenced on breastfed infants (Koletzko et al. 2009). Given the importance of diet during this sensitive period in life course health development and in response to growing demand, the Agricultural Act of 2014 (Farm Bill) officially called for the Dietary Guidelines for Americans to expand to include infants and toddlers (ages 0–2), as well as women who are pregnant, beginning with the 2020 edition (USDA CNPP 2015). The US Department of Agriculture (USDA), in collaboration with Department of Health and Human Services (DHHS), is currently in the evidence-gathering phase (Jan 2015–Jan 2017) prior to developing a technical report to submit to the 2020 Dietary Guidelines Advisory Committee.

The fact that food is related to our health has always been obvious. However, as we have attempted to show, that relationship is very complex, and our understanding of its importance is growing with technological advancements, both in nutritional science and also in the numerous fields of study that have contributed to our knowledge base. That epigenetic mechanisms are so closely linked to the nutrients in our food (Jimenez-Chillaron et al. 2012) suggests that these mechanisms have allowed us to adjust rapidly to changes in our diet over the course of evolution, modifying the expression of our genes to adapt metabolically to a changing environment.

The effect of environmental stressors, other than nutrition, on inheritable epigenetic changes has been recognized and explored perhaps more fully to date (Jablonka 2012), while the importance of nutrition has been underrated, in spite of the rich literature on the subject (Horton 2008; Hanson et al. 2015)). Thus, we would like to echo Horton (2008), quoted at the beginning of the chapter; because of its key role in promoting optimal life course health development, especially for mothers, infants, and children, nutrition should no longer be "neglected." It is time for the attention of the maternal and child health community to turn toward nutrition, as we would argue, along with FIGO (Hanson et al. 2015), the most important environmental factor in the determination of life course health outcomes. As FIGO now recommends for gynecologists and obstetricians, we all need to "Think Nutrition First" (Hanson et al. 2015).

Areas for further study have been alluded throughout the paper. The long-term consequences of periconceptional nutrition to pregnancy outcomes and early development must be recognized; epigenetic changes during periods of rapid health development can have lifelong effects and intergenerational consequences. At the same time, we know that dietary changes at any time during the life course can ameliorate potentially inimical nutritional status.

We have also emphasized that the focus of the "power" of nutrition for life course health development has moved from the centuries-old attention paid to food, to elucidating, during the past century, an understanding of the role of specific nutrients and other bioactive components in food, and now back to food itself as the source of as yet unknown, but potentially important, other health-supporting elements (Fig. 1). The effects of food as translated through the microbiome is an emerging area of research that is likely to affect how we think about the composition and quantity of the food in our diet and the consequences for life course health development at all levels, from physical to mental and emotional health. It is, therefore, essential that access to enough food and the appropriate quality foods be available to all populations to afford the opportunity for optimal health development.

The recognition of nutrition as a central environmental determinant that all investigators should include in their assessment of life course health development and promotion is now becoming more widespread. Therefore, we invite and embrace other disciplines and health professionals to gain a better understanding of the centrality of nutrition and to work together in an effort to optimize population and individual health.

While more extensive than this chapter has space to allow, it bears mention that it is expected that the outcomes of research into the role of nutrition in life course health development would be further translated into priority-setting strategies for both practice and policy development. One current jumping-off point is the recent development of a healthcare system which promises to provide coverage for most Americans. This provides policy-makers, as well as healthcare professionals, an opportunity to switch from a focus on secondary prevention and treatment to a concentration on primary prevention. This should begin, we would argue, with optimizing diets, taking advantage of the current trend among consumers to recognize food as an avenue to health. In addition, recent clinical interventions, such as physicians offering patient's prescriptions to purchase healthy foods, would be a part of such a conversation (Brody 2014), as would the new recommendation by the American Academy of Pediatrics that pediatricians screen families with children for evidence of food insecurity (2015), given the impact of nutrition on health development. Other practice-oriented efforts such as authorizing reimbursement for nutrition services in multiple settings, including those providing primary preventive (e.g., inter-conception care) as well as secondary preventive care (e.g., diabetes) and placing more importance on educating healthcare providers in the basics of nutrition science, would go a long way to improving service delivery and promoting health development across the life course.

With respect to the food industry, broadly speaking, it would be important for those professionals to work collaboratively with academics and governmental agencies to translate academic insights into innovative solutions and agreed-upon regulations, for the benefit of the public's health, with a greater focus on health development as well as food safety. Laws taxing foods containing excessive amounts of sugar and/or fat as well as legislative collaboration between governmental organizations such as USDA, National Institutes of Health (NIH), and Maternal and Child Health Bureau/Health Resources and Services Administration (MCHB/HRSA) around nutrition issues could also support positive changes to the healthcare system as a whole but also to the greater public through crosscutting policy efforts.

5 Key Research Priorities

5.1 Basic Mechanisms

- Identify the genes influenced by the nutrient environment, and translate these findings into improved health with a focus on gaining a better understanding of the contribution of *paternal* diet and lifestyle to epigenetic inheritance.
- Understand the role of maternal nutrition in influencing their children's physiologic pathways, the mechanisms involved, and the long-term health consequences for children.
- Establish the biological/biochemical role of key nutrients, such as folate, iron, and vitamin D, in the epigenomic process.
- Elucidate the mechanisms by which breastfeeding reduces the risk of obesity, and understand the role of nutritional genetics and epigenetics in central and peripheral body weight regulatory mechanisms.
- Identify (1) early biomarkers, more sensitive than growth, that predict later chronic disease and (2) the critical periods for the development of each organ system, and determine the possibility of reversing/attenuating epigenomic changes.

5.2 Clinical Research

- Include data collection relating to nutritional status and diet in all longitudinal studies to better understand the effects of nutrition to life course health development.
- Determine the optimal levels of fortification, supplement doses, and blood levels for women of childbearing age and how these data and concepts translate into population screening for prevention.
- Explore the effects of subclinical nutrient deficiencies, as well as potential effects of supplements exceeding the tolerable upper limits for individual nutrients.

5.3 Population/Epidemiologic Research

- Identify critical periods for nutrition prevention or intervention to prevent later chronic disease.
- Examine the long-term effects of folic acid fortification.
- Understand the genetic/epigenetic contribution to nutrient requirements of specific populations to inform public health policies.
- Maximize the benefits of future research efforts through interdisciplinary birth cohort studies which allow researchers to identify relationships that might otherwise have been overlooked because of the ability to observe outcomes across the life course and across generations.
- Examine the utility of focusing on foods rather than nutrients alone on the life course health development outcomes including the effects of food on the microbiome and its relationship to physical, mental, and emotional health.

5.4 Data and Methods Development

- Refine study design and methods to enhance interdisciplinary collaborations between basic scientists, clinicians, and social scientists to deliver coherent, evidence-based research plans.
- Develop more efficient and feasible methods for recording and evaluating dietary intake to enhance the use of these methods in research studies.
- Develop crosscutting comprehensive data sources that include nutrition indicators to allow for continual quality improvement and consistent performance measurements at the local, state, and national levels.

References

Ahmed, T., Haque, R., Shamsir Ahmed, A. M., Petri, W. A., Jr., & Cravioto, A. (2009). Use of metagenomics to understand the genetic basis of malnutrition. *Nutrition Reviews, 67*(suppl 2), 201–206. doi:10.1111/j.1753-4887.2009.00241.x.

Aihara, K., Azuma, H., Akaike, M., Ikeda, Y., Yaashita, M., Sudo, T., et al. (2004). Disruption of nuclear vitmain D receptor gene causes enhanced thrombogenicity in mice. *Journal of Biological Chemistry, 279*, 35798–35802. doi:10.1074/jbc.M404865200.

Aiyer, H. S., Kichambare, S., & Gupta, R. C. (2008). Prevention of oxidative DNA damage by bioactive berry components. *Nutrition and Cancer, 60*(suppl 1), 36–42.

American Academy of Pediatrics. (2015). Lack of adequate food is ongoing health risk to US children: Nation's pediatricians release policy statement stressing the importance of federal, state and local nutrition programs to help combat the immediate and potentially lifelong impact of food insecurity. *Science Daily*. www.sciencedaily.com/releases/2015/10/151023083717.htm. Accessed 26 Oct 2015.

Annweiler, C., Rolland, Y., Schott, A. M., Blain, H., Vellas, B., Herrmann, F. R., & Beauchet, O. (2012). Higher vitamin D dietary intake is associated with lower risk of alzheimer's disease: A 7-year follow-up. *Journals of Gerontology. Series A, Biological Sciences and Medical Sciences, 67*(11), 1205–1211. doi:10.1093/gerona/gls107.

Annweiler, C., Llewellyn, D. J., & Beauchet, O. (2013). Low serum vitamin D concentrations in Alzheimer's disease: A systematic review and meta-analysis. *Journal of Alzheimer's Disease, 13*(33), 659–674. doi:10.3233/JAD-2012-121432.

Artaza, J. N., Mehrotra, R., & Norris, K. C. (2009). Vitamin D and the cardiovascular system. *Clinical Journal of the American Society of Nephrology, 4*, 1515–1522.

Artaza, J. N., Sirad, F., Ferrini, M. G., & Norris, K. C. (2010). Vitamin D3 inhibits cell proliferation by promoting cell cycle arrest without apoptosis and modifies cell morphology of mesenchymal multipotent cells. *Journal of Steroid Biochemistry and Molecular Biology, 119*, 73–83.

Backhed, F., Ding, H., Wang, T., Hooper, L. V., Koh, G. Y., Nagy, A., et al. (2004). The gut microbiota as an environmental factor that regulates fat storage. *Proceedings of the National Academy of Sciences of the United States of America, 101*, 15718–15723.

Baer, M. T., Harris, A. B., Stanton, R. W., & Haughton, B. (2015). The future of MCH nutrition: A commentary on the importance of supporting nutrition leadership training. *Maternal and Child Health Journal, 19*(2), 229–235.

Barker, D. J. P. (1995). Fetal origins of coronary heart disease. *British Medical Journal, 311*, 171.

Barker, D. J. P., & Thornburg, K. (2013). The obstetric origins of health for a lifetime. *Clinical Obstetrics and Gynecology, 56*(3), 511–519.

Barker, D. J. P., Winter, P. D., Osmond, C., Margetts, B., & Simmonds, S. J. (1989). Weight in infancy and death from ischemic heart disease. *The Lancet, 2*(8663), 577–580.

Barker, D. J. P., Osmond, C., Simmonds, S. J., & Wield, G. A. (1993). The relation of small head circumference and thinness at birth to death from cardiovascular disease in adult life. *British Medical Journal, 306*(6875), 422–426.

Baur, J. A., Pearson, K. J., Price, N. L., Jamieson, H. A., Lerin, C., Kalra, A., et al. (2006). Resveratrol improves health and survival of mice on a high-calorie diet. *Nature, 444*(7117), 337–342.

Beauman, C., Cannon, G., Elmadfa, I., Glasauer, P., Hoffman, I., Keller, M., et al. (2005). The principles, definition and dimensions of the new nutrition science. *Public Health Nutrition, 8*(6A), 695–698.

Beecher, G. R. (1999). Phytonutrients' role in metabolism: Effects on resistance to degenerative processes. *Nutrition Reviews, 57*(9 Pt2), S3–S6.

Behrman, J. R., Calderon, M. C., Preston, S. H., Hoddinott, J., Martorell, R., & Stein, A. D. (2009). Nutritional supplementation in girls influences the growth of their children: Prospective study in Guatemala. *The American Journal of Clinical Nutrition, 90*(5), 1372–1379. doi:10.3945/ajcn.2009.27524.

Berry, R. J., Li, Z., Erickson, J. D., Li, S., Moore, C. A., Wang, H., et al. (1999). Prevention of neural tube defects with folic acid in China. *The New England Journal of Medicine, 341*(20), 1485–1490.

Beurskens, L. W., Schrijver, L. H., Tibboel, D., Wildhagen, M. F., Knapen, M. F., Lindemans, J., et al. (2013). Dietary vitamin A intake below the recommended daily intake during pregnancy and the risk of congenital diaphragmatic hernia in the offspring. *Birth Defects Research Part A-Clinical and Molecular Teratology, 97*(1), 60–66.

Birch, D. G., Birch, E. E., Hoffman, D. R., & Uauy, R. D. (1992). Retinal development in very-low-birth-weight infants fed diets differing in omega-3 fatty acids. *Investigative Ophthalmology & Visual Science, 33*(8), 2365–2376.

Birch, E. E., Castañeda, Y. S., Wheaton, D. H., Birch, D. G., Uauy, R. D., & Hoffman, D. (2005). Visual maturation of term infants fed long-chain polyunsaturated fatty acid supplemented or control formula for 12 mo. *The American Journal of Clinical Nutrition, 81*(4), 871–879.

Blakeborough, P., Gurr, M. I., & Salter, D. N. (1986). Digestion of the zinc in human milk, cow's milk and a commercial babyfood: Some implications for human infant nutrition. *The British Journal of Nutrition, 55*(2), 209–217.

Bodnar, L. M., & Parrott, M. S. (2012). Intervention strategies to improve outcome in obese pregnancies: Micronutrients and dietary supplements. In M. W. Gillman & L. Poston (Eds.), *Maternal obesity* (pp. 199–207). Cambridge: Cambridge University Press.

Brody, J. (2014, December 1). Prescribing vegetables, not pills. *New York Times*. http://well.blogs.nytimes.com/2014/12/01/prescribing-vegetables-not-pills/. Accessed 25 Oct 2015.

Carlsen, S. E. (2009). Early determinants of development: A lipid perspective. *American Journal of Clinical Nutrition, 89*(5), 1523S–1529S.

Carotenoids. (2015). *Linus Pauling Institute, Micronutrient Information Center*. http://lpi.oregonstate.edu/mic/dietary-factors/phytochemicals/carotenoids. Accessed 10 May 2015.

Carpenter, K. J. (2003). A short history of nutritional science: Part 1 (1785–1885). *Journal of Nutrition, 133*(3), 638–645.

Center for Disease Control and Prevention. (2011). *Pediatric and pregnancy surveillance data system, birth outcome and risk factor analysis*. http://www.cdc.gov/pednss/pnss_tables/pdf/national_table2.pdf. Accessed 6 May 2015.

Centers for Disease Control and Prevention. (2015). *Spina bifida data and statistics*. http://www.cdc.gov/ncbddd/spinabifida/data.html. Accessed 17 Apr 2015.

Cerf-Bensussan, N., & Gaboriau-Routhiau, V. (2010). The immune system and the gut microbiota: Friends or foes? *Nature Reviews. Immunology, 10*(10), 735–744. doi:10.1038/nri2850.

Chandler, A. L., Hobbs, C. A., Mosley, B. S., Berry, R. J., Canfield, M. A., Qi, Y. P., et al. (2012). Neural tube defects and maternal intake of micronutrients related to one-carbon metabolism or antioxidant activity. *Birth Defects Research. Part A, Clinical and Molecular Teratology, 94*(11), 864–874. doi:10.1002/bdra.23068.

Chatfield, A., Caglia, J. M., Dhillon, S., Hirs, J., Cheikh Ismail, L., Abawi, K., et al. (2013). Translating research into practice: The introduction of the INTERGROWTH-21st package of clinical standards, tools and guidelines into policies, programmes and services. *British Journal of Obstetrics and Gynaecology, 120*(2), 139–142. doi:10.1111/1471-0528.12416.

Choi, J., Leonard, S. W., Kasper, K., McDougall, M., Stevens, J. F., Tanguay, R. L., et al. (2015). Novel function of vitamin E in regulation of zebrafish (Danio rerio) brain lysophospholipids discovered using lipidomics. *Journal of Lipid Research, 56*(6), 1182–1190. doi:10.1194/jlr.M058941.

Christian, P., & Stewart, C. P. (2010). Maternal micronutrient deficiency, fetal development, and risk of chronic disease. *The Journal of Nutrition, 140*(3), 437–445.

Christianson, A., Modell, B., & Howson, C. (2006). March of Dimes global report on birth defects: The hidden toll of dying and disabled children. *March of Dimes*. http://www.marchofdimes.org/materials/global-report-on-birth-defects-the-hidden-toll-of-dying-and-disabled-children-executive-summary.pdf. Accessed 6 May 2015.

Clifford, M., & Scalbert, A. (2000). Ellagitannins - nature, occurrence and dietary burden. *Science of Food and Agriculture, 80*(7), 1118–1125.

Cole, Z. A., Gale, C. R., Javaid, M. K., Robinson, S. M., Law, C., Boucher, B. J., et al. (2009). Maternal dietary patterns during pregnancy and childhood bone mass: A longitudinal study. *Journal of Bone Mineral Research: the official journal of the American Society for Bone and Mineral Research, 24*(4), 663–668. doi:10.1359/jbmr.081212.

Cordero, A. M., Crider, K. S., Rogers, L. M., Cannon, M. J., & Berry, R. J. (2015). Optimal serum and red blood cell folate concentrations in women of reproductive age for prevention of neural tube defects: World Health Organization guidelines. *Morbidity and Mortality Weekly Report, 64*(15), 421–423.

Corfe, B. M., Harden, C. J., Bull, M., & Garaiova, I. (2015). The multifactorial interplay of diet, the microbiome and appetite control: Current knowledge and future challenges. *Proceedings of the Nutrition Society, 74*(3), 235–244.

Costello, E. K., Lauber, C. L., Hamady, M., Fierer, N., Gordon, J. I., & Knight, R. (2009). Bacterial community variation in human body habitats across space and time. *Science, 326*, 1694–1697.

Crider, K. S., Zhu, J. H., Ling, H., Yang, Q. H., Yang, T. P., Gindler, J., et al. (2011). MTHFR 677C→T genotype is associated with folate and homocysteine concentrations in a large population-based, double-blind trial of folic acid supplementation. *The American Journal of Clinical Nutrition, 93*(6), 1365–1372. doi:10.3945/ajcn.110.004671.

Czeizel, A. E. (2009). Periconceptional folic acid and multivitamin supplementation for the prevention of neural tube defects and other congenital abnormalities. *Birth Defects Research. Part A, Clinical and Molecular Teratology, 85*(4), 260–268. doi:10.1002/bdra.20563.

Czeizel, A. E. (2011). Periconceptional folic acid-containing multivitamin supplementation for the prevention of neural tube defects and cardiovascular malformations. *Annals of Nutrition and Metabolism, 59*(1), 38–40. doi:10.1159/000332125.

Czeizel, A. E., & Bánhidy, F. (2011). Vitamin supply in pregnancy for prevention of congenital birth defects. *Current Opinion of Clinical Nutrition and Metabolic Care, 14*(3), 291–296. doi:10.1097/MCO.0b013e328344b288.

Czeizel, A. E., Dobó, M., & Vargha, P. (2004). Hungarian cohort-controlled trial of periconceptional multivitamin supplementation shows a reduction in certain congenital abnormalities. *Birth Defects Research. Part A, Clinical and Molecular Teratology, 70*(11), 853–861.

da Costa E Silva, O., Knöll, R., & Jager, M. (2007). Personalized nutrition: An integrative process to success. *Genes & Nutrition, 2*(1), 23–25. doi:10.1007/s12263-007-0019-4.

D'Archivio, M., Filesi, C., Di Benedetto, R., Gargiulo, R., Giovannini, C., & Masella, R. (2007). Polyphenols, dietary sources and bioavailability. *Annali dell'Istituto Superiore di Sanità, 43*(4), 348–361.

Darnton-Hill, I., & Mkparu, U. C. (2015). Micronutrients in pregnancy in low- and middle-income countries. *Nutrients, 7*(3), 1744–1768.

de Onis, M., Garza, C., Victora, C. G., Bhan, M. K., & Norum, K. R. (2004). The WHO multicentre growth reference study: Planning, study design, and methodology. *Food Nutrition Bulletin, 25*, S15–S26.

de Onis, M., Onyango, A., Borghi, E., Siyam, A., Blössner, M., & Lutter, C. (2015). WHO multicentre growth reference study group. Worldwide implementation of the WHO child growth standards. *Public Health Nutrition, 15*(9), 1603–1610.

De Quelen, F., Chevalier, J., Rolli-Derkinderen, M., Mourot, J., Neunlist, M., & Boudry, G. (2011). N-3 polyunsaturated fatty acids in the maternal diet modify the postnatal development of nervous regulation of intestinal permeability in piglets. *The Journal of Physiology, 589*(Pt 17), 4341–4352. doi:10.1113/jphysiol.2011.214056.

Dolinoy, D. C., Weidman, J. R., Waterland, R. A., & Jirtle, R. L. (2006). Maternal genistein alters coat color and protects Avy mouse offspring from obesity by modifying the fetal epigenome. *Environmental Health Perspectives, 114*(4), 567–572.

Donkin, I., Versteyhe, S., Ingerslev, L. R., Qian, K., Mechta, M., Nordkap, L., Mortensen, B., Appel, E. V. R, Jørgensen, N., Kristiansen, V. B., Hansen, T., Workman, C. T., Zierath, J. R., & Barrès, R. (2016). Obesity and bariatric surgery drive epigenetic variation of spermatozoa in humans. *Cell Metabolism*, (in press) DOI: 10.1016/j.cmet.2015.11.004.

Duncan, E. J., Gluckman, P. D., & Dearden, P. K. (2014). Epigenetics, plasticity, and evolution: How do we link epigenetic change to phenotype? *Journal of Experimental Zoology. Part B, Molecular and Developmental Evolution, 322*(4), 208–220. doi:10.1002/jez.b.22571.

Dusso, A. S., & Brown, A. J. (1998). Mechanism of vitamin D action and its regulation. *American journal of kindey diseases: the official journal of the National Kidney Foundation, 32*(2 Suppl 2), S13–S24.

Dysken, M. W., Sano, M., Asthana, S., Vertrees, J. E., Pallaki, M., Llorente, M., et al. (2014). Effect of vitamin E and memantine on functional decline in Alzheimer disease: The TEAM-AD VA cooperative randomized trial. *JAMA, 311*(1), 33–44. doi:10.1001/jama.2013.282834.

Erdman, J. W. Jr., Balentine, D., Arab, L., Beecher, G., Dwyer, J. T., Folts, J., et al. (2007). Flavonoids and heart health: Proceedings of the ILSI North America Flavonoids Workshop, May 31–June 1, 2005, Washington, DC. *The Journal of Nutrition, 137*(3 Suppl 1), 718S–737S.

Faldella, G., Govoni, M., Alessandroni, R., Marechiani, E., Salvioli, G. P., Biagi, P. L., et al. (1996). Visual evoked potentials and dietary long chain polyunsaturated fatty acids in preterm infants. *Archives of Diseasein Childhood. Fetal and Neonatal Edition, 75*(2), F108–F112.

Falkenstein, E., Tillman, H. C., Christ, M., Feuring, M., & Wehling, M. (2000). Mulitple actions of steroid hormones – A focus on rapid non-genomic effects. *Pharmacological Reviews, 52*(4), 513–556.

Ferguson, L. R. (2009). Nutrigenomics approaches to functional foods. *Journal of the American Dietetics Association, 109*(3), 452–458. doi:10.1016/j.jada.2008.11.024.

Flores, G. E., Caporaso, J. G., Henley, J. B., Rideout, J. R., Domogala, D., Chase, J., et al. (2014). Temporal variability is a personalized feature of the human microbiome. *Genome Biology, 15*, 531. doi:10.1186/s13059-014-0531-y.

Fontana, L., & Klein, S. (2007). Aging, adiposity, and calorie restriction. *JAMA, 297*(9), 986–994.

Fontana, L., Vinciguerra, M., & Longo, V. D. (2012). Growth factors, nutrient signaling, and cardiovascular aging. *Circulation Research, 110*(8), 1139–1150. doi:10.1161/CIRCRESAHA.111.246470.

Food and Nutrition Board & Institute of Medicine. (1997). *Dietary reference intakes for calcium, phosphorus, magnesium, vitamin D and fluoride*. Washington, DC: National Academies Press.

Food and Nutrition Board, & National Research Council. (1989). *Recommended dietary Allowances* (10th ed.). Washington, DC: National Academies Press.

Ford, E. S., Zhao, G., Tsai, J., & Li, C. (2011). Vitamin D and all-cause mortality among adults in USA: Findings from the National Health and nutrition examination Survey linked mortality study. *International Journal of Epidimiology, 40*(4), 998–1005. doi:10.1093/ije/dyq264.

Frensham, L. J., Bryan, J., & Parletta, N. (2012). Influences of micronutrient and omega-3 fatty acid supplementation on cognition, learning, and behavior: Methodological considerations and implications for children and adolescents in developed societies. *Nutrition Reviews, 70*(10), 594–610. doi:10.1111/j.1753-4887.2012.00516.x.

Garcia-Lafuente, A., Guillamon, E., Villares, A., Rostagno, M. A., & Martinez, J. A. (2009). Flavonoids as anti-inflammatory agents: Implications in cancer and cardiovascular disease. *Inflammation Research, 58*(9), 537–552. doi:10.1007/s00011-009-0037-3.

Gernand, A. D., Simhan, H. N., Klebanoff, M. A., & Bodnar, L. M. (2013). Maternal serum 25-hydroxyvitamin D and measures of newborn and placental weight in a U.S. multicenter cohort study. *Journal of Clinical Endocrinology and Metabolism, 98*(1), 398–404. doi:10.1210/jc.2012-3275.

Gluckman, P. D., Hanson, M. A., Cooper, C., & Thornburg, K. (2008). Effect of in utero and early-life conditions on adult health and disease. *New England Journal of Medicine, 359*(1), 61–73.

Goh, Y. I., Bollano, E., Einarson, T. R., & Koren, G. (2006). Prenatal multivitamin supplementation and rates of congenital anomalies: A meta-analysis. *Journal of Obstetrics and Gynaecology Canada, 28*(8), 680–689.

Gould, J. F., Smithers, L. G., & Makrides, M. (2013). The effect of maternal omega-3 (n-3) LCPUFA supplementation during pregnancy on early childhood cognitive and visual development: A systematic review and meta-analysis of randomized controlled trials. *The American Journal of Clinical Nutrition, 97*(3), 531–544.

Govic, A., Penman, J., Tammer, A. H., & Paolini, A. J. (2016). Paternal calorie restriction prior to conception alters anxiety-like behavior of the adult rat progeny. *Psychoneuroendocrinology, 64*, 1. doi:10.1016/j.psyneuen.2015.10.020.

Grummer-Strawn, L. M., Reinold, C., & Krebs, N. F. (2010). Use of World Health Organization and CDC growth charts for children aged 0-59 months in the United States. *Morbidity and Mortality Weekly Report, 59*(RR09), 1–15.

Hack, M., Klein, N. K., & Taylor, H. G. (1995). Long-term developmental outcomes of low birth weight infants. *The Future of Children, 5*(1), 176–196.

Haider, B. A., & Bhutta, Z. A. (2012). Multiple-micronutrient supplementation for women during pregnancy. *The Cochrane Library*. doi:10.1002/14651858.CD004905.pub3.

Halfon, N., & Forrest, C. B. (2017). The emerging theoretical framework of life course health development. In N. Halfon, C. B. Forrest, R. M. Lerner, & E. Faustman (Eds.), *Handbook of life course health-development science*. Cham: Springer.

Hambidge, M. (2000). Human zinc deficiency. *The Journal of Nutrition, 130*(5), 1344S–1349S.

Hanson, M. A., Bardsley, A., De-Regil, L. M., Moore, S. E., Oken, E., Poston, L., Ma, R. C., McAuliffe, F. M., Maleta, K., Purandare, C. N., Yajnik, C. S., Rushwan, H., & Morris, J. L. (2015). The International Federation of Gynecology and Obstetrics (FIGO) recommendations on adolescent, preconception, and maternal nutrition: "think nutrition first". *International Journal of Gynecology & Obstetrics, 131*(S4), S213–S253.

Hartstra, A. V., Bouter, K. E., Bäckhed, F., & Nieuwdorp, M. (2015). Insights into the role of the microbiome in obesity and type 2 diabetes. *Diabetes Care, 38*(1), 159–165.

Heaney, R. P. (2008). Vitamin D in health and disease. *Clinical Journal of the American Society of Nephrology, 3*(5), 1535–1541.

Herman, D. R., Baer, M. T., Adams, E., Cunningham-Sabo, L., Duran, N., Johnson, D. R., & Yakes, E. (2014). The life course perspective: Evidence for the role of nutrition. *Maternal and Child Health Journal, 18*(2), 450–461.

Heseker, H. B., Mason, J. B., Selhub, J., Rosenberg, I. H., & Jacques, P. F. (2009). Not all cases of neural-tube defect can be prevented by increasing the intake of folic acid. *The British Journal of Nutrition, 102*(2), 173–180. doi:10.1017/S0007114508149200.

Hibbard, E. D., Aberd, M. D., Smithells, R. W., & Lond, M. B. (1965). Folic acid metabolism and human embryopathy. *The Lancet, 285*(7398), 1254.

Hibbeln, J. R., Nieminen, L. R., Blasbalg, T. L., Riggs, J. A., & Lands, W. E. (2006). Healthy intakes of n-3 and n-6 fatty acids: Estimations considering worldwide diversity. *The American Journal of Clinical Nutrition, 83*(6 Suppl), 1483S–1493S.

Honein, M. A., Paulozzi, L. J., Mathews, T. J., Erickson, J. D., & Wong, L. C. (2001). Impact of folic acid fortification of the US food supply on the occurrence of neural tube defects. *The Journal of the American Medical Association, 285*(23), 2981–2986. doi:10.1001/jama.285.23.2981.

Horton, R. (2008). Maternal and child undernutrition: An urgent opportunity. *The Lancet, 371*(9608), 179.

Houston, D. K., Neiberg, R. H., Tooze, J. A., Hausman, D. B., Johnson, M. A., Cauley, J. A., et al. (2013). Low 25-hydroxyvitamin D predicts the onset of mobility limitation and disability in community-dwelling older adults: The health ABC study. *The Journals of Gerentology. Series A, Biological Sciences and Medical Sciences, 68*(2), 181–187. doi:10.1093/gerona/gls136.

Hoyo, C., Murtha, A. P., Schildkraut, J. M., Forman, M. R., Calingaert, B., Demark-Wahnefried, W., et al. (2011). Folic acid supplementation before and during pregnancy in the newborn epigenetics STudy (NEST). *BioMedical Central Public Health, 11*(46). doi:10.1186/1471-2458-11-46.

Huang, C., Li, Z., Wang, M., & Martorel, R. (2010). Early life exposure to the 1959–1961 Chinese famine has long-term health consequences. *The Journal of Nutrition, 140*(10), 1874–1878.

Hujoel, P. P. (2013). Vitamin D and dental caries in controlled clinical trials: Systematic review and meta-analysis. *Nutrition Reviews, 71*(2), 88–97. doi:10.1111/j.1753-4887.2012.00544.x.

Hult, M., Tornhammar, P., Ueda, P., Chima, C., Bonamy, A. E., Ozumba, B., & Norman, M. (2010). Hypertension, diabetes and overweight: Looming legacies of the Biafran famine. *PloS One, 5*(10), e13582.

Huo, Y., Li, J., Qin, X., Huang, Y., Wang, X., Gottesman, R. F., et al. (2015). Efficacy of folic acid therapy in primary prevention of stroke among adults with hypertension in China. *JAMA, 313*(13), 1325–1335.

Hursting, S. D., Lavigne, J. A., Berrigan, D., Perkins, S. N., & Barrett, J. C. (2003). Calorie restriction, aging, and cancer prevention: Mechanisms of action and applicability to humans. *Annual Review of Medicine, 54*, 131–152.

Jablonka, E. (2012). Epigenetic variations in heredity and evolution. *Clinical Pharmacology, 92*(6), 683–688.

Jang, M., Cai, L., Udeani, G. O., Slowing, K. V., Thomas, C. F., Beecher, C. W., et al. (1997). Cancer chemopreventive activity of resveratrol, a natural product derived from grapes. *Science, 275*, 218–220.

Javaid, M. K., Godfrey, K. M., Taylor, P., Robinson, S. M., Crozier, S. R., Dennison, E. M., et al. (2005). Umbilical cord leptin predicts neonatal bone mass. *Calcified Tissue International, 76*(5), 341–347.

Javaid, M. K., Crozier, S. R., Harvey, N. C., Gale, C. R., Dennison, E. M., Boucher, B. J., et al. (2006). Princess Anne hospital study group. Maternal vitamin D status during pregnancy and childhood bone mass at age 9 years: A longitudinal study. *The Lancet, 367*(9504), 36–43.

Jiang, H., Ling, Z., Zhang, Y., Mao, H., Ma, Z., Yin, Y., et al. (2015). Altered fecal microbiota composition in patients with major depressive disorder. *Brain, Behavior, and Immunity, 48*, 186–194. doi:10.1016/j.bbi.2015.03.016.

Jimenez-Chillaron, J. C., Diaz, R., Martinez, D., Pentinat, T., Ramon-Krauel, M., Ribo, S., & Plosch, T. (2012).

The role of nutrition on epigenetic modifications and their implications on health. *Biochimie, 94*, 2242–2263.

Jones, G. (2007). Expanding role of vitamin D in chronic kidney disease: Importance of blood 25-OH-D levels and extra renal I-alpha-hydroxylase in the classical and nonclassical actions of 1-alpha-dihydroxyvitamin D3. *Seminars in Dialysis, 20*(4), 316–324.

Josefson, J. L., Feinglass, J., Rademaker, A. W., Metzger, B. E., Zeiss, D. M., Price, H. E., & Langman, C. B. (2012). Maternal obesity and vitamin D sufficiency are associated with cord blood vitamin D insufficiency. *Journal of Clinical Endocrinology & Metabolism, 98*(1), 114.

Kannan, S., Schulz, A., Israel, B., Ayra, I., Weir, S., Dvonch, T. J., et al. (2008). A community-based participatory approach to personalized, computer-generated nutrition feedback reports: The healthy environments partnership. *Progress in Community Health Partnerships, 2*(1), 41–53. doi:10.1353/cpr.2008.0004.

Kaput, J. (2008). Nutrigenomics research for personalized nutrition and medicine. *Current Opinion in Biotechnology, 19*(2), 110–120. doi:10.1016/j.copbio.2008.02.005.

Kesmodel, U., Bertrand, J., Stoving, H., Skarpness, B., Denny, C., & Mortensen, E. (2012). The lifestyle during pregnancy study group. The effect of different alcohol drinking patterns in early to mid-pregnancy on the child's intelligence, attention, and executive function. *British Journal of Obstetrics and Gynaecology, 19*(10), 1180–1190.

Khan, N., Adhami, V. M., & Mukhtar, H. (2010). Apoptosis by dietary agents for prevention and treatment of prostate cancer. *Endocrine Related Cancer, 17*(1), R39–R52.

Khulan, B., Cooper, W. N., Skinner, B. M., Bauer, J., Owens, S., Prentice, A. M., et al. (2012). Periconceptional maternal micronutrient supplementation is associated with widespread gender related changes in the epigenome: A study of a unique resource in the Gambia. *Human Molecular Genetics, 21*(9), 2086–2101.

Kiecolt-Glaser, J. K., Epel, E. S., Belury, M. A., Andridge, R., Lin, J., Glaser, R., et al. (2013). Omega-3 fatty acids, oxidative stress, and leukocyte telomere length: A randomized controlled trial. *Brain Behavior and Immunity, 28*, 16–24. doi:10.1016/j.bbi.2012.09.004.

Kim, H. W., Choi, Y. J., Dim, K. N., Tamura, T., & Chang, N. (2011). Effect of paternal folate deficiency on placental folate content and folate receptor alpha expression in rats. *Nutrition Research and Practice, 5*(2), 112–116.

King, J. C. (2003). The risk of maternal nutritional depletion and poor outcomes increases in early or closely spaced pregnancies. *The Journal of Nutrition, 133*, 1732S–1736S.

Kirsch, S. H., Herrmann, W., & Obeid, R. (2013). Genetic defects in folate and cobalamin pathways affecting the brain. *Clinical Chemical and Laboratory Medicine, 51*(1), 139–155. doi:10.1515/cclm-2012-0673.

Koletzko, B., von Kries, R., Closa, R., Escribano, J., Scaglioni, S., Giovannini, M., et al. (2009). Can infant feeding choices modulate later obesity risk? *The American Journal of Clinical Nutrition, 89*(5), 1502S–1508S.

Komlos, J. (2008). Stagnation of heights among second-generation U.S.-born Army personnel. *Social Science Quarterly, 89*(2), 445–455. doi:10.1111/j.1540-6237.2008.00541.

Kotelchuck, M., & Fine, A. (2010). *Rethinking MCH: The life course model as an organizing framework*. Washington, DC: Health Resources and Services Administration, Maternal and Child Health Bureau.

Lagouge, M., Argmann, C., Gerhart-Hines, Z., Meziane, H., Lerin, C., Daussin, F., et al. (2006). Resveratrol improves mitochondrial function and protects against metabolic disease by activating SIRT1 and PGC-1alpha. *Cell, 127*(6), 1109–1122.

Lakshminarayanan, B., Stanton, C., O'Toole, P., & Ross, R. P. (2014). Compositional dynamics of the human intestinal microbiota with aging: Implications for health. *The Journal of Nutrition Health & Aging, 18*(9), 773–786.

Lands, W. E. M. (2005). *Fish, omega 3 and human health* (2nd ed.). Champaign: American Oil Chemists' Society Press.

Lang, T., Barling, D., & Caraher, M. (2009). *Food politics: Integrating health, environment & society*. Oxford: Oxford University Press.

Laurence, K. M., Carter, C. O., & David, P. A. (1968). Major central nervous system malformations in South Wales. II. Pregnancy factors, seasonal variation, and social class effects. *Journal of Epidemiology and Community Health, 22*(4), 212–222.

Laurence, K. M., James, N., Miller, M. H., Tennant, G. B., & Campbell, H. (1981). Double-blind randomized controlled trial of folate treatment before conception to prevent recurrence of neural-tube defects. *British Medical Journal (Clinical Research Edition), 282*(6275), 1509–1511.

Lee, H. S., Cho, Y. H., Park, J., Shin, H. R., & Sung, M. K. (2013). Dietary intake of phytonutrients in relation to fruit and vegetable consumption in Korea. *Journal of the Academy of Nutrition and Dietetics, 113*(9), 1194–1199. doi:10.1016/j.jand.2013.04.022.

Ley, R. E., Backhed, F., Turnbaugh, P., Lozupone, C. A., Knight, R. D., & Gordon, J. I. (2005). Obesity alters gut microbial ecology. *Proceedings of the National Academy of Sciences of the United States of America, 102*(31), 11070–11075.

Ley, R. E., Turnbaugh, P. J., Klein, S., & Gordon, J. I. (2006). Microbial ecology: Human gut microbes associated with obesity. *Nature, 444*, 1022–1023.

Ley, R. E., Hamady, M., Lozupone, C., Turnbaugh, P. J., Ramey, R. R., Bircher, J. S., et al. (2008). Evolution of mammals and their gut microbes. *Science, 320*(5883), 1647–1651.

Lillycrop, K. A. (2011). Effect of maternal diet on the epigenome: Implications for human metabolic disease. *The Proceedings of the Nutrition Society, 70*(1), 64–72.

Lin, P. Y., Chiu, C. C., Huang, S. Y., & Su, K. P. (2012). A meta-analytic review of polyunsaturated fatty acid compositions in dementia. *The Journal of Clinical Psychiatry, 73*(9), 1245–1254. doi:10.4088/JCP.11r07546.

Lin, A. L., Zhang, W., Gao, X., & Watts, L. (2015). Caloric restriction increases ketone bodies metabolism and preserves blood flow in aging brain. *Neurobiology of Aging, 36*(7), 2296–2303.

Longo, V. D., & Fontana, L. (2010). Calorie restriction and cancer prevention: Metabolic and molecular mechanisms. *Trends in Pharmacological Sciences, 31*(2), 89–98.

Lopes da Silva, S., Vellas, B., Elemans, S., Luchsinger, J., Kamphuis, P., Yaffe, K., et al. (2013) Plasma nutrient status of patients with Alzheimer's disease: Systematic review and meta-analysis. *Alzheimer's & Dementia*. doi:10.1016/j.jalz.2013.05.1771.

Lu, M. C., & Halfon, N. (2003). Racial and ethnic disparities in birth outcomes: A life-course perspective. *Maternal and Child Health Journal, 7*(1), 13–30.

Manach, C., Scalbert, A., Morand, C., Remesy, C., & Jimenez, L. (2004). Polyphenols: Food sources and bioavailability. *The American Journal of Clinical Nutrition, 79*(5), 727–747.

Mangialasche, F., Solomon, A., Kåreholt, I., Hooshmand, B., Cecchetti, R., Fratiglioni, L., et al. (2013). Serum levels of vitamin E forms and risk of cognitive impairment in a Finnish cohort of older adults. *Experimental Gerontology, 48*(12), 1428–1435. doi:10.1016/j.exger.2013.09.006.

Mariman, E. C. (2008). Epigenetic manifestations in diet-related disorders. *Journal of Nutrigenetics and Nutrigenomics, 1*(5), 232–239. doi:10.1159/000151237.

Martin, F. P., Sprenger, N., Montoliu, I., Rezzi, S., Kochhar, S., & Nicholson, J. K. (2010). Dietary modulation of gut functional ecology studied by fecal metabonomics. *Journal of Proteome Research, 9*(10), 5284–5295. doi:10.1021/pr100554m.

Martorell, R. (1992). Overview of long-term nutrition intervention studies in Guatemala, 1968-1989. *Food and Nutrition Bulletin, 14*(3), 270–277.

Martorell, R., Habicht, J. P., & Rivera, J. A. (1995). History and design of the INCAP longitudinal study (1969-77) and its follow-up (1988-89). *The Journal of Nutrition, 125*(4 Suppl), 1027S–1041S.

Maukonen, J., & Saarela, M. (2015). Human gut microbiota: does diet matter? *Proceedings of the Nutrition Society, 74*(1), 23–36. doi:10.1017/S0029665114000688.

Mayer, E. A., Knight, R., Mazmanian, S. K., Cryan, J. F., & Tillisch, K. (2014a). Gut microbes and the brain: Paradigm shift in neuroscience. *The Journal of Neuroscience, 34*(46), 15490–15496.

Mayer, E. A., Padua, D., & Tillisch, K. (2014b). Altered brain-gut axis in autism: Comorbidity or causative mechanisms? *BioEssays, 36*(10), 933–939. doi:10.1002/bies.201400075.

Maynard, C. L., Elson, C. O., Hatton, R. D., & Weaver, C. T. (2012). Reciprocal interactions of the intestinal microbiota and immune system. *Nature, 489*(7415), 231–241.

McCann, J. C., & Ames, B. N. (2007). An overview of evidence for a causal relation between iron deficiency during development and deficits in cognitive or behavioral function. *The American Journal of Clinical Nutrition, 85*(4), 931–945.

McDonald, S. D., Han, Z., Mulla, S., & Beyene, J. (2010). Overweight and obesity in mothers and risk of preterm birth and low birth weight infants: Systematic review and meta-analyses. *British Medical Journal, 341*, c3428.

McNanley, T., & Woods, J. (2008). Placental physiology. *Global Library of Women's Medicine*. doi:10.3843/GLOWN.10195.

Mente, A., de Koning, L., Shannon, H. S., & Anand, S. S. (2009). A systematic review of the evidence supporting a causal link between dietary factors and coronary heart disease. *Archives of Internal Medicine, 169*(7), 659–669.

Milner, J. A. (2008). Nutrition and cancer: Essential elements for a roadmap. *Cancer Letters, 269*(2), 189–198. doi:10.1016/j.canlet.2008.05.030.

Missmer, S. A., Suarez, L., Felkner, M., Wang, E., Merrill, A. H., Jr., & Rothman, K. J. (2006). Exposure to fumonisins and the occurrence of neural tube defects along the Texas–Mexico border. *Environmental Health Perspectives, 114*(2), 237–241.

Mithal, A., Bonjour, J. P., Boonen, S., Burckhardt, P., Degens, H., Hajj Fuleihan, G., et al. (2012). Impact of nutrition on muscle mass, strength, and performance in older adults. *Osteoporosis International*. doi:10.1007/s00198-012-2236-y.

Montez, J. K., & Eschbach, K. (2008). Country of birth and language are uniquely associated with intakes of fat, fiber, and fruits and vegetables among Mexican-American women in the United States. *Journal of the American Dietetic Association, 108*(3), 473–480. doi:10.1016/j.jada.2007.12.008.

MRC Vitamin Study Research Group. (1991). Prevention of neural tube defects: Results of the Medical Research Council vitamin study. *The Lancet, 338*(8760), 131–137.

Mulvihill, E. E., & Huff, M. W. (2010). Antiatherogenic properties of flavonoids: Implications for cardiovascular health. *Canadian Journal of Cardiology, 26*(suppl A), 17A–21A.

Murphy, M. M., Barraj, L. M., Herman, D., Bi, X., Cheatham, R., & Randolph, R. K. (2012). Phytonutrient intake by adults in the United States in relation to fruit and vegetable consumption. *Journal of the Academy of Nutrition and Dietetics, 112*(2), 222–229.

Murphy, M. M., Barraj, L. M., Spungen, J. H., Herman, D. R., & Randolph, R. K. (2014). Global assessment of select phytonutrient intakes by level of fruit and vegetable consumption. *British Journal of Nutrition, 112*(6), 1004–1018.

Norkus, E. P., Bassi, J., & Rosso, P. (1979). Maternal-fetal transfer of ascorbic acid in the guinea pig. *Journal of Nutrition, 109*(12), 2205–2212.

Olsen, J., Melbye, M., Sørensen, T. I. A., Aaby, P., Andersen, A. M. N., Taxbøl, D., et al. (2001). The Danish National Birth Cohort - its background, structure and aim. *Scandinavian Journal of Public Health, 29*(4), 300–307.

Olson, J. H., Erie, J. C., & Bakri, S. J. (2011). Nutritional supplementation and age-related macular degeneration. *Seminars in Opthamology, 26*(3), 131–136.

Organization for Economic Cooperation and Development (OECD). (2009). *Height. In Society at a Glance 2009: OECD social indicators*. Albany: OECD Publishing.

Painter, R. C., Osmond, C., Gluckman, P., Hanson, M., Phillips, D. I., & Roseboom, T. J. (2008). Transgenerational effects of prenatal exposure to the Dutch famine on neonatal adiposity and health in later life. *British Journal of Obstetrics and Gynaecology, 115*(10), 1243–1249.

Pandey, K. B., & Rizvi, S. I. (2009). Plant polyphenols as dietary antioxidants in human health and disease. *Oxidative Medicine and Cellular Longevity, 2*(5), 270–278. doi:10.4161/oxim.2.5.9498.

Papageorghiou, A. T., Ohuma, E. O., Altman, D. G., Todros, T., Ismail, L. C., Lambert, A., et al. (2014). International standards for fetal growth based on serial ultrasound measurements: The fetal growth longitudinal study of the INTERGROWTH-21st project. *The Lancet, 384*(9946), 869. doi:10.1016/S0140-6736(14)61490-2.

Parker, S. E., Mai, C. T., Canfield, M. A., Rickard, R., Wang, Y., Meyer, R. E., et al. (2010). National Birth Defects Prevention Network. Updated National Birth Prevalence estimates for selected birth defects in the United States, 2004-2006. *Birth Defects Research Part A- Clinical and Molecular Teratology, 88*(12), 1008–1016. doi:10.1002/bdra.20735.

Pollan, M. (2008). *In defense of food: An Eater's manifesto*. New York: Penguin Books.

Poole, K. E., Loveridge, N., Barker, P. J., Halsall, D. J., Rose, C., Reeve, J., & Warburton, E. A. (2006). Reuced vitamin D in acute stroke. *Stroke, 37*(1), 243–245.

Prasad, A. S. (2008a). Clinical, immunological, anti-inflammatory and antioxidant roles of zinc. *Expiremental Gerontology, 43*(5), 370–377.

Prasad, A. S. (2008b). Zinc in human health: Effect of zinc on immune cells. *Molecular Medicine, 14*(5–6), 353–357.

Prasad, A. S. (2009). Impact of the discovery of human zinc deficiency on health. *Journal of the American College Nutrition, 28*(3), 257–265.

Prasad, A. S. (2012). Discovery of human zinc deficiency: 50 years later. *Journal of Trace Elements in Medicine and Biology, 26*(2–3), 66–69.

Qawasmi, A., Landeros-Weisenberger, A., Leckman, J., & Bloch, M. (2012). Meta-analysis: Long chain polyunsaturated fatty acid supplementation of formula and infant cognition. *Pediatrics, 129*(6), 1141–1149.

Qawasmi, A., Landeros-Weisenberger, A., & Bloch, M. H. (2013). Meta-analysis of LCPUFA supplementation of infant formula and visual acuity. *Pediatrics, 131*(1), e262–e272. doi:10.1542/peds.2012-0517.

Rigby, W. F., Denome, S., & Fanger, M. W. (1987). Regulation of lymphokine production and human T-lymphocyte activation by 1, 25-dihydroxyvitamin D3: Specific inhibition at the level of messenger RNA. *Journal of Clinical Inverstigation, 79*, 1659–1654.

Roseboom, T. J., de Rooij, S., & Painter, R. C. (2006). The Dutch famine and its long-term consequences for adult health. *Early Human Development, 82*(8), 485–491.

Rosenfeld, C. S. (2015). Microbiome disturbances and autism spectrum disorders. *Drug Metabolism and Disposition, 43*(10), 1557–1571.

Rostand, S. G., & Warnock, D. G. (2008). Introduction to vitamin D symposium. *Clinical Journal of the American Society of Nephrology, 3*(5), 1534.

Russell, R. M. (1997). New views on the RDAs for older adults. *Journal of the American Dietetic Association, 97*(5), 515–518.

Sachdev, H., Gera, T., & Nestel, P. (2005). Effect of iron supplementation on mental and motor development in children: Systematic review of randomised controlled trials. *Public Health Nutrition, 8*(2), 117–132.

Sandstrom, B., Cederblad, A., & Lonnerdal, B. (1983). Zinc absorption from human milk, cow's milk, and infant formulas. *American Journal of Dieseases of Children, 137*(8), 726–729.

Scalbert, A., & Williamson, G. (2000). Dietary intake and bioavailability of polyphenols. *The Journal of Nutrition, 130*(8S suppl), 2073S–2085S.

Schönbeck, Y., Talma, H., Van Dommelen, P., Bakker, B., Buitendijk, S. E., Hirasing, R. A., & Van Buuren, S. (2012). The world's tallest nation has stopped growing taller: The height of Dutch children from 1955 to 2009. *Pediatric Research, 73*(3), 371–377. doi:10.1038/pr.2012.189.

Schuchardt, J. P., Huss, M., Stauss-Grabo, M., & Hahn, A. (2010). Significance of long-chain polyunsaturated fatty acids (PUFAs) for the development and behaviour of children. *European Journal of Pediatrics, 169*(2), 149–164. doi:10.1007/s00431-1035-8.

Shamim, A., Schulze, K., Merrill, R. D., Kabir, A., Christian, P., Shaikh, L., et al. (2014). First trimester plasma tocopherols are associated with risk of miscarriage in rural Bangladesh. *American Journal of Clinical Nutrition*. doi:10.3945/ajcn.114.094920.

Shaw, G. M., Carmichael, S. L., Yang, W., Selvin, S., & Schaffer, D. M. (2004). Periconceptional dietary intake of choline and betaine and neural tube defects in offspring. *American Journal of Epidimiology, 160*(2), 102–109.

Siklenka, K., Erkek, S., Godmann, M., Lambrot, R., McGraw, S., Lafleur, C., Cohen, T., Xia, J., Suderman, M., Hallett, M., Trasler, J., Peters, A. H. F. M., & Kimmins, S. (2015). Disruption of histone methylation in developing sperm impairs offspring health transgenerationally. *Science*. doi:10.1126/science.aab2006.

Silventoinen, K. (2003). Determinants of variation in adult height. *Journal of Biosocial Science, 35*(2), 263–285.

Simopoulos, A. P. (2002). The importance of the ratio of omega-6/omega-3 essential fatty acids. *Biomedicine & Pharmacotherapy, 56*(8), 365–379. doi:10.1016/S0753-3322(02)00253-6. PMID 12442909.

Simopoulos, A. P. (2010). Nutrigenetics/Nutrigenomics. *Annual Review of Public Health, 31*, 53–68. doi:10.1146/annurev.publhealth.031809.130844.

Smithells, R. W., Sheppard, S., & Schorah, C. J. (1976). Vitamin deficiencies and neural tube defects. *Archives if Disease in Childhood, 51*(12), 944–950.

Smithells, R. W., Sheppard, S., Schorah, C. J., Seller, M. J., Nevin, N. C., Harris, R., et al. (1980). Possible prevention of neural tube defects by periconceptional vitamin supplementation. *The Lancet, 1*(8164), 339–340.

Smithells, R. W., Sheppard, S., Schorah, C. J., Seller, M. J., Nevin, N. C., Harris, R., et al. (1981). Apparent prevention of neural tube defects by periconceptional vitamin supplementation. *Archives of Disease in Childhood, 56*(12), 911–918.

Sourby, A., Schildkraut, J. M., Murtha, A., Wang, F., Huang, X., Bernal, A., et al. (2013). Paternal obesity, is associated with IGF2 hypomethylation in newborns: Results from a newborn epigenetics study (NEST) cohort. *BioMedical Central Medicine*. doi:10.1186/1741-7015/11/29.

Spor, A., Koren, O., & Ley, R. (2011). Unravelling the effects of the environment and host genotype on the gut microbiome. *Nature Reviews Microbiology, 9*, 279–290.

Steckel, R. (1995). Stature and the standard of living. *Journal of Economic Literature, 33*(4), 1903–1940.

Steegers-Theunissen, R. P., Obermann-Borst, S. A., Kremer, D., Lindemans, J., Siebel, C., Steegers, E. A., et al. (2009). Periconceptional maternal folic acid use of 400 microg per day is related to increased methylation of the IGF2 gene in the very young child. *PloS One, 4*(11), e7845. doi:10.1371/journal.pone.0007845.

Stein, A. D., Zybert, P. A., van der Pal-de Bruin, K. M., & Lumey, L. H. (2006). Exposure to famine during gestation, size at birth, and blood pressure at age 59 y: Evidence from the dutch famine. *European Journal of Epidemiology, 21*(10), 759–765.

Szajewska, H., Ruszczynski, M., & Chmielewska, A. (2010). Effects of iron supplementation in non-anemic pregnant women, infants, and young children on the mental performance and psychomotor development of children: A systematic review of randomized controlled trials. *American Journal of Clinical Nutrition, 91*(6), 1684–1690. doi:10.3945/ajcn.2010.29191.

Tinker, S. C., Hamner, H. C., Qi, Y. P., & Crider, K. S. (2015). U.S. women of childbearing age who are at possible increased risk of a neural tube defect-affected pregnancy due to suboptimal red blood cell folate concentrations, National Health and nutrition examination Survey 2007–2012. *Birth Defects Research Part A-Clinical Molecular Teratology*. doi:10.1002/bdra.23378.

Tobi, E. W., Lumey, L. H., Talens, R. P., Kremer, D., Putter, H., Stein, A. D., et al. (2009). DNA methylation differences after exposure to prenatal famine are common and timing- and sex-specific. *Human Molecular Genetics, 18*(21), 4046–4053.

Traber, M. (2014). Vitamin E inadequacy in humans: Causes and consequences. *Advances in Nutrition, 2014, 5*(5), 503–514.

Tremaroli, V., & Backhed, F. (2012). Functional interactions between the gut microbiota and host metabolism. *Nature, 489*, 242–249.

Turnbaugh, P. J., Ley, R. E., Mahowald, M. A., Magrini, V., Mardis, E. R., & Gordon, J. I. (2006). An obesity associated gut microbiome with increased capacity for energy harvest. *Nature, 444*, 1027–1031.

Turnbaugh, P. J., Ley, R. E., Hamady, M., Fraser-Liggett, C. M., Knight, R., & Gordon, J. I. (2007). The human microbiome project. *Nature, 449*, 804–810.

Turnbaugh, P. J., Ridaura, V. K., Faith, J. J., Rey, F. E., Knight, R., & Gordon, J. I. (2009). The effect of diet on the human gut microbiome: A metagenomic analysis in humanized gnotobiotic mice. *Science Translational Medicine, 1*(6), 6ra14.

Tveden-Nyborg, P., Vogt, L., Schjoldager, J. G., Jeannet, N., Hasselholt, S., Paidi, M. D., et al. (2012). Maternal vitamin C deficiency during pregnancy persistently impairs hippocampal neurogenesis in offspring of guinea pigs. *PloS One, 7*(10), e48488. doi:10.1371/journal.pone.0048488.

Ursell, L. K., Metcalf, J. L., Parfrey, L. W., & Knight, R. (2012). Defining the human microbiome. *Nutrition Reviews, 70*(s1), S38–S44.

USDA. (2015). *Center for nutrition policy and promotion*. http://www.cnpp.usda.gov/birthto24months. Accessed 30 Apr 2015.

Vaisman, N., Kaysar, N., Zaruk-Adasha, Y., Pelled, D., Brichon, G., Zwingelstein, G., et al. (2008). Correlation between changes in blood fatty acid composition and visual sustained attention performance in children with inattention: Effect of dietary n-3 fatty acids containing phospholipids. *The American Journal of Clinical Nutrition, 87*(5), 1170–1180.

van Olden, C., Groen, A. K., & Nieuwdorp, M. (2015). Role of intestinal microbiome in lipid and glucose metabolism in diabetes mellitus. *Clinical Therapeutics, 37*(6), 1172–1177.

Verstuyf, A., Carmeliet, G., Bouillon, R., & Mathieu, C. (2010). Vitamin D: A pleiotropic hormone. *Kidney International, 78*(2), 140–145.

Viljakainen, H. T., Saarnio, E., Hytinantti, T., Miettinen, M., Surcel, H., Mäkitie, O., et al. (2010). Maternal vitamin D status determines bone variables in the newborn. *Journal of Clinical Endocrinology and Metabolism, 95*(4), 1749–1757. doi:10.1210/jc.2009-1391.

Villar, J., Papageorghiou, A. T., Pang, R., Ohuma, E. O., Ismail, I. C., Barros, F. C., et al. (2014a). The likeness of fetal growth and newborn size across non-isolated populations in the INTERGROWTH-21st project: The fetal growth longitudinal study and newborn cross-sectional study. *The Lancet Diabetes & Endocrinology, 2*(10), 781–792.

Villar, J., Ismail, L. C., Victora, C. G., Ohuma, E. O., Bertino, E., Altman, D. G., et al. (2014b). International standards for newborn weight, length, and head circumference by gestational age and sex: The newborn cross-sectional study of the INTERGROWTH-21st project. *The Lancet, 384*(9946), 857. doi:10.1016/S0140-6736(14)60932-6.

Vitaglione, P., Sforza, S., Galaverna, G., Ghidini, C., Caporaso, N., Vescovi, P. P., et al. (2005). Bioavailability of trans-resveratrol from red wine in humans. *Molecular Nutrition and Food Research, 49*(5), 495–504.

Walle, T., Hsieh, F., Delegge, M. H., Oatis, J. E., Jr., & Walle, U. K. (2004). High absorption but very low bioavailability of oral resveratrol in humans. *Drug Metabolism and Disposition: The Biological Fate of Chemicals, 32*(12), 1377–1382.

Walravens, P. A., & Hambidge, K. M. (1976). Growth of infants fed a zinc supplemented formula. *American Journal of Clinical Nutrition, 29*, 1114–1121.

Wang, Y., & Kasper, L. H. (2014). The role of microbiome in central nervous system disorders. *Brain, Behavior, and Immunity, 38*, 1–12.

Wang, X., Qin, X., Demirtas, H., Li, J., Mao, G., Huo, Y., et al. (2007). Efficacy of folic acid supplementation in stroke prevention: A meta-analysis. *The Lancet, 369*(9576), 1876–1882.

Wang, T. J., Pencina, M. J., Booth, S. L., Jacques, P. F., Ingelsson, E., Lanier, K., et al. (2008). Vitamin D deficiency and risk of cardiovascular disease. *Circulation, 117*, 503–511. doi:10.1161/CIRCULATION.107.706127.

Waterland, R. A., & Garza, C. (1999). Potential mechanisms of metabolic imprinting that lead to chronic disease. *The American Journal of Clinical Nutrition, 69*(2), 179–197.

Wei, M., Fabrizio, P., Hu, J., Ge, H., Cheng, C., Li, L., & Longo, V. D. (2008). Life span extension by calorie restriction depends on Rim15 and transcription factors downstream of Ras/PKA, tor, and Sch9. *PLoS Genetics, 4*(10), e13. doi:10.1371/journal.pgen.0040013.

Wenzel, E., & Somoza, V. (2005). Metabolism and bioavailability of trans-resveratrol. *Molecular Nutrition and Food Research, 49*(5), 472–481.

Wessells, K. R., & Brown, K. H. (2012). Estimating the global prevalence of zinc deficiency: Results based on zinc availability in national food supplies and the prevalence of stunting. *PloS One, 7*(11), e50568. doi:10.1371/journal.pone.0050568.

Willett, W. C. (2007). The role of dietary n-6 fatty acids in the prevention of cardiovascular disease. *Journal of Cardiovascular Medicine, 8*(Supl), 42S–45S.

Williams, J., Mai, C. T., Mulinare, J., Isenburg, J., Flood, T. J., Ethen, M., et al. (2015). Updated estimates of neural tube defects prevented by mandatory folic acid fortification—United States, 1995–2011. *Morbidity & Mortality Weekly Report, 64*(1), 1–5.

World Health Organization. (2006). *WHO child growth standards: Length/height-for-age, weight-for-age, weight-for-height and body mass index-for-age: Methods and development*. Geneva: World Health Organization. http://www.who.int/childgrowth/publications/technical_report_pub/en/index.html. Accessed 22 Mar 2011.

World Health Organization. (2011). *Anaemia*. http://www.who.int/topics/anaemia/en/. Accessed 22 Mar 2011.

World Health Organization. (2015). Guideline. In *Optimal serum and red blood cell folate concentrations in women of reproductive age for prevention of neural tube defects*. Geneva: World Health Organization. http://www.who.int/nutrition/publications/guidelines/optimalserum_rbc_womenrep_tubedefects/en. Accessed 10 May 2015.

Young, V. B. (2012). The intestinal microbiota in health and disease. *Current Opinion in Gastroenterology, 28*(1), 63–69.

Young, J. K., Giesbrecht, H. E., Eskin, M. N., Aliani, M. N., & Suh, M. (2014). Nutrition implications for fetal alcohol spectrum disorder. *Advances in Nutrition, 5*(6), 675–692. doi:10.3945/an.113.004846.

Yu, X., Jin, L., Zhang, X., & Yu, X. (2013). Effects of maternal mild zinc deficiency and zinc supplementation in offspring on spatial memory and hippocampal neuronal ultrastructural changes. *Nutrition, 29*(2), 457–461.

Zerfu, T. A., & Ayele, H. T. (2013). Micronutrients and pregnancy; effect of supplementation on pregnancy and pregnancy outcomes: A systematic review. *Nutrition Journal, 12*, 20. doi:10.1186/1475-2891-12-20.

How Socioeconomic Disadvantages Get Under the Skin and into the Brain to Influence Health Development Across the Lifespan

Pilyoung Kim, Gary W. Evans, Edith Chen, Gregory Miller, and Teresa Seeman

1 Socioeconomic Disadvantages and Health Across the Lifespan

Socioeconomic disadvantage (SED) has adverse impacts on physical (Adler and Rehkopf 2008; Blair and Raver 2012; Braverman and Egerter 2008; Cohen et al. 2010; Poulton et al. 2002) and psychological (Adler and Rehkopf 2008; Bradley and Corwyn 2002; Grant et al. 2003) health development. SED is similar to low socioeconomic status (SES) which is based on occupation, income, and education or a composite of more than one of these indicators (McLoyd 1998). However, we conceptualize SED more broadly than socioeconomic status to also include subjective perception of social position and contextual indicators of disadvantage, such as neighborhood deprivation. One of the most commonly used SED indicators is poverty, which is calculated using income that falls below an annually adjusted federal poverty line. Some studies suggest independent effects of different SED variables, but each variable tends to be highly correlated with the others; thus, it is often nearly impossible to disentangle independent effects. Therefore, in this chapter, we will review findings on different SED variables but discuss the impact of SED inclusively. In adulthood, SED is assessed based on factors in an individual's own background such as income, occupation, and education level, whereas in childhood, SED is typically assessed based on these factors for the parents.

SED is a widely recognized concern because long-lasting adverse effects on health have been robustly and consistently reported throughout the lifespan (Chen et al. 2007; Chen et al. 2002; Cohen et al. 2010; Evans and Kim 2010; Seeman et al. 2010) . With respect to psychological health development, exposure to SED has been associated with poor language, cognitive deficits, and behavioral problems during childhood (Blair and Raver 2012; Brooks-Gunn and Duncan 1997; Evans 2004; Evans and Kim 2013; McLoyd 1998). In adolescents, SED has been associated

P. Kim (✉)
Department of Psychology, University of Denver, Denver, CO, USA
e-mail: pilyoung.kim@du.edu

G.W. Evans
Department of Design and Environmental Analysis, Department of Human Development, Cornell University, Ithaca, NY, USA
e-mail: gwe1@cornell.edu

E. Chen • G. Miller
Department of Psychology and Institute for Policy Research, Northwestern University, Evanston, IL, USA
e-mail: edith.chen@northwestern.edu; greg.miller@northwestern.edu

T. Seeman
David Geffen School of Medicine, University of California – Los Angeles, Los Angeles, CA, USA
e-mail: tseeman@mednet.ucla.edu

N. Halfon et al. (eds.), *Handbook of Life Course Health Development*,
DOI 10.1007/978-3-319-47143-3_19

with higher rates of psychopathology including substance abuse, disruptive behaviors, and depression (Doan et al. 2012; Fauth et al. 2007; Goodman et al. 2005; Sariaslan et al. 2014). In adulthood, individuals with SED exposure are more likely to exhibit reduced productivity at work, increased involvement in crime, as well as higher rates of mental illness (Duncan et al. 2010; Lorant et al. 2003; Ross 2000).

SED has also been associated with physical health development. In infancy, SED is linked to higher infant mortality and negative birth outcomes (Brooks-Gunn and Duncan 1997; Metcalfe et al. 2011). In childhood and adolescence, SED is associated with higher risk for asthma, dental problems, and physical inactivity (Chen et al. 2004; Miller and Chen 2013). Individuals exposed to SED are more frequently sick, and they die early, with higher morbidity and mortality rates throughout adulthood. Adults exposed to SED have higher rates of cancer, cardiovascular disease, and diabetes (Seeman et al. 2001). Finally, childhood SED exposure has long-lasting impacts on both psychological and physical health development after accounting for adult exposure to SED (Cohen et al. 2010; Danese and McEwen 2012; Evans et al. 2012).

Elevated levels of stress have been identified as a primary mediating mechanism underlying the effects of SED on health development. Childhood SED such as family poverty is associated with greater exposure to stressors such as harsh parenting, exposure to violence, separation from the parent, lower school quality, negative peer relations, substandard housing, pollutants, noise, and crowding (Evans 2004). Neighborhood deprivation is associated with lack of access to physical and cultural resources such as fresh fruits and vegetables, open space and other recreational amenities, libraries, and transportation, as well as greater exposure to violence and crime (Meijer et al. 2012). Adulthood SED is also associated with financial hardship, perceived discrimination, lack of control and reward at work, and job insecurities (Ferrie et al. 2002; Matthews and Gallo 2011). Moreover, one of the distinct characteristics of being exposed to SED is that individuals with SED are far more likely to experience multiple stressors over long periods of time. Chronic and severe levels of stress exposure immobilize the individual's ability to cope with stressors (Blair et al. 2011; Evans and Kim 2013; Wadsworth and Compas 2002).

2 Neurobiological Mechanisms of Stress Regulation

The next step in linking SED and health development is building an understanding of relevant neurobiological mechanisms. Chronic exposure to cumulative risk factors associated with SED can cause dysfunction in the brain and physiological systems, which in turn increases risks for psychological and physical illnesses. Neurobiological mechanisms of stress highlight three brain regions for their key roles in stress perception, appraisal, and regulation – the amygdala, hippocampus, and medial prefrontal cortex. These brain regions regulate the physiological stress systems, particularly the hypothalamus-pituitary-adrenal axis and autonomic nervous system, which lead to physical responses to stress such as "fight or flight" (Ulrich-Lai and Herman 2009).

2.1 Brain

The amygdala is a key region for detecting threats or potentially threatening information from the environment (Rodrigues et al. 2009). When an individual experiences actual or anticipated threats, the amygdala signals the paraventricular nucleus of the hypothalamus which then activates two primary physiological stress systems, the hypothalamus-pituitary-adrenal axis and the autonomic nervous system. Activation of the hypothalamus-pituitary-adrenal axis increases glucocorticoid (cortisol in humans) secretion and autonomic nervous system activation, including release of epinephrine and norepinephrine (Ulrich-Lai and Herman 2009). Long-term exposure to stressors perceived as stress can cause changes in microstructure and function of the amygdala, leading to neurogenesis and synaptogenesis (Davidson and McEwen 2012; Tottenham and Sheridan 2009). These changes may lead to hyperactivity of physiological stress regulation and increased behavioral reactivity to stress (Rodrigues et al. 2009).

The hippocampus is important for memory formation but also for stress regulation (Jacobson and Sapolsky 1991; McEwen 2001). While the amygdala rapidly activates the physiological stress system, the hippocampus plays a regulatory role by decreasing glucocorticoid secretion. This, in turn, leads to recovery of the hypothalamus-pituitary-adrenal axis activation to baseline. The hippocampus has a rich distribution of glucocorticoid receptors; therefore, its structure and function are particularly vulnerable to increased stress hormone level exposure. Exposure to chronic stress injures the microstructure and function of the hippocampus by retraction of apical dendrites and a reduction in spine density (McEwen 2001). The impact is further exacerbated because impaired hippocampal function reduces glucocorticoid negative feedback or regulatory functioning, which in turn leads to higher cortisol levels.

The prefrontal cortex is involved in excitatory and inhibitory physiological stress systems. The prefrontal cortex interacts with the amygdala and hippocampus, with the medial prefrontal cortex inhibiting both hypothalamus-pituitary-adrenal and autonomic stress responses by suppressing amygdala activation (Kalisch et al. 2006; Radley et al. 2006). On the other hand, the orbitofrontal cortex is involved in appraisal of emotional information and activates both hypothalamus-pituitary-adrenal and autonomic stress responses by increasing activity in the amygdala (Milad and Rauch 2007). Exposure to chronic stress impairs the medial prefrontal cortex through structural atrophy and suppression of neurogenesis while increasing dendritic connections of neurons in the orbitofrontal cortex (Davidson and McEwen 2012). Behaviorally, prefrontal cortex dysfunction contributes to difficulty in regulating emotional distress. Indeed, increased amygdala and orbitofrontal cortex activation and decreased hippocampal and medial prefrontal cortex activation are neural risk markers for many mental illnesses such as depression, anxiety, and antisocial behaviors (Coccaro et al. 2007; McEwen 2005; Mervaala et al. 2000; Shin et al. 2006). Similarly, abnormal brain morphometry typically assessed by gray matter volumes, cortical thickness, or white matter structure in the amygdala, hippocampus, and medial prefrontal cortex has also been associated with a range of psychiatric disorders (Phan et al. 2009; Price and Drevets 2012).

The three brain regions discussed above – amygdala, hippocampus, and prefrontal cortex – have been intensely examined in animal studies because of their role in stress regulation and vulnerability to chronic stress exposure. In humans, other brain regions also play an important role in responding to stress, and these too can be affected by chronic stress exposure. Rather than directly influencing human physiological stress responses, these brain areas communicate with and therefore influence the medial prefrontal cortex, hippocampus, and amygdala. The first of these neural networks is the lateral prefrontal cortex and anterior cingulate cortex, which are involved in executive function, decision-making, and self-regulation (Kalisch 2009; Kalisch et al. 2006; Ochsner et al. 2012). Activation in these regions suppresses amygdala activity by supporting cognitive reappraisal strategies and attentional control to help people cope with stressful situations. Chronic stress exposure has been shown to alter microstructure and function in this network, which contributes to difficulties in executive function (Holmes and Wellman 2009).

The second network of neural regions involved in human stress and coping includes the insula, superior temporal gyrus, temporoparietal junction, and posterior cingulate cortex, brain areas which are centrally related to social cognition (Uddin et al. 2007). In humans, most everyday life experiences take place in social contexts, and these brain regions are involved in processing crucial social information such as others' mental states, thoughts, and intentions. Language is also critical for communication during social interactions and likely contributes to coping processes such as cognitive appraisal. Therefore, brain regions involved in language production and comprehension, including Broca's area, Wernicke's area, and the angular gyrus, have also been examined by human stress researchers. Lack of cognitive and social stimulation has been associated with impaired functions in these networks (Adolphs 2001; Hackman and Farah 2009).

In sum, animal and human research consistently highlights the significant role of the amygdala, hippocampus, and medial prefrontal cortex in stress reactivity and regulation. In human research, these three key regions are interconnected with other neural networks integrally involved in higher-level thought, including the executive function network (the lateral prefrontal cortex and anterior cingulate cortex), the social cognition network (insula, superior temporal gyrus, and posterior cingulate cortex), and language regions (Broca's area, Wernicke's area, and the angular gyrus). The three key regions work together with these other networks to process information from positive and negative experience and decide appropriate responses.

2.2 Physiological Systems

When individuals are exposed to stress, information is initially processed and evaluated in the brain, which then activates the primary physiological stress systems, the hypothalamus-pituitary-adrenal axis, and autonomic systems. To activate the hypothalamus-pituitary-adrenal axis, signals from the amygdala cause the paraventricular nucleus of the hypothalamus to release corticotropin-releasing hormone and arginine vasopressin, which trigger secretion of adrenocorticotropic hormone from the pituitary gland. The adrenocorticotropic hormone then causes release of glucocorticoids, cortisol (stress hormone) in humans, by the adrenal cortex. Increased cortisol increases blood pressure and heart rate and stimulates anti-inflammatory and immunosuppressive actions.

The autonomic nervous system includes both the sympathetic and parasympathetic nervous systems. The sympathetic branch of the autonomic nervous system provokes immediate changes such as increased heart rate and blood pressure, representing a "fight-or-flight" response to threat. Neuroendocrine biomarkers for these systems include glucocorticoids (cortisol) for the hypothalamus-pituitary-adrenal axis and epinephrine and norepinephrine for the autonomic nervous system. Increased cortisol levels suppress inflammatory cytokines. Thus hypothalamus-pituitary-adrenal axis dysregulation can lead to inflammatory system dysregulation. Biomarkers of inflammatory system dysregulation include interleukin-6, tumor necrosis factor alpha, C-reactive protein, and insulin-like growth factor-1.

Dysregulation of hypothalamus-pituitary-adrenal axis and autonomic nervous system activation can also suppress and disrupt metabolic processes. Biomarkers of metabolic system dysfunction include low levels of high lipoprotein cholesterol and high levels of low-density lipoprotein cholesterol, triglycerides, glycosylated hemoglobin, glucose, and insulin. Additionally, adiposity as indicated by body mass index and waist-to-hip ratio are potentially downstream indicators of stress dysregulation. The primary stress response systems increase blood pressure and heart rates and thus elevate risk for cardiovascular disease. Biomarkers include systolic and diastolic blood pressure, as well as heart rate (Krantz and Falconer 1995).

The allostatic load model proposes that exposure to chronic stress may cause wear and tear in one or more primary stress regulatory systems (the hypothalamus-pituitary-adrenal axis and autonomic nervous system) and subsequently in secondary physiological stress systems (metabolic processes, inflammatory and immune responses, and cardiovascular responses). Compromised functioning across these multiple physiological systems from chronic environmental demands may lead to long-term damage. Dysregulation of multiple physiological systems, indexed by allostatic load, is a powerful predictor for health development outcomes and adults, including cardiovascular disease, diabetes, as well as cognitive impairment and premature mortality. SED has also been studied for links to allostatic load because SED increases exposure to repeated, severe, and chronic stressors, which elevate allostatic load over the lifespan (Gruenewald et al. 2012; Seeman et al. 2010).

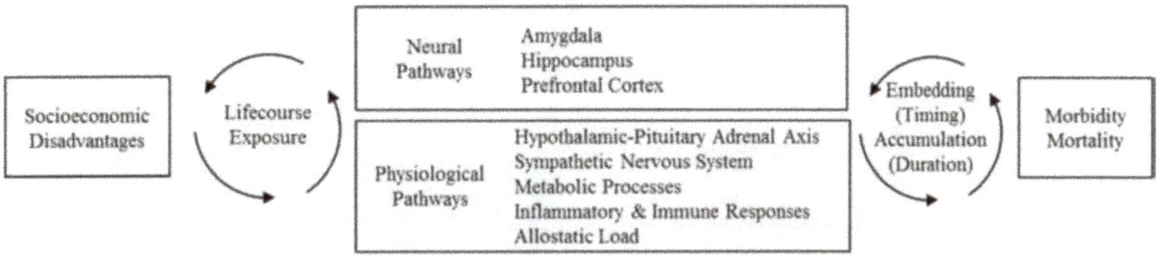

Fig. 1 Conceptual model for chapter

3 Overview of SED and Neurobiological Impacts Over the Life Course

In this section of the chapter, we review current understanding of the effects of SED on neurobiological stress regulatory across the lifespan including (1) how childhood SED affects childhood neurobiological systems, (2) how adulthood SED affects adult neurobiological systems, and (3) how childhood SED affects adult neurobiological systems. Within each temporal focus, we review literature on the brain and physiological systems. Brain regions of interest include the hippocampus, amygdala, prefrontal cortex, and other related regions. We reviewed both structural and functional variations that have been associated with SED. Relevant physiological systems include the hypothalamus-pituitary-adrenal axis, sympathetic nervous system, cardiovascular responses, inflammatory and immune responses, and metabolic processes, as well as allostatic load. When available, the findings on the relations between the brain and physiological systems are also reviewed.

Following this overview of the literature on SED and neurobiological systems, we discuss the literature on life course health development principles (see Halfon and Forrest 2017). In particular, we discuss the multilevel and multidimensional interactions between neurobiological and environmental mechanisms underlying the associations between SED and health development. Finally, we discuss ways in which current scientific understanding of the effects of SED on human biology provides information for interventions and policy from a life course health development perspective (Figs. 1 and 2).

4 Socioeconomic Disadvantages (SEDs) and Neurobiological Mechanisms During Childhood

4.1 Brain: Structure

There is a fast-growing body of literature on the effects of SED on the developing brain suggesting that childhood SED has negative impacts on brain development from infancy to late adolescence. We will discuss recent literature on the development of both brain structure and function in the context of SED exposure in the hippocampus, amygdala, and prefrontal cortex.

In the hippocampus, SED is associated with alterations in its structure across developmental stages (Hanson et al. 2011; Noble et al. 2015). Importantly, these effects have been documented not only in the USA but internationally as well (Jednorog et al. 2012). In a longitudinal study, family income was inversely associated with bilateral hippocampus gray matter volumes in children at age 9. This link was mediated by exposure to stress, both caregiving quality and stressful life events, assessed 3 years earlier (Luby et al. 2013). Another study suggests that reduced hippocampal volume is associated with increased externalizing of

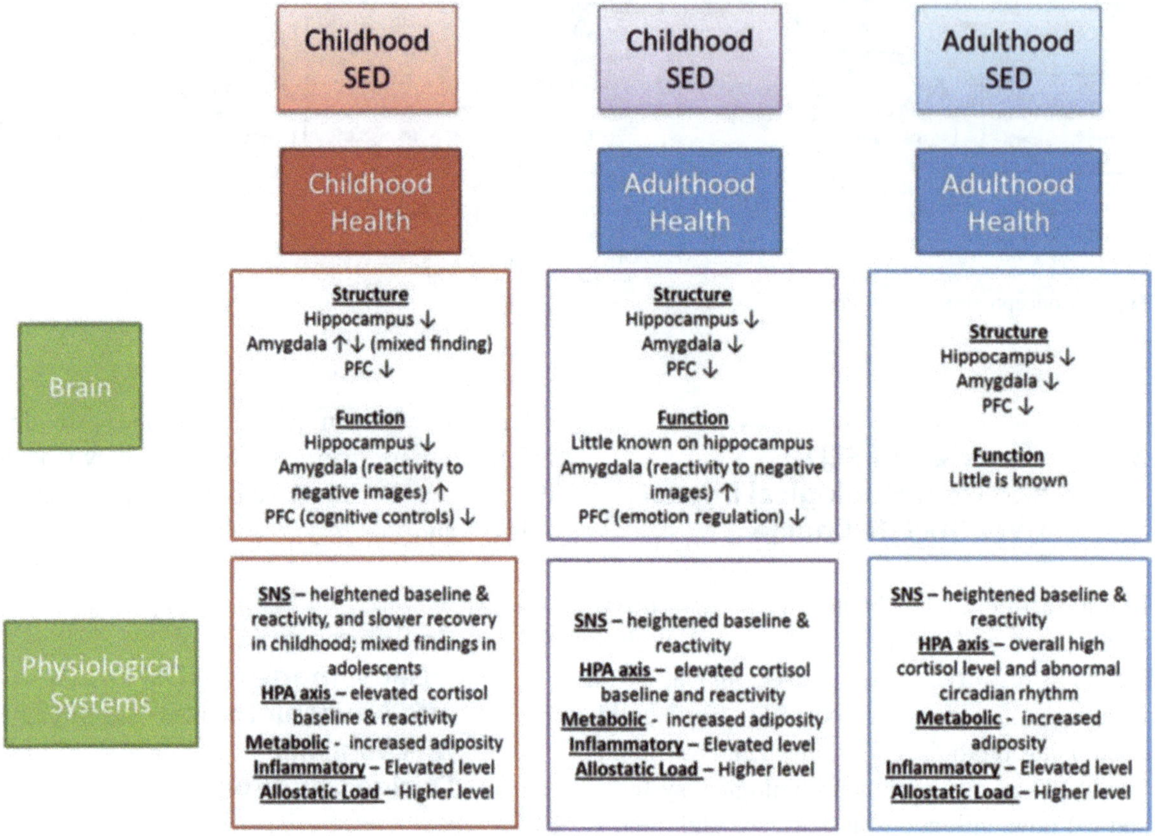

Fig. 2 A summary of socioeconomic disadvantages (SEDs) and neurobiological mechanisms across lifespan (*SEDs* socioeconomic disadvantages; *PFC* prefrontal cortex, *SNS* sympathetic nervous system; *HPA* hypothalamus-pituitary-adrenal)

behavioral problems (Hanson et al. 2014). The reduced volumes in the hippocampus mediated the links between early life adversity and behavioral problems at school including problems with teachers and disruptive behaviors (Hanson et al. 2014).

Amygdala structure has been associated with major chronic stressors in early life such as maternal deprivation (Tottenham and Sheridan 2009). However, the patterns of the associations between early adversity and amygdala structure appear to be more complex compared to the patterns found in the hippocampus. Among children in middle childhood and early adolescence, SED was associated with reduced amygdala gray matter volumes (Hanson et al. 2014; Luby et al. 2013), whereas among children in middle childhood to late adolescence, SED was associated with increased amygdala gray matter volume (Noble et al. 2012). Others have failed to demonstrate the links between SED and amygdala structure (Hanson et al. 2011). More developmental research is needed to identify what SED factors may be associated with different developmental trajectories of the amygdala. Consistent with life course health development principles (see Halfon and Forrest 2017), work to date suggests that both timing and duration of SED exposure are critical for understanding SED impacts on amygdala structure and function.

The prefrontal cortex and other regions for language and social cognition are affected by exposure to SED. Only one study has examined the effects of family income on brain structure in the first years of life (Hanson et al. 2013). Longitudinal analyses revealed that infants from low-income families had lower gray matter volumes in the frontal and parietal lobes compared to their counterparts from mid- and high-income families. Moreover, the low-income infants had more dampened brain growth trajectories compared to mid- and high-income infants: although the brain volumes were comparable during the first year of life, by 3–4 years of age, low-income children showed significantly reduced volumes compared to high- and mid-income children. The reduced volume in the frontal lobe, a brain area involved in cognitive control, was associated with more externalizing behaviors, but not with internalizing behaviors. In another study with children aged 4–18, SED based on income and education was associated with cortical thinning in the prefrontal cortex, particularly in the right anterior cingulate cortex and left superior frontal gyrus, regions that are important for behavioral regulation and executive functions (Lawson et al. 2013). This study also provided evidence that changes due to stress exposure are not linear based on age. In the low SES group, from ages 5–17, gray matter volumes decreased in the inferior and superior temporal gyri, areas involved in language development and cognitive controls. On the other hand, in the high SES group, gray matter volumes in these areas increased over time (Noble et al. Noble et al. 2012b). Given that the pruning process occurs mid- to late adolescence (Giedd 2004), the rapid decline in gray matter volume in the low SES group may limit normal development in the prefrontal cortex. This may be further associated with compromised cognitive functions. In middle childhood, SED was linked to reduced gyrification in the medial prefrontal cortex, indicating delayed maturation (Jednorog et al. 2012).

Finally, a recent study demonstrated a robust association among SED, cortical structure, and cognitive function throughout childhood (age 3–20) (Noble et al. 2015). In the sample of 1099 participants, family income was associated with increased cortical surface area as well as thickness. The gradient relations between family income and cortical surface area were quadratic so that the children of the lower-income families were more affected by income changes compared to the children of the higher-income families. The differences in the cortical surface explained the lower neurocognitive abilities among low-income children. Similar findings that support the role of cortical structure differences in the income-achievement gap were recently reported in a smaller sample of adolescents (Mackey et al. 2015).

4.2 Brain: Function

Existing evidence suggests the effects of SED on whole-brain functioning can start very early in life. A longitudinal study demonstrated that both income and maternal education were positively associated with maturity of the sensorimotor network (primary sensorimotor/auditory) and default mode network at 6 months of age (Gao et al. 2014). At 6 months, babies can sit up and interact more extensively with their environment; therefore, these brain networks may support sensorimotor exploration and a sense of agency. Delayed development in these networks due to exposure to SED during the first year may portend adverse long-term impacts on child health development.

The impact of childhood SED on prefrontal cortex functioning and its role in cognitive development have been examined extensively in the literature, whereas the effects on hippocampal and amygdala functions are less understood. One study focused on the associations between SED and hippocampal function and included both objective measures of SES and maternal subjective ratings of social standing (Sheridan et al. 2013). Interestingly, perceived social standing, but not income or education, was associated with hippocampal function. Among children 8–12 years old, higher perceived social standing was associated with greater hippocampal activation during a memory encoding task. This finding highlights the importance of examining subjective and objective social standing in relation to brain development over the life course.

The role of SED exposure in amygdala functioning is not well understood. In adolescents, low SES was associated with increased amygdala responses to angry faces (Muscatell et al. 2012), which suggests greater neural sensitivity to negative emotional information in social contexts.

In a longitudinal study, early adversity including low family income in infancy was associated with reduced functional connectivity between the amygdala and prefrontal cortex in female adolescents (Burghy et al. 2012). This reduced connectivity, which may be related to difficulties in emotion regulation, was further associated with higher anxiety symptoms.

The impact of SED exposure on the prefrontal cortex and other neural regions associated with cognitive functions has been detected during the first few years of life. Six- to eight-month-old infants from low-income families exhibited reduced gamma band power in the frontal lobe compared to infants from high-income families, after controlling for several covariates such as exposure to smoke (Tomalski et al. 2013). Reduced gamma power may be an early risk marker for poor attentional control and delayed language development, both of which are more prevalent in low SES children (Hackman and Farah 2009; Hoff 2006). This link between SES and frontal lobe development was found in older children as well. Low SES was associated with less mature EEG activity patterns in the frontal lobe across ages 4–6 (Otero et al. 2003; Otero 1997).

In middle childhood, SED exposure was associated with prefrontal cortex activity and executive functioning. Children 7–12 years old performed a target detection task designed to probe cognitive flexibility and working memory, which is related to lateral prefrontal cortex activation (Kishiyama et al. 2009). Lower SES children showed reduced prefrontal cortex activation compared to children of high SES families, indicating delayed prefrontal cortex development and increased risks for delay in executive function. Sheridan et al. (2012) examined the link between SED and neural activation for executive functioning among 8–12-year-old children (Sheridan et al. 2012). Interestingly, low SES children showed greater, rather than reduced, activation in right middle frontal gyrus compared to high SES children. Although there were no behavioral performance differences by SES, in low SES children, increased activation in the right middle frontal gyrus was associated with better accuracy. Therefore, low SES children may have to recruit this region more strongly than high SES children in order to perform at the same level. Additionally, low SED adolescent girls exhibited increased activation in the anterior cingulate cortex during an inhibition control task, which indicated ineffective recruitment of the brain region for behavioral performance (Spielberg et al. 2015).

Neural activations for attention control are also associated with SED exposure in children. In both early childhood (Stevens et al. 2009) and adolescence (D'Angiulli et al. 2008; D'Angiulli et al. 2012), low SES children showed reduced responses to target stimuli and increased responses to distractor stimuli. This pattern of neural activation may contribute to poor suppression of responses to distracting information and less filtering of irrelevant information. In adolescence, low SES was also associated with noisier and inefficient neural responses to auditory stimuli compared to mid-SES (Skoe et al. 2013). Such altered neural responses may require low SES children to exert more effort in order to perform at the same levels as their high SES counterparts, which suggests that SED reduces the overall adaptability and threatens the long-term heath development of these children.

Given consistent evidence of delayed language development in low SES children, the impact of SED exposure on brain regions involved in language development has been examined. Among kindergarteners, neural activations during a phonological awareness task of discriminating rhymed monosyllabic words versus nonwords were assessed (Raizada and Kishiyama 2010). Phonological processing is a critical, underlying process in reading acquisition. Children with high family SES exhibited left inferior frontal gyrus specialization, which is important for language development, while children of low family SES were less likely to exhibit such specialization. On the other hand, in middle childhood (ages 7–11), low SES background was associated with increased, not reduced, activations in left fusiform regions during a reading task, which was further associated with better phonological skills within the low SES group (Noble et al. 2006). Fusiform activation is thought to support visual word recognition, but it is not typically associated with effective phonological skills. Middle SES background was associated with increased activation in the perisylvian and superior frontal regions, typical activation regions for language skills. However, among low SES children, perisylvian and superior frontal region activation was less likely to be shown during a reading task. These results show complex associations between brain activations and development in the context of SED.

4.3 Physiological Systems

The sympathetic nervous system is commonly assessed by resting blood pressure, blood pressure reactivity, and blood pressure recovery in response to an acute stress exposure in children and adolescents. In children, SED is associated with dysregulation of the sympathetic nervous system marked by elevated resting blood pressure and heightened blood pressure reactivity to stress (Chen et al. 2004; Gump et al. 2007; Jackson et al. 1999; Kapuku et al. 2002).

On the other hand, in adolescence, the associations between SED and blood pressure are not consistent or in the opposite direction from childhood. Some researchers have failed to find a consistent association between SED and resting blood pressure during adolescence (Chen et al. 2002). A particularly interesting longitudinal study showed that maternal education was inversely related to childhood resting blood pressure at ages 7 and 9 years, but then had no association among 11- and 15-year-olds (Howe et al. 2013). When exposed to an acute stressor, SED adolescents exhibit dampened rather than elevated blood pressure reactivity (Evans and Kim 2007; Musante et al. 2000). Other studies have failed to reveal any association between SED and blood pressure reactivity in adolescents (Chen et al. 2002). One reason for less consistent findings with blood pressure in adolescence is an increased significance of peer and school environment relative to the family environment during adolescence. For example, neighborhood SED but not family SED was significantly associated with elevated ambulatory blood pressure in adolescents (McGrath et al. 2006). Although it is not consistently found, researchers identified slower blood pressure recovery – blood pressure taking longer to come back to baseline – after lower SES adolescents were exposed to acute stress (Evans et al. 2007; Walter and Hofman 1987). Epinephrine, a hormone that regulates the sympathetic nervous system, was elevated overnight among 9-year-olds exposed to SED (Evans and English 2002; Evans and Kim 2007). SED also reduced expressions of genes regulated by catecholamines in children with asthma, suggesting dysregulation of the sympathetic nervous system (Chen et al. 2009).

Cortisol, a hormone marker of the hypothalamus-pituitary-adrenal axis, is dysregulated in children and adolescents exposed to SED. SED is associated with elevated baseline levels of cortisol during childhood (Essex et al. 2002; Evans and English 2002; Flinn and England 1997; Gustafsson et al. 2006; Lupien et al. 2001; Lupien et al. 2000) and adolescence (Evans and Kim 2007) although Lupien et al. (2001) found that by age 12, SES is no longer related to baseline cortisol levels. The longer children experience poverty, the higher the cortisol level (Blair et al. 2013). In a particularly noteworthy study, Chen et al. (2010) examined salivary cortisol every 6 months for a 2-year period among a group of adolescents. Saliva readings were taken throughout the day. Overall levels were higher among youth from low-income families and, of particular interest, rose faster as the adolescent matured. Children exposed to SED in middle childhood also exhibited heightened reactivity to an acute stressor (Gump et al. 2009). Similar to the findings on blood pressure, neighborhood SES predicted higher cortisol reactivity in adolescent boys (Hackman et al. 2012). These same authors, however, also found a more rapid return of cortisol levels to baseline in relation to residence in more deprived neighborhoods: a result opposite to what one would expect.

Research also suggests that alleviation of SED can improve hypothalamus-pituitary-adrenal axis regulation in early childhood. Fernald and Gunnar

(2009) evaluated the impacts of a conditional cash transfer program on assessments of cortisol during a visit to children's homes. In this experimental program, low-income families are randomly assigned to receive cash in exchange for compliance with better health care for their child (e.g., nutrition supplements, physicals, child health education) plus more school attendance, or they are enrolled in a control group. The amount of cash transfer is considerable, averaging between 20 and 30% of a household's annual income. The results showed that primary school-aged children in the income supplement program had lower overall levels of salivary cortisol if they also had a depressed mother. For low-income families in which the mother was not depressed, there were no impacts of additional income on cortisol levels.

Higher obesity rates are found in children exposed to SED. Obesity is associated with malfunctioning of the metabolism system. Metabolic dysregulation is most commonly indexed by high levels of lipids, low glucose tolerance, and high body mass index (BMI) which is an indicator of adiposity. Children exposed to SED show higher BMI (Shrewsbury and Wardle 2008; Sobal and Stunkard 1989). In an interesting study, Hargreaves et al. (2013) examined childhood obesity (≥ 95th% for age and gender) using four different UK national birth cohorts to illustrate secular trends from 1999 to 2009. Occupational level of the head of household was inversely related to obesity, and the degree of inequality rose 25% over the decade. Some researchers find that the link between SED and adiposity is stronger in younger children, females, and Caucasian children. It is also worth noting that when excess adiposity is defined in terms of obesity (typically >95th percentile for age and gender) rather than by actual BMI, the SES trends are stronger and more consistent.

When metabolic dysregulation was examined across childhood and adolescence, exposure to SED from birth to age 9 years was associated with high BMI at age 9 and also a steeper trajectory of weight gain over the next 8 years (Wells et al. 2010). Howe et al. (2013) tracked the same birth cohort over time and found that whereas there were no differences in BMI in relation to SES prior to age 4, around 60 months of age, clear SES differences emerged and continued to widen up to age 10, the end of their study.

A smaller number of studies have examined weight at different ages during development in relation to childhood SES. Kakinami et al. (2013b) took these early life course analyses a step further by generating poverty trajectory classes from birth to obesity assessments at ages 6, 8, 10, and 12 years among a large, representative sample of children from the province of Quebec. They found four classes: always poor, never poor, increased likelihood of poverty over time, and decreased likelihood of poverty over time. The largest differences occurred between the stable poor and the stable, nonpoor groups, but the effects took time to emerge. For age- and gender-adjusted BMI, the stable poverty group had higher BMI percentiles than the stable, nonpoor group at ages 10 and 12 years. Thus, at 6 and 8 years old, there was no link between duration of early poverty and BMI. For the likelihood of being overweight or obese (≥BMI 85th %), differences emerged by age 8 and continued through to age 12. Two other aspects of their data are noteworthy in thinking about health development. First, the older the child, the greater the impact on weight. Second, they also found elevated risk of greater weight in the group with decreased likelihood of poverty over time (i.e., started out poor but became nonpoor) relative to the stable nonpoor group, but did not find this for the opposite trajectory where children started out nonpoor but became poor. Thus, there is evidence that early poverty exposure has long-lasting impacts, regardless of subsequent upward mobility even among children. All of these effects remained with statistical controls for current income, birth weight, and parental weight.

The effects of SED may begin very early in life. Klebanov et al. (2014) showed that lower-income households have lower-weight infants at birth, a common finding in the literature on SES and birth weight (Spencer 2000). However, Klebanov and colleagues then showed that weight gain was faster in infants from low-income households in comparison to those from middle-income households. Low birth weight babies are at risk for more rapid weight gain because of maternal efforts to help the baby become healthier, leading to overfeeding as well as biological compensatory mechanisms within the baby herself that alter metabolism in order to gain weight.

Glucose metabolism is reduced in children exposed to SED, which contributes to the risk for obesity and metabolic system dysregulation. Several SED variables have been associated with dysregulated glucose metabolism. The National Health and Nutrition Examination Survey (NHANES) data, a nationally representative US dataset, revealed family income was inversely associated with glycosylated hemoglobin levels among children from age 1 to 19 (Seeman et al. 2010). Low parental education was also inversely associated with several metabolic markers including total cholesterol and the ratio of low- to high-density lipoproteins (Leino et al. 1996). Neighborhood deprivation was also associated with dysregulation of the metabolic system including higher low-density lipoproteins, triglycerides, as well as body fat among children aged 9–15 (Gliksman et al. 1990). Kakinami et al. (2013a) conducted a longitudinal study among children beginning at birth until age 10 years old. Poverty exposure was defined in terms of both timing (birth to age 2, 3–6, 7–10 years) and duration (number of age periods [0–3] with poverty exposure). Poverty timing and duration were each linked with elevated triglycerides and insulin with in-depth controls for a host of sociodemographic and physical variables, including family histories of pertinent diseases. Interestingly, for triglycerides, the duration of poverty exposure was most important, whereas for insulin, timing mattered, with exposure from birth to two most consequential. High-density lipids were also reduced by poverty exposure but once the covariates were included in the model, this effect was no longer significant.

Children exposed to SED exhibit elevated inflammatory responses. Chen and colleagues (Chen et al. 2003; Chen et al. 2006) examined the role of childhood SED exposure in inflammation and immune responses particularly among children with asthma. Asthma has a strong association with SED exposure, and the risk of asthma is related to dysregulation of inflammatory response. Among children and adolescents with asthma, low neighborhood SES was associated with increased cytokine responses to allergens (Chen et al. 2003; Chen et al. 2006). On the other hand, in healthy children, no association between neighborhood SES and inflammatory responses was found. Chronic exposure to low SES across ages 1–9 was associated with increased immune responses measured by interleukin-6 production, but a trajectory of initially low SES followed by upward mobility was associated with normal immune responses (Azad et al. 2012).

Inflammatory responses are regulated by gene expression of T cells. Among children with asthma, SED was associated with overexpression of T-cell genes that are involved in chemokine activity and responses to wounds (Chen et al. 2009). This was due to decreased activity of the transcription factors cyclic AMP-binding protein, AP1, and nuclear factor Y as well as increased activity of genes regulated by the proinflammatory transcription factor, nuclear factor kappa-B. Such findings suggest gene and inflammatory pathways linking SED and immune dysfunction among children. Childhood SES was further associated with the genetic mechanisms of inflammatory responses. Low family SES was associated with increased levels of messenger RNA for TLR4, a receptor involved in inflammatory response regulation in adolescence (ages 13–19) (Miller & Chen 2007b). The higher levels of TLR4 suggest leukocyte inflammatory responses to endotoxins, thus greater susceptibility to pathogens such as the cold virus. In addition to objective SED indicators, perceived level of SED was associated with higher proinflammatory biomarkers, IL-6, and TNF-α soluble receptor 2 (sTNFR2) in white, but not black, adolescents (Pietras and Goodman 2013).

When these different physiological systems are considered together in a cumulative fashion, SED is associated with higher allostatic load, indicating chronic wear and tear on physiological stress regulatory systems. Evans and colleagues demonstrated that exposure to chronic stressors including poverty is longitudinally associated with higher allostatic load in middle childhood and early adolescence (Evans 2003; Evans et al. 2007). Longer periods of living in poverty since birth was also associated with high allostatic load at age 13 (Evans 2003; Evans et al. 2007). Although literature on SED and allostatic load in childhood is limited, others have also uncovered significant links between SED and allostatic load in children and adolescents (Goodman et al. Goodman et al. 2005b). In adolescence, neighborhood poverty more significantly predicted higher allostatic load than family poverty (Brody et al. 2014). Using the nationally representative data of the NHANES, researchers also showed that the link between SED and allostatic load is greater in African Americans compared to white and Hispanic adolescents (Rainisch and Upchurch 2013). However, the relative advantages in the white and Hispanic adolescents became smaller as they grew older. The evidence on separate stress systems and allostatic load reveal mechanisms by which SED alters the physiological stress regulatory systems, which may further diminish the ability to cope with stress and increase risks for physical and mental illnesses.

5 SED and Neurobiological Mechanisms During Adulthood

5.1 Brain: Structure

The impact of socioeconomic disadvantage on adult brain structure has been researched less than in children. Existing studies suggest that disadvantages in adulthood are associated with aberrant structure in brain regions involved in language, executive functions, and emotion regulation. It should be noted, however, that while adults living in SED are more likely to have experienced similar disadvantages in childhood, most studies do not control for childhood SES or the trajectories of SED that span childhood, adolescence, and adulthood. Therefore, it is difficult to disentangle the timing effects of SED when understanding the effects on brain and physiological systems. Herein, noting this limitation, we review studies examining the cross-sectional association between adult SED and neurobiological dysfunctions in adulthood.

Exposure to disadvantages, particularly low educational attainment, has consistently been associated with reduced hippocampal volume. Among cognitively healthy seniors, low SES was associated with impaired neural anatomy including reduced white matter integrity in the hippocampus (Piras et al. 2011; Teipel et al. 2009). Among individuals from a wide age range (18–87 years), fewer years of education was also associated with a smaller hippocampus (Noble et al. Noble et al. 2012a). The association between SED and hippocampus structure starts at age 35, showing a decline in this area. Evidence of associations between adult SED and amygdala structure is limited, but SED was related to smaller amygdala structure in adulthood (Noble et al. Noble et al. 2012a), which may also be associated with mood dysregulation among adults exposed to SED.

SED exposure has also been linked to changes in regions involved with cognitive functioning. Among men aged 35–64, high neighborhood deprivation was associated with smaller cortical volume and thinning in the language-related Wernicke's and Broca's areas, as well as smaller cortical surface area in the frontoparietal regions, which are implicated in cognitive control (Krishnadas et al. Krishnadas et al. 2013b). In a sample of more than 300 brains of seniors (average age of 76), low educational attainment was associated with reduced gray matter volumes in the left temporoparietal area and in the bilateral orbitofrontal cortex (Foubert-Samier et al. 2012). In young adult participants, low subjective ratings of social standing using the MacArthur Scale of Subjective Social Status were associated with smaller gray matter volumes in the anterior cingulate cortex, but not in the hippocampus and amygdala (Gianaros et al. 2007). Standard SES, based on objective measures of income, education, and occupation, was not associated with gray matter volume in the anterior cingulate cortex.

The structural integrity of the brain in the context of SED has also been examined. Healthy adults aged 30–50 years were examined for the effects of SED on the fractional anisotropy of white matter tracts, which represents the integrity of neural circuits across different regions (Gianaros et al. 2013). All three SED indicators – education, income, and neighborhood quality – were associated with reduced white matter integrity, assessed by the fractional anisotropy, reflecting axonal caliber, myelin thickness, or fiber coherence (Jung et al. 2010) throughout the brain. In another study, neighborhood deprivation alone was also associated with a less efficient and noisier neural network among men aged 35–64 (Krishnadas et al. 2013a). When both young adults and elders were compared, education attainment was not associated with brain structure in young adults but was positively associated with white matter integrity in seniors age 65 and above (Johnson et al. 2013). Reduced white matter integrity in the bilateral superior frontal gyrus was further associated with poor working memory performance in seniors with low educational attainment.

Several studies examined the role of physiological systems in the link between SED and the adult brain. In particular, the role of inflammation dysfunction has been highlighted as a mediator of the relations between SED and brain. The inflammation factor mediates the links between neighborhood deprivation and reduced cortical thickness in key language regions, including the left Wernicke's area (Krishnadas et al. Krishnadas et al. 2013b). Inflammatory dysfunction (C-reactive protein) and metabolic dysregulation (adiposity) were also examined as a physiological risk marker of cardiovascular diseases. Inflammatory factors mediated the link between SED and adiposity, and adiposity was further associated with reduced integrity of neural circuits (Gianaros et al. 2013).

5.2 Physiological Systems

There is relatively robust evidence on sympathetic nervous system dysregulation in conjunction with adult SED exposure. Several studies have shown that SED is associated with higher resting blood pressure. High resting blood pressure contributes to greater risks for cardiac diseases from young to late adulthood. In developed countries like the USA, Canada, and the UK, evidence is stronger and more consistent than in developing countries (Colhoun et al. 1998; Kaplan and Keil 1993). Neighborhood SED is also associated with higher resting blood pressure among adults in many studies (Chaix et al. 2010; Chaix et al. 2008; Cozier et al. 2007; Cubbin et al. 2000; Diez-Roux et al. 2000; Harburg et al. 1973; McGrath et al. 2006).

Several other markers of sympathetic nervous system dysfunction have been found among adults exposed to SED. SED was associated with dampened blood pressure reactivity to stress (Steptoe et al. 2002a; Steptoe et al. 2003) and reduced heart rate variability (Hemingway et al. 2005; Sloan et al. 2005). Individuals exposed to SED are also less likely to exhibit the normal overnight dip in blood pressure, which is a risk marker for cardiovascular diseases (Spruill et al. 2009; Stepnowsky et al. 2004). One intriguing explanation for these nighttime effects could be sleep disturbance, which appears to be more common among lower SES adults (Buckhalt 2011). In addition, SED was associated with higher norepinephrine and epinephrine levels among adults (Cohen et al. Cohen et al. 2006a; Janicki-Deverts et al. 2007; Seeman et al. 2004).

Cortisol, a hormone index of hypothalamus-pituitary-adrenal axis activation, has a natural diurnal rhythm throughout the day. The level is highest immediately after awakening, and then it sharply decreases and continues to decrease until it gradually increases overnight. Hypothalamus-pituitary-adrenal axis dysregulation is indicated by lower levels of cortisol awakening response and dampened and slower decreases during the day. This has been demonstrated in several developed countries, across different ages of adulthood. Lower levels of awakening cortisol and slower decline during the day both result in overall elevated levels of cortisol in the system (Cohen et al. 2006; Cohen et al. 2006a; Li et al. 2007). SED-exposed adults are more likely to exhibit these circadian patterns (Adam and Kumari 2009; Brandtstädter et al. 1991), indicating dysregulation of the hypothalamus-pituitary-adrenal axis. In the context of low SES, compared to younger adults, older adults exhibited higher circadian levels overall (Karlamangla et al. 2013). In addition, when cortisol level was assessed using overnight urinary sampling, the accumulated level of cortisol was higher in SED-exposed adults compared to non-SED-exposed adults (Gruenewald et al. 2012).

Extensive evidence shows that SED is associated with elevated levels of inflammation among adults. Low socioeconomic status variables such as low education attainment, lower class occupation, and low income have been associated with higher levels of C-reactive protein, interleukin-6, and fibrinogen (Alley et al. 2006; Brunner et al. 1996; Brunner et al. 1997; De Boever et al. 1995; Gruenewald et al. 2009; Hemingway et al. 2003; Ishizaki et al. 2000; Jousilahti et al. 2003; Kivimaki et al. 2005; Koster et al. 2006; Loucks et al. 2006; Lubbock et al. 2005; McDade et al. 2006; Owen et al. 2003; Panagiotakos et al. 2004; Petersen et al. 2008; Pollitt et al. 2007, 2008; Rathmann et al. 2006; Steptoe et al. 2003; Steptoe et al. 2002; Wamala et al. 1999; Wilson et al. 1993). Neighborhood poverty is also associated with higher levels of C-reactive protein and interleukin-6 (Gallo and Matthews 2003). Markers for long-term upregulation of proinflammatory cytokines including tumor necrosis factor-α and interleukin-1 receptor antagonist and hemostatic factors such as factor VII, von Willebrand factor, and plasminogen activator inhibitor-1 have also been identified among SED individuals (Steptoe et al. Steptoe et al. 2002b; Wamala et al. 1999). Elevations in inflammatory markers suggest poor immune response regulation, which increases the risk for greater inflammatory reactions to pathogens and irritants and thus portends eventual morbidity (Gruenewald et al. 2012).

Consistent findings on SED and increased markers of metabolic malfunction, higher fasting/postload glucose, and higher fasting triglycerides were shown in adults with SED (Brunner et al. 1997; Matthews et al. 1989). Higher levels of low-density lipoproteins and lower levels of high-density lipoproteins have also been found in SED adults relative to their more advantaged peers (Matthews et al. 1989; Wamala et al. 1997). Not surprisingly, SED adults have higher rates of diabetes (Everson et al. 2002; Guize et al. 2008; Lidfeldt et al. 2007; Maty et al. 2005; Maty et al. 2008) and other metabolic illnesses including hypertension, obesity, dyslipidemia, and hyperglycemia (Brunner et al. 1997; Chichlowska et al. 2009; Loucks et al. 2007; Wamala et al. 1999).

Taken together, there is evidence for links between SED exposure and physiological stress dysregulation across the adult lifespan. Such evidence is reflected in the association between SED and allostatic load in adulthood. Both individual SED variables such as occupation, income, and education level as well as neighborhood SED exposure have been associated with elevated allostatic load (Bird et al. 2010; Crimmins et al. 2009; Geronimus et al. 2006; Karlamangla et al. 2005; Merkin et al. 2009; Schulz et al. 2012; Seeman et al. 2008; Singer and Ryff 1999). Higher allostatic load predicts elevated morbidity and mortality (Juster et al. 2011; Juster et al. 2010).

6 Childhood SED and Adult Neurobiological Mechanisms

6.1 Brain: Structure

When the effects of childhood SED exposure on adult hippocampus and amygdala were examined, mixed results were reported. It is important to note that in order to be confident that the relationship between childhood SED and adult neural alterations is not simply reflecting concurrent SED status, these life course studies should examine the association of childhood SED and adult brain independently of adult SED. In a sample of over 200 68-year-old adults in England, childhood exposure to SED at age 11 years was prospectively associated with reduced hippocampal volumes after controlling for adulthood exposure to SED at age 65 (Staff et al. 2012). However, another study provides evidence for the opposite result. Among 403 adults in Australia, aged 44–48 years, the impacts of self-reported childhood poverty exposure as well as financial hardship during the past 12 months on hippocampal and amygdalar volumes were examined (Butterworth et al. 2012). Analysis revealed that the current financial hardship, but not childhood poverty exposure, was associated with reduction in gray matter volumes of bilateral hippocampus and amygdala. However, it should be noted that the study sample was predominantly mid- and high-SES individuals and few individuals from low SES were included. The differences between the two studies may be related to the variance of childhood adversity included in the study samples.

Studies examining the prefrontal cortex and other cortical regions demonstrate that stronger evidence exists for the effects of childhood exposure, rather than adulthood exposure, to SED. In a longitudinal study in Germany, brain structure of 134 young adults was assessed. Early life poverty based on family income at 3 months of age was associated with reduced orbitofrontal gyrus gray matter volume at age 25 (Holz et al. 2015). The reduced orbitofrontal cortex volume further mediated the link between early life poverty and conduct disorders. Exposure to current poverty did not predict the orbitofrontal gyrus volume. Other studies have not directly tested the timing effect of childhood SED by controlling for adulthood SED; however, they suggest that childhood SED contributes to reduced structure in the prefrontal cortex (Cohen et al. Cohen et al. 2006b; Narita et al. 2010).

6.2 Brain: Function

The effects of childhood SED on the adult brain are better understood in relation to socio-emotional information processing as compared to cognitive processes. This is different from the literature on the effects of SED in adulthood, which is primarily focused on cognitive functions.

Adults who were exposed to childhood SED exhibited greater neural reactivity to negative emotional information in the amygdala, which may indicate elevated stress reactivity. Low subjective ratings of parental social standing, a retrospective report on childhood SED, were associated with greater amygdala response to angry faces, after controlling for adult SES (Gianaros et al. 2008). Adult SES did not predict amygdala response. Lower social status in childhood may be associated with more negative social interactions such as family conflicts and neighborhood adversity which may lead to greater amygdala sensitivity to angry faces. Childhood SED has also been prospectively associated with neural functions for emotion reactivity and regulation in adulthood. In one study, 49 young adults were asked to regulate negative emotions in response to negative images using cognitive strategies (Kim et al. 2013). Family income at age 9 significantly predicted reduced dorsolateral prefrontal cortex and ventrolateral prefrontal cortex activation during emotion regulation. These results were independent of concurrent adult income. Family income at age 9 years was also positively associated with amygdala activation during emotion regulation, which may suggest inefficient suppression of the amygdala for emotion regulation by dorsolateral prefrontal cortex and ventrolateral prefrontal cortex. Moreover, chronic exposure to stress such as family conflicts, violence, and substandard housing quality mediated the links between family income at age 9 and ventrolateral prefrontal cortex and dorsolateral prefrontal cortex activations.

Effects of childhood SED on brain functions for emotion regulation in a social context were also examined in adults. In young adults, low childhood SES, retrospectively reported, was associated with greater distress and reduced right ventrolateral prefrontal cortex activation in response to social exclusion (Yanagisawa et al. 2013). In another study with young adults, low neighborhood quality at age 13 was associated with greater activations in dorsomedial prefrontal cortex, superior frontal gyrus, and dorsal anterior cingulate cortex during social rejection (Gonzalez et al. 2014). These increased neural activations among individuals from SED backgrounds suggest a need for greater recruitment of these brain regions in order to regulate emotions during social rejection.

Individuals exposed to childhood SED showed neural markers of greater reactivity to negative information and difficulties in regulating emotional distress. They also showed neural indicators for difficulties processing positive information. In a study of African American young adults, individuals were divided into low- and high-SES groups based on both their childhood and current SES (Silverman et al. 2009). Low SES was associated with reduced brain responses to positive pictures (compared to neutral pictures) in insula, anterior cingulate cortex, and caudate compared to high SES. Such reduced neural responses to positive stimuli can be risk factors for depression (Epstein et al. 2006). Childhood exposure to SED was also associated with abnormal neural responses to social support. Low neighborhood quality at age 13 was associated with increased orbitofrontal cortex and insula activation to threats while holding a close friend's hand (Coan et al. 2013), indicating that individuals with early SED experience did not benefit from social support when coping with stress and threats.

6.3 Physiological Systems

The long-lasting effects of childhood SED on the physiological stress systems have been shown in several studies. In the sympathetic nervous system function, low paternal education in childhood was associated with greater blood pressure reactivity to stress (Williams et al. 2008). Low childhood SES was associated with elevated blood pressure reactivity to stress in men but not in women (Taylor et al. 2004b), suggesting the link may be stronger in men. When adolescents experienced both low parental education and low neighborhood SES, SED exposure was also associated with greater reactivity among African Americans as compared to their white counterparts (Wilson et al. 2000). Finally, low SES in childhood is also associated with elevated resting blood pressure in adulthood (Hardy et al. 2003; Lehman et al. 2009). Using data from a nationally representative US longitudinal study, middle-aged adults who were from lower-income families measured during pregnancy through age 2 years had higher incidence of hypertension (Ziol-Guest et al. 2012) independently of concurrent income at middle age. Another important contribution of this study is the authors also had income data for ages 3–5 years and between 6 and 15 years. Only the earliest childhood period of poverty exposure made a difference for middle-aged hypertension. Both Hardy et al. (2003) and Lehman et al. (2009) also showed that increases in adult blood pressure with aging occurred faster among those who grew up in low SES households. In an unusual multigenerational study, adolescents whose parents grew up in a low SES household revealed a pattern of greater elevations in resting blood pressure over a period of one and a half years (Schreier and Chen 2010). Note that SED was measured in terms of their grandparents' SES levels. Thus, not only is resting blood pressure in adults and adolescents elevated by early experiences of SED, but blood pressure rises faster as individuals from low SES backgrounds age. This is a potentially critical finding in thinking about health development and policies to mitigate the effects of childhood poverty.

Childhood SED also influences hypothalamus-pituitary-adrenal axis regulation in later life. Middle-aged men and women exhibited greater awakening cortisol levels when exposed to low SES in adolescence, independent from their adulthood SES (Gustafsson et al. 2010a). Among young adults, low childhood SES was associated with elevated baseline cortisol as well as greater reactivity to stress (Taylor et al. 2004a). One study suggests gender differences in the impact of timing and duration of SED exposure. In middle-aged women, continuous exposure to low SES from childhood to adulthood was associated with elevated cortisol, whereas in middle-aged men, low childhood SES was associated with elevated cortisol independent of adulthood SES (Li et al. 2007). The role of childhood SED has also been revealed in the exploration of genetic mechanisms of the hypothalamus-pituitary-adrenal axis. Lower parental occupational status between ages 0 and 5 was associated with downregulation of genes involved in glucocorticoid receptor expressions, which was further associated with higher levels of salivary cortisol in adults aged 25–40 (Miller & Chen 2007b; Miller et al. 2009b).

Inflammatory responses and immune function in later life are influenced by childhood SED exposure. In a large UK sample, controlling for adult SES, low SES at birth was associated with multiple markers of inflammation over-reactivity – fibrinogen, C-reactive protein, von Willebrand factor antigen, and a tissue plasminogen activator antigen (Tabassum et al. 2008). Similarly, in a large US sample, retrospectively reported low childhood SES was associated with multiple markers of inflammation over-reactivity – C-reactive protein, fibrinogen, white blood cell count, and von Willebrand factor – when adulthood SES was controlled for (Pollitt et al. 2007). Additional studies have identified significant associations between childhood SED, assessed by low parental educational attainment, and inflammation markers in adults (Brunner et al. 1996; Taylor et al. 2006). Similar to the hypothalamus-pituitary-adrenal axis, investigations of genetic mechanisms revealed that childhood SED predicted increased activity of genes regulated by the pro-inflammatory transcription factor, nuclear factor kappa-B, and increased activity of the transcription factor cyclic AMP-binding protein in adults (Miller et al. 2009). The upregulation of such genetic activity markers likely play a role in the links between childhood SED exposure and inflammation. Childhood poverty from the prenatal period to the second year of life significantly predicts rates of immune-mediated chronic diseases in adulthood including arthritis and hypertension, which are associated with reduced productivity at work (Ziol-Guest et al. 2012).

Similar to physiological systems, childhood SED is associated with adulthood metabolic processes. Controlling for SES in adulthood, low childhood SES was linked to higher BMI, (Laaksonen et al. 2004; Langenberg et al. 2003; Moore et al. 1962; Poulton et al. 2002; Power et al. 2005; Power et al. 2003), and low parental occupational status in childhood predicted lower high-density lipoprotein (HDL) levels (Brunner et al. 1999; Wanamethee et al. 1996). The associations between childhood SED and metabolic processes seem to be stronger in women than in men. Low SES at age 15 years was related to the development of obesity in women, but not men, from age 16–21 years (Lee et al. 2008). Additionally, low SES at age 4 years predicted metabolic syndrome as well as low levels of HDL and high body fat in women, but not men (Langenberg et al. 2006).

Given the impact of childhood SED across physiological systems, it is not surprising that childhood SED is associated with allostatic load, the cumulative index of dysregulation in multiple physiological stress systems, in later life. Indeed, studies suggest the long-lasting effects of childhood SED on allostatic load in adulthood (Gruenewald et al. 2012). This does not mean that childhood SED is independent of adulthood SED. Cumulative exposure to SED throughout childhood and adulthood appears to be the most significant predictor of adult allostatic load. For example, growing up in poverty was associated with greater allostatic load at age 60 (Singer and Ryff 1999). However, when both childhood and adulthood incomes were examined, the greatest risk for high allostatic load was related to the combination of childhood and adulthood poverty. The next highest risk was for individuals who did not grow up in poverty, but fell into poverty in adulthood. Adults who were never poor or who were poor in childhood but moved out of poverty as they aged showed the least elevated allostatic load. Another study points to the cumulative effects of SED across the lifespan. At age 42, individuals who were consistently exposed to low SES across ages 16, 21, 30, and 42 had the highest level of allostatic load compared to individuals who were exposed to low SES at one or more time points in life (Gustafsson et al. 2010b).

7 Links to the Life Course Health Development Principles

Some of what we are learning about how SED gets into human brain and biology is related to the seven life course health development principles presented by Halfon and Forrest (2017) and discussed in many other chapters of this handbook. Converging evidence from numerous studies on SED and neurobiological systems demonstrates that SED continuously influences the brain and physiological systems throughout the lifespan. Elder and others suggest that childhood is for developing and acquiring capacities and skills, while older adulthood is for managing losses (Baltes 1987; Elder 1998; Elder et al. 2003). We see from the evidence reviewed in this chapter that SED can disrupt or delay neurobiological development that underlies optimal cognitive and emotional functioning during childhood. In older adulthood, SED can accelerate the loss of neurobiological functions, which is in turn associated with memory loss and physical illness.

Neurobiological responses to SED exposure may support processes of adaptation and increased chances of survival from an evolutionary perspective (Gluckman and Hanson 2004; Worthman and Kuzara 2005). Increased amygdala or cardiovascular reactivity to negative environmental cues may help SED individuals more effectively detect threats in the environment. From a perspective such as the active calibration model (Ellis and Del Giudice 2014), the neurobiological changes due to SED reflect processes to prioritize adaptation to a threatening environment, thereby enabling individuals to maximize their chances of survival.

However, as reviewed above, such neurobiological changes are associated with worse long-term health consequences such as anxiety disorders and cardiovascular diseases, in part through elevated allostatic load. This trade-off in short-term survival strategies and long-term well-being may be related to the principle that optimal health development should enhance thriving and protect against diseases in individuals. Evidence presented in this chapter robustly shows that SED can undermine neurobiological development through the allostatic load; thus, individuals exposed to SED may be more likely to die early and develop illnesses across the lifespan.

Two of the life course health development principles merit particular attention with respect to the question of how SED influences health trajectories: (1) health development is highly sensitive to the timing and social structure of environmental exposures, and (2) health development is a complex, nonlinear process that results from person-environment interactions that are multidimensional, multidirectional, and multilevel.

7.1 Timing Versus Duration of SED Exposure on Neurobiological Systems

Different models have been used to explain how SED exerts its influence. The first model focuses on the timing of SED exposure. In this model, early exposure to SED causes stable and long-lasting adaptive changes in neurobiological systems that have inimical long-term effects. The second model focuses on the duration of SED exposure, with longer exposure generating the greatest impact on neurobiological systems. Empirical findings suggest that the two views are not mutually exclusive and both mechanisms may be operative. Early exposure to SED may have a long-lasting impact, but continuous exposure may further increase the gap between health development trajectories. Additionally, different neurobiological systems may be more influenced by one of the two models. Here, we review the two models and discuss how different neurobiological systems may be affected by SED.

The biological embedding model (Finch & Crimmins 2004; Hertzman 1999) highlights the role of timing of exposure to risks like SED. Critical and sensitive periods are key ideas in this model, meaning that the brain or some other physiological system has a period when it is particularly vulnerable to certain experiences or it requires certain experiences for normal development (Coe & Lubach 2005; Levine 2005; Newport et al. 2002). During a critical or sensitive period, certain experiences will produce adaptive responses that confer some short-term advantage to the individual but leave long-lasting negative influences on health developmental trajectories. In the case of SED, this model suggests that early exposure to SED may lead to epigenetic changes that alter the development of the brain and physiological systems in ways that increase vulnerability to disease across the lifespan. Some argue that the biological embedding model is too deterministic because it implies an individual is programmed to exhibit predicted outcomes when exposed to SED. While the biological embedding model is important for understanding different health developmental trajectories due to SED exposure, it is important to acknowledge considerable interindividual variation. This led some to suggest the term biological conditioning or priming might be more appropriate because it allows room for plasticity that may be influenced by future environments (Hanson and Gluckman 2014).

One example of the biological embedding model is the fetal origins theory (Barker 1990). During the critical prenatal period, a pregnant woman's exposure to extreme physical or psychological stress such as malnutrition or wartime conditions can lead to long-lasting changes in the development of her child's brain as well as the hypothalamus-pituitary-adrenal and sympathetic nervous systems. The changes affected by prenatal events can increase risks in offspring for physical illnesses like diabetes and cardiovascular disease or psychological illnesses like schizophrenia across the lifespan.

Another example of the biological embedding model is epigenetic changes due to early adversity. Animal studies demonstrate that through methylation of DNA or remodeling of the chromatin structure, early adversity such as low quality maternal care can increase expression of the glucocorticoid receptor gene in hippocampal tissue. Such upregulation of the hypothalamus-pituitary-adrenal axis and glucocorticoid levels in the brain then leads to long-term changes in other regions of the brain and in physiological systems (Szyf et al. 2008; Weaver et al. 2004). Animal studies suggest the critical period for early adversity in rodents is the first 8 days, which is equivalent to the first weeks of life in humans. Miller, Chen, and colleagues also have identified associations between early exposure to SED and signaling in leukocyte transcriptome that appear to persist into adulthood (Miller et al. 2009).

The human brain has sensitive periods that differ by region. The brain and biological processes are most plastic in the first few years of life (Lupien et al. 2009). During early childhood, the amygdala and hippocampus develop quickly and are therefore more vulnerable to stress. On the other hand, the prefrontal cortex develops gradually over the course of the entire childhood and young adulthood. Early normative changes include an increase in structure through neurogenesis (increase in number of neurons) and synaptogenesis (increase in dendritic spines of neurons). To promote effective communication within the brain, neurons and connections strengthen through myelination and other mechanisms when they are used and die if unused (Alexander-Bloch et al. 2013). Brain regions are thought to preserve plasticity in adulthood, but changes are more likely driven by gliogenesis (increase in number of glia, nonneuronal cells for supporting neurons) and vascular alterations rather than neurogenesis. Changes based on neurogenesis and synaptogenesis are longer lasting compared to changes driven by gliogenesis and other mechanisms. This explains how childhood SED exposure may have more significant and enduring impacts on the brain than adulthood SED exposure. While the prefrontal cortex and hippocampus seem to preserve plasticity into adulthood and may be able to recover from or reverse the impacts of SED, this does not appear to be true for the amygdala (Tottenham et al. 2010).

A biological embedding model also exists for development of the hypothalamus-pituitary-adrenal axis. SED exposure, indicated by a lack of family home ownership, in early childhood was associated with reduced levels of glucocorticoid receptor RNA in adolescence (Miller and Chen 2007a). When the timing of exposure was further examined, lack of home ownership before age 2 was a stronger predictor than between ages 5 and 9, while home ownership after age 10 had no effects on the outcome. The study demonstrates the role of childhood SED, especially early exposure, in the development of the hypothalamus-pituitary-adrenal axis regulatory system. Another study supports an embedding model for the immune system (Miller et al. 2011). When exposed to the cold virus, adults who were without home ownership from ages 0 to 9 were more likely to develop a cold for the next 5-day period (Cohen et al. 2004). Furthermore, there was a gradient relationship between the age when the parents first owned a home during the first 9 years and the likelihood of developing a cold (Cohen et al. 2004).

The biggest limitation of the biological embedding model is that it does not take later experience into account, which is not consistent with life course health development principles that posit continuous person⇔environment interactions across the life course. It is possible that early adversity leads to modifications in an individual's later environment and behavior, which may further increase the risk for disease.

A second model focuses on the duration and accumulation of SED exposure. According to this model, early adversity can cause "chains of risks" (Kuh and Ben-Shlomo 2004), as individuals and their environments continuously and dynamically influence one another. For example, children living in poverty are more likely to be exposed to chronic stressors like family conflicts and harsh parenting, which may lead them to be more helpless. Less proactive cognitive and behavioral styles give rise to low academic performance and poor social skills, which then lowers the individual's probability of finding and maintaining a good job. As a result, a person is likely to live in poverty as an adult and experience a range of individual and neighborhood deprivation and negative health outcomes. This is the idea that adversity begets negative health development, which begets more adversity. In addition, longer exposure to SED may contribute to an accumulation of chronic stress and lead to more severe damage in neurobiological systems. Indeed, in an earlier section, we explained that allostatic load is affected by SED in an additive fashion. The longer individuals were exposed to low SES, the higher their allostatic load. In addition, cumulative disadvantage is a powerful predictor of many biological markers of mortality and morbidity (Ackerman et al. 1975; Ader et al. 1960; Cameron et al. 2005; Chida et al. 2007; Fenoglio et al. 2006; Kruschinski et al. 2008; Lyons et al. 2009).

Both embedding and accumulative models play a role in predicting health outcomes in SED-exposed individuals. This is true for physiological systems. For example, among women at age 60, the associations among childhood and adulthood SED and metabolic processing including insulin resistance, HDL, and triglycerides were examined. Parental occupation status in childhood was a stronger predictor of metabolic processing than own occupational status in adulthood (Lawlor et al. 2002). However, women who were chronically exposed to low occupational status throughout childhood and adulthood exhibited the worst profile, including a 234% likelihood of being obese compared to women who were never exposed to low occupational status. The results suggest that childhood SED can be embedded in a physiological system to set the developmental trajectory, but accumulative processes may compound these earlier, poorer trajectories leading to worse outcomes throughout the lifespan.

The biggest challenge to understanding exact mechanisms of SED exposure (the embedding versus accumulative model) is that an individual tends to be exposed to poverty early and continuously. Thus, it may be most productive to consider a life course health development model, which examines the relational dynamic person⇔environment interactions, the timing and social patterning of exposures, and evolutionarily determined adaptive plastic responses that unfold during development. It is also difficult to tease apart the role of early exposure versus later exposure to SED because many studies are cross-sectional or measure early exposure to SED retrospectively. Thus, more longitudinal studies are needed to understand how health development is produced over time. Also, intervention studies such as cash transfers to families to improve SED provide opportunities to establish causal and temporal relations between SED and health outcomes.

7.2 Multilevel Neurobiology-Environment Interactions

Interactions between SED and neurobiological systems are highly complex not only because of the multilevel nature of neurobiological systems but also because SED is further associated with multilevel environmental factors (Sameroff 2010). SED is a major risk factor for a host of adverse outcomes because it serves as a proxy for many risk factors that result in psychological and physical illnesses (Chen et al. 2002; Evans and Kim 2010; Repetti et al. 2002). Understanding interactions between multilevel and multidimensional neurobiological and environmental systems is critical for developing effective clinical and community-level interventions to reduce the adverse impact of SED exposure on health.

First, many psychosocial factors have been suggested as mediators. In childhood, threat appraisal and family environment are well-known mediators for the links between SED and physical and psychological outcomes (Repetti et al. 2002). Retrospectively reported elements of the early family environment such as abusive and harsh parenting were associated with direct relationships between amygdala and ventrolateral prefrontal cortex activations, which suggests ineffective suppression of ventrolateral prefrontal cortex on the amygdala (Taylor et al. 2006). Maltreatment and abuse in childhood were also associated with weaker default mode network connectivity and increased connectivity between the amygdala and medial prefrontal cortex (Philip et al. 2013). Lack of maternal warmth in early childhood and early adolescence was associated with less activation in the reward circuits such as the medial prefrontal cortex during loss and winning, which may indicate altered reward processing and more difficulties in handling disappointment (Morgan et al. 2014).

Second, cumulative risk factors including physical environment – noise, crowding, and substandard housing quality – have been identified as strong mediators between SED and neurobiological outcomes across the lifespan (Evans and Cassells 2014; Evans and Kim 2010; Kim et al. 2013; Zalewski et al. 2012). SED exposure is also associated with chaotic home environment and poor quality in social environments outside the home, such as school and neighborhood (Evans et al. in press; Roy et al. 2014; Schreier et al. 2014). Along with these risk factors, it is important to consider factors that protect from the negative effects of SED exposure in childhood. Supportive parenting and support from others and adaptive coping skills have been suggested as protective factors. For example, active coping skills like distraction were associated with better psychological outcomes than avoidance and disengaging coping in children and adolescents (Wadsworth and Berger 2006; Wadsworth et al. in press).

Third, in adulthood, individuals who are exposed to SED are more likely to experience psychological stress, discrimination, negative emotions, and more limited resources such as social support (Cohen et al. 2006a, b; Kubzansky et al. 1999; Kunz-Ebrecht et al. 2004; Marmot et al. 1997). On the other hand, there are protective factors including optimism, mastery, self-esteem, and social support that can help to reduce the negative effects of SED exposure on the neurobiological systems (Kubzansky et al. 2001; Matthews et al. 2010; Taylor et al. 2008).

Fourth, sleep quality, an example of a personal factor, may also play a significant role in the neural and physiological systems throughout the lifespan. Sleep disturbance appears to be more common among lower SES adults (Buckalt 2011) and children (Jarrin et al. 2014). Adults with low income or education levels had significantly shorter sleep duration (Whinnery et al. 2013) and poorer sleep quality and higher levels of daytime sleepiness compared to adults with mid- to high income or education levels (Jarrin et al. 2013). The association between poverty and sleep quality was stronger in white adults than in African American adults (Patel et al. 2010). In children and adolescents, both low subjective social standing ratings and low objective SED indicators including family income and parental education were significantly associated with shorter sleep duration and poorer sleep quality (Jarrin et al. 2014). Sleep duration and quality are a concern because they can significantly influence cognitive functions (Dewald et al. 2010; Steenari et al. 2003; Walker 2008) and mood regulation (Dahl and Lewin 2002; Eidelman et al. 2012; Kahn et al. 2013) in children and adults. Poor sleep has also been associated with physiological stress dysregulation (Jarcho et al. 2013; Rao et al. 1996), brain structure including the hippocampus (Riemann et al. 2007), and brain functions such as risk-taking behaviors in adolescence (Telzer et al. 2013). Thus, examining the role of sleep in the associations between poverty and neurobiological stress regulation is an important future direction for health disparities research.

Furthermore, adding to the complexity of understanding how SED influences health development, there are multiple levels of neurobiological systems including genetic, neural, and physiological stress regulatory systems interacting with each other. While few studies exist, they have identified the significant role of the hypothalamus-pituitary-adrenal axis and immune processes in the associations among SED and brain structure and functions. For example, higher cortisol levels in children mediated the link between childhood SES and prefrontal cortex responses during cognitive tasks (Sheridan et al. 2012). Increased levels of inflammatory markers also mediated the associations between SED and white matter structure integrity in adulthood (Gianaros et al. 2013). Childhood poverty exposure prospectively predicted weaker default mode network activity, which was associated with higher levels of cortisol in response to social stress (Sripada et al. 2014).

In addition, it is important to understand how genes and environment interact in the context of SED across lifespan. Many studies have identified certain genetic variations that may lead individuals to be more susceptible or vulnerable to environmental influences (Ellis et al. 2011). Individuals with such susceptible genetic profiles would likely exhibit greater influence from SED exposure compared to individuals with insusceptible genetic profiles. Thus, the role of genetic profiles in neural and physiological system development throughout the lifespan in the context of SED will be important for refined identification of at-risk individuals (Kim-Cohen et al. 2004). Understanding gene expression, which is known to be affected by person ⇔environment interactions, will also be a fruitful avenue of future investigation.

Last, it is important to pursue understanding of the ways in which these multilevel, multidimensional interactions between the environment and neurobiology are linked to specific health development outcomes, in order to develop effective intervention approaches. Few studies have directly tested the mediating role of neurobiological systems in the relations between SED and health development, largely due to limitations in sample size. Testing mediation requires a large sample size for appropriate statistical power. Cumulative measures of physiological systems such as allostatic load are also useful in building a comprehensive understanding of the effects of SED exposure. While the research has been limited, studies that have included a large number of biological markers have provided evidence for allostatic load as a mediator for the links between SED and health outcomes (Seeman et al. 2004). More research involving large sets of biological markers is needed and will require population-based studies and collaboration across fields.

Population-based studies are also important for statistical power in testing interactions among individual differences such as gender and race/ethnicity. Differences across individuals are likely to be associated with different outcomes and vulnerabilities to SED exposure. For example, some evidence suggests that SED exposure has a greater impact on allostatic load in African American compared to white adults (Geronimus et al. 2006), while others did not find racial differences in the associations between SED exposure and allostatic load (Seeman et al. 2008).

8 Suggestions for Policy and Interventions

This discussion leads to the final part of the chapter on interventions. A greater benefit-cost ratio has been revealed for early intervention (Shonkoff et al. 2009; Heckman 2006). Evidence of the long-lasting effects of early experience also emphasizes the importance of early interventions. Future studies including those we suggested above may help to more clearly identify critical periods when investment would produce the biggest effects and long-term returns (Blair and Raver 2014; Shonkoff 2010).

There are several ways to intervene. The first is to directly intervene with SED, particularly family income. Cash transfer or income increases for a child's parents early in childhood have been shown to improve the physiological stress regulation function as well as cognitive outcomes (Duncan et al. 2011; Fernald et al. 2008). Other ways to intervene would be to target the mediators we discussed above. Interventions for parenting skills, parental psychopathology, health-care quality, as well as a child's cognitive functions have been shown to improve child health outcomes including cognitive and psychological functions and inflammatory regulation (Beeber et al. 2008; Miller et al. 2014; Olds et al. 1997). Third, interventions on protective factors such as coping have also been shown to improve physical and health outcomes in SED children and adults (Wadsworth et al. 2011).

Lastly, given the importance of parents in directly modifying home environments for children, a two-generation approach has received increasing attention (Kim and Watamura 2015). When both parents received a parenting intervention at the same time that children received attention training, children's attentional control and brain functions improved more than when only children received the intervention (Neville et al. 2013). In particular, pregnancy and the first years of a child's life can be an optimal time for the two-generation approach to intervention. Not only is this the period when a child's brain and body are most rapidly developing, it is also a period when a parent's brain undergoes plastic changes to support the parental role (Kim and Bianco 2014; Swain et al. 2014). For example, during the first few months of the postpartum period, both new mothers and fathers exhibit structural growth in brain regions including the striatum and prefrontal cortex that support warm and supportive parenting behaviors (Kim et al. 2010b; Kim et al. 2014). Sensitive neural activations, particularly for one's own baby, have also been consistently identified among new mothers and fathers during these same periods, when parents and infants establish long-lasting emotional relationships (Barrett and Fleming 2011; Mascaro et al. 2013; Musser et al. 2012). At the same time, parents in poverty are far more vulnerable to development of postpartum depression (Boury et al. 2004; U.S. Department of Health and Human Services 2002; Walker et al. 2002), and it is possible that as the result of depression and the stress of living in poverty, they are also more likely to exhibit abusive or harsh parenting (Sedlak and Broadhurst 1996; Widom and Nikulina 2012). Parents who received poor quality of parental care in their own childhood or experienced chronic stress such as poverty are also more likely to show reduced biological and behavioral sensitivity to their own children (Champagne et al. 2003; Kim et al. 2015; Kim et al. 2010a) and to repeat harsh parenting (Belsky et al. 2005; Van Ijzendoorn 1992). Thus, interventions that pay more attention to the well-being of parents with SED backgrounds may ultimately promote optimal development of the next generations and reduce the intergenerational transmission of SED and harsh environments.

Acknowledgments The authors wish to acknowledge Christian Capistrano for literature research assistance and Christina Congleton for editorial assistance.

References

Ackerman, S. H., Hofer, M. A., & Weiner, H. (1975). Age at maternal separation and gastric erosion susceptibility in the rat. *Psychosomatic Medicine, 37*, 180–184.

Adam, E. K., & Kumari, M. (2009). Assessing salivary cortisol in large-scale, epidemiological research. *Psychoneuroendocrinology, 34*, 1423–1436.

Ader, R., Tatum, R., & Beels, C. C. (1960). Social factors affecting emotionality and resistance to disease in animals: I. Age of separation from the mother and susceptibility to gastric ulcers in the rat. *Journal of Comparative and Physiological Psychology, 53*, 446–454.

Adler, N. E., & Rehkopf, D. H. (2008). U.S. disparities in health: Descriptions, causes, and mechanisms. *Annual Review of Public Health, 29*, 235–252.

Adolphs, R. (2001). The neurobiology of social cognition. *Current Opinion in Neurobiology, 11*, 231–239.

Alexander-Bloch, A., Raznahan, A., Bullmore, E., & Giedd, J. (2013). The convergence of maturational change and structural covariance in human cortical networks. *Journal of Neuroscience, 33*, 2889–2899.

Alley, D. E., Seeman, T. E., Ki Kim, J., Karlamangla, A., Hu, P., & Crimmins, E. M. (2006). Socioeconomic status and C-reactive protein levels in the US population: NHANES IV. *Brain, Behavior, and Immunity, 20*, 498–504.

Azad, M. B., Lissitsyn, Y., Miller, G. E., Becker, A. B., HayGlass, K. T., & Kozyrskyj, A. L. (2012). Influence of socioeconomic status trajectories on innate immune responsiveness in children. *PloS One, 7*, e38669.

Baltes, P. B. (1987). Theoretical propositions of life-span developmental psychology: On the dynamics between growth and decline. *Developmental Psychology, 23*(5), 611–626.

Barker, D. J. (1990). The fetal and infant origins of adult disease. *BMJ: British Medical Journal, 301*(6761), 1111.

Barrett, J., & Fleming, A. S. (2011). Annual research review: All mothers are not created equal: Neural and psychobiological perspectives on mothering and the importance of individual differences. *Journal of Child Psychology and Psychiatry, 52*(4), 368–397. doi:10.1111/j.1469-7610.2010.02306.x.

Beeber, L. S., Perreira, K. M., & Schwartz, T. (2008). Supporting the mental health of mothers raising children in poverty - how do we target them for intervention studies? *Reducing the Impact of Poverty on Health and Human Development: Scientific Approaches, 1136*, 86–100.

Belsky, J., Jaffee, S. R., Sligo, J., Woodward, L., & Silva, P. A. (2005). Intergenerational transmission of warm-sensitive-stimulating parenting: A prospective study of mothers and fathers of 3-year-olds. *Child Development, 76*, 384–396.

Bird, C. E., Seeman, T., Escarce, J. J., Basurto-Dávila, R., Finch, B. K., Dubowitz, T., et al. (2010). Neighbourhood socioeconomic status and biological 'wear and tear'in a nationally representative sample of US adults. *Journal of Epidemiology and Community Health, 64*, 860–865.

Blair, C., & Raver, C. C. (2012). Child development in the context of adversity: Experiential canalization of brain and behavior. *American Psychologist, 67*, 309–318.

Blair, C., & Raver, C. C. (2014). Closing the achievement gap through modification of neurocognitive and neuroendocrine function: Results from a cluster randomized controlled trial of an innovative approach to the education of children in kindergarten. *PloS One, 9*, e112393.

Blair, C., Raver, C. C., Granger, D., Mills-Koonce, R., & Hibel, L. (2011). Allostasis and allostatic load in the context of poverty in early childhood. *Development and Psychopathology, 23*, 845–857.

Blair, C., Berry, D., Mills-Koonce, R., & Granger, D. (2013). Cumulative effects of early poverty on cortisol in young children: Moderation by autonomic nervous system activity. *Psychoneuroendocrinology, 38*, 2666–2675.

Boury, J. M., Larkin, K. T., & Krummel, D. A. (2004). Factors related to postpartum depressive symptoms in low-income women. *Women and Health, 39*(3), 19–34. doi:10.1300/J013v39n03_02.

Bradley, R. H., & Corwyn, R. F. (2002). Socioeconomic status and child development. *Annual Review of Psychology, 53*, 371–399.

Brandtstädter, J., Baltes-Götz, B., Kirschbaum, C., & Hellhammer, D. (1991). Developmental and personality correlates of adrenocortical activity as indexed by salivary cortisol: Observations in the age range of 35 to 65 years. *Journal of Psychosomatic Research, 35*, 173–185.

Braverman, P., & Egerter, S. (2008). *Overcoming obstacles to health: Robert Wood Johnson Foundation Commission to build a healthier America.* Princeton: Robert Wood Johnson Foundation.

Brody, G. H., Lei, M.-K., Chen, E., & Miller, G. E. (2014). Neighborhood poverty and allostatic load in African American youth. *Pediatrics, 134*, e1362–e1368.

Brooks-Gunn, J., & Duncan, G. J. (1997). The effects of poverty on children. *The Future of Children, 7*, 55–71.

Brunner, E., Davey Smith, G., Marmot, M., Canner, R., Beksinska, M., & O'Brien, J. (1996). Childhood social circumstances and psychosocial and behavioural factors as determinants of plasma fibrinogen. *Lancet, 347*, 1008–1013.

Brunner, E., Marmot, M., Nanchahal, K., Shipley, M., Stansfeld, S., Juneja, M., & Alberti, K. (1997). Social inequality in coronary risk: Central obesity and the metabolic syndrome. Evidence from the Whitehall II study. *Diabetologia, 40*, 1341–1349.

Brunner, E., Shipley, M. J., Blane, D., Davey-Smith, G., & Marmot, M. (1999). When does cardiovascular risk start? Past and present socioeconomic circumstances and risk factors in adulthood. *Journal of Epidemiology and Community Health, 53*, 757–764.

Buckhalt, J. A. (2011). Insufficient sleep and the socioeconomic status achievement gap. *Child Development Perspectives, 5*, 59–65.

Burghy, C. A., Stodola, D. E., Ruttle, P. L., Molloy, E. K., Armstrong, J. M., Oler, J. A., et al. (2012). Developmental pathways to amygdala-prefrontal function and internalizing symptoms in adolescence. *Nature Neuroscience, 15*, 1736–1741.

Butterworth, P., Cherbuin, N., Sachdev, P., & Anstey, K. J. (2012). The association between financial hardship and amygdala and hippocampal volumes: Results from the PATH through life project. *Social Cognitive and Affective Neuroscience, 7*, 548–556.

Cameron, N. M., Champagne, F. A., Parent, C., Fish, E. W., Ozaki-Kuroda, K., & Meaney, M. J. (2005). The programming of individual differences in defensive responses and reproductive strategies in the rat through variations in maternal care. *Neuroscience and Biobehavioral Reviews, 29*, 843–865.

Chaix, B., Ducimetiere, P., Lang, T., Haas, B., Montaye, M., Ruidavets, J.-B., et al. (2008). Residential environment and blood pressure in the PRIME study: Is the association mediated by body mass index and waist circumference? *Journal of Hypertension, 26*, 1078–1084.

Chaix, B., Bean, K., Leal, C., Thomas, F., Havard, S., Evans, D., et al. (2010). Individual/neighborhood social factors and blood pressure in the RECORD cohort study which risk factors explain the associations? *Hypertension, 55*, 769–775.

Champagne, F. A., Weaver, I. C., Diorio, J., Sharma, S., & Meaney, M. J. (2003). Natural variations in maternal care are associated with estrogen receptor alpha expression and estrogen sensitivity in the medial preoptic area. *Endocrinology, 144*(11), 4720–4724.

Chen, E., Matthews, K. A., & Boyce, W. T. (2002). Socioeconomic differences in children's health: How and why do these relationships change with age? *Psychological Bulletin, 128*, 295–329.

Chen, E., Fisher, E. B., Bacharier, L. B., & Strunk, R. C. (2003). Socioeconomic status, stress, and immune markers in adolescents with asthma. *Psychosomatic Medicine, 65*, 984–992.

Chen, E., Langer, D. A., Raphaelson, Y. E., & Matthews, K. A. (2004). Socioeconomic status and health in adolescents: The role of stress interpretations. *Child Development, 75*, 1039–1052.

Chen, E., Hanson, M. D., Paterson, L. Q., Griffin, M. J., Walker, H. A., & Miller, G. E. (2006). Socioeconomic status and inflammatory processes in childhood asthma: The role of psychological stress. *The Journal of Allergy and Clinical Immunology, 117*, 1014–1020.

Chen, E., Chim, L. S., Strunk, R. C., & Miller, G. E. (2007). The role of the social environment in children and adolescents with asthma. *American Journal of Respiratory and Critical Care Medicine, 176*, 644–649.

Chen, E., Miller, G. E., Walker, H. A., Arevalo, J. M., Sung, C. Y., & Cole, S. W. (2009). Genome-wide transcriptional profiling linked to social class in asthma. *Thorax, 64*, 38–43.

Chen, E., Cohen, S., & Miller, G. W. (2010). How low socioeconomic status effects 2-year hormonal trajectories in children. *Psychological Science, 21*, 31–37.

Chichlowska, K. L., Rose, K. M., Diez-Roux, A. V., Golden, S. H., McNeill, A. M., & Heiss, G. (2009). Life course socioeconomic conditions and metabolic syndrome in adults: The atherosclerosis risk in communities (ARIC) study. *Annals of Epidemiology, 19*, 875–883.

Chida, Y., Sudo, N., Sonoda, J., Hiramoto, T., & Kubo, C. (2007). Early-life psychological stress exacerbates adult mouse asthma via the hypothalamus-pituitary-adrenal axis. *American Journal of Respiratory and Critical Care Medicine, 175*, 316–322.

Coan, J. A., Beckes, L., & Allen, J. P. (2013). Childhood maternal support and social capital moderate the regulatory impact of social relationships in adulthood. *International Journal of Psychophysiology, 88*, 224–231.

Coccaro, E. F., McCloskey, M. S., Fitzgerald, D. A., & Phan, K. L. (2007). Amygdala and orbitofrontal reactivity to social threat in individuals with impulsive aggression. *Biological Psychiatry, 62*, 168–178.

Coe, C. L., & Lubach, G. R. (2005). Prenatal origins of individual variation in behavior and immunity. *Neuroscience and Biobehavioral Reviews, 29*, 39–49.

Cohen, S., Doyle, W. J., Turner, R. J., Alper, C. M., & Skoner, D. P. (2004). Childhood socioeconomic status and host resistance to infectious illness in adulthood. *Psychosomatic Medicine, 66*, 553–558.

Cohen, S., Schwartz, J. E., Epel, E., Kirschbaum, C., Sidney, S., & Seeman, T. (2006a). Socioeconomic status, race, and diurnal cortisol decline in the coronary Artery risk development in young adults (CARDIA) study. *Psychosomatic Medicine, 68*, 41–50.

Cohen, R. A., Grieve, S., Hoth, K. F., Paul, R. H., Sweet, L., Tate, D., et al. (2006b). Early life stress and morphometry of the adult anterior cingulate cortex and caudate nuclei. *Biological Psychiatry, 59*, 975–982.

Cohen, S., Doyle, W. J., & Baum, A. (2006c). Socioeconomic status is associated with stress hormones. *Psychosomatic Medicine, 68*, 414–420.

Cohen, S., Janicki-Deverts, D., Chen, E., & Matthews, K. A. (2010). Childhood socioeconomic status and adult health. *Annals of the New York Academy of Sciences, 1186*, 37–55.

Colhoun, H. M., Hemingway, H., & Poulter, N. R. (1998). Socioeconomic status and blood pressure: An overview analysis. *Journal of Hypertension, 12*, 91–110.

Cozier, Y. C., Palmer, J. R., Horton, N. J., Fredman, L., Wise, L. A., & Rosenberg, L. (2007). Relation between neighborhood median housing value and hypertension risk among black women in the United States. *American Journal of Public Health, 97*, 718–724.

Crimmins, E. M., Kim, J. K., & Seeman, T. E. (2009). Poverty and biological risk: The earlier "aging" of the poor. *The Journals of Gerontology Series A: Biological Sciences and Medical Sciences, 64*, 286–292.

Cubbin, C., Hadden, W. C., & Winkleby, M. A. (2000). Neighborhood context and cardiovascular disease risk factors: The contribution of material deprivation. *Ethnicity & Disease, 11*, 687–700.

Dahl, R. E., & Lewin, D. S. (2002). Pathways to adolescent health sleep regulation and behavior. *Journal of Adolescent Health, 31*, 175–184.

Danese, A., & McEwen, B. S. (2012). Adverse childhood experiences, allostasis, allostatic load, and age-related disease. *Physiology & Behavior, 106*, 29–39.

D'Angiulli, A., Herdman, A., Stapells, D., & Hertzman, C. (2008). Children's event-related potentials of auditory selective attention vary with their socioeconomic status. *Neuropsychology, 22*, 293–300.

D'Angiulli, A., Van Roon, P. M., Weinberg, J., Oberlander, T. F., Grunau, R. E., Hertzman, C., & Maggi, S. (2012). Frontal EEG/ERP correlates of attentional processes, cortisol and motivational states in adolescents from lower and higher socioeconomic status. *Frontiers in Human Neuroscience, 6*, 306.

Davidson, R. J., & McEwen, B. S. (2012). Social influences on neuroplasticity: Stress and interventions to promote well-being. *Nature Neuroscience, 15*, 689–695.

De Boever, E., Braeckman, L., Baele, G., Rosseneu, M., & De Backer, G. (1995). Relation of fibrinogen to lifestyles and to cardiovascular risk factors in a working population. *International Journal of Epidemiology, 24*, 915–921.

Dewald, J. F., Meijer, A. M., Oort, F. J., Kerkhof, G. A., & Bögels, S. M. (2010). The influence of sleep quality, sleep duration and sleepiness on school performance in children and adolescents: A meta-analytic review. *Sleep Medicine Reviews, 14*, 179–189.

Diez-Roux, A. V., Link, B. G., & Northridge, M. E. (2000). A multilevel analysis of income inequality and cardiovascular disease risk factors. *Social Science & Medicine, 50*, 673–687.

Doan, S. N., Fuller-Rowell, T. E., & Evans, G. W. (2012). Cumulative risk and adolescent's internalizing and externalizing problems: The mediating roles of maternal responsiveness and self-regulation. *Developmental Psychology, 48*, 1529–1539.

Duncan, G. J., Ziol-Guest, K. M., & Kalil, A. (2010). Early-childhood poverty and adult attainment, behavior, and health. *Child Development, 81*, 306–325.

Duncan, G. J., Morris, P. A., & Rodrigues, C. (2011). Does money really matter? Estimating impacts of family income on young children's achievement with data from random-assignment experiments. *Developmental Psychology, 47*, 1263.

Eidelman, P., Gershon, A., McGlinchey, E., & Harvey, A. G. (2012). Sleep and psychopathology. In C. M. Morin & C. A. Espie (Eds.), *The Oxford handbook of sleep and sleep disorders* (pp. 172–189). New York: Oxford University Press.

Elder, G. H. (1998). The life course as developmental theory. *Child Development, 69*(1), 1–12.

Elder, G. H., Jr., Johnson, M. K., & Crosnoe, R. (2003). The emergence and development of life course theory. In *Handbook of the life course* (pp. 3–19). New York: Springer.

Ellis, B. J., & Del Giudice, M. (2014). Beyond allostatic load: Rethinking the role of stress in regulating human development. *Development and Psychopathology, 26*(1), 1–20. doi:10.1017/S0954579413000849.

Ellis, B. J., Boyce, W. T., Belsky, J., Bakermans-Kranenburg, M. J., & van Ijzendoorn, M. H. (2011). Differential susceptibility to the environment: An evolutionary-neurodevelopmental theory. *Development and Psychopathology, 23*, 7–28.

Epstein, J., Pan, H., Kocsis, J., Yang, Y., Butler, T., Chusid, J., et al. (2006). Lack of ventral striatal response to positive stimuli in depressed versus normal subjects. *American Journal of Psychiatry, 163*, 1784–1790.

Essex, M. J., Klein, M. H., Cho, E., & Kalin, N. H. (2002). Maternal stress beginning in infancy may sensitize children to later stress exposure: Effects on cortisol and behavior. *Biological Psychiatry, 52*, 776–784.

Evans, G. W. (2003). A multimethodological analysis of cumulative risk and allostatic load among rural children. *Developmental Psychology, 39*, 924–933.

Evans, G. W. (2004). The environment of childhood poverty. *American Psychologist, 59*, 77–92.

Evans, G. W., & Cassells, R. C. (2014). Childhood poverty, cumulative risk exposure, and mental health in emerging adults. *Clinical Psychological Science, 2*(3), 287–296.

Evans, G. W., & English, K. (2002). The environment of poverty: Multiple stressor exposure, psychophysiological stress, and socioemotional adjustment. *Child Development, 73*, 1238–1248.

Evans, G. W., & Kim, P. (2007). Childhood poverty and health: Cumulative risk exposure and stress dysregulation. *Psychological Science, 18*, 953–957.

Evans, G. W., & Kim, P. (2010). Multiple risk exposure as a potential explanatory mechanism for the socioeconomic status-health gradient. *Annals of the New York Academy of Sciences, 1186*, 174–189.

Evans, G. W., & Kim, P. (2012). Childhood poverty and young adults' allostatic load: The mediating role of childhood cumulative risk exposure. *Psychological Science, 23*, 979–983.

Evans, G. W., & Kim, P. (2013). Childhood poverty, chronic stress, self-regulation, and coping. *Child Development Perspectives, 7*, 43–48.

Evans, G.W., & Schamberg, M.A. (2009). Childhood poverty, chronic stress, and adult working memory. *Proceedings of the National Academy of Sciences, 106*, 6545–6549.

Evans, G. W., Kim, P. K., Ting, A. H., Tesser, H. B., & Shanis, D. (2007). Cumulative risk, maternal responsiveness, and allostatic load among young adolescents. *Developmental Psychology, 43*, 341–351.

Evans, G.W., Wells, N.M. & Schamberg, M.A. (2010). The ecological context of SES and obesity. In L. Dube, A. Bechara, A. Dagher, D. Drewnowski, J. LeBel, J., P. James, D. Richard, R.Y. Yada (Eds.). Obesity prevention: The role of society and brain on individual behavior (pp. 713–725). New York: Elsevier.

Evans, G. W., Chen, E., Miller, G. E., & Seeman, T. E. (2012). How poverty gets under the skin: A lifecourse perspective. In V. Maholmes & R. King (Eds.), *The Oxford handbook of poverty and child development* (pp. 13–36). New York: Oxford University Press.

Evans, G. W., Exner-Cortens, D., Kim, P., & Bartholomew, D. (2013). Childhood poverty and late adolescents' blood pressure reactivity and recovery to an acute stressor: The mediating role of family conflict. *Psychosomatic Medicine, 75*, 691–700.

Evans, G. W., Eckenrode, J., & Marcynyszyn, L. A. (in press). Poverty and chaos. In G. W. Evans & T. D. Wachs (Eds.), *Chaos and its influence on children's development: An ecological perspective*. Washington, DC: American Psychological Association.

Everson, S. A., Maty, S. C., Lynch, J. W., & Kaplan, G. A. (2002). Epidemiologic evidence for the relation between socioeconomic status and depression, obesity, and diabetes. *Journal of Psychosomatic Research, 53*, 891–895.

Fauth, R. C., Leventhal, T., & Brooks-Gunn, J. (2007). Welcome to the neighborhood? Long-term impacts of moving to low-poverty neighborhoods on poor children's and adolescents' outcomes. *Journal of Research on Adolescence, 17*, 249–284.

Fenoglio, K. A., Brunson, K. L., & Baram, T. Z. (2006). Hippocampal neuroplasticity induced by early-life stress: Functional and molecular aspects. *Frontiers in Neuroendocrinology, 27*, 180–192.

Fernald, L. C., Gertler, P. J., & Neufeld, L. M. (2008). Role of cash in conditional cash transfer programmes for child health, growth, and development: An analysis of Mexico's *Oportunidades*. *The Lancet, 371*, 828–837.

Fernald, L. C., & Gunnar, M. R. (2009). Poverty-alleviation program participation and salivary cortisol in very lowincome children. *Social Science and Medicine, 68*, 2180–2189.

Ferrie, J. E., Shipley, M. J., Stansfeld, S. A., & Marmot, M. G. (2002). Effects of chronic job insecurity and change in job security on self reported health, minor psychiatric morbidity, physiological measures, and health related behaviours in British civil servants: The Whitehall II study. *Journal of Epidemiology and Community Health, 56*, 450–454.

Finch, C. E., & Crimmins, E. M. (2004). Inflammatory exposure and historical changes in human life-spans. *Science, 305*, 1736–1739.

Flinn, M. V., & England, B. (1997). Social economics of childhood glucocorticoid stress response and health. *American Journal of Physical Anthropology, 102*, 33–53.

Foubert-Samier, A., Catheline, G., Amieva, H., Dilharreguy, B., Helmer, C., Allard, M., & Dartigues, J.-F. (2012). Education, occupation, leisure activities, and brain reserve: A population-based study. *Neurobiology of Aging, 33*(2), 423.e15–423.e25.

Gallo, L. C., & Matthews, K. A. (2003). Understanding the association between socioeconomic status and physical health: Do negative emotions play a role? *Psychological Bulletin, 129*, 10–31.

Gao, W., Alcauter, S., Elton, A., Hernandez-Castillo, C. R., Smith, J. K., Ramirez, J., & Lin, W. (2014). Functional network development during the first year: Relative sequence and socioeconomic correlations. *Cerebral Cortex, 25*(9), 2919–2928.

Geronimus, A. T., Hicken, M., Keene, D., & Bound, J. (2006). "weathering" and age patterns of allostatic load scores among blacks and whites in the United States. *American Journal of Public Health, 96*(5), 826–833.

Gianaros, P. J., Horenstein, J. A., Cohen, S., Matthews, K. A., Brown, S. M., Flory, J. D., et al. (2007). Perigenual anterior cingulate morphology covaries with perceived social standing. *Social Cognitive and Affective Neurosciences, 2*, 161–173.

Gianaros, P. J., Horenstein, J. A., Hariri, A. R., Sheu, L. K., Manuck, S. B., Matthews, K. A., & Cohen, S. (2008). Potential neural embedding of parental social standing. *Social Cognitive and Affective Neurosciences, 3*, 91–96.

Gianaros, P. J., Marsland, A. L., Sheu, L. K., Erickson, K. I., & Verstynen, T. D. (2013). Inflammatory pathways link socioeconomic inequalities to white matter architecture. *Cerebral Cortex, 23*, 2058–2071.

Giedd, J. N. (2004). Structural magnetic resonance imaging of the adolescent brain. *Annals of the New York Academy of Sciences, 1021*, 77–85.

Gliksman, M. D., Dwyer, T., & Wlodarczyk, J. (1990). Differences in cardiovascular disease risk factors in Australian schoolchildren. *Preventive Medicine, 19*, 291–304.

Gluckman, P. D., & Hanson, M. A. (2004). Living with the past: Evolution, development, and patterns of disease. *Science, 305*(5691), 1733–1736. doi:10.1126/science.1095292.

Gonzalez, M. Z., Beckes, L., Chango, J., Allen, J. P., & Coan, J. A. (2014). Adolescent neighborhood quality predicts adult dACC response to social exclusion. *Social Cognitive and Affective Neuroscience*. doi:10.1093/scan/nsu137.

Goodman, E., McEwen, B. S., Dolan, L. M., Schafer-Kalkhoff, T., & Adler, N. E. (2005a). Social disadvantage and adolescent stress. *Journal of Adolescent Health, 37*, 484–492.

Goodman, E., McEwen, B. S., Huang, B., Dolan, L. M., & Adler, N. E. (2005b). Social inequalities in biomarkers of cardiovascular risk in adolescence. *Psychosomatic Medicine, 67*, 9–15.

Grant, K. E., Compas, B. E., Stuhlmacher, A. F., Thurm, A. E., McMahon, S. D., & Halpert, J. A. (2003). Stressors and child and adolescent psychopathology: Moving from markers to mechanisms of risk. *Psychological Bulletin, 129*, 447–466.

Gruenewald, T. L., Cohen, S., Matthews, K. A., Tracy, R., & Seeman, T. E. (2009). Association of socioeconomic status with inflammation markers in black and white men and women in the coronary Artery risk development in young adults (CARDIA) study. *Social Science & Medicine, 69*, 451–459.

Gruenewald, T. L., Karlamangla, A. S., Hu, P., Stein-Merkin, S., Crandall, C., Koretz, B., & Seeman, T. E. (2012). History of socioeconomic disadvantage and allostatic load in later life. *Social Science & Medicine, 74*, 75–83.

Guize, L., Jaffiol, C., Gueniot, M., Bringer, J., Giudicelli, C., Tramoni, M., et al. (2008). Diabetes and socio-economic deprivation. *A study in a large French population. Bulletin de l'Académie Nationale de Médecine, 192*, 1707–1723.

Gump, B. B., Reihman, J., Stewart, P., Lonky, E., Darvill, T., & Matthews, K. A. (2007). Blood lead (Pb) levels: A potential environmental mechanism explaining the relation between socioeconomic status and cardiovascular reactivity in children. *Health Psychology, 26*, 296–304.

Gump, B. B., Reihman, J., Stewart, P., Lonky, E., & Matthews, K. A. (2009). Blood lead (Pb) levels: Further evidence for an environmental mechanism explaining the association between socioeconomic status and psychophysiological dysregulation in children. *Health Psychology, 28*, 614–620.

Gustafsson, P. E., Gustafsson, P. A., & Nelson, N. (2006). Cortisol levels and psychosocial factors in preadolescent children. *Stress and Health, 22*, 3–9.

Gustafsson, P. E., Janlert, U., Theorell, T., & Hammarstrom, A. (2010a). Life-course socioeconomic trajectories and diurnal cortisol regulation in adulthood. *Psychoneuroendocrinology, 35*, 613–623.

Gustafsson, P. E., Janlert, U., Theorell, T., Westerlund, H., Hammarström, A. (2010b). Socioeconomic status over the life course and allostatic load in adulthood: Results from the Northern Swedish Cohort. *Journal of Epidemiology & Community Health*, jech-2010.

Haber, S. N., & Knutson, B. (2009). The reward circuit: Linking primate anatomy and human imaging. *Neuropsychopharmacology, 35*, 4–26.

Hackman, D. A., & Farah, M. J. (2009). Socioeconomic status and the developing brain. *Trends in Cognitive Sciences, 13*, 65–73.

Hackman, D. A., Betancourt, L. M., Brodsky, N. L., Hurt, H., & Farah, M. J. (2012). Neighborhood disadvantage and adolescent stress reactivity. *Frontiers in Human Neuroscience, 6*, 277.

Halfon, N., & Forrest, C. B. (2017). The emerging theoretical framework of life course health development. In N. Halfon, C. B. Forrest, R. M. Lerner, & E. Faustman (Eds.), *Handbook of life course health-development science*. Cham: Springer.

Hanson, M. A., & Gluckman, P. D. (2014). Early developmental conditioning of later health and disease: Physiology or pathophysiology? *Physiological Reviews, 94*(4), 1027–1076. doi:10.1152/physrev.00029.2013.

Hanson, J. L., Chandra, A., Wolfe, B. L., & Pollak, S. D. (2011). Association between income and the hippocampus. *PloS One, 6*, e18712.

Hanson, J. L., Hair, N., Shen, D. G., Shi, F., Gilmore, J. H., Wolfe, B. L., & Pollak, S. D. (2013). Family poverty affects the rate of human infant brain growth. *PloS One, 8*, e80954.

Hanson, J. L., Nacewicz, B. M., Sutterer, M. J., Cayo, A. A., Schaefer, S. M., Rudolph, K. D., et al. (2014). Behavior problems after early life stress: Contributions of the hippocampus and amygdala. *Biological Psychiatry, 77*(4), 314–323.

Harburg, E., Erfurt, J. C., Chape, C., Hauenstein, L. S., Schull, W. J., & Schork, M. A. (1973). Socioecological stressor areas and black-white blood pressure: Detroit. *Journal of Chronic Diseases, 26*, 595–611.

Hardy, R., Kuh, D., Langenberg, C., & Wadsworth, M. E. (2003). Birthweight, childhood social class, and change in adult blood pressure in the 1946 British birth cohort. *The Lancet, 362*, 1178–1183.

Hargreaves, D. S., Marbini, A. D., & Viner, R. M. (2013). Inequality trends in health and future health risk among English children and young people, 1999–2009. *Archives of Disease in Childhood, 98*, 850–855.

Heatherton, T. F. (2011). Neuroscience of self and self-regulation. *Annual Review of Psychology, 62*, 363–390.

Heckman, J. J. (2006). Skill formation and the economics of investing in disadvantaged children. *Science, 312*, 1900–1902.

Hemingway, H., Shipley, M., Mullen, M. J., Kumari, M., Brunner, E., Taylor, M., et al. (2003). Social and psychosocial influences on inflammatory markers and vascular function in civil servants (the Whitehall II study). *American Journal of Cardiology, 92*, 984–987.

Hemingway, H., Shipley, M., Brunner, E., Britton, A., Malik, M., & Marmot, M. (2005). Does autonomic function link social position to coronary risk? The Whitehall II study. *Circulation, 111*, 3071–3077.

Hertzman, C. (1999). The biological embedding of early experience and its effects on health in adulthood. *Annals of the New York Academy of Sciences, 896*, 85–95.

Hoff, E. (2006). How social contexts support and shape language development. *Developmental Review, 26*, 55–85.

Holmes, A., & Wellman, C. L. (2009). Stress-induced prefrontal reorganization and executive dysfunction in rodents. *Neuroscience & Biobehavioral Reviews, 33*, 773–783.

Holz, N. E., Boecker, R., Hohm, E., Zohsel, K., Buchmann, A. F., Blomeyer, D., & Plichta, M. M. (2015). The longterm impact of early life poverty on orbitofrontal cortex volume in adulthood: results from a prospective study over 25 years. *Neuropsychopharmacology, 40*(4), 996–1004.

Howe, L. D., Lawlor, D. A., & Propper, C. (2013). Trajectories of socioeconomic inequalities in health, behaviors and academic achievement across childhood and adolescence. *Journal of Epidemiology and Community Health, 67*, 358–364.

Ishizaki, M., Martikainen, P., Nakagawa, H., & Marmot, M. (2000). The relationship between employment grade and plasma fibrinogen level among Japanese male employees. *YKKJ Research Group. Atherosclerosis, 151*, 415–421.

Jackson, R. W., Treiber, F. A., Turner, J. R., Davis, H., & Strong, W. B. (1999). Effects of race, sex, and socioeconomic status upon cardiovascular stress responsivity and recovery in youth. *International Journal of Psychophysiology, 31*, 111–119.

Jacobson, L., & Sapolsky, R. (1991). The role of the hippocampus in feedback regulation of the hypothalamic-pituitary-adrenocortical axis. *Endocrine Reviews, 12*, 118–134.

Janicki-Deverts, D., Cohen, S., Adler, N. E., Schwartz, J. E., Matthews, K. A., & Seeman, T. E. (2007). Socioeconomic status is related to urinary catecholamines in the coronary Artery risk development in young adults (CARDIA) study. *Psychosomatic Medicine, 69*, 514–520.

Jarcho, M. R., Slavich, G. M., Tylova-Stein, H., Wolkowitz, O. M., & Burke, H. M. (2013). Dysregulated diurnal cortisol pattern is associated with glucocorticoid resistance in women with major depressive disorder. *Biological Psychology, 93*, 150–158.

Jarrin, D. C., McGrath, J. J., Silverstein, J. E., & Drake, C. (2013). Objective and subjective socioeconomic gradients exist for sleep quality, sleep latency, sleep duration, weekend oversleep, and daytime sleepiness in adults. *Behavioral Sleep Medicine, 11*, 144–158.

Jarrin, D. C., McGrath, J. J., & Quon, E. C. (2014). Objective and subjective socioeconomic gradients exist for sleep in children and adolescents. *Health Psychology, 33*, 301.

Jednorog, K., Altarelli, I., Monzalvo, K., Fluss, J., Dubois, J., Billard, C., et al. (2012). The influence of socioeconomic status on children's brain structure. *PloS One, 7*, e42486.

Johnson, N. F., Kim, C., & Gold, B. T. (2013). Socioeconomic status is positively correlated with frontal white matter integrity in aging. *Age, 35*, 2045–2056.

Jousilahti, P., Salomaa, V., Rasi, V., Vahtera, E., & Palosuo, T. (2003). Association of markers of systemic inflammation, C reactive protein, serum amyloid a, and fibrinogen, with socioeconomic status. *Journal of Epidemiology & Community Health, 57*, 730–733.

Jung, R. E., Grazioplene, R., Caprihan, A., Chavez, R. S., & Haier, R. J. (2010). White matter integrity, creativity, and psychopathology: Disentangling constructs with diffusion tensor imaging. *PloS One, 53*, e9818.

Juster, R.-P., McEwen, B. S., & Lupien, S. J. (2010). Allostatic load biomarkers of chronic stress and impact on health and cognition. *Neuroscience & Biobehavioral Reviews, 35*, 2–16.

Juster, R.-P., Bizik, G., Picard, M., Arsenault-Lapierre, G., Sindi, S., Trepanier, L., et al. (2011). A transdisciplinary perspective of chronic stress in relation to psychopathology throughout life span development. *Development and Psychopathology, 23*, 725–776.

Kahn, M., Sheppes, G., & Sadeh, A. (2013). Sleep and emotions: Bidirectional links and underlying mechanisms. *International Journal of Psychophysiology, 89*, 218–228.

Kakinami, L., Seguin, L., Lambert, M., Gauvin, L., Nikiema, B., & Paradis, G. (2013a). Comparison of three life course models of poverty in predicting cardiovascular disease risk in youth. *Annals of Epidemiology, 23*, 485–491.

Kakinami, L., Séguin, L., Lambert, M., Gauvin, L., Nikiema, B., Paradis, G. (2013b). Poverty's latent effect on adiposity during childhood: Evidence from a Québec birth cohort. *Journal of epidemiology and community health*, jech-2012.

Kalisch, R. (2009). The functional neuroanatomy of reappraisal: Time matters. *Neuroscience & Biobehavioral Reviews, 33*, 1215–1226.

Kalisch, R., Wiech, K., Critchley, H. D., & Dolan, R. J. (2006). Levels of appraisal: A medial prefrontal role in high-level appraisal of emotional material. *NeuroImage, 30*, 1458–1466.

Kaplan, G., & Keil, J. (1993). Sociodemographic factors and cardiovascular disease. *Circulation, 88*, 1973–1998.

Kapuku, G. K., Treiber, F. A., & Davis, H. C. (2002). Relationships among socioeconomic status, stress induced changes in cortisol, and blood pressure in African American males. *Annals of Behavioral Medicine, 24*, 320–325.

Karlamangla, A. S., Singer, B. H., Williams, D. R., Schwartz, J. E., Matthews, K. A., Kiefe, C. I., & Seeman, T. E. (2005). Impact of socioeconomic status on longitudinal accumulation of cardiovascular risk in young adults: The CARDIA study (USA). *Social Science & Medicine, 60*, 999–1015.

Karlamangla, A. S., Friedman, E. M., Seeman, T. E., Stawksi, R. S., & Almeida, D. M. (2013). Daytime trajectories of cortisol: Demographic and socioeconomic differences—Findings from the National Study of daily experiences. *Psychoneuroendocrinology, 38*, 2585–2597.

Kim, P., & Bianco, H. (2014). How motherhood and poverty change the brain. *Zero to Three, 34*(4), 29–36.

Kim, P., & Watamura, S. E. (2015). *Two open windows: Infant and parent neurobiologic change*. Retrieved from http://ascend.aspeninstitute.org/pages/two-open-windows-infant-and-parent-neurobiologic-change.

Kim, P., Leckman, J. F., Mayes, L. C., Newman, M.-A., Feldman, R., & Swain, J. E. (2010a). Perceived quality of maternal care in childhood and structure and function of mothers' brain. *Developmental Science, 13*(4), 662–673.

Kim, P., Leckman, J. F., Mayes, L. C., Feldman, R., Wang, X., & Swain, J. E. (2010b). The plasticity of human maternal brain: Longitudinal changes in brain anatomy during the early postpartum period. *Behavioral Neuroscience, 124*(5), 695–700. doi:10.1037/a0020884.

Kim, P., Evans, G. W., Angstadt, M., Ho, S. S., Sripada, C. S., Swain, J. E., et al. (2013). Effects of childhood poverty and chronic stress on emotion regulatory brain function in adulthood. *The Proceedings of the National Academy of Sciences, 110*, 18442–18447.

Kim, P., Rigo, P., Mayes, L. C., Feldman, R., Leckman, J. F., & Swain, J. E. (2014). Neural plasticity in fathers of human infants. *Social Neuroscience, 9*(5), 522–535. doi:10.1080/17470919.2014.933713.

Kim, P., Ho, S. S., Evans, G. W., Liberzon, I., & Swain, J. E. (2015). Childhood social inequalities influences neural processes in young adult caregiving. *Developmental Psychobiology, 57*(8), 948–960.

Kim-Cohen, J., Moffitt, T. E., Caspi, A., & Taylor, A. (2004). Genetic and environmental processes in young children's resilience and vulnerability to socioeconomic deprivation. *Child Development, 75*, 651–668.

Kishiyama, M. M., Boyce, W. T., Jimenez, A. M., Perry, L. M., & Knight, R. T. (2009). Socioeconomic disparities affect prefrontal function in children. *Journal of Cognitive Neuroscience, 21*, 1106–1115.

Kivimaki, M., Lawlor, D. A., Juonala, M., Smith, G. D., Elovainio, M., Keltikangas-Jarvinen, L., et al. (2005). Lifecourse socioeconomic position, C-reactive protein, and carotid intima-media thickness in young adults: The cardiovascular risk in young Finns study. *Arteriosclerosis, Thrombosis, and Vascular Biology, 25*, 2197–2202.

Klebanov, P. K., Evans, G. W., & Brooks-Gunn, J. (2014). Poverty, ethnicity, and risk of obesity among low birth weight infants. *Journal of Applied Developmental Psychology, 35*, 245–253.

Koster, A., Bosma, H., Penninx, B. W., Newman, A. B., Harris, T. B., van Eijk, J. T., et al. (2006). Association of inflammatory markers with socioeconomic status. *Journal of Gerontology: Medical Sciences, 61A*(3), 284–290.

Krantz, D. S., & Falconer, J. (1995). Measurement of cardiovascular responses. In S. Cohen, R. C. Kessler, & L. Gordon (Eds.), *Measuring stress* (pp. 193–212). New York: Oxford University Press.

Krishnadas, R., Kim, J., McLean, J., Batty, G. D., McLean, J. S., Millar, K., et al. (2013a). The envirome and the connectome: Exploring the structural noise in the human brain associated with socioeconomic deprivation. *Frontiers in Human Neuroscience, 7*, 722.

Krishnadas, R., McLean, J., Batty, G. D., Burns, H., Deans, K. A., Ford, I., et al. (2013b). Socioeconomic deprivation and cortical morphology: Psychological, social, and biological determinants of ill health study. *Psychosomatic Medicine, 75*, 616–623.

Kruschinski, C., Skripuletz, T., Bedoui, S., Raber, K., Straub, R. H., Hoffmann, T., et al. (2008). Postnatal life events affect the severity of asthmatic airway inflammation in the adult rat. *Journal of Immunology, 180*, 3919–3925.

Kubzansky, L. D., Kawachi, I., & Sparrow, D. (1999). Socioeconomic status, hostility, and risk factor clustering in the Normative Aging Study: Any help from the concept of allostatic load? *Annals of Behavioral Medicine, 21*(4), 330–338.

Kubzansky, L. D., Sparrow, D., Vokonas, P., & Kawachi, I. (2001). Is the glass half empty or half full? A prospective study of optimism and coronary heart disease in the normative aging study. *Psychosomatic Medicine, 63*, 910–916.

Kuh, D., & Ben-Shlomo, Y. (2004). *A life course approach to chronic disease epidemiology*. New York: Oxford University Press.

Kunz-Ebrecht, S. R., Kirschbaum, C., & Steptoe, A. (2004). Work stress, socioeconomic status and neuroendocrine activation over the working day. *Social Science and Medicine, 58*, 1523–1530.

Laaksonen, M., Sarlio-Lahteenkorva, S., & Lahelma, E. (2004). Multiple dimensions of socioeconomic position and obesity among employees: The Helsinki health study. *Obesity Research, 12*, 1851–1858.

Langenberg, C., Hardy, R., Kuh, D., Brunner, E., & Wadsworth, M. E. (2003). Central and total obesity in middle aged men and women in relation to lifetime socioeconomic status: evidence from a national birth cohort. *Journal of Epidemiology and Community Health, 57*, 816–822.

Langenberg, C., Kuh, D., Wadsworth, E. J., Brunner, E., & Hardy, R. (2006). Social circumstances and education: Life course origins of social inequalities in metabolic risk in a prospective national birth cohort. *American Journal of Public Health, 96*, 2216–2221.

Lawlor, D. A., Ebrahim, S., & Smith, G. D. (2002). Socioeconomic position in childhood and adulthood and insulin resistance: Cross sectional survey using data from British women's heart and health study. *BMJ, 325*, 805.

Lawson, G. M., Duda, J. T., Avants, B. B., Wu, J., & Farah, M. J. (2013). Associations between children's socioeconomic status and prefrontal cortical thickness. *Developmental Science, 16*, 641–652.

Lee, J., Harris, K. M., & Gordon-Larsen, P. (2008). Life course perspectives on the links between poverty and obesity during the transition to adulthood. *Population Research and Policy Review, 28*, 505–532.

Lehman, B. J., Taylor, S. E., Kiefe, C. I., & Seeman, T. E. (2009). Relationship of early life stress and psychological functioning to blood pressure in the CARDIA study. *Health Psychology, 28*, 338.

Leino, M., Porkka, K. V. K., Raitakari, O. T., Laitinen, S., Taimela, S., & Viikari, J. S. (1996). Influence of parental occupation on coronary heart disease risk factors in children. *The cardiovascular risk in young Finns study. International Journal of Epidemiology, 25*, 1189–1195.

Levine, S. (2005). Developmental determinants of sensitivity and resistance to stress. *Psychoneuroendocrinology, 30*, 939–946.

Li, L., Power, C., Kelly, S., Kirschbaum, C., & Hertzman, C. (2007). Life-time socio-economic position and cortisol patterns in mid-life. *Psychoneuroendocrinology, 32*, 824–833.

Lidfeldt, J., Li, T. Y., Hu, F. B., Manson, J. E., & Kawachi, I. (2007). A prospective study of childhood and adult socioeconomic status and incidence of type 2 diabetes in women. *American Journal of Epidemiology, 165*, 882–889.

Lorant, V., Deliege, D., Eaton, W., Robert, A., Philippot, P., & Ansseau, M. (2003). Socioeconomic inequalities in depression: A meta-analysis. *American Journal of Epidemiology, 157*, 98–112.

Loucks, E. B., Sullivan, L. M., Hayes, L. J., D'Agostino, R. B., Larson, M. G., Vasan, R. S., et al. (2006). Association of educational level with inflammatory markers in the Framingham offspring study. *American Journal of Epidemiology, 163*, 622–628.

Loucks, E. B., Magnusson, K. T., Cook, S., Rehkopf, D. H., Ford, E. S., & Berkman, L. F. (2007). Socioeconomic position and the metabolic syndrome in early, middle, and late life: Evidence from NHANES 1999–2002. *Annals of Epidemiology, 17*, 782–790.

Love, J. M., Kisker, E. E., Ross, C. M., Schochet, P. Z., Brooks-Gunn, J., Paulsell, D., et al. (2002). *Making a difference in the lives of infants and toddlers and their families: the impacts of Early Head Start*. U.S. Department of Health and Human Services. Princeton: Mathematica policy research.

Lubbock, L. A., Goh, A., Ali, S., Ritchie, J., & Whooley, M. A. (2005). Relation of low socioeconomic status to C-reactive protein in patients with coronary heart disease (from the heart and soul study). *American Journal of Cardiology, 96*, 1506–1511.

Luby, J., Belden, A., Botteron, K., Marrus, N., Harms, M. P., Babb, C., et al. (2013). The effects of poverty on childhood brain development: The mediating effect of caregiving and stressful life events. *Journal of the American Medical Association Pediatrics, 167*(12), 1135–1142.

Lupien, S. J., King, S., Meaney, M. J., & McEwen, B. S. (2000). Child's stress hormone levels correlate with mother's socioeconomic status and depressive state. *Biological Psychiatry, 48*, 976–980.

Lupien, S. J., King, S., Meaney, M., & McEwen, B. S. (2001). Can poverty can under your skin? Basal cortisol levels and cognitive function in children from low and high socioeconomic status. *Development and Psychopathology, 13*, 653–676.

Lupien, S. J., McEwen, B. S., Gunnar, M. R., & Heim, C. (2009). Effects of stress throughout the lifespan on the brain, behaviour and cognition. *Nature Reviews Neuroscience, 10*, 434–445.

Lyons, D. M., Parker, K. J., Katz, M., & Schatzberg, A. F. (2009). Developmental cascades linking stress inoculation, arousal regulation, and resilience. *Frontiers in Behavioral Neuroscience, 3*, 32.

Mackey, A. P., Finn, A. S., Leonard, J. A., Jacoby-Senghor, D. S., West, M. R., Gabrieli, C. F., & Gabrieli, J. D. (2015). Neuroanatomical correlates of the income-achievement gap. *Psychological Science, 26*(6), 925–933. doi:10.1177/0956797615572233.

Marmot, M. G., Bosma, H., Hemingway, H., Brunner, E., & Stansfeld, S. (1997). Contribution of job control and other risk factors to social variations in coronary heart disease incidence. *Lancet, 350*, 235–239.

Mascaro, J. S., Hackett, P. D., & Rilling, J. K. (2013). Testicular volume is inversely correlated with nurturing-related brain activity in human fathers. *Proceedings of the National Academy of Sciences of the United States of America, 110*(39), 15746–15751. doi:10.1073/pnas.1305579110.

Matthews, K. A., & Gallo, L. C. (2011). Psychological perspectives on pathways linking socioeconomic status and physical health. *Annual Review of Psychology, 62*, 501–530.

Matthews, K. A., Kelsey, S. F., Meilahn, E. N., Kuller, L. H., & Wing, R. R. (1989). Educational attainment and behavioral and biological risk factors for coronary heart disease in middle-aged women. *American Journal of Epidemiology, 129*, 1132–1144.

Matthews, K. A., Gallo, L. C., & Taylor, S. E. (2010). Are psychosocial factors mediators of socioeconomic status and health connections? *Annals of the New York Academy of Sciences, 1186*, 146–173.

Maty, S. C., Everson-Rose, S. A., Haan, M. N., Raghunathan, T. E., & Kaplan, G. A. (2005). Education, income, occupation, and the 34-year incidence (1965-99) of type 2 diabetes in the Alameda County study. *International Journal of Epidemiology, 34*, 1274–1281.

Maty, S. C., Lynch, J. W., Raghunathan, T. E., & Kaplan, G. A. (2008). Childhood socioeconomic position, gender, adult body mass index, and incidence of type 2 diabetes mellitus over 34 years in the Alameda County study. *American Journal of Public Health, 98*, 1486–1494.

McDade, T. W., Hawkley, L. C., & Cacioppo, J. T. (2006). Psychosocial and behavioral predictors of inflammation in middle-aged and older adults: The Chicago health, aging, and social relations study. *Psychosomatic Medicine, 68*, 376–381.

McEwen, B. S. (2001). Plasticity of the hippocampus: Adaptation to chronic stress and allostatic load. *Annals of the New York Academy of Sciences, 933*, 265–277.

McEwen, B. S. (2002). *The end of stress as we know it*. Washington, DC: John Henry Press.

McEwen, B. S. (2005). Glucocorticoids, depression, and mood disorders: Structural remodeling in the brain. *Metabolism, 54*, 20–23.

McGrath, J. J., Matthews, K. A., & Brady, S. S. (2006). Individual versus neighborhood socioeconomic status and race as predictors of adolescent ambulatory blood pressure and heart rate. *Social Science and Medicine, 63*, 1442–1453.

McLoyd, V. C. (1998). Socioeconomic disadvantage and child development. *American Psychologist, 53*, 185–204.

Meijer, M., Röhl, J., Bloomfield, K., & Grittner, U. (2012). Do neighborhoods affect individual mortality? A systematic review and meta-analysis of multilevel studies. *Social Science & Medicine, 74*, 1204–1212.

Merkin, S. S., Basurto-Dávila, R., Karlamangla, A., Bird, C. E., Lurie, N., Escarce, J., & Seeman, T. (2009). Neighborhoods and cumulative biological risk profiles by race/ethnicity in a national sample of US adults: NHANES III. *Annals of Epidemiology, 19*, 194–201.

Mervaala, E., Föhr, J., Könönen, M., Valkonen-Korhonen, M., Vainio, P., Partanen, K., et al. (2000). Quantitative MRI of the hippocampus and amygdala in severe depression. *Psychological Medicine, 30*, 117–125.

Metcalfe, A., Lail, P., Ghali, W. A., & Sauve, R. S. (2011). The association between neighbourhoods and adverse birth outcomes: A systematic review and meta-analysis of multi-level studies. *Paediatric and Perinatal Epidemiology, 25*, 236–245.

Milad, M. R., & Rauch, S. L. (2007). The role of the orbitofrontal cortex in anxiety disorders. *Annals of the New York Academy of Sciences, 1121*, 546–561.

Miller, G., & Chen, E. (2007a). Unfavorable socioeconomic conditions in early life presage expression of proinflammatory phenotype in adolescence. *Psychosomatic Medicine, 69*, 402–409.

Miller, G. E., & Chen, E. (2013). The biological residue of childhood poverty. *Child Development Perspectives, 7*, 67–73.

Miller, G. E., Chen, E., Fok, A. K., Walker, H., Lim, A., Nicholls, S., et al. (2009). Low early-life social class leaves a biological residue manifested by decreased glucocorticoid and increased proinflammatory signaling. *Proceedings of the National Academy of Sciences, 106*, 14716–14721.

Miller, G. E., Chen, E., & Parker, K. J. (2011). Psychological stress in childhood and susceptibility to the chronic diseases of aging: Moving toward a model of behavioral and biological mechanisms. *Psychological Bulletin, 137*(6), 959–997.

Miller, G. E., Brody, G. H., Yu, T., & Chen, E. (2014). A family-oriented psychosocial intervention reduces inflammation in low-SES African American youth. *Proceedings of the National Academy of Sciences, 111*, 11287–11292.

Moore, M. E., Stunkard, A., & Srole, L. (1962). Obesity, social class, and mental illness. *Journal of the American Medical Association, 181*, 138–142.

Morgan, J. K., Shaw, D. S., & Forbes, E. E. (2014). Maternal depression and warmth during childhood predict age 20 neural response to reward. *Journal of the American Academy of Child and Adolescent Psychiatry, 53*(108–117), e101.

Musante, L., Treiber, F. A., Kapuku, G. K., Moore, D., Davis, H., & Strong, W. B. (2000). The effects of life events on cardiovascular reactivity to behavioral stressors as a function of socioeconomic status, ethnicity, and sex. *Psychosomatic Medicine, 62*, 760–767.

Muscatell, K. A., Morelli, S. A., Falk, E. B., Way, B. M., Pfeifer, J. H., Galinsky, A. D., et al. (2012). Social status modulates neural activity in the mentalizing network. *NeuroImage, 60*, 1771–1777.

Musser, E. D., Kaiser-Laurent, H., & Ablow, J. C. (2012). The neural correlates of maternal sensitivity: An fMRI study. *Developmental Cognitive Neuroscience, 2*(4), 428–436. doi:10.1016/j.dcn.2012.04.003.

Narita, K., Takei, Y., Suda, M., Aoyama, Y., Uehara, T., Kosaka, H., et al. (2010). Relationship of parental bonding styles with gray matter volume of dorsolateral prefrontal cortex in young adults. *Progress in Neuro-Psychopharmacology & Biological Psychiatry, 34*, 624–631.

Neville, H. J., Stevens, C., Pakulak, E., Bell, T. A., Fanning, J., Klein, S., & Isbell, E. (2013). Family-based training program improves brain function, cognition, and behavior in lower socioeconomic status preschoolers. *Proceedings of the National Academy of Sciences, 110*, 12138–12143.

Newport, D. J., Stowe, Z. N., & Nemeroff, C. B. (2002). Parental depression: Animal models of an adverse life event. *American Journal of Psychiatry, 159*, 1265–1283.

Noble, K. G., Wolmetz, M. E., Ochs, L. G., Farah, M. J., & McCandliss, B. D. (2006). Brain–behavior relationships in reading acquisition are modulated by socioeconomic factors. *Developmental Science, 9*, 642–654.

Noble, K. G., Grieve, S. M., Korgaonkar, M. S., Engelhardt, L. E., Griffith, E. Y., Williams, L. M., & Brickman, A. M. (2012a). Hippocampal volume varies with educational attainment across the life-span. *Frontiers in Human Neuroscience, 6*, 307.

Noble, K. G., Houston, S. M., Kan, E., & Sowell, E. R. (2012b). Neural correlates of socioeconomic status in the developing human brain. *Developmental Science, 15*, 516–527.

Noble, K. G., Houston, S. M., Brito, N. H., Bartsch, H., Kan, E., Kuperman, J. M., et al. (2015). Family income, parental education and brain structure in children and adolescents. *Nature Neuroscience, 18*(5), 773–778. doi:10.1038/nn.3983.

Ochsner, K. N., Silvers, J. A., & Buhle, J. T. (2012). Functional imaging studies of emotion regulation: A synthetic review and evolving model of the cognitive control of emotion. *Annals of the New York Academy of Sciences, 1251*, E1–E24.

Olds, D. L., Eckenrode, J., Henderson, C. R., Jr., Kitzman, H., Powers, J., Cole, R., et al. (1997). Long-term effects of home visitation on maternal life course and child abuse and neglect. *Fifteen-year follow-up of a randomized trial. The Journal of the American Medical Association, 278*, 637–643.

Otero, G. A. (1997). Poverty, cultural disadvantage and brain development: A study of pre-school children in Mexico. *Electroencephalography and Clinical Neurophysiology, 102*, 512–516.

Otero, G., Pliego-Rivero, F., Fernández, T., & Ricardo, J. (2003). EEG development in children with sociocultural disadvantages: A follow-up study. *Clinical Neurophysiology, 114*, 1918–1925.

Owen, N., Poulton, T., Hay, F. C., Mohamed-Ali, V., & Steptoe, A. (2003). Socioeconomic status, C-reactive protein, immune factors, and responses to acute mental stress. *Brain, Behavior, and Immunity, 17*, 286–295.

Panagiotakos, D. B., Pitsavos, C. E., Chrysohoou, C. A., Skoumas, J., Toutouza, M., Belegrinos, D., et al. (2004). The association between educational status and risk factors related to cardiovascular disease in healthy individuals: The ATTICA study. *Annals of Epidemiology, 14*, 188–194.

Patel, N. P., Grandner, M. A., Xie, D., Branas, C. C., & Gooneratne, N. (2010). "sleep disparity" in the population: Poor sleep quality is strongly associated with poverty and ethnicity. *BMC Public Health, 10*, 475.

Petersen, K. L., Marsland, A. L., Flory, J., Votruba-Drzal, E., Muldoon, M. F., & Manuck, S. B. (2008). Community socioeconomic status is associated with circulating interleukin-6 and C-reactive protein. *Psychosomatic Medicine, 70*, 646–652.

Phan, K. L., Orlichenko, A., Boyd, E., Angstadt, M., Coccaro, E. F., Liberzon, I., & Arfanakis, K. (2009). Preliminary evidence of white matter abnormality in the uncinate fasciculus in generalized social anxiety disorder. *Biological Psychiatry, 66*, 691–694.

Philip, N. S., Sweet, L. H., Tyrka, A. R., Price, L. H., Bloom, R. F., & Carpenter, L. L. (2013). Decreased default network connectivity is associated with early life stress in medication-free healthy adults. *European Neuropsychopharmacology, 23*, 24–32.

Pietras, S. A., & Goodman, E. (2013). Socioeconomic status gradients in inflammation in adolescence. *Psychosomatic Medicine, 75*, 442–448.

Piras, F., Cherubini, A., Caltagirone, C., & Spalletta, G. (2011). Education mediates microstructural changes in bilateral hippocampus. *Human Brain Mapping, 32*, 282–289.

Pollitt, R. A., Kaufman, J. S., Rose, K. M., Diez-Roux, A. V., Zeng, D., & Heiss, G. (2007). Early-life and adult socioeconomic status and inflammatory risk markers in adulthood. *European Journal of Epidemiology, 22*, 55–66.

Pollitt, R. A., Kaufman, J. S., Rose, K. M., Diez-Roux, A. V., Zeng, D., & Heiss, G. (2008). Cumulative life course and adult socioeconomic status and markers of inflammation in adulthood. *Journal of Epidemiology & Community Health, 62*, 484–491.

Poulton, R., Caspi, A., Milne, B. J., Thomson, W. M., Taylor, A., Sears, M. R., & Moffitt, T. E. (2002). Association between children's experience of socioeconomic disadvantage and adult health: A life-course study. *The Lancet, 360*, 1640–1645.

Power, C., Manor, O., & Matthews, S. (2003). Child to adult socioeconomic conditions and obesity in a national cohort. *International Journal of Obesity, 27*, 1081–1086.

Power, C., Graham, H., Due, P., Hallqvist, J., Joung, I., Kuhn, D., & Lynch, J. W. (2005). The contribution of childhood and adult socioeconomic position to adult obesity and smoking behavior: An international comparison. *International Journal of Epidemiology, 34*, 335–344.

Price, J. L., & Drevets, W. C. (2012). Neural circuits underlying the pathophysiology of mood disorders. *Trends in Cognitive Sciences, 16*, 61–71.

Radley, J. J., Arias, C. M., & Sawchenko, P. E. (2006). Regional differentiation of the medial prefrontal cortex in regulating adaptive responses to acute emotional stress. *The Journal of Neuroscience, 26*, 12967–12976.

Rainisch, B. K. W., & Upchurch, D. M. (2013). Sociodemographic correlates of allostatic load among a national sample of adolescents: Findings from the National Health and nutrition examination survey, 1999–2008. *Journal of Adolescent Health, 53*, 506–511.

Raizada, R. D., & Kishiyama, M. M. (2010). Effects of socioeconomic status on brain development, and how cognitive neuroscience may contribute to levelling the playing field. *Frontiers in Human Neuroscience, 4*, 3.

Rao, U., Dahl, R. E., Ryan, N. D., Birmaher, B., Williamson, D. E., Giles, D. E., et al. (1996). The relationship between longitudinal clinical course and sleep and cortisol changes in adolescent depression. *Biological Psychiatry, 40*, 474–484.

Rathmann, W., Haastert, B., Giani, G., Koenig, W., Imhof, A., Herder, C., et al. (2006). Is inflammation a causal chain between low socioeconomic status and type 2 diabetes? Results from the KORA survey 2000. *European Journal of Epidemiology, 21*, 55–60.

Repetti, R. L., Taylor, S. E., & Seeman, T. E. (2002). Risky families: Family social environments and the mental and physical health of offspring. *Psychological Bulletin, 128*, 330–366.

Riemann, D., Voderholzer, U., Spiegelhalder, K., Hornyak, M., Buysse, D. J., Nissen, C., et al. (2007). Chronic insomnia and MRI-measured hippocampal volumes: A pilot study. *Sleep, 30*, 955.

Rodrigues, S. M., LeDoux, J. E., & Sapolsky, R. M. (2009). The influence of stress hormones on fear circuitry. *Annual Review of Neuroscience, 32*, 289–313.

Ross, C. E. (2000). Neighborhood disadvantage and adult depression. *Journal of Health and Social Behavior, 41*(2), 177–187.

Roy, A. L., McCoy, D. C., & Raver, C. C. (2014). Instability versus quality: Residential mobility, neighborhood poverty, and children's self-regulation. *Developmental Psychology, 50*(7), 1891–1896.

Sameroff, A. (2010). A unified theory of development: A dialectic integration of nature and nurture. *Child Development, 81*(1), 6–22. doi:10.1111/j.1467-8624.2009.01378.x.

Sariaslan, A., Larsson, H., D'Onofrio, B., Langstrom, N., & Lichtenstein, P. (2014). Childhood family income, adolescent violent criminality and substance misuse: Quasi-experimental total population study. *British Journal of Psychiatry, 205*(4), 286–290.

Schreier, H. M. C., & Chen, E. (2010). Socioeconomic status in one's childhood predicts offspring cardiovascular risk. *Brain, Behavior, and Immunity, 24*, 1324–1331.

Schreier, H. M. C., & Chen, E. (2013). Socioeconomic status and the health of youth: A multilevel, multidomain approach to conceptualizing pathways. *Psychological Bulletin, 139*, 606–654.

Schreier, H. M., Roy, L. B., Frimer, L. T., & Chen, E. (2014). Family chaos and adolescent inflammatory profiles: The moderating role of socioeconomic status. *Psychosomatic Medicine, 76*, 460–467.

Schulz, A. J., Mentz, G., Lachance, L., Johnson, J., Gaines, C., & Israel, B. A. (2012). Associations between socioeconomic status and allostatic load: Effects of neighborhood poverty and tests of mediating pathways. *American Journal of Public Health, 102*, 1706–1714.

Sedlak, A. J., & Broadhurst, D. D. (1996). *Third National Incidence Study of child abuse and neglect*. Washington, DC: US Department of Health and Human Services.

Seeman, T. E., McEwen, B. S., Rowe, J. W., & Singer, B. H. (2001). Allostatic load as a marker of cumulative biological risk: MacArthur studies of successful aging. *Proceedings of the National Academy of Sciences, 98*, 4770–4775.

Seeman, T. E., Crimmins, E., Huang, M., Singer, B. H., Bucur, A., Gruenewald, T., et al. (2004). Cumulative biological risk and socioeconomic differences in mortality: MacArthur studies of successful aging. *Social Science & Medicine, 58*, 1958–1997.

Seeman, T., Merkin, S. S., Crimmins, E., Koretz, B., Charette, S., & Karlamangla, A. (2008). Education, income and ethnic differences in cumulative biological risk profiles in a national sample of US adults: NHANES III (1988–1994). *Social Science & Medicine, 66*, 72–87.

Seeman, T., Epel, E., Gruenewald, T., Karlamangla, A., & Mc Ewen, B. S. (2010a). Socio-economic differentials in peripheral biology: Cumulative allostatic load. *Annals of the New York Academy of Sciences, 1186*, 223–239.

Sheridan, M. A., Sarsour, K., Jutte, D., D'Esposito, M., & Boyce, W. T. (2012). The impact of social disparity on prefrontal function in childhood. *PloS One, 7*, e35744.

Sheridan, M. A., How, J., Araujo, M., Schamberg, M. A., & Nelson, C. A. (2013). What are the links between maternal social status, hippocampal function, and HPA axis function in children? *Developmental Science, 16*, 665–675.

Shin, L. M., Rauch, S. L., & Pitman, R. K. (2006). Amygdala, medial prefrontal cortex, and hippocampal function in PTSD. *Annals of the New York Academy of Sciences, 1071*, 67–79.

Shonkoff, J. P. (2010). Building a new biodevelopmental framework to guide the future of early childhood policy. *Child Development, 81*, 357–367.

Shonkoff, J. P. (2012). Leveraging the biology of adversity to address the roots of disparities in health and development. *Proceedings of the National Academy of Sciences, 109*, 17302–17307.

Shrewsbury, V., & Wardle, J. (2008). Socioeconomic status and adiposity in childhood. *Obesity, 16*, 275–284.

Silverman, M. E., Muennig, P., Liu, X., Rosen, Z., & Goldstein, M. A. (2009). The impact of socioeconomic status on the neural substrates associated with pleasure. *The Open Neuroimaging Journal, 3*, 58–63.

Singer, B. H., & Ryff, C. D. (1999). Hierarchies of life histories and associated health risks. In N. E. Adler, M. Marmot, B. S. McEwen, & J. Stewart (Eds.), *Socioeconomic status and health in industrial nations* (pp. 96–115). New York: New York Academy of Sciences.

Skoe, E., Krizman, J., & Kraus, N. (2013). The impoverished brain: Disparities in maternal education affect the neural response to sound. *The Journal of Neuroscience, 33*, 17221–17231.

Sloan, R. P., Huang, M.-H., Sidney, S., Liu, K., Williams, O. D., & Seeman, T. (2005). Socioeconomic status and health: Is parasympathetic nervous system activity an intervening mechanism? *International Journal of Epidemiology, 34*, 309–315.

Sobal, J., & Stunkard, A. J. (1989). Socioeconomic status and obesity: A review of the literature. *Psychological Bulletin, 105*, 260–275.

Spencer, N. (2000). *Poverty and child health*. Abingdon: Radcliffe Medical Press.

Spielberg, J. M., Galarce, E. M., Ladouceur, C. D., McMakin, D. L., Olino, T. M., Forbes, E. E., et al.

(2015). Adolescent development of inhibition as a function of SES and gender: Converging evidence from behavior and fMRI. *Human Brain Mapping*. doi:10.1002/hbm.22838.

Spruill, T. M., Gerin, W., Ogedegbe, G., Burg, M., Schwartz, J. E., & Pickering, T. G. (2009). Socioeconomic and psychosocial factors mediate race differences in nocturnal blood pressure dipping. *American Journal of Hypertension, 22*, 637–642.

Sripada, R. K., Swain, J. E., Evans, G. W., Welsh, R. C., & Liberzon, I. (2014). Childhood poverty and stress reactivity are associated with aberrant functional connectivity in default mode network. *Neuropsychopharmacology, 39*(9), 2244–2251.

Staff, R. T., Murray, A. D., Ahearn, T. S., Mustafa, N., Fox, H. C., & Whalley, L. J. (2012). Childhood socioeconomic status and adult brain size: Childhood socioeconomic status influences adult hippocampal size. *Annals of Neurology, 71*, 653–660.

Steenari, M.-R., Vuontela, V., Paavonen, E. J., Carlson, S., Fjällberg, M., & Aronen, E. T. (2003). Working memory and sleep in 6-to 13-year-old schoolchildren. *Journal of the American Academy of Child & Adolescent Psychiatry, 42*, 85–92.

Stepnowsky, C. J., Jr., Nelesen, R. A., DeJardin, D., & Dimsdale, J. E. (2004). Socioeconomic status is associated with nocturnal blood pressure dipping. *Psychosomatic Medicine, 66*, 651–655.

Steptoe, A., Feldman, P. J., Kunz, S., Owen, N., Willemsen, G., & Marmot, M. (2002a). Stress responsivity and socioeconomic status: A mechanism for increased cardiovascular disease risk? *European Heart Journal, 23*, 1757–1763.

Steptoe, A., Owen, N., Kunz-Ebrecht, S., & Mohamed-Ali, V. (2002b). Inflammatory cytokines, socioeconomic status, and acute stress responsivity. *Brain, Behavior, and Immunity, 16*, 774–784.

Steptoe, A., Kunz-Ebrecht, S., Owen, N., Feldman, P. J., Rumley, A., Lowe, G. D., & Marmot, M. (2003). Influence of socioeconomic status and job control on plasma fibrinogen responses to acute mental stress. *Psychosomatic Medicine, 65*, 137–144.

Stevens, C., Lauinger, B., & Neville, H. (2009). Differences in the neural mechanisms of selective attention in children from different socioeconomic backgrounds: An event-related brain potential study. *Developmental Science, 12*, 634–646.

Swain, J. E., Kim, P., Spicer, J., Ho, S. S., Dayton, C. J., Elmadih, A., & Abel, K. M. (2014). Approaching the biology of human parental attachment: Brain imaging, oxytocin and coordinated assessments of mothers and fathers. *Brain Research, 1580*, 78–101. doi:10.1016/j.brainres.2014.03.007.

Szyf, M., McGowan, P., & Meaney, M. J. (2008). The social environment and the epigenome. *Environmental and Molecular Mutagenesis, 49*, 46–60.

Tabassum, F., Kumari, M., Rumley, A., Lowe, G., Power, C., & Strachen, D. (2008). Effects of socioeconomic position on inflammatory and hemostatic markers: A life-course analysis in the 1958 British birth cohort. *American Journal of Epidemiology, 167*, 1332–1341.

Taylor, S., Lerner, J., Sage, R., Lehman, B., & Seeman, T. (2004a). Early environments, emotions, responses to stress and health. *Journal of Personality, 72*, 1365–1393.

Taylor, S. E., Lerner, J. S., Sage, R. M., Lehman, B. J., & Seeman, T. E. (2004b). Early environment, emotions, responses to stress, and health. *Journal of Personality, 72*, 1365–1394.

Taylor, S. E., Eisenberger, N. I., Saxbe, D., Lehman, B. J., & Lieberman, M. D. (2006a). Neural responses to emotional stimuli are associated with childhood family stress. *Biological Psychiatry, 60*, 296–301.

Taylor, S. E., Lehman, B. J., Kiefe, C. I., & Seeman, T. E. (2006b). Relationship of early life stress and psychological functioning to adult C-reactive protein in the coronary Artery risk development in young adults study. *Biological Psychiatry, 60*, 819–824.

Taylor, S. E., Burklund, L. J., Eisenberger, N. I., Lehman, B. J., Hilmert, C. J., & Lieberman, M. D. (2008). Neural bases of moderation of cortisol stress responses by psychosocial resources. *Journal of Personality and Social Psychology, 95*, 197–211.

Teipel, S. J., Meindl, T., Wagner, M., Kohl, T., Bürger, K., Reiser, M. F., et al. (2009). White matter microstructure in relation to education in aging and Alzheimer's disease. *Journal of Alzheimer's Disease, 17*, 571–583.

Telzer, E. H., Fuligni, A. J., Lieberman, M. D., & Galván, A. (2013). The effects of poor quality sleep on brain function and risk taking in adolescence. *NeuroImage, 71*, 275–283.

Tomalski, P., Moore, D. G., Ribeiro, H., Axelsson, E. L., Murphy, E., Karmiloff-Smith, A., et al. (2013). Socioeconomic status and functional brain development – Associations in early infancy. *Developmental Science, 16*, 676–687.

Tottenham, N., & Sheridan, M. A. (2009). A review of adversity, the amygdala and the hippocampus: A consideration of developmental timing. *Frontiers in Human Neuroscience, 3*, 68.

Tottenham, N., Hare, T. A., Quinn, B. T., McCarry, T. W., Nurse, M., Gilhooly, T., et al. (2010). Prolonged institutional rearing is associated with atypically large amygdala volume and difficulties in emotion regulation. *Developmental Science, 13*, 46–61.

U.S. Department of Health and Human Services Administration for Children and Families. (2002). Making a difference in the lives of infants and toddlers and their families: The impacts of early head star. Mathematica Policy Research, Inc. Princeton, NJ Under Contract DHHS-105-95-1936.

Uddin, L. Q., Iacoboni, M., Lange, C., & Keenan, J. P. (2007). The self and social cognition: The role of cortical midline structures and mirror neurons. *Trends in Cognitive Sciences, 11*, 153–157.

Ulrich-Lai, Y. M., & Herman, J. P. (2009). Neural regulation of endocrine and autonomic stress responses. *Nature Reviews Neuroscience, 10*, 397–409.

Van Ijzendoorn, M. H. (1992). Intergenerational transmission of parenting: A review of studies in nonclinical populations. *Developmental Review, 12*(1), 76–99.

Wadsworth, M. E., & Berger, L. E. (2006). Adolescents coping with poverty-related family stress: Prospective predictors of coping and psychological symptoms. *Journal of Youth and Adolescence, 35*, 57–70.

Wadsworth, M. E., & Compas, B. E. (2002). Coping with family conflict and economic strain: The adolescent perspective. *Journal of Research on Adolescence, 12*, 243–274.

Wadsworth, M. E., Santiago, C. D., Einhorn, L., Etter, E. M., Rienks, S., & Markman, H. (2011). Preliminary efficacy of an intervention to reduce psychosocial stress and improve coping in low-income families. *American Journal of Community Psychology, 48*, 257–271.

Wadsworth, M. E., Evans, G. W., Grant, K. E., Carter, J. S., & Duffy, S. (in press). Poverty and the development of psychopathology. In D. Chicchetti (Ed.), *Developmental psychopathology* (3rd ed.). New York: Wiley.

Walker, M. P. (2008). Cognitive consequences of sleep and sleep loss. *Sleep Medicine, 9*, S29–S34.

Walker, L., Timmerman, G. M., Kim, M., & Sterling, B. (2002). Relationships between body image and depressive symptoms during postpartum in ethnically diverse, low income women. *Women and Health, 36*(3), 101–121. doi:10.1300/J013v36n03_07.

Walter, H. J., & Hofman, A. (1987). Socioeconomic status, ethnic origin, and risk factors for coronary heart disease in children. *American Heart Journal, 113*, 812–818.

Wamala, S. P., Wolk, A., Schenck-Gustafsson, K., & Orth-Gomér, K. (1997). Lipid profile and socioeconomic status in healthy middle aged women in Sweden. *Journal of Epidemiology and Community Health, 51*, 400–407.

Wamala, S. P., Murray, M. A., Horsten, M., Eriksson, M., Schenck-Gustafsson, K., Hamsten, A., et al. (1999). Socioeconomic status and determinants of hemostatic function in healthy women. *Arteriosclerosis, Thrombosis, and Vascular Biology, 19*, 485–492.

Wanamethee, G., Whincup, P. H., Shaper, G., & Walker, M. (1996). Influence of father's social class on cardiovascular disease in middle-aged men. *The Lancet, 348*, 1254–1255.

Weaver, I. C. G., Cervoni, N., Champagne, F. A., D'Alessio, A. C., Sharma, S., Seckl, J. R., et al. (2004). Epigenetic programming by maternal behavior. *Nature Neuroscience, 7*, 847–854.

Wells, N. M., Evans, G. W., Beavis, A., & Ong, A. D. (2010). Early childhood poverty, cumulative risk exposure, and body mass index trajectories through young adulthood. *American Journal of Public Health, 100*(12), 2507–2512.

Whinnery, J., Jackson, N., Rattanaumpawan, P., & Grandner, M. A. (2013). Short and long sleep duration associated with race/ethnicity, sociodemographics, and socioeconomic position. *Sleep, 37*, 601–611.

Widom, C. S., & Nikulina, V. (2012). Long-term consequences of child neglect in low- income families. In V. Maholmes & R. B. King (Eds.), *The Oxford handbook of poverty and child development* (pp. 68–85). New York: Oxford University Press.

Williams, R. B., Marchuk, D. A., Seigler, I. C., Barefoot, J. C., Helms, M. J., Brummett, B. H., et al. (2008). Childhood socioeconomic status and serotonin transporter gene polymorphism enhance cardiovascular reactivity to mental stress. *Psychosomatic Medicine, 70*, 32–39.

Wilson, T. W., Kaplan, G. A., Kauhanen, J., Cohen, R. D., Wu, M., Salonen, R., & Salonen, J. T. (1993). Association between plasma fibrinogen concentration and five socioeconomic indices in the Kuopio ischemic heart disease risk factor study. *American Journal of Epidemiology, 137*, 292–300.

Wilson, D. K., Kliewer, W., Plybon, L., & Sica, D. A. (2000). Socioeconomic status and blood pressure reactivity in healthy black adolescents. *Hypertension, 35*, 496–500.

Worthman, C. M., & Kuzara, J. (2005). Life history and the early origins of health differentials. *American Journal of Human Biology, 17*(1), 95–112. doi:10.1002/ajhb.20096.

Yanagisawa, K., Masui, K., Furutani, K., Nomura, M., Yoshida, H., & Ura, M. (2013). Family socioeconomic status modulates the coping-related neural response of offspring. *Social Cognitive and Affective Neuroscience, 8*, 617–622.

Zalewski, M., Lengua, L. J., Kiff, C. J., & Fisher, P. A. (2012). Understanding the relation of low income to HPA-axis functioning in preschool children: Cumulative family risk and parenting as pathways to disruptions in cortisol. *Child Psychiatry & Human Development, 43*, 924–942.

Ziol-Guest, K. M., Duncan, G. J., Kalil, A., & Boyce, W. T. (2012). Early childhood poverty, immune-mediated disease processes, and adult productivity. *Proceedings of the National Academy of Sciences, 109*(Suppl 2), 17289–17293.

Health Disparities: A Life Course Health Development Perspective and Future Research Directions

Kandyce Larson, Shirley A. Russ, Robert S. Kahn, Glenn Flores, Elizabeth Goodman, Tina L. Cheng, and Neal Halfon

1 Introduction

Health disparities on the basis of social class and race/ethnicity are apparent across a broad spectrum of health conditions at all stages of development from birth through older age (Tanner 2015). Historically, much of the research on health disparities has been conducted using cross-sectional data, often in adulthood, with the search for explanatory factors focused on current circumstances that might contribute to health status differentials between individuals in different social groups. Life course theories that seek to explain the developmental origins of and lifespan contributors to health status disparities have gained popularity in recent years, and life course-oriented research has proliferated across diverse disciplines spanning the social, health, and biological sciences (Burton-Jeangros et al. 2015; Kuh and Ben-Shlomo 2004). The goals of this chapter are to describe how an integrated life course health development framework can be applied to better understand health disparities, review examples of the types of life course-oriented research completed to date, identify

K. Larson, PhD (✉)
Department of Research, American Academy of Pediatrics, 141 Northwest Point Boulevard, Elk Grove Village, IL 60007, USA
e-mail: kalarson@aap.org

S.A. Russ, MD, MPH
UCLA Center for Healthier Children, Families, and Communities, Department of Pediatrics, David Geffen School of Medicine, UCLA, Los Angeles, CA, USA

R.S. Kahn, MD, MPH
Division of General and Community Pediatrics, Cincinnati Children's Hospital Medical Center, University of Cincinnati College of Medicine, Cincinnati, OH, USA

G. Flores, MD, FAAP
Medica Research Institute, Division of Health Policy and Management, University of Minnesota School of Public Health, Minneapolis, MN, USA

E. Goodman, MD
Division of General Academic Pediatrics, Mass General Hospital for Children, Department of Pediatrics, Harvard Medical School, Boston, MA, USA

T.L. Cheng, MD, MPH
Department of Pediatrics, Johns Hopkins University School of Medicine, Baltimore, MD, USA

N. Halfon, MD, MPH
Department of Pediatrics, David Geffen School of Medicine, UCLA, Los Angeles, CA, USA

Department of Health Policy and Management, Fielding School of Public Health, UCLA, Los Angeles, CA, USA

Department of Public Policy, Luskin School of Public Affairs, UCLA, Los Angeles, CA, USA

Center for Healthier Children, Families, and Communities, UCLA, Los Angeles, CA, USA

N. Halfon et al. (eds.), *Handbook of Life Course Health Development*,
DOI 10.1007/978-3-319-47143-3_20

gaps in knowledge, and provide recommendations for future research aimed at eliminating health disparities in childhood and through the life course. For the purpose of this chapter, the term "health disparities" is used to refer to differences in health status between members in certain population groups with a primary focus on socioeconomic status (SES) and race/ethnicity.

2 Life Course Health Development Framework

Several articles discuss life course issues applied to health disparities (Alwin and Wray 2005; Braveman and Barclay 2009; DC Baltimore Research Center on Child Health Disparities Writing Group 2009; Wadsworth 1997), but principles, terminologies, and definitions of what constitutes a life course perspective vary across disciplines. Emerging from a synthesis of research across diverse disciplines such as life course sociology, lifespan developmental psychology, neuroscience, chronic disease epidemiology, and epigenetics, the life course health development (LCHD) framework provides an integrated account of the dynamic processes whereby diverse social and environmental exposures interact with biological forces from preconception onward to shape health development trajectories (Halfon and Hochstein 2002; Halfon et al. 2014a). Herein we briefly review how the following basic LCHD principles can be applied to health disparities: (1) health is an emergent developmental capacity of individuals that develops continuously across the lifespan; (2) health development is a dynamic nonlinear process occurring in multiple dimensions and at multiple levels and phases; and (3) health development is sensitive to the timing and social structuring of environmental exposures.

Health is an emergent developmental capacity that develops continuously across the lifespan:

Central to the LCHD theory is the notion that health follows a dynamic trajectory of development that begins before birth and extends through the full lifespan. Drawing on positive notions of health like the Ottawa Charter's definition as a capacity that enables the individual to achieve life's goals, health is conceived as an emergent set of capacities that develops across the life course as a result of transactions between the organism and its internal and external environments (National Research Council & Institute of Medicine 2004). Health develops continuously and progresses through phases beginning with the early formation of the organism in the preconception and prenatal periods, followed by the optimization of health and developmental capacity in early childhood through young adulthood, maintenance of health capacity in middle adulthood, and management of decline in health in late adulthood. At any given time an individual may be moving toward greater or lesser degrees of health.

Applied to health disparities, the LCHD framework underscores the importance of examining how individuals in different SES and racial/ethnic groups may manifest varying trajectories of health development and highlights the need to examine not only differences in ill health and disease, but also subclinical health states, health capacity or potential, and a range of health outcomes that vary from poor to very positive.

Health development is a dynamic nonlinear process occurring in multiple dimensions and at multiple levels and phases:

The LCHD framework incorporates an ecological (Bronfenbrenner 1992, 2005) and relational developmental systems perspective (Overton 2013a, b, 2014) to inform how health development is influenced by complex interactions among risk and protective factors across multiple domains and levels of organization over extended time frames. Physical, biochemical, psychological, social, and cultural domains dynamically interact to shape the health development process. The processes of health development also occur at multiple interacting levels of organization. Factors at the social and geopolitical level (e.g., social policy supports for healthy child development, institutional racism) influence factors at the community, family, and individual levels which, in turn, influence health development at the organ, cellular, molecular, and genomic levels. Processes at the molecular/

genomic level can dynamically interact with each other, as well as with factors at the social and geopolitical level or anywhere in between. The search for explanatory factors for disparities in health associated with SES and race/ethnicity has typically focused on downstream factors such as individual health behaviors and access to health care. By incorporating an ecological perspective, the LCHD framework broadens the focus of potential explanatory factors to also include more upstream determinants like social policy- and community-level factors.

From a relational developmental systems perspective, it is not surprising that health risk and protective factors tend to cluster together for individuals from disadvantaged backgrounds. The relations among risk factors, protective factors, and health outcomes are complex, dynamic, interactive, and nonlinear with exponential effects and tipping points. In contrast to traditional epidemiologic approaches that emphasize single risk factors and single health outcomes, a given risk or protective factor or combination of factors can lead to multiple different health outcomes (multifinality), and there are multiple different pathways to the same outcome (equifinality). Social determinants may be nonspecific such that, for example, poverty and disadvantage elicit exposure to stressors that result in multiple suboptimal outcomes across the physical, cognitive, and socioemotional domains. From an LCHD system view, it may not be possible to isolate the effects of any given risk or protective factor from that of others because their influence may be interactive and dependent on the array of other influences present in the system. Relationships among variables also follow dynamic patterns like feedback loops. For example, health may impact SES and SES may in turn impact health.

Health development is sensitive to the timing and social structuring of environmental exposures:

Although exposures at all points in the life course impact health, those early in life are thought to be particularly important, due to heightened biological plasticity and behavioral sensitivity. This allows early experiences and events to condition biological and behavioral response patterns in ways that can be adaptive or maladaptive, influencing health development pathways into adulthood. The early social environment can impact health development over time through biological conditioning, pathway, and cumulative mechanisms (Hertzman and Boyce 2010).

Biological conditioning occurs when experiences early in life quite literally get "under the skin," altering neural, endocrine, immunologic, and even genetic systems that in turn impact the course of human development (Hanson and Gluckman 2014; Hertzman 2012; Hertzman and Boyce 2010). For example, exposure to specific antigens in utero will stimulate specific immune responses, and exposure to maternal depression during specific developmental phases can lead to alterations in the responsiveness of a child's hypothalamic-pituitary-adrenal (HPA) axis as measured by cortisol output and effects. Although the focus has typically centered on the prenatal and early childhood phases, sensitive periods of heightened biological vulnerability to socially patterned exposures also occur at other stages including preconception and adolescence.

Pathway models represent how exposures at one point in the life course impact exposures at another point which in turn impact health. Cumulative models emphasize the additive impact of risk and protective health exposures over time for individuals in different social groups. Chains of risk models combine elements of both to detail how individuals in different social groups can experience varied social, psychosocial, and biological chains of risk and protection that take a cumulative toll on health development across the life course. These models suggest how patterns of socially arrayed and interacting exposures can channel biological and behavioral adaptations in mutually reinforcing ways. For example, a child growing up in a low-income family might experience less-than-optimal language exposure and a low-quality family childcare experience, where he or she watches television or videos all day. That same child is more likely to attend a low-performing elementary school that is not responsive to his or her already depleted developmental potential. As a consequence of this child's disadvantage, not only do they not arrive at school ready to learn, but a lower trajectory is further reinforced by a low-performing school that does not have the capacity to boost this child into a more promising educational pathway and subsequent life course health development trajectory.

In addition to contributing to health disparity development across a lifetime, biological conditioning, pathway, and cumulative mechanisms can influence the transfer of differential health potential across generations. For example, a mother from lower SES origins may incur an accumulation of health-damaging exposures over a lifetime which increases her risk for gestational diabetes, and this in turn, along with differential feeding and health practices associated with SES, may heighten risk for offspring obesity. Despite the LCHD emphasis on the importance of timing and the social structuring of environmental exposures, the framework also details the potential for developmental plasticity and resilience at all phases of development, thus suggesting a need for research examining protective forces leading to more optimal health outcomes for those from disadvantaged social groups.

3 Brief Overview of Research on Health Disparities from an LCHD Perspective

Life course research that is relevant to understanding SES and racial/ethnic health disparities has expanded rapidly across a diverse set of disciplines. A full review of this literature is beyond the scope of this chapter, but the following examples demonstrate the types of research completed to date that begin to show the value of an LCHD perspective applied to health disparities. In the sections that follow, we briefly review research related to life course social disadvantage and adult health, the biology of social adversity, the intergenerational transfer of health disparities, and early intervention studies.

3.1 Life Course Social Disadvantage and Adult Health

A wide variety of international epidemiological investigations from studies spanning multiple decades have established associations between early life social disadvantage and adult health. Low childhood SES shows an independent association with a range of adverse adult health outcomes, including obesity, diabetes, cardiovascular disease, respiratory illness, cognitive decline, functional limitation, shortened telomere length—an indicator of early aging—and early mortality (Johnson and Schoeni 2011; Kamphuis et al. 2012; Packard et al. 2011; Pudrovska et al. 2014; Robertson et al. 2012; Strand et al. 2011). Studies with multiple indicators of SES at different points across the life course generally find that the risk of ill health and disease increases with more continuous lifetime exposure to lower socioeconomic status (Gustafsson et al. 2011; Luo and Waite 2005). Similarly, research examining racial/ethnic disparities in functional limitation, chronic disease onset, and early mortality demonstrates the important role of life course SES in explaining a portion of the black-white gaps in health (Haas and Rohlfsen 2010; Pais 2014; Warner and Hayward 2006). Studies in early adulthood have shown diverging trajectories of general health, body mass index, blood pressure, and respiratory function for those with different SES and racial/ethnic origins (Albrecht and Gordon-Larsen 2013; Jackson et al. 2004; Janicki-Deverts et al. 2012; Sacker et al. 2011).

The complex associations between early social disadvantage and future health states are becoming better understood as research begins to provide plausible pathways for how childhood SES shapes early cognitive, physical, and behavioral development; future educational attainment; and long-term stressful exposures and health risk behaviors that in turn influence health outcomes (Hertzman et al. 2001; Luo and Waite 2005; Schoon et al. 2003; Van de Mheen et al. 1998). Most studies have examined the role of risk factors in producing poorer health outcomes for those in more disadvantaged social groups, but some recent studies have examined how protective factors such as maternal warmth in childhood can buffer the effects of early social disadvantage and promote more optimal long-term health trajectories for those from lower SES backgrounds (Chen et al. 2011; Miller et al. 2011).

3.2 The Biology of Social Adversity

The underlying biological mechanisms that contribute to health disparities are not clearly delineated, but research suggests possible avenues through exposures known to vary by SES and race/ethnicity, such as early psychosocial stress, maternal nutrition and related preconception health states, and environmental toxicant exposure (Thayer and Kuzawa 2011). A rapidly expanding literature on epigenetics has provided clues to potentially plausible mechanisms that might underlie biological conditioning by demonstrating how gene expression can be modified in response to environmental cues (Cole 2014; Hanson and Gluckman 2014; Meaney 2010; Meloni 2014; Misteli 2013). Although much of the early literature on biological conditioning came from animal studies, several recent epidemiological investigations have examined biomarkers of stress and epigenetic processes in human populations.

Possible stress-related pathways between social adversity and health have received a great deal of attention in the literature. Adverse childhood experiences appear to be associated with enduring changes in the nervous, endocrine, and immune systems (Danese and McEwen 2012). Research has shown that childhood exposure to stressors such as abuse and neglect, maternal depression, and socioeconomic disadvantage shows both short- and long-term associations with future elevated HPA axis and autonomic nervous system reactivity, immune-inflammatory dysregulation, metabolic disturbance, and alterations in the structure and function of the regions of the brain that control emotions, attention, learning, and memory (Brand et al. 2010; Dougherty et al. 2013; Goodman et al. 2005, 2007; Miller and Chen 2007, 2013; Pietras and Goodman 2013; Sheridan et al. 2012). Studies that have examined epigenetic marks and DNA methylation patterns of individuals exposed to these types of stressors in childhood suggest a possible role for epigenetic processes in producing long-term alterations in physiological functioning (Anacker et al. 2014; Oberlander et al. 2008; Perroud et al. 2014; Romens et al. 2014; Tehranifar et al. 2013). Over time, alterations that contribute to repeated chronic activation of stress-responsive systems can lead to what has been termed "allostatic load" or cumulative wear and tear across a variety of physiological systems, thereby increasing susceptibility to many different types of chronic conditions at different stages of life such as asthma, learning disorders, psychiatric disorders, stroke, diabetes, and cardiovascular disease (Danese and McEwen 2012; Seeman et al. 2010).

Early research on nutrition-related biological conditioning examined long-term linkages between low birth weight and future metabolic and cardiovascular disease risk that were thought to be attributable to the impact of undernutrition in utero on blood pressure regulation, cholesterol metabolism, and glycemic control, as well as the mismatch between in utero nutrient scarcity and calorie-dense environments after birth (Barker et al. 1993; Hales and Barker 2001). This work has expanded to investigate the role of a wide variety of specific micronutrients at distinctive phases in preconception, lifetime nutrient stores, and maternal metabolic and cardiovascular functioning and disruptions in the maternal-fetal interface, including placental function, uteroplacental blood flow, and fetal metabolism (Gillman 2005; Shapira 2008). For example, maternal gestational diabetes, which is more common in low-income overweight and obese women, is associated with fetal hyperinsulinemia and a higher risk of obesity and impaired glucose tolerance in the growing child (Gillman et al. 2003). Environmental toxicant exposures include a wide range of factors such as smoking and air pollution. Whereas most research has focused on the biological impact of prenatal and postnatal exposures, new studies are beginning to show possible transgenerational effects through epigenetic changes in the germ-line connected with smoke and toxicant exposure which provides an argument for the importance of the preconception health states of parents (Curley et al. 2011; Laubenthal et al. 2012).

3.3 Intergenerational Health Disparities

A growing line of epidemiologic research examines the early emergence of health disparities in childhood and the possible role of intergenerational mechanisms in contributing to early health disparities. Perhaps most suggestive of a role for intergenerational mechanisms is the fact that beginning at birth, large disparities on the basis of SES and race/ethnicity are already apparent for child outcomes like prematurity and birth weight (Coley and Aronson 2013; Gray et al. 2014). Studies that have examined associations of mother's SES in her own childhood suggest long-term linkages with her future prenatal health, health practices, and reproductive outcomes (Astone et al. 2007; Gavin et al. 2011, 2012).

In 2013, the preterm birthrate for African-Americans was 16%, compared with 10% for white women, with a near doubling of risk for low birth weight (13% vs. 7%) and near tripling of risk for very low birth weight (2.9% vs. 1.1%) (Martin et al. 2015). Although a low-income African-American woman who delivers a child 3 months prematurely might traditionally be assessed in terms of her delayed access to prenatal care, through a life course health development perspective, we would also consider her lifelong health status, her reproductive conditioning, the impact of experiences such as her own mother's depression during her infancy, perceived racism, and other toxic and stressful experiences that potentially impact the structure and function of her HPA axis.

A well-established literature indicates that the cumulative impact of stress-related weathering might have a major impact on the health of African-American mothers (Geronimus 1996; Geronimus et al. 2006; Holzman et al. 2009; Love et al. 2010). The weathering hypothesis, which is similar to allostatic load theory, proposes that, on average, the health trajectory of African-American women may begin to deteriorate early in adulthood as a physical consequence of cumulative socioeconomic disadvantage, stress, and racism. In support of this hypothesis, studies show a near fourfold increase in the risk of low birth weight and very low birth weight with increasing age for African-American women but not for white women (Geronimus 1996). Racial/ethnic disparities in measures of women's health, such as obesity, high blood pressure, high cholesterol, and diabetes, also increase with age (Buescher and Mittal 2006; Geronimus et al. 2010; Miranda et al. 2010). Plausible biological pathways between social and environmental stress and birth outcomes include maternal HPA axis functioning, immune-inflammatory response, and vascular function altering uteroplacental flow (Kramer et al. 2011; Kramer and Hogue 2009). Preliminary research examining diverse biomarkers of risk for preterm birth suggests a possible role for pro-inflammatory pathways for African-American mothers (Brou et al. 2012).

Continuing in early childhood, disparities by SES and race/ethnicity are apparent across a wide range of physical, behavioral, and cognitive measures, and these disparities appear to widen over time as children age (American Academy of Pediatrics Committee on Pediatric Research 2010; Flores et al. 2005; Halle et al. 2009; Larson and Halfon 2009; Martinson et al. 2015). A series of studies examining early child health disparities suggest a possible role for intergenerational transfer of risk through factors like parent SES origins and parent health and health practices. For example, studies have shown a possible contributory role for factors including grandparent social class, maternal psychopathology, maternal stress, and both pre- and postnatal maternal smoking in explaining SES gradients in children's early asthma symptoms (Hafkamp-de Groen et al. 2012; Sternthal et al. 2011; Violato et al. 2009). Early parent health and health practices, including maternal mental health status in particular, have also been associated with SES gradients in children's behavior problems, general health status, and obesity (Kahn et al. 2005;

Khanam et al. 2009; Propper et al. 2007). For cognitive outcomes, health factors like mother's preconception obesity, breastfeeding, and depression appear to make a small contribution to early gradients by SES along with a wide variety of additional early risk and protective factors (Dearden et al. 2011; Larson et al. 2015).

3.4 Early Intervention Studies

A range of studies have examined the short- and long-run impact of early childhood interventions on future health and well-being. For example, early nurse home visiting programs for low-income families show long-term improvements for children including better intellectual functioning, fewer behavioral problems, fewer preventable injuries, and less risky health behaviors in adolescence (Olds et al. 1998, 2004, 2007). Parenting interventions in pregnancy and the first year have been shown to improve parent relationships, decrease family stress, reduce biomarkers of stress, and improve executive function and school performance of children (Feinberg et al. 2014, 2015).

Whereas the focus has been more on social and educational outcomes, a number of preschool early intervention studies have tracked participant well-being into adulthood. For example, the Ypsilanti Perry Preschool study showed that an intensive multicomponent preschool program with teacher home visits for low-income African-American children improved adult educational attainment and literacy scores, employment outcomes, family relationships, and health practices (Schweinhart et al. 2005; Schweinhart and Weikart 1993). Several other educationally focused studies have shown similar results (Campbell et al. 2008; Reynolds et al. 2011). Recent follow-up studies of participants in the Chicago Preschool study, the Brookline Early Education Project, and the Abecedarian Project have shown health-focused benefits like more private health insurance coverage, less disability, less depression, better self-rated health, and less cardiovascular and metabolic risk (Campbell et al. 2014; Palfrey et al. 2005; Reynolds et al. 2007). Studies examining neighborhood-level interventions, such as the Moving to Opportunity study, which randomly assigned some low-income families living in high-poverty neighborhoods to receive free housing in more advantaged neighborhoods, have also shown some future improvements in health for participant parents, children, and youth, although results vary by outcome (Leventhal and Dupéré 2011; Ludwig et al. 2013).

Few studies have examined interventions that begin in the preconception period, although one exception is the Magnolia Project, which targets at-risk African-American women of childbearing age who are not yet pregnant and provides multi-component outreach services, risk reduction, well-woman care, health education, stress resilience services, and community development. Early evaluations demonstrate successful risk reduction with improved family planning and reduced STDs for program participants and marginally statistically significant improvements in low birth weight (Biermann et al. 2006; Livingood et al. 2010). Additional research is needed to determine the impact of social and health interventions beginning before pregnancy.

4 Research Limitations and Gaps in Knowledge and Translation to Policy and Practice

Despite rapid advances in research relevant to understanding health disparities from a life course perspective, there are still many limitations and gaps in the knowledge base and the translation to policy and practice. In this section, we provide an overview of some of the important research challenges.

4.1 Existing Data Sets

Much of the developmental and life course research relevant to understanding health disparities has been conducted on data sources not specifically designed for this purpose. Pregnancy and prepregnancy longitudinal data sources are limited, especially in the USA. Few studies contain three-generational data spanning from grandparent to parent to child health. Research on the early origins of racial/ethnic disparities in health has been particularly hindered by the limited availability of pregnancy and prepregnancy cohort studies in the USA, and studies often exclude important groups and subgroups, such as American Indians/Alaska Natives, multiracial individuals, Mexican Americans, or Puerto Ricans, due to sample size issues. There is also a growing immigrant population who are underrepresented in data sets. Despite the many strengths of US longitudinal studies, such as the Early Childhood Longitudinal Study, the National Longitudinal Survey of Youth, and the Panel Study of Income Dynamics, these surveys do not primarily focus on health and have fairly limited direct physical health assessment. Much of the existing knowledge on the early biological origins of future health problems comes from animal studies, in part owing to the lack of available data sources containing both social and biological measures needed to delineate the complex pathways and interactions leading to health disparities.

4.2 Concepts and Measurement

Understanding health disparities requires having well-defined measures of SES; race/ethnicity; potential explanatory factors across the biological, psychological, social, and cultural domains; and health outcomes (American Academy of Pediatrics Committee on Pediatric Research 2015). Measurement complexity begins with SES and race/ethnicity. Measures of SES are often chosen based on data availability instead of conceptual concerns. Standard approaches to categorizing race/ethnicity may need reconsideration with growing diversity and racial mixing, and many have noted the limitation that self-reported race/ethnicity should not be used as a proxy for genetic ancestry in biological studies (Eisenhower et al. 2014; Mersha and Abebe 2015). Several critical life course concepts such as stress, weathering, and allostatic load lack consistent measurement approaches, and little is currently known about how these concepts might best be operationalized at different stages of life including childhood and adolescence. Much work remains to develop adequate biomarkers for health and disease that can be applied consistently across studies. In the area of stress research, for example, short-term fluctuations in cortisol levels can complicate research findings, and hair cortisol, telomere length, and multifactorial approaches to the choice of biomarkers have been suggested (McEwen 2015; Sauvé et al. 2007). Social contributors to health disparities like discrimination, acculturation, or immigration stress also lack standardized measurement approaches. For health outcome measurement, limited measures of positive health states are available at different life stages. Measures are often not available in diverse languages and have not been tested for equivalence across socioeconomically and culturally diverse groups.

4.3 Statistical Methods

Recent years have seen rapid advancement in the application of sophisticated statistical methods such as longitudinal growth models to examine health status trajectories, multilevel modeling to examine contextual influences on health, and decomposition methodologies to sort through the contribution of multiple risk and protective factors at different life stages to future health status disparities. Despite progress, there are some fundamental limitations with standard statistical approaches that stem from a reductionist approach aimed at isolating the "causal" impact of a given variable. Studies that examine mediators or contributors to health status disparities using standard regression approaches are inherently limited by possible residual confounding and may miss important connections if associations among risk factors, protective factors, and health outcomes are complex, interactive, reciprocal, or nonlinear. New methods of analysis stemming from dynamic systems approaches have the potential to complement more traditional analyses and incorporate many different aspects of the complexity inherent in the LCHD framework, but to date there has been limited application to the field of health disparities (Diez Roux 2007, 2011; Speybroeck et al. 2013). Dynamic systems methods include a range of computational approaches that can be used to model dynamic interactions between individuals and their environments, and complex phenomenon including feedback loops and nonlinear relations.

4.4 LCHD Framework

Comparing the current state of research on the early origins and development of disparities in health with existing life course frameworks reveals several limitations and gaps in knowledge. While the LCHD framework emphasizes the critical importance of structural and upstream policy- and community-level determinants of health status disparities, most research has focused on more downstream factors, such as health behaviors or health care. With the growing popularity of research on toxic stress, epigenetics, and the role of early pre- or postnatal programming of future health states, some have cautioned that the field should not lose sight of the broader structural forces like racism, environmental inequity, and decaying housing structures that can impact health across the life course (Geronimus 2013). There is also limited research available on resilience and the role of protective factors in promoting positive health trajectories for individuals in disadvantaged social groups. Most studies have investigated poor health and disease outcomes rather than functional health trajectories and biomarkers of future health potential. Overall, knowledge of the complex mechanisms whereby biological, environmental, social, and behavioral factors interact over extended time frames to produce disparities in population health is limited, and many critical questions remain unanswered, such as the ongoing debate about the importance of early vs. later events and the timing and mutability of critical or sensitive periods in human development.

4.5 Intervention and Translation

Despite the recent upsurge in research activity on health disparities in the USA, progress toward meeting the US Department of Health and Human Services' Healthy People goals of reducing or eliminating health disparities has been slow, and gaps for socially disadvantaged groups are, in fact, increasing for certain key health indicators such as infant, childhood, and adult mortality (Singh and Kogan 2007; Singh and Siahpush 2002). Indeed, a recent analysis of US data on trends in child health disparities documented that children from ethnic minority families continue to experience multiple disparities in medical and oral health and health care, with most disparities persisting over time and some new disparities arising (Flores and Lin 2013). Currently, few evidence-based practice guidelines are available to address specific health disparities, and there is no fully coordinated national policy effort to address disparities. Although there is a growing trend focusing on translational research to integrate knowledge from basic science studies into practical solutions in the clinical, practice, population health, and policy realms, much of the past research on health disparities has had a greater focus on documenting disparities than providing actionable interventions.

The evidence base on effective health interventions is limited in several ways. Many of the long-term follow-up studies tracking early childhood interventions have primarily been conducted in the field of education and therefore lack a specific focus on health outcomes or on the biological and behavioral adaptive mechanisms that might explain long-term outcomes. Few interventions have been designed to target specific social and health risk and protective factors prior to pregnancy, and we still know very little about the best time to intervene to influence specific health outcomes. Interventions for racial/ethnic health disparities are often not specifically designed to meet the unique needs of individuals in diverse cultural groups, and few studies have examined community-level interventions or the impact of interventions designed to optimize health instead of reverse risk factors. Despite these limitations, a range of early intervention studies demonstrate promise for improving future well-being for children in disadvantaged home environments, and yet these have not been implemented in practice on a broad scale in the USA, indicating a need for policy change and a greater focus on scaling up proven strategies in community-based practice.

5 Recommendations and Considerations for a New Life Course Health Disparities Research Agenda

Addressing disparities in health in the population at large will require attention to the parental, early childhood, and adolescent antecedents of later inequality in health. New research on health disparities from an LCHD perspective will require transdisciplinary collaboration and training in order to advance unified theoretical concepts and measurement approaches and to further research on the complex interplay between social and biological forces in producing health disparities across lifetimes and generations. Similar collaborative efforts are needed to translate knowledge from basic science studies into interventions, programs, and policies that can optimize long-term health development trajectories for individuals from disadvantaged social groups.

Based on our review of the literature related to LCHD and health disparities, we propose the following as priorities for building a new life course health development research agenda:

Research Priorities

Development and funding of studies that:

1. Investigate the underlying biological processes that contribute to health disparities in human populations.
2. Examine protective factors, resilience, and positive health outcomes for individuals from disadvantaged backgrounds.
3. Examine parental preconception health and other intergenerational mechanisms that may contribute to early health disparities.
4. Continue to investigate the dynamic multi-level contributors to health status disparities across the life course with a particular emphasis on upstream determinants.
5. Compare the impact of the timing of intervention at various life stages for selected health outcomes.
6. Shift beyond minimizing risk and preventing poor health with interventions aimed at optimizing health and developmental potential.
7. Address barriers to reliable widespread implementation of evidence-based interventions.
8. Use place-based and community-based participatory research methodologies.
9. Develop and test new policies and policy interventions at the local, state, and national levels to reduce health disparities across the life course.

Data and Methods Development Priorities

1. Shift to focus on longitudinal as opposed to cross-sectional studies.
2. Combine sociodemographic, biologic, and genetic data and link across families.
3. Develop new measures of health and possible contributors to health status disparities validated across different racial/ethnic groups.
4. Adopt a complex systems perspective.
5. Improve training in transdisciplinary research and advanced statistical modeling.

Translational Priorities

1. Identify existing knowledge that is ripe for translation to practice and policy.
2. Align new basic science research with translational approaches to reducing health disparities.

Challenges and Opportunities for Building a New Life Course Health Development Research Agenda to Reduce Health Disparities

1. Need for more funding by NIH, MCHB, and other federal agencies and national foundations for life course-oriented health disparities research.
2. Capitalizing on new momentum, interest, and recognition of the importance of social determinants and toxic stress for health disparities in childhood and across the life course.

Below, we describe these priority areas in greater detail.

5.1 Research Priorities

Development and funding of studies that:

1. Investigate the underlying biological processes that contribute to health disparities in human populations.

Population, regional, and clinic-based studies are needed to examine the underlying biological processes that contribute to health disparities in human populations. Studies should examine biological processes impacting health at all stages including birth outcomes, child and adolescent health, and adult health. Priority research areas include the investigation of novel biomarkers of health and disease for populations that are particularly affected by disparate health outcomes, the contribution of stress and allostatic load to health disparities at various life stages, studies of gene-environment interactions and epigenetic mechanisms of health disparities, identification of genetic susceptibility to disease among minority populations, and studies examining gestational/prenatal physiology and its impact on future health disparities.

2. Examine protective factors, resilience, and positive health outcomes for individuals from disadvantaged backgrounds.

Despite lower economic resources overall, certain racial/ethnic and immigrant groups such as Mexican Americans and blacks born outside the USA show surprisingly good outcomes for certain health indicators like child birth weight and longevity (Buekens et al. 2000; Lariscy et al. 2015; Singh and Hiatt 2006). Likewise, many individuals from lower SES origins manage to overcome the odds and have very good health and well-being in adulthood. More research is needed to not only identify individuals with exceptional health resilience, but also to better understand the health development pathways that lead to a more resilient phenotype. Studies that examine the cultural, social, and psychological resources that can lead to thriving and better-than-expected health outcomes for individuals from disadvantaged social groups should receive priority. Examples of recent research in this area include studies showing long-term benefits of maternal warmth, child optimism, and shift-and-persist strategies for future health and well-being of individuals from lower SES origins (Chen et al. 2011, 2012; Khullar et al. 2011; Miller et al. 2011).

3. Examine parental preconception health and other intergenerational mechanisms that may contribute to early health disparities.

The LCHD framework points to the importance of addressing the early manifestations of health disparities and intergenerational transfer of health risk and potential. Studies are needed to examine the mechanisms contributing to disparities in birth outcomes, biomarkers of future health potential, and early childhood health. Priority areas include three-generation studies that examine how social factors from parent's own childhood may influence their future health, well-being, and parenting practices with consequences for offspring health and the role of parental preconception health status. In the biological realm, an important area of research is the role of the placenta as a regulator of the intrauterine environment and programming agent of future health potential and how this ties in with the social, physiological, and nutritional status of the mother. This might include studies that focus on the potential to boost placental functioning so that the placenta might serve as a resilience generator in what might otherwise be a risky intrauterine environment.

4. Continue to investigate the dynamic multilevel contributors to health status disparities across the life course with a particular emphasis on upstream determinants.

Future research should investigate the multilevel contributors to health status disparities over the life course with a particular emphasis on upstream structural factors and neighborhood-level determinants. Multilevel studies can help examine the impact of neighborhood-level factors on health disparities by SES and race/ethnicity.

Also needed are studies that incorporate longitudinal or life course measures of neighborhood and environmental exposures. At the population level, studies are needed to examine the policy, built environment, and social environment exposures that contribute to geographic differentials in rates of health and disease. To the greatest extent possible, research studies that examine lifelong contributors to SES and racial/ethnic health disparities should investigate the importance of timing of key environmental and social exposures.

In addition to empirical studies that are designed to measure the impact of specific environmental exposures on biological conditioning and health, existing data can be used to develop life course health development models using new agent-based and dynamic systems methods. These modeling approaches can represent dynamic interactions and complex multilevel influences over varying time horizons in ways that may be difficult using standard statistical approaches.

5. Compare the impact of the timing of intervention at various life stages for selected health outcomes.

Longitudinal studies are needed that investigate the impact of interventions at various life stages on future health outcomes. The preconception period is an important area for investigation. Many questions remain about the possible benefit of and best timing for interventions in the preconception period for improving birth outcomes and early childhood health in disparity populations. Studies in childhood should examine social interventions designed to alter specific short-term health outcomes (e.g., asthma or early stress reactivity) in at-risk populations as well as more long-term health and well-being outcomes into adulthood. For example, can population-level interventions, like teaching young children yoga and other mindfulness techniques, serve to "inoculate" them against elevations in allostatic load due to stressful and chaotic family environments? Questions about the best timing for intervention are important. Cost-effectiveness studies can be used to compare the value of interventions at different life stages. In addition to interventions at the individual level, studies that intervene on the multilevel determinants of health (e.g., neighborhood-level interventions) will also be important.

6. Shift beyond minimizing risk and preventing poor health with interventions aimed at optimizing health and developmental potential.

Most prior intervention studies have been designed to alter risk behaviors in disparity populations. Few have examined if interventions designed to build individual, family, or community strengths can optimize health trajectories. As an example, a recent study showed that a psychosocial intervention focused on building family strengths and youth competencies was successful in improving biomarkers of health in early adulthood for African-American youth in lower SES families (Miller et al. 2014). To date, we know very little about the potential of interventions that seek to promote optimal health, nutrition, fitness, parenting, and social, psychological, and community resources in health disparity populations. Intervention studies to address the SES gradient in health will also need to focus on optimizing health across the full SES spectrum, including not just low but also middle SES groups. Prior studies have often focused on the problems of poverty and marginal risk without adequate attention given to individuals in more middle-income groups, who also exhibit suboptimal health outcomes and could benefit from interventions designed to boost their health and developmental potential.

7. Address barriers to reliable widespread implementation of evidence-based interventions.

Some evidence-based interventions for improving health and well-being exist but have not yet been implemented in community-based practice on a broad scale. Some existing health interventions have not yet been tested for specific cultural groups such as Native American populations. Dissemination and implementation research is needed to help spread knowledge about existing evidence-based interventions, adapt interventions for use with specific cultural or regional groups, and test the effectiveness and cost-efficiency of different interventions in community and practice settings.

8. Use place-based and community-based participatory research methodologies.

Community-based participatory research involving collaboration and partnership between community leaders, residents, and academic researchers can be used to help design interventions that are responsive to local needs and promote policy advocacy in disadvantaged neighborhoods. Recently, many place-based efforts have taken a life course approach in attempt to improve cradle-to-career trajectories with attention paid to what works in different kinds of communities and microenvironments. Community-based researchers in Canada have used a new set of measures including the Early Development Instrument (administered from ages 4–6 years) and the Middle Development Instrument (administered at ages 9–11 years) to collect developmentally and dimensionally consistent measures of health development (Janus and Offord 2007; Schonert-Reichl et al. 2013). This life course-oriented population data collection can be used to map and track health and well-being at different developmental stages, and to engage community members in identifying early development outcomes and how they relate with local community services and risk and protective factors, and in turn developing action strategies for systems- and community-level improvements.

9. Develop and test new policies and policy interventions at the local, state, and national levels to reduce health disparities across the life course.

Translational research is needed to transform knowledge from basic science research into new policies designed to reduce health disparities through the life course. As new social and health policies are devised, research will need to monitor impact and outcomes. For new policy development, computer simulation studies provide an important and, to date, underutilized methodology that policymakers can use to test the likely outcomes of policy changes to address the more upstream determinants of health (e.g., changes in income or education) and test what-if scenarios about the likely impact of alternative early intervention strategies targeting different early risk and protective factors for future health outcomes.

5.2 Data and Methods Development Priorities

1. Shift to focus on longitudinal as opposed to cross-sectional studies.

The USA should invest in longitudinal studies that start prior to conception and continue through the life course. Ideally, these longitudinal studies should also collect data on the subsequent generation of children. Despite the difficulties implementing a large-scale study like the US National Children's Study, efforts must continue to investigate new methodologies to make a population-based cohort study like this possible, and smaller-scale regional studies collecting social and biological data on critical life course topics should also receive priority. Existing cross-sectional data sets, such as the National Health and Nutritional Examination Surveys (NHANES) and National Survey of Children's Health (NSCH), could be enhanced by adding longitudinal components, linkages with vital statistics and other available data sources, and retrospective measures of parent's life course health, socioeconomic status, perceived racism, and risk and protective exposures. Ongoing longitudinal studies, such as the Early Childhood Longitudinal Study (ECLS), the National Longitudinal Survey of Youth (NLSY), and Panel Study of Income Dynamics, could be altered to include better health measures. Where possible, researchers should also explore innovative options for expanding and cross-linking data contained in sources like electronic health records.

2. Combine sociodemographic, biologic, and genetic data and link across families.

Longitudinal and cross-generational studies are needed that integrate sociodemographic, biologic, and genetic data. Ongoing and future epidemiologic studies used to investigate health disparities should be examined for opportunities to add biological and genetic data that might contribute to our understanding of life course processes. For example, new studies to investigate social disparities in preterm birth and early childhood health outcomes could add biological information such as maternal blood, DNA, urine, and placenta samples and fetal amniotic fluid and cord blood samples. Likewise, new biorepositories designed to study specific health conditions and built with connections to clinical and questionnaire or epidemiologic data may provide useful opportunities for future health disparities research.

3. Develop new measures of health and possible contributors to health status disparities validated across different racial/ethnic groups.

At present, there are few valid and reliable measures of health not measuring disease, disability, or dysfunction. New measures of health in childhood, adolescence, and adulthood are needed that can be used to study functional health trajectories and positive health outcomes. This will require better conceptualization of health and health development from a measurement implementation standpoint and creation of multimodal health development profiles that include self/parent report, clinical measures, and biomarkers. Research designed to develop standardized measures of critical life course concepts like stress, weathering, and allostatic load at different life stages should also have priority. New measures should be validated for use across different cultural groups.

4. Adopt a complex systems perspective.

Complex systems approaches are gaining popularity in public health. Systems approaches can be used to investigate complex phenomenon including feedback loops, nonlinear dynamics, and macro-level patterns that emerge from the interactions of factors at different levels of organization. Applied to health disparities, complex systems approaches may help broaden our understanding of processes like the reciprocal relations among genes and environments across the life course, feedback mechanisms between health and social standing over time, dynamic interactions between people and places in producing health disparities, and the long-term consequences of intervening on structural determinants of health such as early childhood educational opportunities (Diez Roux 2011).

5. Improve training in transdisciplinary research and advanced statistical modeling.

Advancing life course-focused research on health disparities will require collaboration among researchers from many different specialties and fields of study. Traditional academic training has been discipline specific, but new modes of training are needed to provide exposure to different research methods used across diverse fields of study. Applied researchers will need advanced training in the interpretation and use of sophisticated statistical methods ranging from longitudinal growth modeling to dynamic systems approaches. Social scientists will need to incorporate knowledge of concepts and methods traditionally used in the biological sciences and vice versa.

5.3 Translational Priorities

1. Identify existing knowledge that is ripe for translation to practice and policy.

Application of existing knowledge from life course-oriented health disparities research to practice and policy is still in the early stages of development. Efforts are needed to identify existing knowledge that is ready for translation into concrete practice guidelines, programs, and policies aimed at alleviating disparities in health in childhood and across the life course. For example, life course-oriented research focused on optimizing health development could be used to redesign the health-care system with a greater emphasis on promoting optimal health throughout the life course, from birth through death, instead of focusing on disease management (Halfon et al. 2014b, c). Continued efforts are needed to identify ways in which life course research on health disparities can be integrated into medical, social welfare, education, and public health practice and social and health policies at the local, state, and national levels.

2. Align new basic science research with translational approaches to reducing health disparities.

Historically, research on health disparities has often been conducted in isolated academic institutions without primary attention to how the knowledge gained from basic science studies might be applied in practice or policy. New modes of research involving transdisciplinary collaboration, academic and community partnerships, and new translational research science centers that conduct studies across the continuum from basic science discovery to their application in clinical, practice, and policy settings may help ensure that new discoveries are translated into concrete and practical solutions to promote health for disadvantaged populations.

5.4 Challenges and Opportunities for Building a New Life Course Health Development Research Agenda to Reduce Health Disparities

1. Need for more funding by the National Institutes of Health (NIH), Maternal and Child Health Bureau (MCHB), and other federal agencies and national foundations for life course-oriented health disparities research.

Funding declines and tight competition for federal research grants offer a challenge to moving forward in the many areas needed to advance life course-oriented health disparities research. More funding by NIH, MCHB, and other federal agencies and national foundations is needed for life course-oriented health disparities research with a special emphasis on intervention and translational research designed to reduce health disparities in childhood and through the life course. The LCHD framework emphasizes the importance of addressing disparities from preconception onward; understanding that early exposure to multiple stresses may produce biological changes that are difficult, if not impossible, to eradicate later; and acknowledging that adults who experienced the most extreme disparities as young children are likely to develop the worst health in adulthood and require the most expensive interventions. Life course-oriented health disparities research provides an opportunity for large potential savings associated with the development of strategies to intervene early in optimizing human health.

2. Capitalizing on new momentum, interest, and recognition of the importance of social determinants and toxic stress for health disparities in childhood and across the life course.

Despite challenges, interest in life course-oriented health disparities research has gained rapid popularity in recent years. For example, interest in research on the lifelong health consequences of early adversity has rapidly spread and is currently being translated to changes in medical, public health, education, and child welfare practice including the development and expansion of new trauma-informed systems of care. Several states now track and monitor rates of adverse childhood exposures. Just over a decade ago, life course models were relatively marginal in the Maternal and Child Health (MCH) field but are now foundational in guiding MCH research, practice, and policy (Lu 2014). Within pediatrics, attention to poverty and the social determinants of children's health and development has also grown in response to increasing rates of US family poverty. The emerging research on poverty, toxic stress, and epigenetics has been used to frame new American Academy of Pediatrics (AAP) recommendations concerning screening for early adversity and social risk at primary care visits and building pediatric connections with social and educational services in the community to help promote optimal health and development for all children (American Academy of Pediatrics Committee on Psychosocial Aspects of Child and Family Health, Committee on Early Childhood, Adoption, and Dependent Care, & Section on Developmental and Behavioral Pediatrics 2012). In recent years, both the AAP and the Academic Pediatric Association have placed poverty and child health as a top policy focus.

This growth in attention to social determinants and life course health is encouraging. Research innovation and enhanced support for translational science approaches will be needed to devise and implement practical solutions to address life course health disparities in practice and community settings.

6 Conclusions

Although researchers, policymakers, and clinicians have recognized the existence of health disparities for decades, the importance of social, developmental, and health inequalities in the early years as contributors to lifelong differences in health status has only recently been understood. Attempts to address health disparities in the US population that do not include a strong focus on the early years are, at best, misguided and, at worst, likely to fail. At the national level, difficult conversations are needed to address research priorities and strategies for targeting social inequalities. At the same time, life course health development models suggest that there may be new solutions to long-standing problems. Rather than ever-increasing spending on expensive mid- and late-life therapeutic interventions, many of the answers to persistent disparities in health outcomes could lie in better social conditions and health development services for young children.

References

Albrecht, S. S., & Gordon-Larsen, P. (2013). Ethnic differences in body mass index trajectories from adolescence to adulthood: A focus on Hispanic and Asian subgroups in the United States. *PLOS ONE, 8*(9), e72983. doi:10.1371/journal.pone.0072983.

Alwin, D. F., & Wray, L. A. (2005). A life-span developmental perspective on social status and health. *The Journals of Gerontology Series B: Psychological Sciences and Social Sciences, 60*(2), S7–S14. doi:10.1093/geronb/60.Special_Issue_2.S7.

American Academy of Pediatrics Committee on Pediatric Research. (2010). Technical report – racial and ethnic disparities in the health and health care of children. *Pediatrics, 125*(4), e979–e1020. doi:10.1542/peds.2010-0188.

American Academy of Pediatrics Committee on Pediatric Research. (2015). Race, ethnicity, and socioeconomic status in research on child health. *Pediatrics, 135*(1), e225–e237. doi:10.1542/peds.2014-3109.

American Academy of Pediatrics Committee on Psychosocial Aspects of Child and Family Health, Committee on Early Childhood, Adoption, and Dependent Care, & Section on Developmental and Behavioral Pediatrics. (2012). Early childhood adversity, toxic stress, and the role of the pediatrician: Translating developmental science into lifelong health. *Pediatrics, 129*(1), e224–e231. doi:10.1542/peds.2011-2662.

Anacker, C., O'Donnell, K. J., & Meaney, M. J. (2014). Early life adversity and the epigenetic programming of hypothalamic-pituitary-adrenal function. *Dialogues in Clinical Neuroscience, 16*(3), 321–333.

Astone, N. M., Misra, D., & Lynch, C. (2007). The effect of maternal socio-economic status throughout the lifespan on infant birthweight. *Paediatric and Perinatal Epidemiology, 21*(4), 310–318. doi:10.1111/j.1365-3016.2007.00821.x.

Barker, D. J. P., Godfrey, K. M., Gluckman, P. D., Harding, J. E., Owens, J. A., & Robinson, J. S. (1993). Fetal nutrition and cardiovascular disease in adult life. *The Lancet, 341*(8850), 938–941. doi:10.1016/0140-6736(93)91224-A.

Biermann, J., Dunlop, A. L., Brady, C., Dubin, C., & Brann, A. (2006). Promising practices in preconception care for women at risk for poor health and pregnancy outcomes. *Maternal and Child Health Journal, 10*(1), 21–28. doi:10.1007/s10995-006-0097-8.

Brand, S. R., Brennan, P. A., Newport, D. J., Smith, A. K., Weiss, T., & Stowe, Z. N. (2010). The impact of maternal childhood abuse on maternal and infant HPA axis function in the postpartum period. *Psychoneuroendocrinology, 35*(5), 686–693. doi:10.1016/j.psyneuen.2009.10.009.

Braveman, P., & Barclay, C. (2009). Health disparities beginning in childhood: A life-course perspective. *Pediatrics, 124*, S163–S175. doi:10.1542/peds.2009-1100D.

Bronfenbrenner, U. (1992). Ecological systems theory. In R. Vasta (Ed.), *Six theories of child development: Revised formulations and current issues* (pp. 187–249). London: Jessica Kingsley Publishers.

Bronfenbrenner, U. (2005). *Making human beings human: Bioecological perspectives on human development*. Thousand Oaks: Sage.

Brou, L., Almli, L., Pearce, B., Bhat, G., Drobek, C., Fortunato, S., & Menon, R. (2012). Dysregulated biomarkers induce distinct pathways in preterm birth. *BJOG: An International Journal of Obstetrics & Gynaecology, 119*(4), 458–473. doi:10.1111/j.1471-0528.2011.03266.x.

Buekens, P., Notzon, F., Kotelchuck, M., & Wilcox, A. (2000). Why do Mexican Americans give birth to few low birth-weight infants? *American Journal of Epidemiology, 152*(4), 347–351. doi:10.1093/aje/152.4.347.

Buescher, P. A., & Mittal, M. (2006). Racial disparities in birth outcomes increase with maternal age: Recent data from North Carolina. *North Carolina Medical Journal, 67*(1), 16–20.

Burton-Jeangros, C., Cullati, S., Sacker, A., & Blane, D. (Eds.). (2015). *A life course perspective on health trajectories and transitions*. New York: Springer.

Campbell, F. A., Wasik, B. H., Pungello, E., Burchinal, M., Barbarin, O., Kainz, K., et al. (2008). Young adult outcomes of the Abecedarian and CARE early childhood educational interventions. *Early Childhood Research Quarterly, 23*(4), 452–466. doi:10.1016/j.ecresq.2008.03.003.

Campbell, F. A., Conti, G., Heckman, J. J., Moon, S. H., Pinto, R., Pungello, E., & Pan, Y. (2014). Early childhood investments substantially boost adult health. *Science, 343*(6178), 1478–1485. doi:10.1126/science.1248429.

Chen, E., Miller, G. E., Kobor, M. S., & Cole, S. W. (2011). Maternal warmth buffers the effects of low early-life socioeconomic status on pro-inflammatory signaling in adulthood. *Molecular Psychiatry, 16*(7), 729–737. doi:10.1038/mp.2010.53.

Chen, E., Miller, G. E., Lachman, M. E., Gruenewald, T. L., & Seeman, T. E. (2012). Protective factors for adults from low-childhood socioeconomic circumstances: The benefits of shift-and-persist for allostatic load. *Psychosomatic Medicine, 74*(2), 178–186. doi:10.1097/PSY.0b013e31824206fd.

Cole, S. W. (2014). Human social genomics. *PLOS Genetics, 10*(8), e1004601. doi:10.1371/journal.pgen.1004601.

Coley, S. L., & Aronson, R. E. (2013). Exploring birth outcome disparities and the impact of prenatal care utilization among North Carolina teen mothers. *Women's Health Issues, 23*(5), e287–e294. doi:10.1016/j.whi.2013.06.004.

Curley, J. P., Mashoodh, R., & Champagne, F. A. (2011). Epigenetics and the origins of paternal effects. *Hormones and Behavior, 59*(3), 306–314. doi:10.1016/j.yhbeh.2010.06.018.

Danese, A., & McEwen, B. S. (2012). Adverse childhood experiences, allostasis, allostatic load, and age-related disease. *Physiology & Behavior, 106*(1), 29–39. doi:10.1016/j.physbeh.2011.08.019.

DC Baltimore Research Center on Child Health Disparities Writing Group. (2009). Starting early: A life-course perspective on child health disparities – Research recommendations. *Pediatrics, 124*(3), S257–S261. doi:10.1542/peds.2009-1100O.

Dearden, L., Sibieta, L., & Sylva, K. (2011). The socio-economic gradient in early child outcomes: Evidence from the Millennium Cohort Study. *Longitudinal and Life Course Studies, 2*, 19–40.

Diez Roux, A. V. (2007). Integrating social and biologic factors in health research: A systems view. *Annals of Epidemiology, 17*(7), 569–574. doi:10.1016/j.annepidem.2007.03.001.

Diez Roux, A. V. (2011). Complex systems thinking and current impasses in health disparities research. *American Journal of Public Health, 101*(9), 1627–1634. doi:10.2105/AJPH.2011.300149.

Dougherty, L. R., Tolep, M. R., Smith, V. C., & Rose, S. (2013). Early exposure to parental depression and parenting: Associations with young offspring's stress physiology and oppositional behavior. *Journal of Abnormal Child Psychology, 41*(8), 1299–1310. doi:10.1007/s10802-013-9763-7.

Eisenhower, A., Suyemoto, K., Lucchese, F., & Canenguez, K. (2014). "Which box should I check?": Examining standard check box approaches to measuring race and ethnicity. *Health Services Research, 49*(3), 1034–1055. doi:10.1111/1475-6773.12132.

Feinberg, M. E., Jones, D. E., Roettger, M. E., Solmeyer, A., & Hostetler, M. L. (2014). Long-term follow-up of a randomized trial of family foundations: Effects on children's emotional, behavioral, and school adjustment. *Journal of Family Psychology, 28*(6), 821–831. doi:10.1037/fam0000037.

Feinberg, M. E., Roettger, M. E., Jones, D. E., Paul, I. M., & Kan, M. L. (2015). Effects of a psychosocial couple-based prevention program on adverse birth outcomes. *Maternal and Child Health Journal, 19*(1), 102–111. doi:10.1007/s10995-014-1500-5.

Flores, G., & Lin, H. (2013). Trends in racial/ethnic disparities in medical and oral health, access to care, and use of services in US children: Has anything changed over the years? *International Journal for Equity in Health, 12*, 10. doi:10.1186/1475-9276-12-10.

Flores, G., Olson, L., & Tomany-Korman, S. C. (2005). Racial and ethnic disparities in early childhood health and health care. *Pediatrics, 115*(2), e183–e193. doi:10.1542/peds.2004-1474.

Gavin, A. R., Hill, K. G., Hawkins, J. D., & Maas, C. (2011). The role of maternal early-life and later-life risk factors on offspring low birth weight: Findings from a three-generational study. *The Journal of Adolescent Health, 49*(2), 166–171. doi:10.1016/j.jadohealth.2010.11.246.

Gavin, A. R., Thompson, E., Rue, T., & Guo, Y. (2012). Maternal early life risk factors for offspring birth weight: Findings from the Add Health study. *Prevention Science, 13*(2), 162–172. doi:10.1007/s11121-011-0253-2.

Geronimus, A. T. (1996). Black/white differences in the relationship of maternal age to birthweight: A population-based test of the weathering hypothesis. *Social Science & Medicine, 42*(4), 589–597. doi:10.1016/0277-9536(95)00159-X.

Geronimus, A. T. (2013). Deep integration: Letting the epigenome out of the bottle without losing sight of the structural origins of population health. *American Journal of Public Health, 103*(S1), S56–S63. doi:10.2105/AJPH.2013.301380.

Geronimus, A. T., Hicken, M., Keene, D., & Bound, J. (2006). "Weathering" and age patterns of allostatic load scores among blacks and whites in the United States. *American Journal of Public Health, 96*(5), 826–833. doi:10.2105/AJPH.2004.060749.

Geronimus, A. T., Hicken, M. T., Pearson, J. A., Seashols, S. J., Brown, K. L., & Cruz, T. D. (2010). Do US black women experience stress-related accelerated biological aging? *Human Nature, 21*(1), 19–38. doi:10.1007/s12110-010-9078-0.

Gillman, M. W. (2005). Developmental origins of health and disease. *The New England Journal of Medicine, 353*(17), 1848–1850. doi:10.1056/NEJMe058187.

Gillman, M. W., Rifas-Shiman, S., Berkey, C. S., Field, A. E., & Colditz, G. A. (2003). Maternal gestational diabetes, birth weight, and adolescent obesity. *Pediatrics, 111*(3), e221–e226. doi:10.1542/peds.111.3.e221.

Goodman, E., McEwen, B. S., Huang, B., Dolan, L. M., & Adler, N. E. (2005). Social inequalities in biomarkers of cardiovascular risk in adolescence. *Psychosomatic Medicine, 67*(1), 9–15. doi:10.1097/01.psy.0000149254.36133.1a.

Goodman, E., Daniels, S. R., & Dolan, L. M. (2007). Socioeconomic disparities in insulin resistance: Results from the Princeton School District Study. *Psychosomatic Medicine, 69*(1), 61–67. doi:10.1097/01.psy.0000249732.96753.8f.

Gray, S. C., Edwards, S. E., Schultz, B. D., & Miranda, M. L. (2014). Assessing the impact of race, social factors and air pollution on birth outcomes: A population-based study. *Environmental Health: A Global Access Science Source, 13*(1), 4. doi:10.1186/1476-069X-13-4.

Gustafsson, P. E., Janlert, U., Theorell, T., Westerlund, H., & Hammarström, A. (2011). Socioeconomic status over the life course and allostatic load in adulthood: Results from the Northern Swedish Cohort. *Journal of Epidemiology and Community Health, 65*(11), 986–992. doi:10.1136/jech.2010.108332.

Haas, S., & Rohlfsen, L. (2010). Life course determinants of racial and ethnic disparities in functional health trajectories. *Social Science & Medicine, 70*(2), 240–250. doi:10.1016/j.socscimed.2009.10.003.

Hafkamp-de Groen, E., van Rossem, L., de Jongste, J. C., Mohangoo, A. D., Moll, H. A., Jaddoe, V. W. V., et al. (2012). The role of prenatal, perinatal and postnatal factors in the explanation of socioeconomic inequalities in preschool asthma symptoms: The Generation R Study. *Journal of Epidemiology and Community Health, 66*(11), 1017–1024. doi:10.1136/jech-2011-200333.

Hales, C. N., & Barker, D. J. (2001). The thrifty phenotype hypothesis. *British Medical Bulletin, 60*, 5–20.

Halfon, N., & Hochstein, M. (2002). Life course health development: An integrated framework for developing health, policy, and research. *Milbank Quarterly, 80*(3), 433–479. doi:10.1111/1468-0009.00019.

Halfon, N., Larson, K., Lu, M., Tullis, E., & Russ, S. (2014a). Lifecourse health development: Past, present and future. *Maternal and Child Health Journal, 18*(2), 344–365. doi:10.1007/s10995-013-1346-2.

Halfon, N., Long, P., Chang, D. I., Hester, J., Inkelas, M., & Rodgers, A. (2014b). Applying a 3.0 transformation framework to guide large-scale health system reform. *Health Affairs, 33*(11), 2003–2011. doi:10.1377/hlthaff.2014.0485.

Halfon, N., Wise, P. H., & Forrest, C. B. (2014c). The changing nature of children's health development: New challenges require major policy solutions. *Health Affairs, 33*(12), 2116–2124. doi:10.1377/hlthaff.2014.0944.

Halle, T., Forry, N., Hair, E., Perper, K., Wandner, L., Wessel, J., & Vick, J. (2009). *Disparities in early learning and development: Lessons from the Early Childhood Longitudinal Study – Birth Cohort (ECLS-B)*. Washington, DC: Child Trends.

Hanson, M. A., & Gluckman, P. D. (2014). Early developmental conditioning of later health and disease: Physiology or pathophysiology? *Physiological Reviews, 94*(4), 1027–1076. doi:10.1152/physrev.00029.2013.

Hertzman, C. (2012). Putting the concept of biological embedding in historical perspective. *Proceedings of the National Academy of Sciences, 109*(2), 17160–17167. doi:10.1073/pnas.1202203109.

Hertzman, C., & Boyce, T. (2010). How experience gets under the skin to create gradients in developmental health. *Annual Review of Public Health, 31*(1), 329–347. doi:10.1146/annurev.publhealth.012809.103538.

Hertzman, C., Power, C., Matthews, S., & Manor, O. (2001). Using an interactive framework of society and lifecourse to explain self-rated health in early adulthood. *Social Science & Medicine, 53*(12), 1575–1585. doi:10.1016/S0277-9536(00)00437-8.

Holzman, C., Eyster, J., Kleyn, M., Messer, L. C., Kaufman, J. S., Laraia, B. A., et al. (2009). Maternal weathering and risk of preterm delivery. *American Journal of Public Health, 99*(10), 1864–1871. doi:10.2105/AJPH.2008.151589.

Jackson, B., Kubzansky, L. D., Cohen, S., Weiss, S., & Wright, R. J. (2004). A matter of life and breath: Childhood socioeconomic status is related to young adult pulmonary function in the CARDIA study. *International Journal of Epidemiology, 33*(2), 271–278. doi:10.1093/ije/dyh003.

Janicki-Deverts, D., Cohen, S., Matthews, K. A., & Jacobs, D. R. (2012). Sex differences in the association of childhood socioeconomic status with adult blood pressure change: The CARDIA study. *Psychosomatic Medicine, 74*(7), 728–735. doi:10.1097/PSY.0b013e31825e32e8.

Janus, M., & Offord, D. R. (2007). Development and psychometric properties of the Early Development Instrument (EDI): A measure of children's school readiness. *Canadian Journal of Behavioural Science, 39*(1), 1–22. doi:10.1037/cjbs2007001.

Johnson, R. C., & Schoeni, R. F. (2011). Early-life origins of adult disease: National longitudinal population-based study of the United States. *American Journal of Public Health, 101*(12), 2317–2324. doi:10.2105/AJPH.2011.300252.

Kahn, R. S., Wilson, K., & Wise, P. H. (2005). Intergenerational health disparities: Socioeconomic status, women's health conditions, and child behavior problems. *Public Health Reports, 120*(4), 399–408. doi:10.1177/003335490512000407.

Kamphuis, C. B., Turrell, G., Giskes, K., Mackenbach, J. P., & van Lenthe, F. J. (2012). Socioeconomic inequalities in cardiovascular mortality and the role of childhood socioeconomic conditions and adulthood risk factors: A prospective cohort study with 17-years of follow up. *BMC Public Health, 12*(1), 1045. doi:10.1186/1471-2458-12-1045.

Khanam, R., Nghiem, H. S., & Connelly, L. B. (2009). Child health and the income gradient: Evidence from Australia. *Journal of Health Economics, 28*(4), 805–817. doi:10.1016/j.jhealeco.2009.05.001.

Khullar, D., Oreskovic, N. M., Perrin, J. M., & Goodman, E. (2011). Optimism and the socioeconomic status gradient in adolescent adiposity. *The Journal of Adolescent Health, 49*(5), 553–555. doi:10.1016/j.jadohealth.2011.04.003.

Kramer, M. R., & Hogue, C. R. (2009). What causes racial disparities in very preterm birth? A biosocial perspective. *Epidemiologic Reviews, 31*, 84–98. doi:10.1093/ajerev/mxp003.

Kramer, M. R., Hogue, C. J., Dunlop, A. L., & Menon, R. (2011). Preconceptional stress and racial disparities in preterm birth: An overview. *Acta Obstetricia Et Gynecologica Scandinavica, 90*(12), 1307–1316. doi:10.1111/j.1600-0412.2011.01136.x.

Kuh, D., & Ben-Shlomo, Y. (Eds.). (2004). *A life course approach to chronic disease epidemiology*. New York: Oxford University Press.

Lariscy, J. T., Hummer, R. A., & Hayward, M. D. (2015). Hispanic older adult mortality in the United States: New estimates and an assessment of factors shaping the Hispanic paradox. *Demography, 52*(1), 1–14. doi:10.1007/s13524-014-0357-y.

Larson, K., & Halfon, N. (2009). Family income gradients in the health and health care access of US children. *Maternal and Child Health Journal, 14*(3), 332–342. doi:10.1007/s10995-009-0477-y.

Larson, K., Russ, S. A., Nelson, B. B., Olson, L. M., & Halfon, N. (2015). Cognitive ability at kindergarten entry and socioeconomic status. *Pediatrics, 135*(2), e440–e448. doi:10.1542/peds.2014-0434.

Laubenthal, J., Zlobinskaya, O., Poterlowicz, K., Baumgartner, A., Gdula, M. R., Fthenou, E., et al. (2012). Cigarette smoke-induced transgenerational alterations in genome stability in cord blood of human F1 offspring. *The FASEB Journal, 26*(10), 3946–3956. doi:10.1096/fj.11-201194.

Leventhal, T., & Dupéré, V. (2011). Moving to opportunity: Does long-term exposure to "low-poverty" neighborhoods make a difference for adolescents? *Social Science & Medicine, 73*(5), 737–743. doi:10.1016/j.socscimed.2011.06.042.

Livingood, W. C., Brady, C., Pierce, K., Atrash, H., Hou, T., & Bryant, T. (2010). Impact of pre-conception health care: Evaluation of a social determinants focused intervention. *Maternal and Child Health Journal, 14*(3), 382–391. doi:10.1007/s10995-009-0471-4.

Love, C., David, R. J., Rankin, K. M., & Collins, J. W. (2010). Exploring weathering: Effects of lifelong economic environment and maternal age on low birth weight, small for gestational age, and preterm birth in African-American and white women. *American Journal of Epidemiology*, 127–134. doi:10.1093/aje/kwq109.

Lu, M. C. (2014). Improving maternal and child health across the life course: Where do we go from here? *Maternal and Child Health Journal, 18*(2), 339–343. doi:10.1007/s10995-013-1400-0.

Ludwig, J., Duncan, G. J., Gennetian, L. A., Katz, L. F., Kessler, R. C., Kling, J. R., & Sanbonmatsu, L. (2013). Long-term neighborhood effects on low-income families: Evidence from Moving to Opportunity. *The American Economic Review, 103*(3), 226–231. doi:10.1257/aer.103.3.226.

Luo, Y., & Waite, L. J. (2005). The impact of childhood and adult SES on physical, mental, and cognitive well-being in later life. *The Journals of Gerontology Series B: Psychological Sciences and Social Sciences, 60*(2), S93–S101. doi:10.1093/geronb/60.2.S93.

Martin, J. A., Hamiltion, B. E., Osterman, M. J. K., Curtin, S. C., & Mathews, T. J. (2015). Births: Final data for 2013. *National Vital Statistics Reports, 64*(1), 1–65.

Martinson, M. L., McLanahan, S., & Brooks-Gunn, J. (2015). Variation in child body mass index patterns by race/ethnicity and maternal nativity status in the United States and England. *Maternal and Child Health Journal, 19*(2), 373–380. doi:10.1007/s10995-014-1519-7.

McEwen, B. S. (2015). Biomarkers for assessing population and individual health and disease related to stress and adaptation. *Metabolism, 64*(3 Suppl 1), S2–S10. doi:10.1016/j.metabol.2014.10.029.

Meaney, M. J. (2010). Epigenetics and the biological definition of gene x environment interactions.

Child Development, 81(1), 41–79. doi:10.1111/j.1467-8624.2009.01381.x.

Meloni, M. (2014). The social brain meets the reactive genome: Neuroscience, epigenetics and the new social biology. *Frontiers in Human Neuroscience, 8*, 309. doi:10.3389/fnhum.2014.00309.

Mersha, T. B., & Abebe, T. (2015). Self-reported race/ethnicity in the age of genomic research: Its potential impact on understanding health disparities. *Human Genomics, 9*(1), 1. doi:10.1186/s40246-014-0023-x.

Miller, G. E., & Chen, E. (2007). Unfavorable socioeconomic conditions in early life presage expression of proinflammatory phenotype in adolescence. *Psychosomatic Medicine, 69*(5), 402–409. doi:10.1097/PSY.0b013e318068fcf9.

Miller, G. E., & Chen, E. (2013). The biological residue of childhood poverty. *Child Development Perspectives, 7*(2), 67–73. doi:10.1111/cdep.12021.

Miller, G. E., Lachman, M. E., Chen, E., Gruenewald, T. L., Karlamangla, A. S., & Seeman, T. E. (2011). Pathways to resilience: Maternal nurturance as a buffer against the effects of childhood poverty on metabolic syndrome at midlife. *Psychological Science, 22*(12), 1591–1599. doi:10.1177/0956797611419170.

Miller, G. E., Brody, G. H., Yu, T., & Chen, E. (2014). A family-oriented psychosocial intervention reduces inflammation in low-SES African American youth. *Proceedings of the National Academy of Sciences, 111*(31), 11287–11292. doi:10.1073/pnas.1406578111.

Miranda, M. L., Swamy, G. K., Edwards, S., Maxson, P., Gelfand, A., & James, S. (2010). Disparities in maternal hypertension and pregnancy outcomes: Evidence from North Carolina, 1994–2003. *Public Health Reports, 125*(4), 579–587. doi:10.1177/003335491012500413.

Misteli, T. (2013). The cell biology of genomes: Bringing the double helix to life. *Cell, 152*(6), 1209–1212. doi:10.1016/j.cell.2013.02.048.

National Research Council & Institute of Medicine, Committee on Evaluation of Children's Health, Board on Children, Youth, & Families, Division of Behavioral & Social Sciences & Education. (2004). *Children's health, the nation's wealth: Assessing and improving child health*. Washington, DC: The National Academies Press.

Oberlander, T. F., Weinberg, J., Papsdorf, M., Grunau, R., Misri, S., & Devlin, A. M. (2008). Prenatal exposure to maternal depression, neonatal methylation of human glucocorticoid receptor gene (NR3C1) and infant cortisol stress responses. *Epigenetics, 3*(2), 97–106. doi:10.4161/epi.3.2.6034.

Olds, D. L., Henderson, C. R., Cole, R., Eckenrode, J., Kitzman, H., Luckey, D., et al. (1998). Long-term effects of nurse home visitation on children's criminal and antisocial behavior: 15-year follow-up of a randomized controlled trial. *JAMA, 280*(14), 1238–1244. doi:10.1001/jama.280.14.1238.

Olds, D. L., Kitzman, H., Cole, R., Robinson, J., Sidora, K., Luckey, D. W., et al. (2004). Effects of nurse home-visiting on maternal life course and child development: Age 6 follow-up results of a randomized trial. *Pediatrics, 114*(6), 1550–1559. doi:10.1542/peds.2004-0962.

Olds, D. L., Kitzman, H., Hanks, C., Cole, R., Anson, E., Sidora-Arcoleo, K., et al. (2007). Effects of nurse home visiting on maternal and child functioning: Age 9 follow-up of a randomized trial. *Pediatrics, 120*(4), e832–e845. doi:10.1542/peds.2006-2111.

Overton, W. F. (2013a). A new paradigm for developmental science: Relationism and relational-developmental systems. *Applied Developmental Science, 17*(2), 94–107. doi:10.1080/10888691.2013.778717.

Overton, W. F. (2013b). Relationism and relational developmental systems: A paradigm for developmental science in the post-Cartesian era. *Advances in Child Development and Behavior, 44*, 21–64.

Overton, W. F. (2014). Relational developmental systems and developmental science: A focus on methodology. In P. C. M. Molenaar & R. M. Lerner (Eds.), *Handbook of developmental systems theory and methodology* (pp. 19–65). New York: The Guilford Press.

Packard, C. J., Bezlyak, V., McLean, J. S., Batty, G. D., Ford, I., Burns, H., et al. (2011). Early life socioeconomic adversity is associated in adult life with chronic inflammation, carotid atherosclerosis, poorer lung function and decreased cognitive performance: A cross-sectional, population-based study. *BMC Public Health, 11*, 42. doi:10.1186/1471-2458-11-42.

Pais, J. (2014). Cumulative structural disadvantage and racial health disparities: The pathways of childhood socioeconomic influence. *Demography, 51*(5), 1729–1753. doi:10.1007/s13524-014-0330-9.

Palfrey, J. S., Hauser-Cram, P., Bronson, M. B., Warfield, M. E., Sirin, S., & Chan, E. (2005). The Brookline Early Education Project: A 25 year follow-up study of a family-centered early health and development intervention. *Pediatrics, 116*(1), 144–152. doi:10.1542/peds.2004-2515.

Perroud, N., Dayer, A., Piguet, C., Nallet, A., Favre, S., Malafosse, A., & Aubry, J. (2014). Childhood maltreatment and methylation of the glucocorticoid receptor gene NR3C1 in bipolar disorder. *The British Journal of Psychiatry: The Journal of Mental Science, 204*(1), 30–35. doi:10.1192/bjp.bp.112.120055.

Pietras, S. A., & Goodman, E. (2013). Socioeconomic status gradients in inflammation in adolescence. *Psychosomatic Medicine, 75*(5), 442–448. doi:10.1097/PSY.0b013e31828b871a.

Propper, C., Rigg, J., & Burgess, S. (2007). Child health: Evidence on the roles of family income and maternal mental health from a UK birth cohort. *Health Economics, 16*(11), 1245–1269. doi:10.1002/hec.1221.

Pudrovska, T., Logan, E. S., & Richman, A. (2014). Early-life social origins of later-life body weight: The role of socioeconomic status and health behaviors over the life course. *Social Science Research, 46*, 59–71. doi:10.1016/j.ssresearch.2014.02.007.

Reynolds, A. J., Temple, J. A., Ou, S., Robertson, D., Mersky, J., Topitzea, J., & Niles, M. D. (2007). Effects of a school-based, early childhood intervention on adult health and well-being: A 19-year follow-up of low-income families. *Archives of Pediatrics & Adolescent Medicine, 161*(8), 730–739. doi:10.1001/archpedi.161.8.730.

Reynolds, A. J., Temple, J. A., Ou, S., Arteaga, I. A., & White, B. A. B. (2011). School-based early childhood education and age-28 well-being: Effects by timing, dosage, and subgroups. *Science, 333*(6040), 360–364. doi:10.1126/science.1203618.

Robertson, T., Batty, G. D., Der, G., Green, M. J., McGlynn, L. M., McIntyre, A., et al. (2012). Is telomere length socially patterned? Evidence from the West of Scotland Twenty-07 Study. *PLOS ONE, 7*(7), e41805. doi:10.1371/journal.pone.0041805.

Romens, S. E., McDonald, J., Svaren, J., & Pollak, S. D. (2014). Associations between early life stress and gene methylation in children. *Child Development*. doi:10.1111/cdev.12270.

Sacker, A., Worts, D., & McDonough, P. (2011). Social influences on trajectories of self-rated health: Evidence from Britain, Germany, Denmark and the USA. *Journal of Epidemiology and Community Health, 65*(2), 130–136. doi:10.1136/jech.2009.091199.

Sauvé, B., Koren, G., Walsh, G., Tokmakejian, S., & Uum, S. H. V. (2007). Measurement of cortisol in human hair as a biomarker of systemic exposure. *Clinical & Investigative Medicine, 30*(5), 183–191. doi:10.25011/cim.v30i5.2894.

Schonert-Reichl, K. A., Guhn, M., Gadermann, A. M., Hymel, S., Sweiss, L., & Hertzman, C. (2013). Development and validation of the Middle Years Development Instrument (MDI): Assessing children's well-being and assets across multiple contexts. *Social Indicators Research, 114*, 345–369. doi:10.1007/s11205-012-0149-y.

Schoon, I., Sacker, A., & Bartley, M. (2003). Socio-economic adversity and psychosocial adjustment: A developmental-contextual perspective. *Social Science & Medicine, 57*(6), 1001–1015. doi:10.1016/S0277-9536(02)00475-6.

Schweinhart, L. J., & Weikart, D. P. (1993). Success by empowerment: The High/Scope Perry Preschool Study through age 27. *Young Children, 49*(1), 54–58.

Schweinhart, L. J., Montie, J., Xiang, Z., Barnett, W. S., Belfield, C. R., & Nores, M. (2005). *Lifetime effects: The High/Scope Perry Preschool study through age 40*. Yipsilanti: High/Scope Press.

Seeman, T., Epel, E., Gruenewald, T., Karlamangla, A., & McEwen, B. S. (2010). Socio-economic differentials in peripheral biology: Cumulative allostatic load. *Annals of the New York Academy of Sciences, 1186*, 223–239. doi:10.1111/j.1749-6632.2009.05341.x.

Shapira, N. (2008). Prenatal nutrition: A critical window of opportunity for mother and child. *Women's Health, 4*(6), 639–656. doi:10.2217/17455057.4.6.639.

Sheridan, M. A., Sarsour, K., Jutte, D., D'Esposito, M., & Boyce, T. W. (2012). The impact of social disparity on prefrontal function in childhood. *PLOS ONE, 7*(4), e35744. doi:10.1371/journal.pone.0035744.

Singh, G. K., & Hiatt, R. A. (2006). Trends and disparities in socioeconomic and behavioural characteristics, life expectancy, and cause-specific mortality of native-born and foreign-born populations in the United States, 1979–2003. *International Journal of Epidemiology, 35*(4), 903–919. doi:10.1093/ije/dyl089.

Singh, G. K., & Kogan, M. D. (2007). Widening socioeconomic disparities in US childhood mortality, 1969–2000. *American Journal of Public Health, 97*(9), 1658–1665. doi:10.2105/AJPH.2006.087320.

Singh, G. K., & Siahpush, M. (2002). Increasing inequalities in all-cause and cardiovascular mortality among US adults aged 25–64 years by area socioeconomic status, 1969–1998. *International Journal of Epidemiology, 31*(3), 600–613.

Speybroeck, N., Van Malderen, C., Harper, S., Müller, B., & Devleesschauwer, B. (2013). Simulation models for socioeconomic inequalities in health: A systematic review. *International Journal of Environmental Research and Public Health, 10*(11), 5750–5780. doi:10.3390/ijerph10115750.

Sternthal, M. J., Coull, B. A., Chiu, Y. M., Cohen, S., & Wright, R. J. (2011). Associations among maternal childhood socioeconomic status, cord blood IgE levels, and repeated wheeze in urban children. *The Journal of Allergy and Clinical Immunology, 128*(2), 337–345. e1. doi:10.1016/j.jaci.2011.05.008.

Strand, B. H., Cooper, R., Hardy, R., Kuh, D., & Guralnik, J. (2011). Lifelong socioeconomic position and physical performance in midlife: Results from the British 1946 birth cohort. *European Journal of Epidemiology, 26*(6), 475–483. doi:10.1007/s10654-011-9562-9.

Tanner, V. (Ed.). (2015). *Health disparities and inequalities in the United States: Selected reports*. New York: Nova Science Publishers Inc..

Tehranifar, P., Wu, H., Fan, X., Flom, J. D., Ferris, J. S., Cho, Y. H., et al. (2013). Early life socioeconomic factors and genomic DNA methylation in mid-life. *Epigenetics, 8*(1), 23–27. doi:10.4161/epi.22989.

Thayer, Z. M., & Kuzawa, C. W. (2011). Biological memories of past environments: Epigenetic pathways to health disparities. *Epigenetics, 6*(7), 798–803. doi:10.4161/epi.6.7.16222.

Van de Mheen, H., Stronks, K., Looman, C. W. N., & Mackenbach, J. P. (1998). Does childhood socioeconomic status influence adult health through behavioural factors? *International Journal of Epidemiology, 27*(3), 431–437. doi:10.1093/ije/27.3.431.

Violato, M., Petrou, S., & Gray, R. (2009). The relationship between household income and childhood respiratory health in the United Kingdom. *Social Science & Medicine, 69*(6), 955–963. doi:10.1016/j.socscimed.2009.06.036.

Wadsworth, M. E. (1997). Health inequalities in the life course perspective. *Social Science & Medicine, 44*(6), 859–869.

Warner, D. F., & Hayward, M. D. (2006). Early-life origins of the race gap in men's mortality. *Journal of Health and Social Behavior, 47*(3), 209–226. doi:10.1177/002214650604700302.

Part V
Methodological Approaches

Core Principles of Life Course Health Development Methodology and Analytics

Todd D. Little

The success of life course health development research is tied intimately to the measures and methods used. In this paper, I highlight a number of measurement, design, and analysis issues that researchers must consider in order to execute the highest-quality research possible. Many of the ideas presented here reflect the significant advances in statistical techniques, software functionality, and computational power, all of which afford researchers today with more options and more generalizable procedures than was possible even a decade or so ago.

The face of life course health development research in general is changing at a rapid pace. Because of the advances, teams of researchers with at least one dedicated methodology and analytics expert are needed to manage and integrate the theoretical with the methodological. The advanced techniques, improved estimation algorithms, and user-accessible software/hardware developments signal what I see as a paradigm shift in how life science research will be conducted now and in the future. Although techniques such as structural equation modeling (SEM), multilevel modeling (MLM), and mixture distribution modeling have permeated the research agenda in many fields, the capability of these tools has hardly been fully utilized. In this chapter, I intend to highlight (meaning space won't allow me the luxury of detail) many of the issues that life course health development researchers should be aware of. For more details and examples, I will refer to various sources along the way. More attention and examples to this material can also be found in Little (2013 and in Little et al. 2006a).

1 Measurement Issues

Manifest variable analytics remain popular despite their many flaws and unmet assumptions (e.g., measures are assumed to be without error, measurement invariance is assumed, indirect effects are not possible, items are supposed to be tau-equivalent and locally independent, and so on; McDonald 1999). As a result, scientific progress is mired in these untenable characteristics of classical methods. In order to progress with

Partial support for this project was provided by grant NSF 1053160 (Todd D. Little & Wei Wu, co-PIs) and by the Institute for Measurement, Methodology, Analysis, and Policy (Todd D. Little, director) and Todd Little's Stats Camp (statscamp.org). Correspondence concerning this work should be addressed to Todd D. Little, Institute for Measurement, Methodology, Analysis, and Policy, Texas Tech University, Lubbock, TX 79409. E-mail: yhat@statscamp.org. Web: immap.educ.ttu.edu and statscamp.org. Todd D. Little owns and receives remuneration from Yhat Enterprises (yhatenterprises.com), which runs educational workshops such as Stats Camp (statscamp.org), and processes his royalties and his fees for consulting on statistics and methods with life science researchers.

T.D. Little (✉)
Texas Tech University, Lubbock, TX, USA
e-mail: Todd.D.Little@ttu.edu; yhat@statscamp.org

N. Halfon et al. (eds.), *Handbook of Life Course Health Development*,
DOI 10.1007/978-3-319-47143-3_21

prudent alacrity, life course health development researchers must embrace and leverage the power and sophisticated elegance of latent variable approaches. Structural equation modeling (SEM) is an overarching and general methodology that I will emphasize in this discussion; SEM is predicated on a measurement model that defines and represents latent variables (see Brown 2014, for details of the confirmatory factor analysis measurement model that underlies SEM models).

In this regard, latent variables are represented as the reliable information in a set of indicators – that is, measurement error is removed along with its attenuating and biasing effects. Removing measurement error is desirable because, when not removed, it decreases correlations and effect size estimates (e.g., Cohen's *d*) and inflates measures of dispersion, which biases any statistical tests when tested using classical procedures. When measurement error is removed, the reliable construct-related information about a set of indicators can be tested for measurement (factorial) invariance across age cohorts, measurement occasions, and life contexts. In addition to these positive features of the measurement model, SEM also affords levels of complexity that can be tied directly to theoretical models. For example, models of mediation, moderation, additive effects, and nested dependencies can be specified and easily estimated (see Little 2013, for details, and see below). Before addressing these modeling features of SEM, I turn first to a couple key issues in the measurement model of an SEM: refining measurement, modeling latent variables, factorial invariance and DIF (differential item functioning) testing, and the use of item parcels.

1.1 Refining Measurement

The constructs of life course health development are, for the most part, continuous because they reflect the continuous change across the life span. Unfortunately, researchers seem to disregard this idea when they construct response scales to measure the continuous scaled constructs. The most common scale used in behavioral science research is the Likert scale which was developed over 80 years ago (Likert 1932). It was developed to make measurement of continuous constructs easy to accomplish during the era of paper and pencil administration and laborious data entry. Other methods of measuring constructs are much more efficient and, in fact, can be more intuitive than Likert scaling. Continuous number lines using endpoint anchors (visual analog scales), for example, are easy to understand and typically provide greater information regarding the nature of the construct. Such measures are interval, not ordinal, in nature (Funke and Reips 2012; Reips and Funke 2008; Reips 2006). Such scales have also been around for a long time, but the burden of coding and the error-prone tendency of data entry made Likert scaling more appealing – that is, until now. With computer technology developed to the level that it has become, the use of rich electronically captured responses should become the norm. In this regard, methods for modeling responses, such as item response theory (IRT), will be less useful than continuous variable approaches such as SEM.

A future direction of life course health development is in the area of measurement development. Measures and scales that have been developed in the life sciences are often not designed to optimally measure change processes. The standards of measurement development to establish and model life course trajectories must be modified to include more emphasis on being sensitive to change. Because many scales of constructs such as self-efficacy, self-esteem, well-being, attitudes, and beliefs rely on Likert scales, such scales measure relative levels against an unspecified and unknowable standard. This lack of clarity can easily corrode the foundations of a measure when applied longitudinally.

For example, take a question like "in the past 2 weeks how much have you felt glad?" If I reply 7 on a 1–7 scale, the basis of my rating is unclear. It could be relative to my usual self, relative to my friends, or relative to the particular circumstances of the past 2 weeks. Also, the variability of my happiness in the past 2 weeks is not clear. Am I trending upward, trending downward, or about the same as usual? Such ambiguities of measurement make analyzing life course trajectories for constructs measured in such a way (i.e., with ambiguous referenced Likert scaling) as dubious at best and a fool's errand at worse. New tools for measuring change in such constructs must become a focal point of researchers in the area of life course health development. Modifying existing tools and adapting them to the circumstances of a given study should be encouraged rather than sanctioned.

For objective health measures, the standards for measurement are well established, and changes in them are easily tracked (CO^2, cotinine, cortisol, cholesterol, etc.). For some of these biological gold standards, however, the cost of assessment can be precipitous. Below I will highlight some techniques to reduce cost and yet still yield valid measurements of such constructs. As I intimated above, some of these new techniques for measurement are only possible with the latent variable approaches that I emphasize herein.

1.2 Modeling Latent Variables

A construct is a latent variable. A latent variable cannot be observed directly, but instead its scores are inferred by triangulating across multiple measures that we can directly observe (e.g., responses to a questionnaire scale, reaction time trials, numerous behavioral observations, and so on). When a construct's indicators are measured with four or fewer categories or the items are yes/no or right/wrong in nature, item response theory (IRT) analysis is used to examine the nature of the latent variable. When the construct's indicators are measured with five or more ordinal intervals, IRT analyses are not necessarily needed. Instead, SEM can be used to assess the nature of the latent variable (Rhemtulla et al. 2012). When variables are measured with five or more ordinal intervals, the precision of each item is generalizable across the full range of the latent variable. When four or few ordinal intervals are involved, IRT allows one to adjust and identify the precision of items for where along the latent variable they are most useful to measure the latent variable score well.

As modern measurement tools, both SEM and IRT can be used for advanced statistical features such as test equating, linking scores of the same construct that uses different indicators of it, and the like. The details of how to perform linking are beyond the scope of my discussion here (see Little 2013; McDonald 1999); instead, I simply wish to emphasize that IRT is fundamentally a special case of SEM and that both statistical approaches rely on the idea that latent variables are the level of analysis, that is, the critical level. Multiple measured indicators are the means by which a construct can be assessed. The advantage of SEM over IRT is the ability to measure multiple constructs simultaneously to allow for the idea that health is an integrated set of capacities and an emergent property of humans. IRT and SEM, however, have melded considerably recently. Software programs such as Mplus can now easily allow both categorical and continuous indicators. In this context, DIF testing explicitly becomes testing for factorial invariance.

1.3 Linking Constructs

Figure 1 displays graphically two methods for linking measures of the same construct over time to allow modeling of the growth, change, and trajectory of a construct over time. Note that the model in panel B allows estimation of a bias correction factor for one of the measures of the construct by utilizing a bifactor decomposition (see Little 2013). This model assumes that the measure B in this example is unbiased. Determining whether one measure is biased while the other is not requires strong theory and empirical support. For this example, my main point is that linking construct scores is a relatively straightforward modeling enterprise in the SEM world as well as the IRT world. Linking allows life course health development researchers to be consistent with many of the principles of life course health development by maintaining measurement continuity while allowing for items that are developmentally appropriate.

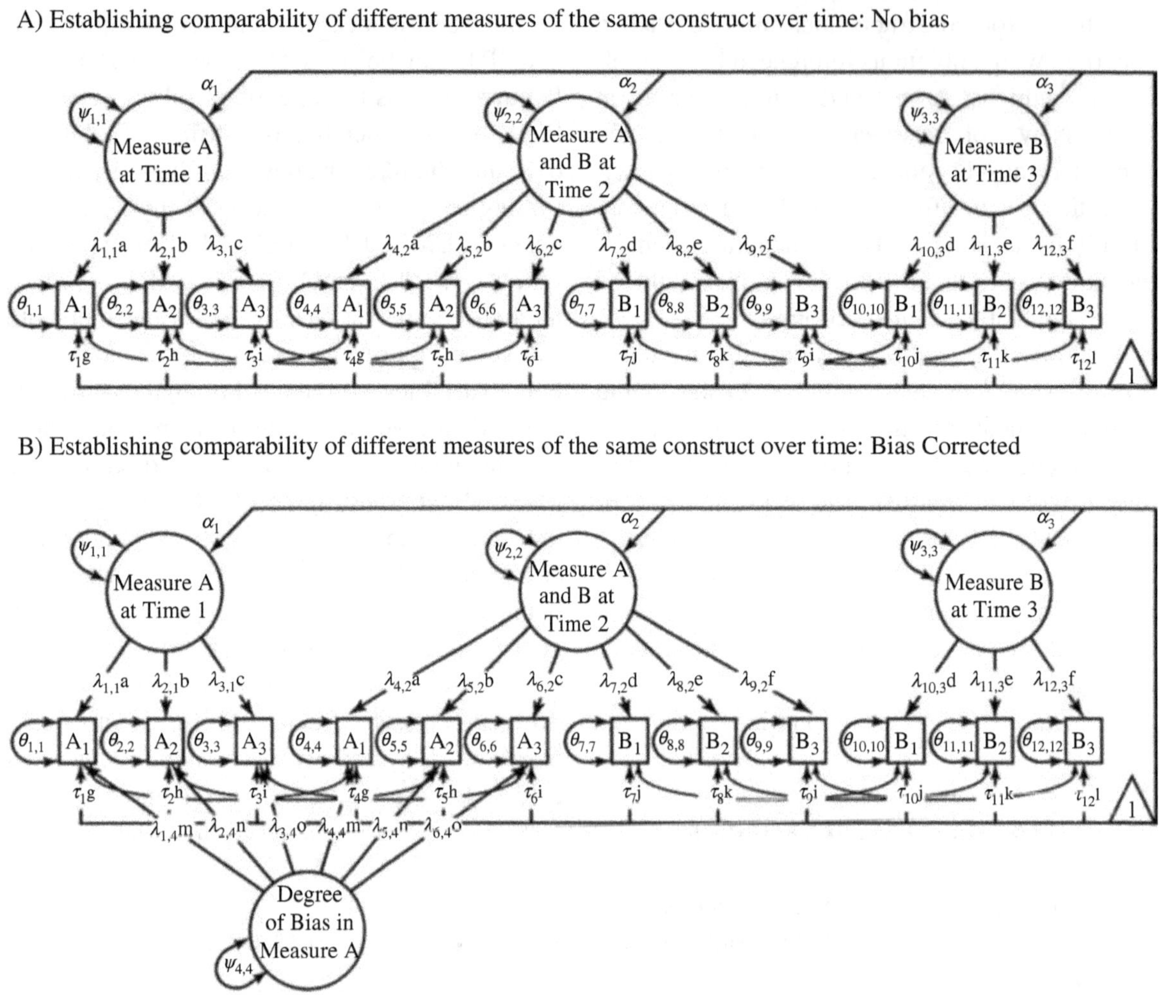

Fig. 1 Two models for establishing comparability of different measures of the same construct over time, with and without a "bias correction" factor. (**a**) Establishing comparability of different measures of the same construct over time: No bias. (**b**) Establishing comparability of different measures of the same construct over time: Bias corrected. (*Note.* The corresponding loadings and intercepts that are equated across time are designated by a superscripted letter (a-o). The residual variances among the corresponding indicators are allowed to associate over time (From Little 2013 and copyright, Todd D. Little. Reproduced with permission))

1.4 Factorial Invariance and Differential Item Functioning

One key assumption of life course health development, which is readily tested in SEM and IRT, is that the core properties of the measurement characteristics for a given construct are invariant across ages, measurement occasions, and contexts. When the measurement "DNA" of a given construct is supported by establishing strong factorial invariance, the certitude of construct comparisons is established. When factorial invariance is established, the interpretation of the observed differences in the constructs is unconfounded by any changes in the underlying psychometric characteristics of the measurement process. Measurement certainty is critical for valid life course research because observed differences across ages or contexts may be due to changes in the measurement of the construct and not changes in the construct itself. In the worlds of SEM and IRT analysis, testing for factorial invariance and differential item function (DIF) is the same thing. They both assess the certitude by which an item is psychometrically valid across different groups and across different ages when conditioned on the latent variable score (McDonald 1999).

More specifically, when indicators of constructs are roughly continuous, establishing measurement certitude involves testing and determining the factorial invariance of the constructs (Meredith 1993) – the basic steps and procedures for which have been well established (Little 1997; Little et al. 2007; Millsap and Cham 2012; Widaman and Reise 1997). In the educational sciences and related literatures, where dichotomous or polytomous item batteries are common, this issue of measurement certainty is addressed through the techniques of DIF testing – the basic steps and procedures for which have also been well established (de Ayala 2007). DIF testing explicitly focuses on item characteristics and often involves item refinements during scale development phases, whereas factorial invariance focuses on the measurement characteristics of constructs to ensure that construct comparisons are veridical during the hypothesis testing phases. A failure of invariance, however, is the continuous variable parallel of finding evidence of DIF. Life course health development research must emphasize measurement certitude for comparing constructs by testing for factorial invariance when the measures are continuous or testing for DIF when the measures or dichotomous or polytomous.

As long as partial strong factorial invariance holds (i.e., where a majority of the loadings and intercepts are proportionally equivalent), then the construct comparisons can proceed with sufficient certainty of comparison. Factorial invariance and DIF are both matters of degree. Within the SEM world, partial invariance is a simple way to allow items with evidence of DIF to not bias the construct's representation. A failure of invariance, if it involves many items however, becomes an exploratory study to determine what may have undermined the ability of the measures to reflect accurately the construct of interest across different ages or groups. Carefully planning and thoughtful measure construction can avoid the disappointment of a lack of invariance or evidence of DIF.

1.5 Parcels

Item parcels, as a measurement approach, are an essential tool for life course health development researchers. The items vs. parcels controversy has been a long-standing debate (Bandalos and Finney 2001; Little et al. 2002). This debate, however, is becoming less about whether or not parcels can be used and more about when and how they can be effective (Little, Rhemtulla et al. 2013a). The use of parcels in SEM is the process of creating a smaller set of more reliable and equally (or more) valid indicators of a construct from the larger pool of items that were used to measure the construct.

Little, Rhemtulla et al. (2013a) detail the covariance algebra of parcels and describe how knowing intimately the item-level information is critical to creating and successfully using parcels in an SEM analysis. Creating parcels that demonstrate factorial invariance is appropriate for life course health development research because the focus of inquiry is on the nature of the constructs and the change relations in and among the constructs of study. Because most longitudinal models that examine changes across the life course can become extremely large, using parcels is a matter of need rather than opinion.

2 Longitudinal Design Issues in Life Course Health Development Research

A number of design concerns arise when best practices in life course health development research are considered. Among these concerns are the timing of measurements, the model of change, and the moderating effect of lag differences. Each of these design issues is consistent with a number of the life course health development principles, particularly continuous change over time and the environmental influences that will impact health development across the life course. I will selectively address each of these issues in turn, even though other issues are certainly germane to this discussion.

2.1 Indexing Change

Life span research generally favors age-related changes, while life course research favors changes related to milestones and contextual influences. To model change well requires that the timing of measurements and the pace of change must by in sync regardless of the change emphasis. Rarely, however, is this synchronization of change with measurement achieved in actual research practice. Researchers need to carefully consider what changes and how fast it changes. In terms of the pace of change, to model change processes adequately requires that the occasions of measurement must be as fast as the fastest-changing process under scrutiny. Note that not all constructs need to be measured at the same pace or at the same occasions because imbalanced measurement intervals are easily handled in modern latent variable analytics.

To model what changes requires a reconsideration of the unit of change that should be used as the index of change. The measurement occasion is a very common index of change, and yet it confounds many factors such as cohort, age, and time of measurement. Sometimes age in years is used as the index of change. As Little (2013) emphasizes, change is a function of time, not necessarily or exclusively age or measurement occasion. Determining the right index of time to capture change is critical to accurately represent life course developmental processes.

2.2 Lag as Moderator

When measurement intervals are not precisely the same for all individuals, the difference in the elapsed interval can impact estimates of a given model. When measurements vary for individuals, this information can be used to represent the unique change processes associated with the varying measurement occasions. One model for representing the varying time lags is the recently introduced lag as moderator (LAM) model (Selig et al. 2012).

The LAM model explicitly incorporates the lag differences at a given measurement occasion to examine the influence that the differences in lag may have on the estimated model parameters. In the empirical data example reported in Selig et al., the influence of early home environment on later cognitive development showed a steeply declined effect as a function of time. When the lag in the measurement occasions was short (3 months), the influence of a rich home environment on intellective functioning was very high ($B = 2.5$), but when the lag was much longer than the intended 10-month interval (17 months), the effect had dropped to essentially zero (see Selig et al., for details of the model and of the empirical example).

One important implication of the LAM model is that lag can be used as a new design feature, with the interval of measurement becoming an element of the design that researchers can control and, with random assignment, allow a much broader universe of generalizability than the traditional longitudinal designs. Variable intervals can also be included in complex growth curve models by using some of the advance features of modern software. For example, Mplus has time scores that allow each person's time of measurement to vary, and OpenMX has definition variables that can accomplish the same goal.

3 Planned Missing Data Designs

Planned missing data designs are, in my estimation, the most underutilized weapon in a modern researcher's arsenal. Because latent variable models and modern approaches to treating missing data are able to provide efficient and unbiased estimates of parameters of interest in a quick and easy manner, not using planned missing data designs is rather difficult to justify. The family of possible planned missing procedures that can be used all provides information that is more valid than traditional ways of collecting data. They are also tremendously cost-effective. The validity component comes into play because planned missing data designs reduce the burden and fatigue on respondents. In life course health development research, the likelihood of selective attrition and other sources of unplanned missingness is also reduced because of the easy nature of responding (Little, Jorgenson et al. 2013b; Little and Rhemtulla 2013; Rhemtulla and Little 2012).

The Missing Data Mechanisms To understand unplanned missing data designs, I need to mention a few words about the mechanisms of missing data and how modern missing data treatments handle them (see Little and Rubin 2002; Enders 2010; van Buuren 2012). Three mechanisms can cause missing data: First, missing completely at random (MCAR) is, as the name indicates, a mechanism whereby their missing scores and their values are unrelated to anything that would impact the validity of inference. MCAR is the preferred mechanism for missing data because the only issue of statistical concern is the loss in power that occurs when data are missing. All missing data produce a loss in power. Only some missing data is unrelated to the observed data or any unobserved process (i.e., MCAR in origin). The second mechanism is termed missing at random (MAR). MAR occurs when the missing data are associated with a linear combination of one or more variables that are contained on the dataset. When MAR is at play, the variables that are observed on the dataset are predictive of the missing data, and, when this information is utilized in a modern treatment procedure, the information that was lost is readily retrieved.

The third mechanism is termed missing not at random (MNAR) and occurs when missing values are associated with one or more variables that are not observed. Large-scale life course research projects can reduce or eliminate the MNAR mechanism from its biasing influence by carefully and systematically including all variables that are known to associate or may likely be associated with missingness into the data collection protocol. If direct measures of these variables are not available, then proxy variables can be included. The goal here is to convert what would have been a MNAR missing data process into a MAR missing data process. The reason for this goal is that MNAR produces biased data that cannot be made unbiased, whereas MAR missing data is a process from which unbiased parameter estimates can be recovered.

The Modern Treatments The two most widely used modern approaches are full information maximum likelihood (FIML) estimation and multiple imputation (MI), which typically will utilize the expectation/maximization algorithm and/or the Markov chain Monte Carlo algorithm. FIML and MI are perfectly suited to handle MCAR missingness, and, unlike classical approaches, they provide an added benefit of restoring most of the power that was lost due to the missing data. FIML and MI are also perfectly well suited to handle data that are MAR and can also handle MNAR missingness when a study is designed to include predictors of missingness or their proxies.

FIML is an estimation procedure whose effectiveness depends on the variables that are included in the analysis model or in the auxiliary data block. If the combination of the variables associated with missingness is included in the analysis model either as a focal variable or as an auxiliary variable, FIML will produce unbiased estimates of all model parameters. MI will give the same answer as FIML when a large number of imputations are conducted (minimum $m = 20$, while 100 is generally recommended; see Enders 2010). The advantage of MI over FIML is that all variables on a dataset are involved in the imputation process. Then the variables associated with missingness are on the dataset, this information will be included in the imputation process, and the missing values will be recovered.

All things being equal, a model fit to imputed data will give the same answer as the FIML estimated model. These two modern approaches to handling missing data are state of the science in the statistical literature (see Enders 2010; van Buuren 2012) and should usurp the biased and ill-informed practices of some fields and disciplines. Techniques such as last or baseline observation carried forward or imputing and then setting the dependent variable as missing again after imputation were deemed effective treatments at one time. These treatments are biased and not recommended anymore (van Buuren 2012). If one of the two modern approaches is used, and when they take full advantage of including variables that are associated with MAR missing, then regardless of the research question, the analytic technique used, or the stakes involved, the best, most generalizable answer will emerge.

Planned Missing Protocols Two of the most effective planned missing protocols are the multiform design and the two-method design (Graham et al. 2001, 2006; Mistler and Enders 2012). The multiform design derives its name from the fact that multiple questionnaire protocols are created. These different forms can be thought of as short forms of the larger data collection protocol. Table 1 displays a layout of the simplest multiform design, the three-form design. The key to the three-form design is assigning items to be in four different blocks of items. The X block is the common block of items that all participants fill out. This block contains demographic variables, marker variables, and other essential elements that logically or theoretically are best collected on all participants. Variables that would be associated with unplanned missing data patterns and that constructs that don't have the multiple indicators of them are good candidates to include in the X block. The A, B, and C blocks each contain the remaining items evenly distributed among them. To enhance the power of this design, creating blocks of items that have high between block correlations is preferred. For longitudinal studies, using a random assignment of form to participant at each measurement occasion also enhances the power of this design. For a detailed simulation studies on the use of the three-form design for longitudinal research, see Jorgensen et al. (2014) and Jia et al. (2014).

The multiform design works so elegantly because the mechanism that produces the missingness for the unassigned items is controlled by the investigator making it an MCAR missing data mechanism. Of course, respondents will also refuse to answer some of the administered items. In such situations, the mixture of MCAR and MAR missingness is simultaneously addressed when FIML or MI is used. There modern treatments make no distinction between these two mechanisms when recovering both the information and the power that is lost due to missing data. Planned missing data designs increase validity by minimizing the fatigue and burden as well as reactivity (Harel et al. 2011). In addition to these validity gains, planned missing data designs reduce the unplanned missing data that occurs (Harel et al. 2011).

As with any design issue, sample size plays a role. As I mentioned at the outset, my focus is on latent variable approaches to modeling life course changes in health development, and as such sample sizes will be larger than many traditional studies of health in this context. Along with the validity gains by reducing respondent burden, fatigue, and reactivity, planned missing protocols allow researchers to redistribute resources to increase the number of participants by reducing the costs associated with each participant. The cost savings may be relatively small for the three-form design because the cost of 45 min vs. 1 h of a participant's reimbursement time may not translate directly into a 25% savings. The cost savings and power enhancement associated with the two-method design, on the other hand, can be dramatic.

The two-method design is based on the fact that many constructs have multiple methods by which they can be assessed. For some of these

Table 1 The general layout of a three-form planned missing data design

Form	Common variables	Variable set A	Variable set B	Variable set C
1	1/4 of Variables	1/4 of Variables	1/4 of Variables	None
2	1/4 of Variables	1/4 of Variables	None	1/4 of Variables
3	1/4 of Variables	None	1/4 of Variables	1/4 of Variables

Note: The distribution and proportions of variables across the different sets do not have to be uniform (From Little (in press))

constructs, one of the methods is considered a gold standard of assessment. Gold standard assessments are usually expensive to collect because they involve highly skilled assessors, copyrighted material, laboratory work, or time on very expensive machinery. Most studies that rely on gold standard assessments often are forced to conduct low-powered research because the costs are prohibitive. These cost barriers to using gold standard assessments, on the other hand, have lead researchers to develop and use less-expensive and easily obtained measures of the same constructs. These less-expensive measures are not as accurate as the gold standard version, but they typically are a reasonable proxy of the construct. Herein lies the beauty and elegance of the two-method design.

Using both the biased proxy measure and the gold standard measure, a given study can increase its sample size three- or more fold! Such increases in sample sizes easily move a given study into the sample size requirements of SEM. In fact, this design can only work when the appropriate SEM measurement model is employed to model the two methods of assessing the same construct. Figure 1 depicts a couple of possible variations of the two-method design. Two notable features of the measurement models shown here are that multiple indicators for each of the methods are included as indicators of the focal construct. In addition, a bifactor method factor is fit to the indicators of the biased proxy measurement tool. This bias factor or method factor extracts all the variance in the biased proxy that is unrelated to the information carried by the gold standard indicators. The indicators from the gold standard measure anchor the construct so that the resulting focal construct is an unbiased measure reflecting the construct centroid defined by the gold standard measurement tool.

This two-method design is ideally suited for researchers in the health sciences. What are the barriers to adopting this design and the associated advantages of SEM models? Lack of understanding on how planned missing designs work and lack of appreciation of the advantages of SEM appear to be the culprits. The statistical theory and the body of research evidence clearly support their use. As I mentioned earlier, research networks must coordinate and include experts in life course analytics (either instead of or in addition to the traditional biostatistics support). If they do, then the research conducted will benefit fully from the advantages and merits of all the techniques that I have outlined in this article.

Wave Missing Designs The simplest wave missing data design is the pre-post design where testing effects and retest effect are of concern. This simple design involves randomly assigning some participants to the pretest only, some to the posttest only, and some to both pre- and posttest. Unlike the flawed ANOVA framework to test the effects using such a design, a simple multiple-group longitudinal SEM with a modern treatment of the missing data provides a powerful way to analyze such data. For longitudinal studies of longer duration, participants can be randomly assigned to participate in different assessment occasions. As with the multiform design, these wave missing designs can be used even when MAR missingness is present. Clearly some participants will drop out of a study and some participants will come and go. These MAR patterns on top of the MCAR patterns are readily handled with modern missing data treatments. In addition, as mentioned, unplanned missing data are often reduced when planned missing is included (Harel et al. 2011s).

The Sequential Designs and the Accelerated Longitudinal Designs Given that MCAR and MAR are readily recoverable missing data mechanisms and MNAR can be minimized by imbuing a dataset with potential predictors of the missingness, using hybrid missing data models is easy and powerful to do. An underutilized model of this nature is the accelerated longitudinal design. To understand the accelerated longitudinal design, I display a graphical rendition of the three sequential longitudinal designs in Fig. 2. The three sequential designs are intended to unconfound two of the three factors that are confounded in a traditional longitudinal model. In a traditional longitudinal design, time of measurement is confounded with the age of the person which is also confounded with the cohort from which the sample is drawn.

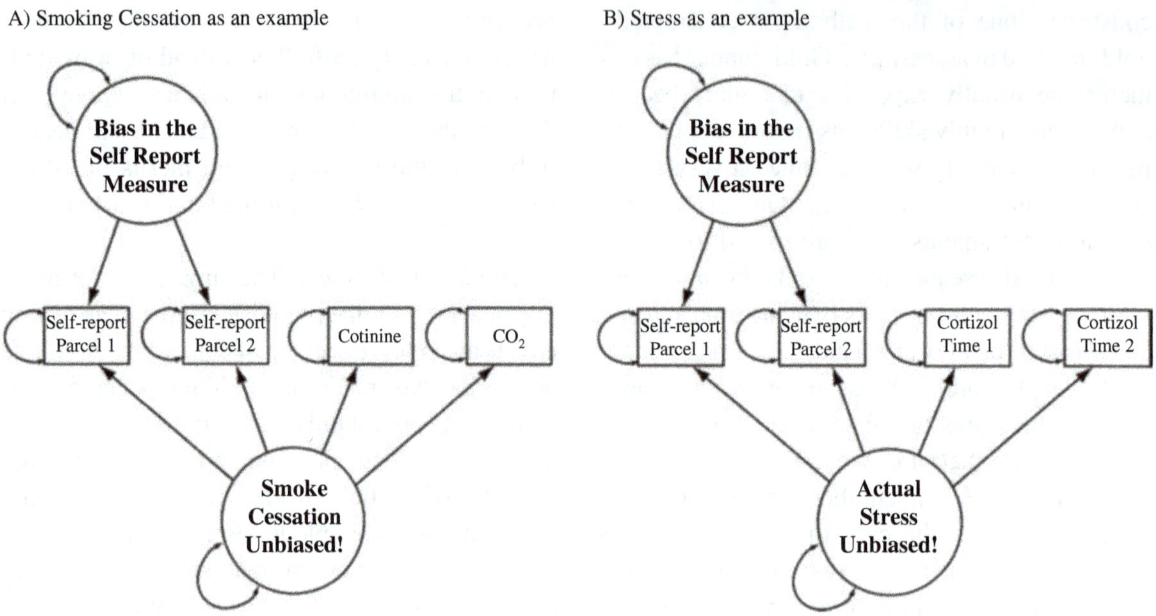

Fig. 2 Two examples of the two-method planned missing data design. (**a**) Smoking cessation as an example (**b**) Stress as an example (*Note*. From Little (2013) and copyright Todd d. Little. Reproduced with permission)

Of the sequential designs, the cross-sequential design is the most popular design. The cross-sequential design (which is commonly mislabeled as the cohort-sequential design) begins with a cross-section design and then follows all individuals for a number of measurement occasions. Here, measurement occasion is confounded with the cohort information, but age effects can be separated from the cohort effects once a sufficient amount of time has passed. The cohort-sequential design examines cohort differences for a specific period of the life course by repeatedly enrolling new individuals at a given age and following them only up to a particular age. In Fig. 3, I have depicted a cohort-sequential design that is optimized for studying the period of adolescence. Finally, the time-sequential design optimizes the ability to estimate effects related to the time of measurement.

Inspired by Bell (1953), modern approaches to the accelerated longitudinal design use the cross-sequential design to transform the collected data into a sparse dataset with many missing cells (see also Duncan and Duncan 2012). This accelerated longitudinal design uses the cohort and time of measurement information to create dummy codes and interaction terms to recover the information that is associated with cohort and time of measurement differences and, in the analysis model, use these dummy codes to estimate and thereby control for the cohort and time of measurement influences. When specified properly, the accelerated longitudinal design provides an unbiased estimate of age-related changes and differences across the total age span represented in the sample. Table 2 shows an example of an accelerated longitudinal model for the period of adolescence.

Another related transformation that life course researchers can utilize is to center the data on a particular event. With a design such as this, the emphasis is on understanding the change processes up to an event and the change processes after an event. Using puberty as an example, Table 3 shows how data can be transformed into a sparse arrangement but where the measurement occasions are either the measurement before the event or after the event. In this example, data from a single age cohort are grouped into the six different possible patterns in which evidence of puberty appears at a given wave of measurement. The letter P refers to puberty. Variables such as age within cohort and gender can be included as time-invariant contextual variables to examine

Cohort (Birth Year)	Time of Measurement														
	1996	1997	1998	1999	2000	2001	2002	2003	2004	2005	2006	2007	2008	2009	2010
1980	16	17	18	19	20	21	22	23	24	25	26	27	28	29	30
1981	15	16	17	18	19	20	21	22	23	24	25	26	27	28	29
1982	14	15	16	17	18	19	20	21	22	23	24	25	26	27	28
1983	13	14	15	16	17	18	19	20	21	22	23	24	25	26	27
1984	12	13	14	15	16	17	18	19	20	21	22	23	24	25	26
1985	11	12	13	14	15	16	17	18	19	20	21	22	23	24	25
1986	10	11	12	13	14	15	16	17	18	19	20	21	22	23	24
1987	9	10	11	12	13	14	15	16	17	18	19	20	21	22	23
1988	8	9	10	11	12	13	14	15	16	17	18	19	20	21	22
1989	7	8	9	10	11	12	13	14	15	16	17	18	19	20	21
1990	6	7	8	9	10	11	12	13	14	15	16	17	18	19	20
1991	5	6	7	8	9	10	11	12	13	14	15	16	17	18	19
1992	4	5	6	7	8	9	10	11	12	13	14	15	16	17	18
1993	3	4	5	6	7	8	9	10	11	12	13	14	15	16	17
1994	2	3	4	5	6	7	8	9	10	11	12	13	14	15	16
1995	1	2	3	4	5	6	7	8	9	10	11	12	13	14	15

Cohort-Sequential

Time Sequential

Cross-Sequential

Fig. 3 Traditional sequential designs (*Note.* Ages are entered in grey in the body of the table. Any given row would be an example of a longitudinal design and any given column would be an example of across-sectional study. A cohort-sequential design would be starting a new cohort at a certain age and then following longituidinally. A cross-sequential design starts with a traditional cross-sectional study and then follows all participants longitudinally. A time-squential design is a repeated cross-sectional design, with some participants followed longitudinally. From Little (2013) and copyright Todd D. Little. Reproduced with permission).

their influence on the change trends that would be modeled after the data transformation.

Life course health development researchers would do very well to incorporate the above design elements into the conduct of life course health development studies. Life course researchers are also keenly interested in the context effects and environmental influences in which the person is engaged. The person ←→ environment interactions across ages are central to life course theory. The various designs described above are also capable of including and modeling the dynamics of contextual interactions. Modeling contextual influences is primarily a measurement issue rather than a statistical or analytics issue.

Contextual influences can be represented analytically in various statistical forms, depending on how the contextual influence is expected to impact the person (Little et al. 2006c). These ways are as (a) direct effects, (b) indirect/mediating effects, (c) reciprocal/feedback effects, (d) moderating effects, and (e) hierarchically nested effects. In the parlance of multilevel modeling (Bickel 2007), the first four ways of including context variables would be as level 1 effects that are measured at the person level and are characterized as features of the person. For example, current health status is an environment of the person. The fifth way of including context variables would be as level 2 (or higher-level) influences if more than one person is measured within that context. For example, family health practices create a health environment that influences the members of the family. Context variables can be considered even higher levels of influence. For example, community health systems that support family health needs can vary across communities and influence family practices differentially, which in turn, influence individual health characteristics.

Hierarchically nested contextual influences can be modeled in an SEM framework using the power and the flexibility of multilevel SEM (Bovaird 2007; Bovaird and Shaw 2012). Multilevel SEM involves specifying any form of a SEM model and adding a multilevel component on top of it. New software such as xxM (Mehta 2013) allows any number of levels of nested data structures. With longitudinal studies of context, person-level contextual variables can also be included as either time-varying or time-invariant influences. The context of gender or race is an example of a time-invariant effect. The size of a

Table 2 Transforming a cross-sequential design into an accelerated longitudinal design

	Age in years; months for each cohort at each assessment					
Age/Cohort	0 Mos	4 Mos	8 Mos	12 Mos	16 Mos	20 Mos
Age 11 yrs	11;0	11;4	11;8	12;0	12;4	12;8
Age 12 yrs	12;0	12;4	12;8	13;0	13;4	13;8
Age 13 yrs	13;0	13;4	13;8	14;0	14;4	14;8
Age 14 yrs	14;0	14;4	14;8	15;0	15;4	15;8
Age 15 yrs	15;0	15;4	15:8	16;0	16;4	16;8
Age 16 yrs	16;0	16;4	16;8	17;0	17;4	17;8

	Full span of the ages covered																				
	11;0	11;4	11;8	12;0	12;4	12;8	13;0	13;4	13;8	14;0	14;4	14;8	15;0	15;4	15;8	16;0	16;4	16;8	17;0	17;4	17;8
Age 11 yrs	W1	W2	W3	W4	W5	W6															
Age 12 yrs				W1	W2	W3	W4	W5	W6												
Age 13 yrs							W1	W2	W3	W4	W5	W6									
Age 14 yrs										W1	W2	W3	W4	W5	W6						
Age 15 yrs													W1	W2	W3	W4	W5	W6			
Age 16 yrs																W1	W2	W3	W4	W5	W6

Note. Multiple cohorts could also be transformed in such a manner. A dummy code to represent age-cohort would be included within each pattern to account for potential cohort differences. The missing data are treated as missing at random and imputed. Mos refers to months, yrs. refers to years, and WB refers to wave of data collection (Copyright Todd D. Little)

Table 3 Transforming a longitudinal design into episodic time

Data Collection Wave Crossed with Episode Occurance											
Pattern	Wave 1	Wave 2		Wave 3	Wave 4		Wave 5	Wave 6			
Pattern 1	P	P + 1		P + 2	P + 3		P + 4	P + 5			
Pattern 2	P – 1	P		P + 1	P + 2		P + 3	P + 4			
Pattern 3	P – 2	P – 1		P	P + 1		P + 2	P + 3			
Pattern 4	P – 3	P – 2		P – 1	P		P + 1	P + 2			
Pattern 5	P – 4	P – 3		P – 2	P – 1		P	P + 1			
Patterns	P – 5	P – 4		P – 3	P – 2		P – 1	P			
	Episodic Occurence Crossed with Data Collection Wave										
	P – 5	P – 4	P – 3	P – 2	P – 1	P	P + 1	P + 2	P + 3	P + 4	P + 5
Pattern 1						W1	W2	W3	W4	W5	W6
Pattern 2					W1	W2	W3	W4	W5	W6	
Pattern 3				W1	W2	W3	W4	Wf	W6		
Pattern 4			W1	W2	W3	W4	W5	W6			
Pattern 5		W1	W2	W3	W4	W5	W6				
Pattern 6	W1	W2	W3	W4	W5	W6					

Note. Multiple cohorts could also be transformed in such a manner. A dummy code to represent age-cohort would be included within each pattern to account for potential cohort differences. The missing data are treated as missing at random and imputed (From Little (2013). Copyright Todd D. Little)

participant's social network is an example of a time-varying context effect. See Little et al. (2007c) for an edited volume dedicated to modeling contextual effects in longitudinal research.

Mediation and Moderation Mediation and moderation are critical statistical concepts for the field of life course health development research. These two concepts are consistently confused and often inappropriately tested. Mediation, for example, is a strict causal model of how one variable imparts its influence on another variable. It addresses the "how" of a causal chain. Like falling dominos, the linkage from one variable to the next as a causal impact must be established. In this regard, the only appropriate test for mediation must be longitudinal in nature (Cole and Maxwell 2003; Little et al. 2007; Maxwell and Cole 2007; Wu and Zumbo 2008).

At a minimum, two measurement occasions are needed to even implicate a mediation effect. Because mediation is a causal hypothesis about change, to implicate mediation involves demonstrating that a predictor, X, is able to predict *changes* in a mediator, M. To show that X is related to the change in M, prior levels of the mediator variable must be controlled. That is, the autoregressive influence of M on itself at a second time point must be estimated in order to show that X can predict changes in M. Similarly, a mediation analysis must be able to show that a mediator can predict changes in the outcome variable, Y. As with the mediator, the prior levels of the outcome variable, Y, must be entered into a model in order to demonstrate that M can predict changes in Y. Figure 3 shows an example of the simplest model for testing mediation. This figure depicts the half longitudinal design for testing mediation. In Fig. 3, the path labeled *a* is the first essential element of a mediation effect. It is the magnitude of the effect of X on the change in M. The second essential element of a mediation effect is labeled *b* in Fig. 3. It is the effect of M on the change in Y. Since mediation is a multiphase process, the joint effect must be calculated and tested for significance. Here, mediation is evident if the product of path *a* and path *b* is significant. To appropriately test with this product term is significant; either bootstrap estimation of the standard error of *ab* or a Monte Carlo simulation approach is used (McKinnnon 2008; Preacher and Hayes 2008a, b; Preacher and Selig 2012) Fig. 4.

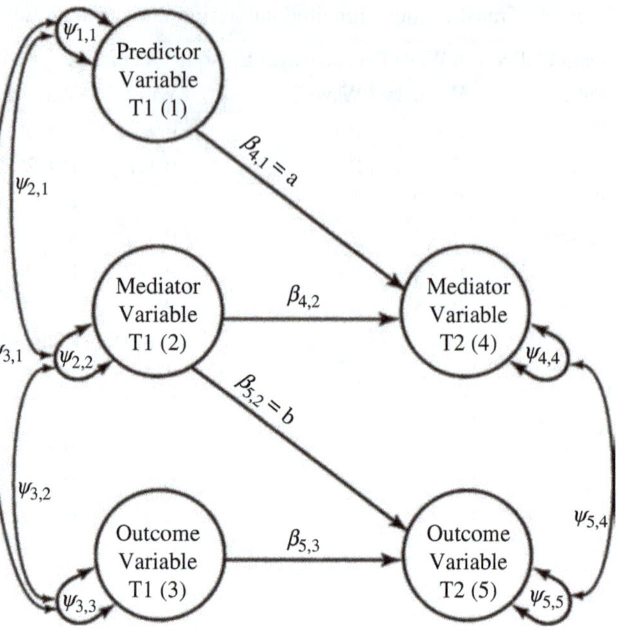

Fig. 4 *The half longitudinal design for testing mediation.* (*Note.* The representation of the measurement model is removed from the diagram. This design is the minimum required in order to empirically demonstrate mediation as a causal hypothesis. From Little (2013) and copyright Todd D. Little. Reproduced with permission)

Moderation is a quintessential context hypothesis. It addresses the conditions in which an effect between two variables is stronger or weaker. Tap water flows from the pipes to the glass at a flow rate determined by the context of the faucet valve. A moderator is like a valve, wide open and water flows freely and partly closed and the flow of water is restricted. Moderation is often confused with multivariate questions, for example, does one glass become fuller than another glass when the same amount of time has passed? The degree to which the water valve is open causes these differences. A question like how did my glass get half full is not a question of moderation. Here, many different liquids can combine or work in isolation to make the glass half full. Mostly juice and some water lead to a half-full glass. Mostly water and some milk also lead to a half-full glass. The type of liquid is not a moderator of the amount of water in the glass. Each liquid is an additive unique contribution to the height of the water in the glass.

Tests of mediation, moderation, and the unique and additive effects of a set of variables are each undermined when measurement error is involved. As I have been emphasizing, a latent variable SEM approach to conducting these tests provides the maximum accuracy and generalizability of inference. Moderation in particular is a notoriously underpowered procedure when tested as a manifest variable interaction term. Testing moderation in the latent space is a bit more complex. Three general approaches exist for testing moderation. A model-based approach is available in the Mplus software (using the LMS approach; Klein and Moosbrugger 2000; Muthén and Asparouhov 2003). Two indicator-based approaches can also be used: the double mean-centering approach forwarded by Marsh and colleagues (see Lin et al. 2010) and the orthogonalizing approach (Little et al. 2006). For more details on testing moderation in general, see Marsh et al.(2012), and for more details on testing both mediation and moderation in longitudinal models, see Little (in press; particularly Chap. 9).

Tests of moderation are also muddied by the fact that a significant interaction term cannot speak to which variable is moderating the other. A significant interaction term only indicates that the regression effect of the outcome on one of the two predictors varies as a function of the other. Although the example of a valve as the moderator of the water flow to a glass seems clear as to its role as a moderating influence, a third variable could potentially confound this conclusion. The amount of water pressure, for example, could cause the value to be open more when pressure is high and open less when the pressure is low.

4 Choice of Analysis Model

Two general types of analysis model dominate longitudinal research (Little 2013). For both of these model types, a mixture distribution approach and/or a multilevel kernel can be included (Masyn and Nylund-Gibson 2012; Mehta 2013). The first analysis model is the traditional cross-lagged panel model. The panel model remains an essential analysis model for life course health development researchers because it addresses key questions about what predicts change controlling for prior levels. Mediation and moderation hypotheses are readily addressed in the basic panel model. The panel model is fundamentally a question about individual differences standings at specific points in time. These models can be made more refined by incorporating lag at each wave as a moderator or using the recent models of continuous time modeling.

The second popular model for the analysis of longitudinal data is the growth curve model. The growth curve model is a model for the mean-level changes. It decomposes the mean and covariance information into a set of constructs to represent the change over time for each of the individuals in the sample. The set of constructs is usually an intercept construct, which usually represents the initial levels of the participants at the first measurement occasion, and a slope construct, which represents the shape of the growth/change over time for the sample. These two constructs have variances that reflect the individual differences in the intraindividual change trajectories. These models and their variants address the change trajectories and what predicts standing in the modeled trajectories.

As should be clear, each of these analysis models addresses distinctly different questions. Life course health development researchers need to be clear to match the correct model with the particular research question at hand. Too often, researchers are tempted to fit the more popular model (i.e., the growth curve model) when the question is fundamentally about the individual differences relationships and changes in those patterns. In the field of life course methodology and analytics, both techniques are undergoing developments and refinements (e.g., Grimm and Ram 2012; Little et al. 2007a; Selig and Little 2012; Wu et al. 2012), and as such, researchers need to stay on top of recent developments in their application to data.

Because life course health development is complex, nonlinear, multidimensional, multidirectional, and multilevel by its nature, the choice of analysis model must accurately correspond to the life course change process under scrutiny. That is, not only are hierarchical nested models (i.e., multilevel models) often needed, but also mixture distribution models bring the ability to discover and model the unobserved heterogeneity inherent in life course health development.

As mentioned the popularity of adding a mixture distribution component to a given model is very attractive to many life course researchers. Such models appeal to the person-centered views of many life course researchers. These techniques, however, are not always appropriate for the data or the research question and should be avoided unless the study and the data were designed to examine archetypes and latent subgroups. Some statisticians would have these techniques buried and a tombstone with R.I.P. placed upon it. Others would have the techniques resurrected and use R.I.P. as the mantra for how the techniques should be used. Namely, replicability, interpretability, and predictability are the three core validity criteria to pass when using these techniques (see Little 2013). For recent discussions of the issues, see Ram et al. (2012), Nagin and Odgers (2012), and Masyn and Nylund-Gibson (2012).

5 Conclusions

The craft of life course health development methodology and analytics requires dedication, sophistication, and a knack for molding the analysis tool to the research question at hand. For life course health development research to be at its most effective, utilizing the expertise of collaborative teams is essential. The days of one person being both expert theoretician and methodologist are waning. Partnering with dedicated experts on the various issues that I have outlined here will bring the needed sophistication and knack to execute research at its finest and most impactful levels.

References

Bandalos, D. L., & Finney, S. J. (2001). Item parceling issues in structural equation modeling. In G. A. Marcoulides & R. E. Schumacker (Eds.), *New developments and techniques in structural equation modeling (chap. 10)* (pp. 269–296). Hillsdale: Lawrence Erlbaum Associates.

Bell, R. Q. (1953). Convergence: An accelerated longitudinal approach. *Child Development, 24*, 145–152.

Bickel, R. (2007). *Multilevel analysis for applied research: It's just regression!* New York: The Guilford Press.

Bovaird, J. A. (2007). Multilevel structural equation models for contextual factors. In T. D. Little, J. A. Bovaird, & N. A. Card (Eds.), *Modeling contextual effects in longitudinal studies* (pp. 149–182). LEA: Mahwah.

Bovaird, J. A., & Shaw, L. H. (2012). Multilevel structural equation modeling. In B. Laursen, T. D. Little, & N. A. Card (Eds.), *Handbook of developmental research methods* (pp. 501–518). New York: Guilford Press.

Brown, T. A. (2014). *Confirmatory factor analysis for applied research* (2nd ed.). New York: Guilford.

Cole, D. A., & Maxwell, S. E. (2003). Testing mediational models with longitudinal data: Questions and tips in the use of structural equation modeling. *Journal of Abnormal Psychology, 112*, 558–577.

de Ayala, R. J. (2007). *The theory and practice of item response theory*. New York: Guilford Press.

Duncan, S. C., & Duncan, T. E. (2012). Accelerated longitudinal designs. In B. Laursen, T. D. Little, & N. A. Card (Eds.), *Handbook of developmental research methods* (pp. 31–45). New York: Guilford Press.

Enders, C. (2010). *Applied missing data analysis*. New York, NY: Guildford Press.

Funke, F., & Reips, U.-D. (2012). Why semantic differentials in Web-based research should be made from visual analogue scales and not from 5-point scales. *Field Methods, 24*, 310–327.

Graham, J. W., Taylor, B. J., & Cumsille, P. E. (2001). Planned missing data designs in the analysis of change. In L. M. Collins & A. G. Sayer (Eds.), *New methods for the analysis of change* (pp. 335–353). Washington, DC: American Psychological Association.

Graham, J. W., Taylor, B. J., Olchowski, A. E., & Cumsille, P. E. (2006). Planned missing data designs in psychological research. *Psychological Methods, 11*, 323–343.

Grimm, K. J., & Ram, N. (2012). Growth curve modeling from a structural equation modeling perspective. In B. Laursen, T. D. Little, & N. A. Card (Eds.), *Handbook of developmental research methods* (pp. 411–431). New York: Guilford Press.

Harel, O., Stratton, J., & Aseltine, R. (2011). Designed missingness to better estimate efficacy of behavioral studies. *Tenth conference on health survey research methods,* pp. 153–158.

Jia, F., Moore, E. W. G., Kinai, R., Crowe, K. S., Schoemann, A. M., & Little, T. D. (2014). Planned missing data design on small sample size: How small is too small? *International Journal of Behavioral Development, 38*, 1–18.

Jorgensen, T. D., Rhemtulla, M., Schoemann, A., McPherson, B., Wu, W., & Little, T. D. (2014). Optimal assignment methods in three-form planned missing data designs for longitudinal panel studies. *International Journal of Behavioral Development, 38*, 397–410.

Klein, A., & Moosbrugger, H. (2000). Maximum likelihood estimation of latent interaction effects with the LMS method. *Psychometrika, 65*, 457–474.

Likert, R. (1932). A technique for the measurement of attitudes. *Archives of Psychology, 22*, 1–55.

Lin, G.-C., Wen, Z., Marsh, H. W., & Lin, H.-S. (2010). Structural equation models of latent interactions: Clarification of orthogonalizing and double-mean-centering strategies. *Structural Equation Modeling, 17*, 374–391.

Little, T. D. (1997). Mean and covariance structures (MACS) analyses of cross-cultural data: Practical and theoretical issues. *Multivariate Behavioral Research, 32*, 53–76.

Little, T. D. (2013). *Longitudinal structural equation modeling*. New York: Guilford Press.

Little, T. D., & Rhemtulla, M. (2013). Planned missing data designs for developmental researchers. *Child Development Perspectives, 7*, 199–204.

Little, R. J., & Rubin, D. (2002). *Statistical analysis with missing data* (2nd ed.). New York: Wiley.

Little, T. D., Cunningham, W. A., Shahar, G., & Widaman, K. F. (2002). To parcel or not to parcel: Exploring the question, weighing the merits. *Structural Equation Modeling, 9*, 151–173.

Little, T. D., Bovaird, J. A., & Slegers, D. W. (2006a). Methods for the analysis of change. In D. K. Mroczek & T. D. Little (Eds.), *Handbook of personality development* (pp. 181–211). Mahwah: LEA.

Little, T. D., Bovaird, J. A., & Widaman, K. F. (2006b). On the merits of orthogonalizing powered and product terms: Implications for modeling interactions among latent variables. *Structural Equation Modeling, 13*, 497–519.

Little, T. D., Bovaird, J. A., & Card, N. A. (Eds.). (2006c). *Modeling contextual effects in longitudinal studies*. Mahwah: LEA.

Little, T. D., Card, N. A., Bovaird, J. A., Preacher, K., & Crandall, C. S. (2007a). Structural equation modeling of mediation and moderation with contextual factors. In T. D. Little, J. A. Bovaird, & N. A. Card (Eds.), *Modeling contextual effects in longitudinal studies* (pp. 207–230). Mahwah, LEA.

Little, T. D., Preacher, K. J., Selig, J. P., & Card, N. A. (2007c). New developments in SEM panel analyses of longitudinal data. *International Journal of Behavioral Development, 31*, 357–365.

Little, T. D., Rhemtulla, M., Gibson, K., & Schoemann, A. M. (2013a). Why the items versus parcels controversy needn't be one. *Psychological Methods, 18*, 285–300.

Little, T. D., Jorgensen, T. D., Lang, K. M., & Moore, E. W. G. (2013b). On the joys of missing data. *Journal of Pediatric Psychology, 39*(2), 151–162. doi:10.1093/jpepsy/jst048.

Little, T. D., Jorgensen, T. D., Lang, K. M., & Moore, E. W. G. (2014). On the joys of missing data. *Journal of Pediatric Psychology, 39*, 151–162.

MacKinnon, D. P. (2008). *Introduction to statistical mediation analysis*. Mahwah: Erlbaum.

Marsh, H. W., Hau, K.-T., Wen, Z., & Nagengast, B. (2012). Moderation. In T. D. Little (Ed.), *The Oxford handbook of quantitative methods* (Vol. 2, pp. 361–386). New York: Oxford University Press.

Masyn, K. E., & Nylund-Gibson, K. (2012). Mixture modeling. In T. D. Little (Ed.), *The Oxford handbook of quantitative methods* (Vol. 2, pp. 551–611). New York: Oxford University Press.

Maxwell, S. E., & Cole, D. A. (2007). Bias in cross sectional analysis of longitudinal mediation. *Psychological Methods, 12*, 23–44.

McDonald, R. (1999). *Test theory: A unified treatment*. Mahwah: Erlbaum.

Mehta, P. (2013). *xxM user's guide, version 1.0*. University of Houston: Author.

Meredith, W. (1993). Measurement invariance, factor analysis and factorial invariance. *Psychometrika, 58*, 525–543.

Milsap, R. E., & Cham, H. (2012). Investigating factorial invariance in longitudinal data. In B. Laursen, T. D. Little, & N. A. Card (Eds.), *Handbook of developmental research methods* (pp. 109–126). New York: Guilford Press.

Mistler, S. A., & Enders, C. K. (2012). Planned missing data designs for developmental research. In B. Laursen, T. D. Little, & N. A. Card (Eds.), *Handbook of developmental research methods* (pp. 742–775). New York: Guilford Press.

Muthén, B., & Asparouhov, T. (2003). *Modeling interactions between latent and observed continuous variables using maximum-likelihood estimation in Mplus*. Mplus Web Notes: No. 6.

Nagin, D. S., & Odgers, C. L. (2012). Group-based trajectory modeling in developmental science. In B. Laursen, T. D. Little, & N. A. Card (Eds.), *Handbook of developmental research methods* (pp. 464–480). New York: Guilford Press.

Preacher, K. J., & Hayes, A. F. (2008a). Asymptotic and resampling strategies for assessing and comparing indirect effects in multiple mediator models. *Behavior Research Methods, 40*, 879–891.

Preacher, K. J., & Hayes, A. F. (2008b). Contemporary approaches to assessing mediation in communication research. In A. F. Hayes, M. D. Slater, & L. B. Snyder (Eds.), *The Sage sourcebook of advanced data analysis methods for communication research* (pp. 13–54). Thousand Oaks: Sage.

Preacher, K. J., & Selig, J. P. (2012). Advantages of Monte Carlo confidence intervals for indirect effects. *Communication Methods and Measures, 6*, 77–98.

Ram, N., Grimm, K. J., Gatzke-Koop, L. M., & Molenaar, P. C. M. (2012). Longitudinal mixture models and the identification of archetypes. In B. Laursen, T. D. Little, & N. A. Card (Eds.), *Handbook of developmental research methods* (pp. 481–500). New York: Guilford Press.

Reips, U.-D. (2006). Web-based methods. In M. Eid & E. Diener (Eds.), *Handbook of multimethod measurement in psychology* (pp. 73–85). Washington, DC: American Psychological Association.

Reips, U.-D., & Funke, F. (2008). Interval level measurement with visual analogue scales in Internet-based research: VAS generator. *Behavior Research Methods, 40*, 699–704.

Rhemtulla, M., & Little, T. D. (2012). Planned missing data designs for research in cognitive development. *Journal of Cognition and Development, 13*, 425–438.

Rhemtulla, M., Brosseau-Liard, P., & Savalei, V. (2012). How many categories is enough to treat data as continuous? A comparison of robust continuous and categorical SEM estimation methods under a range of non-ideal situations. *Psychological Methods, 17*, 354–373.

Selig, J. P., & Little, T. D. (2012). Autoregressive and cross-lagged panel analysis for longitudinal data. In B. Laursen, T. D. Little, & N. A. Card (Eds.), *Handbook of developmental research methods* (pp. 265–278). New York, NY: Guilford Press.

Selig, J. P., Preacher, K. J., & Little, T. D. (2012). Modeling time-dependent association in longitudinal data: A lag as moderator approach. *Multivariate Behavioral Research, 47*, 697–716.

van Buuren, S. (2012). *Flexile imputation of missing data*. Boca Raton: CRC Press.

Widaman, K. F., & Reise, S. P. (1997). Exploring the measurement invariance of psychological instruments: Applications in the substance use domain. In K. J. Bryant, M. Windle, & S. G. West (Eds.), *The science of prevention: Methodological advances from alcohol and substance abuse research* (pp. 281–324). Washington, DC: APA.

Wu, A. D., & Zumbo, B. D. (2008). Understanding and using mediators and moderators. *Social Indicators Research, 87*, 367–392.

Wu, W., Selig, J. P., & Little, T. D. (2012). Longitudinal data analysis. In T. D. Little (Ed.), *The Oxford handbook of quantitative methods* (Vol. 2, pp. 387–410). New York: Oxford University Press.

Epidemiological Study Designs: Traditional and Novel Approaches to Advance Life Course Health Development Research

Stephen L. Buka, Samantha R. Rosenthal, and Mary E. Lacy

1 Introduction

1.1 Goals in Life Course Research

A life course approach to health and human development provides a conceptual and methodological framework to understand the multiple, multilevel, and synchronized (i.e. temporally integrated) determinants of health and disease across the lifespan. Theories underlying life course approaches are varied, but each emphasizes the importance of the occurrence and accrual of life events, plasticity, thriving, or risk over time and how these contribute to the development of particular outcomes of interest, including pathways associated with optimal health (George 1999; Kuh et al. 2003; Ben-Shlomo and Kuh 2002; Halfon et al. 2014). A number of key questions pertinent to the emergence of health development across the lifespan can be addressed using life course frameworks that would otherwise be difficult to ascertain. From furthering our understanding of familial and genetic contributions to the aetiology of health conditions to exploring the natural course of disorders in different populations and to examining the time-specific and cumulative impacts of social and environmental factors, the use of a life course framework has advanced our understanding of the systemic causes and course of multiple health conditions and positive health development.

S.L. Buka (✉) • S.R. Rosenthal • M.E. Lacy
Department of Epidemiology, Brown University, Providence, RI, USA
e-mail: stephen_buka@brown.edu

The goal of the field of epidemiology is to advance the understanding of the determinants of health and disease among human populations. Consistent with the seven principles of LCHD (see Halfon and Forrest, Chap. 2), over the past few decades, there has been a growing recognition of the multiple determinants of most disorders and the need for a life course approach (Kuh et al. 2003; Ben-Shlomo and Kuh 2002; Halfon et al. 2014; Buka 2003; Buka and Lipsitt 1994; Angold and Costello 1995; Susser and Susser 1996). These developments in epidemiology were influenced by earlier and parallel advances in the field of human development (c.f., Baltes, Elder, Magnusson) (Baltes et al. 1998; Giele and Elder 1998; Magnusson 1996; Elder and Rockwell 1979). In epidemiology, as in other disciplines, we have come to understand that few, if any, events occur in isolation (Barker 2004; Elder and Shanahan 2007). Hence, the central focus in life course approaches to health development and life course epidemiology is on the complex process of occurrence and accrual of risks at multiple levels. For example, the probability that two identical twin infants will develop a substance use disorder may differ due to a number of subtle environmental differences

N. Halfon et al. (eds.), *Handbook of Life Course Health Development*,
DOI 10.1007/978-3-319-47143-3_22

that each encounters over the course of their life. In a recent editorial, Stephen Gilman described life course and developmental epidemiology as 'sharing the fundamental principles that health at any given point in time is substantially influenced by prior circumstances, and that disease processes unfold through a combination of risks operating at multiple levels—ranging from genetic inheritance and psychological vulnerability to social conditions' (Gilman 2002).

Epidemiological research shares basic goals with life course development concerning the origins, course, and prevention of health, disease, and disorder and, in turn, through the integration of the perspectives, the promotion of health development. Both advance through a variety of traditional and more recently developed study designs (Aschengrau and Seage 2008; Rothman et al. 2008). Each study design represents a different approach to common research questions and has implications for the ways in which study participants are selected and information is collected and analysed. The design chosen by an investigator is driven by the research question being posed along with considerations of cost, efficiency, and ethical and practical considerations (Aschengrau and Seage 2008; Woodward 2005). While many traditional epidemiological questions can be addressed through a number of alternative designs, some are of limited utility for issues at the core of a life course health development approach.

1.2 Framework for This Chapter

This chapter reviews the major design options for studying health and disease across the life course. The organization is by study design and describes major features of each design approach, key instances of each design, and potential challenges and limitations associated with each design. To limit the scope of this chapter, we take as an example the study of substance use and substance use disorder diagnosis as an instance of a complex health condition warranting investigation from a life course perspective. Study designs included are (i) cohort studies (general prospective cohort studies, perinatal/birth cohorts, twin studies, and high-risk cohort studies); (ii) case–control studies, including nested case–control studies within larger cohorts; (iii) cross-sectional studies; (iv) quasi-experimental designs; and (v) randomized controlled trials (RCTs). Although certain design strategies, namely, cohort studies, lend themselves more readily to the life course approach, we have chosen to describe other study designs that can also be used to further our understanding of health, disorder, and disease from the life course perspective. The chapter concludes with general considerations for designing life course studies, as well as recommendations for future directions of the field.

One frequent topic in life course epidemiology is the initiation, progression, and trajectories following substance use. Given the emphasis in the LCHD principles of the role of synchrony in the timing of developmental processes at multiple levels, ranging from the molecular through the historical (evolutionary), a life course approach has been useful in assessing the timing of substance use onset, the broader contexts that contribute to early use patterns, the progression from use to abuse or dependence, and the identification of intergenerational and early life experiences on substance use patterns (Magnusson 1996; Jablonka and Lamb 2005). One particular research question that has been examined extensively is the relationship between traumatic experience and the development of a substance use disorder. Over the past century, this question has been examined using a variety of different study designs in an effort to more thoroughly probe the potential causal link between trauma and the aetiology of substance use disorder. As the chapter progresses, we use this topic to illustrate the ways in which various threats to the validity of a claim for causality manifest under different study designs. For the purposes of a clear illustration, we focus on diagnosed substance use disorder as our outcome.

2 Major Design Options

In the epidemiological literature, studies are typically grouped into observational and experimental studies (Ahern and Leslie 2014; Pickles et al. 2007).

2.1 Observational

The majority of life course studies are observational studies (Pickles et al. 2007). As compared with experimental studies, in which exposures are randomly assigned to study participants, in observational designs, the investigator observes and records data on a group of people, with no active manipulation of exposure conditions, generating information on the relationships between exposure and disease as they naturally unfold. Whereas the causal inferences that can be derived from observational studies are typically not as strong as those in experimental studies, observational studies are free from the ethical dilemmas associated with allocating exposure in experimental designs. Observational studies typically take two forms, cohort studies or case–control studies; each form has a number of variations.

2.1.1 Cohort Studies

In epidemiology, a prospective cohort study[1] is one in which participants are enrolled before the outcome of interest has occurred and are then followed for a period of time. This is one of the preferred design options for studying substance use disorders across the life course because it allows for direct measurement of both exposures and outcomes as they occur, providing strong evidence for temporality of exposure–outcome relationships. These designs are also useful for illustrating the importance of the LCHD principle regarding the importance of the timing and social structure of exposure to environmental events, both normative and non-normative (Baltes et al. 2006). There remain, however, many important design considerations, challenges, and limitations in the design and conduct of such studies.

In a cohort study, participants are often selected to be representative of a larger population of interest—defining the relevant population of interest is central to designing a maximally informative cohort study. In some instances, the population may be defined by the set of key exposures of interest—e.g. a pregnancy, school-age, or midlife cohort. In others, the most informative population may be those at elevated risk of developing disease, e.g. family history of disorder and certain environmental exposures. If an investigator has multiple outcomes of interest, it can be difficult to identify specific subpopulations at risk of disease, in which case a more general population may be most appropriate.

Data are collected to provide information on the outcomes that are the focus for the study; the implications for this are particularly important in a prospective study because, as the cohort ages, an investigator may wish that additional data had been collected on another exposure or disease (Susser et al. 2000). Additionally, decisions related to study design and data collection are made relative to the science of the field when the study is initiated. This phenomenon is referred to as the scientific period effect (Susser et al. 2000; Wadsworth et al. 2003). Illustrating and reflecting how health development research is embedded in historically defined scientific periods, it has become a truism that many of the greatest discoveries of long-term prospective cohort studies were not anticipated at the time of initiation and that certain data (such as genetic material) that become relevant at a later scientific time may have been overlooked at the onset of earlier projects.

Another key consideration in designing a prospective cohort study is minimizing study dropout and loss to follow-up. Given the long periods of follow-up often involved in prospective cohort studies, it is especially important to consider procedures to minimize study dropout during the

[1]Epidemiology has traditionally made a distinction between prospective cohort studies and retrospective cohort studies, also called historic *cohort* studies, in which the primary outcomes of interest have occurred prior to the initiation of the study, but longitudinal data on both exposures and outcomes exist. Distinctions between prospective, retrospective, and even 'ambispective' cohort studies have become less prominent in more recent epidemiology texts.

planning phase. A number of strategies have been used to minimize study attrition: collection of detailed contact information, sending reminders of follow-up interviews, building rapport, and sharing study findings with participants in the form of newsletters or bulletins (Wadsworth et al. 2003; Stratford et al. 1999).

Challenges and Limitations of Cohort Studies

Cohort studies have contributed greatly to our understanding of the prevalence and distribution of substance use disorders, the course of disorders across time, and information related to utilization of substance use treatment services. They have also been useful in illustrating a number of the challenges and limitations associated with carrying out a long-term prospective cohort study. Considerable human and fiscal resources are needed to enrol, track, and retain participants and to carry out meaningful follow-up for such a long span of time. These challenges are especially prominent in life course studies on substance abuse, due to the time and effort needed to accurately assess outcomes and the multiple potential contributing risk and protective factors that operate at varied levels of influence (from molecular to societal) on the initiation and progression of substance abuse. In addition, as in all observational studies, the designers of cohort studies must anticipate concerns about both imprecisely measured and unmeasured confounding which can undermine the utility of such efforts. Faced with limited resources, investigators must balance the breadth, depth, and size of such cohorts: breadth in terms of the range of contributing conditions and potential confounders assessed, depth regarding the length and intensity of assessment, and size in terms of the number of participants enrolled. Informative cohort studies have ranged from hundreds to hundreds of thousands of participants with commensurate trade-offs between statistical power, on the one hand, and richness of data regarding the multiple complex developmental trajectories that may eventually manifest as disorder, on the other.

Finite resources demand additional trade-offs between cohort enrolment and retention. Successful cohort studies not only need a rich array of data regarding potential risk factors and outcomes, but meaningful inference also requires a high level of retention and protection against threats to validity resulting from attrition and resulting selection bias. While some attrition is inevitable, considerable creative effort and investment in subject retention is necessary to ensure that costly cohort studies yield data of maximal scientific utility. While this applies for cohort studies in general, the close relationship between many disorders and social engagement (such as participation in a prospective cohort study) poses a particularly serious challenge for life course studies. The extent to which attrition is also associated with risk conditions of interest may irrevocably reduce the potential of cohort studies to generate unbiased estimates of interest.

Despite these challenges, however, cohort studies will remain at the forefront of design options to advance the understanding of health development. The strength of a cohort in the LCHD context is primarily the ability to investigate prospectively the synergistic influences of multiple conditions (e.g. genetic, biological, behavioural, social, environmental)—both risk and protective—over time, compare influences at different phases of development, identify potentially sensitive developmental periods, and characterize longitudinal health trajectories as they unfold. They are clearly the method of choice to examine the impact of potentially adverse or risk conditions, which could not be manipulated through a randomized design, due to ethical considerations.

Major Prospective Cohort Studies of Substance Use Disorder

There are several important and well-known general prospective cohort studies examining substance use disorders across the life course. Due to space limitations, we summarize the considerations and decisions made for two of these study designs: Woodlawn Study (2017) and Monitoring the Future Study (2016). These studies serve as excellent examples of the unique type of question that can be answered, as well as the challenges that arise in conducting a prospective cohort study for life course health development. Both studies employed a multi-wave prospective cohort design, and the Monitoring the Future study was designed to enroll a nationally representative sample of the American young adult population. The Woodlawn Study, funded by the National Institute on Drug Abuse (NIDA) and initiated in 1966, recruited a high-risk community of African-American first graders from the same disadvantaged inner city community in Chicago to examine risk factors for substance use disorder. These first graders were followed for a total of four waves: first grade, adolescence, young adulthood, and midlife. This study collected data over the life course—from childhood through adulthood—and initiated data collection prior to the onset of drug use. This design approach allows investigators to compare the onset of substance use disorder and substance use trajectories among children who had similar early roots but disparate pathways to adulthood in terms of family relationships, school, work, peer relationships, religion, and community involvement—a very useful design for a life course health development approach (The Woodlawn Project: A Life Course Study 2017).

Monitoring the Future (MTF) project, also funded by NIDA, began in 1975 using a multistage, stratified random sampling framework to enroll a cohort of participants that were representative of American high school students; each year about 16,000 students in approximately 133 public and private high schools nationwide participate. Though many use this dataset as panel data, or annual cohorts of nationally representative data, there is potential to use MTF as a prospective cohort study. Beginning with the class of 1976, a randomly selected sample from each senior class has been followed up biannually after high school on a continuing basis. Twelve years past high school, participants receive their last young adult questionnaire and then follow-up procedures change to 5-year intervals to cover middle adulthood. This study design allows for investigators to examine (1) changes in particular years such as secular trends or 'period effects', (2) developmental changes that show up consistently for all cohort groups or 'age effects', (3) consistent differences among class cohorts through the life cycle or 'cohort effects', and (4) changes linked to different types of environments or role transitions (Rothman et al. 2008). Both of these cohorts span multiple decades and multiple life stages, providing detailed information on trends in substance use disorder over the life course.

Cohort Example: Trauma and Substance Use Disorder Across the Life Course

Using data from 5 years of follow-up, Chilcoat and Breslau examined the relationship between experiencing a traumatic event and the risk for drug abuse or dependence (Chilcoat and Breslau 1998). They found that participants who had a traumatic event had more than a fourfold increase in risk of drug abuse or dependence compared with those with no history of a traumatic event, after controlling for a number of potential confounders. This study exemplifies the value of prospective cohort studies to advance causal inference in the absence of experimentation: it clearly establishes temporality of exposure (traumatic event) and outcome (drug abuse or dependence), it uses a valid measure to identify diagnoses of drug abuse or dependence (DSM-III-R diagnoses), and it takes into account a number of important factors that could potentially confound the true association between trauma and drug abuse or dependence. However, despite the study's many strengths, because it is an observational study, there remain a number of potential threats to validity. Typically, selection bias is one of the greatest threats to the validity of an observational study. In this case, however, study participants were randomly selected from the membership list of a 400,000 member health maintenance organization in Southeast Michigan. Given all participants were likely from the same region, conclusions may not be generalizable to those in different parts of the

(continued)

(continued)

country. Thus, conclusions should be replicated elsewhere. Information bias is reduced in this example, as diagnoses of drug abuse or dependence were generated independent of knowledge of experiencing trauma. Finally, there remains the potential that there is residual and unmeasured confounding. It would be impossible to measure every potential confounder that occurs over the 5 years that the study spans, and, further, the study was not designed solely to address this particular research question. In any study with such a wide scope and with multiple years of follow-up, there is always the possibility that an important potential confounder was overlooked or was not adequately measured. Prospective cohort studies can span decades, which is very useful for a life course approach, but this comes with additional challenge.

2.1.2 Perinatal and Birth Cohorts

In addition to the general design features of a prospective cohort study, in a birth or perinatal cohort, there are additional challenges involved with recruiting and enrolling participants at or before birth. Parents are the primary target for recruitment, and, depending on the length of follow-up, parents may serve as the primary respondent even though the cohort of interest comprises the offspring generation. In a perinatal cohort study, the emphasis is on factors that occur in the months immediately prior to and following birth. Therefore, studies of this design typically will recruit and enroll parents (usually mothers) who are pregnant or planning to become pregnant in the near future. Data are typically collected on the mother and child throughout the pregnancy, at birth, and for a defined length of time following birth. In a birth cohort, investigators typically design a sampling scheme to target births that occur in a specific geographic region within a specified period of time. For both perinatal and birth cohorts, the length of follow-up is determined by the research questions being posed and the resources available for the study.

Issues related to data collection are another unique concern for perinatal and birth cohorts. While parents may serve as the primary respondent during the child's infancy and toddler years, it is possible to collect data directly on very young children. Special consideration, however, must be given to the length and appropriateness of data collection procedures, training of interviewers, and study consent and assent procedures to ensure adequate protection of human subjects.

Over the years, birth and perinatal cohorts have proved an invaluable source of information in the study of life course health development. Benefiting from the general strengths of cohort studies (e.g. exposure data unbiased by later health status, ability to distinguish cause from effect and temporal sequences), cohorts started at or before birth have the added value of assessing risk, protective variables, and developmental course at the earliest stages of human development. This study design enables investigators to examine the impact of the foetal, infant, and early childhood experience on health development across the life course. We now describe two influential perinatal and birth cohorts, again limiting our scope to studies that have generated substance use disorder diagnoses.

Major Birth Cohort Studies of Substance Use Disorder

There are several important birth cohorts that allow for the study of life course health development and assess substance use disorders. Some of these we describe in detail: the Collaborative Perinatal Project (CPP), New England Family Study (NEFS), and Dunedin Multidisciplinary Health and Development Study (DMHDS).

The CPP was initiated more than 50 years ago to investigate prospectively the prenatal and familial antecedents of paediatric, neurological, and psychological disorders of childhood. The CPP is, in fact, not a birth cohort but rather a prenatal cohort. Across the United States, 12 university-affiliated medical centres participated, including two in New England (in Boston and Providence). More than 50,000 pregnancies were enrolled between 2 January 1959 and 31 December 1965 (16,557 in the NEFS sites) (Broman 1984; Broman et al. 1985). The study followed up 88% of survivors at 1 year, 75% at 4 years, and 79% at 7 years.

Data from examinations and interviews were recorded by trained staff at each site beginning at the time of registration for prenatal care, using standardized protocols, forms, manuals, and codes. At the first prenatal visit, a complete reproductive and gynaecological history, recent and past medical history, socio-economic interview, and family history were recorded. Prenatal clinic visits were scheduled monthly during the first 7 months of pregnancy, every 2 weeks during the 8th month, and every week thereafter. Blood samples were collected for serology and for storage of frozen sera. After admission for delivery, trained observers recorded the events of labour and delivery, and the obstetrician completed labour and delivery protocols. Approximately 75% of subjects had cord blood samples drawn and stored. The neonate was observed in the delivery room, examined by a paediatrician at 24 h intervals in the newborn nursery, and received a neurological examination at 2 days. Study offspring received five subsequent assessments: at ages 4, 8, and 12 months and 4 and 7 years. At each follow-up examination, the mother was interviewed about the child's history, records of medical treatment were obtained if applicable, and physical measurements were taken. Paediatric–neurological examinations occurred at 4 and 12 months and at 7 years and psychological examinations at 8 months and at 4 and 7 years. Family and social history information was obtained from the mother at intake and at 7 years. Diagnostic summaries were prepared by study physicians following the 12-month and 7-year assessments.

Between 2001 and 2004, the New England Family Study was established to locate and interview a sample of the adult CPP offspring in Providence and Boston who lived beyond 7 years of age (15,721)—resulting in a multitude of birth cohort studies spanning more than 40 years. In recent years, this team has extended the follow-up and assessment of three-generation pedigrees in the NEFS, which is still ongoing (i.e. CPP mothers, their offspring who comprise the CPP cohort members, and the offspring of the CPP cohort members). These projects all seek to integrate family designs with early life risk conditions, capitalizing upon the large number of cohort members with multiple offspring. With the increased emphasis on family designs, the overall effort was renamed 'The New England Family Study' (NEFS) (Gilman et al. 2008).

A prominent birth cohort that measures substance use disorder and has taken a life course health development approach is the Dunedin Multidisciplinary Health and Development Study (DMHDS). Investigators enrolled children from 91% of consecutive births from 1 April 1972 through 13 March 1973 in Dunedin, New Zealand. Perinatal data were obtained at delivery, and follow-ups occurred at 3, 5, 7, 9, 11, 13, 15, 18, and 21 years of age. Future assessments are planned for ages 44 and 50 years. At each assessment, study members participated in physical tests, dental examinations, blood tests, and completed computer questionnaires and surveys. At the age 21 year assessment, 94% of cohort members remained in the study, showing no significant attrition effect—a remarkable feat in a longitudinal birth cohort of this nature. Investigators attribute this low attrition rate to aggressive retention measures such as flying participants who had moved away back to New Zealand and using interviewers in other locations such as Australia (Silva and Stanton 1997). Birth cohorts such as the CPP and the DMHDS are incredibly useful for life course health development research because they allow investigators to gain knowledge of developmental processes, as well as multilevel genetic and environmental risk factors.

Birth Cohort Example: Maternal Smoking and Alcohol Use Disorder Across the Life Course

Using the New England Family Study described above, second-generation individuals were followed from birth for more

(continued)

(continued)

than 40 years. Investigators examined the relationship between maternal smoking during pregnancy and lifetime risk for alcohol use disorder (DSM-IV) among 1625 offspring (aged 34–44 years) of 1254 mothers (Nomura et al. 2011). Exposure information was collected from pregnant women at their first prenatal visit, and these questions were repeated at each subsequent prenatal visit up until the time of delivery. Given the robust birth cohort design and long follow-up period, analyses were able to account for maternal mental health during pregnancy, birth weight, neurological abnormality at age 1, childhood behavioural regulation at age 7 years, and academic functioning at age 7 years. Adjusting for these developmental factors and additional demographic variables, results indicated that those with mothers who smoked at least 20 cigarettes per day during pregnancy had a 30% increased risk of lifetime alcohol use disorder. Despite the study's many strengths, there are also limitations inherent to birth cohorts of this type. First, the sample of this particular birth cohort is not representative of a broader population, and therefore external validity is potentially limited. Also, given the long period of follow-up, obstetric care at birth was very different than the modern level of care. Specifically, the mortality rate for those born prematurely was much higher in the late 1960s—thus many children suffering from behavioural regulation problems and poor academic functioning may be offered more effective assistance had they been born today. Finally, as with all observational study designs and those with long follow-up periods, there remains the potential that there is residual and unmeasured confounding. It would be impossible to measure every potential confounder that occurs over the 40 years of that the study.

2.1.3 Twin Studies

Due to their unique genetic status, twins play a valuable role in life course health development research. Using twins as study participants helps investigators advance understanding of genetic and environmental risks, differentiate between genetic influences in different subgroups of people (e.g. males versus females, different age groups, people of different race/ethnicities), and better understand gene–environment interactions. Ultimately, twin studies allow researchers to estimate the proportion of variance in a trait attributable to genetic variation versus the proportion that is due to shared environment or unshared environment (Bundey 1991). Twins are usually recruited from registries, which now exist across the globe. Twin studies can be conducted across study design types, thought the most robust would be longitudinal—similar to a prospective cohort design (Boomsma et al. 2002).

There are several important considerations in twin studies. First, studying twins who grow up in a shared environment does not allow the researcher to consider the effects of both shared environment and gene–environment interaction simultaneously. Rather, this can be addressed by including additional non-twin siblings in the design. Second, results from twin studies cannot be directly generalized to a broader population as there may be genetic factors that lead specifically to a higher incidence of twinning. This raises potential threats to external validity (Bundey 1991). Traditionally, the general consensus was that twin studies represented an optimal study design to examine gene–environment interactions across the life course. Recent criticisms of twin studies and, more generally, 'variation-partitioning' methods employed by behavioural geneticists have emerged, calling into question the extent to which such studies can shed light onto nuanced developmental processes involved in life course development (Tabery 2014; Moore 2015). Tabery (2014) posits that the traditional twin methods offer an overly 'black-box' view of development and are better for general predictions regarding future health outcomes than for nuanced 'mechanism elucidation' of the means by which such developmental processes unfold. This criticism may be unduly harsh as (1) with human populations, observation (rather than experimental manipulation) of gene–environment interactions is the only ethical option and (2) contemporary behavioural geneticists typically avoid simplistic black-box approaches, with hypotheses and analyses informed by other biological and developmental sciences. Recent developments in high-dimensional analysis of both genetic (e.g. GWAS) and environmental (EWAS) factors may help advance traditional approaches to understand the interactive influences of genetic and environmental influences on life course health development (Patel et al. 2010).

Major Twin Studies of Substance Use Disorder

There are many twin registries and twin studies around the world, most of which are in Europe. A few of these have been used to examine substance abuse, two of which we will highlight: the Danish Twin Registry and the Swedish Twin Registry. The Danish Twin Registry was established in the 1950s and is one of the oldest twin registries in the world. The registry now comprises information on almost all twins born in Denmark since 1870. It contains data from church books, the Central Office of Civil Registration, health behaviour and lifestyle variables, and clinical examinations for more than 88,000 twin pairs (Skytthe et al. 2011). Though substance use disorder is one of many outcomes assessed in the registry data, hundreds of other studies using this registry have examined ageing, age-related health, cardiovascular disease, and other rare diseases (Boomsma et al. 2002).

The Swedish Twin Registry contains three cohorts, each differing by ascertainment and extent of data collection. The first cohort was born between 1886 and 1925. Data for the first cohort was ascertained from all parishes across Sweden and contains information on demographics, risk behaviours, cardiovascular health, respiratory health, and environmental exposures. Information on the second cohort, born between 1926 and 1958, was ascertained using nationalized birth registrations and mailed questionnaires. Information covered similar domains as the first cohort and also collected an additional personality inventory. The third cohort, born between 1959 and 1990, was identified by birth registry and has been linked to the Medical Birth Registry. Researchers working with the Swedish Twin Registry have now begun an effort called Screening Across the Lifespan Twin (SALT) study in which investigators have identified subsamples of twins in the registry for more in-depth studies in which blood samples will be obtained; phenotyping and genotyping will be performed; detailed information on health behaviours, clinical diagnoses, and medications will be collected; and linkages will be made to medical records (Lichtenstein et al. 2002). Both of these registries, as well as twin cohorts generally, pose a unique opportunity to examine the multilevel and multidimensional genetic and environmental risks for health development across the life course.

Twin Cohort Example: Childhood Sexual Abuse and Substance Use Disorder

The research literature has consistently suggested a link between childhood sexual abuse and negative health outcomes, but there remain concerns for selection bias and confounding by family environment. To address this question while minimizing confounding by family environment, investigators derived a sample of 1159 female–female twin pairs and 832 male–male twin pairs from a young adult Australian volunteer twin panel. Structured psychiatric telephone interviews were conducted to assess childhood sexual abuse and adverse psychosocial outcomes including alcohol dependence (DSM-IV) and nicotine dependence (DSM-IV). Family background information was elicited including parental fighting, parental conflict, stepparent presence, neglect, and physical abuse. Results suggested that individuals with a history of childhood sexual abuse have increased risk

(continued)

(continued)

of developing alcohol and nicotine dependence. Results also showed that childhood sexual abuse is associated with substantial risk that is not explained by other family background factors. There is, however, a potential for bias. Selection bias may have arisen due to the fact that parents aware of abuse may have been less likely to volunteer their twins for research. Regardless, using a twin study approach allowed researchers to dissect the direct and correlated family background effects of childhood sexual abuse (Nelson et al. 2002).

2.1.4 High-Risk Cohort

The high-risk cohort study is a variation on the general cohort study described above, with the key distinction being that subjects are recruited because they have been selected on the basis of their exposure history. Often, subjects are identified as being at high risk for developing the outcome of interest based on particular behaviours and characteristics or manifestations of previous pathology in their parents.

Studies such as these allow researchers to better examine the natural history of disorders in relation to a particular high-risk population. One potential limitation of high-risk studies, however, is that their results, and, ultimately, the conclusions they draw, may only be applicable for high-risk populations. By contrast, high-risk studies do provide an efficient means of examining relatively rare disorders.

Major High-Risk Cohort of Substance Use Disorder

Though high-risk cohorts of substance use disorder tend to be smaller studies of very specific high-risk populations (e.g. injection-drug users, HIV-infected individuals, or the homeless), veterans have been identified as a high-risk group more likely than others to fall victim to substance abuse as a means of coping. Following the 1991 Gulf War, the US Congress and the Institute of Medicine recommended the US Department of Defense to conduct a high-risk cohort study of military personnel. This initiative was entitled the Millennium Cohort Study and is the largest prospective health study of military personnel including more than 200,000 participants. Data collection for the study began in 2001 with the 77,047 participants enrolled. Every 3 years additional participants are enrolled and an additional wave of data collection is conducted. The very first group recruited has completed five waves of data collection to date. Questionnaires at each wave assess general health, health behaviours, clinical diagnoses, physical symptoms, mental illness, health care utilization, and military life and experience. Many studies have already been conducted using this cohort and many focus on substance disorder and mental health (The Millenium Cohort Study 2010). This high-risk cohort allows researchers to better understand the risk associated with military service and seeing combat, but may not represent health development in the general population.

High-Risk Cohort Example: Posttraumatic Stress Disorder and Substance Abuse

An investigation into the relationship between posttraumatic stress disorder (PTSD) symptoms and substance abuse utilizing a high-risk cohort was conducted by Bremner et al. (1996). These investigators recruited Vietnam combat veterans with PTSD to study the effect of specific PTSD symptoms on substance abuse. Analyses examined the occurrence of substance abuse among veterans with respect to PTSD symptomology. The high-risk design ensured a large number of veterans with and without PTSD symptoms resulting in a powerful method to examine the influence of these symptoms on substance abuse. Analyses revealed a strong and consistent association between onset of PTSD symptoms and onset of substance abuse. Similarly, an increase of PTSD symptoms

(continued)

(continued)

predicted onset of substance abuse. This study allowed researchers to better examine the natural history of substance abuse among Vietnam War veterans with PTSD. However, the conclusions they draw may only be applicable for this high-risk population.

2.1.5 Case–Control Studies

Unlike the study designs we have described up to this point in which participants are recruited into the study and followed over time to ascertain their outcome status, in a case–control study, participants are selected based on the presence or absence of a disorder, and exposure data are obtained after the outcome has been ascertained. Although case–control studies are not the strongest design option for conducting life course research, this particular study design has a number of benefits (Schlesselman and Schneiderman 1982). Because participants are selected after the outcome of interest has occurred, case–control studies are typically extremely cost-effective, especially in studying rare diseases. As compared with cohort studies, in which the investigator may need to follow a large number of participants for years to identify the outcome of interest, in a case–control study, the outcome has already occurred, and the investigator seeks to determine those exposures or conditions that may have contributed to this occurrence.

Challenges and Limitations of Case–Control Studies

In a case–control study, the primary threats to study validity lie in the selection of controls and in the ascertainment of exposure status. Because in a case–control study, the outcome has occurred prior to the investigator's assessment, there is a threat of recall bias (Schlesselman and Schneiderman 1982; Lee et al. 2007; Berney and Blane 1997). Exposures, by definition, occurred in the past, and those collected through participant self-report introduce the possibility of people inaccurately recalling their exposure history. Often, those who have developed the outcome of interest are more likely to examine their past exposures more carefully in an attempt to find an explanation for why they developed the disease. In a case such as this, where cases are systematically reporting exposure differently from controls, recall bias has been introduced into the study, and, because it systematically differs among exposed and unexposed, this bias may potentially skew study findings. The challenge lies in identifying a way to measure past exposures without introducing bias or inconsistencies in their assessment.

In the trauma and substance abuse literature, reports of childhood sexual abuse and physical punishment were shown to be unreliable. Specifically, unreliability arose because those who were subject to abuse often provided false-negative reports. This could cause estimates of abuse prevalence based on a single report to seriously underestimate the true prevalence; however, estimates of the relative risk of psychiatric problems conditional on abuse are robust to the effects of these reporting errors (Fergusson et al. 2000). It is very important when using a case–control design to optimize the reliability of exposure measurements to minimize or avoid the potential of recall bias being introduced into the study.

Another important limitation is the potential for selection bias. In a case–control study, identification of cases is fairly straightforward; it is the identification of controls, however, that presents a challenge (Schlesselman and Schneiderman 1982; Wacholder et al. 1992). Cases and controls must arise from the same study base; if controls were to have developed the outcome of interest, they must have been eligible to be identified as cases. Although this sounds relatively straightforward, in practice it can be quite difficult to ensure that the controls properly represent the study base from which cases have been drawn. This is an especially important point because, in order to estimate accurately the effect of exposure on the outcome, the controls are being used to estimate the exposure distribution in the study population; therefore, a misrepresentative selection of controls could bias study results significantly (Lee et al. 2007).

Given case–control studies are conducted, retrospectively, there are not commonly ongoing examples of case–control studies as there are with cohorts. Therefore, we present a specific example of a case–control study of substance use disorder, but will not highlight any major case–control studies as we did with cohorts.

Case–Control Example: Traumas and Alcohol Abuse and Dependence

Investigators selected cases from area intervention programmes, 132 adolescents with alcohol dependence (DSM-IV) and 51 with alcohol abuse (DSM-IV), and controls by random-digit dialling and advertisement in the broader community, 73 adolescents. Questions were asked concerning lifetime traumatic events such as physical abuse, sexual abuse, violent victimization, witnessing violence, and other miscellaneous traumas. Results found that traumatic events in every category had higher rates of occurrence in the alcohol dependence and abuse groups than in the control group. Some limitations remain in this study: we cannot assume causality, adolescents with disorder may not be representative of all adolescents with disorder, community controls may not be representative of adolescents in the general population, and there may be reporting error in trauma reports (Clark et al. 1997).

2.1.6 Nested Case–Control Designs

A nested case–control study is a variation of the traditional case–control study design. In this study design, cases of a disease that occur in a defined cohort are identified, and often, a specified number of matched controls are selected from among those in the cohort who have not developed the disease. This design is advantageous when the exposure of interest is difficult or expensive to obtain and when the outcome is rare. A nested case–control design is particularly efficient due to reductions in recruitment and data collection costs with relatively minor loss in statistical efficiency (Ernster 1994). Yet, challenges and limitations of this design remain and are similar to those of a traditional case–control design.

Nested Case–Control Example: Trauma and Substance Use Disorder

Cutajar et al. (2010) investigated the relationship between childhood sexual abuse and the occurrence of substance use disorder. In this study, researchers drew cases from a pre-existing cohort of child sexual abuse victims compiled by the Victorian Institute of Forensic Medicine in Australia. This approach is referred to as a nested case–control study design. Researchers identified 2759 sexually abused children from the cohort (verified via forensic medical records assessed between 1964 and 1995). The control group was drawn from a random sample of Victorian residents from the national electoral database. This yielded 2677 age- and gender-matched controls from the general population. Both case and control participants were linked with a public psychiatric database, the Victorian Psychiatric Case Register, between 12 and 43 years later. Control subjects were matched on gender and age groupings drawn from the general population through a random sample of the national electoral database. The use of archival data from childhood to identify victims of sexual abuse lends strength to this study as it minimizes the introduction of recall bias. Yet, there is the potential for selection bias insofar as the comparison group may not be representative of the population from which the cases arose; for instance, there may be something systematically different between those with a history of childhood

(continued)

(continued)

sexual abuse and those in the general population. In a study such as this, where cases are identified from forensic medical records, it can be difficult to define clearly what constitutes the study base, i.e. what group of patients would have eventually been identified by forensic medical records had they experienced childhood sexual abuse. Results from this study suggest those with a history of childhood sexual abuse have almost six times the odds of substance abuse disorder compared to those with no sexual abuse history.

2.1.7 Cross-Sectional Studies

In life course research, cross-sectional studies provide information on both the prevalence of disease and associations between risk factors and disease but typically provide little definitive information to further understanding of causal relationships. In a typical cross-sectional study, participants are sampled and interviewed at a single time point (Gilman 2002). As compared to case–control studies described above, cross-sectional studies typically place less emphasis on reconstructing past exposure; rather they provide a snapshot of prevalence of disease and associations between exposure and disease in a given sample at a given time often limiting the inference we can make regarding the temporal sequence between exposure and disease. Another difference from case–control studies is the sampling framework. In case–control studies, a great deal of effort is placed on sampling an informative set of controls that are representative of the population that gave rise to the case. In cross-sectional studies, participants may include either a sample of convenience (based on their availability and willingness to participate) or they are often based on a representative sample of the general population (which allows for high generalizability). Cross-sectional studies, while not typically considered a strong design option for life course research, provide important insight into the prevalence of disorders in a population and can provide initial evidence as to potential associations that can be investigated further using a more stringent study design (Kraemer et al. 2000). Additionally, retrospective data can be collected from participants either using archival data or during the interview process in an attempt to reconstruct past exposure history.

Challenges and Limitations of Cross-Sectional Studies

Cross-sectional studies have a host of limitations. First, if the sample is a convenience sample, rather than representative of the population, threats to external validity exist. Second, non-response can result in bias of study measures. For example, despite trying to sample for a representative population, many individuals may not respond due to having severe negative health outcomes or being part of a high-risk, transient population; both of these examples would result in a loss of critical study information. Also, due to the cross-sectional nature of data collection, temporality of the exposure and outcome cannot be confirmed. Finally, cross-sectional designs are not suitable for studying rare diseases or diseases with short duration.

Major Cross-Sectional Studies of Substance Use Disorder

There are many publicly available, nationally representative cross-sectional surveys conducted in the United States. Of these, several include measures of substance use disorder. We will describe one of these: the National Survey on Drug Use and Health (NSDUH). The NSDUH provides national- and state-level data on substance use, disorder, and mental health in the United States. It is sponsored by the Substance Abuse and Mental Health Services Administration. The NSDUH is administrated annually to approximately 70,000 randomly selected individuals aged 12 years and older. The goals of NSDUH are to provide accurate prevalence estimates on the level and patterns of substance use and abuse, track trends in substance use, assess the consequences of substance use, and identify groups at high risk for substance disorder. Though this cross-sectional survey assesses different individuals over time, it provides useful information on secular trends of and consistent risk factors for substance use disorder (National Survey on Drug Use and Health 2017).

Cross-Sectional Example: Trauma and Substance Use Disorder

Returning to our examination of the relationship between trauma and substance use disorder, Molnar, Buka, and Kessler conducted a cross-sectional study using a US national household probability sample of 8098 participants aged 15 to 54 years from the National Comorbidity Survey (Molnar et al. 2001). Given the size and relatively low cost of a single cross-sectional assessment, researchers were able to account for age, race, parental divorce, parental psychopathology, parental verbal and physical abuse, and parental substance use problems while examining the association between childhood sexual abuse and substance use disorder (DSM-III-R). Results found those with a history of childhood sexual assault had about a twofold odds of drug dependence and 1.7 times the odds of alcohol dependence compared to those with no history of childhood sexual assault. However, cross-sectional data do not allow for causal inferences to be made about the relationship between being assaulted and substance use disorder; given that all data are from one time point, there is no evidence as to the temporality of the exposure–outcome relationship. Further, information bias can arise depending on how data are collected. In the example above, timing and characteristics of childhood sexual assault and substance use disorder were self-reported, introducing the possibility of reporting bias and recall bias. Cross-sectional studies also have the potential for unmeasured confounding. Given that all data are collected from one time point, many other factors that could be influencing the association of interest are not captured by the one-time assessment.

2.2 Quasi-Experimental Designs

Unlike true experiments, where the investigator manipulates the exposures or conditions affecting research participants, quasi-experiments are characterized by investigator manipulation of observations (not treatments). Given the focus of this chapter, observations would typically be assessments of substance use disorder, implemented after the occurrence of major events of relevance to life course theory—such as natural disasters (e.g. Hurricane Katrina), acts of terrorism, and events resulting from policy changes and the like, such as marijuana legalization. Such quasi- or natural experiments largely differ from traditional observational studies in that participants are largely 'selected' into exposed or unexposed groups by an event that is substantially not within their own control.

2.2.1 Challenges and Limitations of Quasi-Experimental Studies

As natural experiments, these studies are often less subject to selection bias than typical observational studies. However, at the same time, attempts to study the consequences of such quasi-experiments may be hampered by the challenges of responding quickly to initiate an investigation soon after a natural occurrence of interest has taken place. Poorly implemented efforts may introduce problems related to both information bias (where respondents are typically not blind to the event of interest and may provide non-comparable information) and confounding, where the investigation may not be able to assess the full relevant set of potential confounding factors.

Quasi-Experimental Example: Trauma and Substance Use Disorder

Returning to our example on trauma and substance use disorder, Reijneveld et al. found themselves in a position to examine the impact of trauma in a natural experiment (Reijneveld et al. 2003). In 2001, a fire in a café in Volendam, Netherlands, wounded 250 adolescents and killed 14.

(continued)

(continued)

Surprisingly, 15 months prior to the disaster, all students aged 12–15 years from a school in Volendam (of whom 31 had been in the café during the fire), and from two other schools, had been selected as controls for a study. Five months after the disaster, researchers obtained follow-up data from Volendam adolescents and controls from the other two schools. Contrary to previous study designs, which examined the impact of trauma on substance use, Reijneveld et al. were able to examine this relationship in a setting in which trauma, a potentially strong explanatory variable for substance use, was directly manipulated by forces outside the control of the researchers. The exposure (the disaster) was a horrific accident; yet, only adolescents living in Volendam were 'exposed'. Compared with an observational design, in which there are very many interrelated factors impacting an adolescent's likelihood of exposure to trauma, in this study, trauma was controlled by a force outside of the researchers' and participants' control (an 'exogenous' factor). It was not, however, randomly assigned; the exposure to the disaster was correlated with going to school in Volendam, raising potential concerns of remaining confounding. Therefore, any factors related to neighbourhood or town that differ between those exposed to the fire and those not exposed were not addressed. The authors observed that Volendam adolescents who were exposed to the disaster had almost fivefold the odds of excessive alcohol use compared to other adolescents, providing important new evidence supporting the causal relationship between trauma and excessive alcohol use among adolescents.

2.3 Experimental Designs

In experimental studies, such as randomized control trials (RCTs), participants are randomly assigned to receive exposure or not with the exposure being manipulated by study investigators. Given a large enough sample, the implications of this randomization and manipulation of exposure are related to the inferences that may be made about causality. When exposure is truly assigned at random to study participants, it is assumed that, on average, all known and unknown confounders are evenly distributed across the study arms and, therefore, that the two arms of the study are exchangeable. When these and other conditions are fulfilled (adequately large sample, effective randomization, reasonably representative sample, meaningful external validity/generalizability), RCTs provide a unique opportunity to generate evidence of the causal impact of exposures on subsequent health and development. As discussed below, conventionally the major limitations raised regarding experimental studies concerned feasibility and ethics. More recent contributions from the developmental and social sciences raise more fundamental questions regarding the utility of experimental approaches in the context of rich and multifactorial developmental processes such as those involved with life course health development (Lerner and Callina 2014; Sampson 2010).

2.3.1 Challenges and Limitations of Experimental Studies

In substance abuse epidemiology, investigators typically examine the impact of harmful exposures or 'risk factors' on substance use disorders; obviously, the random allocation of harmful exposures to study participants is not ethically permissible. To illustrate, researchers have long wanted to understand the impact of trauma on the development of substance use disorder; nevertheless it would be unethical to randomly assign participants to undergo a traumatic life event so that investigators could study their response. Further, logistic considerations and the high cost associated with the long-term follow-up of subjects further limit the use of RCTs in life course research. As a result, due to the ethical considerations combined with practical constraints, experimental studies (in particular of potentially harmful conditions) are not often used in psychiatric or substance use research. Randomized controlled trials pertaining to trauma and substance use disorders are limited to those that assess the effectiveness of treatments or interventions such as cognitive behavioural therapy or sertraline administration (Cohen et al. 2007; Van Dam et al. 2012).

Randomized Controlled Trial Experimental Example: PTSD and Substance Use Treatment

A recent RCT by Mills et al. aimed to determine whether an integrated treatment for PTSD and substance dependence can achieve greater reductions in PTSD and substance dependence symptom severity compared with usual treatment for substance dependence (Mills et al. 2012). In 2007–2009 in Sydney, Australia, 103 adults with diagnoses of PTSD and substance dependence were recruited from substance use treatment services, media advertisements, and practitioner referrals. Fifty-five participants were randomized to receive Concurrent Treatment of PTSD and Substance Use Disorders Using Prolonged Exposure (COPE) in addition to usual treatment for substance dependence, and 48 were randomized to receive the usual treatment only. Participants were reinterviewed at 6 weeks, 3 months, and 9 months. Results suggested the treatment group had significant reductions in PTSD symptom severity relative to the control group, yet there was no significant difference in prevalence or severity of substance dependence between treatment and control groups. Whereas this study does not perfectly map on to previous examples examining the relationship between trauma and substance use disorder, it does illustrate the strengths of the RCT for life course research. In this study, the randomization of adults diagnosed with PTSD and substance dependence created groups that appear to be exchangeable at baseline. Exchangeability of the groups allows us to make comparisons between the groups under the assumption that the groups are identical with the exception of the treatment. Further, we would expect that randomization would eliminate the potential for selection bias to occur in the allocation of treatment, thus preventing systematic differences between the two groups (i.e. all participants have equal probability of receiving treatment or control). RCTs can be incredibly informative for establishing causation between an exposure and an outcome, though many exposures would be unethical for an investigator to administer. However, in assessing the impact of treatments for disorders throughout the life course, RCTs would be the gold standard.

3 Discussion

We close by revisiting several of the central principles of the life course health development framework introduced at the beginning of this volume (see Halfon and Forrest 2017) and discussing opportunities to advance understanding of the causes and promotion of health development through the various research design alternatives covered in this chapter. The current chapter discusses traditional epidemiologic designs and offers examples of how these have been altered and extended to contribute to our nascent understanding of how health and disease develop across the life course. However, the concept of 'health development' goes beyond traditional and often static definitions of 'health', 'disease', and 'disorder'. Fully integrating the life course health development framework into study design selection requires new thinking and innovation from the epidemiology community. As outlined in Principle 1, health development—the focus of scientific inquiry in this field—is conceptualized as a dynamic process that 'combines both health and development…blends a temporal dimension into our conceptualization of human health…{with} time-dependent and transactional connotations' (p. 15). Designs that are faithful to this view will require new perspectives, measures, and analytic methods. Developments in latent class trajectory modelling (Nagin 2016), behavioural trajectories, and their investigation in multilevel contexts (Cerda et al. 2008) are all contributing to this extension of traditional design approaches.

Principle 3 in the LCHD framework addresses the topic of complexity. Complexity refers to how health development is dependent upon complex reciprocal interactions between individuals and their physical, natural, and social environments. To appropriately study complexity, a broad array of individual and environmental factors must be measured. Epidemiologic methods allow for the assessment of interactions and multiple interactions in studies; however, the number of variables and variable interactions assessed is inversely related to the resulting level of statistical power and directly related to the number of type II or false-positive findings. Similarly, understanding that interactions play an important role in health development, researchers should examine bidirectional relationships between individual and environmental characteristics. Future studies examining interactions should be designed as longitudinal studies (to determine temporality/causality), and large sample sizes should be used to increase power to detect important interactions. New efforts to develop 'environment-wide association study' (EWAS) methods, to parallel genome-wide association studies (GWAS) and new developments in machine learning, may provide additional solutions to the problem of sample size and growing numbers of potential risk and protective factors (Patel et al. 2010). Also, given the complexity of the life course approach, it is unlikely that a single study will definitively advance LCHD theory. Rather, a compilation of studies from different populations (or the same population over time) at different stages in the life course and across different realms of development (e.g. physical, social, environmental, genetic, epigenetic, etc.) and contexts will be necessary for advances regarding health development throughout the life course.

Another fundamental element principle of the LCHD framework is timing. This principle refers to the concept that there are specific developmental stages throughout the life course (e.g. in utero, pubescence) in which the impact of certain exposures on an individual can be greater than during other periods, with the attendant implications of the importance of nurturing children when they are most sensitive to these influences. Reflecting the importance of the time dimension for health development, this principle further underscores the value of prospective cohort designs, not only as these involve the study of time, but also, in contrast to retrospective or cross-sectional designs, they permit more accurate prospective assessment of multiple risk and protective conditions as these occur. For example, the landmark Adverse Child Experiences Survey has documented the association between childhood adversity and a range of poor health outcomes, using adult retrospective reports of child experiences (Felitti et al. 1998). Refined understanding of the impact and timing of such early adverse experiences will, however, require prospective studies that are less subject to potential recall, detection, and selection biases (Widom et al. 2015). Interest in 'timing' does not necessarily always imply the need for longitudinal designs. Cross-sectional studies conducted during particularly sensitive stages of the life course could also be informative, and preferable to cross-sectional studies during other, less impactful periods. Also, in longitudinal cohorts, researchers may want to consider giving more weight to exposures during these sensitive periods. Collaboration across disciplines will help suggest certain stages in the life course that are likely to have particular relevance for long-term health development, for example, due to a propensity for epigenetic alterations or other forms of biologic sensitivity (Moffitt 2013).

In closing, life course approaches to advance understanding of the causes and prevention of disorders are rich in both potential and challenges. Relatively rare disorders and outcomes require large sample sizes; complex conditions require considerable effort and resources for accurate assessment and characterization; multiple contributing factors from the molecular to the societal level require rich exposure assessments; and the complexity of the human condition introduces a range of potential confounding factors. Each of the study designs presented in this chapter has advanced our knowledge of how disorders originate, progress, may be treated, and may diminish over the life course. Yet they have been traditionally used to investigate relative static conditions, disorders, and disease states. Further work applying the principles of life course health development to study design, measurement, and analytic approaches are essential to help realize the goals and aspirations of the life course framework (Buka and Lipsitt 1994; Buka 2003).

References

Ahern, J., & Leslie, H. H. (2014). Life course approach to substance use. In K. C. Koenen, S. Rudenstine, S. Galea, & E. Susser (Eds.), *A life course approach to mental disorders* (pp. 133–140). Oxford: Oxford University Press.

Angold, A., & Costello, E. J. (1995). Developmental epidemiology. *Epidemiologic Reviews, 17*(1), 74–82.

Aschengrau, A., & Seage, G. R. (2008). *Essentials of epidemiology in public health* (2nd ed.). Sudbury: Jones & Bartlett.

Baltes, P. B., Lindenberger, U., & Staudinger, U. M. (1998). Life-span theory n developmental psychology. In W. Damon & R. M. Lerner (Eds.), *Handbook of child psychology volume 1: Theoretical models of human development* (pp. 1029–1143). New York: Wiley.

Baltes, P. B., Lindenberger, U., & Staudinger, U. M. (2006). Life span theory in developmental psychology. In W. Damon & R. M. Lerner (Eds.), *Handbook of child psychology: Vol. 1. Theoretical models of development* (6th ed., pp. 569–664). Hoboken: Wiley.

Barker, D. J. P. (2004). The developmental origins of adult disease. *Journal of the American College of Nutrition, 23*(Suppl 6), 588S–595S.

Ben-Shlomo, Y., & Kuh, D. (2002). A life course approach to chronic disease epidemiology: Conceptual models, empirical challenges and interdisciplinary perspectives. *International Journal of Epidemiology, 31*(2), 285–293.

Berney, L. R., & Blane, D. B. (1997). Collecting retrospective data: Accuracy of recall after 50 years judged against historical records. *Social Science & Medicine, 45*(10), 1519–1525.

Boomsma, D., Busjahn, A., & Peltonen, L. (2002). Classical twin studies and beyond. *Nature Reviews Genetics, 3*, 872–882.

Bremner, J. D., Southwick, S. M., Darnell, A., & Charney, D. S. (1996). Chronic PTSD in Vietnam combat veterans: Course of illness and substance abuse. *The American Journal of Psychiatry, 153*(3), 369–375.

Broman, S. (1984). *The collaborative perinatal project: An overview*. New York: Praeger.

Broman, S., Bien, E., & Shaughnessy, P. (1985). *Low achieving children: The first seven years*. Hillsdale: Lawrence Erlbaum Associates.

Buka, S. L. (2003). Principles of developmental epidemiology. In S. H. White & D. B. Pillemer (Eds.), *Developmental psychology and the social changes of our time*. Cambridge, MA: Harvard University Press.

Buka, S. L., & Lipsitt, L. P. (1994). Toward a developmental epidemiology. In S. L. Friedman & H. C. Haywood (Eds.), *Developmental follow-up: Concepts, domains and methods* (pp. 331–350). San Diego: Academic Press.

Bundey, S. (1991). Uses and limitations of twin studies. *Journal of Neurology, 238*(7), 360–364.

Cerda, M., Sánchez, B. N., Sandro, G., Tracy, M., & Buka, S. L. (2008). Estimating co-occurring behavioral trajectories within a neighborhood context: A case study of multivariate transition models for clustered data. *American Journal of Epidemiology, 168*(10), 1190–1203.

Chilcoat, H. W., & Breslau, N. (1998). Investigations of causal pathways between PTSD and drug use disorders. *Addictive Behaviors, 23*(6), 827–840.

Clark, D. B., Lesnick, L., & Hegedus, A. M. (1997). Traumas and other adverse life events in adolescents with alcohol abuse and dependence. *Journal of the American Academy of Child and Adolescent Psychiatry, 36*(12), 1744–1751.

Cohen, J. A., Mannarino, A. P., Perel, J. M., & Staron, V. (2007). A pilot randomized controlled trial of combined trauma-focused CBT and sertraline for childhood PTSD symptoms. *Journal of the American Academy of Child and Adolescent Psychiatry, 46*(7), 811–819.

Cutajar, M. C., Mullen, P. E., Ogloff, J. R. P., Thomas, S. D., Wells, D. L., & Spataro, J. (2010). Psychopathology in a large cohort of sexually abused children followed up to 43 years. *Child Abuse & Neglect, 34*(11), 813–822.

Elder, G. H., Jr., & Rockwell, R. C. (1979). The life-course and human development: An ecological perspective. *International Journal of Behavioral Development, 2*(1), 1–21.

Elder, G. H., & Shanahan, M. J. (2007). The life course and human development. In *Handbook of child psychology* (6th ed., pp. 665–715). New York: Wiley.

Ernster, V. L. (1994). Nested case-control studies. *Preventive Medicine, 23*(5), 587–590.

Felitti, V. J., Anda, R. F., Nordenberg, D., Williamson, D. F., Spitz, A. M., Edwards, V., Koss, M. P., & Marks, J. S. (1998). Relationship of childhood abuse and household dysfunction to many of the leading causes of death in adults. The Adverse Childhood Experiences (ACE) study. *American Journal of Preventative Medicine, 14*(4), 245–258.

Fergusson, D. M., Horwood, L. J., & Woodward, L. J. (2000). The stability of child abuse reports: A longitudinal study of the reporting behaviour of young adults. *Psychological Medicine, 30*(3), 529–544.

George, L. K. (1999). *Life-course perspectives on mental health* (pp. 565–583). New York: Springer.

Giele, J. Z., & Elder, G. H., Jr. (1998). Life course research: Development of a field. In J. Z. Giele & G. H. Elder Jr. (Eds.), *Methods of life course research: Qualitative and quantitative approaches* (pp. 5–27). Thousand Oaks, CA: Sage.

Gilman, S. E. (2002). Commentary: Childhood socioeconomic status, life course pathways and adult mental health. *International Journal of Epidemiology, 31*(2), 403–404.

Gilman, S. E., Martin, L. T., Abrams, D. B., Kawachi, I., Kubzansky, L., et al. (2008). Educational attainment and cigarette smoking: A causal association? *International Journal of Epidemiology, 37*, 615–624.

Halfon, N., & Forrest, C. B. (2017). The emerging theoretical framework of life course health development. In N. Halfon, C. B. Forrest, R. M. Lerner, & E. Faustman (Eds.), *Handbook of life course health-development science*. Cham: Springer.

Halfon, N., Larson, K., Lu, M., Tullis, E., & Russ, S. (2014). Lifecourse health-development: Past, present and future. *Matern Child Health, 18*(2), 344–365.

Jablonka, E., & Lamb, M. J. (2005). *Evolution in four dimensions: Genetic, epigenetic, behavioral, and symbolic variation in the history of life*. Cambridge, CA: The MIT Press.

Kraemer, H. C., Yesavage, J. A., Taylor, J. L., & Kupfer, D. (2000). How can we learn about developmental processes from cross-sectional studies, or can we? *The American Journal of Psychiatry, 157*(2), 163–171.

Kuh, D., Ben-Shlomo, Y., Lynch, J., Hallqvist, J., & Power, C. (2003). Life course epidemiology. *Journal of Epidemiology and Community Health, 57*(10), 778–783.

Lee, W., Bindman, J., Ford, T., et al. (2007). Bias in psychiatric case—Control studies. *The British Journal of Psychiatry, 190*(3), 204–209.

Lerner, R. M., & Callina, K. S. (2014). Relational developmental systems theories and the ecological validity of experimental designs: Commentary on Freund and Isaacowitz. *Human Development, 56*, 372–380.

Lichtenstein, P., De Faire, U., Floderus, B., Svartengren, M., Svedberg, P., & Pedersen, N. L. (2002). The Swedish twin registry: A unique resource for clinical, epidemiological and genetic studies. *Journal of Internal Medicine, 252*(3), 184–205.

Magnusson, D. (Ed.). (1996). *The lifespan development of individuals: Behavioral, neurobiological and psychosocial perspectives*. Cambridge, CA: Cambridge University Press.

Mills, K. L., Teesson, M., Back, S. E., Brady, K. T., Baker, A. L., et al. (2012). Integrated exposure-based therapy for co-occurring posttraumatic stress disorder and substance dependence. *JAMA, 308*(7), 690–699.

Moffitt, T. E. (2013). Childhood exposure to violence and lifelong health: Clinical intervention science and stress-biology research join forces. *Development and Psychopathology (Cambridge University Press), 25*, 1619–1634.

Molnar, B. E., Buka, S. L., & Kessler, R. C. (2001). Child sexual abuse and subsequent psychopathology: Results from the National Comorbidity Survey. *American Journal of Public Health, 91*(5), 753–760.

Monitoring the Future: a continuing study of American youth (2016). University of Michigan. http://www.monitoringthefuture.org/

Moore, D. S. (2015).The asymmetrical bridge: A review of James Tabery's book "Beyond versus." *Acta Biotheoretica*. doi: 10.1007/s10441-015-9270-z.

Nagin, D. S. (2016). Group-based trajectory modeling and criminal career research. *Journal of Research in Crime and Delinquency, 53*(3), 356–371.

National Survey on Drug Use and Health (2017). Substance Abuse and Mental Health Services Administration. U.S. Department of Health and Human Services. https://nsduhweb.rti.org

Nelson, E. C., Heath, A. C., Madden, P. A., Cooper, M. L., Dinwiddie, S. H., Bucholz, K. K., Glowinski, A., McLaughlin, T., Dunne, M. P., Statham, D. J., & Martin, N. G. (2002). Association between self-reported childhood sexual abuse and adverse psychosocial outcomes: Results from a twin study. *JAMA Psychiatry, 59*(2), 139–145.

Nomura, Y., Gilman, S. E., & Buka, S. L. (2011). Maternal smoking during pregnancy and risk of alcohol use disorders among adult offspring. *Journal of Studies on Alcohol and Drugs, 72*, 199–209.

Patel, C. J., Bhattacharya, J., & Butte, A. J. (2010). An environment-wide association study (EWAS) on type 2 diabetes mellitus. *PloS One, 5*(5), e10746. doi:10.1371/journal.pone.0010746.

Pickles, A., Maughan, B., & Wadsworth, M. (2007). *Epidemiological methods in life course research*. New York: Oxford University Press.

Reijneveld, S. A., Crone, M. R., Verhulst, F. C., & Verloove-Vanhorick, S. P. (2003). The effect of a severe disaster on the mental health of adolescents: A controlled study. *Lancet, 362*(9385), 691–696.

Rothman, K. J., Greenland, S., & Lash, T. L. (2008). *Modern epidemiology* (3rd ed.). Philadelphia: Lippincott Willams & Wilkins.

Sampson, R. J. (2010). Gold standard myths: Observations on the experimental turn in quantitative criminology. *Journal of Quantitative Criminology, 26*(4), 489–500.

Schlesselman, J. J., & Schneiderman, M. A. (1982). Case control studies: Design, conduct, analysis. *Journal of Occupational and Environmental Medicine, 24*(11), 879.

Silva, P. A., & Stanton, W. R. (1997). *From child to adult: The Dunedin Multidisciplinary health and development study*. New York: Oxford University Press.

Skytthe, A., Kyvik, K. O., Holm, N. V., & Christensen, K. (2011). The Danish twin registry. *Scandinavian Journal of Public Health, 39*(7 Suppl), 75–78.

Stratford, R., Mulligan, J., Downie, B., & Voss, L. (1999). Threats to validity in the longitudinal study of psychological effects: The case of short stature. *Child: Care, Health and Development, 25*(6), 401–419.

Susser, M., & Susser, E. (1996). Choosing a future for epidemiology: II. From black box to Chinese boxes and eco-epidemiology. *American Journal of Public Health, 86*(5), 674–677.

Susser, E., Terry, M. B., & Matte, T. (2000). The birth cohorts grow up: New opportunities for epidemiology. *Paediatric and Perinatal Epidemiology, 14*(2), 98–100.

Tabery, J. (2014). *Beyond versus: The struggle to understand the interaction of nature and nurture*. Cambridge: MIT Press.

The Millenium Cohort Study (2010). Department of Defense. https://www.millenniumcohort.org/

The Woodlawn Project: A Life Course Study (2017). Johns Hopkins Bloomberg School of Public Health. http://www.jhsph.edu/research/affiliated-programs/woodlawn-study/

Van Dam, D., Vedel, E., Ehring, T., & Emmelkamp, P. M. G. (2012). Psychological treatments for concurrent posttraumatic stress disorder and substance use disorder: A systematic review. *Clinical Psychology Review, 32*(3), 202–214.

Wacholder, S., Silverman, D. T., McLaughlin, J. K., & Mandel, J. S. (1992). Selection of controls in case-control studies. II. Types of controls. *American Journal of Epidemiology, 135*(9), 1029–1041.

Wadsworth, M. E. J., Butterworth, S. L., Hardy, R. J., et al. (2003). The life course prospective design: An example of benefits and problems associated with study longevity. *Social Science & Medicine, 57*(11), 2193–2205.

Widom, C. S., Zaja, C., & Du Mont, K. A. (2015). Intergenerational transmission of child abuse and neglect: Real or detection bias? *Science, 347*(27), 1480–1485.

Woodward, M. (2005). *Epidemiology: Study design and data analysis* (2nd ed.). Boca Raton: Chapman & Hall/CRC Press.

Using the National Longitudinal Surveys of Youth (NLSY) to Conduct Life Course Analyses

Elizabeth C. Cooksey

1 Introduction

The National Longitudinal Surveys of Youth (NLSY) include two separate youth cohorts in the United States: the NLSY79 that started in 1979 and the NLSY97 that began in 1997. Each is a nationally representative, longitudinal study with high response rates and frequent follow-ups. Also under the NLSY family of studies are the NLSY79 Child and Young Adult surveys, which follow all children born to female NLSY79 respondents. Data from the NLSY are used by researchers from a wide variety of disciplines including sociology, economics, geography, public health, nursing, psychology, statistics, education, maternal and child health, public policy, and political science. Data are free and easy to access and have also been utilized in cross-national research and policy studies.

Another indicator of the importance of the NLSY is the number of publications written by researchers. As of August 2015, 2892 articles, 188 book chapters, and 131 monographs were listed in the NLS bibliography as using at least one of the three NLSY surveys, along with 862 PhD dissertations. In 2014 there were 2250 registered users who downloaded NLSY data, and many others did so as non-registered guests.

In this chapter I begin with a brief history of the National Longitudinal Surveys. I then provide more in-depth information on the three NLSY surveys: the NLSY79, the NLSY79 Child and Young Adult Surveys, and the NLSY97. Next I illustrate some of the ways in which the NLSY provides unique opportunities for researchers. I then present an overview of information pertaining to health that is available in each of the surveys and highlight some of the health-related life course research that has been undertaken using one or more of the NLSY datasets. I conclude with information on how NLSY data may be obtained.

2 A Brief History of the NLS: The Original Cohorts

2016 marked the 50th anniversary of the first National Longitudinal Survey (NLS) interview and 50 years of involvement in the NLS project by the Center for Human Resource Research (CHRR) at The Ohio State University. Sponsored by the US Department of Labor, the first cohort of *Older Men* consisted of 5020 males born

E.C. Cooksey (✉)
Center for Human Resource Research, The Ohio State University, Suite 200, 921 Chatham Lane, Columbus, OH 43221, USA
e-mail: Cooksey.1@osu.edu

N. Halfon et al. (eds.), *Handbook of Life Course Health Development*,
DOI 10.1007/978-3-319-47143-3_23

between 1906 and 1921 who were ages 45–59 when first interviewed by the Census Bureau in 1966. This cohort was selected to enable research on the employment patterns of men as they neared the completion of their careers and answer questions regarding their plans for retirement. An oversample of black respondents was included, and 13 interviews were conducted over a span of 24 years. A total of 2092 Older Men were interviewed in 1990 when they were ages 71–83 years old, and interviews were also conducted with 2206 widows or other family members of deceased respondents. Although primarily focused on aspects of employment income and retirement, the survey also collected information on health and physical condition.

The NLS of *Young Men*, a sample of 5225 males born between 1941 and 1952, was also started in 1966 when they were 14–24 years old. The Young Men's cohort chronicled the employment patterns of men transitioning from school and into the work force or joining the military, i.e., making initial career and job decisions that would impact their employment in the decades to follow. Twelve interviews were conducted between 1966 and 1981 when the study ended. As with the Older Men, young black men were oversampled, and information was collected on health and physical condition.

The following year, 1967, a sample of 5083 *Mature Women* born between 1922 and 1937 was drawn to study the return of women to the labor force as their children grew up, and to investigate how women balanced the roles of homemaker, mother, and labor force participant. A total of 22 surveys were undertaken with these women, with their first interview at ages 30–44 and their last interview in 2003, at ages 63–77. Finally, in 1968, 5159 *Young Women* were interviewed at ages 14–24 as they were completing school, making career and job decisions, and starting families. Twenty-two interviews were undertaken with the Young Women's cohort, ending in 2003. As with both Original Cohorts of males, the two cohorts of female respondents again included oversamples of blacks and survey questions on health and physical condition.

3 The National Longitudinal Surveys of Youth

The *NLSY79* originally comprised a sample of 12,686 men and women born between 1957 and 1964 who were living in the United States when the survey began. When first interviewed in 1979, they were ages 14–22 years. This time CHRR partnered with the National Opinion Research Center (NORC) to undertake the fielding of the survey, which was conducted primarily with funds from the Bureau of Labor Statistics at the US Department of Labor, although other agencies provided funding for various purposes. For example, the National Institute of Child Health and Human Development (NICHD) has supported the collection of a wide range of data in the NLSY79, including marriage and fertility histories for all respondents as well as comprehensive pre- and postnatal data relating to each child born to female NLSY79 respondents and information pertaining to child health and childcare from the early survey years. The Armed Services Vocational Aptitude Battery (ASVAB) was administered to both the civilian and military youth samples interviewed in 1980 ($N = 11{,}914$) with sponsorship from the Department of Defense (DoD). These data include respondent raw scores, standard scores, scale scores, and standard errors for each of the ten test sections, including general science, arithmetic reasoning, work knowledge, mechanical comprehension, and two constructed Armed Forces Qualifications Test (AFQT) scores. The AFQT has been shown to be a significant predictor of later life course outcomes across a whole range of social, economic, educational, and health domains. Support from the DoD also made possible the 1979–1984 interviews of 1280 youth enlisted in the military.

Beginning in 1979, a 5-year collaborative effort between CHRR and the National Center for Research in Vocational Education resulted in a survey of the high schools civilian NLSY79 respondents attended, along with the collection of detailed transcript information, for 8778 NLSY79 respondents expected to complete high school during the 1980–1983 survey years.

Information on up to 64 high school courses, including course descriptions, final grades, and credit received, was collected. Moreover, data were gathered from the record of the last secondary school attended by the NLSY79 respondents. These variables include both respondent-specific and school-specific information on such factors as (a) the respondent's school enrollment status, highest grade attended, remedial classes taken, and scores/percentiles/grade levels for various intelligence and aptitude tests administered during the youth's schooling and (b) each school's total enrollment, grading system, types of curricula offered, dropout rate, student body composition, and staffing characteristics. In addition, the National Institute of Education sponsored a set of time-use questions in 1981, and a self-report supplement to the 1980 survey was funded by the US Department of Justice to collect data on respondents' participation in, and income from, various delinquent and criminal activities. Lastly, funding from the National Institute on Alcohol Abuse and Alcoholism and the National Institute on Drug Abuse has made possible expanded sets of alcohol and substance use questions.

The NLSY79 cohort was selected to replicate the NLS of Young Women and Young Men cohorts and was also designed to help researchers and policymakers evaluate the expanded employment and training programs for youths legislated by the 1977 amendments to the Comprehensive Employment and Training Act. Survey respondents have been interviewed every year through 1994 and every other year since then. The 2014/2015 survey marked the 26th round of data collection, with respondents ages 50–58 at the start of the round.

Interviews are conducted either face to face or by telephone, with telephone mode increasing with each subsequent round as respondents have become more geographically dispersed or expressed a preference for phone interviews. In recent rounds more than 90% have been conducted by telephone.

The initial sample of 12,686 youth interviewed in 1979 comprised a cross-sectional sample of 6111 respondents designed to represent the noninstitutionalized civilian segment of people living in the United States in 1979 and born between January 1, 1957, and December 31, 1964, along with a supplemental sample of 5295 civilian Hispanic or Latino/Latina, black, and economically disadvantaged nonblack/non-Hispanic respondents of the same ages. Also included was a sample of 1280 respondents designed to represent the population serving in one of the four branches of the US military as of September 30, 1978, who were born between January 1, 1957, and December 31, 1961, and who were therefore ages 17–21 as of December 31, 1978. The initial sample was evenly divided by gender and had 7510 nonblack/non-Hispanic respondents, 3174 black respondents, and 2002 Hispanic or Latino/Latina respondents. Due to budget constraints, 1079 members of the supplemental sample of armed forces youth were discontinued after the 1984 survey, and the economically disadvantaged nonblack/non-Hispanic supplemental sample of 1643 individuals was discontinued after 1990. In Round 25 (completed in 2013), over 80% of respondents in the remaining sample types were interviewed; of these respondents, 69% had answered every survey round since 1979 with a further 14% answering all but one.

The oversamples of black and Hispanic respondents and the fact that data have been collected either every year or every other year from the same set of people over such a long period of time, so many of them answering questions at 24 or more separate survey points, make the NLSY79 a remarkable panel study of individuals ideally suited for life course studies. Beginning in their teenage years, these individuals were followed as they left secondary school, entered college or training programs, moved into their first jobs, moved in with partners, got married, had children (although not necessarily in that order), lost jobs, changed jobs, had more children, bought and sold houses, progressed into middle age, began to think that they might like to retire one day, and paid into pension plans. And throughout these years, NLSY79 respondents answered not only questions about work, marriage, and family activities but also about beliefs, hopes, and expectations for the future, mental and physical health, alcohol and drug use, and sexual activity and contraceptive use. Although at its heart the NLSY79 remains a labor survey, its breadth of topics covered ensures that the nuances of people's work lives can be placed into the much larger context within which people actually live their lives. And as I describe later, the NLSY79 has also collected information on a host of healthy and unhealthy behaviors and a range of mental and physical health antecedents and outcomes that are not only important in terms of people's work lives but provide unique opportunities for health researchers who wish to study health over the life course.

Although the NLSY79 is a survey of individuals rather than a survey of households, respondents interviewed in 1979 originated from 8770 unique households out of which 2862 households included more than one NLSY79 respondent. The most common relationships between respondents living in multiple respondent households at this time were those of sibling or spouse: 5863 respondents were members of a household containing multiple interviewed siblings (biological, step, or adopted), and 334 respondents were members of a household in which their spouse was also interviewed (see Table 1).

The NLSY79 Child and Young Adult Surveys The NLSY79 Child study began in 1986 with funding from NICHD; at that time there were 5255 children reported by 2922 interviewed mothers. Designed to obtain comprehensive information on the experiences of children born to female NLSY79 respondents, a battery of cognitive, socioemotional, and physiological assessments has been administered biennially to all children of selected ages through 1992 and to children below the age of 15 since 1994. Some of these assessments directly assess each child's development using nationally normed tests such as the Peabody Picture Vocabulary Test-Revised (PPVT-R) which measures a child's hearing vocabulary; the Digit Span subscale of the Wechsler Intelligence Scale for Children-Revised (WISC-R) which measures short-term memory (Wechsler 1974); the Peabody Individual Achievement Test (PIAT): math, reading recognition, and reading comprehension assessments which measure ability in mathematics, oral reading, and the ability to derive meaning from printed words (Dunn and Dunn 1981); and Harter's Self-Perception Profile for Children (SPPC) that measures a child's perceived competence in academics and sense of general self-worth (Harter 1985). Although all of these tests have been administered to children of the NLSY79 biennially, the ages at which they were given have sometimes changed, and users of the data are advised to check the user's guide at https://www.nlsinfo.org. As shown in Table 2, other tests such as the McCarthy Scale of Children's Abilities: Verbal Memory subscale, Memory for Location Assessment, and Body Parts Assessment were only administered in early rounds of the survey.

Table 1 Number of NLSY79 civilian respondents by type of single/multiple sibling household, 1979

Type of household	Number of respondents	Number of households
Single respondent	5908	5908
Multiple siblings		
Two siblings	3386	1693
Three siblings	1725	575
Four siblings	604	151
Five siblings	130	26
Six siblings	18	3
Total multiple siblings	**5863**	**2448**

The number of children assessed during a given child survey year is a function of the number of children born to interviewed NLSY79 mothers, the number of children living in the homes of those mothers, and, finally, the number of those children actually interviewed. Of the 5842 NLSY79 females eligible for the first child interview in 1986, 2922 mothers and 4971 children were interviewed. From this sample of eligible children, assessment data were collected for 4786 of them.

Each mother also provides reports on her children's temperament, motor and social development, behavior problems, and home environment. Three age-specific versions of the temperament scale assess such factors as activity, predictability, positive affect, fearfulness, compliance, and insecure attachment among young children; the motor and social development scale measures milestones in the areas of motor, cognitive, communication, and social development for children

Table 2 Child assessments by year of survey

Child assessment	1986	1988	1990	1992	1994	1996-2014
Parts of the body: number of body parts child can identify by common names	*	*				
Memory for locations: how long child remembers the location of the doll	*	*				
Verbal memory test: ability to remember and repeat word sequences	*	*	*	*	*	
Peabody Picture Vocabulary Test (PPVT)	*	*	*	*	*	*
Memory for Digit Span test (WISC-R): memory for number order	*	*	*	*	*	*
PIAT math subtest	*	*	*	*	*	*
PIAT reading: recognition and comprehension subtests	*	*	*	*	*	*
SPPC: what child thinks he or she is like, how he or she thinks and feels	*	*	*	*	*	*
Temperament scales	*	*	*	*	*	*
Motor and social development scale (not administered in 2004)	*	*	*	*	*	*
Behavior problems index	*	*	*	*	*	*
Interviewer evaluation of testing conditions	*	*	*	*	*	*
HOME-SF inventory	*	*	*	*	*	*

* Signifies that those questions were asked in that particular survey round

under age four; and one of the most widely used scales in research on children using the NLSY79 is the Behavior Problems Index (BPI) which is completed for all children ages four and over. The BPI consists of an overall behavior problem score that is comprised of six subscales (antisocial, anxious or depressed, hyperactive, headstrong, dependent, and peer conflicts), and individual items may also be classified as internality and externality scales. Interviewer assessments of children's shyness, cooperation, interest, and persistence during the interview, as well as their attitude about and rapport with the interviewer, are also collected. The final measure in Table 2, the Home Observation Measurement of the Environment-Short Form (HOME-SF), is a modification of the HOME inventory (Caldwell and Bradley 1984) and is a unique measure of the quality of the cognitive stimulation and emotional support provided by a child's family. This measure has also been extensively used in research as both an input in helping to explain other child characteristics or behaviors and as an outcome to explain associations between the quality of a child's home environment and earlier familial and maternal traits and behaviors.

The NLSY79 Child surveys have also gathered substantial information about the educational experiences of each child. Mothers have provided information about preschool and regular school attendance, type of school attended, grades skipped or repeated, and how well the child performs in class. Since 1988, children ages 10 and over have supplied information on characteristics of their school, the involvement of their parents in their education, and their educational expectations. In 1995–1996 a one-time school survey—funded by a grant through the National Institute of Child Health and Human Development—was conducted to collect information from school officials at schools attended by NLSY79 child respondents in grades 1 through 12 during either the 1993–1994 or 1994–1995 school year. This effort gathered information about the characteristics of the school and standardized test scores recorded from student transcripts.

Each child survey from 1988 onward has also collected self-reported information from children age 10 and older about child-parent interactions, responsibilities at home, attitudes toward school, time use, employment, religious attendance, alcohol and drug use, sexual activity (at age 13 and older), dating and friendship patterns, and various other attitudes and behaviors.

In 1994, the NLSY79 data collection was again expanded to incorporate extensive interviews with NLSY79 *Young Adults*. This is not a new cohort but rather what NLSY79 Children are called when they turn age 15 (technically, the young adult sample is defined as children who have their 15th birthday in the year they are interviewed; thus, some of them are still age 14 when interviewed as young adults). In 1994, 6109 children under age 15 and 980 young adults reported by 3464 mothers were interviewed. In 1994 and 1996, the young adult data collection effort was part and parcel of the child data collection effort under a contract with the US Department of Labor with funds provided by NICHD. In 1998, because of funding constraints, interviews were limited to young adults under age 21. Since 2000, however, CHRR has obtained separate funds through the NICHD grant process to continue to interview young adults aged 21 and over and hence expand the analytical value of these data. All young adults ages 15–30 are interviewed biennially, and after age 30, they are interviewed every other survey round or roughly every 4 years.

In 1994, 1996, and 1998, the interviews were mainly conducted in person and included two parts. First was a computer-assisted personal interview that largely paralleled the main NLSY79 data collection but with a greater focus on youth issues. This included detailed employment, education, and family/relationship profiles, income, training, military service, and attitudinal measures and assessments such as the Rosenberg Self-Esteem Scale and the CESD depression scale. Second, young adults completed a confidential self-report questionnaire which focused on more sensitive issues including sexual activity, contraception, expectations for the future, dating and relationship experiences, political attitudes, pro-social behaviors, substance use, and risk-taking attitudes.

Other questions continued or were parallel to questions from the Child survey such as data on routine health checks, accidents and injuries, dating behaviors, the respondent's relationship with his or her parents, risk-taking behaviors, and school experiences and satisfaction.

The 2000 and later data collection efforts shifted to focus more heavily on recent mainstream employment and family experiences for the older grant-age young adults, many of whom had completed their schooling. Examples of more tailored questions for this older age group include the timing of and reasons for leaving home, the contact young adults had with their parents when they left home, their marriage and cohabitation histories, and (as they entered parenthood) the different kinds of childcare facilities they used and how much their childcare arrangements cost. In 2004 a series of questions on asthma was added, and the Ten-Item Personality Inventory (TIPI) was included in 2006. In 2008 the survey incorporated a six-item anger scale and questions on whether or not respondents had seen action in combat zones, with whom their biological children lived at the time of their birth, and more details about healthy activities. Also, building from qualitative research done by Wendy Manning and Pamela Smock (2005), new questions were designed to get a better handle on the types of relationships and dating activities that youth engaged in during their teens and twenties. Additional health-related questions were included between 2010 and 2014 and these are described in more detail in the health section.

At the start of the 2014 field period for round 26 of the NLSY79, female respondents were ages 50–57 and had essentially completed their fertility. At this time a total of 11,512 children were known to have been born to the original 6283 NLSY79 female respondents. Most of these births occurred during the years this cohort has been interviewed although a modest number of children were born prior to 1979. An unknown number of additional children will have been born to women who have left the survey (mostly as a result of being part of the economically disadvantaged oversample that was dropped after 1990) subsequent to their attrition. Fifty-one percent are sons and 49% are daughters, and based on the race/ethnicity of their mothers, 53% would be classified as nonblack/non-Hispanic, 28% as black, and 19% as Hispanic. The oldest child was born in 1970 to a teenage mother. The youngest child was born in 2011 to a mother in the older childbearing years. At the time of the first interview in 1986, child ages ranged from 0 to 15 years of age. In 2014/2015 NLSY79 Children were 0–14 years old and Young Adults were ages

14–44 years. Finally, retention rates have again been very high: at the end of fielding in 2013, 81% of young adults and 90% of children eligible to be fielded during this survey round had been interviewed. Of these respondents, close to 77% of young adults had been interviewed either every time or all but once which translates into 13 or 14 different data points over a 28-year period.

The *NLSY97* is the newest survey in the NLS program and comprises a sample of 8984 young men and women born between 1980 and 1984 who were ages 12–17 when first interviewed in 1997. As with the NLSY79, the NLSY97 also had a cross-sectional sample of respondents designed to be representative of people at those ages and living in the United States at the time ($N = 6748$) and a supplemental sample of 2236 black and Hispanic respondents, which resulted in a total sample that was 52% nonblack/non-Hispanic, 26% black, 21% Hispanic or Latino/Latina, and just under 1% mixed race. Because all household residents in the appropriate age range were selected, again some households included more than one NLSY97 respondent, the most common relationship being that of siblings. The original sample in 1997 was 51% male and 49% female.

CHRR and NORC again partnered to undertake the study which was also primarily funded by the BLS. Other agencies have contributed to the project over the years, however. For example, in Round 1, a computer adaptive version of the Armed Services Vocational Aptitude Battery (ASVAB) was given to NLSY97 respondents with sponsorship by the Department of Defense. Various questions in the self-administered portion of the questionnaire, including questions on health, fertility, and social relationships, have been funded by the NICHD. School surveys were undertaken in 1996 and 2000 to collect information from all high schools with a 12th grade in the 147 NLSY97 primary sampling units as well as the collection and coding of high school transcripts, and this work was funded by the Department of Education. Questions on crime and criminal activities have been sponsored by the Department of Justice, Office of Juvenile Justice and Delinquency Prevention.

The NLSY97 cohort was designed to enable research on youths' transition from school to the labor market and into adulthood for a generation born into a very different time period than youth in the '79 cohort who had transitioned into adulthood during the 1980s: NLSY79 respondents are younger baby boomers, whereas NLSY97 respondents are the oldest of the millennial generation. These two cohorts have moved into early adulthood under very different educational, employment, and family building circumstances. Current population survey time trend data (www.census.gov/hhes/socdemo/education/data/cps/historical/index.html) show that in 1990, when the youngest NLSY79 cohort member was 25, the percentages of youth ages 25 and over who had completed high school or college were 23.7% for men and 22.8% for women. In 2009 when the youngest member of the NLSY97 cohort was age 25, the percentage for males had increased only slightly to 26.6%, but for women, the rise was substantial to 34.8%. Based on figures from the March 2013 current population survey, 38% of older millennial females ages 25–32 had a bachelor's degree. The corresponding figure for their male counterparts was 31%. Higher education has become increasingly important for successful labor force participation for millennials. According to a report from the Pew Research Center (2013), women accounted for 43% of the US labor force in 1980, and this rose to 47% in 2012. Among young women (ages 25–34), 74% were in the labor force in 2012, up from 66% in 1980. Labor force participation among men on the other hand has declined over the past 30 years, from 78% in 1980 to 70% in 2012. Furthermore, each new wave of adult men younger than age 35 has been less active in the labor market than the preceding wave. Living arrangements have also changed over time. For example, in 1987 when NLSY79 respondents were ages 22–29 years old, the percentage of 25–29-year-olds who had ever cohabited was 41%. In 2009–2010 when NLSY97 cohort members were 25–30, this percentage had risen to 66% (Bumpass and Sweet 1989; Bumpass and Lu 2000; Kennedy and Bumpass 2008).

The NLSY97 cohort is also ongoing and has been surveyed every year from 1997 through 2011 and biennially since. In 2015, 16 survey rounds had been completed and respondents were ages 28–34. Up until 2015, data collection has been primarily via in-person interviewing. Beginning in round 18, set to start in late fall of 2017, there will be a shift to mostly phone interviewing. As with the NLSY79 and the NLSY79 Child and Young Adult surveys, oversamples of black and Hispanic respondents, very high retention rates, and the fact that the same people have been interviewed so frequently make the NLSY97 another remarkable panel that is highly appropriate for longitudinal and life course studies, especially during the life course stages from adolescence through early adulthood when frequent education, employment, fertility, and living arrangement transitions occur. And again, response rates have been exceedingly high: in Round 16 which was completed in 2014, 81% of respondents not known to be deceased were interviewed. Of these interviewed respondents, 69.5% had answered all 16 surveys since 1997, and a further 12% had answered 15 of them.

4 The Uniqueness of the NLSY

Many factors make the NLSY datasets a unique source of data for researchers interested in studying the life course. First, there have been many rounds of data collection at very frequent intervals: NLSY79 respondents have been interviewed up to 26 times between when they were teens in 1979 and their late forties to mid-fifties in 2015; children born to NLSY79 females have been assessed and interviewed up to 15 times, most of them from birth onward; and NLSY97 respondents have been interviewed up to 16 times from their early to mid-teens into their thirties. Such a wealth of data can seem overwhelming at times, but they also lend themselves to a better understanding of important life course trajectories and how change in one area of life can lead to both short-term and longer-term change in other realms.

The length of time that these studies have been ongoing, and the extraordinarily high response rates achieved from so many individuals who have been prepared to share of their lives round after round, means that researchers can explore potential consequences of events that happen at early stages in the life course many years later, while still being able to account for a broad array of occurrences in the intervening years. In 2004, Hayward and Gorman published a paper in *Demography* titled "The Long Arm of Childhood: The Influence of Early-Life Social Conditions on Men's Mortality" in which they drew on the NLS Older Men's cohort to study links between various childhood conditions and mortality in adulthood. Although they had to rely on retrospective reports from men in their forties and fifties about their childhood years, their results showed that men's mortality was indeed associated with an array of childhood conditions including socioeconomic status, family living arrangements, mother's work status, rural residence, and parents' nativity. With information from multiple interviews to draw from, they were then able to demonstrate how, with the exception of parental nativity, these associations were mediated by various lifestyle factors, particularly body mass and socioeconomic achievement processes in adulthood. They concluded that their findings highlighted the idea that economic and educational policies targeted at children's well-being are implicitly health policies with effects that reach far into the adult life course. As the NLSY79 cohort ages into their retirement years and beyond, it will be possible to replicate this research with prospective rather than retrospective data, and the NLSY79 Child and Young Adult data will enable researchers to go back to the earliest years of childhood and even include prenatal conditions as reported by mothers.

The United States does not have birth cohort studies as other countries, such as the United Kingdom, do. However, data on the children of the NLSY79 do provide information on children from birth. With input from child development experts, the child study was designed to gather information from their mothers during infancy and early childhood, to assess children in their elementary and middle school years and to interview them from middle school onward into adolescence and adulthood.

As illustrated in Fig. 1 below, given the wealth of data that have been collected on these children

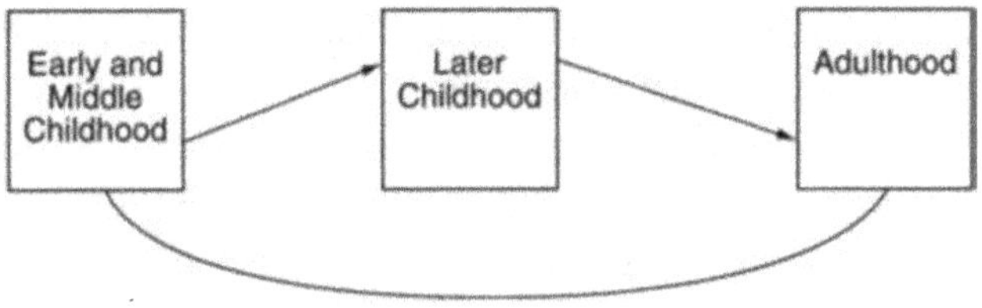

Fig. 1 Research possibilities using the NLSY79 Child and Young Adult data

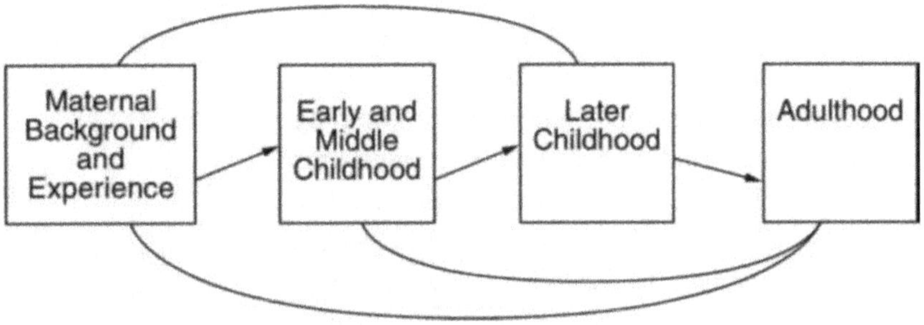

Fig. 2 Cross-generational research possibilities using the NLSY79 Maternal, Child, and Young Adult data

every other year, the NLSY79 Child and Young Adult data present researchers with enormous possibilities to link information ascertained when the child was quite young to outcomes in later childhood and beyond, plus to see how potential predictors from early or middle childhood of certain behaviors or outcomes in early adulthood or later might or might not be mediated by events and occurrences in later childhood or adolescence.

Of course, the 11,512 children of the NLSY do not constitute a birth cohort themselves as they were born between 1970 and 2011. However, they were all born to a cohort of women, and the NLSY79 Child/Young Adult files can be easily combined with information from the complete longitudinal record of their NLSY79 mothers. In addition, the Child/Young Adult dataset contains a number of created variables providing information on the mother with respect to the child's life situation. These constructed variables, drawn from the mother's record, include: family background, household composition, quarterly maternal work histories before and after each child's date of birth, educational background of members of the household, maternal health history, and information on childcare experiences during the first 3 years of life for all children of at least 1 year of age. Also available for each child are data regarding gestation and birth weight, as well as breastfeeding practices, other infant feeding practices, illnesses and injuries, and well-baby care in the first year of life. NLSY79 mothers also provide prenatal information for all births including data on their use of prenatal care, alcohol, cigarettes, marijuana, cocaine and dietary supplements and whether they had sonograms or amniocentesis during pregnancy.

As shown in Fig. 2, the availability of comprehensive child data, coupled with a wealth of longitudinal information on the background, and well-being of their NLSY79 mothers, provide researchers with a unique opportunity to undertake intergenerational research and examine linkages between maternal family behaviors and attitudes on the one hand and multiple aspects of their children's development on the other hand.

As an example, one might be interested not only in how deviancy develops from childhood into the young adult years but also in how the evolution of deviant behaviors might relate to behaviors and experiences in the prior generation—in this case among the youths' mothers. Further, as mentioned earlier, not only are similar data collected from both mothers and their children but retrospective reporting need not be relied on to link maternal reports of behaviors with those of their child, since data were collected from the NLSY79 mothers on their behaviors at, for example, ages 16 or 18 when they were 16 or 18, and then again from their children when they were 16 or 18 years old. The fact that many questions were asked of NLSY79 females and of their children when they were the same ages makes these data especially distinctive.

The information presented earlier in Table 1 provides another example of how the NLSY79 provides opportunities for life course research in ways not necessarily expected from cohort studies. Because information is collected for all children born to female respondents, and some of those NLSY79 female respondents were themselves sisters, the NLSY79 Child/Young Adult data not only offer opportunities for comparing developmental and other outcome measures between siblings but also between *cousins*. The relatively large sample of siblings and cousins permits researchers to explore both within- and cross-family effects to a greater extent than is typically possible. Over the course of the survey years, more than 3000 children in the sample have been identified as having an aunt in the NLSY79 main youth sample. Most of these children have one aunt, but there are also some child respondents with multiple aunts. The number of children who are cousins is also considerable.

More typically, researchers have tended to utilize the large number of child sibling sample cases that have been born to the female respondents. As shown in Table 3, 78.5% of NLSY79 women had at least one child, and most of them have had more than one, including a fairly large sample of women who have had three or more children by the end of their childbearing years. In addition to multiple births, there are many family units where two or more children are widely spaced in age. This enables exploring the impact of childbearing on children born to the same mother at different maternal life cycle stages.

A number of articles published in recent years have used either sibling data from the NLSY79 main youth sample or the Child and Young Adult sample or cousin data from this second generation (see, e.g., D'Onofrio et al. 2008, 2009a, b; Rodgers et al. 2008; Mendle et al. 2009; Jaffe et al. 2011; Goodnight et al. 2012 and Donahue et al. 2014).

Because there is considerable overlap in questions asked of NLSY97 and NLSY79 participants, intergenerational comparisons can be made using information from these two cohorts. Furthermore, a significant number of NLSY79 Young Adults were born in the same years as NLSY97 respondents, and hence members of these two datasets can be compared with each other when overlap of questionnaire design allows. One of the drawbacks of the NLSY79 Young Adult data is that although young adults were born to women who were part of a nationally representative sample of youth living in the United States in 1979, due to immigration and fertility differentials by various background variables (e.g., race/ethnicity), the NLSY79 Young Adults are by no means nationally representative in nature. The NLSY97 respondents are, however, representative of teenagers who were living in the United States in 1997 and hence are a more generalizable sample. Although immigration since 1997 has changed the racial/ethnic makeup of the US population so that NLSY97 respondents are also no longer representative of all Young Adults in their thirties living in the US today, they are still closer than the NLSY79 Young Adults of the same ages.

On the other hand, the NLSY79 Young Adults of comparable age to the NLSY97 respondents have the strong advantage of having been followed since birth, plus in-depth information was gathered from their mothers over many years. Comparisons of research using the Young Adults with research utilizing the NLSY97 can therefore provide insights concerning the importance of

Table 3 NLSY79 women by number of children and race/ethnicity

Number of households				
Type of household (female)	Hispanic	Black	White	Total
Females with no children	**158**	**285**	**908**	1351
Mothers with 1 or more child	**844**	**1276**	**2812**	**4932**
Mothers with 1 child	147	278	750	1175
Mothers with 2 children	310	457	1204	1971
Mothers with 3 children	222	315	591	1128
Mothers with 4 or more children	165	226	267	658
Total	**1002**	**1561**	**3720**	**6283**

non-representativeness in the Young Adult sample and potential selectivity bias in the NLSY97 due to the failure to include important prenatal or early childhood information. In other words, the strengths of one dataset can be used to evaluate potential weaknesses in the other.

Lastly, geographic residence information is available in all three datasets and the county and state of residence are provided in a separate restricted-access geocode CD that can be matched with other data sources to investigate community characteristics and contextual variables.

A number of design decisions make the NLSY97 the preferred choice of dataset to study certain behavioral choices and life events. For example, more in-depth data related to crime and delinquency are available in the NLSY97 than in the NLSY79, and a full cohabitation history also exists in the NLSY97 whereas the information available from NLSY79 respondents does not enable a complete record of living arrangements to be constructed. However, the linked NLSY79 and NLSY79 Child and Young Adult files are more ideally suited for the study of maternal and child health, since NLSY79 women have now aged through their fertile years and detailed information has been collected on all of their biological children. It is therefore the NLSY79 data that I primarily focus on in the next sections of this chapter.

5 Health Data in the NLSY Surveys

NLSY79 health sections are divided into two periods. Between 1979 and 1996, although the specific questions that were asked varied at times, most questions focused on health concerns that restricted or inhibited the respondent's ability to work. From 1998 on, as respondents reached middle age, the health section was expanded to provide a baseline profile of the respondent's overall health as they turned 40 years old. From 2008 onward, respondents have been asked another set of health questions when they turn 50.

Although the pre-1998 health questions provide a picture of the respondents' health restrictions at the time of interview, they offer little insight into chronic health problems that might affect their labor force activity in the future. For example, a serious ailment with slow development would not be picked up by the regular health questions until a respondent actually dropped out of the labor market. The extended *40-and-over health module* was therefore created to provide a baseline health profile for each respondent to facilitate research of the interrelationship of health and labor market activity in the advancement of retirement ages. Questions are not restricted to work-related health problems, and all questions are asked irrespective of the respondent's labor force status. Full information is available on www.nlsinfo.org but questions include items from the Center for Epidemiological Studies Depression Scale (CES-D), information on when respondents last saw a health care professional, and reports about the health and life status of the NLSY79 respondents' biological parents designed to improve researchers' understanding of hereditary health problems. The module also reproduces the SF-12 scale, a 12-question health survey designed by John Ware of the New England Medical Center Hospital that provides a measure of the respondents' mental and physical health irrespective of their proclivity to use formal health services (Ware et al. 1995). Finally, respondents are asked if they suffer from an extensive list of health conditions including asthma, back problems, problems with their feet and legs, kidney or bladder, stomach or intestinal ulcers, high cholesterol, chest pain, heart trouble, low blood pressure, sinus infections, joint swelling or pain, leg cramps, painful shoulders, elbows or knees, frequent headaches, severe tooth or gum trouble, skin diseases, and thyroid problems.

The *50-and-over health module* was included beginning in 2008 at which time the module was administered to respondents born in 1957–1958. In 2010, it was administered to those born in 1959–1960, and anyone who skipped the 2008 interview, and so on. This module contains many of the same questions as the 40-and-over health module. Some questions therefore provide a second decennial point of reference for general health information and many others provide updates on previously reported conditions.

Questions about diagnosis of skin cancer and other types of cancer, various heart disease-related conditions, and stroke were also asked.

50-and-over respondents are again administered the CES-D items and the SF-12 question series, as well as questions about the life and health status of their parents if they were previously reported as living. In addition, 50-and-over respondents update information on previously reported conditions such as hypertension/high blood pressure, diabetes/high blood sugar, asthma and non-asthma breathing problems, depression and other emotional/psychiatric problems, and arthritis. Questions have also been included on diagnosis of osteoporosis and the use of special equipment needed to accomplish usual activities, as well as a scale of functionality and the respondent's sleep habits.

In addition to the two health modules asked around age 40 and around age 50, other health questions have been incorporated into the NLSY79 questionnaire as mini-modules or small groups of questions to capture retrospective accounts of health in the childhood years prior to 1979, baseline measures of general health and cognition, information on the use of particular medications, and reports of head injuries. For example, in 2012 all respondents were asked a series of new questions on childhood health including overall health, major hospitalizations, or long periods of home recovery. Questions on childhood adversity that dealt with family mental health, alcohol abuse, physical abuse, and amount of parental affection were also added as researchers believe that questions such as these are predictive of adult obesity and other health-related outcomes.

Beginning in 2006, respondents ages 48 and 49 were given a battery of exercises designed to capture cognitive capabilities. Similar to the 50-and-over health module, this cognition module has also been administered to progressive 2-year birth year cohorts in the survey year during which they would turn at least age 48. This module solicits the respondent's own assessment of his/her general health, a word recall exercise using randomly assigned sets of ten words, and exercises requiring the respondent to count backward from a starting point by a specified number.

In 2004 a series of questions about asthma were added to the survey, and starting in 2008, respondents were asked if they were taking any statin drugs or heart medications. In 2012 all respondents were asked if they had experienced a serious head injury or loss of smell. Because traumatic head injury and loss of smell have been found in numerous studies to be linked to subsequent dementia, these questions were included to augment ongoing efforts to track respondents' cognitive function as they advance through middle age and beyond.

As mentioned in the section above, NLSY79 mothers have also provided a variety of information about their prenatal and postnatal activities relating to each child since 1983. Table 4 below summarizes some of the other health-related data available on *children born to NLSY79 mothers* and collected since the advent of the child survey in 1986:

Starting in 1996, mothers have additionally been asked to rate their child's health on a 4-point scale from "poor" to "excellent." Detailed information is available in the User's Guide at www.nlsinfo.org/content/cohorts/nlsy79-children/topical-guide/health.

Health questions continue as children become *Young Adults*. In some areas, questions closely parallel the health history obtained for all children of NLSY79 mothers (e.g., height and body weight, types of limitations, number of accidents and injuries in the last 12 months, hospitalizations resulting from these accidents/injuries, and insurance coverage). Young Adult respondents who do not live with their mother are also asked about illnesses and routine medical care. For younger Young Adults who do live with their mother, comparable questions are asked of the mother. Items from the CES-D depression scale are also asked of Young Adults in multiple survey rounds.

In 2004, respondents received two new series of questions. The first focused on health-related behaviors such as fruit and vegetable consumption, hours of sleep per night, and level of exercise. The second series was centered on asthma with detailed questions designed to track the onset of asthma and the persistence and severity of related symptoms. This series also includes two questions about whether anyone has smoked cigarettes in the respondent's home in the last 2 weeks and whether the respondent has routinely spent time somewhere in the last 2 weeks where they can smell cigarette smoke.

Table 4 Health-related data available on children of the NLSY79

Child health	1986	1988–1992	1994	1996–2002	2004–2012
Rating of child's health				M	M
Does health limit school or play	M	M	M	M	M
Physical, emotional, or mental condition requiring: treatment, medicine, or special equipment	M	M	M	M	M
Type/duration of limiting health conditions	M	M	M	M	M
Accidents/injuries needing medical attention in last 12 months	M	M	M	M	M
Accidents/injuries needing hospitalization since last interview/ since birth		M	M	M	M
Number of illnesses requiring medical attention or treatment	M	M	M	M	M
Date of last routine health checkup	M	M	M	M	M
Date of last dental checkup/work	M	M	M	M	M
Source of health insurance, if any	M	M	M	M	M
Behavioral, emotional, or mental problems; did insurance cover doctor visit	M	M	M	M	M
Any medications or prescription drugs taken to help control activity/behavior	M	M	M	M	M
Menarche; age at first menses for female child (and mother)	M	M	M	M	M
Right-/left-handedness				M	M
Height and body weight of child	M-I	M-I	M-I	M-I	M-I
Healthcare during pregnancy leading to child's birth	M	M	M	M	M
Postnatal infant healthcare and feeding	M	M	M	M	M
Asthma					M/C

C child report, *M* mother report, *M-I* mother report or interviewer measurement

In 2006, a series of questions concerning catastrophic events that might adversely affect the health and well-being of respondents, such as death or imprisonment of a close relative, was included in the health section. These questions are a modified version of the catastrophic events series used in the NLSY97 questionnaire. Initially all respondents were asked about any such events that had occurred since they were 10 years old. Beginning in 2008, respondents who had previously answered this series are asked only about events since the date of last interview.

In 2010, several additional questions about healthy behaviors and routine checkups were included, and a *health and cognition module for respondents aged 29* and over was added. This module was modeled after the age 29 module from the NLSY97 with some adjustments and additions to also maintain comparability to the health modules in the NLSY79. For 2010 and 2012, this module was asked of all respondents ages 29 and older in order to get baseline information for all Young Adults. Thereafter, it has been asked only of respondents who are 29/30 or Young Adults who are over that age but have not yet completed the module. In 2012, a series of questions about head injuries, based on questions asked of NLSY79 respondents and described above, was incorporated into the health module.

The NLSY97 also collects information on the general health status of respondents in all rounds; for example, they report their height and weight and also describe how they would characterize their weight (very underweight, slightly underweight, etc.) and if they currently wish to lose or gain or stay at the weight they are. Information on health insurance coverage is collected in various rounds as are questions forming a five-item short version of the Mental Health Inventory (MHI-5), developed by Veit and Ware (1983). Information on various health conditions, medical treatments and visits, and out-of-the-ordinary stressors such as being a victim of a violent crime or being homeless is also collected in various survey rounds. In rounds 13–15, respondents who were 29 years of age answered a special series of health questions as a *Health-At-Age-29 health module*. These included questions about a family history of diseases (including detailed questions about diabetes), parents' mortality, respondents' health limitations (including limitations on moderate activities, climbing stairs, social activities, and productivity), energy level, and mood. Other questions were asked about whether the respondent had had a flu shot, a cholesterol test, diabetes test, pap smear, and blood pressure check at some point during the past 2 years. More information on health-related questions included in the NLSY97 can be found at https://www.nlsinfo.org/content/cohorts/nlsy97/topical-guide/health.

6 Health Research Using the NLSY Surveys

Considerable health-related research has been undertaken using the three NLSY surveys. In this section I highlight a sample of published studies and focus primarily on studies published since 2000 and those that center on child health. The NLS online bibliography (NLSinfo.org) provides a much more complete list of health focused studies. Of note, however, is the wide range of health topics studied, as well as the diversity of disciplinary backgrounds drawn upon. As the examples below illustrate, the surveys provide a great resource for examining aspects of life course health development.

Returning to Fig. 1, the first set of studies I feature use data from the NLSY79 Child and Young Adult surveys to look at health during childhood and adolescence. For example, Atkins and Matsuba (2008) use maternal ratings of childhood personality for over 1000 5- and 6-year-olds to derive resiliency, undercontrol and overcontrol prototypical profile scores. They then extend their analyses to later in childhood and examine whether childhood personality is associated with the likelihood and the timing of an unintentional injury requiring hospitalization or medical attention before the child turned age 13. Their findings suggest an inverse association between the likelihood of childhood unintentional injury and the overcontrolled prototype score. A recent paper by Cheadle and Goosby (2010) focuses on the complex interplay between childhood health and educational development over the early life course by estimating the relationship between birth weight, cognitive development, and timely high school completion. Their models therefore spanned childhood, adolescence, and early adulthood. Especially notable about this paper is the fact that they were able to adjust for fixed-family characteristics and aspects of the home environment by making use of information from siblings. Among several findings from this study, the authors noted that lower birth weight was associated with decreased cognitive skills at age 5 and marginally significantly slower growth rates into adolescence. They also showed that low birth weight increased the risk of not graduating by age 19. The authors concluded that their pattern of findings painted a multifaceted picture of disadvantage that begins in the womb and extends over the life course.

Reflecting the reality that childhood obesity is a major public health problem in the United States, many studies using the NLSY79 Child data focus on how obesity develops over the life course. For example, Huang and colleagues (Huang et al. 2013) identified developmental trajectories of obesity between ages 6 and 18 and classified four distinct categories: chronically obese, decreasing, increasing, and nonobese. They then studied associations between the various obesity trajectories and a number of risk behaviors and psychosocial health in adolescence. Although obesity trajectories were not found to be associated with greater trends in alcohol use or marijuana use, they did find that youth who became obese between childhood and adolescence had poorer psychosocial health compared to youth who followed other trajectories. Other potential effects of childhood overweight on health development have also been studied. For example, Richard Strauss (Strauss 2000) compared 9- and 10-year-old children who were obese and nonobese to see if they differed on global self-esteem scores. He found no significant difference at these ages between the two groups but by 13–14 years of age, significantly lower levels of self-esteem were observed in obese boys, obese Hispanic girls, and obese white girls compared with their nonobese counterparts. More recently, Averett and Stifel (2010) looked at the effect of obesity on cognitive development and uncovered significant effects when the relationship was examined separately by race and gender.

Other studies focusing on obesity in childhood and adolescence have incorporated maternal and family data into their analyses by merging data from NLSY79 mothers with data on their children as outlined in Fig. 2. The range of inputs varies considerably from breastfeeding versus bottle-feeding (Li et al. 2005; Salsberry and Reagan 2005; Seipel and Shafer 2013), food choices offered to young children (Faith et al. 2003), family income (Chia 2013), parental marital disruption and divorce (Arkes 2012), maternal prenatal behaviors such as smoking (Huang et al. 2014; Li et al. 2003; Salsberry and Reagan 2005, 2007; Seipel and Shafer 2013), maternal prepregnancy weight (Li et al. 2005; Salsberry and Reagan 2005, 2007), weight gain during pregnancy (Seipel and Shafer 2013), and other background factors such as parental engagement in children's daily activities, maternal age, and maternal education (Huang et al. 2014).

The relationship between various aspects of maternal employment and children's obesity has also gained attention. In a 2003 publication, Anderson, Butcher, and Levine suggest that increasing child obesity might be related to an increase in mothers working outside the home and posit that working mothers may not have time to prepare nutritious low-calorie meals and supervise their children's outdoor play that tends to expend calories. Using data on siblings to hold constant all of the family characteristics that might be correlated both with children's weight and mothers' hours worked, study results indicated that although children were more likely to be overweight if their mothers worked more hours per week over the child's life, it was higher socioeconomic status mothers whose work intensity was particularly deleterious for their children's overweight status. Others have also examined the relationship between maternal work hours and child obesity and found longer hours worked to be positively related to children's overweight (Courtemanche 2009; Liu et al. 2009). Other studies have found a more nuanced relationship, however. For example, Miller (2011) found that the timing of maternal work during a child's life mattered to the relationship and that effects of maternal work were confined to relatively low income families and to children who grew up with single mothers. Stewart et al. (2012) also found that unemployment events and the type of support that a mother received during unemployment spells were related to changes in children's weight.

Additional studies have examined various parental and family background influences on a range of child health development outcomes aside from child obesity. Some of these include how income and family structure impact routine medical and dental care provision for children (Berger 2004), the association between unwanted pregnancy and prenatal and postpartum maternal behaviors that adversely affect infant and child health (Joyce et al. 2000), the relationship between dark and cluttered home environments and the incidence of home injuries among children (Mott 1999), the distance between a child's home and a hospital and the probability of utilizing preventive care (Currie and Reagan 2003), length of maternity leave and children's immunizations (Berger et al. 2005), the effects of breastfeeding on long-term child health and well-being (Colen and Ramey 2014), various measures of economic disadvantage on intrauterine growth restriction (Reagan et al. 2007), household income histories, and changes in child depression levels (Strohschein 2005). Finally, a recent paper by Wolfe (2015) unpacked the components of socioeconomic status and found that children's health was more vulnerable to their families' wealth whereas adolescents' health was more sensitive to the current income of their families.

This brief and selected review of past studies provides a glimpse of the ways the NLSY data can be used to explore important aspects of life course health development. As the maternal and child health research community continues to explore how health develops across the life course, the NLSY can continue to be a rich source of data to answer important research questions.

7 Obtaining and Using NLSY Data

The NLSY public datasets (along with the data from the Original Cohorts) can be accessed free of charge through the NLS Investigator (www.nlsinfo.org/investigator), the data retrieval system used for obtaining public NLS data. In NLS Investigator, cohort-specific datasets can be searched by Area of Interest, Word in Title, Question Text, Question Name, Reference Number, and Survey Year. Also available at www.nlsinfo.org are cohort-specific Users Guides with an introduction to each sample, information on how to use and understand the data, topical guides, tutorials on various topics such as how to merge the NLSY79 Mother and Child data, and questionnaires for all rounds. Data can be downloaded into SAS, STATA, SPSS, and R. In addition to the public data, geocode data variables are available on a restricted basis: researchers interested in using the restricted data must complete an accessing agreement and be approved. Users with questions may also contact NLS User Services at usersvc@chrr.osu.edu for assistance with data use.

References

Anderson, P., Butcher, K., & Levine, P. (2003). Economic perspectives on childhood obesity. *Economic Perspectives, 27*(3), 30–49.

Arkes, J. (2012). Longitudinal association between marital disruption and child BMI and obesity. *Obesity, 20*(8), 1696–1702.

Atkins, R., & Matsuba, M. K. (2008). Association of personality and the likelihood of serious unintentional injury during childhood. *Journal of Pediatric Nursing, 23*(6), 451–459.

Averett, S., & Stifel, D. (2010). Race and gender differences in the cognitive effects of childhood overweight. *Applied Economics Letters, 17*(17), 1673–1679.

Berger, L. (2004). Income, family structure, and child maltreatment risk. *Children and Youth Services Review, 26*(8), 725–799.

Berger, L., Hill, J., & Waldfogel, J. (2005). Maternity leave, early maternal employment and child health and development in the US. *Economic Journal, 115*(501), F29–F47.

Bumpass, L., & Sweet, J. (1989). National estimates of cohabitation. *Demography, 26*(4), 615–625.

Bumpass, L., & Lu, H. (2000). Trends in cohabitation and implications for children's family contexts in the United States. *Population Studies, 54*, 29–41.

Caldwell, B., & Bradley, R. (1984). *Home observation for measurement of the environment*. Little Rock: University of Arkansas at Little Rock, Center for Child Development and Education.

Cheadle, J., & Goosby, B. (2010). Birth weight, cognitive development, and life chances: A comparison of siblings from childhood into early adulthood. *Social Science Research, 39*(4), 570–584.

Chia, Y. F. (2013). Dollars and pounds: The impact of family income on childhood weight. *Applied Economics, 45*(14), 1931–1941.

Colen, C., & Ramey, D. (2014). Is breast truly best? Estimating the effects of breastfeeding on long-term child health and wellbeing in the United States using sibling comparisons. *Social Science and Medicine, 109*, 55–65.

Courtemanche, C. (2009). Longer hours and larger waistlines? The relationship between work hours and obesity. *Forum for Health Economics and Policy, 12*(2). doi:10.2202/1558-9544.1123.

Currie, J., & Reagan, P. (2003). Distance to hospital and children's use of preventive care: Is being closer better, and for whom? *Economic Inquiry, 41*(3), 378–392.

D'Onofrio, B., Goodnight, J., Van Hulle, C., Rodgers, J., Rathouz, P., Waldman, I., & Lahey, B. (2009a). A quasi-experimental analysis of the association between family income and offspring conduct problems. *Journal of Abnormal Child Psychology, 37*(3), 415–429.

D'Onofrio, B., Goodnight, J., Van Hulle, C., Rodgers, J., Rathouz, P., Waldman, I., & Lahey, B. (2009b). Maternal age at childbirth and offspring disruptive behaviors: Testing the causal hypothesis. *Journal of Child Psychology and Psychiatry, 50*(8), 1018–1028.

D'Onofrio, B., Van Hulle, C., Waldman, I., Rodgers, J., Harden, K. P., Rathouz, P., & Lahey, B. (2008). Smoking during pregnancy and offspring externalizing problems: An exploration of genetic and environmental confounds. *Development and Psychopathology, 20*(1), 139–164.

Donahue, K., Van Hulle, C., Rodgers, J., & D'Onofrio, B. (2014). Psychosocial predictors of adolescent sexual risk behavior: A quasi-experimental analysis in a nationally representative sample of american youths. *Journal of Adolescent Health, 54*(2), S15–S16.

Dunn, L., & Dunn, L. (1981). *PPVT-R revised manual*. Circle Pines, Minnesota: American Guidance Service, Inc..

Faith, M., Heshka, S., Keller, K., Sherry, B., Matz, P., Pietrobelli, A., & Allison, D. (2003). Maternal-child feeding patterns and child body weight: Findings from a population-based sample. *Archives of Pediatrics and Adolescent Medicine, 157*(9), 926–932.

Goodnight, J., Lahey, B., Van Hulle, C., Rodgers, J., Rathouz, P., Waldman, I., & D'Onofrio, B. (2012). A quasi-experimental analysis of the influence of neighborhood disadvantage on child and adolescent conduct problems. *Journal of Abnormal Psychology, 121*(1), 95–108.

Harter, S. (1985). *Manual for the self-perception profile for children*. Denver, Colorado: University of Denver.

Hayward, M., & Gorman, B. (2004). The long arm of childhood: The influence of early-life social conditions on men's mortality. *Demography, 41*(1), 87–108.

Huang, D., Lanza, H. I., Wright-Volel, K., & Anglin, M. D. (2013). Developmental trajectories of childhood obesity and risk behaviors in adolescence. *Journal of Adolescence, 36*(1), 139–148.

Huang, D., Lanza, H. I., & Anglin, M. D. (2014). Trajectory of adolescent obesity: Exploring the impact of prenatal to childhood experiences. *Journal of Child and Family Studies, 23*(6), 1090–1101.

Jaffee, S., Van Hulle, C., & Rodgers, J. (2011). Effects of nonmaternal care in the first 3 years on children's academic skills and behavioral functioning in childhood and early adolescence: A sibling comparison study. *Child Development, 82*(4), 1076–1091.

Joyce, T., Kaestner, R., & Korenman, S. (2000). The effect of pregnancy intention on child development. *Demography, 37*(1), 83–94.

Kennedy, S., & Bumpass, L. (2008). Cohabitation and children's living arrangements: New estimates from the United States. *Demographic Research, 19*, 1663–1692. doi:10.4054/DemRes.2008.19.47.

Li, C., Mayo, M. S., & Ahluwalia, J. (2003). Maternal smoking during pregnancy, birth weight, and childhood overweight: A suppression effect model. *Annals of Epidemiology, 13*(8), 569.

Li, C., Kaur, H., Choi, W., Huang, T., Lee, R., & Ahluwalia, J. S. (2005). Additive interactions of maternal prepregnancy BMI and breast-feeding on childhood overweight. *Obesity Research, 13*(2), 362–371.

Liu, E., Cheng, H., Matsumoto, T., & Chou, S. (2009). Maternal full-time employment and overweight children: Parametric, semi-parametric, and non-parametric assessment. *Journal of Econometrics, 152*(1), 61–69.

Manning, W. D., & Smock, P. (2005). Measuring and modeling cohabitation: New perspectives from qualitative data. *Journal of Marriage and the Family, 67*(4), 989–1002.

Mendle, J., Harden, K. P., Turkheimer, E., Van Hulle, C., D'Onofrio, B., Brooks-Gunn, J., Rodgers, J., Emery, R., & Lahey, B. (2009). Associations between father absence and age of first sexual intercourse. *Child Development, 80*(5), 1463–1480.

Miller, D. (2011). Maternal work and child overweight and obesity: The importance of timing. *Journal of Family and Economic Issues, 32*(2), 204–218.

Mott, J. (1999). Personal and family predictors of children's medically attended injuries that occurred in the home. *Injury Prevention, 5*(3), 189–193.

Reagan, P., Salsberry, P., & Olsen, R. (2007). Does the measure of economic disadvantage matter? Exploring the effect of individual and relative deprivation on intrauterine growth restriction. *Social Science and Medicine, 64*(10), 2016–2029.

Rodgers, J., Bard, D., Johnson, A., D'Onofrio, B., & Miller, W. (2008). The cross-generational mother–daughter–aunt–niece design: Establishing validity of the MDAN design with NLSY fertility variables. *Behavior Genetics, 38*(6), 567–578.

Salsberry, P., & Reagan, P. (2005). Dynamics of early childhood overweight. *Pediatrics, 116*(6), 1329–1338.

Salsberry, P., & Reagan, P. (2007). Taking the long view: The prenatal environment and early adolescent overweight. *Research in Nursing and Health, 30*(3), 297–307.

Seipel, M., & Shafer, K. (2013). The effect of prenatal and postnatal care on childhood obesity. *Social Work, 58*(3), 241–252.

Stewart, L., Liu, Y., & Rodriguez, E. (2012). Maternal unemployment and childhood overweight: Is there a relationship? *Journal of Epidemiology and Community Health, 66*(7), 641–646.

Strauss, R. (2000). Childhood obesity and self-esteem. *Pediatrics, 105*(1), N1–N5.

Strohschein, L. (2005). Household income histories and child mental health trajectories. *Journal of Health and Social Behavior, 46*(4), 359–375.

Veit, C., & Ware, J. (1983). The structure of psychological distress and well-being in general populations. *Journal of Consulting and Clinical Psychology, 51*(5), 730–742.

Ware, J., Jr., Kosinski, M., & Keller, S. (1995). *SF-12: How to score the SF-12 physical and mental health summary scales.* New England Medical Center, Boston, MA: The Health Institute.

Wechsler, D. (1974). *Wechsler intelligence scale for children-revised.* New York: Psychological Corporation.

Wolfe, J. (2015). The effects of socioeconomic status on child and adolescent physical health: An organization and systematic comparison of measures. *Social Indicators Research, 123*(1), 39–58.

Using the Panel Study of Income Dynamics (PSID) to Conduct Life Course Health Development Analysis

Narayan Sastry, Paula Fomby, and Katherine McGonagle

1 Introduction

The Panel Study of Income Dynamics (PSID) is a nationally representative, longitudinal study of families in the USA that began in 1968—nearly 50 years ago. It is the longest-running household panel survey in the world, and has been the model for similar studies launched in a number of other countries. Data from PSID are widely used by researchers for scientific and public policy research. The study is a unique resource for answering many questions that can be answered with no other data source.

PSID data are a cornerstone of social science research in the USA. To date, approximately 3800 publications have used PSID data, including over 700 dissertations. Nine US federal agencies use the data in fulfilling their missions. Each year, nearly 25,000 data extracts are downloaded by over 2500 different users, and there are nearly five million visits to the PSID web site. As an indicator of its significance, the study's lead sponsor, the National Science Foundation (NSF), named PSID one of the 60 most important innovations that NSF played a key role in creating.

N. Sastry (✉) • P. Fomby • K. McGonagle
Survey Research Center, Institute for Social Research, University of Michigan,
426 Thompson Street, Ann Arbor, MI 48106, USA
e-mail: nsastry@umich.edu

PSID's innovative design, broad content, and long duration have been central to understanding many key research and policy issues, including income and poverty dynamics; demographic behavior such as marriage and cohabitation, teen childbearing, and migration; child health and development; cyclical behavior of wages, labor supply, and consumption; savings and wealth accumulation; disparities in health and health behaviors including obesity, exercise, and smoking; the intergenerational transmission of socioeconomic status; and the effects of neighborhoods. PSID data have shaped a new and still emerging definition of economic well-being by transforming research in this area from a static and narrow view of rich and poor to a dynamic one in which families experience episodes of poverty or affluence (e.g., Brooks-Gunn and Duncan 1997; Hirschl et al. 2003; Sandoval et al. 2009; Rank and Hirschl 2014) and shocks to wealth (e.g., Stephens 2001; Conley and Thompson 2013). The growing number of three- and four-generation families is now supporting important new analyses of multigenerational associations in socioeconomic status attainment (e.g., Sharkey and Elwert 2011; Hertel and Groh-Samberg 2014; Pfeffer 2014; Wightman and Danziger 2014).

Across these and other topics, research based on PSID data has demonstrated the importance of a life course approach, in which factors much earlier in life have lasting influences on outcomes

N. Halfon et al. (eds.), *Handbook of Life Course Health Development*,
DOI 10.1007/978-3-319-47143-3_24

later in life. The PSID data allow researchers unique opportunities to test specific hypotheses that emerge from the seven principles of life course health development (see Halfon and Forrest 2017). In particular, by spanning the entire life course from conception to death, the study allows researchers to focus on multiple specific life course functional phases for individuals within their social and economic context. Researchers can examine *generativity* by examining the family and socioeconomic context of mothers during the preconception and prenatal period; *acquisition of capacity*, through components of the study that focus on health and development during childhood; *maintenance of capacity*, by examining how individuals function across the prime adult years; and *managing decline*, through focused components of PSID that examine how individuals manage, adjust, and adapt to old age (see Halfon and Forrest 2017: Principle 2, health development evolves over the life course).

Beginning in the late 1990s, several developments further increased the research potential of the PSID archive for studying life course health development. Most notably, content was expanded in the areas of health, wealth, expenditures, philanthropy, development, the transition to adulthood, and time use. Two important supplements were also added to the study, focusing on child health and development and the young adult years.

In this chapter we provide a profile of PSID and its recent supplemental studies, highlighting features that support life course health development research. In the next section, we describe the origins of PSID. We then provide an overview of the design and evolution of PSID. This is followed by a description of the content of the PSID interviews and the unique features of PSID for life course health development analysis. Next, we provide an introduction to PSID supplements that focus on children and young adults—the Child Development Supplement and the Transition into Adulthood Supplement. We then provide illustrations of topics of life course health development research using PSID, highlighting prominent studies that have used the PSID data. This is followed by a description of PSID's companion international studies. Finally, we explain how to obtain data from PSID and its supplements and end the chapter with an outline of future plans for the PSID project.

2 Origins of PSID[1]

PSID started with the "War on Poverty," which President Lyndon B. Johnson launched in the 1960s. Although the Social Security Retirement, Unemployment Insurance, and the Aid to Dependent Children programs were established in the mid-1930s at the height of the Great Depression, welfare programs were greatly expanded in the mid-1960s with the establishment of the Food Stamp Program in 1964, Medicare and Medicaid in 1965, and the School Lunch and Breakfast Programs in 1966. In order to assess the effectiveness of these new programs, the US Office of Economic Opportunity directed the US Bureau of the Census to design and field a survey that was later named the Survey of Economic Opportunity (SEO). In 1966 and 1967, SEO conducted interviews with approximately 30,000 households.

There was subsequently an interest at the Office of Economic Opportunity in extending the duration of the SEO study, in order to better understand the dynamics of poverty. However, there was also a desire to avoid the bureaucratic difficulties associated with conducting the study through the Census Bureau. These circumstances led the Office of Economic Opportunity to the Survey Research Center (SRC) at the University of Michigan and to commissioning SRC to conduct a 5-year follow-up survey with approximately 2000 low-income households from SEO.

The goal of the SEO follow-up study was to understand a number of crucial and highly policy-relevant issues related to poverty dynamics. A key question was tracking the reasons for changes in household poverty over time. In particular, if

[1]This section draws on previous descriptions of the history of PSID, including publications by McGonagle et al. (2012), Brown et al. (1996), and Hill (1992).

household poverty rates were estimated at 20% each year over the 5-year study period, were the same 20% of households in poverty in each of those 5 years, or were households entering and leaving poverty during that time? In order to answer this question and other similar questions, it was essential for the study to include not just low-income households, but also to include a representative sample of nonpoor households. SRC researchers convinced the Office of Economic Opportunity to launch the study with a nationally representative sample by adding 3000 households from the SRC national sampling frame to the 2000 households from the SEO sample. The 5000 households that comprised PSID at its launch in 1968 were representative of the entire US population, while also including a large oversample of low-income households.

A second major design innovation at the launch of the study was to incorporate into the sample the family members who "split off" from study households to form their own independent households. These split-off households were largely comprised of adult children of the original sample members who were forming their own nuclear families. This design feature allowed the study to remain representative over time of all (nonimmigrant) households and, combined with the study's high wave-to-wave response rates, led to substantial growth in the study's sample size and supported research on outcomes across multiple generations of the same family.

Although the study was planned to last for just 5 years, at the end of this initial period its considerable value became clear, and there was support for its continuation. At the same time, responsibility for PSID was shifted from the Office of Economic Opportunity to the Office of the Assistant Secretary for Planning and Evaluation in the US Department of Health, Education, and Welfare. As the study continued, its prominence grew steadily as a major data source for analyzing changes in poverty over time, over the life course, and across generations, as well as for studying a wide range of additional topics. In the early 1980s, the NSF became the primary sponsor for PSID. NSF currently initiates funding for PSID and provides the majority of support for the Core PSID component, although the National Institute on Aging and the *Eunice Kennedy Shriver* National Institute of Child Health and Human Development also provide major support for the Core PSID and additional funding comes from other sponsors and agencies such as the Food and Nutrition Service of the US Department of Agriculture. Since 1982, PSID has had an NSF-sponsored Board of Overseers that provides input to the study from a national and international community of researchers and survey research experts.

3 Design and Evolution of PSID

The Core PSID survey was conducted annually from 1968 through 1997 and has been conducted biennially since 1997. As of 2015, a total of 39 waves of data have been collected over 47 years. In 1997, because of the escalation in costs driven by the doubling of the sample size during its 30-year history, PSID was forced to drop some families from the study. The cuts were made from the SEO sample. Between 1997 and 1999, an immigrant refresher added to the PSID sample a total of 441 families who had moved to the USA between 1968 and 1997. Because some of the 441 immigrant families created split-off families, by 2013 the number of post-1968 immigrant families increased to 685. In 2013, the PSID sample comprised 9063 family units with 13,693 heads and spouses and 9747 other family members, for a total of 23,440 individuals. Table 1 shows the age composition in 2013 of PSID heads and spouses and other family members. Heads and spouses are largely prime-aged adults. Other

Table 1 PSID sample members (heads and spouses and other family members), by age, 2013

	Heads and spouses		Other family members	
Age group	N	%	N	%
≤18 years	20	0.1	7485	76.8
19–39	5917	43.2	1778	18.2
40–59	5009	36.6	285	2.9
60+	2747	20.1	199	2.0
All ages	13,693	100.0	9747	100.0

family members are largely composed of children and young adults—almost all of whom are the children of the heads and spouses. The 2013 interview was about 82 min in length, which is slightly higher than the average length of the post-1997 biennial interviews but about twice as long as the pre-1997 annual interviews.

Core PSID includes a telephone interview with a single respondent in each household, using computer-assisted interview software. Interviews are conducted by SRC's Survey Research Operations group, and households receive a financial incentive for completing the interview. The PSID respondent is typically the head or the spouse of the head, but may be another adult household member. An attempt is made to interview the same family member in each wave in order to maximize the consistency of respondent reports over time; approximately 95% of families that appear in successive waves have the same respondent for both interviews. The respondent provides information on himself or herself, the spouse or partner, other household members, and characteristics of the household. Individuals in PSID households are classified as other family members if, at the time of interview, they are members of the respondents' family and either residing in an interviewed family unit or temporarily away in an institution (e.g., college, jail, hospital, or the military). Family members are individuals who are related to the head or spouse by blood, marriage, or adoption, although unrelated individuals are included in the family unit if they are permanently living together and share income and expenses. PSID's tracking rules call for following the sample members' children, who are themselves classified as sample members and are eligible for tracking as separate family units when they set up their own economically independent households. Adult sample members who move out of PSID family units are tracked to their new family units (see Hill 1992). Two strengths of the PSID sample are the large representation of African-Americans and families below the poverty line. Across all ages, approximately one-third of individuals in PSID families are African-American, and 14% reside in families below the poverty line; among children, 41% are black and over 20% are in poor families.

Consistently achieving high response rates is critical to the success of a long-term panel study such as PSID. Although most cross-sectional surveys and other telephone surveys have experienced major declines in response rates over the past several years (Curtin et al. 2005; National Research Council 2013), PSID has experienced no such decline (Schoeni et al. 2013). In fact, the study's response rates in the most recent waves have been as high as any in its nearly 50-year history. PSID has achieved reinterview response rates of 96–98% in virtually every wave. In 2003 and later, the 1997 immigrant sample's reinterview response rate increased to more than 93% on average. These high rates are attributable to a number of factors, including incentive payments, experienced interviewers matched with the same families, use of tailored techniques to address respondents' concerns, and inter-wave communications with respondents.

Despite PSID's extremely high wave-to-wave response rates, the cumulative loss to follow-up after nearly 50 years now exceeds 40%. Attrition has been higher for certain groups—in particular, for men and low-income individuals. However, PSID's weights are designed to adjust for attrition (Gouskova et al. 2009), after incorporating the original sampling probabilities (see Heeringa and Connor 1999). Weighted PSID estimates show close agreement with estimates based on corresponding samples from benchmark studies, including income to the Current Population Survey (Gouskova et al. 2010), wealth to the Survey of Consumer Finances (Bosworth and Anders 2008; Pfeffer et al. 2014), expenditures to the Consumer Expenditure Survey (Li et al. 2010; Andreski et al. 2014), health behaviors and outcomes to the National Health Interview Survey (Andreski et al. 2009), and children's demographic characteristics to the American Community Survey (Sastry and Duffy 2012). Moreover, research suggests that attrition is random within families (Wiemers et al. 2010), does not account for health-wealth relationships (Meer et al. 2003) or the substantial intergenerational correlations in income (Schoeni and Wiemers forthcoming), and does not consistently bias sibling models (Fitzgerald 2011).

4 PSID Interview Content

PSID interviews collect information on a wide range of economic, demographic, social, and health topics. However, a considerable focus is on individual and household economic status, with detailed information collected on employment, earnings, income from other sources, consumption expenditures, welfare program participation, borrowing and saving, and wealth. Table 2 summarizes the PSID instrument content in PSID's most recent wave, which was fielded in 2013. Many of these content domains, and many specific questions, have been included in the instrument since 1968.

PSID has collected an increasing amount of health content over the years. Beginning in 1968, information was collected on work and activity limitations, health insurance, smoking and alcohol use, and mortality. Data were later added on workers' compensation (1977), hospital and nursing care (1982), general health status and Social Security Disability Insurance (1984), and exercise, height, and weight (1986). A major increase in health content in the 1990s added information on activities of daily living and instrumental activities of daily living (1992) and health conditions, health expenditures, and general health status in childhood (1999).

Table 2 Core PSID instrument content in 2013

Section	Description of content
Roster	Family composition update, split-off information, location of family unit members
A	Housing, utilities, computer use
B, C, D, E	Employment
F	Housework, child care, food expenses, and food assistance
F	Transportation, education expenses, other expenditures
G	Income
G	Education updates for other family unit members
H	Health status and behavior, health insurance, health-care use and expenditures
J	Marriage, fertility, and newborn children
K and L	New head or spouse background and existing head and spouse updates, including education
M	Philanthropic giving, volunteering, religiosity, help received
P	Pensions
R	Off-year income and welfare receipt
W	Wealth and active savings; intergenerational transfers of time and money

Two Core PSID modules offer special opportunities for life course health development research. First, the childhood health calendar, which was added in 2007, asks a series of retrospective questions for the household head and spouse about health conditions that arose during their own childhood including asthma, diabetes, respiratory disorders, speech impairment, depression, drug or alcohol problems, and other emotional problems. These data appear to have high validity (Smith 2009) and allow researchers to examine the effects of health conditions on life course health development by providing markers very early in the life span. Second, beginning in 2009, new questions were added to Core PSID about mortgage distress, including foreclosure activity, falling behind in payments, mortgage modifications, and expectations about payment difficulties in the coming year. These data support research on the medium-term effects of the recent economic recession for family formation and dissolution, childbearing, and educational attainment. Researchers can examine, for instance, whether higher unemployment rates and declines in income and wealth have led young adults to postpone or avoid higher education, marriage and cohabitation, and childbearing.

5 Unique Features of PSID for Life Course Analysis

The extended time series and high response rates of PSID provide substantial analytic power to study the antecedents of a range of social, economic, and health factors as well as their effects on life course health development. PSID's design supports research based on several different analytical perspectives. First, PSID provides a nationally representative cross-sectional sample of families and of children and adults of all ages. Cross-sectional analyses based on PSID data are able to draw on a rich set of covariates that describe individual and family background characteristics, behavior, and outcomes. The vast majority of PSID respondents are themselves—or have family members who were—part of the original 1968 sample (the remainder come from the 1997 immigrant refresher samples), providing information (as of 2015) from 39 waves of data collection. Moreover, PSID now collects retrospective childhood health measures for all household heads and their partners and obtains them for new entrants (who marry into or split from a family unit) making this content available irrespective of timing of entry into the study.

Second, PSID provides prospective panel data for conducting longitudinal analyses of individuals and families. PSID follows adults over the entire life course, and hence, the number of observations for an individual is related to his or her current age and age at entry into the sample. However, individuals who were born into PSID families also have information on their childhood circumstances from their parents' reports. This combination of information on childhood circumstances and later adult behavior and outcomes represents a major analytical strength of PSID that supports a variety of different analyses. Moreover, these analytical samples are large—for instance, over 2700 children who were under 18 years of age in 1968 and were residing in the original PSID families have been followed for 43 years by the 2011 wave.

Third, PSID provides rich intergenerational and intragenerational samples. The intergenerational sample is composed of adult children of respondents who split off from their parents to form their own households and who are recruited into the study. In the 2011 wave of PSID, there were 4800 parent-child pairs in which both the parent and the adult child completed a core interview. This sample supports analyses of concurrent effects of one (or more) generations on another—for example, how current parental or grandparental circumstances affect adult children's outcomes (and vice versa). In 2011, PSID interviewed over 1200 triples that included grandparents, parents, and adult children. These data provide unique opportunities for research on the equality or inequality in opportunity and the extent to which the life prospects of youth in the USA are shaped by their parents' and grandparents' social and economic status. For many PSID families, self-reported information is currently available on up to four generations within the same family at various points in their life course. Intragenerational analyses using PSID have focused on outcome comparisons among siblings (and, to a lesser extent, among cousins) as a means to control for, or examine, unmeasured family effects. In PSID in 2011, there were 3647 pairs of siblings in which both were interviewed as a head or partner. As the size of PSID's three-generation sample increases, so too does the number of first cousins (who share a common grandmother and grandfather). In 2011, there were 4330 first-cousin pairs in PSID participating as a head or partner.

6 PSID Supplements Focusing on Children and Young Adults

From its inception, the Core PSID interview has collected information primarily about the activities and characteristics of adult household members, with the largest share of data pertaining to the head of household and his spouse or partner. As a result, PSID supports research on intragenerational and intergenerational mobility in adulthood, but has historically lacked direct, prospective measures of childhood experience to operationalize theoretically informed models of the role of early life events and circumstances in shaping adult status attainment and mobility.

6.1 Original PSID Child Development Supplement

To address this limitation, in 1997 PSID launched the Child Development Supplement (CDS) to gather longitudinal information on children in PSID families. The original CDS sample included up to two randomly selected children aged 0–12 years ($N = 3563$ at Wave I of CDS) and their primary caregivers (who were usually the children's mother). Eligible CDS participants were descended by blood or adoption from the original 1968 PSID lineage or the 1997 PSID immigrant refresher sample. In most cases, this means that the child's father or mother is the child or grandchild of an original 1968 PSID respondent. Following a longitudinal cohort design, the same children and their caregivers were reinterviewed in 2002/2003 and again in 2007/2008 with a child-based response rate of approximately 90% in each wave.

The content of CDS is shaped by the theoretical perspective that child development is determined by financial, time, and social-psychological resources. Research in this area generally views resources very broadly, defining them to include purchased resources, time, interpersonal connections, and institutions that parents, schools, and communities may use to promote the development of children (e.g., Bronfenbrenner 1979; Bronfenbrenner and Morris 2006). Access to and use of these resources shape the future health, cognitive ability, and productive social behavior of children, with development at each age building upon levels attained in previous periods (Kail 2006; Shonkoff and Phillips 2000). The design of the CDS instrument also incorporates the main pathways through which the intergenerational transmission of social, economic, and health status is theorized to operate—such as wealth, human capital, learning at home and at school, kin, local institutions, social interactions, and genetic factors.

To build a comprehensive portrait of family resources and child development, CDS collected information from multiple reporters in a variety of modes. Table 3 provides an overview of the measures collected in CDS. At each wave, primary caregivers completed a telephone interview about their own and their children's characteristics and home, school, and neighborhood environments.

Table 3 Domains and measures in the original CDS and in the new CDS

Domain	Measures
Child health status and behavior	*PCG*: Child's general health rating; chronic conditions; limitations; health-care use and expenditures *Child*: General health rating; nutrition; exercise; sleep; smoking; sexual behavior; height and weight for BMI; and weight status (underweight, normal, risk for overweight, and overweight)
Child psychological and social well-being	*PCG*: Child's internalizing and externalizing behavior problems index (BPI); positive behaviors scale; social well-being; closeness with parents, absent parent, and siblings *Child*: Relationship with parents, siblings, friends, peers, and romantic partners; depression, self-esteem, worry, social well-being; risky behaviors, thrill seeking, antisocial behaviors; drug and alcohol abuse/dependence; dating behaviors; parental psychological control; initiative; languishing and flourishing; non-cognitive skills such as self-regulation, optimism, conscientiousness, and coping
Family environment	*PCG*: Child's *home* environment; conflict with father and mother; financial training; whether child has an allowance and savings; whether child has own bank account; parental warmth; involvement in daily activities and school; household tasks; parental aggravation; disagreement in parenting
Parental monitoring	*PCG*: Caregivers' knowledge of the child's whereabouts, activities, and associations *Child*: Child disclosure of activities, family rules, and limits
Child education	*PCG*: Child's enrollment; type of school; tuition; attendance; participation in federal lunch and breakfast programs; participation in special class/school for gifted students; classified as needing special education; repeated grade; dropped out; parental expectations for future schooling *Child*: Goals and expectations for own future schooling and academic success; attitudes toward and connectedness with school; ability self-concepts for reading and math; peer bullying

(continued)

Table 3 (continued)

Domain	Measures
School environment	*NCES-CCD* and *PSS*: School type; student racial/ethnic composition; other enrollment characteristics; pupil/teacher ratio; completion rates; expenditures per child; other school resources *Child*: Perceived characteristics of school and classroom; discrimination experience by race, sex, etc.
Cognitive achievement	*Child*: Courses and grades; rewards, including awards and honors received *Assessment*: WISC-III Digit Span short-term memory; forward and backward scores
Child care	*PCG*: Child's type of care, frequency of use, and costs of arrangements
Child time use	*PCG*: Child's stylized time use on structured and unstructured extracurricular activities; costs and frequency of participation; activities with parents *Child*: Stylized time use on sport; extracurricular, community, religious, and part-time work activities; frequency of participation and peer group involvement *Time diary*: Child's type, number, duration, location of activities for 1 weekday and 1 weekend day; social context of activities describing who participated with child
Religiosity	*Child*: Comfort, importance of religious affiliation, or spirituality
Future work, family, and schooling expectations	*Child*: Negative economic expectations; achieved occupational certainty and identity; job values, career orientation, and expectations for future; ideal age at marriage and birth of children; attitudes toward marriage and childbearing out of wedlock; understanding of the implications of having a child, of leaving school
Sib relationships	*Child*: Type and frequency of cooperation with sibs, kindness, and helping behaviors toward sibs
PCG sociopsychological characteristics	*PCG*: Rosenberg self-esteem; Pearlin self-efficacy; psychological distress and well-being; social support; parenting attitudes and styles; family conflict; economic strain; work schedules; community involvement
Child expenses and savings	*PCG*: Child's expenses; savings mechanisms for child, including savings for future postsecondary education
Absent parents	*PCG*: Frequency/types of activities absent parents are involved with their children; conflict between resident and absent parent

During a home visit, children aged 8–17 years completed an interviewer-administered questionnaire, and older children (ages 12–17 years) responded to an audio computer-assisted self-interview covering more sensitive topics such as sexual behavior and drug and alcohol use. Children and primary caregivers also completed cognitive tests from the Woodcock-Johnson Revised battery that assessed reading and math skills and provided height and weight measurements during the home visit. A restricted-use data file includes school identifiers that analysts may link to administrative data to incorporate information about CDS participants' school composition and quality.

CDS is unique among national child health development studies for its inclusion of diaries of children's time use. At each wave, time diary instruments were mailed to households prior to the interviewer's home visit. Children (or caregivers acting on behalf of younger children) were assigned to complete diaries on one randomly selected weekday and weekend day. Each time diary provides a chronological report of a child's activities over a specified 24-hours period, beginning at midnight. It collected information about the flow of activities, such as what the child was doing at that time, when the activity began and ended, and what else they were doing (if they were engaged in multiple activities), as well as asking questions about who was doing the activity with the child and who else was present. These questions provide information on the extent and nature of both parent/child interactions and the more general availability of parents. These questions also provide unbiased estimates about activities that children do with their siblings, their peers, and nonfamily adults. The time diaries include specific questions about media use whenever it is mentioned, yielding information about the total time spent using media, the timing of media use during the day, the content of media used (e.g., names of television programs, movies, web sites, and electronic games), and the social context of media use (e.g., who was participating with the child).

6.2 The PSID Transition into Adulthood Supplement

In recognition that the early years of adulthood (ages 18–26 years) are critical for life span development, PSID began a new study in 2005 designed to follow the children from CDS who had turned age 18 years and had completed or left high school and had families still active in PSID, called the Transition into Adulthood Supplement (TAS). The primary scientific aim of TAS was to understand the causes and consequences of social, economic, and health transitions of young adults. To describe significant milestones in the transition to adulthood in their developmental context, TAS bridges substantive content from the CDS and the Core PSID survey instruments, in addition to introducing new age-appropriate content areas. Information is collected about educational pursuits, employment, occupational choices, education and career expectations, family responsibilities, skills and abilities, intimate relationships, and more. TAS respondents who also respond to the Core PSID interview (with eligibility based on establishing their own independent household) have a shorter TAS instrument because many of the questions of interest (e.g., employment and income) are already asked in the Core PSID interview.

Across CDS and TAS, detailed information is available about development from early and middle childhood through adolescence and into adulthood. Additional information will be collected on this cohort over its life course as these youth transition to economic independence and become Core PSID respondents. TAS data have been collected biennially for 2005–2013 and will be collected through 2015 at which time all children from CDS will have been observed at least once in the study. For 2017 and beyond, a successor study to TAS is planned. As of 2013, 2571 young adults had participated in at least one wave of TAS. The response rate for TAS was 90% in the most recent wave.

6.3 2014 Child Development Supplement

By 2013, all children in the original CDS cohort had aged into adulthood. A new round of CDS began in 2014 to collect information on the next generation of children in PSID families. The new CDS includes all children who were aged 0–17 years during the 2013 Core PSID interview and their primary caregivers (approximately 5800 children and 3300 primary caregivers). This universe represents two design changes compared to earlier rounds of CDS: first, the sample includes all eligible children in a household, rather than a limit of two children; and, second, the age range has been expanded to include all years in childhood and adolescence. In the future, CDS will adopt a steady-state model in which previously recruited children and their caregivers will be reinterviewed every 5 years until children reach adulthood and children born since the last round of the study will be added to the sample. This will produce a longitudinal data resource that is also cross-sectionally representative of children of all ages at each wave.

Primary caregivers in the new CDS participate in a computer-assisted 75-min telephone interview. Children aged 12–17 years complete a 30-min interviewer-administered questionnaire by telephone and then transition to a computerized telephone interview administered by interactive voice response (IVR) technology to answer questions on sensitive topics. The IVR approach was adopted in order to protect respondent privacy and confidentiality and to maximize data validity. To permit analysis of changes over time and across cohorts, all of the content domains from the original CDS are maintained in the new CDS caregiver and child interviews. Changes in the instrument reflect theoretical and methodological advancements in the relevant disciplines and the goal of a shorter overall instrument length. One significant addition is the expansion of questionnaire content about computer and media use. Children and primary caregivers report on the number and types of computers and other electronic devices used in the household; the types of online educational, social, and entertainment activities in which children engage; and household rules governing the use of computers and mobile devices. To date, no other nationally representative study of child development in the USA or elsewhere includes a similar level of detail about children's computer and media use. The new CDS provides a unique opportunity to study how health and social behavior correlate with children's use of digital technologies across the early life course.

The new CDS introduces two additional components of interest to health researchers. First, primary caregivers and children aged 5–17 years were asked to contribute saliva samples using an Oragene OG-500 DNA Genotek saliva kit for subsequent genetic analysis. This is the first effort to collect genetic material from two generations of family members in a large-scale nationally representative study. Second, primary caregivers were asked to complete administrative record linkage consent forms providing access to children's and caregivers' birth records and to children's school records including transcripts and state-standardized test scores for children aged 8 years and older. Birth record data provide objective, detailed information on children's health status at birth, and information from both the child and caregiver generation permit study of the intergenerational transmission of early health risk factors. State-standardized test scores obtained through school records data will provide objective measures of students' academic achievement, and school transcripts will summarize students' course taking and course performance, which are important predictors of eventual college readiness.

Finally, a randomly selected 50% of CDS 2014 households received supplemental home visits from interviewers. During these visits, children aged 3–17 years and caregivers completed the Woodcock-Johnson cognitive assessments used in previous rounds of CDS. Interviewers also reviewed and collected children's completed weekday and weekend time diaries and record home and neighborhood observations. Finally, during the in-person visits by interviewers, children aged 8–11 years complete an abbreviated version of the child questionnaire. Due to methodological constraints, these study components were not administered to families that were not selected for the supplemental home visit. Fieldwork for CDS 2014 began in October 2014 and is scheduled to end in April 2015. We expect to release final data from the study to researchers through the PSID Online Data Center in April 2016.

6.4 Life Course Health Development Analysis with CDS-TAS-PSID

With the addition of CDS and TAS to the PSID suite of studies, researchers have a comprehensive, nationally representative, prospective database of young children and their families for studying the dynamic process of child health development. Embedded in the context of PSID, CDS and TAS provide a unique framework for considering how long-range family background factors influence children's health development. As shown in Fig. 1, the value of these supplements continues to increase as sample children

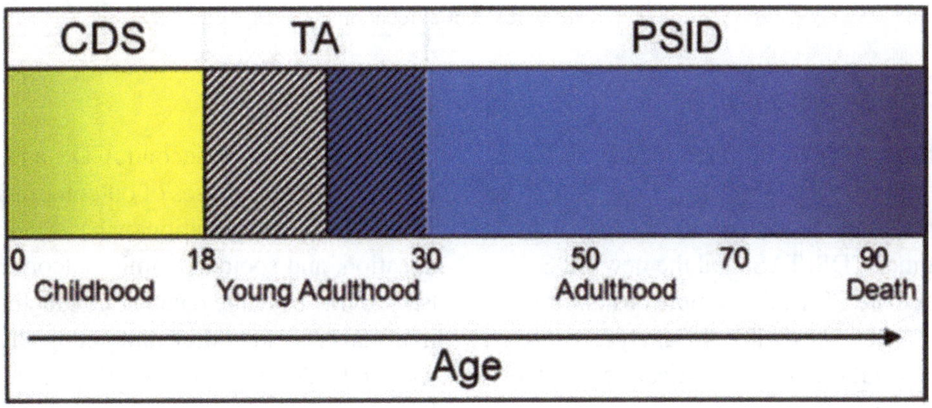

Fig. 1 Life course data from CDS-TAS-Core PSID

Table 4 Summary of key features of the original CDS, TAS, and the new CDS

	Child Development Supplement I–III (1997–2007)	Transition into Adulthood Supplement (2005–2015)	Child Development Supplement 2014
Sample eligibility	Up to two PSID children ages 0–12 years in 1997 and their primary (PCGs) and other caregivers (OCGs)	CDS children who finished or left high school and were ages 18–26 years	All PSID children ages 0–17 years in 2013 and their primary caregivers (PCGs)
Sample size	3563 children and 2394 PCGS/OCGs at Wave I	765 in 2005; 2000 in 2013	5300 children and 3000 caregivers (projected)
Response rate	Child-centered response rate of 88% at Wave I, 90% at Wave III	90% in most recent wave (2013)	Child-centered response rate of 88% (projected)
Interview mode and length	PCG: 35-min telephone or in-person Child: 20-min in-person OCG: mailback questionnaire Follow-up home visit to full sample	74-min telephone interview (for non-heads/spouses) or 51 min (for heads/spouses)	PCG: 75-min telephone Child (age 12–17 years), 30-min telephone + 15-min IVR; child (age 8–11 years, home visit sample only), 15-min in-person Follow-up home visit to half of sample
Cognitive assessments	PCG (Wave I only) and children ages 3–17 years (all waves): Woodcock-Johnson assessments of reading and math; WISC Digit Span	None	PCG and children ages 3–17 years (in-home sample): Woodcock-Johnson assessments of reading and math
Time diaries	Child: random weekday and weekend day		Child (in-home sample): random weekday and weekend day
Anthropometry	PCG and children: height and weight	Self-reported height and weight	PCG and children ages 2–17 years: height and weight
Biological samples	None	None	PCG and children (ages 5–17 years): saliva samples (Oragene OG-500 DNA Genotek saliva kit)
Administrative linkages (restricted data)	School characteristics from the National Center for Education Statistics' Common Core of Data and Private School Universe Survey Neighborhood characteristics based on residential location	Characteristics of postsecondary education institutions from the National Center for Education Statistics' Integrated Postsecondary Education Data System Neighborhood characteristics based on residential location	School characteristics from the National Center for Education Statistics' Common Core of Data and Private School Universe Survey. Future linkages to child and PCG birth records and child (age 8–17) school records Neighborhood characteristics based on residential location

age and form their own economically independent households and join the Core PSID as respondents. Table 4 summarizes the key features of the original CDS, TAS, and the new CDS.

As with Core PSID, the sample design of CDS and TAS makes it possible to analyze the data based on several different analytical perspectives. First, CDS and TAS provide nationally representative cross-sectional sample of children and young adults at each wave. Second, CDS and TAS support prospective analyses of outcomes using previously collected information on basic demographic, education, and socioeconomic outcomes, but will also provide baseline data for conducting longitudinal analyses of children and young adults. Third, CDS and TAS provide samples for conducting intergenerational and intragenerational analyses focused on childhood and the young adult years.

Almost all children in CDS and TAS have parents and grandparents who have been followed over many years in Core PSID. Approximately one-quarter of the new CDS children—a total of about 1500 children—will have a parent who participated in the original CDS and, subsequently, in the TAS study, providing extremely rich information about parent-child pairs that includes detailed developmental and behavioral data from both members of the dyad. These unique data will support innovative intergenerational analysis of key outcomes such as educational achievement, the acquisition of non-cognitive skills (e.g., self-regulation, conscientiousness, social competency, coping skills, and optimism), and behavioral problems when both individuals were children. The CDS and TAS intragenerational samples comprise of siblings and cousins. In both the original and new CDS, approximately 70% of children had a sibling in the study.

7 Topics of Life Course Research Using PSID

PSID data provide opportunities for conducting life course health development research on a variety of topics, including the dynamic process of early human capital formation; the intergenerational transmission of human capital and social capital, as well as health development assets; the historical family and contextual processes that may underlie both cohort and generational differences in children's health development; and issues related to continuity and change across generations in a wide variety of indicators of adaptive and maladaptive functioning. These data support studies of the ways in which time, social capital, and economic resources at the family, school, and neighborhood levels, as well as parenting practices and characteristics of caregivers, grandparents, extended family members, and siblings, are linked to health development over the full range of childhood, adolescence, and early adulthood. This section provides a small number of illustrations of the ways that PSID data have been used for life course health development research.

7.1 Fertility and Birth Outcomes

PSID is an important data source for understanding the causes and consequences of fertility and birth outcomes. The study has been a leading data source for understanding the causes and consequences of teen childbearing, with several articles published recently (e.g., Meadows et al. 2013; Sullivan et al. 2011; South and Crowder 2010; Wodtke 2013) that build on numerous PSID-based studies from the 1990s and early 2000s (Geronimus and Korenman 1992, 1993; Haveman et al. 1997, 2001; Corcoran and Kunz 1997; Hoffman et al. 1993; Foster and Furstenberg 1998; Foster et al. 1998). Studies of the determinants of fertility among women of all ages have examined the effects of child support (Anderson 2011), family wealth shocks (Lovenheim and Mumford 2013), and neighborhood poverty (South and Crowder 2010). PSID has become a key source of data to understand the effects of birth outcomes and health in early childhood on later health and well-being (Johnson and Schoeni 2011a, b; Johnson 2012; Johnson et al. 2012; Delaney and Smith 2012; Haas 2007; Smith 2009), reflecting the theoretical and empirical advances provided by Barker and colleagues (Barker 1998; Barker and Osmond 1986; Barker et al. 2001), by Wadsworth (1987, 1991), and by others (Kuh and Ben-Shlomo 1997; Kuh and Shlomo 2004; Hertzman and Power 2003).

7.2 Neighborhood Effects

The design of PSID and its supplements recognizes the theoretical perspective that human health development is determined by a broad set of family, social, cultural, and community resources (e.g., Bronfenbrenner 1979; Bronfenbrenner and Morris 2006). A major research focus based on this paradigm is the study of neighborhood effects on a variety of outcomes. The availability across the life course of PSID individuals' census tract of residence (and census block beginning in 2009) through a restricted-use contract permits the study of neighborhood effects. PSID has been used extensively to examine migration and the effects of neighborhoods, as evidenced by more than 400 publications on these topics with about half published in the past decade. PSID was one of the earliest data sources for studying contextual effects on socioeconomic status (Corcoran et al. 1990; Dachter 1982) and remains one of the most important and widely used sources across multiple disciplines for examining neighborhood effects on a variety of outcomes including child, adolescent, and young adult health development (Dearing et al. 2009; Jackson and Mare 2007; Timberlake 2009a, b; Wimer et al. 2008; Sharkey and Elwert 2011), health (Do and Finch 2008; Halliday 2007; Halliday and Kimmitt 2008; Johnson and Schoeni 2011b; Do et al. 2013; Wen and Shenassa 2012), education (Brooks-Gunn et al. 1993; Crowder and South 2003; Galster et al. 2007; Harding 2003; Crowder and South 2011; Galster et al. 2013; Wodtke et al. 2011), income and earnings (Islam and Tonmoy 2013; Sharkey 2008; Sharkey 2012), the intergenerational transmission of neighborhood context (Dawkins 2005a; Sharkey 2008; Sharkey and Elwert 2011; Solon et al. 2000), family migration and labor force outcomes (Blackburn 2010; Shauman 2010), and fertility behavior (South and Crowder 2010; South 1999, 2001a, b; South and Crowder 2010; Wodtke 2013). Because of its oversample of African-American families, the data have been used to examine levels and trends in racial equality in neighborhood economic status and migration (Sharkey 2008; Dawkins 2005b, 2006; Freeman 2005a, b, 2008; South and Crowder 2005; Timberlake 2007; White et al. 2005; Vartanian et al. 2007; Crowder and South 2005; Bruch 2014; Pais et al. 2012, 2014; Sharkey 2012; South et al. 2011; Wagmiller 2013).

7.3 Outcomes Across Generations of the Same Family

Because PSID follows adult children as they form their own households, it is uniquely positioned to investigate outcomes across generations of the same family. Recent studies have examined correlations across generations in health (Fitzgerald 2011; Vandewater et al. 2014; Lê-Scherban et al. 2014; Li 2015; Johnson and Schoeni 2011a), income (Bloome 2015; Chau 2012; Shore 2011), education (Roksa and Potter 2011; Torche 2011; Wightman and Danziger 2014), socioeconomic status (Eberharter 2014; Gouskova et al. 2010; Hertel and Groh-Samberg 2014), consumption expenditures (Charles et al. 2013), and cognitive ability (Sharkey and Elwert 2011). This recent research builds on the extensive work that began in the early 1990s (e.g., Corcoran et al. 1992; Solon 1992; Charles and Hurst 2003). In fact, because of the length of the panel, PSID has been used to estimate changes over time in the intergenerational transmission of economic status (Lee and Solon 2009; Mayer and Lopoo 2008). Researchers are also beginning to use the health data in conjunction with the socioeconomic data to examine the extent to which transmission of health across generations within the same family accounts for the transmission of socioeconomic status and vice versa (Johnson and Schoeni 2011b). Studies have used the CDS and TAS data in combination with the Core PSID data to examine associations across multiple generations. For example, a highly cited article in the *American Economic Review* examines the effect of parents' income on children's health to explain the intergenerational transmission of socioeconomic status (Case et al. 2002). The CDS child height and weight data were the basis of the first national study to examine the intergenerational transmission of body weight over three generations, finding an association of childhood obesity with grandparental obesity distinct from parental obesity (Davis et al. 2008).

7.4 Time Use

The CDS time diary data in particular have been the basis of a large and influential body of research examining the relationships among time spent in various activities, the family environment, and outcomes related to achievement, social and behavioral development, and health development. A frequently cited article in the *Journal of Marriage and Family* showed marked differences in child time use associated with poverty and maternal employment, with poor children spending substantially less time with fathers and more time with extended kin such as grandmothers; among poor children, those whose mothers were employed spent more time per week watching television, in daycare, and less time in sport activities (Yeung et al. 2001). Using the rich codes for television program content in CDS, an article in *JAMA Pediatrics* found that violent television programming was associated with an increased risk for antisocial behavior for boys but not for girls; neither educational nor nonviolent programming was associated with increased risk for boys or girls (Zimmerman and Christakis 2007). Several studies have used the time diary data to provide national portraits of time use among American children in various domains. A recent article in *JAMA Pediatrics* used the data to establish nationally representative sleep duration norms for US children (Williams et al. 2013). The CDS data were also featured in an article in the journal *Child Development* to document time spent by American children aged 6–12 years playing video games, using the computer, and watching TV in 1997 and 2003 and the association of early media use with academic achievement and behavior in adolescence and differences in outcomes by race (Hofferth 2010).

8 PSID's Companion International Surveys

PSID has a set of companion international studies with comparable samples and harmonized measures that allow researchers to conduct comparative international analysis of health and well-being outcomes across a range of key domains and across the life course. These companion studies are based in the UK (British Household Panel Survey/Understanding Society), Germany (Socio-Economic Panel), Canada (Survey of Labor and Income Dynamics), Australia (Household, Income and Labour Dynamics in Australia Survey), Switzerland (Swiss Household Panel), South Korea (Korea Labor and Income Panel Study), and South Africa (National Income Dynamics Study). Future studies that are planned or recently underway in China, Israel, and elsewhere will further enhance researchers' ability to conduct international comparative research that includes the USA. The Cross-National Equivalent File (CNEF) facilitates comparisons between PSID and many of these studies by providing a set of equivalently defined and constructed variables measuring income and other household attributes.

9 Obtaining Data from PSID and Its Supplements

The majority of PSID data and documentation is freely and publicly available on the Internet through the PSID Data Center (www.psidonline.org). Information is currently available on more than 70,000 variables, on approximately 75,000 individuals, and for all waves of the main PSID and its supplements. Users can create customized data extracts from any set of waves by searching or browsing for variables, obtain customized codebooks specific to their data extract, and archive data extracts for shared and later use. Data carts may be saved, allowing specific extracts to be shared with colleagues, reviewers, and students. A range of file formats is available when the user is ready to "check out," including widely used statistical software formats such as SAS, STATA, and SPSS. For researchers wishing to create genealogical samples, an application on the PSID web site called the Family Identification Mapping System (FIMS) automatically creates a customized file containing identifiers for PSID respondents' relatives (including biological and adoptive children, parents, grandparents, great-grandparents, and siblings). Online PSID courses, or webinars, are available to users on demand through the PSID web site to introduce the sample design and facilitate hands-on use of the PSID data for a variety of research purposes. PSID provides support to users through the PSID help desk, accessible by email at psidhelp@umich.edu.

PSID provides restricted data to authorized users under contract. Restricted data contain sensitive or potentially identifying information, and must be used in a secure data environment under a research plan approved by the user's institutional review board and by PSID administrators. Restricted data resources include a geocode-matched data file that provides the census tract and block codes for each dwelling occupied by PSID householders since 1968 and links PSID households to aggregated decennial census data (1970–2000) and American Community Survey data (2005 to the present). These data permit analyses of changing neighborhood context and the influence of neighborhood characteristics on health and well-being over time.

PSID has also developed links to administrative data sources in recent waves to expand opportunities for life course health development research on social context, health care, and outcomes. Since 2005, PSID has tracked known study decedents in the National Death Index (NDI). There are now nearly 6000 individuals from PSID families included in the PSID-restricted mortality files, which contain information on date of death, location of death, and International Statistical Classification of Diseases and Related Health Problems (ICD) codes for cause of death. In a separate Medicare claims file, up to 20 years of claims data (1991–2010) are available for approximately 2000 age-eligible PSID respondents and decedents. Claims data begin with a respondent's first service after Medicare entitlement, which is at age 65 or when qualification for disability insurance is met. Claims files include short-stay inpatient, skilled nursing facilities, hospital outpatient, physician/supplier, home health, and hospice services. Health plan enrollment files provide exact dates of respondent enrollment in Medicare health maintenance organizations. Although utilization information has not been reported for HMO enrollees in the past, characteristics of respondent health plans are reported. Summary files are compiled annually and by quarter.

Other external data sources provide information on housing and education. An assisted housing data file indicates whether each PSID family in every year through 2009 (except 1969, for which the addresses are not available) was living in a housing unit subsidized by the US Department of Housing and Urban Development, the Farmers Home Administration, through tax credits administered by the Department of Treasury, or state housing programs (Newman et al. 2009). PSID has also created linkable files for several data sources from the National Center for Education Statistics (NCES). Information from the Integrated Postsecondary Education Data System (IPEDS) describing the characteristics of post-secondary education institutions has been linked to the names of colleges that PSID heads and wives reported attending for all waves since 1975. Common Core of Data (CCD), Private School Universe Survey (PSS), and IPEDS data have also been linked to the CDS and TAS data and made available to users under restricted data use contract. Together, CCD and PSS provide general descriptive information on schools and school districts, data on students and staff, and fiscal data for nearly the entire universe of elementary and secondary schools attended by US students.

10 Conclusions and Future Plans

The history and evolution of PSID have resulted in a unique data set that spans 50 years, 10,000 households, and multiple generations of each family in the sample. These data have provided valuable insights into numerous topics related to life course research—most notably, the dynamics of poverty, its consequences for health development, childhood well-being, and its transmission across generations.

In this final section, we briefly discuss future plans for PSID that will likely enhance the value of the study for life course health development research. The main element of future planning for PSID is to continue the core interview every 2 years. In 2018, between the planned waves for Core PSID in 2017 and 2019, the study will mark its 50th anniversary—a major milestone for the study.

Plans for the next two waves of Core PSID include an addition to the study of a sample of post-1997 immigrants—that is, families who moved to the USA after 1997 (when PSID last added an immigrant refresher sample) and who would otherwise not be captured in the study. Screening and recruitment for this new immigrant refresher sample is planned for 2016 and 2017, with a target sample size of approximately 750 families. The proportion of the Core PSID sample these families would represent (approximately 7.5%) is similar to their representation among all US families (approximately 6.5%).

Adding a new immigrant refresher sample to PSID will provide many new research opportunities. The addition will increase the coverage of PSID's national representative sample, which is particularly salient for studying children's outcomes; expand diversity within the PSID sample, particularly by race and ethnicity; and support research that examines outcomes for new immigrant families. Hispanics are estimated to comprise 47% of the new immigrant refresher sample, Asians 26%, whites 16%, blacks 9%, and others 2%. We expect to conduct interviews with new immigrants in either English or Spanish (as is the case for Core PSID); due to cost constraints, we will likely exclude families who are unable to complete an interview in either English or Spanish. The new immigrant refresher sample will lead to virtually complete coverage by PSID of the national population of US families in 2017. The new immigrant refresher will also lead to PSID capturing the increasing diversity of the US population, especially by race and ethnicity and by immigration status. In 2017, we estimate that 12% of PSID's approximately 10,000 households will be Hispanic—a substantial increase from the current 8%. Researchers will be able to use these new data to study how the life course trajectories of individuals from recent immigrant families compare to those from nonimmigrant families and from immigrant families who arrived in earlier periods.

A second major future goal for PSID is to obtain genetic markers for all sample members. This effort has already begun, through the collection of saliva samples for children and primary caregivers in the new CDS. We expect in the future to expand the collection of saliva samples to other family members and families. Obtaining genetic markers for PSID individuals is among our top priorities because of the high scientific impact of new research on the genetic basis of social, economic, and health behavior. PSID's rich genealogical structure will allow researchers to investigate, and adjust for, the influence of gene-environment correlation by controlling for parents' and grandparents' genetic characteristics. It will allow for sharper gene-environment interaction estimates by using sibling differences—leading to better causal estimates. Among numerous topics, the data could be used to understand how genes interact with economic shocks in models that exploit both within-family and cross-time variation. Collecting genetic markers from all PSID sample members would distinguish PSID as the only national source in the USA for genetic data over multiple generations. Linking genetic information with life course data will open new opportunities to test theories that involve epigenetic and biological mechanisms (Jayasinghe 2011; Davey Smith 2012).

Future data collection activities include plans to repeat the CDS every 5 years. Future waves of CDS will collect data on all children from the previous wave who are still under age 18 years and will add all new children who were subsequently born or adopted into PSID households. We plan to field the next wave of the new CDS in 2019, on the heels of the Core PSID data collection for that year. PSID is also planning a separate initiative to directly interview all sample family members aged 18–26 years, whether they are primary respondents, spouses/partners, or other household members. This new project will build on the original TAS and will continue to focus on understanding the demographic, health, psychological, and socioeconomic development of young adults. The new CDS and the TAS successor together will offer researchers a unique opportunity to study pathways and outcomes from early and middle childhood through adolescence and into adulthood. Furthermore, the new CDS and TAS will allow researchers to study differences in early life course trajectories across cohorts, beginning with the original CDS cohort (born from 1985 to 1996) and continuing through to the most recent birth cohorts. Comparisons of life course trajectories across cohorts will provide insights into the effects of important period factors on child, adolescent, and young adult health development. For example, researchers will be able to examine the effects of the Great Recession on family behavior and outcomes and on children's health development and well-being, such as, whether parents' experience of unemployment and declines in income and wealth have led to lower investments in children (such as less schooling, a shift between private and public schools, less frequent visits to health-care providers, and changes in the time children and parents spend together and in their specific activities during this shared time).

Acknowledgment This document was supported by funding from the *Eunice Kennedy Shriver* National Institute of Child Health and Human Development (R01-HD069609; R01 HD059779; R01-HD072493; R01-HD052646).

References

Anderson, K. G. (2011). Does paying child support reduce Men's subsequent marriage and fertility? *Evolution and Human Behavior, 32*(2), 90–96.

Andreski, P., McGonagle, K. A., & Schoeni, R. F. (2009). Analysis of the quality of the health data in the panel study of income dynamics. Panel Study of Income Dynamics Technical Paper Series, #09-02.

Andreski, P., Li, G., Samancioglu, M. Z., & Schoeni, R. (2014). Estimates of annual consumption expenditures and its major components in the PSID in comparison to the CE. *The American Economic Review, 104*(5), 132–135.

Barker, D. J. P. (1998). *Mothers, babies and health in later life*. Edinburgh: Churchill Livingstone.

Barker, D. J., & Osmond, C. (1986). Infant mortality, childhood nutrition, and ischaemic heart disease in England and Wales. *Lancet, 1*(8489), 1077–1081.

Barker, D. J. P., Forsen, T., Uutela, A., Osmond, C., & Eriksson, J. G. (2001). Size at birth and resilience to effects of poor living conditions in adult life: Longitudinal study. *British Medical Journal, 323*(7324), 1273.

Blackburn, M. L. (2010). Internal migration and the earnings of married couples in the United States. *Journal of Economic Geography, 10*(1), 87–111.

Bloome, D. (2015). Income inequality and intergenerational income mobility in the United States. *Social Forces, 93*(3), 1047–1080.

Bosworth, B. B., & Anders, S. (2008). Savings and Wealth Accumulation in the PSID 1984–2005. Center for Retirement Research at Boston College Working Paper 2008–2.

Bronfenbrenner, U. (1979). *The ecology of human development*. Cambridge, MA: Harvard University Press.

Bronfenbrenner, U., & Morris, P. A. (2006). The bioecological model of human development. In R. M. Lerner & W. Damon (Eds.), *The handbook of child psychology, Vol. 1: Theoretical models of human development* (6th ed., pp. 793–828). Hoboken: Wiley.

Brooks-Gunn, J., Duncan, G. J., Klebanov, P. K., & Sealand, N. (1993). Do neighborhoods influence child and adolescent development? *American Journal of Sociology, 99*, 353–395.

Brooks-Gunn, J., & Duncan, G. J. (1997). The effects of poverty on children. *Children and Poverty, 7*(2), 55–71.

Brown, C., Duncan, G. J., & Stafford, F. P. (1996). Data watch: The panel study of income dynamics. *Journal of Economic Perspectives, 10*(2), 155–168.

Bruch, E. E. (2014). How population structure shapes neighborhood segregation. *American Journal of Sociology, 119*(5), 1221–1278.

Case, A., Lubotsky, D., & Paxson, C. (2002). Economic status and health in childhood: The origins of the gradient. *The American Economic Review, 92*, 1308–1334.

Charles, K. K., & Hurst, E. (2003). The correlation of wealth across generations. *Journal of Political Economy, 111*(6), 1155–1182.

Charles, K. K., Hurst, E., & Killewald, A. (2013). Marital sorting and parental wealth. *Demography, 50*(1), 51–70.

Chau, T. W. (2012). Intergenerational income mobility revisited: Estimation with an income dynamic model with heterogeneous age profile. *Economics Letters, 117*(3), 770–773.

Conley, D., & Thompson, J. (2013). The effects of health and wealth shocks on retirement decisions. *Federal Reserve Bank of St. Louis Review, 95*, 389–404.

Corcoran, M., & Kunz, J. P. (1997). Do unmarried births among African-American teens lead to adult poverty? *Social Service Review, 71*(2), 274–287.

Corcoran, M., Gordon, R., Laren, D., & Solon, G. (1990). Effects of family and community background on economic status. *The American Economic Review, 80*(2), 362–366.

Corcoran, M., Gordon, R., Laren, D., & Solon, G. (1992). The association between men's economic status and their family and community origins. *Journal of Human Resources, 27*(4), 575–601.

Crowder, K. D., & South, S. J. (2003). Neighborhood distress and school dropout: The variable significance of community context. *Social Science Research, 32*, 659–698.

Crowder, K. D., & South, S. J. (2005). Race, class and changing patterns of migration between poor and nonpoor neighborhoods. *American Journal of Sociology, 110*, 1715–1763.

Crowder, K. D., & South, S. J. (2011). Spatial and temporal dimensions of neighborhood effects on high school graduation. *Social Science Research, 40*(1), 87–106.

Curtin, R., Presser, S., & Singer, E. (2005). Changes in telephone survey nonresponse over the past quarter century. *Public Opinion Quarterly, 69*, 87–98.

Dachter, L. (1982). Effects of community and family background on achievement. *Review of Economics and Statistics, 64*, 32–41.

Davey Smith, G. (2012). Epigenesis for epidemiologists: Does evo-devo have implications for population health research and practice? *International Journal of Epidemiology, 41*(1), 236–247.

Davis, M., McGonagle, K., Schoeni, R., & Stafford, F. (2008). Grandparental and parental obesity influences on childhood overweight: Implications for primary care practice. *Journal of American Board of Family Medicine, 21*, 549–554.

Dawkins, C. J. (2005a). Evidence on the intergenerational persistence of residential segregation by race. *Urban Studies, 42*, 545–555.

Dawkins, C. J. (2005b). Racial gaps in the transition to first-time homeownership: The role of residential location. *Journal of Urban Economics, 58*, 537–554.

Dawkins, C. J. (2006). Are social networks the ties that bind families to neighborhoods? *Housing Studies, 21*, 867–881.

Dearing, E., Wimer, C., Simpkins, S. D., Lund, T., Bouffard, S. M., Caronongan, P., Kreider, H., & Weiss, H. (2009). Do neighborhood and home contexts help explain why low-income children miss opportunities to participate in activities outside of school? *Developmental Psychology, 45*, 1545–1562.

Delaney, L., & Smith, J. P. (2012). Childhood health: Trends and consequences over the life course. *The Future of Children, 22*(1), 43–63.

Do, D. P., & Finch, B. K. (2008). The link between neighborhood poverty and health: Context or composition? *American Journal of Epidemiology, 168*, 611–619.

Do, D. P., Wang, L., & Elliott, M. R. (2013). Investigating the relationship between neighborhood poverty and mortality risk: A marginal structural modeling approach. *Social Science and Medicine, 91*, 58–66.

Eberharter, V. V. (2014). The intergenerational dynamics of social inequality: Empirical evidence from Europe and the United States. *Global Journal of Human Social Science, 14*(1), 95–108.

Fitzgerald, J. M. (2011). Attrition in models of intergenerational links using the PSID with extensions to health and to sibling models. *The B.E. Journal of Economic Analysis and Policy, 11*(3), 3444.

Foster, E. M., & Furstenberg, F. F. (1998). Most disadvantaged children: Who are they and where do they live? *Journal of Poverty, 2*(2), 23–47.

Foster, E. M., Jones, D., & Hoffman, S. (1998). The economic impact of nonmarital childbearing: How are older, single mothers faring? *Journal of Marriage and the Family, 60*(1), 163–174.

Freeman, L. (2005a). Black homeownership: The role of temporal changes and residential segregation at the end of the 20th century. *Social Science Quarterly, 86*, 403–426.

Freeman, L. (2005b). Displacement or succession? Residential mobility in gentrifying neighborhoods. *Urban Affairs Review, 40*, 463–491.

Freeman, L. (2008). Is class becoming a more important determinant of neighborhood attainment for African-Americans? *Urban Affairs Review, 44*, 3–26.

Galster, G., Marcotte, D. E., Mandell, M., Wolman, H., & Augustine, N. (2007). The influence of neighborhood poverty during childhood on fertility, education and earnings outcomes. *Housing Studies, 22*, 723–751.

Galster, G., Marcotte, D. E., Mandell, M., Wolman, H., & Augustine, N. (2013). The influence of neighborhood poverty during childhood on fertility, education and earnings outcomes. In J. Blasius, J. Friedrichs, & G. Galster (Eds.), *Quantifying neighbourhood effects: Frontiers and perspectives* (pp. 95–123). New York: Routledge.

Geronimus, A. T., & Korenman, S. (1992). The socioeconomic consequences of teen childbearing reconsidered. *Quarterly Journal of Economics, 109*(4), 1187–1214.

Geronimus, A. T., & Korenman, S. (1993). The socioeconomic costs of teenage childbearing: Evidence and interpretation. *Demography, 30*(2), 281–290.

Gouskova, E., Heeringa, S. G., McGonagle, K. A., Schoeni, R., & Stafford, F. (2009). Construction and Evaluation of the Longitudinal Sample Weights, Panel Study of Income Dynamics, Working Paper, Institute for Social Research, University of Michigan.

Gouskova, E., Chiteji, N., & Stafford, F. (2010). Estimating the intergenerational persistence of lifetime earnings with life course matching: Evidence from the PSID. *Labor Economics, 17*, 592–597.

Haas, S. A. (2007). The long-term effects of poor childhood health: An assessment and application of retrospective reports. *Demography, 44*(1), 113–135.

Halfon, N., & Forrest, C. B. (2017). The emerging theoretical framework of life course health development. In N. Halfon, C. B. Forrest, R. M. Lerner, & E. Faustman (Eds.), *Handbook of life course health-development science*. Cham: Springer.

Halliday, T. J. (2007). Business cycles, migration and health. *Social Science and Medicine, 64*, 1420–1424.

Halliday, T. J., & Kimmitt, M. (2008). Selective migration and health in the USA, 1984–1993. *Population Studies, 62*, 321–334.

Harding, D. (2003). Counterfactual models of neighborhood effects: The effect of neighborhood poverty on high school dropout and teenage pregnancy. *American Journal of Sociology, 109*(3), 676–719.

Haveman, R., Wolfe, B., & Wilson, K. (1997). Childhood poverty and adolescent schooling and fertility outcomes: Reduced-form and structural estimates. In G. J. Duncan & J. Brooks-Gunn (Eds.), *Consequences of growing up poor* (pp. 419–460). New York: Russell Sage Foundation.

Haveman, R., Wolfe, B., & Pence, K. (2001). Intergenerational effects of nonmarital and early childbearing. In L. L. Wu & B. Wolfe (Eds.), *Out of wedlock: Causes and consequences of nonmarital fertility* (pp. 287–316). New York: Russell Sage Foundation.

Heeringa, S. G., & Connor, J. H. (1999). 1997 Panel Study of Income Dynamics Analysis Weights for Sample Families and Individuals. Panel Study of Income Dynamics, Technical Report, Institute for Social Research, University of Michigan.

Hertel, F. R., & Groh-Samberg, O. (2014). Class mobility across three generations in the U.S. and Germany. *Research in Social Stratification and Mobility, 35*, 35–52.

Hertzman, C., & Power, C. (2003). Health and human development: Understandings from life-course research. *Developmental Neuropsychology, 24*(2–3), 719–744.

Hill, M. S. (1992). *The panel study of income dynamics: A user's guide*. Newbury Park: Sage Publications.

Hirschl, T. A., Altobelli, J., & Rank, M. R. (2003). Does marriage increase the odds of affluence? Exploring the life course probabilities. *Journal of Marriage and the Family, 65*(4), 927–938.

Hofferth, S. L. (2010). Home media and children's achievement and behaviour. *Child Development, 81*, 1598–1619.

Hoffman, S., Foster, E. M., & Furstenberg, F. F. (1993). Reevaluating the costs of teenage childbearing. *Demography, 30*(1), 1–13.

Islam, T., & Tonmoy, M. (2013). Childhood neighborhood conditions and the persistence of adult income. *Regional Science and Urban Economics, 43*(4), 684–693.

Jackson, M. I., & Mare, R. D. (2007). Cross-sectional and longitudinal measurements of neighborhood experience and their effects on children. *Social Science Research, 36*, 590–610.

Jayasinghe, S. (2011). Conceptualising population health: From mechanistic thinking to complexity science. *Emerging Themes in Epidemiology, 8*(1), 2.

Johnson, R. C. (2012). Health Dynamics and the Evolution of Health Inequality over the Life Course: The Importance of Neighborhood and Family Background. *The B.E. Journal of Economic Analysis and Policy, 11*(3).

Johnson, R. C., & Schoeni, R. F. (2011a). Early-life origins of adult disease: National longitudinal population-based study of the United States. *American Journal of Public Health, 101*(12), 2317–2324.

Johnson, R. C., & Schoeni, R. F. (2011b). The influence of early-life events on human capital, health status, and labor market outcomes over the life course. *The B.E. Journal of Economic Analysis and Policy, 11*(3).

Johnson, R. C., Schoeni, R. F., & Rogowski, J. A. (2012). Health disparities in mid-to-late life: The role of earlier life family and neighborhood socioeconomic conditions. *Social Science and Medicine, 74*(4), 625–636.

Kail, R. (2006). *Children and their development*. New York: Prentice Hall.

Kuh, D., & Ben-Shlomo, Y. (1997). Introduction: A life course approach to the aetiology of adult chronic disease. In *Life course approach to chronic disease epidemiology* (pp. 3–14). Oxford: Oxford University Press.

Kuh, D., & Shlomo, Y. B. (Eds.). (2004). *A life course approach to chronic diseases epidemiology* (2nd ed.). Oxford: Oxford University Press.

Lê-Scherban, F., Diez Roux, A. V., Yun, L., & Morgenstern, H. (2014). Associations of grandparental schooling with adult grandchildren's health status, smoking, and obesity. *American Journal of Epidemiology, 180*(5), 469–481.

Lee, C. I., & Solon, G. (2009). Trends in intergenerational income mobility. *Review of Economics and Statistics, 91*, 766–772.

Li, M. (2015). Chronic exposure of grandparents to poverty and body mass index trajectories of grandchildren: A prospective intergenerational study. *American Journal of Epidemiology, 181*(3), 163–170.

Li, G., Schoeni, R. F., Danziger, S., & Charles, K. K. (2010). New expenditures in the PSID: Comparison with the CE. *Monthly Labor Review, 133*(2), 29–39.

Lovenheim, M. F., & Mumford, K. J. (2013). Do family wealth shocks affect fertility choices? Evidence from the housing market. *Review of Economics and Statistics, 95*(2), 464–475.

McGonagle, K. A., Schoeni, R. F., Sastry, N., & Freedman, V. A. (2012). The panel study of income dynamics: Overview, recent innovations, and potential for life course research. *Longitudinal and Life Course Studies, 3*(2), 268–284.

Mayer, S. E., & Lopoo, L. M. (2008). Government spending and intergenerational mobility. *Journal of Public Economics, 92*(1–2), 139–158.

Meadows, S. O., Beckett, M. K., Elliott, M. N., & Petersen, C. (2013). Maternal health status and early childbearing: A test of the weathering hypothesis. In N. Hoque, M. A. McGehee, & B. S. Bradshaw (Eds.), *Applied demography and public health*. New York: Springer.

Meer, J., Miller, D. L., & Rosen, H. S. (2003). Exploring the health-wealth nexus. *Journal of Health Economics, 22*(5), 713–730.

National Research Council. (2013). *Developing new national data on social mobility: A workshop summary*. Amy Smith, Rapporteur. Washington, DC: The National Academies Press.

Newman, S. J., Holupka, C. S., & Harkness, J. M. (2009). The long-term effects of housing assistance on work and welfare. *Journal of Policy Analysis and Management, 28*(1), 81–101.

Pais, J., Crowder, K., & Downey, L. (2014). Unequal trajectories: Racial and class differences in residential exposure to industrial hazard. *Social Forces, 92*(3), 1189–1215.

Pais, J., South, S. J., & Crowder, K. (2012). Metropolitan heterogeneity and minority neighborhood attainment: Spatial assimilation or place stratification? *Social Problems, 59*, 258–281.

Pfeffer, F. T. (2014). Multigenerational approaches to social mobility. A multifaceted research agenda. *Research in Social Stratification and Mobility, 1*(35), 1–12.

Pfeffer, F. T., Schoeni, R., Kennickell, A., & Andreski, P. (2014). Measuring wealth and wealth inequality: Comparing two U.S. surveys. PSID Technical Paper #14-03.

Rank, M. R., & Hirschl, T. A. (2014). Economic security and the American dream. In M. Crain & M. Sherraden (Eds.), *Working and living in the shadow of economic fragility* (pp. 140–156). Oxford: Oxford University Press.

Roksa, J., & Potter, D. (2011). Parenting and academic achievement: Intergenerational transmission of educational advantage. *Sociology of Education, 84*(4), 299–321.

Sandoval, D. A., Rank, M. R., & Hirschl, T. A. (2009). The increasing risk of poverty across the American life course. *Demography, 46*(4), 717–737.

Sastry, N., & Duffy, D. (2012). *An assessment of the national representativeness of children in the 2007 panel study of income dynamics* (pp. 12–01). Ann Arbor: Panel Study of Income Dynamics Technical Paper.

Schoeni, R. F., & Wiemers, E. (Forthcoming). The implication of selective attrition for estimates of intergenerational elasticity of family income. *Journal of Economic Equality*.

Schoeni, R. F., Stafford, F. P., McGonagle, K. A., & Andreski, P. (2013). Response rates in national panel surveys. *The Annals of the American Academy of Political and Social Science, 645*(1), 60–87.

Sharkey, P. (2008). The intergenerational transmission of context. *American Journal of Sociology, 113*, 931–969.

Sharkey, P. (2012). Temporary integration, resilient inequality: Race and neighborhood change in the transition to adulthood. *Demography, 49*(3), 889–912.

Sharkey, P., & Elwert, F. (2011). The legacy of disadvantage: Multigenerational neighborhood effects on cognitive ability. *American Journal of Sociology, 116*(6), 1934–1981.

Shauman, K. A. (2010). Gender asymmetry in family migration: Occupational inequality or interspousal comparative advantage? *Journal of Marriage and the Family, 72*(2), 275–392.

Shonkoff, J. P., & Phillips, D. (2000). *From neurons to neighborhoods: The science of early childhood development*. Washington, DC: National Academies Press.

Shore, S. H. (2011). The intergenerational transmission of income volatility: Is riskiness inherited? *Journal of Business and Economic Statistics, 29*(3), 372–381.

Smith, J. P. (2009). The impact of childhood health on adult labor market outcomes. *Review of Economics and Statistics, 91*(3), 478–489.

Solon, G. (1992). Intergenerational income mobility in the United States. *The American Economic Review, 82*, 93–408.

Solon, G., Page, M. E., & Duncan, G. J. (2000). Correlations between neighboring children in their subsequent educational attainment. *Review of Economics and Statistics, 82*(3), 383–392.

South, S. J. (1999). Historical changes and life course variation in the determinants of premarital childbearing. *Journal of Marriage and the Family, 61*, 752–763.

South, S. J. (2001a). The variable effects of family background on the timing of first marriage: United States, 1969–1993. *Social Science Research, 30*, 606–626.

South, S. J. (2001b). Time-dependent effects of wives' employment on marital dissolution. *American Sociological Review, 66*, 226–245.

South, S. J., & Crowder, K. D. (2005). Exiting and entering high-poverty neighborhoods: Latinos, Blacks and Anglos compared. *Social Forces, 84*, 873–900.

South, S. J., & Crowder, K. D. (2010). Neighborhood poverty and nonmarital fertility: Spatial and temporal dimensions. *Journal of Marriage and the Family, 72*(1), 89–104.

South, S. J., Crowder, K. D., & Pais, J. (2011). Metropolitan structure and neighborhood attainment: Exploring intermetropolitan variation in racial residential segregation. *Demography, 48*, 1263–1292.

Stephens, M., Jr. (2001). The long-run consumption effects of earnings shocks. *Review of Economics and Statistics, 83*(1), 28–36.

Sullivan, K., Clark, J., Castrucci, B., Samsel, R., Fonseca, V., & Garcia, I. (2011). Continuing education mitigates the negative consequences of adolescent childbearing. *Maternal and Child Health Journal, 15*(3), 360–366.

Timberlake, J. M. (2007). Racial and ethnic inequality in the duration of children's exposure to neighborhood poverty and affluence. *Social Problems, 54*, 319–342.

Timberlake, J. M. (2009a). "Scratchin' and surviving" or "movin' on up?" Two sources of change in children's neighborhood SES. *Population Research and Policy Review, 28*, 195–219.

Timberlake, J. M. (2009b). Effects of household and neighborhood characteristics on children's exposure to neighborhood poverty and affluence. *Social Science Research, 38*, 458–476.

Torche, F. (2011). Is a college degree still the great equalizer? Intergenerational mobility across levels of schooling in the United States. *American Journal of Sociology, 117*(3), 763–807.

Vandewater, E. A., Park, S. E., Carey, F. R., & Wilkinson, A. V. (2014). Intergenerational transfer of smoking across three generations and forty-five years. *Nicotine and Tobacco Research, 16*(1), 11–17.

Vartanian, T. P., Buck, P. W., & Gleason, P. (2007). Intergenerational neighborhood-type mobility: Examining differences between blacks and whites. *Housing Studies, 22*(5), 833–856.

Wadsworth, M. E. J. (1987). Follow-up of the first national birth cohort: Findings from the Medical Research Council National Survey of Health and Development. *Paediatric and Perinatal Epidemiology, 1*(1), 95–117.

Wadsworth, M. E. J. (1991). *The imprint of time: Childhood, history, and adult life*. Oxford: Oxford University Press.

Wagmiller, R. L. (2013). Blacks' and whites' experiences of neighborhood racial and ethnic diversity: Intercohort variation in neighborhood diversity and integration in early and early middle adulthood. *Urban Affairs Review, 49*(1), 32–70.

Wen, X., & Shenassa, E. (2012). Interaction between parenting and neighborhood quality on the risk of adolescent regular smoking. *Nicotine and Tobacco Research, 14*(3), 313–322.

White, K. J. C., Crowder, K. D., Tolnay, S. E., & Adelman, R. M. (2005). Race, gender, and marriage: Destination selection during the great migration. *Demography, 42*, 215–241.

Wimer, C., Simpkins, S. D., Dearing, E., Bouffard, S. M., Caronongan, P., & Weiss, H. B. (2008). Predicting youth out-of-school time participation: Multiple risks and developmental differences. *Merrill-Palmer Quarterly: Journal of Developmental Psychology, 54*, 179–207.

Wiemers, E., Schoeni, R. F., & Andreski, P. (2010). Attrition of second generation sample members in the PSID. Paper presented at the 2nd Panel Survey Methods Workshop, Mannheim Germany, July, 2010.

Wightman, P., & Danziger, S. (2014). Multi-generational income disadvantage and the educational attainment of young adults. *Research in Social Stratification and Mobility, 35*, 53–69.

Williams, J. A., Zimmerman, F. J., & Bell, J. F. (2013). Norms and trends of sleep time among US children and adolescents. *JAMA Pediatrics, 167*, 55–60.

Wodtke, G. T. (2013). Duration and timing of exposure to neighborhood poverty and the risk of adolescent parenthood. *Demography, 50*(5), 1765–1788.

Wodtke, G. T., Harding, D. J., & Elwert, F. (2011). Neighborhood effects in temporal perspective the impact of long-term exposure to concentrated disadvantage on high school graduation. *American Sociological Review, 76*(5), 713–736.

Yeung, W. J., Sandberg, J., Davis-Kean, P., & Hofferth, S. L. (2001). Children's time with fathers in intact families. *Journal of Marriage and Family, 63*, 136–154.

Zimmerman, F. J., & Christakis, D. A. (2007). Associations between content types of early media exposure and subsequent attentional problems. *JAMA Pediatrics, 120*, 986–992.

Using the Fragile Families and Child Wellbeing Study (FFCWS) in Life Course Health Development Research

Amanda Geller, Kate Jaeger, and Garrett Pace

1 Background

1.1 Policy and Scholarly Debates

Of the many potential determinants of child health development throughout the life course, one of the most contentiously debated has been the role of marriage and nonmarital childbearing. The now-famous Moynihan Report (1965), titled *The Negro Family*, highlighted family structure, along with the legacy of slavery and sustained discrimination, and inadequate employment opportunities, as key determinants of intransigent poverty among African-Americans of the time (Massey and Sampson 2009). Moynihan's primary policy recommendation was for increased federal efforts toward economic opportunity, and he was initially praised by black leaders for focusing such high-level attention on the wellbeing of black families. However, a more enduring legacy of his report, particularly in the context of the civil rights and feminist movements of the 1960s, was his reference to the "pathological" nature of mother-headed households (ibid.) and the controversy it engendered.

In the subsequent decades, scholars and policymakers debated whether nonmarital childbearing was the result of a "culture of poverty," which encouraged choices that undermined African-American children's life chances, or of structural factors such as racial discrimination, which trapped families in circumstances of intergenerational poverty and social disadvantage (Wilson 1988). The nature and causes of poverty, and the racialized discourse about social welfare programs, single-parent families, and their implications for child wellbeing, played a significant role in policy debates as well. This rhetoric was particularly notable in passage of the 1996 welfare reform law, the Personal Responsibility and Work Opportunity Reconciliation Act (Cherlin et al. 2009).

At the same time, the prevalence of nonmarital births has grown considerably, both among blacks and other racial and ethnic groups (McLanahan 2009). This growth, illustrated in Fig. 1, engendered further debate about the nature of nonmarital childbearing and whether its widespread increase should be cause for concern.

However, in the 1990s, empirical data on unmarried parents and their children was limited

A. Geller (✉)
New York University, New York, NY, USA
e-mail: amanda.geller@nyu.edu

K. Jaeger
Princeton University, Princeton, NJ, USA

G. Pace
Doctoral Student, School of Social Work, Department of Sociology, University of Michigan, Ann Arbor, MI, USA

N. Halfon et al. (eds.), *Handbook of Life Course Health Development*,
DOI 10.1007/978-3-319-47143-3_25

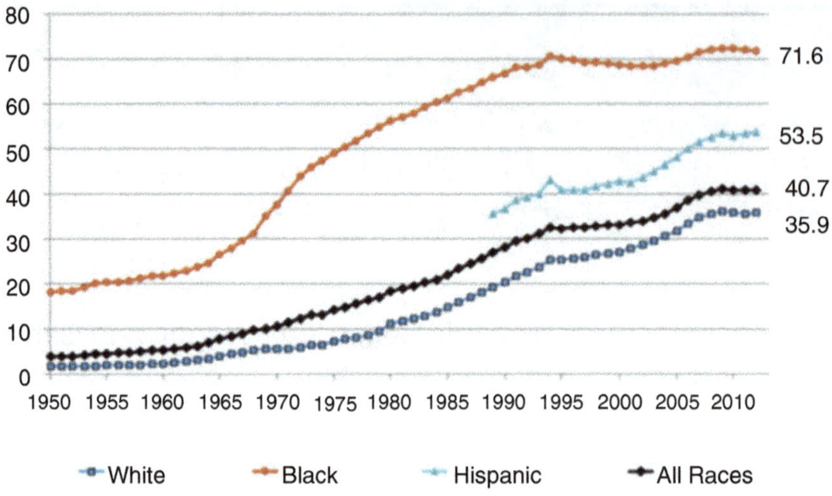

Fig. 1 Unmarried births as a percent of US births, 1950–2013 (National Center for Health Statistics; National Vital Statistics System). Note: Hispanics can be of any race. "*Black*" data from 1950 to 1969 refers to all non-whites

(McLanahan 2009). Scholars and analysts alternately posited that children born to unmarried parents were the result of encounters so casual that mothers might not know who the fathers were, or that nonmarital childbearing in the United States might resemble that in other Western industrialized countries in which committed, cohabiting parents raised children within the same stable unions as a married couple, "lacking only the piece of paper." Still others suggested that while unmarried parents might be committed to each other and their children, the American welfare state did not provide the support of those in other Western industrialized countries, leaving the family units at risk (McLanahan et al. 2010).

At the point when these debates were most salient, the literature on single parenthood and father absence focused predominantly on widows and divorced families (McLanahan and Sandefur 1994), who researchers suspected differed significantly from parents who never married. Some basic demographic information was available about the women who gave birth while unmarried, but very little was known about the fathers of their children or about the social and cultural environments in which their children grew up (McLanahan 2009). Still less was known about the health development outcomes of children born outside of marriage or the role of the family and social environment in their development.

1.2 Development of the Fragile Families and Child Wellbeing Study

To build a sound evidence base on the causes and consequences of nonmarital childbearing, a team of researchers at Columbia and Princeton Universities developed and implemented a large national survey, the Fragile Families and Child Wellbeing Study (FFCWS). The "Fragile Families" moniker was carefully chosen and derived from the Ford Foundation's "Strengthening Fragile Families" initiative of the 1990s (Sorensen et al. 2002). Although a variety of family transitions carried the potential for resulting instability – divorce and parental death, among others – the term "Fragile Families" referred specifically to families in which parents were not married at the time a child was born (ibid.). The word "fragile" referred to the risks that unmarried parents faced in terms of their economic and relationship stability, while the word "families" was used in recognition that unmarried partners with children represent a cohesive family unit (ibid.).[1]

The FFCWS was designed to address four key questions raised by the Moynihan Report and subsequent public discourse (Reichman et al. 2001).

[1] To avoid potential stigma associated with the term "fragile," families participating in the FFCWS were approached using more neutral terms and asked to participate in the "Survey of Parents."

1. What are the capabilities of unmarried parents (especially fathers) when their child is born? How many of the fathers hold steady jobs? How many want to be involved in raising their children?
2. What is the nature of parental relationships in fragile families at birth? How many couples are involved in stable, long-term relationships? How many expect to marry? How many experience high levels of conflict or domestic violence? How do relationships change over time?
3. What factors push new unwed parents together? What factors pull them apart? How do public policies affect parents' behaviors and living arrangements or child wellbeing? What are the long-term consequences of new welfare regulations, stronger paternity establishment, and stricter child support enforcement? What roles do childcare and healthcare policies play? How do these policies play out in different labor market environments?
4. How do parents and children fare in fragile families, and how does family structure and stability affect child wellbeing and development?

The study has since expanded to become a key source of information about family relationships and the broader social environment and their effects on child health development and wellbeing. At time of writing, the FFCWS is in the middle of its sixth wave of data collection, and the children born at the study baseline are turning 15 years old. The study is a joint effort by the Princeton University Center for Research on Child Wellbeing (CRCW) and Center for Health and Wellbeing, the Columbia Population Research Center (CPRC), and the National Center for Children and Families (NCCF) at Columbia University. The Principal Investigators of the Fragile Families Study are Sara McLanahan, Dan Notterman, Janet Currie, and Christina Paxson[2] at Princeton University and Irwin Garfinkel, Jeanne Brooks-Gunn, Ron Mincy, and Jane Waldfogel at Columbia University. The study's funding has come from the Eunice Kennedy Shriver National Institute of Child Health and Human Development, as well as a variety of other government and private funders, listed in Appendix A. More than 730 scholarly articles, theses, books, and abstracts have used the FFCWS data, which has also been used to inform testimony to policymakers at the national, state, and local levels (e.g., Sorensen et al. 2002; Geller 2011).

1.3 The FFCWS and Life Course Health Development Research

The FFCWS has several features that make it ideally suited for life course health development research on children. The Life Course Health Development (LCHD) model (see Halfon and Forrest 2017) views health as a "dynamic, emergent capacity that develops continuously over the lifespan, in a complex, nonlinear process" forming health development trajectories that are influenced by physical and social environmental as well as personal and genetic factors. Specifically, the model lays out seven principles of health development (ibid.):

1. Health is an emergent set of developmental capacities.
2. Health develops continuously over the life span.
3. Health development is a complex, nonlinear process occurring in multiple dimensions and at multiple levels and phases.
4. Health development is sensitive to the timing and social structuring of environmental exposures and experience.
5. Health development is an adaptive process that has been engendered by evolution with strategies to promote resilience and plasticity in the face of changing and often constraining environmental contexts.
6. Optimal health development promotes survival, enhances thriving, and protects against disease.
7. Health development is sensitive to the timing and synchronization of molecular, physiological, behavioral, social, and cultural function.

[2]Since the start of the FFCWS, Dr. Paxson has left Princeton University and at time of writing is the President of Brown University.

Health is a broad set of developmental capacities that are in constant and dynamic transactions with individuals' biological, physical, and social environments (National Research Council and Institute of Medicine 2004). The FFCWS measures children's environments across all of these domains: the study contains biological indicators of children's wellbeing from the time of their birth, including low birthweight (Reichman and Teitler 2006) and overweight and obesity (Kimbro et al. 2007), among others (e.g., Holt et al. 2013). In many cases the FFCWS is even able to study children's prenatal environments through their mothers' hospital records (Reichman and Nepomnyaschy 2008; Smulian et al. 2005). More recently, the study has also started to collect genetic data, to enable examination of gene-environment interactions (Mitchell et al. 2014).

The FFCWS also contains rich information on children's physical environments, examining factors with significant influence on health development throughout the life course. The study collects data on the homes and neighborhoods in which children live, exposure to lead (Boutwell et al. 2014), access to food (Corman et al. 2014), and other neighborhood conditions.

One of the richest contributions of the FFCWS is its measurement of the social environment in which children are raised. According to the theoretical principles of life course health development, health development is a multilevel construct, and the FFCWS measures children's social environments at many of the levels that influence their health development throughout the life course: the family (both biological parents and the social unit that comprises the household) (Jackson et al. 2012; Pilkauskas 2014), childcare settings (Rigby et al. 2007), schools (Razza et al. Forthcoming), neighborhoods (Suglia et al. 2013), and broader contexts such as states or local labor markets (Rigby et al. 2007; Pilkauskas et al. 2012).

In addition to the rich multilevel data contained in the FFCWS, another significant contribution the study makes to life course research is its unique sampling strategy (detailed below in Sect. 2.1). Given the study's focus on unmarried parents and nonmarital childbearing, the study systematically oversamples unmarried couples, who face disproportionate socioeconomic challenges (McLanahan 2011). The FFCWS permits the observation of these challenges on a population level, and enables the identification of factors that might exacerbate risk or promote resilience among children. By nature of the FFCWS sampling plan, the data also contain large samples of racial and ethnic minority families, who are often underrepresented in population-based surveys (Reichman et al. 2001).

Another contribution of the FFCWS is the longitudinal nature of its data collection. The study contains rich information on children's environments, health status throughout infancy, early childhood, school entry, and middle childhood, which permits the construction of health development trajectories. As important as these periods are for long-term health and wellbeing (Shonkoff and Phillips 2000; Heckman 2006), very few population-based American datasets track birth cohorts or begin in infancy or early childhood (though see Flanagan and West 2004 for information on the Early Childhood Longitudinal Study, a notable exception).

The longitudinal birth cohort structure of the FFCWS, coupled with the rich data it collects on multiple domains of health and health determinants, permits the joint analysis of children's physical and emotional health development, both of which develop continuously over the life span. Health development and environmental constructs are tracked over time, with indicators either measured repeatedly or updated to be age-appropriate, as needed. These measures are therefore able to capture the time-sensitive nature of child development. Children (and adults) experience several key transitions throughout the life course (e.g., school entry, puberty, etc.), which require new modes of adaptation to biological, psychological, or social changes (Elder 1985; Graber and Brooks-Gunn 1996). Events they experience – both positive and negative – may also serve as turning points that alter their life course trajectories (Elder 1985; Sampson and Laub 1990). The effects of turning points and other key exposures on life course trajectories may further be linked to the timing of these exposures with respect to developmental transitions (Graber and Brooks-Gunn 1996). An important strength of the FFCWS is its observation of exposures to key influences, and measurement of children's risk and resilience, throughout their health developmental trajectories.

1.4 Road Map

The rest of this chapter proceeds as follows. Section 2 lays out the sampling plan and study design of the FFCWS. Section 3 provides an inventory of the data available at time of writing. Section 4 provides greater detail on how the FFCWS data may be used for life course health development research. Section 5 lays out future plans for the FFCWS. Section 6 concludes with resources available for FFCWS data users.

2 Study Design

The FFCWS was designed to provide information on unmarried couples and their newborn children (McLanahan et al. 2010). Previous efforts to describe these "fragile families" were limited by the challenges in collecting data on unmarried fathers (Reichman et al. 2001). What little was known about men who fathered children outside of marriage suggested that they were younger and less educated than men who father children within marriage, with lower incomes and fewer attachments to the labor market (Reichman et al. 2001; Garfinkel et al. 1998). These fathers also reported more disability, more depression, and a greater prevalence of risky health behaviors such as drinking and substance use (ibid.). These factors create challenges in recruiting and retaining them in population-based surveys (Aday and Cornelius 2006). Unmarried fathers also are less likely to be their children's legal guardians and to have fewer formal ties to their families, and may be harder to locate as a result. Accordingly, it is also likely that data obtained from prior household surveys understated the disadvantage faced by families with unmarried fathers.

The FFCWS focused its study design around the objective of obtaining information about previously understudied, unmarried, and often nonresident fathers. Early pilot studies suggested that unmarried fathers were often present at the birth of their child, and that both parents were willing to be interviewed at this time (Reichman et al. 2001). Baseline data collection was designed around this "magic moment," and both mothers and fathers were initially contacted for interview while in the hospital, shortly after their child's birth. Sampling from hospitals also provided a spatial clustering of new parents that both improved response rates and kept recruitment and interview costs manageable.

2.1 Sampling Strategy

The FFCWS was based on a multistage stratified random sample: cities were sampled, then hospitals within cities, and then births within hospitals. The sampling of cities was based on all cities in the United States with populations of 200,000 or more. Some of the cities in the sampling frame had a population of over 200,000 only when outlying suburban areas were included, while some cities were considered only in terms of their inner city – the definition of each city was drawn from its vital statistics (Reichman et al. 2001). These cities were then characterized by their policy environments, as defined by three variables: the welfare generosity, the strength of the local labor market, and the strength of local child support enforcement. (See Reichman et al., at 310–311, for further details on the scoring of policy environments.)

Each city's welfare, labor market, and child support regimes were scored on a three-point scale: low, medium, or high welfare generosity and strong, medium, or weak labor markets and child support enforcement policies. Cities were then sorted into two groups: those with only extreme values (low or high) for all three dimensions (leaving 8 different "extreme cells") and cities with at least one middle value (19 remaining cells). One city was sampled from each of the 8 extreme cells, and 8 additional cities were

Table 1 Fragile Families and Child Wellbeing Study cities and sample sizes

Oakland, CA: $N = 330^a$	Philadelphia, PA: $N = 337$	New York, NY: $N = 384$	Jacksonville, FL: $N = 100$
Austin, TX: $N = 326$	Richmond, VA: $N = 327$	San Jose, CA: $N = 326^a$	Toledo, OH: $N = 101$
Baltimore, MD: $N = 338$	Corpus Christi, TX: $N = 331$	Boston, MA: $N = 99$	San Antonio, TX: $N = 100$
Detroit, MI: $N = 327^a$	Indianapolis, IN: $N = 325$	Nashville, TN: $N = 102$	Pittsburgh, PA: $N = 100$
Newark, NJ: $N = 342^a$	Milwaukee, WI: $N = 348$	Chicago, IL: $N = 155$	Norfolk, VA: $N = 99$

[a]Newark, Oakland, Detroit, and San Jose were strategically selected due to funder interest and therefore are not part of the FFCWS "national sample"

randomly sampled from the 19 remaining cities, with selection probability based on city populations. In the 8 "extreme policy" cities, the plan was to collect data on 250 nonmarital births and 75 marital births, for a total of 325. In the other 8 cities, the plan was to sample a total of 100 births. The "large sample" cities provided an ability to understand the social and policy environment and social processes within cities, as well as differences between cities. The eight "small sample" cities, selected from the cells with at least one middle value, improved the ability to observe nonlinearities in the effects of welfare, child support, and labor markets.

The 16 cities randomly selected along the systematic stratified sampling plan comprise the "national sample" of the FFCWS.[3] Four additional cities were added to the study, given their special substantive interest to funders. Table 1 lists the cities sampled in the FFCWS, whether they were selected as part of the national (i.e., random) sample and their baseline sample sizes.

The FFCWS is not only designed to be nationally representative of births in large cities but to offer detailed case studies of the included cities themselves. Hospitals were systematically sampled in order to increase coverage of nonmarital births, which led to a full sample of 75 hospitals (see Reichman et al. 2001, for the full list of included hospitals). Within each hospital, mothers of new babies were sampled from maternity ward lists. Once sampled, mothers were asked to complete a screening instrument to determine marital status and eligibility for participation in the study. Quotas were set at each hospital for the number of unmarried and married births, based on sample cities' 1996/1997 unmarried birth rates. Marital and nonmarital births were randomly sampled until preset quotas were reached for each hospital. If a mother was determined to be above the set quota for a given marital status, the case was coded "over quota," and the mother was not interviewed. In the rare cases that surveyed parents had had twins or a higher-order multiple birth, one child was designated the "focal child," the child to whom answers to the FFCWS refer.

The FFCWS oversample of nonmarital births, coupled with the significantly higher rates of nonmarital childbearing among blacks and Hispanics noted in Fig. 1, provided a study sample with a significantly higher representation of non-white families than most household surveys. Racial and ethnic classification of the mothers and fathers in the survey are provided in Table 2.

Several subgroups of parents were not included in the study: those who did not speak English or Spanish well enough to complete the interview, those who planned to place the child for adoption, those for whom the father of the baby was deceased, those whose baby died before the interview could take place, those mothers who were too ill to complete the interview (or

[3]Two cities (Baltimore and San Jose) were selected in a second round of sampling, when the research team was unable to gain access to hospitals in two of their initially sampled cities (Birmingham, AL and Santa Ana, CA).

Table 2 Racial and ethnic composition, FFCWS sample

	Mothers (%)	Fathers (%)
White, non-Hispanic	21	18
Black, non-Hispanic	47	49
Hispanic (all races)	27	28
Other races and ethnicities	4	4
Race/ethnicity unknown	<1	1
Total	100	100

Note: Mothers' race-ethnicity are based on self-reports. Fathers' race-ethnicity are based on a mix of self-reports and mother reports

whose babies were too ill for the mother to complete the interview), and, in many hospitals, parents who were under 18 and therefore prohibited by the hospital from being interviewed (Reichman et al. 2001). Because the study was designed to examine the roles of mothers and fathers in families, the study is also limited to births to heterosexual couples. As the sample is hospital-based, home births and births in other venues are also not represented. With these and other slight exceptions, the FFCWS sample is representative of the nonmarital births taking place in each city. However, the marital sample is not necessarily representative of marital births in each city because in many cities, births were purposively sampled from hospitals with the highest rates of nonmarital births. It is also important to note that the sample is representative of nonmarital births taking place in each city rather than of births to residents of each city (Reichman et al. 2001), since parents giving birth within the city may live elsewhere.

2.2 Sampling Weights

Due to the complex sampling design of the FFCWS, the data are provided with sampling weights to make the data representative of the sample cities and of urban births nationally. These weights account for the stratified random sample of cities, the sample of hospitals, and the sample of births, as well as the clustering of births by hospital, the oversample of nonmarital births, the underrepresentation of teen births, and mothers' marital status, education, race/ethnicity, and age. The survey includes six sets of weights: to make the data nationally representative and representative of sample cities, for couples and for mothers and fathers separately. These weights are provided for the five waves of data currently available, to account not only for design but for baseline nonresponse and attrition over time (Carlson 2008; CRCW 2008a, b).

2.3 Timing of Interviews

Baseline interviewing for the FFCWS took place over 3 years, between 1998 and 2000. Couples were subsequently contacted for re-interview in four additional waves, reflecting various developmental stages of the focal child's life. Interviews took place when the focal children were 1, 3, 5, and 9 years of age, and a sixth wave of the study is currently in the field (interviewing the families while the focal children are 15 years old.) Due to the short time that elapsed between the early interviews, some families were interviewed for their Year 1 (Y1) follow-up before baseline interviewing was completed for all families, for their Year 3 (Y3) follow-up before Y1 interviewing was completed, and for Year 5 (Y5) follow-up before Y3 interviewing was completed.

Because interviews were carried out over approximately 3 years in each wave, many of the early interviews provided valuable information to improve the survey while it was ongoing. Interviews took place in the first two cities (Oakland, CA and Austin, TX) approximately a full year before interviewing began in the remaining 18 cities, and the early interviews served as a form of pilot test. If questions were not well understood by the respondents, or responses did not have sufficient variation to permit meaningful analysis, these questions were revised before interviewing in the remaining 18 cities.

It also bears noting that considerable time may elapse between father and mother interviews within the same family. Of the families in which both mothers and fathers were interviewed at baseline, more than half (55%) of couples were interviewed on the same day. However, in more than 10% of families, parents were interviewed more than 1 month apart. By Year 9 (Y9), only 15% of parents who both participated were interviewed on the same day. More than 30% were interviewed more than 1 month apart from their partners, with a small number interviewed over a year apart. It is quite possible that discrepancies in mothers' and fathers' reports of family circumstance reflect differences in timing as well as differences in perspective and other traditional sources of measurement error.

2.4 Attrition and Retention

The FFCWS has been unusually successful in collecting data on its generally hard-to-reach target population. Core response rates are provided in Table 3 for mothers and fathers, by their baseline marital status. Mothers' baseline response rates are computed as the percent of mothers approached for interview who agreed to participate. Fathers' results at baseline are computed as the percent of mothers interviewed at baseline whose partners agreed to participate. Response rates in subsequent waves are computed as a percent of the couples interviewed at baseline who participated in subsequent waves. Even among the hardest-to-reach population, unmarried fathers, the majority of the sample was retained in the survey at the 9-year follow-up wave. Nearly all fathers (96% of fathers married at baseline and 87% of unmarried fathers) were interviewed at least once.

2.5 Couple Data

Another way in which the FFCWS provides unique information into its hard-to-reach target population is by the collection of couple data. Not only does the "magic moment" of the focal child's birth provide an opportunity to identify fathers who might not otherwise be located, information on these fathers is not only provided through personal interviews but also through the data collected from their partners. Mothers report not only on their own background and behavior and their personal perception of the couple relationship, but they also report detailed information on their partners' own background and behavior. This information includes the fathers' racial and ethnic background, place of residence, and educational attainment, as well as behavioral information such as labor market activity, incarceration history, parenting behavior, and other aspects of father involvement (e.g., child support payment and visitation). Likewise, fathers are asked to report on similar domains of the mothers' background and behavior.

Couple data provides value in two important ways. When both parents are interviewed, concordance or disagreement between the two parents' responses can be used to assess many domains of their relationship, subject to differences in the phrasing of some questions and the timing of each parent's interview. When only one parent is interviewed, responses about their partner provide information not directly obtainable. This is particularly important given the factors likely to influence attrition and retention. If the fathers least involved with their partners and

Table 3 Response rates, FFCWS core biological parent survey

	Mother		Father	
	Unmarried (%)	Married (%)	Unmarried (%)	Married (%)
Baseline	87	82	75	89
Year 1	90	91	71	82
Year 3	88	89	69	82
Year 5	87	86	67	78
Year 9	76	75	58	70
Ever			87	96

children are the most likely to leave the survey, analyses based only on those retained are likely to be affected by selection bias. Collecting mothers' reports of father characteristics helps to reduce this bias.

3 Current Data Availability

3.1 Data Access

As noted, five waves of FFCWS data collection have been completed as of time of writing. A sixth wave of data collection is ongoing. Baseline, Y1, Y3, Y5, and Y9 core follow-up data are available to the public through the data archive at the Office of Population Research (OPR) at Princeton University. These data, excluding Y9, are also available through the Inter-university Consortium for Political and Social Research (ICPSR). In-home data from the Y3, Y5, and Y9 waves are also available for a subset of core respondents. Additional data, described below, are available to the public via a restricted use contract.

The FFCWS restricted-use dataset (also known as the "contract data") contain more sensitive information such as geographic identifiers (i.e., the city where the focal child was born and state of respondent residence), census tract characteristics, local macroeconomic measures, genetic data, medical records data, and school characteristics. More information on these measures is provided in Appendix B. While these indicators are invaluable for researchers who are interested in children's local or school environments, gene-environment interactions, or detailed information about maternal health, it bears noting that the vast majority of FFCWS research is done using the public-use dataset.

Access to the FFCWS contract data is limited to researchers who agree to the terms and conditions contained in the Contract Data Use License. Access is limited to faculty and research personnel at institutions which have an institutional review board (IRB) or human subjects review committee registered with the US Office for Human Research Protections (OHRP) or the National Institutes of Health (NIH). Researchers must obtain IRB approval of their research and data protection plans. Students may use the FFCWS contract data for dissertation research; however, a faculty advisor must serve as the investigator and complete the application process, with the student signing a Supplemental Agreement with Research Staff form. The faculty advisor and the institution bear full responsibility for ensuring that all conditions of the license are met by the student. Further information about the data access process for both the public- and restricted-use files is available in Appendix B.

3.2 Data Modules

In every wave, participating mothers and fathers each completed a "core" survey, administered in-person for most baseline interviews and by phone in most subsequent interviews. For both mothers and fathers, each core interview included questions on household and family characteristics (including a household roster and parents' marital and coresidence status, as well as contact between nonresident parents and the focal child); sociodemographic and background characteristics; information on parenting behavior; romantic relationships (with the focal biological child's other biological parent or, where relevant, with new partners); details about each parent's health, education, employment, and income; as well as indicators of the focal child's health development and wellbeing. Many of the indicators in the core are collected using the same survey questions at each wave, enabling longitudinal analyses of family trajectories. Details on the data collected in the FFCWS core are provided in Sect. 4. In addition to the data available in the core, both the FFCWS public- and restricted-use files contain several other modules with additional information. These include in-home observations, supplemental surveys, official records, and genetic data.

3.2.1 In-Home Module (Public and Restricted Use)

In addition to the data collected by phone from both mothers and fathers in the FFCWS core data, both the public- and restricted-use files include an in-home module in the Y3, Y5, and Y9 waves. The in-home module includes several assessments of the child and his or her home environment and a survey of the child's primary caregiver (PCG), defined as person the focal child lives with at least half the time. The PCG, who can be either the biological mother or father, or a nonparental figure such as a grandparent, is interviewed in the Y3, Y5, and Y9 survey waves. Interviews include a mix of in-person and self-administered questionnaires conducted in the home and questions asked over the phone.

The PCG survey covers information about the child's home and neighborhood environment, including questions of neighborhood safety, the availability of household resources, parenting behaviors, and childcare arrangements. The PCG also provides details of the focal child's health development, which are best reported by the person the focal child spends the most time with. It is notable, however, that which questions are answered in the PCG survey and which are answered by the biological parents in the core survey vary by wave.

In addition, the in-home module in all three waves includes several systematic assessments by the interviewer, including the focal child's general health and cognitive health development, the PCG's health and cognitive abilities, and assessments of the home and neighborhood environment. These include measures of the height and weight of both the PCG and child, cognitive tests of both the PCG and child, and recorded observations of interactions between the PCG and child.

In the most recent wave (Y9), the in-home assessment also includes an interview of the focal child. In the "child survey," the focal child provides his or her perspective on the home environment, including relationships with each of their biological parents, as well as any new partners that the parents are married to or living with. The child also reports on the extent of discipline and monitoring provided by their primary caregiver and discipline provided by each of their biological parents and any new partners. The focal child also reports on relationships with his or her siblings and how and with whom he or she spends time. He or she provides self-reports of personal information that might not be accurately assessed by the parents or PCG, including health, personal safety, his or her school environment, school connectedness, bullying and bully victimization, and several aspects of behavior, including early delinquent behavior.

3.2.2 Childcare Provider and Teacher Surveys (Public and Restricted Use)

In the Y3 survey, families using nonparental childcare for at least 7 hours per week, and one consistent childcare arrangement for at least 5 hours per week, were asked if a representative of the childcare program could be interviewed. A subset of these parents and childcare providers consented to be interviewed and observed. The childcare provider survey included information on the focal child's behavior, social skills, and learning, as well as characteristics of the program. In many cases the interviewer also observed interactions between the provider and the child.

In Y5 and Y9, the focal child's teachers were also asked to participate in the survey. Teachers who agreed completed a self-administered questionnaire and provided characteristics of their classroom, the school climate, and their assessment of the child's behavior, social skills, and learning, as well as the parents' involvement. The teacher surveys did not include administrative details of the school itself; further information provided on the child's school is provided in the restricted-use file and described in Sect. 2.4.

3.2.3 Medical Records (Restricted Use Only)

Approximately 75% of the mothers interviewed at the FFCWS baseline gave permission for their medical records to be abstracted for analysis. These records contain detailed quantitative and qualitative data on the mother's health and healthcare history, including details of her reproductive history, such as how many previous pregnancies she had had before the focal child was born, and how much weight she gained during the pregnancy. The FFCWS medical records data also contain other anthropomorphic measures (such as the mother's weight and the child's birth weight), indicators of chemical substances in the body at the time of the birth, and diagnoses, including both physical and mental health. The medical records data provides a rich narrative of the mother's health at the time of the birth and serves to identify inconsistencies in maternal self-reports.

3.2.4 School Characteristics File (Restricted Use Only)

At the Y9 follow-up survey, data on the focal child's school was collected by the National Center for Education Statistics (NCES). Although the names and locations of the school are not released in the restricted-use file, a unique identifier is provided for each school in the file, so that children attending the same school can be identified. The NCES data include information on whether the school is a public or private school, the school's grade span (i.e., the grades taught in the school), the racial composition of the student population, Title I funding and eligibility (United States Department of Education 2014), an indicator of socioeconomic disadvantage among the students, and the percent of the student body eligible for free or reduced price lunches.

3.2.5 "Neighborhood" Contextual Data File (Restricted Use Only)

Neighborhood data for both mothers and fathers are measured at each wave. "Neighborhoods" in the FFCWS are defined as each parent's census tract of residence, though to protect respondent privacy, the tract identifiers are coded, and respondents cannot be matched to a specific tract in the restricted-use files. In addition, some random noise has been introduced into the data to ensure that respondents' census tracts cannot be identified from the data. This noise should have no impact on analyses. The contextual data file is based on the US Census and contains information on the tracts' racial composition, local employment and income levels, housing characteristics and rent, and receipt of public assistance.

3.2.6 Macroeconomic Data File (Restricted Use Only)

In addition to tract-level contextual data, the FFCWS has recently released broader contextual data for restricted use. The macroeconomic data file contains information on the national and local economic climate facing both mothers and fathers in the month of their interview. This file is based on MSA-level data from the US Bureau of Labor Statistics, on employment, unemployment, and labor force participation in the MSA containing their sample city, as well as monthly population data in both the MSA and sample state. The file also contains national-level data from the Survey of Consumers on the Consumer Sentiment Index in the month of interview. These data, coupled with the fact that Y9 data collection in the FFCWS took place between August 2007 and March 2010, permit unique analyses of the Great Recession and the effects of economic downturns on families and children (Pilkauskas et al. 2012).

3.2.7 Genetic Data (Restricted Use Only)

In the Y9 wave of data collection, in addition to the survey data collected from parents, children, and teachers, and the administrative data collected to supplement the surveys, the in-home module included the collection of genetic data. More than half of families in the study – and more than 75% of families participating in the Y9 in-home survey – provided noninvasive saliva samples for genotyping. The goal of the genetic data collection was to allow researchers to directly incorporate genetic information into their models of family relationships and child development and to test hypotheses about the relationships between genes, environment, and child health development. Saliva samples were sealed into containers with a liquid preservative and mailed to the survey subcontractor, where they were in turn shipped to the Princeton

University Molecular Biology laboratory, where genetic information was extracted and quantified into genetic markers such as single nucleotide polymorphisms (SNPs) and telomere length (CRCW 2013).

The genetic data file includes results from the genotyping of several candidate polymorphisms hypothesized to influence child health development through their interactions with children's social environments. These candidate polymorphisms include serotonin transporters, dopamine transporter, dopamine D2 receptor, dopamine D4 receptor, catechol-O-methyltransferase, melanocortin 4 receptor, transmembrane protein, and tryptophan hydroxylase. Further information on the specific polymorphisms included in the data file, the genotyping process and quality control mechanisms for each, and valuable references for the study of gene-environment interactions, are available through the Center for Research on Child Wellbeing (2015). At the time of writing, additional data are being developed in conjunction with active research programs, for future release. Data users are encouraged to check the FFCWS home page for up-to-date information.

3.3 Module Participation Rates

Although not all of the data collection modules were completed for each family at each wave, the majority of modules were completed for a substantial majority of families at the waves they were offered. Table 4 provides the participation rates for each of the data collection modules by wave.

4 Using the FFCWS

As noted in Sect. 3.1, FFCWS data can be obtained through two different processes: public access and the contract process for accessing restricted-use data. The access details described in this section apply only to the public-use file. The remainder of this section lays out details of the FFCWS data, which apply to both the public- and restricted-use data.

4.1 Data Access

The FFCWS public-use files can be accessed through a two-step process: users must first register with the data archive at the Princeton University Office of Population Research and then sign up for access to the FFCWS. Registration applications are usually reviewed within one business day. Public-use files, not including Y9, are also available through the Inter-university Consortium for Political and Social Research (ICPSR); however, the Princeton archive has the most current data files and is preferential for scientific research. Access protocols for the

Table 4 Participation rates, FFCWS modules by wave

	Baseline	Year 1	Year 3	Year 5	Year 9
Primary caregiver survey			3258 (67%)	2981 (61%)	3630 (74%)
In-home assessments			2618 (53%)	2376 (49%)	3346 (68%)
Child survey					3375 (69%)
Childcare provider/teacher survey			810 (17%)	1039 (21%)	2254 (46%)
Medical records data file	3684 (75%)				
School data file					3595 (73%)
Neighborhood contextual data file	4725 (96%)	4261 (87%)	4078 (83%)	4251 (87%)	3744 (76%)
Macroeconomic data file	4897 (100%)	4456 (91%)	4365 (89%)	4295 (88%)	3735 (76%)
Genetic data file					2908 (59%)

restricted-use file are available from the Center for Research on Child Wellbeing at Princeton University (CRCW 2009a).

4.2 Data Structure

In both the public- and restricted-use datasets, the FFCWS data are structured with one record per child and identified with a unique family identifier, a string variable called *idnum*. At each wave, mother and father data are stored in separate files and can be merged using the *idnum* variable to match members of the same family. The other modules described in Sect. 3 can also be merged to the core data using the *idnum* variable. Each core dataset has records for all 4898 families, regardless of whether each parent was interviewed. Flag variables indicate whether or not a mother or father was interviewed at a given wave, and cases who didn't participate in a given interview/wave are coded as "not in wave" on all other variables.[4]

4.3 Variable Documentation

The complete merged FFCWS dataset contains more than 10,000 variables, covering a wide variety of domains used in life course health development research. These include parents' demographic information, parental relationships, relationships the parents may form with new partners, relationships between each parent and the focal child, relationships between parents' new partners and the focal child, child wellbeing, health, behavior, and other aspects of health development. The data also contain information on the focal child's physical and social environments, including parental employment, household income and economic wellbeing, parental health and behavior, parental incarceration, social support and other family relationships, housing and neighborhood quality, and access to government programs. Not all domains are covered in each wave of the FFCWS and where each domain appears in the survey varies across waves. Each topic can be located within the five available waves using the FFCWS Core Question Map (CRCW 2009b), which lists in which waves a given topic appears; whether a topic is covered by mothers, fathers, or both; and in which section of the survey. Additionally, there is an In-Home Questionnaire Map for Y3 and Y5. Complete questionnaires are also available on the documentation page of the FFCWS website.

4.3.1 Variable Structure and Construction

Other than the variable *idnum*, which identifies families across data modules, core FFCWS variables are named according to a consistent convention. Core variable names begin with either an *m* or an *f*, depending on whether it was reported by the mother or father, respectively, followed by an indicator of the wave in which it was asked (1 = baseline, 2 = 1 year, 3 = 3 years, 4 = 5 years, and 5 = 9 years), followed by a letter and number to indicate the section and question where it appears in the survey instrument. For example, the variable *m1a12* refers to the mother's baseline survey and the 12th question of section *a*. Variables from the in-home survey are stored in separate modules and are numbered only with a letter and number to indicate section and question.[5] The Y9 dataset includes several additional variable prefixes to accommodate the additional modules described in Sect. 3.2 (CRCW 2011).

Variables in the FFCWS data are also characterized by a consistent schema for responses and

[4]In Y9, there were several types of interviews a PCG may have participated in, so it was possible for them to be coded as "not in wave" for one interview but to participate in a different interview, technically in the same wave. For example, a mother who is the PCG might have participated in the mother core survey but not completed the PCG self-administered questionnaire.

[5]It is important to note that many variable names are used in both the Y3 and Y5 in-home modules, and will need to be renamed for unique identification, usually by adding prefixes (i.e., ih3, ih4), if the variables are used together in a single data file. Future data updates may correct for this by including variable prefixes.

Table 5 Missing data codes in the FFCWS

Numeric code	Meaning	Explanation
-9	Not in wave	Respondent was not interviewed in wave
−8	Out of range	Rare code suggests the response was not appropriate for the question
−7	Did not apply	Also indicated at times by −10 or −14
−6	Skipped question	Question skips are usually dictated by survey design, indicating that a given question did not apply to a given respondent or the answer could be inferred from information already provided
−5	Not asked	This code is most often used when a question was added or taken away following the Oakland and Austin "pilot" interviews. Respondents not receiving the new (or removed) question are coded −5
−3	Missing	Missing for some reason not otherwise listed
−2	Don't know	
−1	Refuse	

Note: In the Y9 survey, a PCG could be coded as "not in wave" for a portion of the survey, but present for other components – if, for example, the PCG participated in the core survey but not the in-home.

missing data. All substantive responses appear in the data as positive numbers. Nonnumeric variables are also coded as positive integers, and their substantive meaning is indicated in the questionnaires and embedded variable labels. (For example, "Yes" answers are usually coded as 1, and "No" answers are usually coded as 2.) Missing responses are indicated with negative numbers, with different negative values indicating different reasons that the data are missing. Details on the missing data codes are provided in Table 5.

The FFCWS dataset also includes numerous variables constructed by CRCW staff to ensure that commonly used concepts are coded consistently by all users. At baseline, examples of constructed variables include the baby's sex, whether or not the birth was of multiple children (i.e., twins), whether the baby had low birth weight (i.e., less than 2500 grams), the ethnicity and race of both parents, and each parent's educational attainment at baseline. At Y1, additional variables were constructed to note the mother's age when she first had a baby and the total number of biological children she had. At Y3, variables were constructed to indicate each parent's cognitive ability (Wechsler 1981). Several other variables were constructed to indicate household composition (along with a second variable to indicate whether the child's grandparents lived in the household), fathers' incarceration histories, whether each parent reported depression and anxiety, and several details of the interview itself – whether it was conducted in Spanish, whether each parent was interviewed, and whether the primary caregiver participated in the in-home study.

4.3.2 Variable Content

The FFCWS data, collected through multiple methods, contains a rich set of child health and behavioral indicators, measures of parental resources and behavior, as well as indicators of parents' physical mental health, health behaviors, incarceration histories, and relationship stability before and since the focal birth. A summary of information collected to date is provided in Table 6, along with the modes of collection used for each class of data.

4.3.3 Tracking Constructs Over Time

One of the strengths of the FFCWS for life course health development research is the consistent measure of multiple substantive constructs across waves of the study. Many of the questions on child health were asked in each wave: parents or primary caregivers are asked to report the focal child's general health status, whether he or she has any physical disabilities, and whether he or she has had any experience with asthma – a diagnosis or an attack, with particular attention to whether the attack required a visit to the emergency room. Parents and caregivers are also asked to report children's medical visits at each wave, including doctor's visits for preventive care, illnesses, and accidents, as well

Table 6 Summary of data collected, FFCWS baseline through year 9 waves

Construct	Data collection method
Child health and development	
Child physical health: health status, developmental milestones, medical conditions, injuries, dental hygiene, exposure to tobacco smoke, physical and developmental disabilities, child height and weight at Y3, Y5, Y9	Interview and assessment
Child mental health: Child Behavioral Checklist (internalizing, externalizing, and various subscales such as aggression, withdrawal, and anxious/depressed) at Y3, Y5, and Y9. Somatic symptoms at Y9, child's report of early delinquency, task completion, sibling relationships, and emotional wellbeing at Y9. Adaptive Social Behavior Inventory at Y9	Interview and assessment
Child's use of medical care: doctor's visits, emergency care, hospitalizations	Interview
Child's health at birth: gestational age, APGAR score, weight and length	Medical records
Child's nutrition: foods consumed, frequency of snacking, use of vitamin supplements	Interview
Daily routines: TV and videogame use, hours of sleep, meals with family	Interview
Cognitive development: Peabody Picture Vocabulary Test (Y3, Y5, Y9), Woodcock-Johnson (Y5, Y9), Forward-Backward Digit Span (Y9)	Assessment
Child relationships: Attachment Q-Sort (Y3), 5-Min Speech Sample (Y5, Y9), mother-child relationship, mothers' perceptions of the father-child relationship	Interview and assessment
Household characteristics	
Household roster: current members, characteristics of new household members	Interview
Child's living arrangements: history between survey waves	Interview
Economic status: employment, earnings, income, public/private transfers, material hardship	Interview
Housing and neighborhoods: Mobility, quality, safety	Interview and observation
Incarceration: current status and history of parents and new partners	Interview
Family relationships	
Bio-parents' relationship and new partners: quality of romantic relationship, cooperation, co-parenting, violence	Interview
Social support: relatives, friends, church attendance, civic participation	Interview
Parental health and cognitive ability	
Physical health: self-rated health, height and weight, smoking, drug and alcohol use, pregnancy risk factors, obstetrical information, and information on delivery of focal child (mothers only)	Medical records
Mental health: anxiety and depression, impulsivity, mental health history, perceived stress	Interview
Cognitive ability: Wechsler Adult Intelligence Scale (Y3); Peabody Picture Vocabulary Test (primary caregiver, English dominant), Testo de Vocabulario en Imagenes Peabody (primary caregiver, Spanish dominant)	Assessment
Parenting	
Nurturance and discipline: HOME, Conflicts Tactics Scales, emotional closeness, supervision	Interview and observation
Cognitive stimulation: reading, materials for cognitive stimulation in home (from HOME assessment)	Interview and observation
Child protective services involvement: whether reported to CPS; disposition of the report	Interview
Childcare/schooling	
Childcare use: time spent in childcare, types and stability of childcare arrangements, cost of care, parents' involvement in childcare centers/kindergarten, connections to other parents	Interview
Childcare/kindergarten: ratings of daycare (Y3), kindergarten (Y5), classroom size, type of instruction, school climate	Observation
Elementary school (Y9): school, classroom, and teacher characteristics, child's behavior, special education services, comparative academic performance, parental involvement, connectedness to school	Interview

as any visits to the hospital or emergency room. Many indicators of the family's social environment were also asked in similar formats across waves, such as parents' reports of relationship quality and co-parenting.

Other family characteristics differ slightly from one wave to the next; for example, parents are asked to report on between 8 and 14 indicators of material hardship in each of the Y1, Y3, and Y5 waves. These measures may be reconciled by analyzing only the eight indicators that appear in all three waves or can be used in their differing format. Still other characteristics, particularly those related to child health development, would be inappropriate to measure in the same way in all waves (e.g., questions on child behavior, cognitive development, and puberty onset). The FFCWS measures are selected and designed to be age-appropriate at the time they are asked. Researchers maintain considerable flexibility in ways to model child cognitive and behavioral health trajectories over time.

5 Looking Ahead

In addition to the rich data that has been collected in the FFCWS to date, the study is currently in the field for a new round of data collection. This data collection is timed around the focal child's 15th birthday (hereafter "Year 15" or "Y15") and designed to improve understanding of how children's experiences in early and middle childhood influence adolescent behaviors. Adolescence is a critical period in human development when children engage in both positive and negative behaviors with lasting consequences for future health and wellbeing. The new wave of the FFCWS will provide new information about how children's adolescent outcomes are influenced by their experiences in infancy and early childhood.

Data in the Y15 wave is being collected through a series of new measures, as well as measures from existing waves that have been expanded to capture children's experiences directly from their self-report. Key areas of expansion include sexual activity (and particularly risky sexual activity), school performance and engagement, delinquency, civic and extracurricular participation, pro-social behaviors, pubertal development, substance use and abuse, sleep, physical activity, eating, multimedia exposure, and a variety of other measures of adolescent health and wellbeing. The Y15 survey is also collecting data on the focal child's relationships with both his or her biological parents, any new partners, and siblings, in order to understand how family complexity and instability influence family interactions and adolescent wellbeing. Finally, the Y15 wave will include new collection of genetic information through additional saliva samples.

The new data will facilitate research on topics related to adolescent risk; the role of the family in shaping adolescent outcomes; racial and ethnic, gender, and income disparities in adolescent health development; and the role of gene-environment interactions in adolescent development. Data collection is scheduled to be completed by 2017, and the data will be cleaned and released for limited and public use in the coming years.

6 Key Resources for Users

In addition to the rich data resources available in the FFCWS, Princeton's Center for Research on Child Wellbeing (CRCW) and the Columbia Population Research Center (CPRC), as the home institutions of the study, devote considerable material and intellectual resources to the community of data users. In addition to the data and extensive documentation available online, CRCW staff maintain an online database of working papers and publications using the FFCWS. Data users are encouraged to publish their working papers and submit their publications for inclusion in the database. CRCW also publishes a series of research briefs based on FFCWS publications, which are both available from the FFCWS website and distributed to a broad audience of researchers, policymakers, and advocates. Finally, CRCW staff are available to answer questions about the study. In addition,

FFCWS researchers host an annual 3-day workshop at CPRC to train new users of the data on the capabilities and use of the dataset. A complete list of FFCWS resources is available in Appendix C.

Fragile Families and Child Wellbeing Study Funders

Government Agencies

R01-HD-36916 from the Eunice Kennedy Shriver National Institute of Child Health and Human Development

5P30-HD-32030 from the Eunice Kennedy Shriver National Institute of Child Health and Human Development through the Office of Population Research, Princeton University

National Science Foundation

US Department of Health and Human Services (ASPE and ACF)

Foundation Support

California HealthCare Foundation

The Center for Research on Religion and Urban Civil Society at the University of Pennsylvania

Commonwealth Fund

Ford Foundation

Foundation for Child Development

Fund for New Jersey

William T. Grant Foundation

Healthcare Foundation of New Jersey

William and Flora Hewlett Foundation

Hogg Foundation

Christian A. Johnson Endeavor Foundation

Kronkosky Charitable Foundation

Leon Lowenstein Foundation

John D. and Catherine T. MacArthur Foundation

A.L. Mailman Family Foundation

Charles Stewart Mott Foundation

David and Lucile Packard Foundation

Public Policy Institute of California

Robert Wood Johnson Foundation

St. David's Hospital Foundation

St. Vincent Hospital and Health Services

Accessing the FFCWS Contract Dataset

The FFCWS restricted-use data includes six add-on files:

- A geographic file with variables for the focal child's birth city, mother's and father's state of residence at each interview, and the family's stratum and primary sampling unit
- Medical records data for mothers and children from the birth hospitalization record (see Sect. 3.2.3 for further information)
- A school characteristic file based on National Center for Education Statistics data (see Sect. 3.2.4 for further information)
- A set of contextual characteristics of each parent's census tract at each wave (see Sect. 3.2.5 for further information)
- A labor market and macroeconomic file with data on local employment and national consumer confidence data (see Sect. 3.2.6 for further information)
- A genetic file for mothers and children drawn from saliva samples (see Sect. 3.2.7 for further information)

To be given access to the contract data, researchers meeting the terms described in Sect. 3.1 must submit two copies of the following items to the Center for Research on Child Wellbeing at Princeton University:

- An extended abstract describing the project and what the Principal Investigator hopes to accomplish, including a one-paragraph justification for why the public-use data will not be sufficient to complete the project.
- Written assurance by the Principal Investigator that his or her institution has an Institutional Review Board (IRB) for Human Subjects which has a Multiple Project Assurance (MPA) or Federalwide Assurance (FWA) from the National Institutes of Health (NIH). The MPA or FWA number must be submitted with the application.
- A data protection plan detailing how the researcher will protect the files while they are

being used, both electronically and any printouts.

- Proof of IRB approval for both the final research plan (the extended abstract in #1) and the final data protection plan (in #3).
- An application fee of $250, payable by check or money order to CRCW.
- A signed Contract Data Agreement by the Principal Investigator.
- A signed Contract Data Agreement by a senior university official who binds the university or institution. This refers to an individual who has the authority to represent the organization in agreements of this sort, such as a Vice President, Dean, Provost, Center Director, or similar official.
- A signed Supplemental Research Agreement with Research Staff for every person who will have access to the data.
- A curriculum vitae for each person who will be accessing the information.
- A copy of the Protecting Human Research Participants web-based training completion certificate from NIH for all research staff who will access the contract data. Proof of equivalent training is also acceptable.

Links to necessary paperwork are available from the Center for Research on Child Wellbeing at Princeton University (CRCW 2009c).

Resources for FFCWS Data Users

Study website

www.fragilefamilies.princeton.edu

Data downloads

www.opr.princeton.edu/archive/ff/

Email questions to

ffdata@princeton.edu

Information on Summer Data Workshops

http://cupop.columbia.edu/research/research-areas/fragile-families-data-workshops

Searchable publications database

http://cupop.columbia.edu/research/research-areas/fragile-families-data-workshops

Includes abstracts, citations, complete working papers, and full articles if the viewing institution has access

Documentation page

www.fragilefamilies.princeton.edu/documentation.asp

Includes questionnaires, guide to the public-use file, core scales documentation, weights documentation and design paper, codebooks including tabulations of all variables, and in-home user's guide

References

Aday, L., & Cornelius, L. J. (2006). *Designing and conducting health surveys* (3rd ed.). San Francisco: Jossey-Bass.

Boutwell, B. B., Beaver, K. M., & Barnes, J. C. (2014). The Association of Parent-Reported Lead Exposure with language skills and externalizing behavioral problems in children. *Journal of Geography & Natural Disasters, 4*(2). doi:10.4172/2167-0587.1000124.

Carlson, B. L. (2008). Fragile families & child wellbeing study: Methodology for constructing mother, father, and couple weights for core telephone public survey data waves 1–4. http://www.fragilefamilies.princeton.edu/documentation/core/weights/const_ffwgts.pdf. Accessed 14 Feb 2015.

Center for Research on Child Wellbeing. (2008a). Fragile families & child wellbeing study: A brief guide to using the mother, father, and couple replicate weights for core telephone surveys waves 1–4. Princeton University Bendheim-Thoman Center for Research on Child Wellbeing. http://www.fragilefamilies.princeton.edu/documentation/core/weights/_vti_cnf/using_ffwgts_rev0709.pdf. Accessed 14 Feb 2015.

Center for Research on Child Wellbeing. (2008b). Fragile families & child wellbeing study: Methodology for constructing mother, father, and couple weights for core telephone public survey data waves 1–4. Princeton University Bendheim-Thoman Center for Research on Child Wellbeing. http://www.fragilefamilies.princeton.edu/documentation/core/weights/const_ffwgts.pdf. Accessed 10 Mar 2015.

Center for Research on Child Wellbeing. (2009a). Fragile families and child wellbeing study restricted use data. http://www.fragilefamilies.princeton.edu/restricted.asp. Princeton University Bendheim-Thoman Center for Research on Child Wellbeing. Accessed 1 Feb 2015.

Center for Research on Child Wellbeing. (2009b). Map of items included in four waves of the fragile families telephone interview. http://www.fragilefamilies.princeton.edu/documentation/core/coreFFqmap.pdf. Princeton University Bendheim-Thoman Center for Research on Child Wellbeing. Accessed 1 Feb 2015.

Center for Research on Child Wellbeing. (2009c). Guide to accessing the fragile families contract data. http://www.fragilefamilies.princeton.edu/documents/restricted_agreement.pdf. Princeton University Bendheim-Thoman Center for Research on Child Wellbeing. Accessed 16 Feb 2015.

Center for Research on Child Wellbeing. (2011). Data user's guide for the nine-year follow-up wave of the fragile families and child wellbeing study. http://www.fragilefamilies.princeton.edu/documentation/year9/year9wave_ff_public.pdf. Princeton University Bendheim-Thoman Center for Research on Child Wellbeing. Accessed 1 Feb 2015.

Center for Research on Child Wellbeing. (2013). *Genetic component of the fragile families and child wellbeing study: Year 9 DNA file*. Princeton: Bendheim-Thoman Center for Research on Child Wellbeing.

Center for Research on Child Wellbeing. (2015). Fragile families genetic component/DNA restricted use data appendage documentation: 9-year follow-up wave. http://www.fragilefamilies.princeton.edu/documentation/collaborative/genetic/ff_gen_9y_pub1.pdf. Princeton University Bendheim-Thoman Center for Research on Child Wellbeing. Accessed 30 June 2015.

Cherlin, A., Frogner, B., Ribar, D., & Moffitt, R. (2009). Welfare reform in the mid-2000s: How African American and Hispanic families in three cities are faring. *Annals of the American Academy of Political and Social Sciences, 621*, 178–201.

Corman, H., Noonan, K., & Reichman, N. E. (2014). Effects of infant health on family food insecurity: Evidence from two US birth cohort studies. *Social Science & Medicine, 123*, 18–25.

Elder, G. H., Jr. (1985). Perspectives on the life course. In G. H. Elder Jr. (Ed.), *Life course dynamics: Trajectories and transitions. 1968–1980* (pp. 23–49). Ithaca: Cornell University Press.

Flanagan, K. D., & West, J. (2004). Children born in 2001: First results from the base year of the Early Childhood Longitudinal Study, Birth Cohort (ECLS-B). http://nces.ed.gov/pubSearch/pubsinfo.asp?pubid=2005036. National Center for Education Statistics. Accessed 14 Feb 2015.

Garfinkel, I., McLanahan, S. S., & Hanson, T. L. (1998). A patchwork portrait of non-resident fathers. In I. Garfinkel, S. S. McLanahan, D. Meyer, & J. Seltzer (Eds.), *Fathers under fire: The revolution in child support enforcement* (pp. 31–60). New York: Russell Sage Foundation.

Geller, A. (2011). Testimony to the New York City Council Committees on General Welfare, Youth Services, Public Safety, Fire and Criminal Justice Services. New York, NY. April 13, 2011.

Graber, J. A., & Brooks-Gunn, J. (1996). Transitions and turning points: Navigating the passage from childhood through adolescence. *Developmental Psychology, 32*(4), 768–776.

Halfon, N., & Forrest, C. B. (2017). The emerging theoretical framework of life course health development. In N. Halfon, C. B. Forrest, R. M. Lerner, & E. Faustman (Eds.), *Handbook of life course health-development science*. Cham: Springer.

Heckman, J. J. (2006). Skill formation and the economics of investing in disadvantaged children. *Science, 312*(5782), 1900–1902.

Holt, E. W., Theall, K. P., & Rabito, F. A. (2013). Individual, housing, and neighborhood correlates of asthma among young urban children. *Journal of Urban Health, 90*(1), 116–129.

Jackson, M., McLanahan, S., & Kiernan, K. (2012). Nativity differences in mothers' health behaviors a cross-national and longitudinal lens. *The Annals of the American Academy of Political and Social Science, 643*(1), 192–218.

Kimbro, R. T., Brooks-Gunn, J., & McLanahan, S. (2007). Racial and ethnic differentials in overweight and obesity among 3-year-old children. *American Journal of Public Health, 97*(2), 298–305. doi:10.2105/AJPH.2005.080812.

Massey, D. S., & Sampson, R. J. (2009). Introduction: Moynihan Redux: Legacies and Lessons. *Annals of the American Academy of Political and Social Sciences, 621*, 6–27.

McLanahan, S. S. (2009). Fragile families and the reproduction of poverty. *Annals of the American Academy of Political and Social Sciences, 621*, 111–131.

McLanahan, S. S., Garfinkel, I., Mincy, R. B., & Donahue, E. (2010). Introducing the issue. *Future of Children, 20*(2), 3–16.

McLanahan, S. S. (2011). Family instability and complexity after a nonmarital birth: Outcomes for children in fragile families. In M. J. Carlson & P. England (Eds.), *Social class and changing families in an unequal America* (pp. 108–133). Stanford, CA: Stanford University Press.

McLanahan, S. S., & Sandefur, G. (1994). *Growing up with a single parent: What hurts, what helps*. Cambridge, MA: Harvard University Press.

Mitchell, C., Hobcraft, J., McLanahan, S. S., Siegel, S. R., Berg, A., Brooks-Gunn, J., Garfinkel, I., & Notterman, D. (2014). Social disadvantage, genetic sensitivity, and children's telomere length. *Proceedings of the National Academy of Sciences, 111*(16), 5944–5949.

Moynihan, D. P. (1965). *The negro family: The case for national action*. Washington, DC: Office of Policy Planning and Research. U.S. Department of Labor.

National Research Council and Institute of Medicine. (2004). *Children's health, the nation's wealth: Assessing and improving child health*. Committee on

Evaluation of Children's Health. Board on Children, Youth, and Families, Division of Behavioral and Social Sciences and Education. Washington, DC: The National Academies Press.

Pilkauskas, N. V. (2014). Breastfeeding initiation and duration in coresident grandparent, mother and infant households. *Maternal and Child Health Journal, 18*(8), 1955–1963.

Pilkauskas, N. P., Currie, J. M., & Garfinkel, I. (2012). The great recession, public transfers, and material hardship. *Social Service Review, 86*(3), 401–427.

Razza, R., Martin, A., & Brooks-Gunn, J. (Forthcoming). Are approaches to learning in Kindergarten associated with academic and social competence similarly? *Child & Youth Care Forum*. doi: 10.1007/s10566-015-9307-0.

Reichman, N. E., & Nepomnyaschy, L. (2008). Maternal pre-pregnancy obesity and diagnosis of asthma in offspring at age 3 years. *Maternal and Child Health Journal, 12*, 725–733.

Reichman, N. E., & Teitler, J. O. (2006). Paternal age as a risk factor for low birthweight. *American Journal of Public Health, 96*(5), 862–866. doi:10.2105/AJPH.2005.066324.

Reichman, N. E., Teitler, J. O., Garfinkel, I., & McLanahan, S. S. (2001). Fragile families: Sample and design. *Children and Youth Services Review, 23*(4/5), 303–326.

Rigby, E., Ryan, R. M., & Brooks-Gunn, J. (2007). Child care quality in different state policy contexts. *Journal of Policy Analysis and Management, 26*(4), 887–908.

Sampson, R. J., & Laub, J. H. (1990). Crime and deviance over the life course: The salience of adult social bonds. *American Sociological Review, 55*(5), 766–779.

Smulian, J., Teitler, J., Nepomnyaschy, L., Anath, C., & Reichman, N. (2005). Intrapartum fever and newborn complications. *American Journal of Obstetrics and Gynecology, 193*(6), S193. doi:10.1016/j.ajog.2005.10.782.

Shonkoff, J. P., & Phillips, D. A. (2000). *From neurons to neighborhoods: The science of early child development*. Washington, DC: National Academy Press.

Sorensen, E., Simms, D. R., Mincy, R. Jones, B., Johnson, J., Garrison, P. J., & Garfinkel, I. (2002). *Recommendations on TANF reauthorization from the strengthening fragile families initiative*. Statement before the U.S. House of Representatives Ways and Means Committee, Subcommittee on Human Resources. http://www.urban.org/publications/900508.html. Accessed 18 Dec 2014.

Suglia, S. F., Solnick, S., & Hemenway, D. (2013). Soft drinks consumption is associated with behavior problems in 5-year-olds. *The Journal of Pediatrics, 163*(5), 1323–1328.

United States Department of Education. (2014). Programs: Improving Basic Programs Offered by Local Educational Agencies (Title I, Part A). http://www2.ed.gov/programs/titleiparta/index.html. Accessed 31 Jan 2014.

Wechsler, D. (1981). *Wechsler adult intelligence scale – Revised (WAIS-R manual)*. New York: Harcourt Brace Jovanovich, for the Psychological Corporation.

Wilson, W. J. (1988). *The truly disadvantaged*. Cambridge, MA: Harvard University Press.

Part VI

Future Directions

Life Course Research Agenda (LCRA), Version 1.0

Neal Halfon, Christopher B. Forrest, Richard M. Lerner, Elaine M. Faustman, Ericka Tullis, and John Son

1 Introduction

A rapidly growing number of research studies show that experiences and exposures in the early years can influence health development throughout life. This research also shows that suboptimal experiences and higher rates of early risk exposures can result in a cascading array of poor health outcomes, with compounding effects across subsequent life stages. This emerging life course health science has fundamentally challenged older models of how health develops and how diseases manifest over the lifecourse. It has also challenged thought leaders, researchers, policymakers, and service providers to redefine the role of health programs and policies as a platform to organize strategies that improve immediate health outcomes for children and their mothers, while also enhancing the health development of the adults those children will become (Wise 2016).

Authors' note: In 2010, the Maternal and Child Health Bureau of the Health Resources and Services Administration created the Maternal and Child Health Life Course Research Network (LCRN) and charged it with creating a new infrastructure for catalyzing progress and enhancing funding to support basic, theoretical, applied, and translational life course health development research of relevance to practice and policy. In addition to undertaking a variety of other activities and projects aimed at advancing the emerging field, the LCRN initiated an inclusive agenda-setting process that resulted in the Handbook of Life Course Health Development, including this chapter and the research agenda it contains. For a more detailed description of the development and history of the LCRN, the Handbook, and the research agenda, please see the Preface and Introduction to this volume.

N. Halfon (✉)
Department of Pediatrics, David Geffen School of Medicine, UCLA, Los Angeles, CA, USA

Department of Health Policy and Management, Fielding School of Public Health, UCLA, Los Angeles, CA, USA

Department of Public Policy, Luskin School of Public Affairs, UCLA, Los Angeles, CA, USA

Center for Healthier Children, Families, and Communities, UCLA, Los Angeles, CA, USA
e-mail: nhalfon@ucla.edu

C.B. Forrest
Applied Clinical Research Center, Children's Hospital of Philadelphia, Philadelphia, PA, USA

R.M. Lerner
Tufts University, Medford, MA, USA

E.M. Faustman
Institute for Risk Analysis and Risk Communication, Department of Environmental and Occupational Health Sciences, School of Public Health, University of Washington, Seattle, WA 98105, USA

E. Tullis • J. Son
Center for Healthier Children, Families and Communities, UCLA, Los Angeles, CA, USA

N. Halfon et al. (eds.), *Handbook of Life Course Health Development*,
DOI 10.1007/978-3-319-47143-3_26

Life course health science research is "connecting the dots" between child health development, adult patterns of premature morbidity and mortality, and more integrated notions of healthy aging. It is also starting to inform new ways of controlling costs by limiting the prevalence of chronic health conditions. One indication of how fertile, important, and interconnected this research is becoming is the growing number of research studies that are spawning in this nascent field. There are not only many outstanding questions about the relationship between early experiences and lifelong health and well-being, but a growing need to understand how emerging knowledge can be applied to the development of evidence-based practice and policy that can reduce risks, minimize exposures, and optimize lifelong health. As major national research initiatives advance clinical translational research and precision medicine, the life course health sciences can play an important role in informing research questions, leveraging life course informed health development focused strategies, and advancing translational activities from laboratories to patients to communities. Life course health science can play an important role in pinpointing key molecular leverage points, linking those processes to higher-level (body system, organism, family, or social) influences, and illuminating the often overlooked relationship between the individual and population manifestations of underlying health development processes. The findings from life course health science research will also shape the organization, design, and financing of emerging and future healthcare systems (Halfon et al. 2014a, b).

Although this Handbook is far from comprehensive, in that there are numerous health conditions and issues it does not address, it does offer state-of-the-art reviews and analyses of life course health development research focused on key life stages and a variety of specific health conditions. Based on their analysis of existing research, the authors of each chapter have suggested how life course health development research can be supported and advanced. In developing this concluding chapter, we synthesized their findings and recommendations in order to propose an integrated set of research priorities and strategies that can advance the entire field of life course health development research.

The resulting transdisciplinary research agenda focuses on foundational research types and topics, including research that addresses life course epidemiology, research that elucidates life course health development (LCHD) processes (e.g., sensitive periods, epigenetics), and research that identifies effective interventions, with a special emphasis on health disparities research and research on high priority conditions (e.g., obesity and mental health conditions) and specific vulnerable populations (e.g., children in foster care, premature infants, and children with medical complexity). Next, we consider essential research capacity-building activities focused on data, data systems, and methods, as well as strategies for building the human, technical, cultural, and financial capacity required to carry out this challenging work. Lastly, we discuss the importance of translational and intervention research that can speed the application of concepts and findings to the practice and policy arenas. We conclude with a discussion of advancing the overall life course health development research paradigm, including the framework and principles that have emerged from the research thus far, and that are helping to define a robust explanatory and theoretical LCHD framework.

2 Rationale: Why a Life Course Research Agenda?

Until recently, a strong US-based life course focused research and data infrastructure has been lacking. There have also been limits on funding currently available in the US to support the development of new methodologies and collaborative approaches to life course health development research. This has hampered the production of the transformative research that is needed to advance the emerging field of life course health development. The recently aborted National Children's Study is a major example of an unsuccessful attempt to launch a cohort study and research infrastructure that would have allowed the US to start catching up with the many other nations that have launched one or more national cohorts in the past, are in the process of conducting millennium cohort studies, or already have well developed national data systems that permit exploration into life course specific health development questions. Nonetheless, the move toward multidisciplinary LCHD research is advancing in the U.S. as research continues to break out of discipline-specific silos that have often constrained rapid transdicsiplinary progress. Over time, we believe that life course health development will become an increasingly productive and impactful transdisciplinary field.

Current and future production, dissemination, and application of life course health development research can improve our understanding of the origins, development, and manifestation of health and disease. This research must also be strategically aligned with and responsive to ongoing and emerging trends that are important influences on health development research. Because the epidemiology of human health and the capacity of the health system to respond to challenges are constantly changing, a robust LCHD research strategy must be informed by and responsive to emerging trends and shifts. These include but are not limited to:

- The ongoing epidemiologic shift in diseases and disease burdens, from infectious diseases of the past to chronic, preventable, noncommunicable diseases.
- The recognition that health is not the absence of disease, and that health as an outcome is a key target for healthcare systems.
- The "new" epidemics of obesity, several mental health conditions, and multi-morbidity, particularly in older adults.
- The growing recognition that contributing to the US's dubious distinction as the sickest of rich nations is the fact that it spends more on healthcare late in life, compared to nations with better health outcomes that invest in social and education services early in the life course.
- The World Economic Forum's recent focus on what they have termed as "inflection points" across the life course that serve as strategic targets for intervention and present opportunities to leverage population health improvement goals. These inflection points of health development suggest that life course health development research can be translated into effective policy frameworks.
- The transition in how healthcare services are organized and paid for, including the focus on preventing disease and designing payment methodologies that pay for health instead of services. These major system-level changes can use the new science of health development to define the value of healthcare, align payments with health development time frames, and establish overall health system goals.
- A range of different research organizing strategies—from those focused on translating research into action at a patient, community, or health system level to the Clinical Translation Science Institutes, to the National Institutes of Health's new efforts focused on precision medicine—can potentially benefit from new insights from the life course health sciences and can also help advance this type of basic, clinical, applied, and translational research.

The research revolution that gave birth to the life course health sciences is now about four decades old. Several disciplines, fields, and seminal research studies have contributed to the emergence of the field. These converging, interacting, and interdependent empirical and analytic trends are important to recognize and to strategically leverage as we advance the life course health sciences through a robust research agenda.

Longitudinal cohort studies that have allowed for direct empirical interrogation of the role of early life factors on adult health behaviors and outcomes contributed to the emergence of the field, as did the recognition that the impact of early adversity on lifelong health was not being captured by prevailing biomedical and biopsychosocial models that ignored the timing and influences of social and environmental factors on health development. David Barker et al.'s (1989) pathbreaking research describing the long-term associations between perinatal health conditions, such as birthweight, and adult chronic disease decades later provided an important empirical nudge for considering a new form of life course epidemiological research.

More recently, chronic disease epidemiologists have teamed up with neurobiologists and molecular biologists to elucidate the biological mechanisms for the effects of early childhood exposures and experiences on later and lifelong health. While these largely biomedical research studies were being done, a parallel set of investigations in sociology and psychology examined how mental health develops over the life course in response to interpersonal and environmental interactions. The convergence of life course epidemiology, biology, life course sociology, and life span human development psychology has established the contours of a multidisciplinary field of life course health development (Kuh and Ben-Shlomo 2004; Ben-Shlomo and Kuh 2002; Halfon et al. 2014a) that is in the process of maturing into a unified, transdisciplinary field with a unique set of theoretical constructs, frameworks, models, and methodologies.

By integrating evolutionary and developmental perspectives, the life course health development framework also spans the gap between these two fields of research that emerged with the post-Darwinian synthesis of evolution and heredity, coupled with advances in human genetics and epigenetics. As the LCHD framework began to take shape, it helped support the growing recognition that (1) health development is a complex adaptive process that emerges out of the dynamic coactions between an organism and its environments, (2) this emergent process is mediated by different types and levels of plasticity that evolution has engineered into the human developmental process to optimize a range of adaptive responses to diverse environments, and (3) the synchronization and harmonization of different embedded time frames must be considered, assessed, and understood (Hochberg 2009).

LCHD as a discrete, multidisciplinary field of inquiry is young. Irrespective of how conceptually attractive constructs such as sensitive periods or biological conditioning might be, it is important that the field be appropriately self critical in determining how strong the evidence really is for these notions. The biological plausibility of many of the LCHD hypotheses about the role and impact of different types of plasticity on the development of health and disease needs to be tested and strengthened by carefully designed and implemented research. The tension between advancing the field and ensuring sufficient awareness and reflection about whether and how it challenges the prevailing orthodoxy of biomedical research requires more careful analysis.

Hanson and Gluckman have highlighted the reasons behind the delayed acceptance of the concept of the Developmental Origins of Health and Disease (DOHaD), including a lack of conceptual framework, confusion between factors correlated with disease risk and those involved with causation, assumptions that all of the DOHaD effects were operating only through the pathway of lower birthweight, lack of plausible biological mechanisms, failure to recognize the importance of the DOHaD concept under normal developmental conditions as opposed to extreme conditions, lack of evidence of its relative importance in relation to other risk factors (i.e., population attributable risk analysis), and lack of plausible ways to use the concept clinically and in public health (Hanson and Gluckman 2014). Many of the barriers that Hanson and Gluckman describe are part of the impetus and genesis for further developing the LCHD framework so that DOHaD concepts—including notions of sensitive periods, biological priming and conditioning, life histories, and evolutionary constraints—can be used to further empirical, analytic, translational, health services, policy, and conceptual research.

The LCHD framework that has been articulated in this volume by Halfon and Forrest (2017), while not a fully developed paradigm, provides a new approach for linking health and developmental processes. The framework challenges the explanatory power of older and more linear biomedical models, as well as multidimensional biopsychosocial approaches. The LCHD framework is portrayed as a dynamic network of interactive and interdependent concepts that are coming of age and formulating this new investigative approach. In spite of the challenges for moving life course health research forward, the amount of consistent evidence, the convergence of several fields of inquiry, and the recognition of common principles are providing the opportunity—and need—for not only a more coherent explanatory framework but for the second generation of priority research topics, questions, activities, and strategies that are presented in the next section.

3 Recommendations

The following recommendations are presented in four main sections: (1) priority research types and topics, (2) priority research capacity-building activities, (3) translational priorities pertaining to the application of current knowledge to practice and policy, and (4) strategies for refining the LCHD theoretical framework.

3.1 Section I: Priority Research Types and Topics

3.1.1 Priority Research Types

Epidemiological Research

There is a growing recognition of the value of life course chronic disease epidemiologic research and its application to understanding the origins, distribution, and patterns of various diseases and health conditions. LCHD epidemiology has benefited from a better appreciation for the timing and time-specific interactions of numerous multilevel factors that influence health development. As the importance of what has been called the exposome (i.e., the set of environmental factors that influence health) become more salient and new measures and approaches for assessing environmental influences are created, a demand will be generated for multilevel epidemiologic studies (Robinson et al. 2015). Better epidemiologic measures, modeling, and analysis will all be needed to understand how different kinds of adversity interact with one another and impact health development (see Buka et al. 2017; Little 2017).

A better, more systematic, and useful understanding of how social adversity stimulates different stress responses, how the development of those stress reactivity patterns are biologically conditioned by other stimuli, and how they cascade, or play forward, requires studies using longitudinal cohorts. Such studies will need to further refine the characterization and measurement of different and specific kinds of environments. This includes better measurement of specific components, experiences, and exposures but also how different elements of that environment are contextually linked and expressed both independently and synergistically. Understanding the interplay of genes and environment, and how different contexts influence the emergence of different trajectories, requires that epidemiologic studies focus on proximal neurobiological processes, including the epigenetic influences on the emergence of behaviors that manifest as endophenotypes and how environmental context influences the progression to full-fledged behavioral or psychiatric disorders (see Boyce and Hertzman 2017). This raises a number of measurement challenges, especially concerning how to assess changes in interacting and interdependent influences from the cellular to the social level.

A new fruitful area of LCHD epidemiologic research will focus on better characterizing the role and impact of the places where children and families live, grow, learn, work, and play (Pearce 2014; Dunn et al. 2015). With the expanding number of place-based interventions that attempt to improve the organization and functioning of entire community ecosystems, there is a mounting interest in how place as an organizing force influences health development at both the individual and population levels. The notion that multiple risk and protective factors are uniquely organized and deployed by a particular place provides new ways of understanding how to design and implement place-based interventions that strategically aggregate services, programs, and systems into a more coordinated approach to optimizing health development (Pearce et al. 2016).

Given the role that different mediators and modifiers can play at different ages and with different subgroups, more research is needed to determine how both normal and disordered development unfolds in relationship to nested exposures and experiences. Such research should also include a more strategic focus on how mutable these relationships might be. Specific interventions have been developed to modify family relationships, including interventions focused on parent-child relational content, maternal and infant bonding, or the capacity of mothers and fathers to co-parent (Leslie et al. 2016). How these interventions transform the ecosystem in which the child is developing, and how these alterations track over chronological and developmental time frames, requires further study.

While developmental trajectories are routinely used by developmental psychologists to describe the patterns and contours of developmental pathways and how they change over time, the measurement of health development trajectories in relationship to different proximal (maternal depression) and distal (violent neighborhood) risks, as well as different proximal (supportive grandmother) and distal (strong faith community) protective factors, is sorely lacking. A better understanding of how these different risk and protective factors interact and influence, both individually and in combination, health development requires different measurement and study design strategies than are routinely incorporated into cohort studies where exposures are evaluated as independent influences and causal attribution is often oversimplified (Dunn et al. 2014).

LCHD epidemiologic studies should also focus on better characterization of the role that differential timing of exposures to risk and protective factors has on the emergent quality and function of developmentally contingent hormonal systems and on the development of superordinate behavioral capacities including executive functioning, empathy, and perseverance. In addition, there is also a great need to focus on how multitiered pathways emerge, how they are influenced by different interventions, and how those influences affect outcomes over years and decades.

Mechanism Research

As the life course health sciences mature, they are more fully embracing the complexity of health development. There is a growing realization that health development is a complex adaptive nonlinear, multilevel, and multidirectional process in which the timing, patterning, and interactions of exposures and experience play out against a set of evolutionarily influenced developmental processes, each with its own sequencing and time signature. Throughout this volume, the need for better and more precise mechanism research has been emphasized, such as:

- Elucidating the nature and role of, and the mediators that influence, how sensitive periods emerge, develop, and manifest
- Developing a better understanding of how family- and community-level factors interact and influence each other over time
- Evaluating how the health capital that mothers bring to conception influences prenatal as well as postnatal child health development
- Assessing how biological sensitivity to context emerges and is modified by different signals and cues from both slowly and rapidly changing environmental influences

Biological conditioning—also sometimes referred to as biological priming or, more deterministically, biological embedding—includes the various ways in which environmental influences either exert transitory or more long-lasting impacts on developing biobehavioral regulatory systems. This is a high-value target for future research. Key questions include: What are the specific biological, neurologic, epigenetic, and physiologic mechanisms that are most important for altering biobehavioral regulatory systems? What is the mutability of these mechanisms? Do certain key factors act as "triggers," setting in motion a cascade of future biological response patterns? Biological conditioning processes can range from the exposure to a specific nutrient like folate and its influence on epigenetic methylation based on availability in indigenous diets (see Herman and Taylor Baer 2017) to the role that different patterns of sleep and sleep duration have on cycling of neuroendocrine hormones that serve to prime other factors related to growth, metabolism, and the biological underpinning of behavioral response systems (see Mummert et al. 2017; Hawkins et al. 2017).

Given worldwide rising rates of neurological, mental health, developmental, and substance abuse (NMDS) disorders, the international health community has prioritized developing a better understanding of the epigenetic effects of nutrition, infections, a range of environmental exposures, and psychosocial factors on developing nervous systems, especially the role early exposures and experiences have on later onset neurological conditions (Silberberg et al. 2015). Included in this prioritization is the recognition that adolescents are particularly at risk for developing neurocognitive deficits and mental health problems. Given that 50–75% of lifetime mental health disorders have their onset before age 24, a focus on better understanding the mechanisms that create this long-lasting vulnerability and how it can be addressed is also a high priority (Davidson et al. 2015). The life course health sciences should capitalize on worldwide interest in NMDS by highlighting the importance of life course approaches to understanding how NMDS develops (Birbeck et al. 2015).

Several chapters in this book emphasized the role of biological and behavioral transitions as sensitive periods and how they may afford leverage to alter developmental trajectories (see DelGiudice 2017; Boyce and Hertzman 2017; Wood et al. 2017). Similarly, interactions between the hypothalamic-pituitary-adrenal axis and basic energy metabolism that are also controlled by the hypothalamus may be relevant to the development of both physical and mental health, and understanding these interactions holds promise in better understanding why conditions like attention-deficit hyperactivity disorder (ADHD) and obesity cluster together (Halfon et al. 2013).

The way in which one sensitive period emerges and influences the development of subsequent sensitive periods also bears further investigation. This includes how the preconception period serves as an important platform for the creation and management of health development capital, and how the preconception period organizes and influences the prenatal and subsequent postnatal periods, each with its own defining characteristics, functions, and sensitivities. As more attention focuses on the prevention of adverse birth outcomes and the promotion of equity from the start of life, our understanding of the role and function of the preconception and prenatal periods in lifelong health will become all the more important. As capacity improves to identify, measure, differentiate, and understand the relationships between different sensitive periods of health development, our ability to devise and test more longitudinally integrated health-optimizing interventions will also assume greater importance.

Many of the chapters emphasized the need for research designs that specifically target multilevel influences, multilevel measurement, and analytic techniques that focus on multilevel interactions and modifications. They also suggested extant data limitations and methodological challenges that pose barriers to measuring and modeling the complexity of these influences and interactions. A whole new set of analytic tools and modeling techniques are emerging from the world of complex systems science. Their adaptation and application to the complex multilevel and life course health development processes is likely to be very fruitful and illuminating (Osypuk 2013; El-Sayed et al. 2013).

Evolutionary perspectives on how adversity, stress, and complex evolving cultural structures (e.g., educational and religious institutions) have shaped selection of human development priorities are also ripe for further cross-disciplinary research. The chapters by Boyce and Hertzman (2017) and DelGiudice (2017) in this volume emphasize the importance of how environmental stressors can lead to diverse adaptive responses that can manifest at different levels of impact depending on other contextual factors. They suggest that in advancing life course health development research, we recognize the value of cross-species, comparative studies that can shed light on the relationship between evolutionary biology and social environments and their consequences on human developmental adaptation and environmental mismatches.

Lastly, the evidence reviewed in several of the chapters suggest the potential value of a more integrative developmentally nuanced systems-physiology approach to understanding how co-occurring risks manifest in developmentally comparable changes across multiple physiological systems (Singer and Ryff 2001). For example, while it is well established that exposure to aminoglycoside antibiotics early in life can have detrimental and potentially devastating effects on both auditory and renal function, the chapters in this volume by Russ and colleagues (Russ et al. 2017) on hearing and Brophy and colleagues (Brophy et al. 2017) on chronic kidney disease (CKD) suggest that there are ways that the developing sensory apparatus in the ear and the developing filtration apparatus in the kidney may share other potential vulnerabilities across the life course. Future research on how risks and protective factors influence multiple systems will potentially lead to multi-solving interventions that can optimize health development across several discreet physiological systems. Better modeling of how seemingly distinct biological and behavioral systems develop holds promise to understanding how they develop their inherent robustness, where they share similar vulnerabilities, and how they might be buffered and protected from undesirable insults and risks (Kitano 2004; Cohen 2016).

Intervention Research

Our understanding of the impact of life course risks will be improved by better intervention research that targets key developmental processes and time periods. Throughout this volume, authors have highlighted the important role of intervention research for better understanding not only how to intervene, but also when. For example, the chapter by Hawkins and colleagues (Hawkins et al. 2017) suggests that a key to reducing childhood obesity is finding the right level and time in the life course to intervene for the maximal effectiveness and efficiency of interventions. However, the challenge of mounting programs designed to modify obesogenic health development pathways may be quite complex, involving multiple settings (e.g., medical care, homes, child care, school) (Taveras, Blackburn, et al. 2011a; Taveras, Gortmaker, et al. 2011b; Taveras et al. 2012), or components (e.g., system redesign, individual behavior change strategies including e-technology) (Lubans et al. 2010; Taveras et al. 2012), and targeting single or multiple factors (Taveras, Gortmaker, et al. 2011b; Vesco et al. 2012).

The chapter in this volume by Kim and colleagues (Kim et al. 2017) highlights how new insights into multilevel influences on health development pave the way for a range of different interventions that will further clarify these relationships. New research on pregnancy and the first years of a child's life indicate not only that this is a sensitive period for child neurological development but that it is a period when a parent's brain may demonstrate higher levels of plasticity and undergo changes to support the parental role (Kim et al. 2016). Given that parental brains are being remodeled at the same time that children's brains are developing, there are several potential ways to intervene so that parents modify home environments in developmentally optimizing ways for both their children and for themselves. Many potential interventions that span from cells to society have been studied in isolation, ranging from those that attempt to modify socioeconomic position via cash transfers to those that focus on harmonizing parenting approaches via co-parenting skills training (see Kim et al. 2017; Duncan et al. 2011; Feinberg et al. 2009). Less research has been done to better understand how best to combine interventions into a more integrated, sustained, and sustainable developmentally optimizing strategy.

The chapter in this volume by Boyce and Hertzman (2017) suggests that more effective prevention science demands new and innovative intervention designs that are responsive to the emerging science of health development. Highlighting how the Nurse Family Partnership broke new ground when it was first conceived and launched, the authors point to the need for ambitious and "more radical departures … from the conventions of traditional early development programs, including careful consideration of how complex dynamic systems thinking might be wed to novel, preventive interventions."

The chapter in this volume by Larson and colleagues (Larson et al. 2017) similarly focuses on the importance of intervention research to better understand the origins, impact, and mutability of health disparities that arise from different health development pathways. They argue that a multilevel intervention research strategy is needed. Intervention research on decreasing disparities in health development could focus on a range of possible sensitive periods, examining the possible and potential benefit of and best timing for interventions in the preconception period for improving birth. They also suggest that new social interventions, designed to alter specific short-term health outcomes (e.g., asthma or early stress reactivity) in at-risk populations, should be designed and tested in relation to how they modify long-term health and well-being outcomes in adulthood. For example, can population-level interventions like teaching young children yoga and other mindfulness techniques serve to "inoculate" them against elevations in allostatic load due to stressful and chaotic family environments?

Questions about the best timing for intervention are important. Cost-effectiveness studies can be used to compare the value of interventions at different life stages. In addition to interventions at the individual level, interventions focused on the multilevel determinants of health (e.g., neighborhood-level interventions) will also be important. Lastly, the chapter by Larson and colleagues (Larson et al. 2017) suggests that research should focus on the impact of new policies and programs at the local, state, and national levels to reduce health disparities across the life course. The authors also make an important distinction between research focused on minimizing risk and preventing poor health and interventions aimed at optimizing health and developmental potential.

3.1.2 Priority Research Topics

The Impact of Adverse Experiences on Health Development and the Origins and Implications of Health Disparities

Because of growing and persistent income inequality, high rates of child poverty, and associated levels of adversity, there is a pressing need to better understand the impact of adversity on health development, as well as ways of mediating and modifying its influence. Recent data from the National Survey of Children's Health reveals that the experience of adversity is not confined solely to children living below the federal poverty level, but extends up the income ladder (Halfon et al. 2014c). With nearly half of all children living in low income families with earnings below 200% of the Federal Poverty Level, these are concerns that now affect a majority of children. Related to the greater prevalence and experience of adversity in children from low income families is the relationship that the experience of adversity has to the development of a range of phenotypic responses.

Research on childhood adversity has been highly influenced by the conceptualization of adversity advanced by Felitti et al. (1998) in the original Adverse Childhood Experiences (ACE) Study. This retrospective cohort study of patients attending a weight reduction clinic at a southern California Kaiser Permanente facility in the 1990s has provided important information on the relationship between adversity early in life and the subsequent occurrence of a range of chronic diseases. However, it has also limited the conceptualization of adversity and how it is measured. Moving forward, it will be important to refine our definition and measurement of adversity, as well as the patterns and variations in its occurrence. The recognition and description of how specific types of adversity can be traumatic, and how that trauma can in turn lead to different kinds of stress response patterns, also call for a better understanding of the relationship between adversity, trauma, and stress. Given that all adversities are not equal, and that not all adversity is experienced as trauma, it is important to develop better measures of the experience of adversity, as well as to examine how that adversity is transduced by the brain and other body systems, including behavioral response patterns, proximal neurobiological processes, and epigenetic and other molecular changes (Hane and Fox 2016).

The chapter by DelGiudice (2017) in this volume warns that researchers should exercise caution in assuming that undesirable developmental outcomes reflect dysregulation of biological systems, and should remain open to the possibility that those outcomes may be part of adaptive (or formerly adaptive) strategies for survival and reproduction. He argues here and elsewhere (Del Giudice 2014b, c) that a life history framework is especially useful in teasing out the logic of potentially adaptive combinations of traits, highlighting critical factors in the environment, and bridging behavioral development with physical growth trajectories. A similar observation is made in the chapter in this volume by Lerner et al. (2017) in their analysis of adolescent health development, highlighting the context dependency of adaptive developmental regulation and how such regulation may vary by specific social situations, times, and places.

Related to the experience of adversity is the capacity for resilience among individuals and populations that experience it. The chapter by Larson and colleagues (Larson et al. 2017) suggests that additional research is needed to not only identify individuals with exceptional health resilience but to better understand the health development pathways that lead to more resilient phenotypes. Studies that examine the cultural, social, and psychological resources that can lead to thriving and better-than-expected health outcomes for individuals from disadvantaged social groups should also receive priority consideration, along with studies that lead to a better understanding of how those resources affect entire populations.

A basic notion of the life course health development framework is that the balance and interplay of risk and protective factors influence health development trajectories. Children living in environments with many more risk factors than protective factors will have a greater propensity for delayed or disordered health development trajectories, while those growing and developing in environments with more protective and health-promoting factors will achieve more optimal developmental pathways and trajectories. However, this simple characterization of the distribution of risk and protective factors in low- versus high-income communities obscures more complex and dynamic processes, a high degree of variability, and other deeper dynamics that might not be readily apparent and need to be considered and measured more directly. As the chapter in this volume by Mummert et al. (2017) points out, the ecosystems in which today's children are developing are novel when conceptualized across evolutionary timescales, with our manmade environments posing additional biological and behavioral challenges to developing humans that can both mediate and exacerbate other forms of more readily observable and measurable adversity.

While the experience of adversity has been directly related to the onset and development of different health outcomes that range from heart disease to depression, the relationships and variability at a population level is less well defined. The chapter in this volume by Larson and colleagues (Larson et al. 2017) suggests that it is important to continue to investigate the underlying biological processes that contribute to health disparities in human populations, and to better understand the role of protective factors and resilience on positive health outcomes for individuals from disadvantaged backgrounds. They also suggest more attention to parental preconception health and other intergenerational mechanisms that may contribute to early health disparities. To inform public policy and further elucidate the link between adversity and health disparities, they suggest additional investigations of the dynamic multilevel contributors to health status disparities across the life course.

The Impact of Family- and Community-Level Factors on Health Development

The LCHD framework highlights how the importance of understanding how health development processes is influenced by multiple factors at multiple levels in dynamic, transactional ways. Of particular salience to practitioners is the role that family- and community-level factors may have on health development. Related to the independent impact of these factors is their combined impact, as well as the impact that comes when these factors are considered in relationship to a particular ecosystem or place. This kind of multilevel and integrative analysis is important in a world where place-based strategies aimed at creating multiple potential opportunities for health improvement are routinely deployed.

Several of the chapters emphasize the importance of multilevel contributors to health status disparities over the life course, with a particular emphasis on upstream structural factors and neighborhood-level determinants. Multilevel studies can help examine the impact of neighborhood-level factors on health disparities by socioeconomic status, race, and ethnicity. Also needed are studies that incorporate longitudinal or life course measures of neighborhood and environmental exposures. At the population level, studies are needed to examine the natural environment, built environment, and social environment exposures that contribute to geographic differentials in rates of health and disease, as well as how variation in health policies contribute to disparities. To the greatest extent possible, research studies that examine lifelong contributors to sociodemographic health disparities should investigate the importance of the timing of key environmental and social exposures.

There is also a need to better understand the role that family and community risk and protective factors play in mediating influences at different levels. For example, how do positive health development enhancing family routines and other family-centric protective factors insulate or buffer a child's response patterns in a community where violence, social chaos, and family isolation are the norm? Evaluating the contribution of family capacities and routines—as well as social isolation, social relationships, and social support—is a fertile and strategically important area for further research. This kind of research is particularly important for a health-care arena in which "care bundles" are being developed to address both the medical and non-medical social, family, and behavioral influences on health.

The Impact of Specific Exposures and Experiences, the Importance of Various Life Stages, and the Development of Health Conditions

There are dynamic developmental relationships between different kinds of experiences and exposures that can be better understood from a life course perspective. For example, the chapter in this volume by Lerner and colleagues (Lerner et al. 2017) suggests profiling how different patterns of nutrition develop and influence a range of related behaviors and outcomes during adolescence. How do adolescents' diets influence their cardio-metabolic risk as adolescents and adults? Do adolescents maintain a healthy diet across different settings involving peers and family members? Is there age-associated variation in answers to this question, for instance, variation associated with pubertal development or pubertal status/stage (e.g., early, on time, or late)? Do answers to these questions vary in relation to gender? As well, do they vary in relation to normative social transitions (e.g., moving from elementary school to middle school)? How do peer social networks influence these behaviors or family mealtime behaviors? Are answers moderated or changed by the socioeconomic, cultural, religious, or national contexts of youth? In turn, do answers here vary in relation to media exposure about eating and about desirable body types that may be prevalent for youth living in particular settings at particular times in history? Given the synchronization issues raised by the seventh life course health development principle (see Halfon and Forrest 2017), how are all these answers moderated or changed by what may be nonnormative life events in the lives of adolescents? Examples here may be the death of a parent or deployment in the military (Cozza and Lerner 2013), family disruption due to divorce or separation, or family challenges in the face of environmental tragedies such as weather.

Important New Epidemics or Emerging Changes in Population Epidemiology

Rapidly changing environmental conditions and exposures have resulted in a variety of epidemiological transitions that yield new patterns of health and disease. Perhaps the most dramatic epidemiologic transition is the one that took place as a result of improvement in sanitation and public health—from mortality due to infectious or communicable disease to mortality due to non-communicable chronic health conditions like diabetes, hypertension, heart disease, and cancer. This transition has been well described and appreciated, although not without controversy as to its origins and drivers. In the past several decades, we have witnessed increased rates of child obesity and child and adolescent mental health disorders. While there have been relatively simple notions about the origins and drivers of the obesity epidemic, the chapter by Hawkins and colleagues in this volume (Hawkins et al. 2017) highlights the developmental complexity underlying this major epidemiologic change.

There has been far less focus and research on the developmental origins and patterns of manifestation of a range of mental health problems that appear to be rapidly increasing in children and adolescents. Recent epidemiologic surveys suggest that over 20% of adolescents now have a mental health disorder with impaired functioning (Merikangas et al. 2010). A better understanding of the mechanisms, causal factors, mutability, and lifelong consequences of these disorders is sorely needed. While there has been some research on whether mental health disorders arising in adolescence persists into adulthood, there is evidence that when they do, the impact on functioning and lifelong success can be more debilitating than the lifelong impact of chronic medical conditions (Moffitt 1993; Currie and Stabile 2006). While there have been studies that have begun to link increasing rates of media and television exposures to the development of attentional problems, the nature and impact of this rapidly changing epidemiology calls out for better life course health development research (Zimmerman and Christakis 2007).

The Health Development of Particularly Vulnerable Populations

The health development of particularly vulnerable populations of children demands more life course focused research. The chapter in this volume by Msall and colleagues (Msall et al. 2017) highlights the impact of socioeconomic-associated risks on the health development of premature infants. While there have been many longitudinal follow-up studies of premature infants, few have adopted a health development perspective or examined the role that other risk and protective factors play in shaping the developmental trajectories of this very vulnerable population. The same can be said for individuals with autism spectrum disorder, CKD, or most other chronic health conditions. In their chapter on autism spectrum disorder (ASD), Drmic, Szatmari, and Volkmer highlight how little that is known about the trajectories of children and adolescents with ASD and how studies focused on optimizing the health development of individuals with ASD could provide critical information. They highlight how adolescents with ASD who are clearly benefiting from participating in school and other educationally related activities experience a functional downturn once the developmental scaffolding that school provides is no longer available. The suggestion that individuals with ASD have delayed maturation of key developmental processes also argues for a more developmentally attuned and integrated understanding of how to optimize outcomes. The chapter on CKD by Brophy and colleagues (Brophy et al. 2017) also connects the dots between prematurity and other insults that may lead to decreased number of functional kidney filtration units (nephrons) and the time-specific and cumulative insults that are increasingly understood as the life course developmental pathway to CKD.

There are several other vulnerable populations of children where a life course health development perspective could be very illuminating and more importantly could shape the services and interventions that are provided. For example, it is well known that children who are abused, neglected, and placed into the foster care system can experience dramatically altered life course trajectories (Zlotnick et al. 2012; Tyler and Schmitz 2013; Patterson et al. 2015). Initial studies examining the impact of adversity, institutional placement, and out-of-home care have suggested how such experiences can alter neurobiological functioning and cellular processes associated with the regulation of cellular aging and longevity (Drury et al. 2012; Karatsoreos and McEwen 2013). Life course health development research could improve these interventions in regard to their capacity to improve long-term trajectories for children in foster care and other vulnerable populations, including young people involved in the juvenile justice system and children with chronic and debilitating medical conditions and impairments (Zlotnick et al. 2012). In each case, better understanding the health, growth, and developmental trajectories—and the factors and experiences associated with optimal health development outcomes—is sorely needed.

3.2 Section II: Priority Research Capacity-Building Activities

3.2.1 Advance LCHD Measurement Capacity and Improve Study Design to Provide Useful Data and Promote Greater Collaboration Across Disciplines

Throughout this volume, the authors have emphasized the importance of new and better measures of health and health development, with specific reference to developing and aging body systems (e.g., kidney health, hearing health). Closely related to measurement research are new and better analytic strategies that utilize data in more creative ways. Several chapters emphasize the need for better measures of "positive health." For example, Russ and colleagues' chapter on hearing (Russ et al. 2017) suggests that researchers need operational measures of positive hearing health to enable better measurement of treatment outcomes and functional hearing ability. Measures of positive health—including oral health, nutritional health, and mental health - as well as measures of positive health trajectories in these and other areas provide an empirical way of measuring both general and targeted health-optimizing strategies. Such measures might be composed of several different related measures and biomarkers that could be used to profile a specific health development capacity.

Measures of positive health development are not only important for assessing the health status and trajectories of individuals but also for use in assessing populations. The Early Development Index is a measurement tool that is used in Canada, Australia, and the USA to assess healthy development and school readiness for 4–6-year-olds (Janus et al. 2016). The EDI is composed of 110 items that span 5 dimensions and 16 subdomains of functioning. It is routinely collected and mapped at the neighborhood level to provide a population measure of health development. It has been used to predict early language and cognitive development and to examine differences in cognitive and emotional development in populations of children (Brownell et al. 2016). It is part of an evolving set of population health development measurement tools that now includes the Middle Development Index that was designed to measure similar dimensions in 9–11-year-olds (Schonert-Reichl et al. 2013; Guhn et al. 2016a). The same Canadian team that created the EDI and MDI is in the process of developing health development indices covering the entire child span, using the EDI to develop a pan-Canadian population health monitoring system (Guhn et al. 2016b). In addition, the EDI has also been used as a measure in "cells to society" research that is examining the impact of social gradients and how that manifests in relationships to social epigenetics (Hertzman and Boyce 2010).

Enhanced data collection of individual behaviors, traits, and biomarkers is now possible using low-cost, readily available technologies like smartphones and self-reported questionnaires. The National Institutes of Health have invested millions of dollars into the creation of state-of-the science self-reported measures of physical, mental, and social health as part of its program called the Patient Reported Outcome Measurement Information System (PROMIS, see www.healthmeasures.net for more information). These assessments of health can be combined with a wide array of environmental sensor assessments that can measure macro and micro fluctuations in the local environments, as well as clinical data stored in electronic health records and other molecular data such as genetics and epigenetics.

Aggregation of large amounts of data of these types can be done to create *big health development data* resources that can be mined and used to elucidate novel, unanticipated associations to inform future causal modeling and interventions.

Advances in life course health sciences have depended on the creation of longitudinal data collection efforts over the past century, most of which have been undertaken in countries located in Europe and Oceania. Recognizing the value of these longitudinal studies, several nations launched millennial cohort studies. This volume profiles several existing longitudinal surveys that can be used for examining life course impacts of different social and environmental factors (see Geller et al. 2017; Sastry et al. 2017; Cooksey 2017).

Longitudinal life course studies are important for capturing the dynamics of intra-individual health development trajectories and their environmental influences and epigenetic profiles. Because longitudinal cohort studies capture temporal relationship between exposures and outcomes, they can assist in defining causality and also in identifying predictive epigenetic biomarkers that may be used clinically and for targeted and more precise public health interventions.

There is also growing recognition that existing longitudinal and disease focused cohorts could be more effectively used to investigate specific questions by increasing sample sizes to enhance statistical power to examine interactions. Work is underway both in the USA and Europe to align and link cohorts, recognizing that the heterogeneity of the different studies will require conceptual and analytic harmonization to allow data to be pooled. Existing cohort studies are being encouraged to not only collect genetic information but to obtain detailed phenotype data—along with broader and more detailed information on environmental, behavioral, and lifestyle measures—in order to improve the capacity to link data sets for new kinds of analysis. Given the growing prevalence of a range of neurodevelopmental disorders in adults, there is an increasing interest collecting early cognitive, behavioral, metabolic, and epigenetic markers that might herald the onset and development of these diseases.

3.2.2 Develop and Apply New and Improved Methodologies to Reflect a Complex Systems Approach and Enable Causal Inference

As an emerging transdisciplinary field, LCHD research is typically done with scientific teams that include several methodologists and analysts to address the complex and multifaceted biological variation that epitomizes human health, but also the many and multilevel relational influences that are interacting and inducing changes in this continuously unfolding biological matrix. The complex and interconnected relationships of factors contributing to the development of obesity, mental health disorders, and other conditions with multiple complex causes typify the challenges that confound many common analytic approaches. Conventional longitudinal analyses, even those that account for multiple levels of influence, are often not powerful enough to account for the complexity and interconnectedness of obesity. Little's chapter in this volume (Little 2017) explains that several new techniques are available to improve estimation and causal inference for study designs with a multitude of time-varying covariates that interact across multiple levels. These include, among others, longitudinal structural equation modeling which can model hierarchically nested contextual influences on health over time. In addition, an emerging set of analytic tools from the systems sciences including agent-based and system dynamics modeling can be utilized to examine longitudinal relationships over multiple levels and, at the same time, account for more complex features of relationships like nonlinearity, path dependence, loops, and tipping (Hammond 2009; Huang, Drewnoski, Kumanyika, and Glass 2009).

Several authors reference the need for better community-based participatory research involving collaboration and partnership between community leaders, residents, and academic researchers. This kind of research can be used to help design assessments of living conditions (i.e., risk factors and influences) that are richer in content and more appropriately reflect the complex interactions that take place in family and community settings. It can also help to design interventions that are responsive to local needs and promote policy advocacy in disadvantaged neighborhoods. As place-based efforts attempt to transform the basic conditions in a community, they have often taken a life course approach to improve cradle-to-career trajectories with attention paid to what works in different kinds of communities and microenvironments.

3.2.3 Build, Strengthen, and Improve Institutional Capacity to Conduct LCHD Research

Increasing our capacity to conduct life course health science research requires a systematic and purposeful effort that focuses on human skills and talent, infrastructure, and institutional capacity, as well as state-of-the-art life course research tools and methods. Capacity building at the individual level requires mentoring, career guidance, research opportunities, and research pathways that are transdisciplinary and designed to promote optimal development of a life course health development researcher. At an institutional level, advancing life course health science research requires an appreciation for its importance, as well as prioritization of resources allocated for integrative approaches that characterize LCHD research.

Current major research infrastructure building and reform efforts like the Clinical Translational Science Institutes (CTSIs) permit institutions to use life course health development as an integrating strategy for building cross-disciplinary research teams and for focusing research priorities on key health development strategies. The CTSIs have also encouraged approaching diseases and health conditions in a more holistic manner, moving beyond traditional clinic-based models to engage individuals and families in the context of their own lives and life course goals. Similarly, the Patient-Centered Outcome Research Initiative has spearheaded research from a patient's perspective that also lends itself to life course consideration, including challenges presented by specific life course transitions. Life course health science requires team-based, often multi-institutional approaches to research, which is rapidly becoming the norm in the natural, biomedical, and social sciences.

3.3 Section III: Translational Priorities

Efforts are needed to identify existing knowledge that is ready for translation to concrete practice guidelines, programs, and policies aimed at improving health trajectories and alleviating disparities in health. Bringing this life course health development lens to the current healthcare system permits a critical review of how medical care clinics are organized, how healthcare systems organize care pathways, and more. Perhaps the greatest practical clinical and programmatic realization coming from LCHD research is the value of care delivery pathways and systems that are purposeful in their horizontal integration across all of the social ecological domains that influence health development and that are inclusive of all of the sectors and potential influencers on the whole person's health. The other important integration strategy is one that focuses on longitudinal or life course integration, not only anticipating future needs and concerns but designed to optimize life course-organized transitions and challenges. For example, life course-oriented research focused on optimizing health development could be used to redesign the healthcare system with a greater emphasis on promoting optimal health throughout the life course from birth through death, instead of focusing on disease management alone (Halfon et al. 2014b, c). Continued efforts are needed to identify ways in which life course research on health disparities can be integrated into medical, social welfare, education, and public health practice, as well as social and health policies at the local, state, and national levels.

There is also a great need to begin to explore how different periods of the life course have been underappreciated for their potential influence and leverage on downstream outcomes. For example, the chapter in this volume by Del Giudice (2017) calls attention to the juvenile transition and how this underappreciated and virtually unexplored period may be an important developmental window for intervention. The author suggests that interventions focused on optimizing transitions and occurring during these grammar school years can have an important priming and long-term influence on adolescent development. The idea that intervening *during* a biological transition may afford more leverage to alter developmental trajectories resonates with recognizing the nonlinearity of developmental processes and their time sensitivity.

Several of the chapters focused on better screening and assessment tools and approaches that attempt to capture key emergent characteristics and needs so that families can be provided with information about the consequences of decisions being made for a child early in his or her life. Local, state, and national governments also need policies in place that enhance child health development throughout childhood.

Improving public health messaging regarding health development across the life course with specific messaging about healthy hearing trajectories, healthy growth and nutrition trajectories, healthy teeth, and healthy family trajectories can all begin to build awareness and insights into the importance of health development goals, pathways, and trajectories. These include providing growth standards to help individual families implement health-promoting activities, exercise standards, sleep standards, and the like. Such an effort could include both family- and practitioner-based education programs to promote more robust efforts surrounding nutrition and exercise recommendations.

Better ways of sharing life course health development information should also extend to communities so that the optimizing health development of children can be built into the community ethos and appropriate educational materials and policy initiatives developed. Many communities have launched initiatives to promote health development and well-being across the life course. For example, the city of Santa Monica, California, has a lifelong learning system in place and a well-being index that is designed to highlight life course specific health data (Warner and Kern 2013). These kinds of initiatives can promote the importance of life course health science and can mobilize ingenuity and resourcefulness at local and national levels.

3.4 Section IV: Refinement of the LCHD Theoretical Framework

As the chapter by Halfon and Forrest (2017) in this volume indicates, the LCHD framework is an initial version of what may become a new scientific paradigm. As such, LCHD is synthesizing research from a range of different disciplines in ways that will guide the development and testing of new theories of health development and organize future research based on principles established by the field. As the field matures, it will be important to update the framework and its principles, and to consider research approaches, methods, and questions that will further elaborate the framework, moving toward the creation of a model that helps guide future hypothesis-driven research. Important considerations are further developing the explanatory power of the overall framework and interrogating the veracity of the principles that structure the network of ideas, theories, hypotheses, and research questions.

Halfon and Forrest present seven principles that structure the contours of the LCHD framework. They have conceived of these principles not as a linear sequence of defining characteristics but as network of high-level, interconnected generalizations that are empirically supported, logically consistent, and holistically justified. The network presentation suggests that these different principles are distinct but not independent of each other and that judging their explanatory robustness often requires that we consider not the principle in isolation but in relationship to other principles. In keeping with our systems approach to understanding human health development, the system of interconnected and interdependent explanatory principles suggests a dynamic and flexible network of concepts that can be used to build and test theories of causation, interactions, and relational importance. Because some of the principles are not as well supported by a robust empirical literature, some priority should be given to focusing research that addresses areas where additional research is needed.

Further development of the LCHD framework, using it to define the scope and level of life course health development inquiry, and applying it as an organized approach to theory testing will all require continued knowledge synthesis. Because the LCHD framework incorporates a diverse set of factors which interact with each other over significant and variable time horizons, there is a growing need to more systematically analyze and synthesize this information with reference to the overall framework. Greater synthesis of existing cross-disciplinary knowledge of different aspects of LCHD is also necessary for more precise investigation of pathophysiologic mechanisms.

3.4.1 The LCHD Framework, Precision Medicine, and Population Health

As the chapter by Halfon and Forrest suggests, the LCHD framework grew out of recognition that health development is a complex adaptive response of a dynamic, multidimensional, and multilevel system comprising individuals and their contexts codeveloping over time. Adopting the holism of systems biology and other systems sciences, the LCHD framework places more emphasis on the relationship between different components of the system (holism) than on describing the component parts (reductionism). In keeping with emerging notions of precision medicine and precision population health, not only are the insights from systems biology important but also understanding and integrating panomics—the interdependent interactions between the genome, epigenome, microbiome, virome, and exposome. The dynamics, patterns, and predictability of these panomic relationships are not only important for better targeting cancer therapy or customizing the treatment of inflammatory bowel disease but also for creating more effective, efficient, and responsive prevention and health promotion strategies at the population level that are not based on simple notions of risk and dependent on one-size-fits-all interventions (Halfon 2016).

The LCHD framework not only provides a powerful process and tool for knowledge integration but importantly introduces novel and important considerations of emergent developmental processes and developmentally contingent time frames that are important for the synchronization and integration of particular influence, as well as the interactions, flexibility, and dynamics of these relationships across the different combined influences. As the healthcare system focuses more on precision medicine and precision population health, there will be a growing interest in better characterizing health development processes at the individual and population level.

As research using the LCHD framework gallops forward, attention should be paid to how to further develop this framework. Is there an emergent and adaptive strategy to enable the LCHD framework to grow, develop, mature, and evolve as the field of LCHD research moves forward? As LCHD evidence accumulates, is analyzed, and is synthesized, the number of LCHD principles may grow or shrink, and the relationship of the LCHD principles between the principles should become clearer and more useful as a more fully articulated LCHD paradigm emerges. Halfon and Forrest have conceptualized the principles as a network of conceptual nodes whose explanatory utility and robustness is only fully realized in relationship to each other. Modeling and more fully exploring the relationships between the principles can also help test whether this conceptualization of how the principles manifest has explanatory value. As an overarching meta-framework, it will also be useful to examine how the LCHD framework can inform new notions of precision medicine and emerging notions of precision population health.

3.4.2 LCHD and Health System Transformation

Halfon and Forrest also suggest that the LCHD framework is not only strategically responding to a large body of empirical work that challenges long held notions of the causal mechanism responsible for disease causation and the production of different levels of health, but that by focusing on how to optimize health development, it includes considerations of the complex health influencing ecosystem and how that health development ecosystem evolves and changes over time. The framework suggests that health development does not occur solely within an individual or even as a result of an individual's exposure to certain environmental factors, but rather results from continuous coactions between persons and their environments, which we have represented as P⇔E. Thus, individuals are affected by their environments, but they also shape their environments, and the focus on health development is on individual's health assets, their environmental influences, and the ⇔ as well—that is, the relational mechanisms by which persons influence and are influenced by their environments (and vice versa). These insights not only challenge the simpler biomedical and biopsychosocial models of health and disease causation, but challenge the appropriateness, utility, effectiveness, and efficiency of a healthcare system that is largely built on a biomedical chassis and is just now in the process of upgrading its engine to accommodate psychosocial "upstream influences."

The LCHD framework implies that this new and more evolved paradigm of health development and disease causation provides the explanatory rational for how the healthcare delivery system evolves and is organized. The simple linear biomedical framework underwrote the rational for much of the 1.0 acute care focused medical care system with its focus on providing time-limited and rescue care for specific medical conditions over short time horizons. Similarly, the scientific advances and research that led to the development of the more dynamic and multilevel biopsychosocial framework begin to underwrite the upgrade and reengineering of the 2.0 chronic disease system with its greater focus on managing behavioral and lifestyle influences on chronic disease over longer time horizons. The emergence of the LCHD framework is already providing a way of underwriting the need for a more horizontally and longitudinally integrated, anticipatory, and developmentally primed health system (3.0 health system) that is structured to optimize health and health-promoting environments over the life span (Halfon et al. 2014b). Moving forward, it will be important to consider how the LCHD framework can be more fully exploited to inform healthcare innovations and health systems transformation. By fortifying a 3.0 operating system, can LCHD principles be translated into new healthcare system design concepts and innovation strategies? For example, does a better understanding of the potential vulnerability associated with the transition from homecare to preschool suggest a way in which services and supports should be developmentally organized to optimize this transition and support necessary adaptation on the part of the child as well as those in the family?

3.4.3 The LCHD Framework and the Measurement of Health Development

Health in the LCHD framework is defined as an emergent adaptive response to environmental (e.g., biological, behavioral, family, social, physical) challenges. The dynamics of health development and the emergence of diseases, dysfunction, or disintegration depend on dynamic processes and patterns of responses that typically span from the cellular to the whole person level. Because no component of this cluster of interdependent processes and purposeful relationships is ever standing still but is in a constant state of dynamic fluctuations, health is recognizable in the organism's dynamic developmental adaptability and their capacity to strategically respond to different environmental challenges. Because health is conditional on these different environments, measures of health development must be able to capture an individual and populations capacity to dynamically respond when an individual, population, or ecosystem is "out of balance." It also suggests the importance of capturing levels (cellular to ecosystem) of flexibility and resilience that are necessary and manifest to rebalance and achieve not only renewed level of health but an optimal level of health development. Our current measures of health and health development at an individual level are sorely lacking the capacity to sense and integrate signals from the cellular to the whole person level, across physiological systems and response patterns, and across developmentally significant time horizons. At a population level, there are similar conceptual and measurement gaps in how health development is measured and how to capture the developmentally contingent aspects of health development for different populations in facing different ecosystem contexts.

4 Conclusions and Next Steps

This volume has attempted to highlight the importance of the rapidly evolving field of life course health science and its potential impact on improving the lifelong health trajectories. We have used the life course health development framework as a way of organizing inquiry and understanding the relationship between a diverse but converging set of empirical findings. We have proposed a set of LCHD principles that are emerging and, we contend, on their way to describing a new paradigm of scientific investigation and can be used to organize and explain what has been learned and to guide and organize future inquiry (Ostrom 2009; Gatzweiler and Baumuller 2014). This volume has also begun to link and network related areas of inquiry, utilizing these common principles and what they illuminate about deeper and more complex processes of health development. Lastly, we have attempted to relate LCHD research to the field of maternal and child health and to explore how life course enlightened knowledge of health development can be used to improve the health of mothers and children and achieve greater health equity from the start of life.

In this volume, different teams of scholars have analyzed and synthesized the current state of knowledge and research progress in a range of important areas of health development. Spanning topics as diverse as hearing health, kidney health, metabolic health, and oral health across different developmental stages from preconception to emerging adulthood, the chapters examine the health development contribution of different life stages, revealing new considerations for how to prevent losses in health potential, as well as how to optimize lifelong health development. Through the process of writing their chapters, the authors have analyzed and synthesized what is currently known and have begun to shine a light on the way forward by identifying specific research questions and strategies intended to advance research productivity and impact, as well as translation to programs, policy, and practices.

4.1 What's Next?

There are several important national trends that make life course health science and future research on life course health development particularly salient and important at the present time (McGinnis et al. 2016). First are the growing concerns about persistent and structural inequalities in the USA. The life course health sciences have already contributed to the growing recognition of the lifelong health, social, and economic impacts of poverty-associated adversity early in life. Additional research focused on the impact of the early years on future health development will continue to play an important role in refocusing policy, programs, and practices on addressing and leveraging what is at stake in these early years (Halfon et al. 2014c).

Second are the opportunities provided by the implementation of the Affordable Care Act (ACA) and related initiatives designed to move healthcare upstream and to focus more attention and resources on prevention and population health. The life course health sciences are illuminating how such upstream strategies must focus not only on the social and environmental causes of health outcomes but in particular on the upstream influences on costly and preventable adult health outcomes (Wise 2016). As post-ACA policy attempts to steer healthcare financing from a focus on volume (outputs) to value (outcomes), there is a real opportunity to demonstrate how health development value chains begin early in life and how investments in health development capital can be leveraged into significant long-term value results (McGinnis et. al. 2016). ACA-stimulated health system reform is also accelerating the consideration of transformational strategies that are challenging the dominant 2.0 operating logic, structure, and organization that arose to address the diagnosis, treatment, and management of adult chronic health conditions. What is now emerging is a new 3.0 operating logic aimed at optimizing lifelong health by leveraging the new science of life course health development (Halfon et al. 2014b). The findings from the life course health sciences can continue to support this transition from 2.0 to 3.0 by providing the empirical basis for justifying healthcare systems that are more horizontally integrated to address multiple interacting dimensions and influences on health development, as well as longitudinally integrated to anticipate future health development scenarios and build long-term pull strategies into the structure and design of health and health-related social and educational services.

Third are the opportunities and challenges posed by major federal research initiatives, like those focused on precision medicine and clinical translational science and the lag from discovery to wide scale implementation. While both of these National Institutes of Health (NIH)-funded efforts begin with a biomedical orientation—with precision medicine focused on specifying the biological characteristics (phenotype) that will assist in pinpointing pharmacological interventions with greater accuracy and translational science focused on moving from the discovery of a new molecule in a laboratory and more rapidly and efficiently testing it at the hospital bedside and in the clinic making it widely available on a population basis—there is a critical need to inform these and other traditionally biomedically oriented research efforts with life course health science thinking and approaches.

Fourth is the fact that the national health policy focus on improving population health and reducing health disparities can benefit from the LCHD framework and life course health science results. As Larson and colleague (Larson et al. 2017) argue in this volume, "the LCHD framework emphasizes the importance of addressing disparities from preconception onward; understanding that early exposure to multiple stresses may produce biological changes that are difficult, if not impossible, to eradicate later; and acknowledging that adults who experienced the most extreme disparities as young children are likely to develop the worst health in adulthood and require the most expensive interventions. Life course-oriented health disparities research provides an opportunity for large potential savings associated with the development of strategies to intervene early in optimizing human health." Real headway in not only addressing health disparities but reducing these inequalities in health development will arise by taking advantage of the life course health science along with the opportunities afforded by ACA-induced health system transformation to focus greater attention and the role of the early years in reducing disparities, decreasing the prevalence and impact of chronic illness, and saving healthcare costs.

As a product of the Life Course Research Network (LCRN) that is funded by the Department of Health and Human Services (DHHS) Health Resources and Services Administration (HRSA) Maternal and Child Health Bureau (MCHB), this volume is meant—in addition to serving as a catalyst and tool for advancing the LCHD field—to inform MCHB's thinking, planning, and funding of future research. To this end, the content of this chapter will be used to create a more traditionally structured research agenda containing specific research questions that the members of the LCRN (see lcrn.net to learn more and join) and the broader community of LCHD stakeholders will be invited to participate in refining and prioritizing among. Over time, the LCRN—which was recently awarded another 3 years of funding from MCHB—will produce, commission and/or solicit additional research agenda-setting papers on topics missing from the present volume in order to enable the periodic updating of the LCRA and enhance the dissemination and synthesis of emerging findings. Taken together, these efforts will help to advance both the life course health sciences and our understanding of their importance for optimizing life course health development.

References

Barker, D. J., Osmond, C., Winter, P. D., Margetts, B., & Simmonds, S. J. (1989). Weight in infancy and death from ischaemic heart disease. *The Lancet, 334*(8663), 577–580.

Ben-Shlomo, Y., & Kuh, D. (2002). A life course approach to chronic disease epidemiology: Conceptual models, empirical challenges and interdisciplinary perspectives. *International Journal of Epidemiology, 31*(2), 285–293.

Birbeck, G. L., Meyer, A.-C., & Ogunniyi, A. (2015). Nervous system disorders across the life course in resource-limited settings. *Nature, 527*(7578), S167–S171.

Boyce, W. T., & Hertzman, C. (2017). Early childhood and the life course: The state of the science and proposed research priorities. In N. Halfon, C. B. Forrest, R. M. Lerner, & E. Faustman (Eds.), *Handbook of life course health-development science*. Cham: Springer.

Brophy, P. D., Charlton, J. R., Carmody, J. B., Reidy, K. J., Harshman, L., Segar, J., Askenazi, D., & Shoham, D. (2017). Chronic kidney disease: A life course health development perspective. In N. Halfon, C. B. Forrest, R. M. Lerner, & E. Faustman (Eds.), *Handbook of life course health-development science*. Cham: Springer.

Brownell, M. D., Ekuma, O., Nickel, N. C., Chartier, M., Koseva, I., & Santos, R. G. (2016). A population-based analysis of factors that predict early language and cognitive development. *Early Childhood Research Quarterly, 35*, 6–18.

Buka, S. L., Rosenthal, S. R., & Lacy, M. E. (2017). Epidemiological study designs: Traditional and novel approaches to advance life course health development research. In N. Halfon, C. B. Forrest, R. M. Lerner, & E. Faustman (Eds.), *Handbook of life course health-development science*. Cham: Springer.

Cohen, A. A. (2016). Complex systems dynamics in aging: New evidence, continuing questions. *Biogerontology, 17*(1), 205–220.

Cooksey, E. (2017). Using the National Longitudinal Surveys of Youth (NLSY) to conduct life course analyses. In N. Halfon, C. B. Forrest, R. M. Lerner, & E. Faustman (Eds.), *Handbook of life course health-development science*. Cham: Springer.

Currie, J., & Stabile, M. (2006). Child mental health and human capital accumulation: The case of ADHD. *Journal of Health Economics, 25*(6), 1094–1118.

Davidson, L. L., Grigorenko, E. L., Boivin, M. J., Rapa, E., & Stein, A. (2015). A focus on adolescence to reduce neurological, mental health and substance-use disability. *Nature, 527*(7578), S161–S166.

DelGiudice, M. (2017). Middle childhood: An evolutionary-developmental synthesis. In N. Halfon, C. B. Forrest, R. M. Lerner, & E. Faustman (Eds.), *Handbook of life course health-development science*. Cham: Springer.

Drury, S. S., Theall, K., Gleason, M. M., Smyke, A. T., De Vivo, I., Wong, J. Y., Fox, N. A., Zeanah, C. H., & Nelson, C. A. (2012). Telomere length and early severe social deprivation: Linking early adversity and cellular aging. *Molecular Psychiatry, 17*(7), 719–727.

Duncan, G. J., Morris, P. A., & Rodrigues, C. (2011). Does money really matter? Estimating impacts of family income on young children's achievement with data from random-assignment experiments. *Developmental Psychology, 47*(5), 1263.

Dunn, E. C., Masyn, K. E., Yudron, M., Jones, S. M., & Subramanian, S. V. (2014). Translating multilevel theory into multilevel research: Challenges and opportunities for understanding the social determinants of psychiatric disorders. *Social Psychiatry and Psychiatric Epidemiology, 49*(6), 859–872.

Dunn, E. C., Richmond, T. K., Milliren, C. E., & Subramanian, S. V. (2015). Using cross-classified multilevel models to disentangle school and neighborhood effects: An example focusing on smoking behaviors among adolescents in the United States. *Health & Place, 31*, 224–232.

El-Sayed, A. M., Seemann, L., Scarborough, P., & Galea, S. (2013). Are network-based interventions a useful antiobesity strategy? An application of simulation models for causal inference in epidemiology. *American Journal of Epidemiology, 178*(2), 287–295.

Feinberg, M. E., Kan, M. L., & Goslin, M. C. (2009). Enhancing coparenting, parenting, and child self-regulation: Effects of family foundations 1 year after birth. *Prevention Science, 10*(3), 276–285.

Felitti, V. J., Anda, R. F., Nordenberg, D., Williamson, D. F., Spitz, A. M., Edwards, V., Koss, M. P., & Marks, J. S. (1998). Relationship of childhood abuse and household dysfunction to many of the leading causes of death in adults: The adverse childhood experiences (ACE) study. *American Journal of Preventive Medicine, 14*(4), 245–258.

Gatzweiler, F. S., & Baumuller, H. (2014). Marginality-a framework for analyzing causal complexity of poverty. In J. von Braun & F. W. Gatzweiler (Eds.), *Marginality: Addressing the nexus of poverty, exclusion, and ecology*. Dordrecht: Springer.

Geller, A., Jaeger, K., & Pace, G. (2017). Using the Fragile Families and Child Wellbeing Study (FFCWS) in life course health development research. In N. Halfon, C. B. Forrest, R. M. Lerner, & E. Faustman (Eds.), *Handbook of life course health-development science*. Cham: Springer.

Guhn, M., Gadermann, A. M., Almas, A., Schonert-Reichl, K. A., & Hertzman, C. (2016a). Associations of teacher-rated social, emotional, and cognitive development in kindergarten to self-reported wellbeing, peer relations, and academic test scores in middle childhood. *Early Childhood Research Quarterly., 35*, 76–84.

Guhn, M., Janus, M., Enns, J., Brownell, M., Forer, B., Duku, E., Muhajarine, N., & Raos, R. (2016b). Examining the social determinants of children's developmental health: Protocol for building a pan-Canadian population-based monitoring system for early childhood development. *BMJ Open, 6*(4), e012020.

Halfon, N. (2016). More precisely targeting the coal mine of social adversity. *JAMA Pediatrics, 170*(11), e162523.

Halfon, N., & Forrest, C. B. (2017). The emerging theoretical framework of life course health development. In N. Halfon, C. B. Forrest, R. M. Lerner, & E. Faustman (Eds.), *Handbook of life course health-development science*. Cham: Springer.

Halfon, N., Larson, K., & Slusser, W. (2013). Associations between obesity and comorbid mental health, developmental, and physical health conditions in a nationally representative sample of US children aged 10 to 17. *Academic Pediatrics, 13*(1), 6–13.

Halfon, N., Larson, K., Lu, M., Tullis, E., & Russ, S. (2014a). Lifecourse health development: Past, present and future. *Maternal and Child Health Journal, 18*(2), 344–365.

Halfon, N., Long, P., Chang, D. I., Hester, J., Inkelas, M., & Rodgers, A. (2014b). Applying a 3.0 transformation framework to guide large-scale health system reform. *Health Affairs, 33*(11), 2003–2011.

Halfon, N., Wise, P. H., & Forrest, C. B. (2014c). The changing nature of children's health development: New challenges require major policy solutions. *Health Affairs (Millwood)., 33*(12), 2116–2124.

Hammond, R. A. (2009). Peer reviewed: complex systems modeling for obesity research. *Preventing Chronic Disease, 6*(3), A97.

Hane, A. A., & Fox, N. A. (2016). Early caregiving and human biobehavioral development: A comparative physiology approach. *Current Opinion in Behavioral Sciences, 7*, 82–90.

Hanson, M. A., & Gluckman, P. D. (2014). Early developmental conditioning of later health and disease: Physiology or pathophysiology? *Physiological Reviews, 94*(4), 1027–1076.

Hawkins, S. S., Oken, E., & Gillman, M. W. (2017). Early in the life course: Time for obesity prevention. In N. Halfon, C. B. Forrest, R. M. Lerner, & E. Faustman (Eds.), *Handbook of life course health-development science*. Cham: Springer.

Herman, D., & Taylor-Baer, M. (2017). From epidemiology to epigenetics: Evidence for the importance of nutrition to optimal health development across the life course. In N. Halfon, C. B. Forrest, R. M. Lerner, & E. Faustman (Eds.), *Handbook of life course health-development science*. Cham: Springer.

Hertzman, C., & Boyce, T. (2010). How experience gets under the skin to create gradients in developmental health. *Annual Review of Public Health, 31*, 329–347.

Hochberg, Z.'e. (2009). Evo–devo of child growth II: Human life history and transition between its phases. *European Journal of Endocrinology, 160*(2), 135–141.

Huang, T. T., Drewnowski, A., Kumanyika, S. K., & Glass, T. A. (2009). A systems-oriented multilevel framework for addressing obesity in the 21st century. *Preventing Chronic Disease, 6*(3), A82.

Janus, M., Harrison, L. J., Goldfeld, S., Guhn, M., & Brinkman, S. (2016). International research utilizing the early development instrument (EDI) as a measure of early child development: Introduction to the special issue. *Early Childhood Research Quarterly., 35*, 1–5.

Karatsoreos, I. N., & McEwen, B. S. (2013). Annual research review: The neurobiology and physiology of resilience and adaptation across the life course. *Journal of Child Psychology and Psychiatry, 54*(4), 337–347.

Kim, P., Strathearn, L., & Swain, J. E. (2016). The maternal brain and its plasticity in humans. *Hormones and Behavior, 77*, 113–123.

Kim, P., Evans, G. W., Chen, E., Miller, G., & Seeman, T. (2017). How socioeconomic disadvantages get under the skin and into the brain to influence health-development across the lifespan. In N. Halfon, C. B. Forrest, R. M. Lerner, & E. Faustman (Eds.), *Handbook of life course health-development science*. New York: Springer.

Kitano, H. (2004). Biological robustness. *Nature Reviews Genetics, 5*, 826–837.

Kuh, D., & Shlomo, Y. B. (2004). *A life course approach to chronic disease epidemiology*. Oxford: Oxford University Press.

Larson, K., Russ, S. A., Kahn, R. S., Flores, G., Goodman, E., Cheng, T. L., & Halfon, N. (2017). Health disparities: A life course health development perspective and future research directions. In N. Halfon, C. B. Forrest, R. M. Lerner, & E. Faustman (Eds.), *Handbook of life course health-development science*. Cham: Springer.

Lerner, R. M., Brindis, C. C., Batanova, M., & Blum, R. W. (2017). Adolescent health: A relational developmental systems perspective. In N. Halfon, C. B. Forrest, R. M. Lerner, & E. Faustman (Eds.), *Handbook of life course health-development science*. Cham: Springer.

Leslie, L. K., Mehus, C. J., Hawkins, J. D., Boat, T., et al. (2016). Primary care: Potential home for family focused interventions. *American Journal of Preventive Medicine, 51*(4), S106–S118.

Little, T. D. (2017). Core principles of life course health development methodology and analytics. In N. Halfon, C. B. Forrest, R. M. Lerner, & E. Faustman (Eds.), *Handbook of life course health-development science*. Cham: Springer.

McGinnis, J. M., Diaz, A., & Halfon, N. (2016). Systems strategies for health throughout the life course. JAMA, 316(16), 1639–1640.

Merikangas, K. R., He, J. P., Burstein, M., Swanson, S. A., Avenevoli, S., Cui, L., Benjet, C., Georgiades, K., & Swendsen, J. (2010). Lifetime prevalence of mental disorders in US adolescents: Results from the National Comorbidity Survey Replication–Adolescent Supplement (NCS-A). *Journal of the American Academy of Child and Adolescent Psychiatry, 49*(10), 980–989.

Moffitt, T. E. (1993). Adolescence-limited and life-course-persistent antisocial behavior: A developmental taxonomy. *Psychological Review, 100*(4), 674.

Msall, M. E., Sobotka, S. A., Dmowska, A., Hoga, D., & Sullivan, M. (2017). Life course health development outcomes after prematurity: Developing a community, clinical, and translational research agenda to optimize health, behavior and functioning. In N. Halfon, C. B. Forrest, R. M. Lerner, & E. Faustman (Eds.), *Handbook of life course health-development science*. Cham: Springer.

Mummert, A., Schoen, M., & Lampl, M. (2017). Growth and life course health development. In N. Halfon, C. B. Forrest, R. M. Lerner, & E. Faustman (Eds.), *Handbook of life course health-development science*. Cham: Springer.

Ostrom, E. (2009). A general framework for analyzing sustainability of social-ecological systems. *Science, 325*(5939), 419–422.

Osypuk, T. L. (2013). Invited commentary: Integrating a life-course perspective and social theory to advance research on residential segregation and health. *American Journal of Epidemiology, 177*(4), 310–315.

Patterson, M. L., Moniruzzaman, A., & Somers, J. M. (2015). History of foster care among homeless adults with mental illness in Vancouver, British Columbia: A precursor to trajectories of risk. *BMC Psychiatry, 15*(1), 1.

Pearce, J. (2014). Invited commentary: history of place, life course, and health inequalities—historical geographic information systems and epidemiologic research. *American Journal of Epidemiology, 181*(1), 26–29.

Pearce, J., Shortt, N., Rind, E., & Mitchell, R. (2016). Life course, green space and health: Incorporating place into life course epidemiology. *International Journal of Environmental Research and Public Health, 13*(3), 331.

Robinson, O., Basagaña, X., Agier, L., et al. (2015). The pregnancy exposome: Multiple environmental exposures in the INMA-Sabadell birth cohort. *Environmental Science & Technology, 49*(17), 10632–10641.

Russ, S. A., Tremblay, K., Halfon, N., & Davis, A. (2017). A life course approach to hearing health. In N. Halfon, C. B. Forrest, R. M. Lerner, & E. Faustman (Eds.), *Handbook of life course health-development science*. Cham: Springer.

Sastry, N., Fomby, P., & McGonagle, K. (2017). Using the Panel Study of Income Dynamics (PSID) to conduct life course health development analysis. In N. Halfon, C. B. Forrest, R. M. Lerner, & E. Faustman (Eds.), *Handbook of life course health-development science*. Cham: Springer.

Schonert-Reichl, K. A., Guhn, M., Gadermann, A. M., Hymel, S., Sweiss, L., & Hertzman, C. (2013). Development and validation of the middle years development instrument (MDI): Assessing children's well-being and assets across multiple contexts. *Social Indicators Research, 114*(2), 345–369.

Silberberg, D., Anand, N. P., Michels, K., & Kalaria, R. N. (2015). Brain and other nervous system disorders across the lifespan [mdash] global challenges and opportunities. *Nature, 527*(7578), S151–S154.

Singer, B. H., & Ryff, C. D. (Eds.). (2001). *New horizons in health: An integrative approach* (Vol. 277). Washington, D.C.: National Academies Press.

Taveras, E. M., Blackburn, K., Gillman, M. W., Haines, J., McDonald, J., Price, S., & Oken, E. (2011a). First steps for mommy and me: a pilot intervention to improve nutrition and physical activity behaviors of postpartum mothers and their infants. *Maternal and Child Health Journal, 15*(8), 1217–1227.

Taveras, E. M., Gortmaker, S. L., Hohman, K. H., Horan, C. M., Kleinman, K. P., Mitchell, K., & Gillman, M. W. (2011b). Randomized controlled trial to improve primary care to prevent and manage childhood obesity: The high five for kids study. *Archives of Pediatrics & Adolescent Medicine, 165*(8), 714–722.

Taveras, E. M., McDonald, J., O'Brien, A., Haines, J., Sherry, B., Bottino, C. J., & Koziol, R. (2012). Healthy Habits, Happy Homes: Methods and baseline data of a randomized controlled trial to improve household routines. *Preventive Medicine, 55*(5), 418–426.

Tyler, K. A., & Schmitz, R. M. (2013). Family histories and multiple transitions among homeless young adults: Pathways to homelessness. *Children and Youth Services Review, 35*(10), 1719–1726.

Warner, K., & Kern, M. (2013, December). A City of Wellbeing: The what, why & how of measuring community wellbeing. The City of Santa Monica Office of Wellbeing.

Wise, P. H. (2016). Child poverty and the promise of human capacity: Childhood as a foundation for healthy aging. *Academic Pediatrics, 16*(3), S37–S45.

Wood, D., Crapnell, T., Lau, L., Bennett, A., Lotstein, D., Ferris, M., & Kuo, A. (2017). Emerging adulthood as a critical stage in the life course. In N. Halfon, C. B. Forrest, R. M. Lerner, & E. Faustman (Eds.), *Handbook of life course health-development science*. Cham: Springer.

Zlotnick, C., Tam, T. W., & Soman, L. A. (2012). Life course outcomes on mental and physical health: The impact of foster care on adulthood. *American Journal of Public Health, 102*(3), 534–540.

Erratum to: Handbook of Life Course Health Development

Neal Halfon, Christopher B. Forrest, Richard M. Lerner, and Elaine M. Faustman

Erratum to:
N. Halfon et al. (eds.), *Handbook of Life Course Health Development*, https://doi.org/10.1007/978-3-319-47143-3

Name and affiliation details for Claire D. Brindis have been updated throughout the book. In addition, acknowledgment section by Dr. Brindis was inserted.

Affiliation details for Ashley Bennett have been updated throughout the book.

The book was published with typos in Chapter 7. The typos have been updated.

The updated online version of these chapters can be found at
https://doi.org/10.1007/978-3-319-47143-3_6
https://doi.org/10.1007/978-3-319-47143-3_7
https://doi.org/10.1007/978-3-319-47143-3

N. Halfon et al. (eds.), *Handbook of Life Course Health Development*,
https://doi.org/10.1007/978-3-319-47143-3_27

Index

N. Halfon et al. (eds.), *Handbook of Life Course Health Development*,
DOI 10.1007/978-3-319-47143-3

Q

T

U

V

W

www.ingramcontent.com/pod-product-compliance
Lightning Source LLC
LaVergne TN
LVHW082007200926
848481LV00010B/2817
* 9 7 8 1 0 1 3 2 6 9 1 0 3 *